The Cambridge Handbook of International Prevention Science

The Cambridge Handbook of International Prevention Science offers a comprehensive global overview on prevention science with the most up-to-date research from around the world. Over 100 scholars from 27 different countries (including Australia, Bhutan, Botswana, India, Israel, Mexico, Singapore, South Korea, Spain, and Thailand) contributed to this volume, which covers a wide range of topics important to prevention science. It includes major sections on the foundations of prevention, as well as examples of new initiatives in the field, detailing current prevention efforts across the five continents. A unique and innovative volume, *The Cambridge Handbook of International Prevention Science* is a valuable resource for established scholars, early professionals, students, practitioners, and policy-makers.

MOSHE ISRAELASHVILI is Associate Professor at the Tel Aviv University (Israel) School of Education. He has extensive experience in prevention programs' development, implementation and evaluation, especially in the context of children and youth resilience promotion and substance abuse prevention. He is a consultant to major institutions in Israel, such as the Israel Ministry of Education/Psych-Counseling Services, Israel Anti-Drug Authority, Israel Internet Association, and Israel Defence Forces and is a member of the Society for Prevention Research (SPR), American Psychological Association (APA), and the Society for Stress and Anxiety Research (STAR). A visiting professor in Canada and the United States, he also serves on the editorial boards of international journals.

JOHN L. ROMANO is Professor Emeritus at the University of Minnesota, United States. His scholarship emphasizes prevention science and international psychology. The author of *Prevention Psychology: Enhancing Personal and Social Well-Being* (APA, 2015), he is a Fellow of the American Psychological Association (APA). The awards he has received include Prevention Section (APA's Society of Counseling Psychology) Inaugural Lifetime Achievement Award, Distinguished Contributions to Counseling Psychology (Society of Counseling

Psychology), APA's International Psychology Division International Mentoring Award, and the American Counseling Association Research Award. He has been a visiting professor, consultant, and external evaluator/assessor at universities in several countries. He has disseminated research/scholarship through international journals and conferences and serves on the editorial boards of international journals. He is a former U.S. Peace Corps Volunteer (Nigeria) and has been a Visiting Professor in Malaysia and Thailand.

The Cambridge Handbook of International Prevention Science

Moshe Israelashvili
Tel Aviv University
John L. Romano
University of Minnesota

CAMBRIDGE
UNIVERSITY PRESS

CAMBRIDGE
UNIVERSITY PRESS

One Liberty Plaza, 20th Floor, New York NY 10006, USA

Cambridge University Press is part of the University of Cambridge.

It furthers the University's mission by disseminating knowledge in the pursuit of education, learning, and research at the highest international levels of excellence.

www.cambridge.org
Information on this title: www.cambridge.org/9781107087972

First published 2017

Printed in the United States of America by Sheridan Books, Inc.

A catalogue record for this publication is available from the British Library.

Library of Congress Cataloguing-in-Publication Data
Names: Israelashvili, Moshe, editor. | Romano, John L., editor.
Title: The Cambridge handbook of international prevention science / edited by Moshe Israelashvili, John L. Romano.
Description: New York, NY : Cambridge University Press, 2017. | Series: Cambridge handbooks in psychology | Includes bibliographical references and index.
Identifiers: LCCN 2016015774| ISBN 9781107087972 (Hardback) | ISBN 9781107458321 (Paperback)
Subjects: LCSH: Mental illness–Prevention. | Preventive mental health services. | Mental health promotion. | BISAC: PSYCHOLOGY / Applied Psychology.
Classification: LCC RA790 .C483 2016 | DDC 616.89–dc23 LC record available at https://lccn.loc.gov/2016015774

ISBN 978-1-107-08797-2 Hardback
ISBN 978-1-107-458321 Paperback

To our families, that directly and indirectly supported our global journey to promote prevention science, and to scholars, practitioners, and policy makers who are bringing the science of prevention to their countries, cultural groups, and disciplines to improve the health and well-being of children, youth, and adults across the globe

Contents

Figures

Tables

Contributors

BOLANLE E. ADETOUN, ECOWAS, Nigeria.

MODUPE ADEWUYI, Lenoir-Rhyne University, United States.

ADEBOWALE (DEBO) AKANDE, IRC, South Africa.

TITILOLA AKANDE, Dublin University, Ireland, and Malmö University, Sweden.

PAULA ALLEN-MEARES, University of Michigan, United States.

MIRIAM ÁLVAREZ, University of La Laguna, Spain.

JOAN AMER, University of the Balearic Islands, Spain.

DELIL ATHIÉ, Instituto Mexicano de Investigación de Familia y Población, A.C. (Yo quiero Yo puedo-IMIFAP), Mexico.

LLUÍS BALLESTER, University of the Balearic Islands, Spain.

JOSIPA BAŠIĆ, University of Zagreb, Croatia.

K. A. BATES, Yale University, United States.

CADY BERKEL, Arizona State University, United States.

MARTINA BRAASCH, University of Wuppertal, Germany.

PETRA BUCHWALD, University of Wuppertal, Germany.

SONIA BYRNE, University of La Laguna, Spain.

AMADOR CALAFAT, European Institute of Studies on Prevention (IREFREA), Spain.

GIOVANNA CAMPELLO, United Nations Office on Drugs and Crime (UNODC), Austria.

CHEUNG-MOON CHO, National Information Society Agency, Korea.

WAN HAR CHONG, Nanyang Technological University, Singapore.

MILENA CLAUDIUS, Boston College, United States.

MADELINE A. COHEN, Columbia University, United States.

ROBERT CONYNE, University of Cincinnati, United States.

BARBARA DE LARM, Indiana University, United States.

SEAN C. DEMARTINO, Springfield College, United States.

ANNAMARIA DI FABIO, University of Florence, Italy.

TSHERING DOLKAR, Counseling Services, RENEW, Bhutan.

GRANT ELLISON, Eastern Michigan University, United States.

KARIN ENGSTRÖM, Karolinska Institutet, Sweden.

DOROTHY L. ESPELAGE, University of Florida, United States.

ZELDE ESPINEL, University of Miami Miller School of Medicine and Jackson Memorial Hospital, United States.

MARIA ESPINOLA, University of Cincinnati College of Medicine, United States

BARRY EYE, Eastern Michigan University, United States.

LEA FERRARI, University of Padova, Italy.

PERRY FIRTH, Seattle University, United States.

YVONNE FORSELL, Karolinska Institutet, Sweden.

ERICA FRYDENBERG, University of Melbourne, Australia.

MARIA ROSARIA GALANTI, Karolinska Institutet, Sweden.

ABIGAIL H. GEWIRTZ, University of Minnesota, United States.

DANIEL GOLDBERG, Indiana University, United States.

BETHANY GOURLEY, Eastern Michigan University, United States.

BRANDON J. GRIFFIN, Virginia Commonwealth University, United States.

SALLY M. HAGE, Springfield College, United States.

NADIA HASAN, Texas A&M University at Kingsville, United States.

HANNA HEIKKILA, United Nations Office on Drugs and Crime (UNODC), Austria.

ANNA-EMILIA HIETANEN, Universidad Nacional Autónoma de México (UNAM), Mexico.

JUN SUNG HONG, Wayne State University, United States, and Sungkyunkwan University, Korea.

JI SU HONG, Affinia Healthcare, St. Louis, Missouri, United States.

SAJID HUMAYUN, University of Greenwich, United Kingdom.

MOSHE ISRAELASHVILI, Tel Aviv University, Israel.

SARAH JONES, Arizona State University, United States.

MONTSE JUAN, European Institute of Studies on Prevention (IREFREA), Spain.

MAUREEN E. KENNY, Boston College, United States.

ELYSSA KLANN, Indiana University, United States.

DOUGLAS KNUTSON, Oklahoma State University, United States.

ELLEN KOCH, Eastern Michigan University, United States.

JULIE M. KOCH, Oklahoma State University and Grand Canyon University-College of Doctoral Studies, United States.

AI LENG PATRICIA KOH, KK Women's & Children's Hospital, Singapore.

GENOMARY KRIGBAUM, Marian University–College of Osteopathic Medicine, United States.

KATHERINE KULICK, Virginia Commonwealth University, United States.

CAROLINE R. LAVELOCK, Virginia Commonwealth University, United States.

ELIZABETH LETOURNEAU, Johns Hopkins Bloomberg School of Public Health. and Moore Center for the Prevention of Child Sexual Abuse, Johns Hopkins University, United States.

WADIH MAALOUF, United Nations Office on Drugs and Crime (UNODC), Austria.

ANNA MÅNSDOTTER, Karolinska Institutet, Sweden.

MARTÍ MARCH, University of the Balearic Islands, Spain.

ANNE MAURICIO, Arizona State University, United States.

DAVID V. MCQUEEN, Global Consultant in Health Promotion, United States.

JULIANA MEJÍA-TRUJILLO, Nuevos Rumbos Corporation, Colombia.

JETTE MÖLLER, Karolinska Institutet, Sweden.

STEFANIE MORGENROTH, University of Wuppertal, Germany.

NEHA NAVSARIA, Washington University School of Medicine in St. Louis, United States.

LAURA NOTA, University of Padova, Italy.

K. M. NYAMA, UW University, South Africa.

CARMEN ORTE, University of the Balearic Islands, Spain.

KRZYSZTOF OSTASZEWSKI, Institute of Psychiatry and Neurology in Warsaw, Poland.

TEBATSO PAUL, Institute of Development Management, Botswana.

ANTHONY A. PEGUERO, Virginia Tech University, United States.

AUGUSTO PÉREZ-GÓMEZ, Nuevos Rumbos Corporation, Colombia.

SUSAN PICK, Universidad Nacional Autónoma de México, Yo quiero Yo puedo-IMIFAP, Mexico.

AGNIESZKA PISARSKA, Institute of Psychiatry and Neurology in Warsaw, Poland.

ANDREAS RECHKEMMER, Graduate School of Social Work, University of Denver, United States.

SOLOMON RENATI, K B P College, Vashi, Navi Mumbai, India.

ARTHUR REYNOLDS, University of Minnesota, United States.

MARÍA JOSÉ RODRIGO, University of La Laguna, Spain.

JOHN L. ROMANO, University of Minnesota, United States.

DARKO ROVIŠ, University of Rijeka, Croatia.

KYLE RUNDLES, Emerson College, United States.

IRWIN N. SANDLER, Arizona State University, United States.

JONATHAN SCHWARTZ, University of Houston, United States.

STEPHEN SCOTT, King's College, London, United Kingdom.

TERESA MARIA SGARAMELLA, University of Padova, Italy.

DANIEL T. L. SHEK, The Hong Kong Polytechnic University, Hong Kong.

RYAN T. SHIELDS, Johns Hopkins University, United States.

JAMES M. SHULTZ, Center for Disaster and Extreme Event Preparedness, University of Miami Miller School of Medicine, United States.

SKULTIP SIRIKANTRAPORN, Alliant International University, United States.

SHREELETHA SOLOMON, Institute for Child and Adolescent Health Research, Mumbai, India.

SALVATORE SORESI, University of Padova, Italy.

REX STOCKTON, Indiana University, United States.

HANAKO SUZUKI, University of Tsukuba, Japan.

CHOO SYLVIA HENN TEAN, KK Women's and Children's Hospital, Singapore.

HUI NEE TANG, KK Women's and Children's Hospital, Singapore.

JENN-YUN TEIN, Arizona State University, United States.

JUDITH A. TEMPLE, University of Minnesota, United States.

JOHN W. TOUMBOUROU, Deakin University, Australia.

M. M. TSERERE, King of Kings Globe, South Africa.

ARUNYA TUICOMEPEE, Chulalongkorn University, Thailand.

ELLEN L. VAUGHAN, Indiana University, United States.

MARGA VIVES, University of the Balearic Islands, Spain.

NATHANIEL G. WADE, Iowa State University, United States.

NANCY WIGTON, Applied Neurotherapy Center, Scottsdale, Arizona, United States.

EMILY WINSLOW, Arizona State University, United States.

SHARLENE WOLCHIK, Arizona State University, United States.

Y. JOEL WONG, Indiana University, United States.

EVERETT L. WORTHINGTON, Jr., Virginia Commonwealth University, United States.

ADRIANA M. YOUSSEF, University of Minnesota, United States.

Foreword

Historically, the prevention of problem behaviors and the promotion of positive behaviors have received extensive commentary and scientific study. However, in more recent years, newer theoretical approaches, rigorous research methodologies, intensive explorations of efficacy and effectiveness models, and careful implementations of prevention/promotion programs served as accumulating components for the establishment of knowledge on prevention into the relatively new interdisciplinary professional domain of prevention science.

Currently, the domain of prevention science is characterized by increasing groups of scientists and practitioners who focus on prevention as their main field of expertise. The establishment of such groups was the natural result of the enlarging and crystalizing body of knowledge on the science of prevention. This knowledge is presented and exchanged in various vivid professional forums, both oral (e.g., conferences, workshops) and written (e.g., journals, books). Moreover, an increasing number of stakeholders and decision makers are gradually getting to know the power of early interventions as an essential component in the prevention of behavioral disorders and diseases as well as in the promotion of health and well-being. Yet, one of the major limitations of existing knowledge of prevention science is its concentration in a relatively narrow spectrum of countries, as the more developed prevention interventions are often designed and implemented in higher-income countries. This does not suggest that prevention interventions are not developed in other parts of the world (as demonstrated in this *Handbook*), nor that prevention programs that have been developed and implemented in some countries are not applicable for implementation in other countries. Rather, the *Handbook* emphasizes the need for a more global perspective of prevention science as an important step in widening the scope of knowledge and relevance of this academic and professional domain. This broader perspective may include how problems and understandings of prevention are conceptualized globally and how best to use theoretical and applied knowledge from prevention science across different countries and cultural contexts.

Therefore, the major purposes of this *Handbook* are to strengthen communication among prevention scholars from across the globe and to provide updated knowledge about prevention science to researchers and practitioners in different parts of the world. It is believed that this global exposure will lead not only to more intensive international exchanges of ideas and collaborations but also to assist in the crystallization of already existing knowledge in prevention science.

Accordingly, the *Handbook* includes two main parts. The first part contains chapters that represent the current state of knowledge on important topics and paradigms of prevention science. The second part includes chapters that were written by prevention scholars from various parts of the world. Each scholar, or group of scholars, wrote about his or her nation and how prevention has been applied in their given country or region.

The call for chapter proposals for this *Handbook*, the first of its kind, attracted many authors from across the globe from various disciplines. As a final publication, the *Handbook* includes descriptions, commentaries, and lessons learned by more than one hundred scholars from twenty-seven different countries. While the scope of the countries is not balanced across all parts of the world, the rich and varied group of authors presents a wide range of prevention topics and methodologies. The authors describe not only behaviors to be prevented (e.g., drug and alcohol abuse) but also behaviors to be enhanced and strengthened (e.g., promoting health and well-being). In addition, challenges associated with prevention work in various countries, most notably the lack of funding for prevention activities, limited training opportunities, and the need to empirically validate implemented prevention interventions, are especially highlighted.

Naturally, it was impossible to cover all the prevention efforts conducted in each and every nation of the world. Nevertheless, we trust the *Handbook* will be a valuable resource for both experienced and novice prevention scholars, practitioners, and policy makers. Finally, in pursuit of the promotion of prevention science, we hope that the *Handbook* offers inspiration and future increased collaboration among scholars throughout the world.

Acknowledgments

As editors, we give much thanks and appreciation to the many people who contributed to this *Handbook* in various ways. Perhaps most important are the scholars from across the globe who contributed their knowledge and expertise and joined us in the journey to see this volume to completion. Their commitment to prevention science is inspirational.

We also acknowledge the staff at Cambridge University Press, who gave encouragement during the early stages of this project and worked to make the published *Handbook* a reality. While several people assisted us throughout the publication process, we want to specifically acknowledge the assistance of David Repetto, who guided us throughout the early stages of the *Handbook*, and Alexandra Poreda, Claudia Bona-Cohen, and Emma Collison for their editorial assistance. We also want to acknowledge the international prevention scholars who reviewed our initial proposal for the *Handbook*, supported the project, and gave us valuable insights on how best to strengthen the *Handbook* to meet our goals and objectives. Finally, we especially want to thank members of our families, who continuously supported and encouraged us and supplied help throughout the long process of bringing the published *Handbook* to completion.

The Nature of Prevention Science

1 The Emergence of Prevention Science

Moshe Israelashvili & John L. Romano

The history and development of prevention has been described in various publications (e.g., Mrazek & Haggerty, 1994; Romano, 2015; Spaulding & Balch, 1983). Some of these reviews addressed general aspects of prevention, such as the process of formalizing prevention efforts in the United States (U.S.; Romano, 2015), whereas others have addressed specific aspects of prevention, such as society's changing attitude toward problem behavior (e.g., illicit drugs; Jonnes, 1999), the societal benefits of promoting positive behaviors (e.g., breastfeeding; Renfrew et al., 2012) as a way of preventing disease, or the early childhood antecedents of major health problems that should be prevented (e.g., obesity; Morris, Skouteris, Edwards, & Rutherford, 2015). The purpose of this chapter is neither to describe nor to review the field of prevention, but rather to suggest a descriptive analysis of how the ancient idea of prevention has become a vivid scientific discipline in recent years. In line with this analysis, the chapter will advocate the notion that globalization – that is, broadening the perspective of prevention scientists and practitioners to include the efforts, effectiveness, and efficacy of preventive interventions that are taking place around the globe – is the next necessary step that *prevention* as a *science* needs to address. Naturally, along this general description, only part of the information will be outlined, and hence the reader is encouraged to explore further the details – and especially additional, and maybe alternative, approaches – in order to get an even more comprehensive picture of the emergence of prevention science.

Biblical and Ancient Times

Prevention is the oldest human problem known in history. Moreover, it is a question with which many people around the globe, consciously or often unconsciously, are still preoccupied. An explanation for these claims can be found in the Bible (the Old Testament). It does not matter whether one believes in God or not, nor whether the Bible was written by God or by a human being; in any case, the Bible is well accepted as one of the most ancient books ever written. Interestingly, the first three events that open the Bible are all related to human beings dealing with issues that are associated with the prevention of sexual behavior, aggression, and alcohol use.

Firstly, it was Eve who disobeyed God's restriction not to eat from the Tree of Knowledge, and she surrendered to the snake's "temptations" to taste it. Why is the story of Adam and Eve, living in Heaven and then breaking God's command, one of the first events of human history? This question gains more importance when we explore the details of the story; that is, what arguments did the snake use in order to convince Eve? Why did Eve listen to the snake rather than ignore it? Why did Adam follow suit and taste the fruit from the Tree of Knowledge as well? And, the most interesting question of all: what knowledge did Eve and Adam gain from eating from the Tree of Knowledge? Welcome to the debate on *healthy sexuality* – that is, once Adam and Eve ate the fruit, they realized they were naked and tried to cover their bodies. Billions of words have been spoken and written about this story and its interpretations, each one shedding light on it from a difference perspective. However, one common shortcoming of all existing references is the difficulty in explaining what should have been done (by Adam?) or have occurred (as an act of God?) in order to prevent Eve from disobeying the order and its devastating result – the exile from heaven. Alternatively, it is possible that the message that this story tries to convey is the ultimate truth regarding human nature – that is, that nothing can prevent a human being from experiencing the "un-permitted."

The biblical story goes on to tell us about Cain's aggression against Abel. Cain was too jealous of Abel, who was favored by the father/leader figure (God), and finally turned his jealously into aggression, murdering Abel and hiding the body. No one existed except for these two brothers and their parents – that is, no gang, violent television, electronic games, or movies, and no previous murder to imitate. Nevertheless, Cain couldn't control himself and committed the first ultimate aggression ever. Why? Welcome to the debate on healthy (or adaptive) *aggression*. Not much later in the Bible comes the description of Noah's departure from the Ark. Astonished by his survival of the flood, probably overwhelmed by his feelings and thoughts regarding his extraordinary experience, and yet almost the first thing he did was to get drunk (Genesis, 9, 21); welcome to the debate on *(healthy) alcohol consumption.*

Interestingly, these three stories are well known to people around the world, unrelated to their religiosity or belief. This is especially the case in regard to the story about Eve and "The Ancient Sin" and the glorification of returning (once "passing away…") to heaven, which three major religions highlight: in Judaism, the wish to return to heaven is a leading theme – for example, it is mentioned in every Jewish wedding; in Christianity, the wish to go away from sins and return to heaven is discussed in the New Testament several times (e.g., Lucas, XIII, 43); in Islam, it is widely discussed in the Koran (in Sora 47, 15; 56, 15–22; etc.), and returning to heaven (جنة عدن) is presented as approaching the ultimate place of physical and spiritual pleasures.

In light of the intensive preoccupation with the story of "The Ancient Sin," the question of why Eve – and since then, many other people – could not prevent herself from being involved in "forbidden activities" is challenging.

This is why prevention can be regarded as one of the most ancient problems that human beings address and an issue that is relevant to everyone's life.

The importance of prevention is also emphasized in Greek mythology as well as in Roman mythology. In Roman mythology, one of Asclepius's children, the god of medicine, was Hygeia (currently, Hygiene), the goddess of health and cleanliness. Hygeia had several sisters and brothers, among them Iaso, the goddess of recovery from illness; Aceso, the goddess of the healing process; and Panacea, the goddess of remedy. Yet, there are several indications of Hygeia's exceptional importance in ancient times: (a) the intensive documentation of ordinary people's belief in the power of sleeping in one of the temples that were named after her; (b) the Pythagorean philosophers' nomination of their five-angles-star symbol of greeting with the five (Roman) letters of her (Roman) name; and (c) the placement of her statue – along with the statue of her Greek duplication, Athena Hygeia – in the entrance to the Acropolis of Athens. Hygeia's importance represents the power that has been attributed to prevention on ancient times.

Beyond these ancient examples, it seems that for the ordinary person the idea of prevention is very appealing and somehow encouraging: everything would be fine if we were able to conduct a program that prevents disease, risk behavior, natural disasters, and so on. This is why, since ancient times and up to these days, the idea of prevention has actually been the guideline of many well-known and well-established concepts, values, and duties, such as "(Good) Parenthood" as a way to prevent problems in children's development; "Education" as a way to prevent societal and personal problems as a child matures into adulthood and beyond; "Special Education" as a way to prevent greater problems among children with special needs; "driving license" as a way to prevent car accidents; medical inoculation (e.g., polio vaccines) as a way to prevent personal and familial suffering along with public health costs; and so forth. However, it should be noted that prevention is also a very irritating idea, as no one likes to think that a problem could have been prevented had she or he – that is, the individual, the community, the company, the nation, the world – behaved differently and intervened. For example, for some parents it may be easier to claim that their child suffers from an organic/neurological problem (e.g., ADD/ADHD) rather than confront the notion that their parenthood is problematic and might be the cause of their child's problem behavior (e.g., Singh, 2004). Another example is the case for decision makers who have to make decisions and develop policies regarding what potential terrorist attack should be addressed – the one that is more normative or the one that might expose them to greater public blame in case of a failure to prevent it (McGraw, Todorov, & Kunreuther, 2011). Practically speaking, since ancient times people did try to prevent maladaptive behaviors; however, it was considered to be only secondary in importance to healing those who were already suffering from a disease or already suffering from the outcomes of maladaptive behavior. However, in recent years, gradually the situation has been changed and a new science has emerged: *prevention science*.

Several Historical Notes

Throughout history, occasional references to the importance of prevention have been made by various individuals and under various circumstances. Several of these references were highlighted by Martin Bloom, during his term as the editor of the *Journal of Primary Prevention* (2000–4), under the title of "An historical note." Bloom mentioned, among others, the businessman Robert Owen (1771–1858), who believed that society and education – rather than the person himself or herself – mold people's character. Based on this belief, he advocated for the improvement of the educational, communal, familial, and industrial circumstances within which (his) workers were occupied, in order to prevent them from becoming ill and ignorant; the educator Maria Montessori (1870–1952), who tried to promote effective learning in preschool children, in hopes of improving their lives; and the U.S. physician and epidemiologist Joseph Goldberger (1874–1929), who was ready to be infected by pellagra during his trials to prevent it. Bloom's homage to these people represents the notion that prevention has always existed as a possibility, but only a few people actively pursued its large-scale implementation.

Moving forward to modern history, at the beginning of the twentieth century, the idea of prevention was significantly promoted by the personal experience, personal dedication, and personal resources of Clifford Beers (1864–1929). Beers, a wealthy person who had been hospitalized due to a mental breakdown, wrote the milestone book *A Mind that Found Itself* (1908). In this autobiography, Beers described his and others' dehumanized personal experiences as mental health patients and wrote in support of the need to prevent mental health problems. However, Beers was not only a person of words and conclusions but also a person of acts; right after the strong and positive public response to his book, the National Committee for Mental Hygiene was established in the United States (1909) by him and another one hundred attendees (see Long, 1986), followed by the establishment of a mental hygiene clinic (1913) and the publication of the interdisciplinary journal *Mental Hygiene* (established 1917). Beers' legacy is still influential, with the Clifford-Beers Foundation's (United Kingdom [UK]) significant contribution to today's global efforts to promote mental health and prevent mental illness (www.claifordbeers.org.uk).

Since the beginning of the twentieth century, the idea of prevention has gained greater prominence, with cascading movements toward the establishment of prevention as a science. Many people and numerous events were part of this journey and paved the way to the increasing importance of prevention science. A random and extremely short list of examples of acts, events, institutions, and people – together with numerous others who were as significant as these examples are – would include the following:

- Based on Darwin's theory of evolution, the "eugenic movement" advocated the idea of improving the quality of human beings *born* into the world (e.g., by early intervention among those parents-to-come). Yet, it should be mentioned here that this pro-prevention movement, which was popular in the 1900s through the 1930s, was also the birthplace of racial discriminations, such as that of Ernst Rüdin, who used eugenics as a justification for the racial policies of Nazi Germany (Joseph & Wetzel, 2013).

- Alfred Adler's (1927, 1928) interest in the prevention on neurosis later initiated his development of the strategy for preventative education (Ansbacher, 1990).
- The establishment of the U.S. National Institutes of Health (NIH) and Communicable Disease Center (CDC), both in 1946, played an influential role in shaping the contents of research in both health sciences and social sciences, such as grant competitions as well as the later (1963) support in establishing National Institute of Mental Health (NIMH) community mental health centers across the United States.
- U.S. President Dwight Eisenhower's administration's Joint Commission on Mental Illness and Health (1961) was headed by George Albee, who later postulated the idea that both "risk factors" and "protective factors," as well as the relationship between these factors, are important in understanding the intensity and the nature of prevention (Albee, 1980).
- G. Caplan (1964) noted the well-known differentiation among primary, secondary, and tertiary prevention. It should be noted that originally Caplan's differentiation referred to the prevention of problems that might arise due to mental health hospitalization problems; however, later on it was adopted by others to represent the three general domains of prevention, until replaced by the current differentiation among universal, indicative, and selective prevention (Gordon, 1983; Mrazek & Haggerty, 1994);
- Albee's later contributions in collaboration with colleagues declared that "Primary prevention works" (Albee & Gullotta, 1997).
- Emory Cowen (1970), one of the founders of prevention as a science, undertook innovative and extensive prevention studies and initiations, including setting "baby-steps to prevention."
- Price, Cowen, Lorion, and Ramos-McKay's (1998) eye-opening book, *14 Ounces of Prevention: A Casebook for Practitioners*, was one of the first publications to pose a demand on people who are dealing with prevention to establish their interventions on solid, theoretical, and evidence-based grounds, as well as one of the first publications to present well-established prevention interventions – although only fourteen at the time – that work.
- The U.S. Surgeon General's Office Report on Healthy People (Healthy People, 1979) widened the scope of the perspective on health and living by suggesting goals and recommendations to improve the health of U.S. citizens across the life span.
- The World Health Organization (WHO, 1999) redefined health as "a state of complete physical, mental and social well-being and not merely the absence of disease or infirmity"
- The Melbourne Charter for Promoting Mental Health and Preventing Mental and Behavioural Disorders (2008) provides a framework that

recognizes the influence of social and economic determinants on mental health and mental illness and identifies the contribution that diverse sectors (including, but not exclusive to, health sectors) make to influencing those conditions that create or ameliorate positive mental health.

- The Society for Prevention Research (SPR) (www.preventionscience.org/) was established in 1991 and the SPR official journal *Prevention Science* began publication in 2000.
- The European Society for Prevention Research (EUSPR) (euspr.org) was established in 2010 and was formally approved and registered by the Polish authorities as an international not-for-profit organization, based at the Institute of Psychiatry and Neurology in Warsaw.
- The discussion paper on "Unleashing the Power of Prevention" (Hawkins et al., 2015) proposes "to mobilize across disciplines and communities to unleash the power of prevention on a nationwide scale" (p. 1).

In addition, several chapter authors in this *Handbook* describe prevention organizations and government initiatives that highlighted prevention in the latter part of the twentieth century and early-twenty-first century (e.g., in this volume, see the chapters by Basic and Rovǐs [Croatia]; Pérez-Goméz and Mejía-Trujillo [Latin America]; and Campello, Heikkila, and Maalouf). As mentioned previously, this list of institutions, declarations, and people includes neither the most important nor the most representative components of the antecedents of prevention science. Rather, these are examples of the rich and diverse milestones of the modern history of prevention. However, what is more important is to analyze which processes underlie these milestones, leading to the emergence of prevention as a science and the demand "to unleash" its power.

For example, a closer look at the list of the aforementioned milestones, and the institutional and professional affiliations of the people who propelled the transition from one milestone to another, reveals that scholars and institutions from various professional domains were involved in the study of prevention. This large scope of professional affiliation represents the multidisciplinary nature that characterizes the field of prevention science. In a retrospective analysis of the emergence of prevention science, it seems that such interdisciplinary development served as a fertilizing power toward the emergence of this new science.

Interdiscipline Facilitates Prevention

Some people argue that prevention is not a subject matter in itself but rather a domain in which knowledge and discoveries from other scientific fields are applied. A very similar argument has frequently been directed toward the domain of education that some people see as the umbrella under which prevention should also be categorized as a subsection. Actually, in both domains (i.e., prevention and education) one may find scholars who have conducted their research on a wide selection of subjects, not to mention people who are dealing with prevention, for example, and who are faculty members of various departments, such as psychology (e.g., cultural competence), social work (e.g., social advocacy and social justice), family studies, criminology, medicine (e.g., HIV prevention), psychiatry (e.g., prevention of mental health disorders), sociology, political science (e.g., prevention and public policy), mathematics (e.g., prevention of math anxiety), physics (e.g., prevention of community disaster), business administration (e.g., burnout prevention), labor studies (e.g., prevention of unemployment), economy (prevention of unemployment and economics of prevention), and so on. In relation to prevention as an interdisciplinary science, while some may view prevention as a subset of scholarship of many fields, perhaps it is more accurate to propose that prevention science is not an accumulation of partial knowledge and contributions from various fields, but rather a specialty in itself that includes different specialties and disciplines. The multidisciplines that comprise prevention science have certainly contributed in many ways to better theoretical understandings, research and evaluations methods, and strategies for interventions. Thus, the contributions are much stronger than what might be gained without the multidisciplines that contribute to prevention science. However, the multidisciplinary orientation of prevention exists not only in the academic affiliation of those who focus on this domain, but also, and more profoundly, in the mutual enrichment of prevention and other related domains of the behavioral sciences, such as developmental psychopathology, community psychology, public health, counseling psychology, counseling, and counselor education.

Prevention science's growing interdisciplinary orientation occurred in a time (i.e., since the mid-1990s) of increasing awareness of another emerging interdisciplinary scientific domain, namely developmental psychopathology (DP). Developmental psychopathology – that is, the exploration of personal, biological, situational, communal, as well as other determinants of children's positive development versus psychopathology (e.g., Moffitt, 2005) – is currently a dominant and somehow revolutionary field in the behavioral sciences. One of the major assumptions of DP is that "normal" development is neither simple nor something that can be taken for granted; rather, during every child's development, there are potentially many risks and obstacles that may lead the child to develop problematically (e.g., Garmezy, 1985). However, another major assumption is that over time, every child – even the one who enters the world with "a problematic heredity" (e.g., a child of schizophrenic parents) – could potentially encounter many positive opportunities and fostering events that could lead to the child's positive development, development that *overcomes the odds* (Werner, 1992). These two assumptions are extremely challenging, as they postulate that child's development should not be taken for granted – that is, (many times) negative development is preventable and (many times) positive development is a kind of ordinary magic (Masten, 2001) that results from proper preliminary fostering interventions. The link between these postulations of DP and the basic notions of prevention science is clear. Yet, the scope of interests and goals of each domain is not identical, rather only partially overlapping, although the accumulating knowledge within each field is mutually enriching. As one might expect, many of the leading researchers in the field of DP graduated from psychology programs in which the concept of prevention was integrated into graduate training (Cicchetti, & Rogosch, 2002).

In terms of the emergence of prevention science, one of the general influences of DP on both scientists and practitioners was the encouragement to readdress preliminary assumptions regarding the power to change children's development. Probably the most representative example of the departure from the old assumptions regarding child development and prevention of problem behavior is the emergence of the term (child) *resilience* (e.g., Garmezy, 1987; Rutter, 1987) and the continuing extensive explorations regarding its antecedents. Such a growing openness to consider the possible contributions of well-designed interventions further paved the way to the establishment of prevention science.

Another field of scientific exploration that to some degree is related to prevention science is positive psychology. The basic notion of those promoting positive psychology (e.g., Kobau, 2011; Snyder & Lopez, 2007) is that psychology is too preoccupied with the treatment of psychopathology while paying much less attention to people's strengths and assets. Thus, positive psychology's demand to enlarge the scope of (dependent) variables that need further scientific understanding would be followed by professional interventions to enhance a person's strengths (e.g., protective factors). Interventions that contribute to those people who are not yet in a serious problematic situation (e.g., selective and indicated prevention) deserve attention as much as interventions that help people who are already in an extreme situation (e.g., those clinically diagnosed). Once the scope of a possible relevant intervention was enlarged also to include interventions that help people who are not in an extreme position, many of the already existing prevention interventions became relevant and acceptable, such as interventions to promote resilience (Cutuli et al., 2013). In this context, it is worth mentioning Cowen's suggestion of the term "wellness," saying that it is time to coin this term in relation to the goals of prevention (1984); this term was later a unifying concept in exploring the nature and scope of prevention in various fields (Cicchetti, Rappaport, Sandler, & Weisberg, 2000) and, recently was presented and reinforced through Conyne's book on counseling for wellness and prevention (Conyne, 2015).

In relation to wellness, or well-being, it is important to mention that to a significant degree there is a resemblance among several of the postulations of positive psychology, especially the goals and interventions that counseling psychology (CP) and counselor education (CE) address. For example, researchers in the field of CP have long been preoccupied with questions relating to issues that are in the scope of positive psychology, such as the promotion of happiness and well-being, career choice job satisfaction, and positive adaptation. As one might expect, researchers in the field of CP also address the issues of prevention, which has led to significant insights and practices in prevention science. One example of this work are the Guidelines for Prevention in

Psychology, that were initiated by a workgroup of mainly American Psychological Association (APA) Division 17 (Society of Counseling Psychology) members and have been approved and adopted by the APA Council (APA, 2014). See the final chapter of this *Handbook* for a summary of the guidelines.

Finally, cognitive-behavioral therapy (CBT) as a theoretical foundation is often used in prevention applications (e.g., Romano, 2015). There are many examples of CBT conceptualizations and models that are relevant to prevention science, of which two examples will be mentioned here: (1) Stress inoculation training (SIT; Meichenbaum, 1985) is a general framework for the prevention of future negative responses to stressful encounters. Originally, SIT was proposed as a demonstration of the implementation of CBT in the context of stress management, including a special emphasis on the need to promote clients' (a) cognitive conceptualization of the problem, (b) skills that are relevant to stress management in a specific situation, and (c) exposure to and experiences in future related situations. This approach has been implemented widely in various contexts (Meichenbaum, 2007), most of which are related to topics that the prevention literature addresses. However, while only a few references to SIT exist in the prevention literature (e.g., Gullotta, 1997), analysis of the strategy and components of prevention efforts that have been published (e.g., Griffin, Scheier, Botvin, & Diaz, 2001) show a basis for incorporating SIT into prevention contextualizations and applications. (2) CBT's concern for relapse prevention (e.g., Rose, Skelly, Badger, Naylor, & Helzer, 2012) could be more effectively elaborated and implemented should knowledge from prevention science be applied to these types of efforts.

The Emergence of Prevention Science

The preceding description of boundaries and mutual influences between prevention science and other fields of psychology can further be extended to present other interdisciplinary connections that facilitated the emergence of prevention science, such as its connections with developments in public health, social work, medicine, public policy, and economics. However, the somewhat associative mentioning of prevention science, developmental psychopathology, positive psychology, counseling psychology, counselor education, and finally clinical psychology is not incidental. Rather, it represents the interactive nature of the gradual emergence of prevention science as a prominent scientific domain. For example, one of the most profound shifts in prevention paradigms (see Israelashvili, 2002) that has taken place over the years is the increasing comprehension that efforts to promote and foster various aspects of the individual and/or the situation (e.g., skills acquisition) are frequently more powerful in dealing with potential risks for negative behavior than are efforts to eliminate or destroy problematic issues that may lead to problem behavior or disease. In addition, there has been a shift from only focusing on the individual to acknowledging and trying to influence institutional and systemic changes needed to empower people and reduce problematic behaviors that stem from larger societal and institutional problems (e.g., poverty, discrimination, and social inequities) (APA, 2014; Kenny & Hage, 2009; Prilleltensky, 2001).

In addition to the many *people* and *circumstances* that have contributed to the emergence of prevention science – that is, the shift that gradually took place from previous beliefs to current scientifically based knowledge on the need and techniques to prevent maladaptive, risk, and problematic behaviors and conditions – several additional *insights*, gained by prevention scholars, should be mentioned:

(1) *The adoption of a rigorous methodology*: Solid and expanded scientific paradigms, that supply hard-core facts regarding the contributions of prevention interventions have been widely disseminated. These scientific paradigms include intensive use of controlled designs that essentially refer to the Solomon Four-Group Design (e.g., Iphofen, 2011). In addition, an extensive awareness and practical explorations of both moderating and mediating variables (e.g., Dawson-McClure, Sandler, Wolchik, & Millsap, 2004) frequently and significantly contribute to increasing the percentage (level) of the variance of the (dependent) intervention goals. Another feature of the advanced scientific paradigms in prevention studies is the expanded spectrum of measurements (i.e., dependent variables), aiming to include those measures that explore various positive changes that might have occurred, in contrast with the previous tendency to focus on the measurement of risk indicators and to prove that their level is significantly lower due to the preventive intervention.

(2) *The incorporation of sociopolitical concerns as a legitimate component in prevention efforts*: This involves the awareness of politicians (and policy makers), who are not only those who control the budget and decline/enable the implementation of prevention interventions, but rather those with significant and legitimate roles in the prevention activities. These other stakeholders (e.g., politicians, school principals, parents) have their own and institutional needs, different perspectives on the situation, and other ways of interpreting the results of evaluation studies that have been conducted by a distinguished researcher, who is unaware of the possible negative implications of the recommendations listed in an evaluation report (e.g., possible implications in terms of the results of future local elections; negative changes in the school image as a result of conducting a prevention program on a "tender issue"). Moreover, prevention researchers and scientists may not realize their underestimated dependency on policy makers and the need to coordinate their goals and objectives with stakeholders early on in the development of prevention interventions. A powerful example of political influences on the development and implementation of prevention efforts was given by Humphreys and Rappaport (1993), in their paper "From the Community Mental Health Movement to the War on Drugs: A Study in the Definition of Social Problems." In this paper, Humphreys and Rappaport suggested that, in an effort to enact new social control policies in the 1980s, the U.S. administration replaced funding for community mental health

programs with support for substance abuse treatment agencies, while claiming that substance abuse is primarily the result of a defect in the abuser's character and disposition. Though this specific example is invalid today, the prominent impact of political considerations on policy makers regarding prevention (as well as other issues) is internationally evident and hence has been internalized by prevention researchers and practitioners (e.g., Charo, 2014; Roumeliotis, 2015).

(3) *The dominant focus on matters of utility*: Speaking "the language of economy" (i.e., incorporation of utility calculations) is not just a welcomed outcome of prevention interventions but rather the essence and basic justification for investing more money in the implementation of what seems potentially to be a promising prevention intervention (see Temple & Reynolds, this volume). However, the last notion needs further clarification: utility, economy, and budget are terms that should be seriously taken into account. Yet, their interpretation shouldn't be narrowly defined. Rather, the use of financial resources (i.e., money) is only one aspect of economical calculation. Another utility-related resource that should sometimes be incorporated into utility calculations could be freedom, that is, the extent to which a prevention program facilitates feelings of and possibilities for freedom and liberty. For a politician, as well as to any other ordinary person, feelings of freedom – that is, the capability of speaking your true opinion, the ability to manage one's life without fear, and the knowledge that one's loved ones are safe – are all significant examples of utility that justify investment in a prevention programs (against violence, crime, discrimination, etc.).

(4) *Realization of the multifaceted nature of prevention*: While early approaches tended to focus the preventive intervention on the person who is at risk of conducting the problem behavior that should be prevented, awareness of the need to intervene also in the surrounding forces gradually increased. Namely, the focus of prevention shifted from concentration on either the person, or the family, or the community, or the organization, or the nation into a comprehensive approach that recommended a need for multifaceted interventions, that is, among the person, the family, the community, and so forth. Therefore, studies are conducted to measure whether focusing on one of the facets, or conducting the interventions in a certain order, would lead to better results, such as (a) focusing on the divorced mother only rather than conducting parallel interventions for the child and the mother together (Wolchik et al., 2000) or (b) focusing firstly on community leaders in order to gain their collaboration, which is essential to the success of future preventive interventions among a community's children (Fagan, & Hawkins, 2015).

(5) *Attention and consideration to social justice*: In more recent years, prevention research and applications have given much more attention to issues of social advocacy and social justice as motivations to guide prevention science (e.g., Kenny, Horne, Orpinas, & Reese, 2009; Kenny & Merdvide, 2013; Pieterse, Hanus, & Gale, 2013). This *Handbook* has also included chapters that incorporate these concepts within their areas of scholarship (e.g., see Hage, Schwartz, & DeMartino; Wong, Vaughan, & Klann, this volume).

(6) *Cultural awareness and cultural adaptation*: There has also been increased attention to the cultural context in which prevention interventions are delivered. Taking the term *culture* in its broader meaning (rather than ethnicity only), prevention scholars realized and started to incorporate cultural-adaptive approaches into their prevention studies and programs. This notion is not that easy to address, especially in light of the possible tension (Barrera, Castro, Strycker, & Toobert, 2013) between the will to keep the general guidelines that have been scientifically developed to prevent a given problem behavior and the need to adapt these guidelines into the language, examples, circumstances, and so on of various cultural groups (e.g., this volume, see Galanti et al; Gewirtz & Youssef; Orte et al.; Tein).

As mentioned previously in this chapter, the list of people, episodes, and processes is not a comprehensive description of prevention history; nor is it an analysis of the most influential figures in the field. Rather, it is a partial list of examples of those milestones that promoted the process that finally led to the emergence of prevention science. However, it should be noted that the emergence of prevention science has been a long and gradual process in which various people and experiences have been accumulated into a large body of knowledge. During the twenty-first century, prevention science will be greatly impacted by forces and innovations that offer enormous opportunities and challenges; among them are developments in neuroscience, technology, and population demographic shifts (Romano, 2013).

Thus, in terms of the sociology of science, consider indications such as the following:

- The *establishment of the Society for Prevention Research* (SPR)
- The 2014 *APA formal confirmation of the prevention guidelines*
- The publication of the *Journal of Primary Prevention* (Impact Factor: 1.018) and *Prevention Science* (Impact Factor: 3.153) as the major journals in the field of prevention

These three indications were the signs of the successful "formal" birth and growth of prevention science. Additional steps in the transition from birth to maturity, included the following:

- The *formal establishment of graduate programs and training* for those who wish to gain a degree or specialized training in prevention science (e.g., Harvard Graduate School of Education; the University of Minnesota; the University of Wisconsin– Madison; Washington State University; the University of Oregon; Pennsylvania State University; the University of Miami; the University of Zagreb, Croatia).
- Recent *advertisements of job opportunities* for experts in prevention science, as published in the SPR website, are another representation of the current academic status of prevention science among other domains of human knowledge.

The following is another significant and necessary step in the establishment of a comprehensive scientific field of prevention:

- *The globalization of prevention* entails further documentation of the prevention activities taking place in various parts of the world, followed by an exploration of the generalizations and the limitations that may be suggested to prevention scientists and practitioners all over the world. Currently, the scope of such documentation and exploration that has been done is very limited. While several Western prevention programs and initiatives have been implemented in other nations, an accumulation of reports and evidence to support their use in different contexts is limited (Romano et al., 2014; Tein, & Israelashvili, 2014). Similarly, there is a need to incorporate lessons learned from non-Western nations into existing prevention models of intervention, implementation, and evaluation. Therefore, the need to address the globalization of prevention is critically important, and offers a major challenge to prevention science.

This *Handbook* intends to promote the last item – that is, the globalization of prevention – both by enabling the reader to learn about the current general issues that prevention science is addressing and by describing prevention activities that are being conducted by scholars in various parts of the world.

Potential readers of the *Handbook* are prevention scientists, practitioners, students, and policy makers from all over the world. It is our hope that exposure to the different conditions, strategies, limitations, and successes of prevention efforts across different nations, with different mentalities and different circumstances, will facilitate a better understanding of both the global and local challenges, opportunities, and successes of prevention science.

The *Handbook* includes two main parts: Part I includes chapters that represent the current state of knowledge on the essential topics and paradigms of prevention science. Part II includes chapters that were written by prevention scholars from various parts of the world. Each scholar (or group of scholars) wrote about his or her nation (e.g., major characteristics of the state, society, and traditions) and about a specific or several prevention intervention(s) or topics salient in in the country (e.g., what is relevant to better understand issues that are related to prevention interventions and topics in this nation; what lessons have been learned in the course of developing and/or implementing prevention programs; etc.).

We trust the *Handbook* will be a valuable text and resource for those who are interested in prevention, that is, well-trained prevention experts as well as novices who want to become familiar with prevention. Naturally, it is impossible to cover all of the prevention efforts conducted in each and every nation in the world within the framework of this *Handbook*. Hence, once the reader has finished reviewing and reading this *Handbook*, and raises his or her eyes from the text, much more remains to be learned about international prevention science.

Reference

Adler, A. (1927). The cause and prevention of neuroses. *Journal of Mental Science* 73: 1–8.

Adler, A. (1928). The cause and prevention of neuroses. *Journal of Abnormal and Social Psychology* 23(1): 4–11. dx.doi.org/10.1037/h0074804

Albee, G. W. (1980). A competency model must replace the defect model. In Bond, L. A., & Rosen, J. C. (eds.), *Competence and Coping during Adulthood* Hanover, NH: University Press of New England, (pp. 75–104.

Albee, G. W., & Gullotta, T. P. (1997). *Primary Prevention Works*. Thousand Oaks, California: Sage

Ansbacher, H. L. (1990). Alfred Adler, pioneer in prevention of mental disorders. *Journal of Primary Prevention* 11: 37–68.

APA (American Psychological Association) (2014). Guidelines for prevention in psychology. *American Psychologist* 69 (April): 285–96. dx.doi.org/10.1037/a0034569

Barrera, M., Castro, F. G., Strycker, L. A., & Toobert, D. J. (2013). Cultural adaptations of behavioral health interventions: a progress report. *Journal of Consulting and Clinical Psychology* 81: 196–205. dx.doi.org/10.1037/a0027085

Caplan, G. (1964). *Principles of Prevention Psychiatry*. Oxford, UK: Basic Books.

Charo, R. A. (2014). Physicians and the (woman's) body politic. *New England Journal of Medicine* 370: 193–5. dx.doi.org/10.1056/NEJMp1313499

Cicchetti, D., Rappaport, J., Sandler, I., & Weisberg, R. P. (eds.) (2000). *The Promotion of Wellness in Children and Adolescents*. Washington, DC: CWLA Press.

Cicchetti, D., & Rogosch, F. A. (2002). A developmental psychopathology perspective on adolescence. *Journal of Consulting and Clinical Psychology* 70: 6–20. dx.doi.org/10.1037/0022–006X.70.1.6

Conyne, R. K. (2015). *Counseling for Wellness and Prevention: Helping People Become Empowered in Systems and Settings*. New York: Routledge

Cowen, E. L. (1977). Baby-steps toward primary prevention. *American Journal of Community Psychology* 5: 1–22.

Cowen, E. L. (1994). The enhancement of psychological wellness: challenges and opportunities. *American Journal of Community Psychology* 22: 149–79.

Cutuli, J. J., Gillham, J. E., Chaplin, T. M., Reivich, K. J., Seligman, M. E. P., Gallop, R. J., ... Freres, D. R. (2013). Preventing adolescents' externalizing and internalizing symptoms: effects of the Penn Resiliency Program. *International Journal of Emotional Education* 5: 67–79.

Dawson-McClure, S. R., Sandler, I. N., Wolchik, S. A., & Millsap, R. E. (2004). Risk as a moderator of the effects of prevention programs for children from divorced families: a six-year longitudinal study. *Journal of Abnormal Child Psychology* 32: 175–90. dx.doi.org/10.1023/B:JACP.0000019769.75578.79

Fagan, A. A., & Hawkins, J. D. (2015). Enacting preventive interventions at the community level: the Communities that Care Prevention System. In Scheier, L. M. (ed.), *Handbook of Adolescent Drug Use Prevention: Research, Intervention Strategies, and Practice*. Washington, DC: American Psychological Association, pp. 343–60. http://dx.doi.org/10.1037/14550-020.

Garmezy, N. (1985). Stress-resistant children: the search for protective factors. In Stevenson, J. E. (ed.), *Recent Research in Developmental Psychopathology*. Oxford: Pergamon, pp. 213–33.

Garmezy, N. (1987). Stress, competence, and development: continuities in the study of schizophrenic adults, children vulnerable to psychopathology, and the search for stress-resistant children. *American Journal of Orthopsychiatry* 57: 159–74. dx.doi.org/10.1111/j.1939-0025.1987.tb03526.x.

Gordon, R. (1983). An operational classification of disease prevention. *Public Health Reports* 98: 107–9.

Griffin, K. W., Scheier, L. M., Botvin, G. J., & Diaz, T. (2001). Protective role of personal competence skills in adolescent substance use: psychological well-being as a mediating factor. *Psychology of Addictive Behaviors* 15(3): 194–203. dx.doi.org/10.1037/0893–164X.15.3.194

Gullota, T. P. (1997). Operationalizing Albee's incidence formula. In Albee, G. W., & Gullota, T. P. (eds.), *Primary Prevention Works*. Thousand Oaks, CA: Sage, pp. 23–40.

Hawkins, J. D., Jenson, J. M., Catalano, R., Fraser, M. W., Botvin, G. J., Shapiro, V., Hendricks Brown, C., … et al. (2015). *Unleashing the Power of Prevention*. Washington, DC: National Academy of Medicine (NAM), June 22. nam.edu/perspectives-2015-unleashing-the-power-of-prevention/

Healthy People (1979). *The Surgeon General's Report on Health Promotion and Disease Prevention 1979*. Washington, DC: U.S. Department of Health, Education, and Welfare, Public Health Service, Office of the Assistant Secretary for Health and Surgeon General (PHS). Publication No. 79-55071. profiles.nlm.nih.gov/ps/access/NNBBGK.pdf

Humphreys, K., & Rappaport, J. (1993). From the community mental health movement to the war on drugs: a study in the definition of social problems. *American Psychologist* 48: 892–901. dx.doi.org/10.1037/0003–066X.48.8.892

Iphofen, R. (2011). Ethical decision making in qualitative research. *Qualitative Research* 11: 443–6. dx.doi.org/10.1177/1468794111404330

Israelashvili, M. (2002). Inoculation as a third paradigm in mental health promotion. *International Journal for Mental Health Promotion* 4: 34–40.

Joint Commission on Mental Illness and Health, Eisenhower administration (1961). Action for mental health: final report of the Joint Commission on Mental Illness and Health. See Grob, G. N. (1991). *From Asylum to Community: Mental Health Policy in Modern America*. Princeton, NJ: Princeton University Press.

Jonnes, J. (1999). *Hep-Cats, Narcs, and Pipe Dreams: A History of America's Romance with Illegal Drugs*. Baltimore, MD: Johns Hopkins University Press.

Joseph, J., & Wetzel, N. A. (2013). Ernst Rüdin: Hitler's racial hygiene mastermind. *Journal of the History of Biology* 46, 1–30. doi: 10.1007/s10739-012–9344-6.

Kenny, M. E., & Hage, S. M. (2009). The next frontier: prevention as an instrument of social justice. *Journal of Primary Prevention* 30: 1–10.

Kenny, M. E., Horne, A. M., Orpinas, P., & Reese, L. E. (2009). *Realizing Social Justice: The Challenge of Preventive Interventions*. Washington, DC: American Psychological Association.

Kenny, M. E., & Medvide, M. (2013). Prevention in pursuit of social justice. In Vera, E. M. (ed.), *The Oxford Handbook of Prevention in Counseling Psychology*. New York: Oxford University Press, pp. 125–40.

Kobau, R., Seligman, M. E. P., Peterson, C., Diener, E., Zack, M. M., Chapman, D., & Thompson, W. (2011). Mental health promotion in public health: perspectives and strategies from positive psychology. *American Journal of Public Health* 101: e1–e9. dx.doi.org/10.2105/AJPH.2010.300083

Long, B. B. (1986). The prevention of mental-emotional disabilities: a report from a National Mental Health Association Commission. *American Psychologist* 41: 825–9. dx.doi.org/10.1037/0003–066X.41.7.825

Masten, A. S. (2001). Ordinary magic: resilience processes in development. *American Psychologist* 56: 227–38.

McGraw, A. P., Todorov, A., & Kunreuther, H. (2011). A policy maker's dilemma: preventing terrorism or preventing blame. *Organizational Behavior and Human Decision Processes* 115: 25–34.

Meichenbaum, D. (1985). *Stress Inoculation Training*. New York: Pergamon.

Meichenbaum, D. (2007). Stress inoculation training: a preventative and treatment approach. In Lehrer, P. M., Woolfolk, R. L., & Sime, W. E. (eds.), *Principles and Practice of Stress Management*. New York: Guilford Press, pp. 491–516.

Melbourne Charter for Promoting Mental Health and Preventing Mental and Behavioural Disorders (2008). www.vichealth.vic.gov.au/media-and-resources/publications/melbourne-charter.

Moffitt, T. E. (2005). The new look of behavioral genetics in developmental psychopathology: gene-environment interplay in antisocial behaviors. *Psychological Bulletin* 131: 533–54. dx.doi.org/10.1037/0033–2909.131.4.533

Morris, H., Skouteris, H., Edwards, S., & Rutherford, L. (2015). Obesity prevention interventions in early childhood education and care settings with parental involvement: a systematic review. *Early Child Development and Care* 185(8): 1283–1313. dx.doi.org/10.1080/03004430.2014.991723

Mrazek, P. J., & Haggerty, R. J. (eds.). (1994). *Reducing Risks for Mental Disorders: Frontiers for Preventive Intervention Research*. Washington, DC: National Academy Press.

Pieterse, A. L., Hanus, A. E., & Gale, M. M. (2013). Advocacy and prevention: dismantling systems of oppression. In Vera, E. M. (ed.), *The Oxford Handbook of Prevention in Counseling Psychology*. New York: Oxford University Press, pp. 109–24.

Price, R. H., Cowen, E. L., Lorion, R. P., & Ramos-McKay, J. (eds.). (1998). *14 Ounces of Prevention: A Casebook for Practitioners*. Washington, DC: American Psychological Association.

Prilleltensky, I. (2001). Value-based praxis in community psychology: moving toward social justice and social action. *American Journal of Community Psychology* 29: 747–78. doi: 10.1023/A:1010417201918.

Renfrew, M. J., Pokhrel, S., Quigley, M., et al. (2012). Preventing disease and saving resources: the potential contribution of increasing breastfeeding rates in the UK. UNICEF UK 2012. www.unicef.org.uk/Documents/Baby_Friendly/Research/Preventing_disease_saving_resources.pdf?epslanguage=en

Romano, J. L. (2013). Prevention in the 21st century. In Vera, E. M. (ed.), *The Oxford Handbook of Prevention in Counseling Psychology*. New York: Oxford University Press, pp. 36–50.

Romano, J. L. (2015). *Prevention Psychology: Enhancing Personal and Social Well-being*. Washington, DC: American Psychological Association. dx.doi.org/10.1037/14442-002

Romano, J. L., Israelashvili, M., Nair, E., Nota, L., Soresi, S., & Horne, A. M. (2014). Global applications of prevention psychology to enhance health and well-being. Invited symposium in the 28th International Congress on Applied Psychology, Paris, France.

Rose, G. L., Skelly, J. M., Badger, G. J., Naylor, M. R., & Helzer, J. E. (2012). Interactive voice response for relapse prevention following cognitive-behavioral therapy for alcohol use disorders: a pilot study. *Psychological Services* 9(2): 174–84. dx.doi.org/10.1037/a0027606

Roumeliotis, F. (2015). Politics of prevention: the emergence of prevention science. *International Journal of Drug Policy* 26: 746–54. dx.doi.org/10.1016/j.drugpo.2015.03.011

Rutter, M. (1987). Psychosocial resilience and protective mechanisms. *American Journal of Orthopsychiatry* 57: 316–31. dx.doi.org/10.1111/j.1939-0025.1987.tb03541.x

Singh, I. (2004). Doing their jobs: mothering with Ritalin in a culture of mother-blame. *Social Science & Medicine* 59: 1193–1205. dx.doi.org/10.1016/j.socscimed.2004.01.011

Snyder, C. R., & Lopez, S. J. (2007). *Positive Psychology: The Scientific and Practical Explorations of Human Strengths.* Thousand Oaks, CA: Sage.

Spaulding, J., & Balch, P. (1983). A brief history of primary prevention in the twentieth century: 1900–1980. *American Journal of Community Psychology*, 11: 59–80.

Tein, J-Y., & Israelashvili, M. (2014). Cultural adaptation of an existing evidence-based program. Paper presented in the 28th International Congress on Applied Psychology, Paris, France.

Werner, E., & Smith, R. S. (1992). *Overcoming the Odds: High Risk Children from Birth to Adulthood.* Ithaca, NY: Cornell University Press.

WHO (World Health Organization) (1999). Definition of health. www.who.int/about/definition/en/print.html

Wolchik, S. A., West, S. G., Sandler, I. N., Tein, J. Y., Coatsworth, D., Lengua, L., . . . & Griffin, W. A. (2000). An experimental evaluation of theory-based mother and mother–child programs for children of divorce. *Journal of Consulting and Clinical Psychology* 68: 843–56. doi: 10.1037/0022–006X.68.5.843

PART I

The Essence of Prevention Science

Foundations

2 Policy Development and Decision Making in Prevention Science

David V. McQueen

A Brief Orientation

Public health has always been a broad area of work. While it may be seen by many in the general public as well as many within the field of medicine as an area of work that is part and parcel of the medical world, those who work in public health recognize the broad diversity of the enterprise. As now practiced, public health cuts across all sectors of society. Recent movements, such as "health in all policies" (HiAP), have argued that public health is a concern for all ministers in government; that, indeed, no area of daily life is free of health concerns. Furthermore, health is not just an issue for individuals, but the whole of society, from communities to governments, is engaged in the concern for health. Public health has been recognized globally in the academic world both as an area of expertise within the university curricula and also in brick-and-mortar institutions devoted primarily to public health, such as the schools of public health in the United States (U.S.) as well as the older institutions such as the London School of Hygiene and Tropical Medicine. In the academic world of public health, there is an acceptance that public health is not just the application of epidemiology as a field of work but that other sciences from the biological to the social have a powerful role to play in the field of public health. In the past four decades of research and practice, there has been a growth in concern with health promotion, evidence, and policy. Each of these concerns has brought some of its own special characteristics. Health promotion has championed the role of values in public health decision making, arguing that social justice and equity are part and parcel of the public health enterprise. Evidence, partly as a response to the evidence-based medicine movement, has also entered the realm of public health in a powerful way. The evidence debate has argued for hard scientific evidence for prevention as well as alternative approaches to evaluate the complicated issues that arise in prevention science. In the area of health policies, discussions have taken on large aspects of society and brought health into discussions of development at the highest levels in the United Nations (UN). Taking all of this into account has meant that the science of prevention is now viewed as far more diverse and complicated than in earlier days with its narrower focus on such areas as risk taking at the individual level. We now assume that prevention science lies inside a broad context of human and social reality. Despite this broad reality of current thinking and the relationship that exists among health promotion, health policy, and evidence, the road to understanding the complexity that has arisen is difficult, time consuming, and now a concern for worldwide health organizations.

This chapter explores several aspects of current efforts to address policy related to public health. By necessity, it will cross over many key issues that have arisen in the discussions on policy in recent years. For the purposes of this chapter, these key issues are the social determinants of health (SDOH); social justice and equity; governance; values; HiAP; health promotion; institutions; and evidence. These areas all relate to each other but are often treated as separate entities in discussion. This separation often leads to mixed efforts and mixed messages, providing a somewhat confusing picture for those interested in the topic of policy and health. Nonetheless, it is the current state of the art, and although the individual areas may reflect the highest of current prevention science efforts, the combination still remains a complicated area to understand. Please refer to the author's note at the end of this chapter for further comments on some of the terms used in this chapter.

There is a tendency by some to regard these recent areas of public health work as primarily a Western phenomenon of interest. In part, this is an artifact of the dominance of relevant publications in Western languages, notably English. Nonetheless, global organizations such as the World Health Organization (WHO) have taken a major lead in addressing these areas. This lead has been followed by the regional offices of the WHO taking up these causes prominently. Indeed, the Pan American Health Organization (PAHO) region of the Americas has taken a very strong approach in these areas, with strong efforts in South American countries. In addition, member nations of the UN have taken up development goals that deal both indirectly and directly with the efforts to address the SDOH and HiAP areas. It is instructive for the reader to consider a document such as *Health in All Policies: Report on Perspectives and Intersectoral Actions in the Western Pacific*, a regional report from the Western Pacific Region Organization (WPRO, 2013). The five sections are titled, respectively, "Assembling the Evidence," "An Environment Conducive to Intersectoral Action on the Social Determinants of Health and Health Equity in the Western Pacific Region," "Building Blocks for the Development and Implementation of Intersectoral Action on the Social Determinants of Health and Health Equity," "Intersectoral Action That Addresses the Social Determinants of Health and Health Equity," and "Sustaining Intersectoral Action on the Social Determinants of Health and Health Equity." The titles alone illustrate the role of these emergent areas in public health. Many such documents from around the world are available on the Internet.[1]

For purposes of this chapter, these areas are here very briefly summarized; more background and detail on each area are found in much of the extensive

1 www.wpro.who.int/topics/social_determinants_health/health_in_all_policy_report.pdf.

literature cited throughout this chapter. The area that is termed the "social determinants of health" is an ancient pursuit in public health, but has risen to more prominence in recent years through the concerted efforts of the WHO Commission on the Social Determinants of Health (WHOCSDOH, 2008) and the work of scholars and institutions following the Commission's work. It remains largely a highly epidemiologically focused approach. Given the attention to the SDOH area and its centrality to policy and other areas of concern, a few more comments are in order. The SDOH area arises out of the notion that risk factors outside of the individual relate to, correlate with, or actually cause health and illness at the population level. The topic of these contextual factors that lie outside the individual and relate to health and illness is an enormous area of consideration, and in recent years much of the relevant research has been carried out under the rubric of the SDOH.

A comment on the word "factor" is in order. It is a problematic word. It is word that often implies causality and is used often to describe a variable in a scientific model. It implies agency, that is, it acts on other components in any model. In short, its meaning is quite interpretable. It is used here because it is a weaker word than "determinant" with respect to causality; the term "determinant" implies a greater certainty of causality and rigor of proof than can rarely be met in multifactorial public health applications and conveys a notion of complexity and a degree of uncertainty appropriate in most of the discussions related contextually to health and illness. More critically, SDOH conveys an image of an important relationship between context and health and illness. In addition, the idea of context specificity is highly relevant in discussions of HiAP.

The areas of social justice and equity are here linked together, reflecting the manner in which they are generally explored and treated in the public health literature. Social justice is, of course, a broad area going far beyond the health sector, but has entered into the public health sector as a value and driver to address the concerns revealed by the inequities in health outcomes globally. "Equity" is a present-day word used often when referring to issues of inequality, disadvantage, and disparities in health outcomes faced by individuals and/or groups. A summary review of the literature on equity often reveals very different biases and positions taken by different national government agencies; a universal agreement on the equity perspective remains elusive. "Governance" is a term that has become very prominent in the public health policy area. This follows from the fact that most policy is the result of the process of governments conducting their business. Nonetheless, the understanding of that process remains complicated, and for many in the health sector, untrained in political science, policy making may appear distal. In particular, the field of health promotion has introduced "values" into the discussions of policy and public health. It is a central focus of the area, and thus, by example, embraces concepts such as equity and social justice. This changing picture of public health has brought about significant changes in the institutions of public health in the academic, government, and nongovernmental sectors. Thus the concerns with

SDOH and HiAP equity are mirrored in the research, funding, and work of these institutions. Importantly, evidence is a common scientific theme that lies behind all these endeavors. Thus there is an ongoing search for the scientific evidence of what works to change the SDOH, make healthy policy happen, and address social justice and inequalities related to health.

Understanding what is evidence in this complex, emergent, multicausal way of thinking in public health has led to many challenges. Important factors are the lack of (consensus about) research evidence; competing sources of evidence; a social environment not favorable to policy change; and other social, strategic, and financial goals of policy makers besides clinical effectiveness (Black, 2001). Some assert that policy is rather evidence informed than evidence based, as has been asserted in Bowen and Zwi, 2005 and further cited in Lomas and Brown, 2009). Reflecting on the connection between areas of concern, Lomas (2000) gave a framework for understanding the policy- and decision-making process in which he points to a diversity of factors involved: the role of institutional structure (formal and informal); information (from different sources); and values (ideologies, beliefs, and interests). The argument is also made that the perspective one takes on policy making influences the role of science and evidence in policy. Thus we are faced today with multiple interactions around the components of public health and prevention science. Part of the complexity in understanding the role of evidence in policy related to health is the need to understand how the institutions of public health create evidence, use evidence, and in general apply the science of public health to policy making.

Role of Institutions in Prevention Policy

While it is a function of institutions to carry out policy, it is individuals and groups active in the institutions that help form these policies. Policies are made and carried out at different types and levels of institutions. For example, governmental institutions make and carry out policies. In the United States, public health policy is made and taken through a complex relationship between elected government (e.g., Congress) and agencies of the executive branch of government such as the Centers for Disease Control and Prevention (CDC), National Institutes of Health (NIH), and other agencies. This is, however, unique to the United States; other countries, such as Canada, Britain, and others, have differing approaches. Global agencies such as the WHO (Geneva) and the WHO regional offices engage in health policy formation. Nongovernmental organizations (NGOs) are often involved in setting policy, ranging from national disease foundations, such as the American Heart Association and American Cancer Society, to global foundations in health promotion NGOs, such as the International Union for Health Promotion and Educations (IUHPE). Globally, there a multitude of such organizations that represent the role of civil society in framing health-related policies. Finally, the UN itself functions as an international agency that deals with policies across all areas of society and may be seen as an obvious agency to carry out the idea of HiAP.

In public health policy discussions, the term "governance" is widely used today. It should be noted, however, that there are many definitions of governance from a wide range of sources, (cf. Bevir, 2013; Dodgson, Lee, & Drager, 2002; Finkelstein, 1995; Hufty, 2011; Rosenau, 1995, 1999; World Bank, 1991). Discussions and definitions are best understood by a perusal of the Internet on this topic, (e.g., Council on Foreign Relations).[2] Independent of the definition, a key consideration is that the related word "government" is a noun that expresses the structural aspect of government and may be considered an institutional word. Governance is a word expressing action or process and is a verbal concept; it is what a government does. Furthermore, "government" is a broad term, and although we often think of it as a geopolitical entity (nation-state), it may also be a corporate government (business entity), a sociopolitical entity (tribe, family, etc.), or any number of different kinds of governmental structures. In contrast, governance is the physical exercise of power and policy within a governmental structure. Often the term "government" is used more abstractly as a synonym for governance, as in the phrase, "Peace, Order and Good Government" found in Section 91 of the 1867 Canadian Constitution Act. In general, "governance" relates to how decisions are made, how political authority is exercised, and how the institutions of government collaborate and delegate resources. From its beginnings, public health has been involved with governance, and it remains a key area for public health research and understanding (McQueen, Wismar, Lin, Jones, & Davis, 2012).

A comment should be made on the idea of health governance, a term that one also encounters. As a broad idea, governance for health is an old concept; however, as a modern concept, it is relatively recent as argued clearly in the work of Kickbusch (2007, 2010). A recent WHO study considered the concept in detail and tied it to many of the key issues in today's public health. Many of the challenges faced globally have significant health impacts. The challenges include natural disasters, urbanization, epidemiological and demographic transitions, food insecurity, climate change, and widening economic disparities. More than ever, these synergistic large-scale challenges may require interdependent solutions. The complexity calls for systems approaches at all levels and will force policy makers to move out of their silo compartments, an approach championed by the European Office of WHO (WHO [EURO], 2011a).

The recognition of this complexity has given rise to new approaches to address the complicated causality of preventable, postponable, or manageable noncommunicable diseases (NCD). "The whole of government and the whole of society must become more familiar with the complex dynamics of health and its determinants in order to govern better" (WHO [EURO], 2011a, p. 73). This approach makes the development of policies to address NCD and in particular

2 www.cfr.org/issue/global-governance/ri23.

the social determinants of health much more plausible because it implies the necessity for change in the institutions of health themselves. Not only do internal governmental institutional structures, such as departments, agencies, bureaus, and civil service structures, need to be changed, but also the relationships between these institutional structures and the organizational entities residing outside of the governmental institutions, such as NGOs, civil society (individuals and organizations in a society independent of the government), and the business sector. Health policy for governance now becomes a whole-of-society approach that requires a major shift from twentieth-century approaches (McQueen et al., 2012).

The whole discussion of governance and health now includes all the dimensions of governance, ranging from ethical considerations, to ideas about leadership, and ultimately to a comprehension of global health systems. Thus health governance is faced not only with complexity but is also intertwined with all the other difficult problems in contemporary public health. There are considerable scholarly materials on global health governance available at blogs.shu.edu.[3] A seminal article in this domain was published by Ng and Ruger (2011) titled *Global Health Governance at a Crossroads*. This extensive review covers many of the issues found in global health governance. They note that global health governance is more complex than the older notion of international health governance because of the influence of globalization and the declining relevance of national boundaries. They also emphasize that global health governance has not been well defined conceptually. Also notable is that the traditional international players have moved into the global concept even as their institutional structures, bound by national politics, often remain locked in a nationalistic past. This is particularly true for the major global health organizations that maintain organizational structures tied to national member states, as found in many NGOs with an organizational structure based on nation-states or the regions of the WHO.

One may assert that the structural models of many global organizations are now outmoded and in fact inhibit health promotion and prevention efforts. Also, NGOs and civil society may be faster than more established organizations and governmental entities in responding to new structural needs. New roles are being sought by nongovernmental organizations and civil society. These groups are less constrained by what part of the institutionalized governmental structure must be worked with when addressing public health issues. They have more degrees of freedom in approaching specific health issues. For example, such groups are not necessarily constrained by national or other geopolitical boundaries. Examples of such NGO work are abundant, such as the Carter Center's work to eliminate malaria and lymphatic filariasis in the Caribbean,[4] CARE's work on maternal health Programs in sub-Saharan Africa,[5] or the many

3 blogs.shu.edu/ghg/about-global-health-governance.

4 www.cartercenter.org/health/hispaniola-initiative/index.html.

5 www.care.org/campaigns/mothersmatter/index.asp.

preventive health programs funded by the Gates Foundation. Nonetheless, despite the many success stories and the changing nature of global health governance, Ng and Ruger (2011) note that there are remaining major issues. Perhaps the major issue involves the way for all the various institutions and governments to cooperate with each other. Cooperation generally depends upon mechanisms to make this possible, and historically most institutions, whether governments or NGOs, have little experience in creating or managing such mechanisms. Other nontechnical problems are commonplace. For example, many organizations work in their own silos, as do government agencies and much of academia.

We observe this in seemingly successful public health programs globally and locally that are single disease or single risk factor oriented. Unfortunately, the success of vertical programs may be diverting resources away from more comprehensive multifactorial or multidisease approaches both within and outside medicine. Further, the silo approach moves research away from addressing the complexities of the public health enterprise. Nonetheless, there are efforts that concentrate on underlying broad-based concerns. Ng and Ruger (2011) note that "Non-communicable diseases (NCDs) are receiving more attention now that the globalization of unhealthy diets and sedentary lifestyles is making them both more common and more deadly . . . . Observers urge action, particularly through multisectoral partnerships" (p. 13).

It is the broad concept of public health and prevention science that links to the emerging efforts on HiAP. Nonetheless, it could be argued that the theoretical foundation of HiAP, and in particular the evidence base stemming from theory that would show its efficacy, is still in development. In essence, HiAP remains largely a question of political will and is as much more driven by values than based on any sound hard evidence of efficacy. As with so much political action that rests on political power, there is a difficult task ahead to delineate clearly the effects of such an approach. HiAP is an ideologically based framework for action on health because the idea that health needs to be incorporated throughout all political processes is an assertion that rings true with the underlying moral approach of public health. Statements such as "all ministers are health ministers" echo the sentiments of the great nineteenth-century German public health champion and founder of social medicine Rudolph Virchow and others who injected politics into the health arena (Silver, 1987). It is also clear that the concept of HiAP is a move away from the individual-centered, biomedical view of public health that dominated much of the twentieth century.

If one considers the notion of HiAP as representative of an emerging broader scope for public health, then one should also note the emergence of the recognition of contextual factors, both social and cultural, as helping to define this as an area of legitimacy for public health. Once contextual factors are seen as a legitimate area for public health action, the political implications follow. They follow because most of the contextual factors lie outside of the traditional medical realm. And it follows that issues such as equity become important both politically and from a health standpoint. It also follows that health promotion as an activity of public health becomes salient; one does not prevent inequity, one promotes equity.

The relationship between HiAP and governance – that is, the underlying processes of governing – is seen in advanced economies where it operates at all levels of government from national to local. Most areas of governance that relate to health are commonplace and routine governmental functions (e. g., sewers, transportation, energy, education). While politics plays a role in these activities, one does not expect the supply of potable water to be dependent on whether the government is politically left leaning, centrist, or right wing. Nonetheless, the politically formed institutions of government related to HiAP play a role in the public's health. They comprise the institutions for action in the HiAP approach. Furthermore, some seemingly mundane areas such as housing policy may become controversial political items. Health considerations may then enter into the controversy. How these considerations enter may be highly contextual, variable, parochial, local, or national. For example, potable drinking water may seem rather nonpolitical until it becomes an issue of water resources and supplies that may cross over political boundaries to obtain access. When controversy arises, values are not far behind.

Role of Values in Public Health

Public health has always operated on a values base. It was the curmudgeon H. L. Mencken who wrote: "*Hygiene is the corruption of medicine by morality. It is impossible* to find a hygienist who does not debase his theory of the healthful with a theory of the virtuous" (Menken, 1922, p. 269, emphasis added). In recent years, the discussion of values has been central in health promotion (Gostin, Boufford, & Martinez, 2004; Gostin & Madison, 2006; Mayes & Oliver, 2012). Much of the discussion often lacks definitional clarity, perhaps because many of the discussants are not well versed in philosophy or logic. Fortunately, a recent treatise by Michael Shermer (2015), *The Moral Arc: How Science and Reason Lead Humanity toward Truth, Justice, and Freedom*, adds much clarity to this area of thought.

Within the public health discussion, the principal value concepts are equity, social justice, dignity, and human rights. These values are reflected in numerous documents and notably in those associated with the WHO Commission on the Social Determinants of Health (WHOCSDH, 2008). While the philosophical discussion of values is ancient, their presence in academic discourse on public health is more recent; fortunately, there is an extensive historical account that has been provided by writers such as Joas (2000) and Kuhn (1975).

When values are involved, the discussion of ethics also arises. Most ethical considerations in public health involve normative ethics. Normative ethics is concerned with how to act taking into account value concepts. Normative ethics is largely a prescriptive effort or, as some would term it, applied ethics. Ethical decisions are seldom straightforward. It is complex to judge what is right or wrong in actions, and this in turn has led to considerations of partial rightness, a concept that was historically quite developed in ethical writings. However, the influence of the work of John Rawls (1971), in particular, with its emphasis on each person in society having an equal claim to basic equal liberties, was picked up by the health sector and linked to the health equity and justice argument, and tended to move the focus in health directly to moral arguments underpinning action. Of course, this is a simplification of both Rawls' position over time as well as to those with differing philosophical approaches. Nonetheless, it seems to be Rawls' position that was picked up by the public health social justice proponents.

In public health, when actions are taken to protect the population's health – to prevent the spread of disease, to promote the community health, to reduce poverty, to increase health literacy – then ethical, value-laden efforts are being undertaken. These efforts to effect change link values and ethics directly to governance. It may be argued that these efforts are tied to concerns of public health prevention and health promotion arising chiefly out of a Western philosophical tradition. This tradition is made explicit with the use of value concepts such as equity and social justice in the efforts to address the SDOH in the work of the WHO Commission on SDOH (WHOCSDOH, 2008). This discussion on SDOH was, of course, at a high level of governance. Policy discussions of health at the highest levels may be viewed as aspirational or visionary. Major policy documents of international organizations (e.g., UN agencies such as WHO) and those stemming from the ministries of governments belong to this category (UNGA, 2011; WHO, 2009). Of course, in reality they are generally statements derived from the collective work of staffers, bureaucrats, and political appointees. As such, they are usually crafted after many hours of debate and dialogue among the writers and assigned no explicit authorship beyond that of the institution itself. The policy documents produced are given titles such as "statement," "resolution," "charter," or "agreement." They draw on value principles rather than ethics because they are primarily visionary and rarely state the ethical means by which the vision is to be carried out. Because the statements are at such a visionary level, those outside the visionary process may consider them somewhat vague. The challenge for policy at this level is how to translate this vision into collective action. That process is generally left to others, often lower-level bureaucrats, and to broader collectives such as civil society. The bureaucrats may be well positioned within governmental institutions and charged with the governance responsibility implied by the policy, whereas civil society, residing outside direct government, generally must argue policy from its direct merits to those whom they would wish to take action.

The process of taking high-level policy to action is hardly simple and often lacks specificity for application. Those framing policy are seldom the same people who would put policy into action. In addition, substantive resources for action, particularly monetary resources, are often lacking. In recent years, the role of civil society in creating the impetus for visionary statements has been well recognized and appreciated by those studying policy; the extensive literature on this is well documented in many sources but notably summarized in the Canadian government's foreign affairs document.[6] That recognition has been often less understood by institutionally based policy makers. Nonetheless, civil society, particularly NGOs comprising part of civil society, has pushed back at governmental institutions with its own sets of values. Indeed, sometimes an NGO will be organized specifically around a value that directly relates to health or health promotion. That is, the NGO's raison d'être is in itself to persuade standing governmental institutions to adopt value-based visionary statements in their area of interest. Often it is difficult to distinguish when the primary operation is one of policy or governance, but the expressions of governance and policy within government are found in the day-to-day operations of management, legislation, procurement, resource allocation, communication, and the other categorical operations of the institution we call government. In brief, policy, governance, and the institutions of government ultimately lead back to the value concepts that underlie the functioning of government. In essence, the role of government is to make values explicit to the governed.

Evidence and Policy in Public Health and Prevention

When one moves to a broad policy perspective such as HiAP, one is no longer just in the health arena. All the dimensions of policy, how it is developed and carried out, become part of the discussion. What is revealed is a large literature of relevance, and the broad area of policy supersedes the narrow field of health policy in general. The question of evidence takes on new dimensions. That is, what is the evidence basis for making broad policy? What is the evidence basis that policy, particularly broad policy, makes any difference in health outcomes? If there is a scientific basis for advocating HiAP, what is that basis? Those in public health may be comfortable with the ideological and value basis for HiAP, but the comfort level for the evidence of the effectiveness of health in all policy is much more questionable (cf. Brownson, Chriqui, & Stamatakis, 2009; Macintyre, 2012).

This is not a new concern. In the United States, a 1978 National Research Council (NRC) report, *Knowledge and Policy: The Uncertain Connection* (NRC, 1978), argued that the state of knowledge with regard to systematic evidence of policy effectiveness was not good. As a result, more recently the Committee on the Use of Social Science Knowledge in Public Policy (U.S.) was charged by the NRC "to review the knowledge utilization and other relevant literature to assess what is known about how social science knowledge is used in

6 www.international.gc.ca/development-developpement/cs-policy-politique-sc.aspx?lang=eng.

policy making ... [and] to develop a framework for further research that can improve the use of social science knowledge in policy making" (NRC, 2012, p. 2). Remarkably, this 2012 report, *Using Science as Evidence in Public Policy*, also showed that the evidence base is weak or nonexistent, concluding that a research approach leading to a better understanding of how policy is developed needs attention by researchers. One summation from the report applies particularly to health:

> Science has five tasks related to policy: (1) identify problems, such as endangered species, obesity, unemployment, and vulnerability to natural disasters or terrorist acts; (2) measure their magnitude and seriousness; (3) review alternative policy interventions; (4) systematically assess the likely consequences of particular policy actions – intended and unintended, desired and unwanted; and (5) evaluate what, in fact, results from policy. Across all of these tasks, there are political and value considerations that are outside the scope of science (p. 4).

HiAP faces significant challenges when it comes to reviewing alternative policy interventions that address the broader social factors related to health. To date, many of the policy-oriented statements still reflect interventions that address individual behavioral factors in the causation of NCDs. Alternative policy areas have been proposed for some time. Labonte (2012) has made the case in detail with regard to issues related to globalization and has provided specific alternative proposals, and Graham (2009) has made a case for addressing inequalities. Although many have proposed broadening policy areas, the key element is what policies global institutions take up.

When systematically assessing the consequences of particular policy actions, intended and unintended, desired and unwanted, and evaluating what actually results from policy, the public health area is on very weak ground. There are recent efforts (McQueen, et al., 2012) that provide insight into some of the specific processes and institutional and organizational mechanisms that tie structure to agency in policy actions, as well as the excellent report from the expert group on how can the health equity impact of universal policies be evaluated (WHO [EURO], 2011b). Following extensive discussions to delineate the challenges in policy evaluation, the expert group noted several promising approaches, such as systems approaches; innovative uses of natural experiments; crossnational comparative policy analyses using policy typologies; historical analyses; and insights drawn from complexity theory. There are other laudable efforts to assess policy such as discussed by Rütten, Abu-Omar, Frahsa, & Gelius (2013), but there is a need for many more studies to more fully understand the complex evaluative dimensions of policy. Significant challenges remain if we are to fully understand the impact of policies systematically. Unfortunately, at present, with regard to how policy translates into results on the ground, locally, nationally, or globally, there is relatively little available good evaluation. Until greater resources are given to evaluation of health policy, health policies will continue to be based largely on persuasion rather than on any scientific evidence basis.

Role of Institutions

The word "institution" denotes many different ideas; the meaning of the term can be either structural or functional, having both a physical and personnel structure as well as an acting or agency component. For example, the CDC is a U.S. federal agency under the Department of Health and Human Services, headquartered near Atlanta, Georgia. As such, the CDC has many buildings, bricks and mortar, with thousands of employees working in many centers, divisions, and branches charged with the mission to be an agency for public health in the United States. It is notable that this institution is regarded as an agency, because that wording means that it is designed for intervention. Geoffrey Hodgson (2006), in his definitive article "What Are Institutions?" defines them as such: "... systems of established and prevalent social rules that structure social interactions" (p. 2). This is a very broad and conceptual definition that seems distant from the actual brick-and-mortar agency. In common public health parlance, the use of the word institution is as an organization. Hodgson describes organizations as "special institutions that involve (a) criteria to establish their boundaries and to distinguish their members from nonmembers, (b) principles of sovereignty concerning who is in charge, and (c) chains of command delineating responsibilities within the organization" (p. 18).

In recent years, the debates in political science and sociology around the nature of institutions have led to a critical discussion of what is termed the "new institutionalism." For the public health researcher concerned with prevention, this discussion of new institutionalism may be somewhat arcane; however, it reveals some of the key considerations that operate in public health institutions and/or organizations. Ellen Immergut (1998), in her work on "The Theoretical Core of the New Institutionalism," delineated some of the chief ideas that one has to keep in mind with regard to institutions. First, institutions may be seen as collective organizing bodies to carry out political will through actions. This is at the heart of the agency idea and ties into discussions of governance. Second are what Immergut calls the "contextual logics of causality" (p. 15); this notion relates to the idea that institutions themselves determine the specific variables that are chosen for action. In a most comprehensive review of the new institutionalism, Hall and Taylor (1996) discuss the various forms of institutionalism and give examples in organizational entities. They review the work on the sociological perspective on institutions; one quotation seems particularly pertinent to health institutions dealing with NCDs and health promotion:

> ... the problematic that sociological institutionalists typically adopt seeks explanations for why organizations take on specific sets of institutional forms, procedures or symbols; and it emphasizes how such practices are diffused through organizational fields or across nations. They are interested, for instance, in explaining the striking similarities in organizational form and practice that Education Ministries display throughout the world, regardless of the differences in local conditions ... (p. 947).

It seems very appropriate to extend the arguments of Hall and Taylor to health ministries. The point here is that there are many dimensions of institutionalism that are relevant to understanding why institutions in public health act as they do. This multidimensionality reveals the need to better understand the role of the varied institutional interpretations found in the discussions of health policy. But above all, it reveals a need to understand why our institutions address the contextual factors in health as they do.

The literature related to governance, policy, and institutions related to public health is vast and undoubtedly increasing at a rapid rate as global institutions, academic and governmental, take on this topic. Consider just one subcomponent of these intersections, the area of intersectoral governance and its relation to HiAP. This has been explored extensively by institutions such as IUHPE, WHO (EURO), and the European Observatory on Health Systems and Policies (McQueen, et al, 2012). The European Observatory document concentrates just on the structures, actions, and experiences inside of governmental institutions in developing HiAP. The revealed structures and actions are highly complex, highly cultural, and in many cases highly related to national political structures. The point is that the whole policy area of public health is very complex. A response to this complexity by the Canadian government was the establishment of the National Collaborating Centre for Healthy Public Policy, located in the Province of Quebec, whose mission is to increase the expertise of public health actors across Canada in healthy public policy.[7]

Values, Equity, and Policy in Public Health and Prevention Science

Equity has become a central value in three key areas of present-day prevention science: (a) the social determinants of health (SDOH), (b) health in all policies (HiAP), and (c) health promotion. Why and how the idea of equity entered into these three areas is a lengthy story. Fortunately, much of this story is well documented and in the broad academic literature, if not specifically in the health-related literature. As mentioned earlier, much of the general discussion on values has been reviewed well by writers such as Joas (2000), Kuhn (1975), and Schnaedelbach (1983). Relevant to the values discussion are the earlier works of key German figures such as Hermann Lotze and Immanual Kant and in particular the works of Friedrich Nietzsche, mainly because they emphasized the contextual nature of values. In turn, this view originates in the older philosophical discourse on realism and nominalism, which, in turn, relied on debates between an Aristotelian or a Platonic position. The discourse centers on the question of whether values are fundamental ideas (the Platonic position) that exist independently of humans perceiving them, or whether they are highly

7 www.ncchpp.ca/en/.

contextual (the nominalist Aristotelian position) and bound to changing human perspectives. With regard to prevention science and health promotion, it is the nominalist position that has triumphed. The predominant position is that the context in which values are found is the key to understanding the role of values. However, there is a remnant of a more Platonic position in the idea that health itself is a value. Allowing for health as a value opens the door for public health and the promotion of health to fully incorporate the idea of values as fundamental to an understanding of public health. Once values are accepted as part of the public health position, then nominalist ideas such as equity as a value and social justice as a value become by default part of the discussion. This evolution is rarely specifically laid out but is implied in many public health statements and documents. A prime example is the Ottawa Charter for Health Promotion (WHO, 1986), a largely European-based document, which states that health promotion is driven by values and not just from biomedical approaches to health.

Equity may be a public health value; however, health equity requires some further clarification. There has been considerable discussion on the topic (e.g., Braverman, 2006); however, a precise definition of health equity remains elusive. Equity has been a key component in global discussions on health disparities and the unequal health resources in populations. The WHO (2015) sums up the idea of equity:

> Equity is the absence of avoidable or remediable differences among groups of people, whether those groups are defined socially, economically, demographically, or geographically. Health inequities therefore involve more than inequality with respect to health determinants, access to the resources needed to improve and maintain health or health outcomes. They also entail a failure to avoid or overcome inequalities that infringe on fairness and human rights norms. Reducing health inequities is important because health is a fundamental human right and its progressive realization will eliminate inequalities that result from differences in health status (such as disease or disability) in the opportunity to enjoy life and pursue one's life plans.

In such a statement, the concept of equity is transformed into a political concept by a global health institution that itself is shaped by government policies. At the nation-state level, health inequities are highly related to decisions by government actors to distribute resources equally or unequally in the population. In doing so, they favor some components of the population over others. The prevention science that evolves from this is shaped by such policies in the allocation of resources for public health.

The present-day concept of health equity owes much to the writings of Amartya Sen (1979), who in his Tanner Lecture laid out some the essential components of equity in terms of moral philosophy. In critiquing then-predominant types of equality – namely utilitarian equality, utility equality, and John Rawls' notion of equality – Sen, as an economist, introduced concepts of equality that stemmed from welfare economics. This moved equality out of the more classical philosophical realm and into the world of economics. This would be ultimately adapted in to the world of public health, health economics, health promotion, and prevention. In the same decade that health promotion was embracing crossdiscipline thinking in health, Sen moved to what is termed a "capabilities approach" that began to tie resources to the individual and group efforts to distribute these resources in an ethically driven effort toward equitable distribution. At the same time, these efforts created a paradigm shift that would tie together equity with human and economic development. This shift in thinking ultimately was linked to ideas of development found in the UN Millennium Goals[8] and early in the current century tied to the SDOH that included equity as a primary component of action. Thus it can be argued that current values of health equity have inherited an ideological base from earlier moral philosophy that leads to the integration of health equity into concrete policy related to development. This is how the concept moved from a value to an institutional concern in health. In September 2000, 189 heads of state adopted the UN Millennium Declaration and endorsed a framework for development. The plan was for countries and development partners to work together to reduce poverty and hunger and tackle ill health, lack of education, gender inequality, lack of access to clean water, and environmental degradation.[9]

- Eight Millennium Development Goals (MDGs) were established, with targets for 2015, and indicators to monitor progress.
- Three MDGs relate directly to health; to reduce child mortality by two-thirds (MDG 4); to reduce maternal deaths by three-quarters and achieve universal access to reproductive health (MDG 5); and to halt and reverse the spread of HIV/AIDS, achieve universal access to treatment for HIV/AIDS by 2010, and halt and reverse the incidence of malaria and other major diseases (MDG 6).
- Other MDGs have an indirect influence on health; MDG 1 has a target of halving the proportion of people who suffer from hunger; MDG 7 includes a target of halving the proportion of the population without sustainable access to safe drinking water and basic sanitation; and MDG 8 has a target to provide access to affordable essential drugs in developing countries. Primary education (MDG 2) and empowering women (MDG 3) also lead to health gains.

There is an additional component to the equity issue around the notion of social justice, a concept that has been heavily embraced personally by Michael Marmot as head of the WHO Commission Report on the Social Determinants of Health (WHOCSDOH, 2008). As mentioned previously, Rawls had a strong influence on the health equity arguments in public health. The critical point arising from Rawls, and seemingly taken up by the SDOH work, is that social justice and hence equity are tied to agency – that is, one's capacity to act

8 www.who.int/topics/millennium_development_goals/en/.
9 www.who.int/topics/millennium_development_goals/MDG-NHPS_brochure_2010.pdf?ua=1.

independently – and the very actions that would be carried out in a public health perspective. From a sociological perspective, a value concept such as health equity readily results in a discussion of structural change (e.g., distribution of government resources) versus agency (e.g., actors, individuals, and civil society). The debate often centers on which approach may be more effective. Furthermore, the structure versus agency discussion introduces the question of whether those concerned with health equity should focus on values or on how to improve human health. Ruger (2004, 2010) has taken up this discussion of social justice in detail and successfully linked it to health and health care.

Variation in Values in Prevention Science

If indeed one argues that values are contextual, then one can entertain the question: "How do European values related to health differ from, say, North American values?" There are aspects that are peculiarly European and that distinguish that perspective from other geographic regions of the world. In addition, there is variation on values within and across Europe. By analogy, we could assert that values with regard to health in a North America containing Canada, the United States, and Mexico might have considerable variation. Much has been written about the particular role of values in health in the Canadian context (Giacomini, Hurley, Gold, Smith, & Abelson, 2001), where the health care system itself is seen as a core Canadian value. In an opposite way of thinking, in the United States there has been an ongoing debate for decades over whether health, and by implication health care, is a human right or a privilege, a debate that continues with marked disputes in the U.S. Congress over the Affordable Care Act that political opponents label "Obamacare." In any case, the European context appears in line with a WHO perspective of health as a human right and a public good.

What are the specific components of this value (i.e., health as a fundamental right), and are these components recognized in policies, documents, programs, and advocacy statements? With regard to components, the European discussions generally have a tacit agreement that the components are dignity, liberty, democracy, equality, the rule of law, human rights, pluralism, tolerance, justice, solidarity, and nondiscrimination. These components are found in the European Constitution in the Preamble, Article 2, Article 3, and implied in many other parts of the document. Of course, it must be noted that the European Constitution is not a short, explicitly framed document; in contrast to the brief U.S. Constitution, it is open to considerable interpretation that is often bound to the current context of political thinking. Despite agreement on value fundamentals, European values about health are subject to possible value conflicts when working on health across sectors. This includes possible value trade-offs in the policy translation process. It is this trade-off and translation that moves the value-based ideology into the realm of ethical actions regarding health, health prevention, and health promotion. Further, these potential value conflicts lead inevitably to confrontation with parallel values such as accountability and civil participation.

Unfortunately, for decision making and policy efforts, healthy choices are often not transparent. The emerging importance of healthy choices, aroused by the *WHO Commission Report on Social Determinants* (WHOCSDOH, 2008), directly addresses conflicting value approaches. In the document, the scientific, epidemiologically based evidence clearly lays out the causal connections between health-related values such as health equity, social justice, education, and human dignity and good health. Despite a long history in public health of knowing the strong relationship between social and cultural factors and good health, it was the *Commission Report* that solidified this knowledge to a position beyond doubt scientifically. However, knowledge is not enough for effective action on the value-related causes of poor health. It is only the precursor to action. The science of how effectively to address these causes is highly problematic, and in reality significant changes in the attributable causes may imply political philosophies that are themselves tied to values that may not be in concert with those of the underlying values that relate to good health. Very basic value concepts such as freedom of choice and public democracy may in themselves be inimical to addressing some key causal values. It is not the point to debate this here, but merely to lay out why governance and ethical considerations to deal with such problems of health inequities face such extraordinary challenges.

Values, Ethics, and Practical Actions

Ethics and values are obviously related. Ethics is concerned with the decisions to take action on values and the underlying principles for these decisions. Most of the ethical considerations in the health field deal with what is generally termed normative ethics. Normative ethics is the part of historical ethical philosophy that is concerned with how to act taking into account value concepts. It views ethical considerations as largely a prescriptive effort. However, in recent decades value-based thinking related to health became more complex with judging what is right or wrong in actions, and this in turn has led to considerations of partial rightness, a concept that is historically quite developed in ethical writings.

Values are turned into ethical considerations when they become stated, when they appear explicitly in documents – that is, when stated efforts are taken to protect the health of a population; to prevent the spread of disease: to promote the health of a community; to reduce poverty that leads to poor health; to increase health literacy; and so on. It is this verbalization of efforts to effect change that is based on values that ties values and ethics directly to governance, which in sum can be imagined as the action component of government structure.

Given the current interest in the idea of HiAP, it is useful to characterize policy as used in discussions of health. At the highest levels, policy may be seen as aspirational or visionary, residing outside direct government and mainly in NGOs, which must argue for policy implementation to those who would be taking action. In recent years, the role of civil society in creating the impetus for visionary statements has been well recognized and appreciated chiefly by those examining policy. That recognition has been often less understood by institutionalized policy makers. Nonetheless, civil society and in particular those more formal NGOs comprising part of civil society have pushed back at governmental institutions with their own sets of values.

Final Thought for Prevention Science Policy

Public health today is faced with the challenges of weaving together the areas of HiAP; the SDOH; issues of social justice; and evidence of what works to prevent disease and illness in an increasingly urbanized, globalized world. It is perhaps the chief task of policy development and decision-making institutions to address these challenges. It is not easy, in part because of the huge dimension of the task, but also because the component fields and personnel of public health who would assist in taking action with regard to policy remain somewhat in their own silos. This is an area that requires considerable thinking across areas within public health and beyond, especially areas that lie outside the scope of traditional public health work. Interdiscipinarity, while praiseworthy and sought, is rarely a feature of the actual day-to-day work of people working in public health and prevention science. This chapter has presented some of the broad challenges in which we are currently engaged, but the chapter also reveals how much more broadly one must think in the future. As scientists, we have been taught to reduce a problem down to its solvable elements, and now we are told to be all-inclusive and embrace complexity. Without strong and highly convincing evidence on how we should do it, we are encouraged to bring social justice into the health arena and thus more successfully prevent disease and promote health globally. The challenges are scientific, moral, and political all at the same time.

Author's Note

This chapter uses a number of general terms, such as "values," "ethics," "structure," "agency," "policy," "governance," and "concepts." All of these terms as currently used in the public health sector are open to considerable discussion as to meaning and indeed may also have much variation when they, or their equivalents, are used in other languages. It is wholly impossible to define many such terms in a manner that would yield consensus among those who regularly employ such terms. My understanding of these terms is heavily influenced by my own doctoral training in the history, sociology, and philosophy of science, as well as by a public health career in academia and government of over four decades. Thus, many terms do have particular meaning and nuance to the author, and I will briefly note them. For example, the term "values" is a largely conceptual idea that often gets translated into cultural values, political values, moral values, and so on. However defined, values tend to be broad, enduring constructs that are regarded as fundamental to being human. They can often be contextual, but many would regard some values as beyond context. Health is a fundamental value. Ethics, on the other hand, relates much more to moral philosophy and is related to how an individual or a collective acts in relation to values. Ethics is about how one takes a course of action; it is more contextual than values and relates highly to concepts of justice. With regard to structure and agency, there is an excellent starter discussion in Wikipedia that argues that the primacy of either structure or agency with regard to human behavior is a central ontological concern in sociology, political science, and the other social sciences. Many recent books have explored many dimensions of the discussions in this chapter in greater depth. In particular, I would note the excellent summaries and presentation of many of these issues in Michael Shermer's (2015) book, *The Moral Arc: How Science and Reason Lead Humanity toward Truth, Justice, and Freedom.*

References

Bevir, M. (2013). *Governance: A Very Short Introduction*. Oxford, UK: Oxford University Press.

Black, N. (2001). Evidence-based policy: proceed with care. *British Medical Journal* 323: 275–9.

Bowen, S., & Zwi, A. B. (2005). Pathways to "evidence-informed" policy and practice: a framework for action. *PLoS Med* 2(7): e166. doi:10.1371/journal.pmed.0020166.

Braverman, P. (2006). Health disparities and health equity: concepts and measurement. *Annual Review of Public Health* 27: 167–94.

Brownson, R. C., Chriqui, J. F., & Stamatakis, K. A. (2009). Understanding evidence-based public health policy. *American Journal of Public Health* 99: 1576–83.

CSDH (Commission on Social Determinants of Health) (2008). Closing the gap in a generation: health equity through action on the social determinants of health. Final Report of the Commission on Social Determinants of Health. Geneva, World Health Organization.

Dodgson, R., Lee, K., & Drager, N. (2002). *Global Health Governance: A Conceptual Review*. London: WHO/London School of Hygiene & Tropical Medicine. Discussion Paper No. 1. (www.bvsde.paho.org/texcom/cd050853/dodgson.pdf)

Dworkin, R. (2011). *Justice for Hedgehogs*. Cambridge, MA: Belknap Press of Harvard University Press.

Finkelstein, L. (1995). What is global governance? *Global Governance*, 1: 367–72.

Gasparishvili, A., Smolentseva, A., & Tumanov, S. (2009). In Mansurov, V. A. (ed. in chief), *European Society or European Societies: A View from Russia*. (www.isras.ru/files/File/publ/Russia%20and%20Europe.pdf).

Giacomini, M., Hurley, J., Gold, I., Smith, P., & Abelson, J. (2001). *"Values" in Canadian Health Policy Analysis: What Are We Talking About?* Ottawa: Canadian Health Services Research Foundation.

Gostin, L. O., Boufford, J. I., & Martinez, R. M. (2004). The future of the public's health: vision, values, and L.O. strategies. *Health Affairs* 23 (4): 96–107.

Gostin, L. O., & Madison, P. (2006). What does social justice require for the public's health? Public health ethics and policy imperatives. *Health Affairs* 25 (4): 1053–60.

Graham, H. (2009). Tackling health inequalities: the scope for policy. In Graham, H. (ed.), *Understanding Health Inequalities*. New York: McGraw Hill. pp. 199–218.

Hall, P. A., & Taylor, R. C. R. (1996). Political science and the three new institutionalisms. *Political Studies* 44: 936–57. Article first published online: 22 DEC 2006.DOI: 10.1111/j.1467–9248.1996.tb00343.

Hodgson, G. M. (2006). What are institutions? *Journal of Economic Issues* 40: 1–25.

Hufty, M. (2011). Investigating policy processes: the Governance Analytical Framework (GAF). In Wiesmann, U., & Hurni, H. (eds.) *Research for Sustainable Development: Foundations, Experiences, and Perspectives*. Perspectives of the Swiss National Centre of Competence in Research (NCCR) North-South, University of Bern, Vol. 6. Bern, Switzerland: Geographica Bernensia, pp. 403–24.

Immergut, E. (1998). The theoretical core of the New Institutionalism. *Politics and Society* 26: 5–34.

Joas, H. (2000). *The Genesis of Values*. Chicago: University of Chicago Press.

Joas, H. (2008). Entstehung der Werte (28.5.2008). Köln: Karl Rahner Akademie. www.kath.de/akademie/rahner/04Vortraege/02audio/audio-body.html

Kickbusch, I. (2007). Health governance: the health society. In McQueen, D., & Kickbusch, I. (eds), *Health and Modernity: The Role of Theory in Health Promotion*. New York: Springer.

Kickbusch, I. (2010). Health in all policies: the evolution of the concept of horizontal governance. In Kickbusch, I., & Buckett, K. (eds.), *Implementing Health in All Policies*. Adelaide: Government of South Australia, pp. 11–22.

Kuhn, H. (1975). Werte – eine Urgegebenheit. In Gadamer, H-G., & Vogler, P. (eds.), *Neue Anthologie*. Vol. 7. Stuttgart: Thieme, pp. 343–73.

Labonte, R. (2012). The austerity agenda: how did we get there and where do we go next? *Critical Public Health* 22(3): 257–65.

Lee, K. (2006). Global health promotion: how can we strengthen governance and build effective strategies? *Health Promotion International* 21(suppl 1): 42–50.

Lomas, J. (2000). Using "linkage and exchange" to move research into policy at a Canadian foundation. *Health Affairs* 19: 3236–40. doi: 10.1377/hlthaff.19.3.236.

Lomas, J., & Brown, A. (2009). Research and advice giving: a functional view of evidence-informed policy advice in a Canadian Ministry of Health. *Milbank Quarterly* 87(4): 903–26.

Macintyre, S. (2012). Evidence in the development of health policy. *Public Health* 126: 217–9.

Mayes, R., & Oliver, T. R. (2012). Chronic disease and the shifting focus of public health: is prevention still a political lightweight? *Journal of Health Politics, Policy and Law* 37: 181–200.

McKee, M. (2002). Values, beliefs, and implications. In Marinker, M. (ed.), *Health Targets in Europe: Polity, Progress and Promise*. London: BM, p. 181.

McQueen, D. V. (2012). Value base, ethics and key challenges of health governance for health protection, prevention and promotion. Expert background paper for the WHO/EURO document *Governance for Health in the 21st Century: A Study Conducted for the WHO Regional Office for Europe*. Copenhagen: WHO Regional Office for Europe. /RC61/Inf.Doc./6.

McQueen, D V., & Jones, C. (2007). *Global Perspectives on Health Promotion Effectiveness*. New York: Springer Science.

McQueen, D. V., Wismar, M., Lin, V., Jones, C. M., & Davis, M. (eds). (2012). *Intersectoral Governance for Health in All Policies: Structures, Actions and Experiences*. Copenhagen: WHO Regional Office for Europe on behalf of the European Observatory on Health Systems and Policies.

Mencken, H. L. (1922). *Prejudices: Third Series*. New York: A. Knopf.

Ng, N. Y., & Ruger, J. P. (2011). Global health governance at a crossroads. *Global Health Governance* 3 (2): 1–37.

NRC (National Research Council) (1978). *Knowledge and Policy: The Uncertain Connection*. Washington, DC: National Academies Press.

NRC (National Research Council), Committee on the Use of Social Science Knowledge in Public Policy (2012). *Using Science as Evidence in Public Policy*. Prewitt, K., Schwandt, T. A., & Straf, M. L. (eds.), Division of Behavioral and Social Sciences and Education. Washington, DC: National Academies Press.

Ottawa Charter.(1986). *Health Promotion International* 1(4): 405.

Rawls, J. (1971). *A Theory of Justice*. Cambridge, MA: Belknap Press of Harvard University Press.

Rosenau, J. N. (1995). Governance in the twenty-first century. *Global Governance* 1, 13–43.

Rosenau, J. N. (1999). Toward an ontology for global governance. In Hewson, M., & Sinclair, T. (eds.), *Approaches to Global Governance Theory*. Albany: SUNY Press, pp. 296–6.

Rütten, R., Abu-Omar, K., Frahsa, A., & Gelius, P. (2013). Physical inactivity and health promotion: evidence and challenges. In McQueen, D. V. (ed.), *Global Handbook on Noncomminicable Diseases and Health Promotion*. New York: Springer, pp. 159–69.

Ruger, J. P. (2003). Health and development. Lancet. 362678.

Ruger, J. P. (2004a). Ethics of the social determinants of health. Lancet. 3641092–1097. [PubMed]

Ruger, J. P. (2004b). Health and social justice. Lancet. 3641075–1080. [PubMed]

Ruger, J. P. (2006a). Ethics and governance of global health inequalities. *Journal of Epidemiol Community Health* 60(11): 998–1002.

Ruger, J. P. (2006b). Health, capability, and justice: toward a new paradigm of health ethics, policy and law. *Cornell Journal of Law and Public Policy* 15(2): 403–82.

Ruger, J. P. (2010). *Health and Social Justice*. New York: Oxford University Press, pp. 276.

Schnädelbach, Herbert. (1983). *Werte im Widerstreit – Werte als "Glühbirnen" am platonischen Ideenhimmel(14.5.2008)*. Köln: Karl Rahner Akademie. www.kath.de/akademie/rahner/04Vortraege/02audio/audio-body.html

Sen, A. K. (1979). "Equality of what?" The Tanner Lecture on Human Values, delivered at Stanford University, May 22.

Sen, A. K. (1999). *Development as Freedom*. New York: Knopf.

Shermer, M. (2015). *The Moral Arc: How Science and Reason Lead Humanity toward Truth, Justice, and Freedom*. New York: Henry Holt.

Silver, G. A. (1987). Virchow, the heroic model in medicine: health policy by accolade. *American Journal of Public Health* 77(1): 82–8.

Ståhl, T., Wismar, M., Ollila, E., Lahtinen, E., & Leppo, K. (eds.). (2006). *Health in All Policies: Prospects and Potentials*. Helsinki: Ministry of Social Affairs and Health.

UNGA (United Nations General Assembly) (2011). *Political Declaration of High Level Meeting of the General Assembly on the Prevention and Control of Noncommunicable Diseases*. Rep noA/66/L. New York: United Nations General Assembly.

Whitehead, M., Dahlgren, G., & Gilson, L. (2001). Developing the policy response to inequities in health: a global perspective. In Evans, T., Whitehead, M., Diderichsen, F., Bhuiya, A., & Wirth, M. (eds). *Challenging Inequities in Health: From Ethics to Action*. London: Oxford University Press, pp. 309–24).

WHO (World Health Organization) (1986). *The Ottawa Charter for Health Promotion*. Geneva: WHO. www.who.int/healthpromotion/conferences/previous/ottawa/en/WHO

WHO (World Health Organization) (2009). *Milestones in Health Promotion: Statements from Global Conferences*. Geneva: WHO. (cf. www.who.int/healthpromotion/Milestones_Health_Promotion_05022010.pdf)

WHO (World Health Organization) (2011). *Global Status Report on Noncommunicable Diseases 2010*. Geneva: World Health Organization.

WHO (World Health Organization) (2015). Health systems: equity. www.who.int/healthsystems/topics/equity/en/

WHO (EURO) (2011a). *Governance for Health in the 21st Century: A Study Conducted for the WHO Regional Office for Europe*. EUR/RC61/Inf.Doc./6. Copenhagen: WHO EURO.

WHO (EURO) (2011b). *How Can the Health Equity Impact of Universal Policies Be Evaluated? Insights into Approaches and Next Steps: Synthesis of Discussions from an Expert Group Meeting*. Milton, B., Moonan, M., Taylor-Robinson, D., & Whitehead, M. (eds.). A joint publication between the WHO European Office for Investment for Health and Development, Venice, Italy, and the Liverpool WHO Collaborating Centre for Policy Research on Social Determinants of Health. Held at the University of Liverpool, November 2010. Copenhagen: WHO EURO.

WHOCSDOH (WHO Commission on the Social Determinants of Health) (2008). *Closing the Gap in a Generation: Health Equity through Action on the Social Determinants of Health*. Geneva: WHO.

Wismar, M., McQueen, D., Lin, V., Jones, C. M., & Davies, M. (2012). Intersectoral governance for health in all policies. *Eurohealth* 18(4): 3–7.

World Bank (1991). *Managing Development: The Governance Dimension*. Discussion Paper No. 34899. Washington, DC: World Bank.

3 New Developments in the Economics of Prevention

Social Impact Borrowing to Finance Cost-Effective Interventions

Judy A. Temple & Arthur J. Reynolds

Overview

Numerous policies or programs promote the well-being of individuals and society by reducing the incidence of unhealthy or undesirable behaviors. A growing number of these preventive interventions have been subjected to economic evaluations that have demonstrated that their benefits far exceed their costs in dollar terms. Cost-benefit analyses may reveal that an additional dollar spent on prevention programs may generate benefits of two, seven, or even more than ten dollars. Moreover, these economic evaluations are often able to distinguish between the existence of private benefits that accrue mostly to the targeted individuals and public benefits that spill over to other individuals and society as a whole. For example, policies to reduce smoking may make the program or policy's intended participants better off as they experience better health. But in addition to that private benefit, other members of society benefit from the reduction in secondhand smoke and from the reduction in publicly funded health care costs. The existence of these spillover benefits is a major justification for government involvement.

A basic tenet in the field of prevention science is that expenditures made early to prevent health, educational, or behavioral problems may lead to even larger savings later due to the reductions in costs associated with remediation. Interest in the use of cost-benefit analysis to evaluate preventive interventions and social policies more generally is growing (Karoly, 2012; Vining &Weimer, 2010). Benefit-cost analysis aids prevention scientists by helping them understand the magnitude of program effects relative to program costs. Moreover, benefit-cost analysis may help prevention advocates gain crucial allies among policy makers and taxpayers in efforts to promote the expansion of promising cost-effective social, education, or health services.

This chapter provides an overview of the economic approach to assessing program effectiveness. The basic approaches to estimating costs and benefits are outlined. Examples are then provided of cost-benefit analyses applied to a preventive intervention in the area of early childhood education in the United States (U.S.). Early childhood programs involve costs that are incurred in the early years and benefits that possibly may be realized for decades. While some of the benefits of this intervention take the form of higher participant incomes and higher tax revenues consequently received by government, a large portion of the benefits take the form of averted governmental costs due to lower crime, reduced need for school remedial services, and reductions in welfare program participation. Of course, early childhood programs are only one type of preventative intervention, and others will be discussed as well.

Coinciding with the growth in the number of economic evaluations of preventive interventions, in the last five years these studies of costs and benefits have started to serve as the academic foundation for a new type of private–public partnership devoted to providing funding from private investors to expand promising preventive interventions. Social impact borrowing is a new funding mechanism in which private investors are providing funds ranging from \$5 million to over \$20 million (U.S.) to local providers of effective services to scale up the most promising interventions. Private investors work together with nonprofit intermediaries, program evaluators, and state or local public finance analysts to identify which promising interventions to fund. Once services are delivered, evaluators determine whether the services are effective or not in terms of the estimated cost savings to government. If the program meets its prespecified targets for success, then the government pays back the investors using revenues made available due to the reduction in the need for costly remediation of social problems.

This chapter describes the concept of social impact borrowing, sometimes called pay-for-success or pay-for-performance, or human capital performance bonds, as a means of raising funds from the private sector to expand promising prevention programs. To the extent that these services are found to generate cost savings to the public sector, a state, local, or provincial government is obligated to make payments to the private investors based on the estimated cost savings. Economic evaluation is crucial both in determining the suitability of intervention programs to be financed in this manner and in determining the magnitude of the "success" payments. Advocates of social impact borrowing argue that this innovative private–public financing mechanism can promote the realignment of government expenditure portfolios from costly interventions to forward-looking preventative interventions.

While the first social impact bond was issued in 2010 in the United Kingdom (U.K.), interest in leveraging private investments to promote preventative interventions has spread to many countries across the globe. A recent comprehensive report by the Brookings Institute in the United States (Gustafsson-Wright, Gardiner, & Putcha, 2015) identifies and describes several dozen social impact bonds that have been launched in a number of developed countries to expand services to promote educational attainment, increase employment, reduce recidivism, and promote health and well-being of disadvantaged individuals. Interest in expanding preventative interventions is a high priority in lower-income countries as well. In all of these settings, economic analyses of program or policy costs and societal benefits serve as the foundation of the private-public endeavors.

Economic Analysis of Program Costs

While program evaluators often focus on the question of whether or not the intervention has an effect on outcomes, cost studies are needed to understand whether the intervention is affordable given budget constraints. Cost studies also provide valuable information for a comparison of the resources needed to implement various alternative interventions and ultimately can be used in a comparison of the program benefits and costs for a particular program. Economists take a broad view of the concept of costs and believe that a cost estimate should reflect the value of all resources used to deliver services.

A number of texts and other reports in the area of cost-benefit analysis and economic program evaluation describe the general process to estimating and reporting costs. The estimation of costs typically is described in a series of steps. A valuable guide to the process of conducting and reporting cost analyses for prevention programs was written by the late E. Michael Foster and colleagues. In the following, we reproduce and paraphrase the list of six steps outlined in Foster, Porter, Ayers, Kaplan, and Sandler (2007, p. 263). The steps to conceptualizing, conducting, and reporting estimates of program costs include the following:

1. State clearly the intervention for which the costs are to be estimated.
2. Establish the perspective and scope of the study.
3. Create a list of program inputs of ingredients.
4. Measure the use of program inputs.
5. Value the inputs used in monetary terms.
6. Conduct sensitivity analyses as a way of recognizing uncertainty in the estimates of program costs.

Regarding the issue of stating the specific intervention for which the costs are to be estimated, Foster et al. (2007) suggest that a key issue is the need to ensure that the costs of the program are estimated for the program that was actually delivered. Prevention advocates often want to see promising interventions moved from research settings into the community and might want to know how the costs would be different from those of the project delivered within the community. While cost analysts are free to speculate on how costs might differ in a community versus research setting or how costs might differ if the program is brought to scale, it is important to use measures of costs for the intervention as delivered in the research setting (but to ignore the costs of the research itself). For consumers of the cost analysis to understand the broader context of the intervention, ideally the cost study would include details of the intervention such as the dates of service delivery, location, names of organizations providing the services, and the characteristics of the participant pool.

While bringing programs to scale might entail lower costs per person served if economies of scale can be exploited, in some cases the scaling up of programs may lead to larger per capita costs. For example, if a large-scale intervention is expected to employ a great share of a particular resource that is available in the community or region, then the costs of this resource may rise as the intervention requires more and more of it. Two examples include a statewide implementation of small class sizes in elementary grades or a national policy greatly expanding funding for nurse home-visiting programs. In these cases, the tremendous increase in demand for teachers or nurses may lead to an overall increase in their market wages, and this additional cost would need to be included in estimating the costs of bringing a program to scale.

Establishing the perspective and scope of the study is the second step needed in the cost evaluation. Perspective refers to the issue of whose costs are being included. Choices may include only the costs of the nonprofit or governmental organization that delivers the services or an expanded notion of costs that includes costs incurred by participants as well as those due to the time and travel costs of participating in the intervention. Some participants may need to arrange for child care, which is an additional cost. Sometimes resources are being contributed by various levels of government or multiple organizations and it might be of interest to one of the organizations to report the costs of only their part of the provided services. But to better understand the costs from a societal perspective, the reported costs of the intervention should include all of the resource costs incurred by all of the service partners (including various levels of government) and program participants.

Scope often refers to the definition of the relevant geographic area or jurisdictional boundaries. Sometimes the public or private clients requesting the cost studies specifically request that only costs incurred within a state or region are included. In discussing how federal agencies estimate costs and benefits of U.S. policies, Dana (2010, p. 1) quotes a U.S. Office of Management and Budget directive that directs each federal agency to "focus on benefits and costs that accrue to citizens of the United States." Economists prefer that all costs be included regardless of where they are incurred or who incurs them.

Scope also may refer to the overall types of costs observed in the delivery of an intervention. Often sizable research costs exist for services that are being evaluated as part of a research study. While researchers may get large external grants to fund pilot projects, research costs should not be included in the cost estimates associated with the intervention. The importance of excluding research costs is emphasized by Foster, Dodge, & Jones (2003). Related to the topic of pilot projects and research, it may be the case that the costs of a relatively small-scale pilot project will be greater on a per-participant basis than it will be for successive cohorts. Foster et al. (2003) suggests reporting costs separately for different program cohorts if this is a concern.

The third step in conducting a cost study involves putting together a list of inputs or ingredients used to deliver the intervention. Interventions use personnel, building, materials, and equipment. These resources are described as ingredients. The ingredients approach to estimating program costs is advocated by Henry Levin, an expert in cost-effectiveness studies in the area of elementary, secondary, and postsecondary education, and is described in more detail in

Levin and McEwan (2001). It is important to realize that each ingredient has value whether used to produce the intervention or devoted to some alternative use. Economists use the phrase "opportunity costs" to describe the true economic value of inputs or ingredients as measured by the value of the resources that must be given up when an input is used to produce an intervention.

While the ingredients approach of Levin and McEwan (2001) has general appeal to economists and underlies the conceptualization of program costs for many types of education, social, and medical costs, an alternative framework for cost analysis called cost-procedure-process-outcome analysis (CPPOA) has been developed by Brian Yates (2009). As described in Long, Brown, Jones, Alber, and Yates (2015), Yates embeds the importance of measuring resources used as part of a larger model that attempts to "quantify relationships between the resources, procedures, processes and outcomes" of the intervention. Yates' model explicitly encourages evaluators to express costs in terms of the costs for each procedure that makes up the larger intervention. Both the ingredients framework and the CPPOA model use the same basic approaches to measuring costs. A recent discussion of how the two approaches compare is provided by Long et al. (2015) in a detailed cost analysis of a social and emotional learning intervention. The CPPOA model can be viewed as providing a more explicit view of the connection among various program inputs, the input costs, and the specific outcomes they are intended to affect.

The fourth step in the cost analysis involves measuring the use of program inputs. Once the list of ingredients has been constructed, the analyst then attempts to estimate the quantity of these inputs used. How many personnel of various types were involved? How many hours of training, coaching, or therapy did the participants receive? How many meals were served or how many immunizations delivered? How much driving was involved, and how many minutes or hours were spent setting up home-visiting appointments? Organization budgets can be consulted for this purpose, but the analyst should try to develop an understanding of what types of inputs might not be well described in the budgets. Ideally, organizations should keep track of the quantity of inputs used prospectively rather than trying to obtain this information after the intervention has already been delivered. For example, in the United States the state legislature in Tennessee authorized and funded a randomized trial of small class sizes called Tennessee STAR. This experiment, which was implemented in the mid-1980s, did not collect information on the costs of small class sizes, so researchers later had to make attempts to generate their own crude estimates of personnel and infrastructure costs (e.g., Krueger, 2003).

A critical next step for estimating costs involves taking information on the quantity of inputs used and attempting to value them in dollar (or monetary) terms. Certainly, a sizable amount of the cost information is likely to be found in organization budgets. The expenditures on personnel frequently account for the largest category of costs, and information on this expenditure frequently is available. The organization budgets may contain accurate information on the dollar value of materials used to deliver the intervention. However, there are likely to be several complications in using budget outlays as the key source for cost data. These complications include (1) the allocation of overhead costs; (2) the possible need to adjust the reported cost information in the budget in the case of market imperfections; and (3) the need to estimate or impute costs for donated, subsidized, or otherwise unpriced inputs. Regarding (1), the allocation of overhead costs can be done on a per-participant basis. In the case of an organization that is providing the intervention and engaging in other activities as well, the overhead costs can be allocated to the project using the share of total organization personnel expenditures devoted to the intervention as a guide. For example, if the intervention accounts for 40 percent of the personnel costs for the organization, the analyst can allocate 40 percent of the overhead costs to the intervention as well. As an example of the possible need to adjust budgetary cost data for market imperfections, one could consider the cost of hiring workers subject to the minimum wage or a living wage in communities that require that higher-than-market-rate wages be paid. If workers would have been willing to work for less, then the observed wage ends up being an overstatement of the true value of the resources used. In practice, however, the budgeted labor costs are included without major alteration as the economic cost of the labor input.

Certain inputs or ingredients in the provision of the interventions may not be included in program budgets. Organizations may make use of donated or subsidized resources and may also depend heavily on volunteer labor. Although these donations are useful because they help keep the expenditures low for the organization, economic evaluation requires that the measurement of the value of resources needs to include the market value of all inputs, including those that were donated or purchased. Nonprofit organizations frequently keep track of the value of donated inputs or the number of hours of volunteer time and use this information to communicate to funders about their abilities to attract such contributions in kind. The value of time of volunteers or program participants often is measured by the wages that the volunteers could be earning in paid work. For some populations, this wage could be assumed to be the minimum wage. For other volunteers and participants who may be drawn from the population at large, it might be more relevant to use the average county or state wage.

A final consideration needs to be given to estimating the value of facilities space used to provide the intervention. If this space is rented, then the organization's budget may contain the relevant information on rental costs. If the space is donated, then estimates of the opportunity cost of the space could be gathered from information on the fees that are charged to other organizations for similar spaces. For services provided by governmental organizations, the government budgets may not contain information on rental costs if the space is publicly owned. Levin and McEwan (2001) provide a very useful discussion of different ways of estimating the costs of space used to provide services in public schools. These cost estimates reflect not only the opportunity cost of the original investment in infrastructure expressed as a foregone annual rate of return in an alternative investment but also take into account the depreciation of the building.

As an example of how cost information is reported, Table 3.1 shows the costs separately for each ingredient of an early childhood program in the United States called the Child–Parent Centers (CPC). The CPC early education program is an ongoing education intervention that is offered in public school sites in some of the most economically disadvantaged neighborhoods in Chicago. The CPC program consists of a preschool through third-grade intervention offering small class sizes, staff and school space devoted to parent involvement activities, and an aligned curriculum taught by public school teachers with four-year degrees. This table showing the costs of the preschool portion of the CPC intervention only was included in an economic evaluation by Reynolds, Temple, Robertson, and Mann (2002). In the current table, the consumer price index has been used to update the dollar amounts here so that they represent the value of a U.S. dollar in 2007. Note that the majority of the costs listed in Table 3.1 come directly from school district budgets. The largest cost category, instructional services, was listed separately along with the costs of the parent program staff in the original district budget for teachers and staff in the CPC program. Several other categories, including administrative services, operations and management, and schoolwide services, were listed as broad aggregates in the district budget, so these figures were allocated on a per-pupil basis to all students in the district.

The next two categories in Table 3.1, parental participation and depreciation/interest, were not listed in the district's budget and needed to be imputed so that all resources used in the intervention are assigned a value. Parent participation was assumed to be 2.5 hours a week valued at the minimum wage. Levin and McEwan (2001) were consulted about how to value facilities space in the public school system. That dollar amount reflects both the annual depreciation of the

Table 3.1 *Costs of the Child–Parent Center Preschool Program (2007 Dollars)*

Category	Amount ($)	Percent of total
Instructional staff	9,987,566	43.4
Parent program staff	2,216,080	9.6
Administration	2,905,954	12.6
Operations & maintenance	2,419,745	10.5
Schoolwide services	990,474	4.3
Parent program participation	1,805,553	7.9
Capital depreciation/interest	2,098,194	9.1
Other	563,681	2.5
Total	22,987,246	100
Number of children in 25 sites	4,114	
Average cost per child for 1 year	5,588	
Present value of average cost per child (for 1.55 years of preschool)	8,512	

Note: Updated from Reynolds et al. (2002).

CPC buildings and a measure of the interest that could have been earned on an annual basis if the funds to finance the building were invested in bonds instead.

In Table 3.1, the total costs spent in a particular year on the preschool portion of the CPCs are reported and then are expressed in per-pupil terms. The final step recognized that the average child had one and a half years of preschool (actually 1.55 years). All students were assumed to have participated for one year at age 4 and then 0.55 percent of the sample was assumed to have started at age 3. The $8,512 cost of preschool to the typical student is the combined cost of 0.55 years of preschool at age 3 plus the cost of a full school year at age 4, where the cost of the second year was discounted by 3 percent to generate its present value at age 3. Discounting to allow dollar values from different time periods to be added together will be discussed later in this chapter.

Finally, the sixth step in conducting a cost study is to acknowledge uncertainty in the estimation of costs if it exists. Cost data collected retrospectively may be more inaccurate than data gathered prospectively. Some cost studies are based on detailed budgetary information in which the costs of the intervention program are clearly separated from costs of other projects of the same organization, but some budgets aggregate costs for various projects, requiring analysts to make more assumptions about intervention-specific costs. Importantly, a standard recommendation in cost-benefit analysis is to focus relatively more attention on the careful estimation of the largest categories of costs or benefits for each particular project (Boardman, Greenberg, Vining, & Weimer, 2010). In the example of the CPC preschool component, the largest categories of costs seemed well measured, as they were taken from school district budgets. On the other hand, estimates of the quantity of parents' time spent participating in school activities are based on a general impression from teachers rather than detailed record keeping, but fortunately this category accounted for less than 10 percent of the total cost of the preschool program. More discussion of accounting for uncertainty will be provided in the following section.

Economic Analyses of Program Benefits

The discussion of the steps to estimating the benefits of an intervention follows in a parallel fashion the steps used to estimate costs. This section outlines the process. Many of these steps are familiar to analysts who regularly conduct impact evaluations. A key difference is the need to transform estimates of program impact into monetary terms. The estimation of benefits often, but not always, can require more research efforts on behalf of the analysts due to the critical need for designing and executing a research evaluation that generates estimates of the effects of the intervention rather than estimates that are correlational in nature.

1. State clearly the intervention for which the benefits are to be estimated
2. Establish the perspective and scope of the study

3. Create a list of outcomes that credibly could be affected by the intervention
4. Employ a rigorous study design that allows for the identification of the causal impact of the program on the outcomes
5. Value the outcomes achieved by the intervention in monetary terms.
6. Conduct sensitivity analyses as a way of recognizing uncertainty in the estimates of program benefits

The first two steps involve issues of identifying the specific intervention, its perspective, and scope that are similar to earlier discussions on the cost side. The specific intervention being studied may differ from an intervention that might be later brought to scale. Researchers need to be clear about the specificities about the intervention offered and the population treated so that consumers of the study can understand that the benefits of a larger, community-based program may not necessarily be the same.

There are two primary perspectives that can be taken by a benefit-cost analyst. The typical approach that is of most interest to economists involves determining the benefits that accrue to everyone in society. As before, the scope in terms of the geographic or governmental boundaries may be specified by a client requesting the study, but economists prefer to analyze all of the benefits of an activity or project no matter who is affected. This is the social benefits perspective. The second perspective that is relevant for some purposes is the governmental or guardian approach, in which only benefits and costs that affect governmental budgets are included (Boardman et al., 2010). Using this second perspective, social programs are desirable only to the extent that the fiscal benefits (in terms of higher tax revenues and lower costs of welfare programs, criminal justice, and public health expenditures) exceed the publicly funded costs of the program. Packard, Delgado, Fellmeth, and McCready (2008) is a recent example of a cost-benefit analysis of a preventive intervention that provides guardian support and other funding to help foster children in the United States more successfully make the transition from high school into early adulthood. Although this intervention was expected to increase the educational attainment and earnings of foster children, only the projected added tax revenues (and averted welfare costs) arising from this additional income were included as benefits. Under the social perspective, the added income received by the program participants would be included as a benefit.

The list of outcomes that could be affected by the intervention is informed by program theory as well as by the literature on program effectiveness of preventative interventions. Certain outcomes tend to be used in multiple studies because of their relative ease of measurement. For some types of outcomes, such as health status, earnings, test scores, and arrest records, it might be possible to obtain information observed both before and after the intervention, while for others, such as high school graduation or age at death, obviously repeated measures are not observed. Some studies might focus on a single outcome, while others might attempt to ascertain program effectiveness across multiple outcomes.

The fourth item on the list typically requires designing a study involving a comparison group and using either random assignment or a carefully controlled nonexperimental study design. In order to obtain a causal estimate of the effect of participation in the intervention, the observed outcomes of program participants ideally would need to be compared to the outcomes these same participants would experience if they had *not been assigned* to the intervention. In reality, of course, this comparison is not possible. Well-implemented, randomized control trials yield causal estimates. Other study designs involving careful matching or making use of a regression discontinuity perhaps due to strict administrative cutoffs for program eligibility can also generate credible estimates of program impact. Nonexperimental approaches require close scrutiny to make sure that any causal inferences generated are not arising due to alternative explanations unrelated to the program.

Once credible estimates of the effects of a preventive intervention are obtained as a result of the impact evaluation, then analysts attempt to transform these estimated effects into monetary terms. While the impact evaluations may suggest, for example, that a preschool program may reduce duration in special education by seven months, the analyst then attempts to determine the cost of an academic year (nine months) of special education and could then multiply that by 7/9 to determine the benefit in terms of cost savings. Similarly, programs to help children in foster care make the transition to adulthood may lead to an increase in the high school completion rate by 20 percentage points (as assumed by Packard et al., 2008). Using information on earnings associated with different levels of educational attainment from the U.S. Bureau of Labor Statistics, for example, the lifelong earnings impact of this increase in the probability of high school completion can be estimated in dollar terms.

A sizable literature exists (e.g., Aos, Lieb, Mayfield, Miller, & Pennucci, 2004; Foster, Johnson-Shelton, & Taylor, 2007; Heckman, Moon, Pinto, Savelyev, & Yavitz, 2010; Reynolds, Temple, White, Ou, & Robertson, 2011b; Vining & Weimer, 2010) that can help inform ways that analysts can try to monetize certain program impacts. Importantly, the feasibility of transforming estimates of program impacts into monetary terms is more apparent in some program areas than others. For example, economists regularly assign a monetary value to the social benefits resulting from one additional student graduating from high school instead of dropping out (e.g., Reynolds and Temple, 2011b). Programs that improve cultural sensitivity among human service personnel, for example, are hard to monetize unless assumptions are made that these improvements can lead to realized reductions in some type of government expenditures. Child maltreatment is an example of a social problem for which researchers have estimated its associated costs (e.g., Fang, Brown, Florence, & Mercy, 2012). Analysts studying crimes such as murder, assault, and rape have taken the estimation of costs even further by incorporating estimates of the pain and suffering of crime victims along with the standard costs involving the criminal justice system (e.g., McCollister, French, & Fang, 2010).

The process of translating program impacts into monetary terms is likely to involve multiple assumptions. The final step in estimating program benefits involves conducting some type of sensitivity analysis to assess the robustness of estimates to varying assumptions within a reasonable range. Boardman et al. (2010) recommend conducting sensitivity analysis by reporting result estimates ranging from a possible best-case scenario to a more conservative set of assumptions or using Monte Carlo simulations to account for uncertainty in key factors affecting the determination of benefits or costs. Monte Carlo simulations can be used to take into account uncertainty in the estimation of either program benefits or costs by conducting multiple trials in which a random variable is added to the cost or benefit calculation to reflect uncertainty. More detail on allowing for uncertainty in reporting results is discussed in the following section.

Comparing Benefits and Costs and Reporting Findings

Benefits and costs often accrue in different time periods. In preventative interventions, costs may be realized in the early time periods, but benefits may accrue in later time periods, even in future decades. Analysts need to correct for inflation using the U.S.-based consumer price index or the gross domestic product (GDP) deflator. As a result, financial amounts are then reported in terms of dollars of a particular year. In Table 3.1, for example, the costs are described as being in terms of 2007 U.S. dollars. But even after the inflation correction, or if inflation didn't exist, it still needs to be recognized that consumers do not view receiving or paying a dollar today to be equivalent to receiving or paying a dollar in a future time period. The "time value of money" refers to the fact that a dollar today could be invested at an interest rate "r," and so the dollar today would be worth (1 + r) times a dollar next year. Alternatively, the promise of receipt of a dollar in the future is worth less than a dollar in the present time period, as 97 cents could be invested today to generate that future dollar. *Discounting* is the term financial analysts use to describe the corrections to future dollar amounts that need to be made to obtain an estimate of a future dollar's present value. A typical value to use for the discount rate is 3.0 percent or 3.5 percent. Moore, Boardman, Vining, Weimer, and Greenberg (2004) discuss the choice of the discount rate in more detail. Researchers often conduct sensitivity analyses allowing the discount rate to vary. Reynolds et al. (2011b) show how the estimated benefit-cost ratio varies as the interest rate is assumed to vary between 0 percent and 7 percent.

In cost-benefit analysis, both costs and benefits in future time periods need to be converted or discounted into dollars (or other currency) in an earlier time period. For preschool interventions beginning at age three, for example, all future costs and benefits need to be discounted and brought back to age three. For prevention programs beginning in high school, the costs and benefits may be discounted back to the child's age fifteen years or so. In this way, recommendations can be made about whether the interventions represent a good use of resources as measured at the time that the decision is made to enroll participants in the intervention. All standard cost-benefit analysis texts, including Boardman et al. (2010), contain discussion of how to implement discounting of future benefits and costs to obtain present value estimates for a particular year.

Reporting calculations of benefits and costs can be done in any of three ways. The most common is the ratio of the present value of the benefits divided by the present value of the costs. For an intervention to be considered attractive, the ratio should be greater than one. Aos et al. (2004) list results for over thirty cost-benefit analyses of interventions for youth, and approximately ten of these interventions show a benefit-cost ratio of less than 1.0. For these interventions, the present value of the benefits is less than the present value of the costs, and therefore the interventions probably should not be undertaken. Packard et al. (2008) report a ratio of 1.5:1 for a foster care intervention, indicating that benefits exceed costs, and, therefore, the intervention is "admissible" or worthy of consideration as an efficient use of public resources.

The second way of reporting and comparing benefits and costs is to report the net benefit. The net benefit is the present value of the benefits minus the present value of the costs. This method is recommended by Boardman et al. (2010). There are two advantages. First, reporting the net benefit, especially for the entire intervention, is a better way of taking into account the scope of the project. The second rationale takes into account that some of the benefits realized by the intervention take the form of averted future costs, such as reductions in criminal justice costs or health care costs. Sometimes analysts subtract these averted costs from the estimated costs of the intervention rather than add them to the benefit calculation. The reported ratio is sensitive to whether averted costs are added to the numerator or subtracted from the denominator. However, the net benefit is not affected by this decision. Aos et al. (2004), Reynolds and Temple (2008), and Temple and Reynolds (2007) are examples of studies that report both the benefit-cost ratio and the net benefit.

A recently popular third way of reporting results is to estimate the social return on investment or the internal rate of return. This rate of return, which is commonly calculated in corporate finance, is an interest rate that equates the present value of the benefits to the present value of costs. The rate of return for a cost-effective project might be anywhere between 3 percent to 18 percent or more. Rolnick and Grunewald (2003) were among the first to report this social rate of return for a social program. They took existing findings from the Perry Preschool program in the United States and estimated the annual rate of return to be 18 percent. Since then, many analysts have reported social return on investment (SROI) or return on investment (ROI) estimates. Heckman et al. (2010), for example, report various estimates of the ROI ranging from 5.3 percent to 11.1 percent for the Perry Preschool program depending on various assumptions used. Given the possibility of receiving a 3 percent rate of return on alternative investments, for example, an ROI over 3 percent suggests that the project should be considered.

Table 3.2 provides an illustration of the three ways of reporting results from a cost-benefit analysis. Consistent with Table 3.1, the findings here are for the

Table 3.2 *Indicators of Economic Returns per Child for Chicago Child-Parent Center Early Education Program (2007 U.S. Dollars)*

Component	Benefit ($)	Cost ($)	B–C ($)	B/C	IRR (%)
Preschool (PS)	92,220	8,512	83,708	10.83	17.8
School age (SA)	15,064	3,792	11,273	3.97	9.8
Extended intervention (PS + 2–3 years of SA)	42,520	5,163	37,357	8.24	18.0

Note: IRR = internal rate of return (annually, %). Extended intervention is participation for four to six years. The cost is relative to less extensive participation ($12,719–$7,556) rather than to no participation in the program. Thus benefits are relative to children with less extensive participation (zero to three years). Benefits and costs are reported in present value terms discounted at 3 percent back to the child's age three. See Reynolds et al. (2011b) for more information.

benefits and costs of participation in the CPC education program, a preschool-through-third-grade intervention offered in schools in high-poverty neighborhoods. While Table 3.1 reported the cost data for participation in the preschool portion of the CPC program only, Table 3.2 contains estimates of the economic effects of participation in the preschool portion, the elementary grade portion through third grade, or extended participation, which is defined as five or six years out of a possible six years in total. To obtain estimates of the benefits of program participation, the impact evaluation was conducted using a quasi-experimental study design in which approximately one thousand children who participated in the CPC preschool program have been followed for approximately thirty years. More than twenty entire kindergarten classrooms in CPC sites were matched to similar schools that did not offer the CPC program containing approximately six hundred children for the control group. Estimates of program impact for the preschool component, grade school component, and extended intervention were obtained through regression analyses as described in Reynolds et al. (2011a, 2011b).

Table 3.2 reports the present value of the benefits and costs discounted back to the child's age three and reported in 2007 dollars. Participation in the preschool portion of the intervention for one or two years generated benefits per child of $92,220 (U.S.). As explained in Reynolds et al. (2011b), these benefits consisted of reduced crime costs to society, higher earnings for participants, and a number of other benefits arising from better school performance. Compared to a cost of $8,512 for an average of approximately 1.5 years of preschool, the net benefit for participation in preschool is $83,708. The benefit-cost ratio for preschool participation is then $10.83. The other components of the intervention also have estimated benefits that exceed costs by a significant margin.

In the final column of Table 3.2, the IRRs (or ROIs) for these various components of the intervention are reported. As previously explained, the use of a spreadsheet helps the analyst identify the estimated rate of return that produces a present value amount for the benefits that equals the present value amount for the costs. All three components of this intervention generate a high return on investment. The preschool rate of return is very similar to that estimated by Rolnick and Grunewald (2003) in their study of the Perry Preschool program.

Social Impact Borrowing to Expand Preventive Interventions

Cost-benefit analyses of preventive interventions play a crucial role in motivating the feasibility of a new kind of private–public collaboration to promote investments in social programs that ultimately save governments more than they cost. Social impact borrowing is a new approach to financing certain governmental activities that generate cost savings to state or local governments. Social impact bonds, sometimes called human capital bonds, pay for performance bonds, or pay for success bonds, are actually not bonds but are loans in which repayments of the loan plus interest depend on whether a service provider (such as a nonprofit organization or a school) is able to meet performance targets (Liebman & Sellman, 2013). For job training programs, performance targets might include placing participants in jobs with employment continuing for a specified time. For recidivism-prevention programs targeting prison inmates or recently released ex-offenders, the key success indicator might be the number of days of jail avoided.

Social impact borrowing hinges on the ability of analysts to conduct a cost-benefit analysis of a program with a specific focus on estimating the magnitude of government savings as the key benefit. An outside evaluator is hired to conduct an impact evaluation of the effectiveness of the government project. This requires a formal study design, perhaps involving a randomized trial or a different quasi- or nonexperimental study with a matched comparison group or/ and data on individual participants both before and after the intervention is offered.

Cost-benefit analysis is central to existence and implementation of these social impact borrowing initiatives because only those services that generate benefits greater than costs will be candidates for financing. Not only must the benefits be greater than costs, but the benefits must take the form of averted future government spending or higher government tax revenues as a result of participation in the intervention. In identifying which projects could be funded by social impact bonds, policy makers and analysts often look for ideas by understanding which avoidable social problems generate high costs that could be avoided to governments. Recidivism is an obvious choice, but other preventative interventions targeting costly conduct behaviors among youth are worthy of consideration (e.g., Scott, Knapp, Henderson, & Maughan, 2001) if impact evaluations demonstrate that interventions exist that can reduce problem behaviors. Programs that have a primary benefit of increasing incomes to participants will be of interest only if it can be shown that these higher incomes generate significant new tax revenues to the government or if the higher incomes of participants make them less likely to rely on public welfare or health programs or engage in criminal behavior. The role of the evaluator in a social impact borrowing initiative is not only to determine whether the program had a desired effect or not, but to calculate the amount of the benefit in terms of government savings, as the governments need to realize these cost savings in order to repay the investors.

The process of social impact borrowing starts with a private investor such as an investment bank like Goldman Sachs or a private foundation. Often several funders work together to help finance the expansion of promising interventions. An intermediary such as the United Way or other similar nonprofit organization receives the funds and arranges with a nonprofit service provider to expand the number of clients, students, or program participants served. The funds from the investors serve as the working capital to pay for the program expansion. The evaluator then determines whether or not the services provided by the nonprofit or school have actually led to government savings. If so, then this government savings is used to pay back the private investors. The payments made by the state or local government are called "success payments." In the social impact borrowing initiatives currently in operation around the United States, the investors themselves bear the risk if the service providers fail to generate government savings.

While the first social impact bond or loan was issued in 2010 in the United Kingdom for a prison recidivism program (Disley, Rubin, Scraggs, Burrowes, & Culley, 2011), immediately following in quick succession were a number of state or local governments in Europe, Australia, and several other countries (Gustafsson-Wright et al. 2015), including the United States. Since then, there has been a flurry of activity around the world in discussing and implementing similar types of financing arrangements for preventive interventions.

Table 3.3 lists the first seven social impact borrowing initiatives in the United States. The first U.S. social impact bond was financed by Goldman Sachs investment bank to expand services for youthful offenders at the U.S. Rikers Island correctional facility. This innovative financing mechanism is described in detail in Olson and Phillips (2013). More details on all of these borrowing initiatives can be found on the www.payforsuccess.org website as well as in Gustafsson-Wright et al. (2015). Once the evaluator has determined that the services have generated benefits in the form of government savings, then the City of New York will repay Goldman Sachs' investment where the success payment is based on the program's reduction in jail days for the intervention group compared to a control group.

Recidivism is a popular policy area for social impact borrowing, accounting for three of the first seven social impact bond initiatives. Programs to serve the homeless also have been attractive to public-private financing entrepreneurs, as preventive interventions to help homeless populations are likely to generate government savings in terms of lower police costs and lower health care costs. For example, the social impact borrowing initiative in Cuyahoga County in Ohio focuses on improving housing conditions for homeless families, and the success payments are conditioned entirely on preventing the number of days

Table 3.3 *Selected Recent Social Impact Borrowing Initiatives in the United States*

Initiatives and policy area	Private investment	Outcomes triggering success payments
1. New York City ABLE Project for Incarcerated Youth (Rikers Island) August 2012 Policy area: recidivism	$9.6 million	Number of jail days avoided
2. Utah High Quality Preschool Program June 2013 Policy area: early childhood education	$4.6 million	Reductions in rates of placement in special education
3. New York State Increasing Employment and Improving Public Safety June 2013 Policy areas: recidivism and job training	$13.5 million	Increase in employment rates Number of jail days avoided Increase in placement rates in transition jobs
4. Massachusetts Juvenile Pay for Success Initiative January 2014 Policy areas: recidivism and employment	$18 million	Number of jail days avoided Increase in job readiness Increases in employment rates
5. Massachusetts Chronic Homelessness Pay for Success Initiative December 2014 Policy areas: homelessness	$3.5 million	Achievement of stable housing for one year
6. Cuyahoga Partnership for Family Success Program December 2014 Policy areas: homelessness and child welfare	$ 4 million	Reductions in days spent in foster care
7. Chicago Child–Parent Centers December 2014 Policy area: early childhood education	$16.9 million	Reduction in special education placement Increase in kindergarten readiness Increase in third-grade test scores

Based on information from www.payforsuccess.org.

that children from homeless families spend in foster care. Two early childhood interventions also are in the list of the first seven social impact borrowing initiatives (Temple & Reynolds, 2015). Both of these social impact bonds were initiated by Goldman Sachs in recognition that high-quality early educational interventions can lead to significant reductions in special education placement.

Research on the connection between early intervention and special education savings has been reported in numerous studies (e.g., Reynolds et al., 2011a, 2011b; Temple & Reynolds, 2007), but the funders behind these initiatives believe that the cost savings arising from preschool interventions may be even larger than these previous studies suggest. In both the Utah and Chicago borrowing initiatives listed in Table 3.3, a government such as the state in Utah or the school district in Chicago will repay the investors for each child assumed to have avoided special education. In the case of the Chicago social impact bond, the City of Chicago also will help repay the investors with success payments tied to the number of children who participate in the CPC intervention who are ready for kindergarten as determined by a readiness assessment and the number of children who are proficient in reading in grade three. The research by Reynolds et al. (2011b) served as the foundation for the Chicago borrowing initiative.

Social Impact Borrowing to Expand Preventative Interventions around the World

Dozens of social impact bond initiatives supporting preventative interventions are either in operation or in the discussion stage in various countries outside of the United States. The work of Gustaffson-Wright et al. (2015) contains a very detailed list describing these initiatives, mostly in the United Kingdom and the United States, but also including funding projects to support social welfare, employment, and education programs in Australia, the Netherlands, Belgium, Canada, Germany, and Portugal. For example, in Saskatchewan, Canada, a relatively small project funds a "Sweet Dreams House" for single mothers and their young children. Participants living in this house will receive support services and education intended to improve parenting and help the mothers become employed. In the Netherlands, social impact borrowing will help expand programming for unemployed young adults so that they can create their own businesses or other local paid employment. Both of these projects and others will be evaluated using the methods of cost-benefit analysis to determine whether the governments involved will ultimately be making payments to pay back the private investors.

Much attention also is being paid to ways of expanding preventative services in developing countries. In the developing country context, social impact bonds (SIBs) are referred to as developmental impact bonds (DIBs) (Social Finance, 2013). While social impact borrowing in the United States and the United Kingdom, for example, involves performance risks due to the fact that investors do not know whether the intervention services will be successful or not, other types of risks may be of concern in developing countries (Burand, 2013). Whether or not a government will abide by the contract might be a concern, especially since some countries have inadequate tax systems that make future revenues uncertain and turnover or upheaval in leadership may lead investors to worry whether the long-term contracts are credible. Given additional risks involved in enforcing pay-for-success contracts in developing countries, donors may be less likely to ever be paid back. There may be less interest among investment bankers, for example, but in developing countries charitable donor organizations are likely to be a more important source of funding. Despite these difficulties, however, efforts are under way to expand funding for health and education programs such as projects that will reduce the prevalence of HIV or malaria or provide local schools in areas where these services are lacking (Social Finance, 2013).

Conclusion

As a systematic approach to evaluating the benefits and costs of a program or policy, benefit-cost analysis can help identify ways of targeting scarce public revenues. Prevention researchers and advocates of preventative programs can use benefit-cost analysis to their advantage by using this evaluation method to help gain important allies among taxpayers and policy makers in efforts to expand prevention programming and help alter government spending priorities from intervention to prevention in the areas of human services, education, or health services.

While many preventative interventions may ultimately save taxpayers money to the extent that the benefits associated with reducing certain social problems are greater than the intervention costs, careful analysis is required to first quantify and then compare the benefits and the costs. Some interventions may not generate strong enough effects to offset costs. Moreover, interventions that are not well targeted often end up expending resources on those who would not ultimately develop the problem of interest, such as dropping out of high school, becoming addicted to drugs, or engaging in other unhealthy and costly behaviors (Foster, 2010). These participants receive costly intervention services, but ultimately their behavior may not be affected by the intervention. Hence prevention is not always cost effective, and the use of cost-benefit analyses can help program providers and policy makers identify not only programs that work but programs that work and save money.

In just a few short years, private funders have taken the results of cost-benefit analyses of preventive interventions and have used these results as the basis for an innovative new type of financing mechanism that is lauded by advocates for its ability to bring proven and promising preventive interventions up to scale. As described by Liebman and Sellman (2013), this new way of financing social services can help governments expand interventions even in the face of tight fiscal constraints. In a time when raising new public revenues is difficult, social impact borrowing can expand needed services, encourage a focus on "what works" in the area of preventive interventions, and promote innovation in service delivery. Future developments in this area are likely to experiment with alternative ways of risk sharing because most of the funded projects under way do not involve any risk put on the service provider or the government.

In addition, the currently high administration costs associated with these contracting arrangements are likely to fall in the future as more experience is gained and information about contracting and evaluation is shared. As private funders, nonprofit service providers, and governments learn more about social impact borrowing, these types of contractual arrangements may evolve and change. What is clear about the future of preventive interventions is that the economic analysis of prevention programs will be central to their growth.

References

Aos, S., Lieb, R., Mayfield, J., Miller, M., & Pennucci, A. (2004). *Benefits and Costs of Prevention and Early Intervention Programs for Youth* (Publication no. 04–07-3901). Olympia: Washington State Institute for Public Policy.

Boardman, A., Greenberg, D., Vining, A., & Weimer, D. (2010). *Cost-Benefit Analysis*, 4th ed. Upper Saddle River, NJ: Prentice Hall.

Burand, D. (2013). Globalizing social finance: how social impact bonds and social impact performance guarantees can scale development. *NYU Journal of Law & Business* 9: 447–502.

Center for Global Development and Social Finance (2013). Investing in social outcomes: Development impact bonds. Summary report of the Developmental Impact Bond Working Group.

Dana, D.A. (2010). Valuing foreign lives and settlements. *Journal of Benefit-Cost Analysis* 1: 1–26.

Disley, E., Rubin, J., Scraggs, E., Burrowes, N., & Culley, D. M. (2011). Lessons learned from the planning and early implementation of the social impact bond at HMP Peterborough. Research Series 5/11. Report prepared by RAND Europe for the Ministry of Justice.

Fang, X., Brown, D. S., Florence, C. S., & Mercy, J. A. (2012). The economic burden of child maltreatment in the United States and implications for prevention. *Child Abuse and Neglect* 36: 156–65.

Foster, E. M. (2010). Costs and effectiveness of the Fast Track Intervention for anti-social behavior. *Journal of Mental Health Policy and Economics* 13: 101–19.

Foster, E. M., Dodge, K. A., & Jones, D., (2003). Issues in the economic evaluation of mental health programs. *Applied Developmental Science* 7: 76–86.

Foster, E. M., Johnson-Shelton, D., & Taylor, T. K., (2007). Measuring time costs in interventions designed to reduce behavior problems in children and youth. *American Journal of Community Psychology* 40: 64–81.

Foster, E. M., Porter, M. M., Ayers, T. S., Kaplan, D. L., & Sandler, I. (2007). Estimating the costs of preventive interventions. *Evaluation Review* 31: 261–86.

Gustafsson-Wright, E., Gardiner, S., & Putcha, V. (2015). *The Potential and Limitations of Impact Bonds: Lessons from the First Five Years of Experience Worldwide*. Washington, DC: Brookings Institution.

Heckman, J. J., Moon, S. H., Pinto, R., Savelyev, P. A., & Yavitz, A. (2010). The rate of return to the High/Scope Perry Preschool program. *Journal of Public Economics* 94: 114–28.

Karoly, L. A., (2012). Toward standardization of benefit-cost analysis of early childhood interventions. *Journal of Benefit-Cost Analysis* 3: 1–45.

Krueger, A. B., (2003). Economic considerations and small class sizes. *Economic Journal* 113: F34–F63.

Levin, H. M., & McEwan, P. J. (2001). *Cost-effectiveness Analysis: Methods and Applications*, 2nd ed. Thousand Oaks, CA: Sage.

Liebman, J., & Sellman, A., (2013). *Social Impact Bonds: A Guide for State and Local Governments*. Cambridge, MA: Harvard Kennedy School Social Impact Bond Technical Assistance Lab.

Long, K., Brown, J. L., Jones, S. M., Aber, J. L., & Yates, B. T. (2015). Cost analysis of a school-based social and emotional learning and literacy intervention. *Journal of Benefit Cost Analysis* 6: 1–17.

McCollister, K. E., French, M. T., & Fang, H. (2010). The cost of crime to society: new crime-specific estimates for policy and program evaluation. *Drug and Alcohol Dependence* 108: 98–109.

Moore, M. A., Boardman, A. E., Vining, A. R., Weimer, D. L., & Greenberg, D. H., (2004). Just give me a number! Practical values of the social discount rate. *Journal of Policy Analysis and Management* 23: 789–812.

Olson, J., & Phillips, A., (2013). Rikers Island: the first social impact bond in the US. *Community Development Investment Review* 9 (1): 97–101.

Packard, T., Delgado, M., Fellmeth, R., & McCready, K., (2008). A cost-benefit analysis of transitional services for emancipating foster youth. *Child and Youth Services Review* 20: 1267–78.

Reynolds, A. J., & Temple, J. A. (2008). Cost-effective early childhood development programs from preschool through third grade. *Annual Review of Clinical Psychology* 4: 109–39.

Reynolds, A. J., Temple, J. A., Ou, S. R., Arteaga, I., & White, B. A. B. (2011a). School-based early childhood education and age-28 well-being: effects by timing, dosage, and subgroups. *Science* 333 (July 15): 360–4.

Reynolds, A. J., Temple, J. A., Robertson, D. L., & Mann, E. A. (2002). Age 21 cost-benefit analysis of the Title I Chicago Child Parent Centers. *Education Evaluation and Policy Analysis* 24: 267–303.

Reynolds, A. J., Temple, J. A., White, B. A. B., Ou, S. R., & Robertson, D. L. (2011b). Age 26 cost benefit analysis of the Chicago Child Parent Center early education program. *Child Development* 82: 379–404.

Rolnick, A., & Grunewald, R. (2003). Early childhood development: Economic development with a high public return. *Region* 17: 6–12.

Scott, S., Knapp, M., Henderson, J., & Maughan, B. (2001). Financial cost of social exclusion: followup study of antisocial children into adulthood. *British Medical Journal* 323: 191–4.

Temple, J. A., & Reynolds, A. J. (2007). The benefits and costs of investments in preschool. *Economics of Education Review* 26: 126–44.

Temple, J. A., & Reynolds, A. J. (2015). Using social-impact borrowing to expand preschool through third grade programs in urban public schools. *Journal of Education for Students Placed at Risk* 20: 280–92.

Vining, A., & Weimer, D. L., (2010). An assessment of important issues concerning the application of benefit-cost analysis to social policy. *Journal of Benefit-Cost Analysis* 1: 1–40.

Yates, B. T. (2009). Cost-inclusive evaluation: a banquet of approaches for including costs, benefits, and cost-effectiveness and cost-benefit analysis in your next evaluation. *Evaluation and Program Planning* 32: 54–6.

4 International Issues in the Ethics of Prevention

Sally M. Hage, Jonathan P. Schwartz, &
Sean C. DeMartino

The need for prevention on an international level is compelling. A significant portion of the global disease burden is attributed to mental health (Murray & Lopez, 1996). Mental health issues are a significant contributor to the global disease burden, and the impact is growing (Collins et al., 2011). The supply–demand imbalance for mental health disorders in relation to investment in prevention and treatment is significant in every country (WHO, 2005). Within the supply–demand imbalance, mental health disparities exist internationally. For example, Europe has two hundred times as many psychiatrists as does Africa (WHO). This supply–demand has been referred to as the treatment gap, leaving greatly untreated (often over 50 percent) and poorly treated mental health issues, particularly in low- and middle-income countries (Saxena, Thornicroft, Knapp, & Whiteford, 2007).

The impact of untreated or poorly treated mental health issues is significant. For example, by 2020, an estimated 1.5 million people will die each year by suicide, and between 15 and 30 million will make the attempt (Bertolote & Flieschmann, 2002). In addition, mental health issues are inextricably linked to overall health (Chapman, Perry, & Strine, 2005; Kubzansky, Sparrow, Vokonas, & Kawachi, 2001) and myriad other issues, including substance abuse and school and employment failure (Mrazek, Biglan, & Hawkins, 2004; Vogelzangs et al., 2008). Since prevention seeks, among other issues, to reduce or eliminate mental health issues before they occur, it has been referred to as a more humane approach to exclusive reliance on treatment (Albee, 1990; Prilleltensky, 1997).

As evidence of the individual, social, and economic impact of mental health issues globally has grown, attention has focused on prevention and health promotion as a potential answer (Chatterji, Caffray, Crowe, Freeman, & Jensen, 2004; Smith et al., 2002). The World Health Organization Comprehensive Mental Health Action Plan (CMHAP; 2013–20) proposes the implementation of universal prevention interventions to reduce the mental health burden (WHO, 2013). In general, the utility and cost effectiveness of prevention have been well supported (e.g., Kumpfer, Alvarado, & Smith, 2004; O'Connell, Boat, & Warner, 2009). Thus, there is compelling international need for prevention and solid evidence that prevention is both socially and economically viable (Zechmeister, Kilian, & McDaid, 2008). As noted by Vera and Shin (2006), prevention and outreach services are a critical supplement to therapy services, as those who are most in need are often those least likely to access and enter therapy. Increasing the international focus on prevention raises numerous issues. Foremost, it emphasizes the need to conduct prevention that works and practice that is ethical.

This chapter reviews the major ethical issues currently faced by prevention researchers and practitioners across the globe. In addition, the authors will present a set of guidelines to assist researchers and practitioners with the successful resolution of ethical dilemmas in prevention work. Finally, the implementation of these guidelines will be illustrated through a case application of an ethical problem in a global context. Before beginning a review of major ethical issues faced by that undertaking prevention work, we provide a definition of prevention.

Definition of Prevention

In providing ethical guidance for international prevention work, it is important to define what is meant by the term "prevention." The expansiveness of the field of prevention is evident in the definition proposed by Romano and Hage (2000). They define "prevention" as including one or more of the following five dimensions: (1) stopping problem behavior before it occurs (primary prevention); (2) delaying the onset of problem behavior (secondary prevention); (3) reducing the negative impact of current problem behavior (tertiary prevention); (4) promoting strengths to reduce risks; and (5) promoting structural policies that promote well-being.

Current Status of Prevention Ethics

The major ethical dilemmas faced by international prevention researchers and practitioners are generally similar. The only difference is that global prevention brings some of the core prevention ethical issues to the forefront. In this section, we will explicate the ethical issues in prevention work internationally (i.e., the imposition of cultural values, informed consent, and competence).

Utility of Prevention Ethics Internationally

As prevention is applied in an international context, fundamental questions need to be ethically addressed. One of the core issues is what empirical evidence exists that a specific intervention will work with a specific population in a specific context. Although there is a sound empirical basis for many approaches to prevention (i.e., Catalano, Berglund, Ryan, Lonczak, & Hawkins, 2004; Nation et al., 2003), these evidence-based programs have not been widely used and assessed internationally (Bumbarger, Perkins, & Greenberg,

2010; Kumpfer & Alvarado, 2003; McCall, 2009; Ringwalt et al., 2011). Thus it is vital to find an appropriate balance between fidelity to evidence-based approaches and the imperative to adopt culturally relevant prevention.

Cultural Relevance

The idea of cultural relevance takes on even more importance on an international level. The success of prevention is linked to the context of the target population (Trickett, 1992; 1998). To further complicate prevention work, impactful prevention typically addresses multiple systems (i.e., individual, family, community; Conyne, 2015; Durlak, 2003). Thus the cultural relevance of prevention practice is vital to successful prevention practice. It has been argued that prevention programs are inherently value-laden, and the values stem from the cultural context of the practitioner (Trickett, 1998). There is danger in prevention programs that are applied without an understanding of the context of the targeted behavior (Trickett, 1998). For example, prevention that does not account for social forces may blame individuals who are victims of social inequalities (Prilleltensky, 1997; Vera & Reese, 2000). A key component relevant to prevention is understanding and addressing the danger of value imposition (Vera & Reese, 2000).

Within an international context, understanding cultural assumptions, worldviews, and biases that may be imposed may be more complicated, particularly when applying an existing program in a new context. This may be a particular danger when practitioners attempt to apply existing programs to international cultural contexts without making adaptations to that culture. For example, a practitioner who is attempting to address violence in a country and culture different from his or her own may misunderstand the multiple contexts that sustain the violent behavior. If the purpose of violence is to protect family members or to provide food, interventions designed in other contexts will not work and may actually do damage. Additionally, cultural communication differences may impede finding ways to mediate the violence.

Informed Consent

To avoid imposing one's values, careful attention to the process of a person's/participant's agreement to be exposed to the prevention intervention, such as by getting informed consent, is an additional and necessary ethical issue to emphasize. Informed consent is one of the bedrocks of ethical mental health practice (Welfel, 2013), as it leads to respecting the autonomy of clients or consumers and communities. This practice is complicated in prevention practice and may face additional complications in global practice, due to language, social norms, and contextual differences. In the preceding section, the balance between empirically validated prevention programs with a strong theoretical base was contrasted with the need for cultural relevant prevention. As practitioners find this balance, clearly communicating the empirical support and theoretical base in informed consent becomes more complicated (Schwartz & Hage, 2009).

Since prevention programs are often provided to a group as opposed to an individual and focus on impacting multiple systems, the informed consent process becomes more challenging. In universal prevention, there is no clearly defined client and often multiple ecological points of impact (Bloom, 1996; Pope, 1990). Additionally, the target population is often not directly soliciting help (Conyne, 2010), further complicating the informed consent process. Thus, imposing an intervention on a community or group (i.e., school) has the potential to exacerbate the already existing power differential between the practitioner and the target population (Danish, 1990; Trickett, 1998). In a global context, comprehensive familiarity with the culture of the targeted group and understanding of the theoretical and empirical base are key issues to communicate in informed consent. For example, if a Western practitioner was attempting to conduct a prevention program in a non-Western country. It would be vital to understand potential cultural bias in the theoretical and empirical base and communicate how that bias will be addressed with risks and benefits.

Competence

Due to the unique aspects of prevention work, the training and resultant knowledge and skills needed are vital for competent and ethical practice. The myriad professionals who conduct prevention work along with the global differences in training and availability of competent practitioners further complicates this issue. An example of this is prevention interventions that are conducted in school settings, as teachers may be required to take part in a prevention intervention against their will, not understanding their role, and/or feel incompetent to carry out their tasks. Unfortunately, little has been written on the competencies necessary for ethical prevention practice (Schwartz, Hage, & Gonzalez, 2013). Recently there has been increased attention to addressing competent prevention practice (Hage et al., 2007; O'Neil & Britner, 2009) resulting in the American Psychological Association (APA) *Guidelines for Prevention in Psychology* (APA, 2014).

Guidelines for the Resolution of Ethical Dilemmas in Prevention

Further multidisciplinary and cross-cultural dialogue is needed to establish a clear set of ethical guidelines to govern prevention research, practice, and training across the globe. Traditional ethical codes stop short of providing the necessary guidance for prevention work. The evolution of the field of prevention and the formulation of a framework to guide prevention efforts are important steps to the eventual establishment of ethical guidelines for prevention. This section provides recommendations to assist the field of prevention in the resolution of ethical dilemmas in prevention (Hage, Schwartz, & Murray, 2013; Schwartz & Hage, 2009). These principles are meant to provide direction and guidance to prevention practitioners and researchers in the development of an ethics of prevention.

Focus on Ecological Contexts

Given the number and complexity of variables with an impact on prevention, the first principle meant to guide ethical decision making in global contexts is the need to incorporate multiple ecological contexts, including families, schools, industry, communities, and government, into prevention work. Programs that focus solely on individual change and ignore multiple ecological influences fail to account for the broader context of behavior and may place undue blame and responsibility on the individual (Prilleltensky, 1997; Vera & Reese, 2000).

Addressing both individual and contextual factors is associated with successful prevention programs (Vera & Reese, 2000). One example is the Communities That Care (CTC) prevention program (Jane-Llopis, Barry, Hosman, & Patel, 2005), which operates in or is in being implemented in several countries, including the United States, the Netherlands, England, Scotland, and Wales. The CTC is a prevention initiative to activate communities to implement evidence-based community violence and aggression prevention interventions. Using local assessment data related to risk and protective factors, communities develop action plans that fit the needs of the community at multiple ecological levels, including the community (e.g., media, policy change), the school (e.g., school management or teaching practices), the family (e.g., parent training), and the individual (e.g., social competence) (Hawkins, Catalano, & Arthur, 2002; Jane-Llopis et al., 2005).

Further, it is imperative that ethical prevention programs create a means for assessing procedures and outcomes at multiple ecological levels (Conyne, 2010). Systematic methods must be developed for identifying possible harm before it is produced. The many advantages of attending to multiple causative factors include avoiding the pathologizing of participants and communities, a focus on building client and community strengths, and respect for the influence of contextual factors. One example of an ecologically focused intervention is the Gatehouse Project in Australia (Bond et al., 2004; Patton et al., 2000), which involved 3,623 middle school students over a three-year period. Researchers implemented a districtwide intervention to promote adolescent emotional well-being and to reduce health risk behaviors. Each participating school was provided with local social climate and risk profiles in order to create individualized interventions addressing multiple levels of the school environment, including overall school climate, the classroom climate, and the school curriculum.

A planning team served to coordinate systemic and sustainable changes at these different ecological levels. Results from these interventions suggest the positive potential of a multilevel approach to affect individual-level outcomes. Differences of 3 percent to 5 percent for alcohol, smoking, and friends' drug use were found between the intervention and control groups (Bond et al., 2004).

In sum, efforts to determine the effect of environmental influences on behavior are empowering in that they do not stigmatize participants and encourage the use of existing community resources to succeed.

Culturally Responsive Prevention

Prevention programs in global contexts must be collaborative, empowering, and culturally relevant (Hage et al., 2007; Vera & Kenny, 2013). The cultures of the communities affected by a preventive intervention vary enormously. Those engaged in prevention work need to understand their own cultural values and biases and avoid imposing them on the targeted population (Reese & Vera, 2007; Sanson-Fisher & Turnbull, 1987). The most effective prevention programs include program participants in the planning, implementation, and evaluation of the prevention intervention (Kenny & Romano, 2009; Reiss & Price, 1996). In the process of designing a prevention intervention, practitioners and researchers need to clearly communicate their own values and beliefs and understand the values and cultural of the target population (Trickett, 1992), as well as use culturally sensitive evaluation measurements in search of evidence-based interventions. For example, Wainberg et al. (2007) adapted a U.S.-designed HIV prevention intervention for Brazilian adults with severe mental illness, using a four-step process: (1) optimizing fidelity; (2) optimizing fit; (3) balancing fidelity and fit; and (4) pilot testing and refining the intervention. The bicultural research team included both U.S. and Brazilian clinicians and researchers. This diversity facilitated the development of an intervention that reflected Brazilian values of social responsibility, sexual expression, and self-expression (Wainberg et al., 2007).

Competent prevention work involves a process of interaction between the values and assumptions related to the prevention program and that of the targeted population (Kumpfer, Alvarado, Smith & Bellamy, 2002; Kumpfer, Pinyuchon, Teixeira de Melo, & Whiteside, 2008). Behaviors that may seem unhealthy from one contextual perspective may serve an important purpose in another context. Context includes nuances related to culture, politics, economy, history, geography, and community organizations and institutions (Patton, 2014). For example, in India, some families kept their children from a polio vaccine, and researchers who studied the area discovered that Muslim mothers has heard rumors of a plot to sterilize their children and were simply acting to protect them (Renwick, 2015).

Understanding this possibility prevents imposition of one's own values and avoids pathologizing individuals or a community based on contextual behavior.

Ethical practice involves adapting programs to fit the cultural and community norms and values of participants (Nation et al., 2003; Vera & Kenny, 2013). One example of an evidence-based culturally relevant prevention program is the Strengthening Families Program (SFP), which has been culturally adapted for use in seventeen countries (Kumpfer et al., 2008). The SFP is an evidence-based family skills training intervention developed and found efficacious for substance abuse. For example, the cultural adaptation process in countries such as Spain and Portugal included materials development and translation into Spanish, staff training, on-site and online Web-based supervision and technical assistance, and evaluation services to assure quality implementation and process evaluation feedback for improvements (Kumpfer et al., 2008). Parents were taught, for example, the importance of talking about drugs and sex with their children, topics that are often thought of as taboo in the culture. In Portugal, meals were delivered at the end of the SFP sessions instead of at the beginning to accommodate preferred dining hours. In sum, the SFP prevention program illustrates the importance of a collaborative approach so that integral aspects of the prevention program are culturally relevant and focused on facilitating the empowerment of communities rather than imposing program values in multiple ecological contexts.

Evidence-Based Approaches

Prevention programs need to be developed from a sound theoretical base, be supported by evidence, and address issues of replicability as well as long-term outcomes or effects (Raczynski, Waldo, Schwartz, & Horne, 2013). Many prevention programs have found short-term success only to have long-term results return to the original level or below (Brown & Liao, 1999). Designing programs that are supported by a strong generative base, when such a base exists, is a protective factor against value imposition (Heller, 1996) and allows for evidence-based informed consent. A strong evidence base also contributes to the progression of the field of prevention science as it leads to replicable programs that are efficacious, and ready for dissemination.

This focus does not preclude pilot interventions and exploratory prevention work, especially prevention work that meets the contextual needs of culturally diverse groups and addresses issues of power and oppression. While a tension may appear to exist between fidelity and adaptation, both are essential components of effective prevention intervention program design, and they may be addressed by a planned, organized, and systematic approach (Castro, Barrera, & Martinez, 2004).

Toward this aim of balancing fidelity with the need for cultural adaptation, an innovative program design strategy is to develop hybrid prevention programs that "build in" adaptation to enhance program fit while also maximizing fidelity of implementation and program effectiveness. The ethical progression of research on prevention programs includes formative research that identifies core components of change, thus addressing issues of replicability as well as cultural relevance (Raczynski et al., 2013). Adapting an evidence-based approach to a new cultural context involves an effort to meet the cultural characteristics of the new context, as well as fidelity to the successful components of the intervention. For example, in adapting an evidence-based HIV prevention program in rural Kenya, Poulsen et al. (2010) conducted a community needs assessment and then thoughtfully adapted the program to meet the context of rural Kenya, finally piloting the program with community collaboration. Cultural adaptations were made to the program using feedback from local stakeholders. For example, parenting strategies and skills to increase effective parent–child communication related to sexuality were culturally adapted, implemented, and evaluated. This program example highlights the importance of careful adaptation of evidence-based programs in other cultures.

Attending to Power and Privilege

In all prevention work, dynamics of privilege and power, and the potential for exploitation, exist among prevention researchers, practitioners, and community members (Hage & Kenny, 2009). Prevention research needs to involve the community in determining the research goals and methods to ensure both that programs are developed to meet the community's specific needs as well as to encourage the community members' commitment to the programs that are being implemented. In typical prevention programs, the participants are not actively seeking help, and the intervention is designed to prevent a problem that may or may not happen. Additionally, prevention interventions have the potential to create changes not only in the individual but also at multiple ecological levels (Conyne, 2015). With an understanding of these issues, it is imperative to protect the autonomy of participants (APA, 2002) and to engage in collaborative planning, implementation, and evaluation of prevention efforts. Such efforts need to be aimed at building the "capacity for all individuals and groups, to participate fully in all aspects of society, to foster equity in social and political power, and to promote strengths and copings skills for responding to societal stress and oppression" (Vera & Kenny, 2013, p. 40).

This effort to address power dynamics in prevention work also involves actively addressing the dangers of exploitation and undue influence. Ethical practice involves creating collaborative egalitarian relationships, safeguarding against inappropriate dual relationships, providing alternatives to participation in prevention programs, and providing ongoing informed consent. For example, participatory action research (PAR) involves forming a collaborative relationship with members of the target group (Kidd & Kral, 2005). Thus, the participants are encouraged to become involved and empowered, leading to relevant ethical prevention interventions (Cohen & Wolfe, 2007). PAR is a form of research in which researchers operate as full collaborators with members of a community or organizations in studying and transforming those organizations. It emphasizes co-learning, participation, and organizational transformation (Greenwood, Whyte, & Harkavy, 1993). Furthermore, a focus on building competency rather than addressing risk factors has been conceptualized as being less stigmatizing and more empowering.

An example of PAR is Fine and Torre's (2006) collaborative program with United States (U.S.) prison inmates, which included a prison-based college program with a public policy focus. An additional example, taken from an international context, is a PAR project involving Black gay men and lesbian women in post-apartheid South Africa (Graziano, 2004). The researcher joins with participants as collaborators in recognizing the validity of their voices, which are signs of strength and hope in the midst of oppression and despair. These PAR projects utilize methods of empowerment evaluation. Empowerment evaluation uses evaluation concepts, techniques, and findings to foster community improvement and self-determination and to increase the capacity of program participants to plan, implement, and evaluate their own programs (Fetterman & Wandersman, 2007).

Environmental Change

When designing and implementing prevention programs, practitioners and researchers need to focus on transformative preventive interventions with the aim of long-term systemic change that empowers both individuals and communities. In addition, the allocation of prevention services should be fair, equal, and free of discrimination. An understanding of the central and contributing effects of oppression in mental health services as well as the disparity of these services for poor and diverse communities underscores the ethical imperative to make prevention in these communities a priority. Additionally, prevention programs should focus on changing societal structures, policies, and systemic barriers that limit equal access to resources (Kenny & Hage, 2009; Toporek & Williams, 2006).

Furthermore, prevention should facilitate participants' empowerment to reach their full capacity (Prilleltensky & Nelson, 2002). Ignoring the multiple effects of oppression and the resulting contextual barriers, such as poverty, will limit the effectiveness of preventive interventions and ultimately limit the potential of those involved. For example, in some areas of Ecuador, like in many low- and middle-income countries, more than half of the population live below the poverty level and 20 percent live in extreme poverty. Poverty is a significant risk factor for mental illness, and thus in order to address and prevent social issues such as alcohol and drug use, domestic violence, and teen pregnancy, the general lack of resources among the community must also be addressed (Salerno et al., 2009).

Application of Guidelines for the Resolution of Ethical Dilemmas in Prevention

The World Health Organization (WHO, 2013) has identified suicide prevention as an integral part of its Mental Health Action Plan with the hopes of decreasing suicide rates by 10 percent by 2020. Due to the sensitive nature of suicide (e.g., suicide is illegal in some countries), it is likely that rates of suicide attempts and completions are underreported. However, suicide is the second leading cause of death globally for fifteen- to twenty-nine-year-olds as well as accounts for 50 percent and 71 percent of all violent deaths for men and women, respectively. In addition, up to 75 percent of suicides occur in low- and middle-income countries (WHO, 2013). The reasons and methods used in suicides vary across populations and settings, making it challenging to develop prevention programs across cultures without a set of international ethical guidelines. In the following section, we will apply the recommended guidelines to a fictional case study that was created for the purposes of this chapter.

Case Study: Suicide Prevention in Japan

As a part of a newly formed WHO task force to implement suicide prevention programs, a local community in Japan is identified as a potential area for a new program. The community has seen a rise in its suicide rates, especially among adult men, since the beginning of the global recession in 2008. Many of the adults in the area have lost or are at risk of losing their job. After completing a needs assessment, it is determined that it is important to provide a one-day workshop during the workday for community members to learn how to identify the warning signs of suicide and how to intervene if someone they know demonstrates the warning signs, as well as provide information on local resources that can help.

After reviewing the literature and developing the workshop, it is learned that community members are resistant to the program and do not want to become actively involved. In consulting with community members, they state that they do not find the program to be relevant and would prefer to work. It is later learned that many Japanese communities have a history of "honorable suicides" in order to prevent bringing shame or becoming a burden on one's family. The local government has identified suicide prevention as a goal and is eager to intervene, but is unsure of how to proceed. Based on the situation described, what would be an appropriate next step?

Discussion of Application

Using the guidelines discussed earlier, there are five steps to be taken. First, it is important to identify the different ecological contexts that can be integrated into the program. A one-day workshop allows for participation from an individual experiencing suicidal ideation, his or her friends, and family, but fails to take into consideration other ecological influences, such as cultural norms, the influence of work, the media, and social policy. After researching Japanese cultural values regarding family and community norms, it is learned that there is a cultural value of not bringing shame or burdening one's family (Traphagan, 2004). Many members of the community value hard work and are working fourteen-to-sixteen-hour days in order to provide for their family. They often experience guilt and shame when they lose their job and are unable to provide for their family. To identify ways to adjust the program to better address the ecological contexts involved, key community leaders are identified in order to form a collaborative partnership in moving forward.

The second step involves working with the community leaders to identify values, beliefs, and content in order to develop a culturally responsive suicide prevention program. Information is learned that suicide was once considered to be an acceptable means of removing burden or bringing prestige to the family, especially among older generations. Group interdependence is also an important social value, and suicide in Japan has also been related to social isolation. Several names have given to different forms of suicide, such as *ikkanshinjû* (family suicide), *shinjû* (double suicide), *kamikaze*, or *harakiri* (ritual self-killing typically completed by samurais; Traphagan, 2004).

Program developers learn that about 46 percent of suicides in Japan are committed due to health problems, while about another 25 percent are due to financial or lifestyle problems (Ono et al., 2008). *Karōshi,* also known as "death from overwork," is common in the area for those who are working (Motohaski, Kaneko, & Sasaki, 2004). Community leaders share that community members feel compelled to work long hours for fear of losing their job. An understanding begins to develop that community members are not interested in attending the workshop and it is recognized that a greater understanding about the social and cultural context of Japan is needed.

Having a better understanding of the cultural values of the community, the next objective is to find research support for the program. Information is sought about evidenced-based programs targeted toward suicide prevention. Details are learned about a government-initiated program named Healthy Akita 21, after the capital city of Akita Prefecture, which previously had the highest rates of suicide in Japan (Motohaski et al., 2004). The program focuses on raising awareness through, for example, the use of media, including news articles on different topics regarding suicide, such as features of suicide, family backgrounds of victims, recent trends, reader's opinions, and community activities for prevention. The program also incorporates other action such as increasing opportunities for mental health consultation, promoting the prevention of depression, and creating a supportive environment for mental health promotion.

Healthy Akita 21 seeks to decrease the rate of suicide across all generations by also incorporating the family, school, workplace, and community settings. The program saw a decrease of suicide rates by 27 percent during the four-year implementation (Ono et al., 2008). A similar program implemented in a rural Japanese community that expanded on the Healthy Akita 21 multimodal model also was effective in decreasing suicide rates for men and elderly in the community (Ono et al., 2013). Community leaders are identified in order to begin developing and implementing a new, similar program, based on the supporting evidence from the Health Akita 21 initiative that is culturally sensitive to the local community.

In addition, recognition of potential power dynamics should be considered during the planning process. While suicide has been a problem for the community, it is not a problem for which the community was actively seeking help. Intervening can create change on several levels. Considering the impact the suicide prevention program can potentially have on the community, the relationship with community leaders should be a collaborative and equal relationship. Government and work officials also hold a certain level of power with community members, as they can determine policies for the community and workplace, respectively. Local leadership involvement can be critical to the long-term commitment to the program in the community (Ono et al., 2013).

For some in the community, having access to mental health resources may be a privilege, perhaps because they have financial resources to access mental health care or because they are not impacted by the stigma associated on mental health services. Creating opportunities for all to access mental health services as well as getting community members involved in efforts to decrease stigma is important (Motohaski et al., 2004). In order to empower community members to recognize and support each other, training for local gatekeepers and primary care providers will be an important intervention in the process of implementing the program.

Two important concepts to be considered in this program are informed consent and competence. While it is imperative to ensure that the program is culturally relevant to the local community, it is also important to avoid imposing one's own values (Welfel, 2013). Informed consent is one way to prevent the imposition of one's values. The Japanese Psychological Association (JPA, 2012) code of ethics states that all participants must be fully informed of the details related to psychology-related activities and give written consent, with the ability to suspend or terminate participation at any point. Several challenges to informed consent exist. Community members may feel compelled to participate in program events due to the power that government officials and employers have. This subtle pressure may challenge their desire to provide for their families and prevent bringing guilt and shame. The language of the informed consent documents would need to be carefully worded to communicate the voluntary nature of participation in the program, with no repercussions for nonparticipation. Participants would also need to know that the program has been developed based on the Akita 21 program and that the local community's values and cultures have been taken into consideration in the development of the program.

The idea of competence is complex. Professionals must be trained to implement prevention activities, but they also need to be culturally competent (APA, 2014). Cultural competence consists of professional attitudes or beliefs, knowledge, and skills to intervene with a particular cultural group (Sue, 2001). To be competent in implementing the suicide prevention program, program developers must maintain an awareness of their own cultural values, experiences, and biases. Techniques such as the use of self-reflective journaling may assist them with exploring their values and biases. While new knowledge and information has been gained on the local community and on the topic of suicide in Japan, recognition of the limitations of one's knowledge and competencies is necessary, with assistance sought from other professionals and community members to gain further understanding. The inclusion of community leaders in the development and implementation of the program provides some assurance that the community's practices and values will be respected, while also facilitating education to the community on the knowledge and skills that support the success of the program.

Incorporating a multimodal prevention model (Ono et al., 2013), an evidence-based intervention (Motohaski et al., 2004), and collaboration with community leaders, a new prevention program is developed that is culturally relevant. On the governmental level, the program will publicize messages from local leaders, such as the mayor, to engage in self-care and suicide prevention and form a committee to raise awareness and collaborate with government offices on suicide preventions activities. This level of intervention can begin to address the community's values toward working hard professionally and experiencing shame and guilt for being unable to do so. It is imperative for the program to address these cultural values to be considered relevant and effective for members of the community (Vera & Reese, 2000).

For the community, public educational events and training sessions are organized to discuss warning signs, treatment options, causes and risk factors, and associated mental illness with suicide. Additionally, trainings are provided to teach community members to identify individuals at risk and to provide appropriate resources. For those who are identified as being at risk, screening tools to identify those at risk and provide resources are developed, home visits with health care providers are organized, supports to maintain self-help activities are implemented, and regional social gatherings are held to build the individual's support network. Based on the evidence from similar suicide prevention programs in other similar communities, it is anticipated that the community will be effectively engaged and the rate of suicide will decrease.

Conclusion

The development of prevention interventions has been shown to have great promise in promoting the health and well-being of individuals and communities across the world. International cultural adaptation of prevention interventions presents unique ethical challenges to the prevention researcher and practitioner. Thoughtful action to reduce the burden of mental disorders worldwide and to enhance the ability of countries' to respond to this rising challenge is imperative. Without concerted and systematic action, the health of millions of people across the globe is at risk.

References

Albee, G. W. (1990). The futility of psychotherapy. *Journal of Mind and Behavior* 11: 369–84.

APA (American Psychological Association). (2002). Ethical principles of psychologists and code of conduct. *American Psychologist* 57: 1060–73.

American Psychological Association (2014). Guidelines for prevention in psychology. *American Psychologist* 69: 285–96. doi: 10.1037/a0034569.

Bertolote, J. M., & Fleischmann, A. (2002). Suicide and psychiatric diagnosis: a worldwide perspective. *World Psychiatry 1*, 181.

Bloom, M. (1996). *Primary Prevention Practices*. Thousand Oaks, CA: Sage.

Bond, L., Patton, G., Glover, S., Carlin, J. B., Butler, H., Thomas, L., & Bowes, G. (2004). The Gatehouse Project: can a multilevel school intervention affect emotional wellbeing and health risk behaviours? *Journal of Epidemiology and Community Health* 58: 997–1003.

Brown, C. H., & Liao, J. (1999). Principles for designing randomized preventive trails in mental health: an emerging developmental epidemiology paradigm. *American Journal of Community Psychology* 27: 677–714.

Bumbarger, B., Perkins, D. F., & Greenberg, M. (2010). Taking effective prevention to scale. In Doll, B., Pfohl, W., & Yoon, J. (eds.), *Handbook of Youth Prevention Science*. New York: Routledge, pp. 433–44.

Castro, F. G., Barrera, M., & Martinez, C. R. (2004). The cultural adaptation of prevention interventions: resolving tensions between fidelity and fit. *Prevention Science: The Official Journal of the Society for Prevention Research* 5: 41–5.

Catalano, R. F., Berglund, M. L., Ryan, J. A., Lonczak, H. S., & Hawkins, J. D. (2004). Positive youth development in the United States: research findings on evaluations of positive youth development programs. *Annals of the American Academy of Political and Social Science* 591: 98–124.

Chapman, D. P., Perry, G. S., & Strine, T. W. (2005). The vital link between chronic disease and depressive disorders. *Prevention of Chronic Disease* 2: A14.

Chatterji, P., Caffray, C. M., Crowe, M., Freeman, L., & Jensen, P. (2004). Cost assessment of a school-based mental health screening and treatment program in New York City. *Mental Health Services Research* 6: 155–66.

Cohen, L., & Wolfe, A. (2007). Working collaboratively to advance prevention. In Cohen, L., Chavez, V., & Chihimi, S. (eds.). *Prevention Is Primary: Strategies for Community Wellbeing*. San Francisco, CA: Jossey-Bass, pp. 141–60.

Collins, P. Y., Patel, V., Joestl, S. S., March, D., Insel, T. R., & Daar, A. S. (2011). Grand challenges in global mental health. *Nature* 475: 27–30.

Conyne, R. (2010). *Preventive Program Development and Evaluation: An Incidence Reduction, Culturally Relevant Approach*. Thousand Oaks, CA: Sage.

Conyne, R. K. (2015). *Counseling for Wellness and Prevention: Helping People Become Empowered in Systems and Settings*, 3rd ed. New York: Brunner-Routledge.

Danish, S. J. (1990). Ethical considerations in the design, implementation, and evaluation of developmental interventions. In Fisher, C. B., Tryon, W. W., Fisher, C. B., & Tryon, W. W. (eds.), *Ethics in Applied Developmental Psychology: Emerging Issues in an Emerging Field*. Westport, CT: Ablex, pp. 93–112.

Durlak, J. A. (2003). The long-term impact of preschool prevention programs: a commentary. *Prevention & Treatment* 6. doi:10.1037/1522-3736.6.1.632c.

Fetterman, D. M., & Wandersman, A. (2007). Empowerment evaluation: yesterday, today, and tomorrow. *American Journal of Evaluation* 28, 179–98. doi: 10.1177/1098214007301350

Fine, M., & Torre, M. E. (2006). Intimate details: participatory action research in prison. *Action Research* 4: 253–69. doi: 10.1177/1476750306066801

Graziano, K. J. (2004). Oppression and resiliency in a post-apartheid South Africa: unheard voices of black gay men and lesbians. *Cultural Diversity and Ethnic Minority Psychology* 10, 302–16. dx.doi.org/10.1037/1099-9809.10.3.302

Greenberg, M. T., Domitrovich, C., & Bumbarger, B. (2000). *Preventing Mental Disorders in School-age Children: A Review of the Effectiveness of Prevention Programs*. University Park: Prevention Research Center for the Promotion of Human Development, College of Health and Human Development, Pennsylvania State University.

Greenwood, D. J., Whyte, W. F., & Harkavy, I. (1993). Participatory action research as a process and as a goal. *Human Relations* 46: 175.

Hage, S. M., & Kenny, M. (2009). Promoting a social justice approach to prevention: future directions for training, practice, and research. *Journal of Primary Prevention* 30: 75–87. doi: dx.doi.org/10.1007/s10935-008-0165-5

Hage, S. M., Romano, J., Kenny, M. E., Matthews, C. R., Schwartz, J. P., & Waldo, M. (2007). Best practice guidelines on prevention practice, research, training, and social advocacy for psychologists. *Counseling Psychologist* 35: 493–566.

Hage, S. M., Schwartz, J., & Murray, M. (2013). Best practice guidelines on prevention: improving the well-being of individuals and communities. In Vera, E. (ed.). *Handbook of Prevention in Counseling Psychology*. New York: Oxford University Press, pp. 51–64.

Hawkins J. D., Catalano R. F., & Arthur, M. (2002). Promoting science-based prevention in communities. *Addictive Behavior* 90, 1–26.

Heller, K. (1996). Coming of age of prevention science: comments on the 1994 National Institute of Mental Health-Institute of Medicine prevention reports. *American Psychologist* 51: 1123–7.

Jane-Llopis, E., Barry, M., Hosman, C., & Patel, V. (2005). Mental health promotion works: a review. *International Journal of Health Promotion & Education* (supplement): 9–25.

JPA (Japanese Psychological Association) (2012). *Ethical Principles of Psychologists.* Retrieved from http://www.psych.or.jp/english/ethical.html.

Kenny, M., & Hage, S. M. (2009). The next frontier: prevention as an instrument of social justice. *Journal of Primary Prevention,* 30: 1–10. doi: http://dx.doi.org/10.1007/s10935-008-0163-7.

Kenny, M. E., & Romano, J. I. (2009). Promoting positive development and social justice through prevention: a legacy for the future: the challenge of prevention interventions. In Kenny, M. E., Horne, A. M., Orpinas, P., & Reese, L. E. (eds.), *Realizing Social Justice: The Challenge of Prevention Interventions.* Washington, DC: American Psychological Association, pp. 17–35.

Kid, S. A., & Kral, M. J. (2005). Practicing participatory action research. *Journal of Counseling Psychology* 52: 187–95.

Kubzansky, L. D., Sparrow, D., Vokonas, P., & Kawachi, I. (2001). Is the glass half empty or half full? A prospective study of optimism and coronary heart disease in the normative aging study. *Psychosomatic Medicine* 63: 910–16.

Kumpfer, K. L., & Alvarado, R. (2003). Family-strengthening approaches for the prevention of youth problem behaviors. *American Psychologist* 58: 457–65. doi:10.1037/0003-066X.58.6-7.457.

Kumpfer, K. L., Alvarado, R., & Smith, P. (2004). Drug abuse prevention tools and programs. In Coombs, R. H. (eds.), *Addiction Counseling Review: Preparing for Comprehensive, Certification, and Licensing Exams.* New York: Lahaska Press, Houghton Mifflin, pp. 467-86.

Kumpfer, K. L., Alvarado, R., Smith, P., & Bellamy, N. (2002). Cultural sensitivity and adaptation in family-based prevention interventions. *Prevention Science* 3: 241–6.

Kumpfer, K. L., Pinyuchon, M., de Melo, A., & Whiteside, H. (2008). Cultural adaptation process for international dissemination of the Strengthening Families Program (SFP). *Evaluation and Health Professions* 33: 226–39.

McCall, R. B. (2009). Evidence-based programming in the context of practice and policy. *Social Policy Report* 23: 3–18.

Motohaski, Y., Kaneko, Y., & Sasaki, H. (2004). Community-based suicide prevention program in Japan using a health promotion approach. *Environmental Health and Preventive Medicine* 9: 3–8.

Mrazek, P., Biglan, A., & Hawkins, J. D. (2004). *Community-monitoring Systems: Tracking and Improving the Well-being of America 's Children and Adolescents.* Falls Church, VA: Society for Prevention Research. Retrieved from www.preventionresearch.org

Murray, C. J., & Lopez, A. D. (1996). *The Global Burden of Disease and Injury Series, Volume 1: A Comprehensive Assessment of Mortality and Disability from Diseases, Injuries, and Risk Factors in 1990 and PROJECTED to 2020*. Cambridge. MA: World Health Organization.

Nation, M., Crusto, C., Wandersman, A., Kumpfer, K., Seybolt, D., & Morrissey-Kane, E., et al. (2003). What works in prevention: principles and effective prevention programs. *American Psychologist* 58: 449–56.

O'Connell, M. E., Boat, T., & Warner, K. E. (eds.) (2009). *Preventing Mental, Emotional, and Behavioral Disorders among Young People: Progress and Possibilities*. Washington, DC: National Academies Press.

O'Neil, J. M., & Britner, P. A. (2009). Training primary preventionists to make a difference in people's lives. In Kenny, M. E., Horne, A. M., Orpinas, P., Reese, L. E. (eds.), *Realizing Social Justice: The Challenge of Preventive Interventions.* Washington, DC: American Psychological Association, pp. 141–62. doi: 10.1037/11870-007

Ono, Y., Awata, S., Iida, H., Ishida, Y., Ishizuka, N., Iwasa, H., ... Watanabe, N. (2008). A community intervention trial of multimodal suicide prevention program in Japan: a novel multimodal community intervention program to prevent suicide and suicide attempt in Japan, NOCOMIT-J. *BMC Public Health* 8: 315–23.

Ono, Y., Sakai, A., Otsuka, K., Uda, H., Oyama, H., Ishizuka, N., ... Yonemoto, N. (2013). Effectiveness of a multimodal community intervention program to prevent suicide and suicide attempts: a quasi-experimental study. *PLoS ONE* 8: e74902.

Patton, M. Q. (2014). *Qualitative Research and Evaluation Methods: Integrating Theory and Practice*, 4th ed. Thousand Oaks, CA: Sage.

Patton, G. C., Glover, S., Bond, L., Butler, H., Godfrey, C., Di Pietro, G., & Bowes, G. (2000). The Gatehouse Project: a systematic approach to mental health promotion in secondary schools. *Australian and New Zealand Journal of Psychiatry* 34: 586–93.

Pope, K. S. (1990). Identifying and implementing ethical standards for primary prevention. *Prevention in Human Services* 8: 43–64. doi: 10.1300/J293v08n02_04

Poulsen M. N., Vandenhoudt H., Wyckoff S. C., Obong'o, C. O., Ochura, J., Njika G., et al. (2010). Cultural adaptation of a U.S. evidence-based parenting intervention for rural western Kenya: from parents matter! To families matter! *AIDS Education and Prevention* 22: 273–85.

Prilleltensky, I. (1997). Values, assumptions, and practices: assessing the moral implications of psychological discourse and action. *American Psychologist* 52: 517–35.

Prilleltensky, I., & Nelson, G. (2002). *Doing Psychology Critically: Making a Difference in Diverse Settings*. New York: Palgrave Macmillan.

Raczynski, K., Waldo, M., Schwartz, J. P., & Horne, A. M. (2013). *Evidence-Based Prevention*. Thousand Oaks, CA: Sage.

Reese, L. E., & Vera, E. M. (2007). Culturally relevant prevention: the scientific and practical considerations of community-based programs. *Counseling Psychologist* 35: 763–78. doi: 10.1177/0011000007304588

Reiss, D., & Price, R. H. (1996). National research agenda for prevention research: the National institute of Mental Health. *American Psychologist* 51: 1109–15.

Renwick, D. (2015). Global efforts to eradicate polio. In Council on Foreign Relations (eds.), *CFR Backgrounders*. www.cfr.org/public-health-threats-and-pandemics/global-efforts-eradicate-polio/p36122

Ringwalt, C., Hanley, S., Ennett, S. T., Vincus, A. A., Bowling, J. M., Haws, S. W., & Rohrbach, L. A. (2011). The effects of no child left behind on the prevalence of evidence-based drug prevention curricula in the nation's middle schools. *Journal of School Health* 81: 265–72. doi: 10.1111/j.1746-1561.2011.00587.x

Romano, J., & Hage, S. M. (2000). Prevention and counseling psychology: revitalizing commitments for the 21st century. *Counseling Psychologist* 28: 733–63. doi: http://dx.doi.org/10.1177/0011000000286001

Salerno, A., Carroll C., Cruz, M., Jue, K., Silvestri, F., & Culebras, M. (2009). Developing comprehensive community mental health services in developing countries. *International Journal of Mental Health* 38: 87–99.

Sanson-Fisher, R., & Turnbull, D. (1987). "To do or not to do?": Ethical problems for behavioral medicine. In Fairbairn, S., & Fairbairn, G. (eds.), *Psychology, Ethics and Change*. New York: Routledge, pp. 191–211.

Saxena, S., Thornicroft, G., Knapp, M., & Whiteford, H. (2007). Resources for mental health: scarcity, inequity, and inefficiency. *Lancet* 370: 878–89.

Schwartz, J., & Hage, S. M. (2009). Prevention: ethics, responsibility, and commitment to public well-being. In Kenny, M. E., Horne, A., Orpinas, P., & Reese, L. E. (eds.), *Realizing Social Justice: The Challenge of Preventive Interventions*. Washington, DC: American Psychological Association Press, pp. 123–40. doi: dx.doi.org/10.1037/11870-006

Schwartz, J., & Hage, S. M., & Gonzalez, D. (2013). Ethical principles for the practice of prevention. In Vera, E. (ed.). *Handbook of Prevention in Counseling Psychology*. New York: Oxford University Press, pp. 65–75.

Smith, J. L., Rost, K. M., Nutting, P. A., Libby, A. M., Elliott, C. E., & Pyne, J. M. (2002). Impact of primary care depression intervention on employment and workplace conflict outcomes: Is value added? *Journal of Mental Health Policy and Economics* 5: 43–50.

Sue, D. W. (2001). Multidimensional facets of cultural competence. *Counseling Psychologist* 29: 790–821.

Toporek, R. L., & Williams, R. A. (2006). Ethics and professional issues related to the practice of social justice in counseling psychology. In Toporek, R. L., Gerstein, L. H., Fouad, N. A., Roysircar, G. S., & Israel, T. (eds.) *Handbook for Social Justice in Counseling Psychology: Leadership, Vision, & Action*. Thousand Oaks, CA: Sage, pp. 17–34.

Traphagan, J. W. (2004). Interpretations of elder suicide, stress, and dependency among rural Japanese. *Ethnology* 43: 315–29.

Trickett, E. J. (1992). Prevention ethics: explicating the context of prevention activities. *Ethics & Behavior* 2: 91–100. doi: 10.1207/s15327019eb0202_2

Trickett, E. J. (1998). Toward a framework for defining and resolving ethical issues in the protection of communities involved in primary prevention projects. *Ethics & Behavior* 8: 321–37. doi: 10.1207/s15327019eb0804_5

Vera, E. M., & Kenny, M. (2013). *Social Justice and Culturally Relevant Prevention*. Thousand Oaks, CA: Sage.

Vera, E. M., & Reese, L. E. (2000). Preventive interventions with school-age youth. In Brown, S. D., Lent, R. W., Brown, S. D., & Lent, R. W. (eds.), *Handbook of Counseling Psychology*, 3rd ed. Hoboken, NJ: John Wiley & Sons, pp. 411–34).

Vera, E. M., & Shin, R. Q. (2006). Promoting strengths in a socially toxic world: supporting resiliency with systemic interventions. *Counseling Psychologist* 34: 80–9.

Vogelzangs, N., Kritchevsky, S. B., Beekman, A. T., Newman, A. B., Satterfield, S., Simonsick, E. M., & Penninx, B. W. (2008). Depressive symptoms and change in abdominal obesity in older persons. *Archives of General Psychiatry* 65: 1386–93.

Wainberg, M. L., McKinnon, K., Mattos, P. E., Pinto, D., Mann, C. G., de Oliveira, C. S., & . . . Cournos, F. (2007). A model for adapting evidence-based behavioral interventions to a new culture: HIV prevention for psychiatric patients in Rio de Janeiro, Brazil. *AIDS and Behavior* 11: 872–83.

Welfel, E. R. (2013). *Ethics in Counseling and Psychotherapy: Standards, Research, and Emerging Issues*, 5th ed. Belmont, CA: Brooks/Cole.

World Health Organization. Department of Mental Health & Substance Abuse (2005). *Mental Health Atlas 2005*. Geneva: World Health Organization.

World Health Organization (2013). Comprehensive Mental Health Action Plan 2013–2020. www.who.int/mental_health/publications/action_plan/en

Zechmeister, I., Kilian, R., & McDaid, D. (2008). Is it worth investing in mental health promotion and prevention of mental illness? A systematic review of the evidence from economic evaluations. *BMC Public Health* 8: 20.

5 Effectiveness Trial of the New Beginnings Program for Divorcing Parents

Translation from an Experimental Prototype to an Evidence-Based Community Service

Irwin Sandler, Sharlene Wolchik, Cady Berkel, Sarah Jones, Anne Mauricio, Jenn-Yun Tein, & Emily Winslow

This chapter presents a case study of an effectiveness trial of the New Beginnings Program (NBP) for divorced families (developed and implemented in the United States [U.S.]), a program that has demonstrated efficacy to reduce mental health and substance abuse problems in two randomized experimental trials (Wolchik et al., 2002, 2013). The program has considerable implications for the public health in the United States because divorce impacts between 30 and 50 percent of U.S. children (National Center for Health Statistics, 2008) and is associated with multiple problem outcomes (Amato, 2001). The program may have significant benefits in other countries as well because the divorce rate in other developed countries is comparable to that of the United States (United Nations Statistical Division, 2012).

The perspective of this case study is that there are two major functions of effectiveness trials. One function is to demonstrate that a program has positive impact on defined outcomes for the intended population when it is delivered under natural service delivery conditions (Gottfredson et al., in press). This function is important for understanding the potential public health implications of preventive interventions. Much of the evidence on the effects of preventive interventions comes from efficacy trials that test programs under ideal, "hot house" conditions. Although a large number of efficacy studies have shown positive effects of preventive interventions (National Research Council/Institute of Medicine, 2009; Sandler, Schoenfelde, Wolchik, & MacKinnon, 2011), there is growing evidence that these programs may not have positive effects when delivered under real-world conditions (Eisner, Nagin, Ribaud, & Malti, 2012; Gottfreson et al., 2006).

The second function of an effectiveness trial is to serve as a bridge between the experimental prototype tested in the efficacy trial and a community service that can be widely disseminated. We conceptualize a community service to include the program being implemented; the procedures for recruiting participants to the program; the providers of the program; the methods to train, supervise, and maintain quality of program implementation; the funding stream that supports the program; and the setting in which it occurs. There are multiple conceptual frameworks to guide research on the translation of evidence-based experimental prototypes into community services (e.g., Aarons, Hurlburt, & Horwitz, 2011; Spoth et al., 2013). In this chapter, we describe the methods we employed to translate the NBP prototype into a community service, the design of a randomized effectiveness trial to evaluate the effects of the NBP community service, and some preliminary evidence on the population that we recruited and the fidelity of implementation. Finally, we discuss steps that were taken to plan for the sustainability of the NBP following the randomized trial. Before describing the translation of NBP into a community service and the effectiveness trial, we will briefly describe the NBP and the extensive evidence of its efficacy.

Establishing the Efficacy of a Theory-Based Program to Promote Resilience of Children from Divorced Families

The NBP has been evaluated in two randomized efficacy trials (Wolchik et al., 1993, 2000). The program has been extensively described elsewhere (Wolchik, Sandler, Weiss, & Winslow, 2007), so only a brief program description is provided here. The program is designed to change empirically supported risk and protective factors that are associated with child outcomes following divorce, primarily parental warmth (i.e., positive exchanges and active listening), effective discipline, and interparental conflict (Kelly, 2012). The program focuses on the parent acquiring and using effective skills to change each of these risk and protective factors. Sessions are highly structured and include both didactic and experiential components. Parents are assigned weekly practice of program skills with their children. In the efficacy trial, the NBP consisted of eleven weekly group sessions (1.75 hours each) and two individual, in-person sessions (one hour each) designed to tailor the program skills to the family's needs. Eight to ten mothers participated in each group. The steps involved in implementation of the NBP in the efficacy trial are presented in Table 5.1, including the recruitment method, eligibility criteria, and the methods of training and supervising group leaders.

Multiple eligibility criteria were used to ensure that families would be likely to participate fully in the program and assessments and that the effects of the NBP would not be confounded with other treatments. Intensive training and supervision were implemented to ensure high levels of fidelity. Because at the time of the study mothers were the primary residential parent following divorce (Parkinson, 2011) and a pilot study indicated that the dynamics of mixed-gender groups were problematic, the program was tested with mothers only. As shown in Table 5.2, the sample recruited through these methods was primarily White (non-Hispanic) and included only mothers with 50 percent or greater parenting time.

The NBP has been evaluated in two randomized experimental trials. The first randomized efficacy trial (N = 70) used a wait-list control design and involved mothers with children between ages eight and fifteen years. The second

Table 5.1 *Delivery of New Beginnings Program during Efficacy Trial and during Effectiveness Trial*

NBP Efficacy Trial	NBP Service Effectiveness Trial
New Beginnings Program • 11 sessions (1.75 hours each) • 2 individual in person sessions • Small groups 8-10 • 2 group leaders	**New Beginnings Program** • 10 sessions (1.75 hours each) • 2 individual telephone sessions • Small groups 8-10 • 1 group leader
Recruitment of parents • Identify eligible families in court records • Mail letter of invitation • Follow-up phone call • Home visit to explain program and study • Community referrals and media	**Recruitment of parents** • Invitational video shown to all parents in mandatory parent education program • Parents indicate interest • Contact interested parents by phone • Court and community referrals and media
Eligibility criteria • Divorce decree in past 2 years • Child age 9–12 • Reside with primary residential mother 50% of time or greater • Neither mother or any child currently in treatment for psychological problems • Mother not married or planned to marry during the trial; no live-in partner • Family resided within 1-hour drive of the program • Child not in a special education program for mentally challenged or learning disabled; if the child had a diagnosis of ADHD, he or she was taking medication • Mother and child could complete assessment measures in English	**Eligibility criteria** • Divorced, separated, or some relitigation of divorce in the prior 2 years • Nonmarried separating families included • Child age 3–18 • Contact with parent of 3 hours per week or 1 overnight every other week • Mother or father both invited • Parent and child could complete the assessment in English
Selection training and supervision of leaders • Leaders screened and selected by program developers • 30 hours of initial training • 1.5 hours training prior to every session • 1.5 hours per week supervision following every session • Training and supervision continue at same level throughout the trial	**Selection, training and supervision of leaders** • Leaders from community agencies selected through normal request for service solicitation • 30 hours of initial training • Weekly online training • Weekly 1.5 hours of combined weekly training and supervision • Training and supervision decrease following "outstanding delivery" to proactive consultation
Setting in which NBP delivered • University-based research center • Schools in the community	**Setting in which NBP delivered** • Agency facilities

Table 5.2 *Characteristics of the Sample in the Efficacy and Effectiveness Trial of New Beginnings*

NBP Efficacy Trial[1]	NBP Service Effectiveness Trial
Total sample 240 parents 240 children (one child per family)	**Total sample** 830 parents 1638 children (multiple children per family)
Gender of parent Mother = 240 (100%)	**Gender of parent** Mother = 474 (57.1%) Father = 356 (42.9%)
Parent ethnicity White (non-Hispanic) = 211 (87.9%) Hispanic = 18 (7.5%) Other = 11 (4.6%)	**Parent ethnicity** White (non-Hispanic) = 491 (59.2%) Hispanic = 261 (31.4%) Other = 78 (9.3%)
Parent education High school or less = 37 (15.4%) Some college or technical = 129 (53.7%) College graduate or above = 74 (30.8%)	**Parent education** High school or less = 161 (19.4%) Some college or technical = 423 (51%) College graduate or above = 246 (29.6%)
Age of children Mean = 10. 35 (range = 9–12).	**Age of children** Mean = 8.84 (range = 3–18)
Parent age $\leq$ 25 = 0 (0%) 26–35 = 96 (40%) 36–45 = 128 (53.3%) >46 = 16 (6.6%)	**Parent age** $\leq$25 = 50 (6%) 26–35 = 351 (42.2%) 36–45 = 322(38.7%) $\geq$46 = 139 (16.7%)

[1] The demographics describe the sample in the second and larger efficacy trial of the NBP.

randomized efficacy trial (N = 240) was designed to assess whether the positive program effects in the first trial could be replicated, whether the program effects persisted over time, and whether adding a child coping program led to greater benefits than the mother program alone. Because a prerequisite for the child coping groups was a narrow age range, the trial included only families with children between the ages of nine and twelve years. Families were randomly assigned to the mother-only program, the mother-plus-child program, or a literature control program. Mothers and children in the literature control program received three books on children's divorce adjustment. Analyses for both trials found positive effects of the NBP at posttest to reduce children's behavior problems and improve parenting (Wolchik et al., 1993, 2000) and that the benefits were greater for families with poorer pretest functioning.

The child program tested in the second trial did not lead to additive effects on child outcomes at posttest or at six-month follow-up. Thus, to provide a parsimonious view of the program effects assessed in the follow-ups, the mother program and mother-plus-child program were combined and compared to the literature control condition. At the six-year follow-up, 91 percent of the families were reinterviewed. As shown in Table 5.3, the NBP had positive effects on a wide range of problem outcomes, including reductions in child mental health problems, substance use, and the number of sexual partners (Wolchik et al., 2007). The NBP also increased multiple competencies of the children, including grade point average, active coping, coping efficacy, self-esteem, educational goals, and job aspirations (Sigal, Wolchik, Tein, & Sandler, 2012; Vélez, Wolchik, Tein, & Sandler, 2011). The breadth of these effects and the effects on outcomes that have important implications for concurrent and future functioning, such as grade point average and diagnosis of mental disorder, provide evidence of the clinical significance of the findings. Illustratively, the program led to a 37 percent reduction in the number of adolescents who met diagnostic criteria for a mental disorder (23.5 percent literature control, 14.8 percent NBP). For several effects, program benefits were greater for youth with higher risk at program entry, as assessed by an index comprised of baseline indicators of risk (Dawson-McClure, Sandler, Wolchik, & Millsap, 2004).

At the fifteen-year follow-up, data were collected from 89.6 percent of the families randomly assigned to condition. As shown in Table 5.3, the NBP had positive effects on a broad range of indices of child adjustment, including reductions in mental disorder, mental health service use, and criminal justice system involvement, and for males, reductions in substance use and substance abuse disorder (Herman, Mahrer, Wolchik, Jones, & Sandler, 2015; Wolchik et al., 2013). The findings indicate meaningful benefits of the NBP. For example, there was a 69 percent decrease in the incidence of developing an internalizing disorder (e.g., major depression) in the NBP versus literature control groups (24.4 percent literature control, 7.5 percent NBP) from mid-to-late adolescence to emerging adulthood assessed at the fifteen-year follow-up. Also, males in the NBP had fewer substance-related disorders between mid-to-late adolescence and emerging adulthood than those in the literature control condition. A positive cost-benefit was found in terms of savings of $1,077 (discounted over fifteen years) in the one-year period prior to the fifteen-year follow-up. Reductions in criminal justice system involvement and mental health service use by the emerging adults (who were age nine to twelve years when they entered the study) and their parent accounted for the cost savings (Herman et al., 2015). Mediation analyses tested factors that account for program long-term outcomes. These analyses showed that the program effects to strengthen parenting partially accounted for effects of the NBP to reduce problem outcomes (Tein, Sandler, MacKinnon & Wolchik, 2004; Zhou, Sandler, Millsap, Wolchik, & Dawson-McClure, 2008) and improve coping efficacy (Vélez et al., 2011) six years later. A developmental cascade model was supported in which the short-term program effects to strengthen parenting mediated reductions in externalizing and internalizing in childhood, which in turn accounted for the

Table 5.3 *Program Effects in the NBP Efficacy Trial*

Constructs	Posttest	6-year follow-up	15-year follow-up
Behavior problems			
Externalizing problems	Prog × baseline[1]	Prog × risk[2]	-
Internalizing problems	Prog main	Prog × risk[2]	-
Number of drug abuse or dependence diagnoses	na	-	Prog × gender[3]
Alcohol use	na	Prog x risk[2]	Prog × gender[4]
Polydrug use	na	Prog x risk2	Prog × gender[3]
Other drug use	na	Prog x risk2	Prog × gender[3]
Substance use problems	na	na	Prog × gender[3]
Number of sexual partners	na	Prog main	Not analyzed
Diagnosis of mental disorder		Prog main	Prog main
Days in jail last year	na	Na	Prog main
Mental health service use last year	na	na	Prog main
Health outcomes			
Cortisol reactivity	na	na	Prog × age[5]
Competencies			
Grades	na	Prog main	na
Coping efficacy	na	indirect	not analyzed
Active coping	ns	indirect	not analyzed
Self-esteem	ns	Prog × risk	not analyzed
Occupational aspirations	na	Prog × risk	na
Educational goals	na	Prog × risk	na
Work competence	na	na	Prog × risk[2]
Job success	na	na	Prog × risk[2]
Attitudes toward parenting-warmth	na	na	Prog × risk[2]
Attitudes toward parenting-harsh discipline	na	na	Prog × risk[2]

Note: ns = nonsignificant; na= not assessed.

[1] Prog × baseline = program by baseline interaction. Program benefits were greater for those who entered the program with higher levels of externalizing problems.

[2] Prog × risk = program × risk at program pretest. Risk index is a composite of child baseline problems, poor parenting, interparental conflict, parent mental health problems, and missed visits with nonresidential parent. All interactions showed program benefits were greater for those who entered the program at higher risk.

[3] Interactions indicated significant positive program effects for males.

[4] Interactions were significant for females but not for males. Females in the program had higher levels of use than those in the control condition.

[5] Older offspring in the control group had higher reactivity relative to the intervention group, and younger offspring in the control group exhibited a decline across the task relative to younger offspring in the intervention group.

program effects on substance use, mental disorder, grades, and self-esteem in adolescence (McClain et al., 2010).

The replication of the positive program effects and the finding that the NBP had lasting effects on a wide array of children's outcomes provided strong support for conducting an effectiveness trial to evaluate the program as a community service delivered under natural service delivery conditions. Because the child coping component did not have an additive effect, the effectiveness trial tested whether the parenting program alone would have positive benefits when delivered as a community service. The findings about which targeted risk and protective factors were changed and the results of the mediational analyses guided program revision. More specifically, mediation analyses indicated that parent–child relationship quality and effective discipline should be considered core components of the program. Because the program had no effects on program components designed to increase contact with the nonresidential parent and increase support from nonparental adults, we deleted these components. Although neither efficacy trial found changes on exposure to interparental conflict, we retained a focus on conflict as a core program component because of its significant impact on children's postdivorce outcomes and strengthened the program activities on conflict. In the next section, we discuss the other changes that we made to translate the experimental prototype of the NBP tested in the efficacy trials into a viable community service to be tested in the effectiveness trial.

Translating the NBP Prototype into a Community Service

Because we viewed the effectiveness trial as a bridge to a sustainable community service, we redesigned the program to address issues that had implications for later adoption and implementation as part of the process of translating the NBP from an experimental program to a service that would be tested in our randomized effectiveness trial. Based on conceptual models of dissemination of evidence-based programs (Spoth et al., 2013), this process addressed five key issues in translating the program into a community service: (1) identification of the collaborating organizations that would deliver the program, (2) study of the organizational preferences that might influence adoption of the program, (3) identification of the program design features that would enable high-quality implementation by community organizations, (4) redesign of the program delivery features to fit community organization needs, and (5) study of the factors that would influence ability of the program to recruit divorcing parents effectively. This systematic, iterative approach was implemented over six years.

Identification of the Organizational Homes for the NBP

The first and probably most significant step in translating an experimental prototype into a community service is to develop collaborative relationships with the organizations that would provide the service. We selected the domestic relations court as one of our collaborating organizations for three reasons. First, from a public health perspective, collaborating with the family court potentially provides access to the full population of legal divorces and separations. Second, in many jurisdictions, the court's mission has evolved from administering justice solely in an adversarial model to including nonadversarial dispute resolution services and parent education services (Kierstead, 2011; Salem, Sandler, & Wolchik, 2013; Singer, 2009). Third, we had a twenty-year history of working with the local court to conduct our research and were thus familiar with the culture of the court and the ways that the NBP might contribute to its mission and functioning (Sandler, Knox, & Braver, 2012). Because the NBP is much lengthier than the programs offered through the courts, we believed that it should be delivered by community-based organizations with experience delivering similar parenting programs and thus selected community-based family mental health and child service agencies as another collaborating organization. Court–community agency collaborations for the delivery of parent-education courses are quite common, and the administrative procedures for setting up such systems are well developed in many courts. We developed a three-way collaboration for the effectiveness trial in which the research team secured the funds to support the trial and provided training and support for all aspects of parent recruitment and program implementation, the court implemented the major method of recruiting parents into the program, and the community agencies delivered the NBP (see Figure 5.1). This collaborative interagency model of service delivery is distinct from the service delivery context in the efficacy trial where all functions were conducted at a university-based research center.

Marketing Study of Court Preferences

Because we wanted our effectiveness trial to evaluate a program that had a good chance of being widely disseminated through family courts, it was necessary to address basic market research questions about court needs, preferences, and practices prior to designing the NBP service. These questions include the following: What other parenting programs are currently being provided by the court? What changes are being considered for future services? What factors might encourage or hinder adoption of the program? A national survey of courts reported that parent-education courses were offered in forty-six U.S. states (Pollet & Lombreglia, 2008). The programs are typically short in duration (Braver, Salem, Pearson, & DeLuse, 1996), and there is considerable variability in their intended goals (e.g., information about children's divorce adjustment, conflict resolution skills). Although parent satisfaction with these programs is high, little is known about their actual impact on parent or child outcomes (Sigal, Sandler, Wolchik, & Braver, 2011). To assess the degree to which courts would be interested in adopting the NBP, which was much lengthier than their typical programs, we developed a stratified random sample of 154 courts that were currently offering a parent-education program and interviewed a key

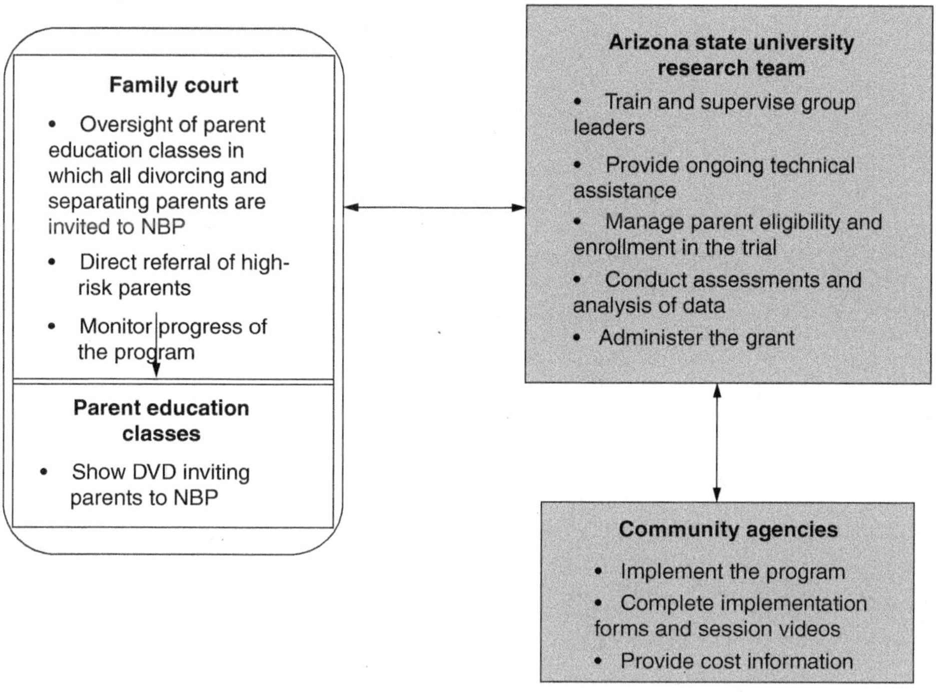

Figure 5.1. *Collaborative service delivery model for the New Beginnings Program.*

informant who was knowledgeable about the program in each court (Cookston, Braver, Sandler, & Genalo, 2002). Sixty-one percent of courts reported that they were considering changing their programs for parents in the next three years, with 19 percent reporting that they were considering a lengthier program; 75 percent reported that lengthy evidence-based parent-education programs should be offered and would be supported by key stakeholders. The two biggest barriers to adopting such programs were seen as funding and parent attendance. Consistent with theory on the dissemination of innovations (Rogers, 1995), the presence of stakeholder champions for the innovation was the strongest predictor of interest in adopting a lengthier program and finding funds to support it (Cookston, Braver, Griffin, De Luse, & Miles, 2007).

Identification of Program Design Features to Maximize Fit with Key Stakeholder Needs

A community service has to meet the needs of key stakeholders who will provide the service as well as its consumers. We modified design features of the NBP to maximize its fit with the needs of three stakeholder groups: family courts, community service providing agencies, and divorced parents. We used methods from quality function deployment (QFD; Akao & Mazur, 2003), an approach commonly used in business for developing new products, to guide the redesign of

NBP. QFD uses a set of tools to identify stakeholder needs, prioritize those needs, and use these priorities to develop goals for program design.

To assess the preferences of the courts, we developed a national court advisory board that consisted of three family court judges, four professionals with extensive experience in court-related conciliation services or court administration, and the executive director of the Association of Family and Conciliation Courts, a national interdisciplinary organization of court professionals (Smith-Daniels, Sandler, & Wolchik, 2008). Perceived needs were generated by the group using a set of "revealed preference" techniques in which participants responded to hypothetical scenarios (e.g., "You intend to respond to an RFP [request for proposal] that would fund a parent-education program. Two proposals ... are contenders and you must select one. ... What factors are likely to make you select one program over another?"). Participants identified sixty-five issues that might affect a court's decision to adopt the NBP. These issues were grouped into six needs and ordered in terms of how much they would affect adoption decisions using methods commonly applied in QFD (e.g., affinity diagrams). The highest priority need was program fit with court funding and resource investment, which included the need that the program fit with the court structure so that it was easy to implement, maintain, and monitor and did not put a burden on court resources. The second highest priority was perceived program efficacy, which included that the program could meet the needs of culturally diverse families, could be delivered to a large number of families, and had a broad base of support by professionals and citizens.

We used a similar process to assess the needs of agency providers of parenting programs. Three focus groups were conducted with providers who had experience running the NBP or other parenting groups. Participants were asked what they liked and disliked about the NBP "package" (i.e., leader manual, teaching aids [e.g., posters, handouts], training program, monitoring of implementation, and supervision) and then generated ideas about program features, materials, and formats that would improve the program. This process resulted in 241 "verbatims" (e.g., features, desires) that were categorized and prioritized by 27 other agency administrators and 27 other providers. The seven highest ranked needs were that the program should (1) fit with agency priorities, needs, and resources; (2) be held in a welcoming and comfortable environment; (3) utilize and respect providers' clinical skills; (4) make reasonable time demands on providers; (5) be appropriate for and accessible to a broad range of families; (6) involve parents and meet families' needs; and (7) use materials and delivery formats that are engaging, professional-looking, and easy to use.

Redesign of the NBP as a Community Service That Meets Court, Agency, and Program Developer Needs

The redesign of the NBP as a community service had to meet the program developers' needs to have the core program components delivered with fidelity and quality to the targeted population, and the needs of the two organizations who would host the NBP as a community service. The needs of the court and the community agencies and the design modifications that were developed to meet these needs are shown in Figure 5.2. The court need that the service fit with its resources was met by defining the court's role to include three activities; (1) recruitment of families through a DVD shown in the parent-education class, (2) judicial referral of parents in need of a parenting class (Kierstead, 2011), and (3) solicitation of provider agencies through a request-for-services procedure. Conducting the groups at the community agencies met the agency's need to use their welcoming facilities and the court's need not to provide the service.

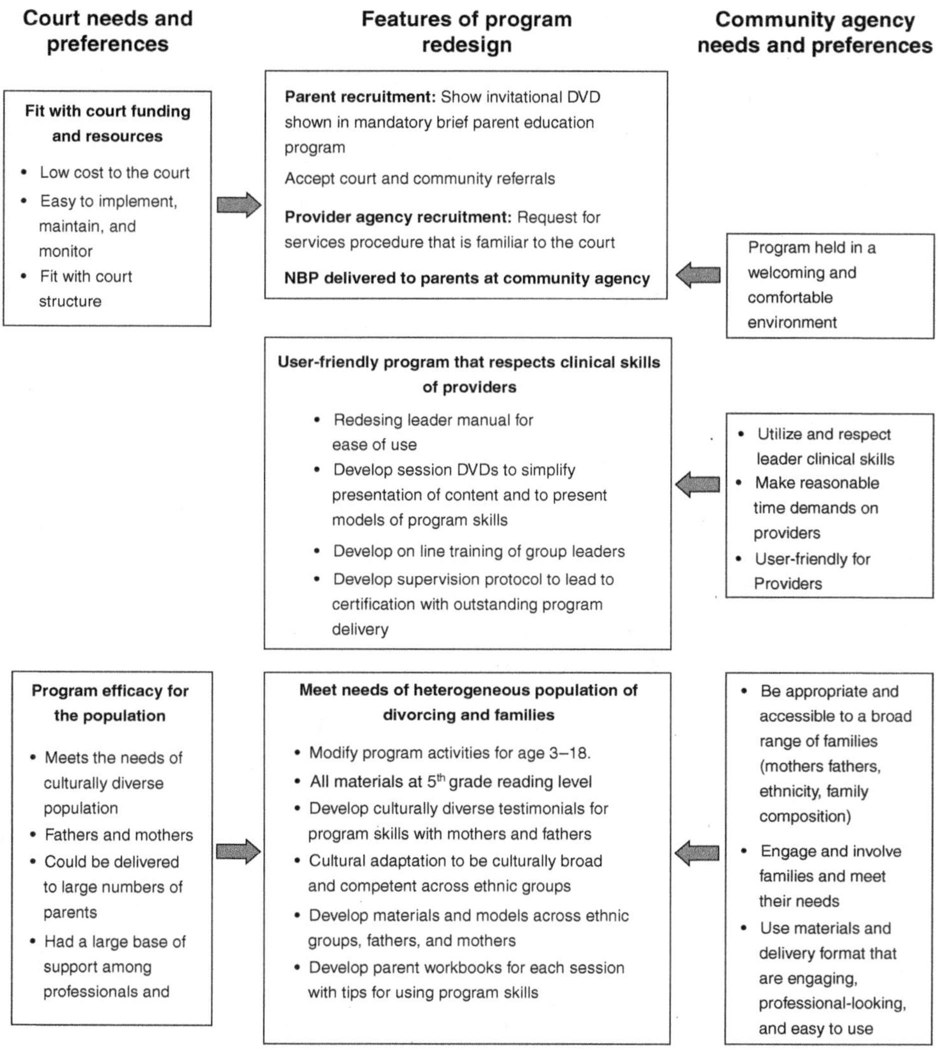

Figure 5.2. *Program redesign informed by needs and preferences of the court and community agencies.*

We made the following changes to meet agency needs. To increase user-friendliness, we redesigned the leader manual and developed an extensive training and supervision program, including online supervision using Skype for each program session. Supervision and training focused on mastery of program material and ways in which providers use their clinical skills to individualize parent use of program skills to meet the needs of their children. We developed DVDs of the major content points of each session (with twenty-five to thirty slides per session, including video modeling of program skills) in order to reduce leader burden and increase likelihood of high fidelity of program implementation. This design feature also enabled us to decrease cost by enabling delivery by one rather than two providers.

Extensive revisions were also made in the areas of training and supervision in order to reduce leader burden and decrease costs while maintaining high levels of fidelity and quality. Training was modified to consist of two phases. The initial phase was a four-day workshop that includes a detailed overview of the program, including roleplay of selected activities, presentation of the research on the NBP's effects, and an intensive focus on quality and fidelity of delivery of the program. At the completion of the workshop, leaders take a quiz to assess their mastery of the program content. The second phase of training occurs during their first delivery of the program. Prior to delivering each session, leaders review the program manual and observe an online training video that reviews the session and provides models of good program delivery. Leaders then participate in a one-and-a-half-hour small-group supervision using Skype that consists of a brief overview of the upcoming session and discussion of issues that arose in the prior session. Prior to supervision, the supervisor views a section of a video of the prior session and provides feedback on strengths of delivery and delivery issues that require additional work. At the end of a leader's first program delivery, the supervisor, in consultation with the program developers, assesses the leader's level of competence as outstanding, satisfactory, or unacceptable. The level of supervision following this initial training depends on the level of competence and may include periodic proactive consultation once the leader has achieved outstanding provider status and is certified.

We modified several design features to make the program sensitive to the preferences and needs of the population of divorced families served by the court who are heterogeneous in the ethnicity, gender, and educational level of the parent and the age of children. First, we modified the program activities to ensure that they were appropriate for a broad age range of children, three to eighteen years old, providing tips to parents and training for leaders on age-appropriate use of the skills. We decided on the lower age bound of three because of the heavy focus on listening skills. We evaluated these adaptations in a clinical pilot that included parents' response to questions about the developmental appropriateness of the program activities. Second, to ensure that reading comprehension would not be a barrier to learning the program skills, we modified all program materials (e.g., handouts, slides) to be at a fifth-grade reading level. Two fifth-grade teachers suggested replacements for words above a fifth-grade reading level, and one of the program developers assessed whether these changes altered the intended meaning of the information. Third, we developed a program for fathers. We chose to offer separate programs for mothers and fathers rather than mixed-gender groups on the basis of pilot tests and our judgment that parents would be more able to focus on improving their parenting skills in same-gender groups. The mother and father programs are identical in the skills they teach based on research indicating that the same aspects of parenting quality by both mothers and fathers are predictive of outcomes for children following divorce (Sandler et al., 2012). However, separate gender-specific program materials (e.g., modeling videos, father testimonials) are provided for mothers and fathers. To maximize the degree to which the program engages parents, we developed parent workbooks that provide tips for using each program skill. We also developed testimonials from prior participants attesting to the value of each program skill and identifying strategies to overcome barriers to using the program skills.

One of the most extensive revisions involved changes to ensure that the program would be competent for delivery across ethnic groups. In making these adaptations, we focused on three major ethnic groups in the United States: African Americans (AA), Latino Americans (LA), and Asian Pacific Americans (APA). We realized that additional cross-cultural adaptations may be necessary for international applications of this program. As the largest Latino subgroup, Mexican Americans (MA) were selected to circumvent problems associated with assuming that various Latino subgroups are equivalent. We elicited insider points of view from several groups of cultural informants to guide our revisions (i.e., prevention scientists with experience in adapting prevention programs for MA, AA, and APA families; providers who worked with ethnic minority families; and ethnic minority parents who participated in the NBP). Five prevention scientists and eight providers reviewed each session, assessing whether the language was familiar, easily understood, and comfortable for MA, AA, and APA families; whether the values in the program (e.g., concepts, program goals) and methods (e.g., roleplays, home practice) were compatible with the values, customs, beliefs, and traditions of each cultural group; and whether the program goals, activities, and skills took into account the social and economic contexts in which families live (e.g., financial strain, family size). Although this procedure resulted in numerous suggestions for "surface structure" changes, such as using people and language familiar to the group, the scientists and providers consistently noted that with some revision, the NBP would fit well with the needs, values, and preferences of AA and MA parents. Examples of adaptations that were made include offering rationales and explanations of program skills that were compatible with goals and values of ethnic minority parents; acknowledging potential cultural barriers to program skills and recommendations, such as the recommendation against spanking (which might be incompatible with some AA and MA parents' views about physical discipline); and providing more opportunities for parents to consider ways to make program skills more compatible with their own cultural style.

After making the recommended surface structure adaptations, we conducted six NBP groups that consisted mostly or exclusively of ethnic minority mothers (two groups for each of the three ethnic groups). Multiple methods (e.g., weekly feedback forms, surveys at program completion, focus groups) were used to collect data on the NBP's cultural appropriateness from mothers and group leaders. The data indicated that the overall themes and core components of the NBP were generally consistent with the values and preferences of MA, AA, and APA families, and that the program seemed acceptable to and engaging for these parents. Like the other types of cultural informants, mothers and group leaders suggested changes in rationales and examples used to teach skills rather than changes in the skills. Although we were able to make adaptations to address the concerns raised by our AA and MA cultural informants, we were not able to address all the concerns raised by APA cultural informants without substantially changing some core skills. To address this concern, one member of our team developed a culturally tailored version of the NBP for low-acculturated APA families, which she plans to evaluate in an efficacy trial.

Design of a System for Parent Recruitment and Engagement

An effective and efficient method of recruiting participants is an important component of a community service. Both our U.S. national survey of courts and QFD assessment of court needs indicated that reaching large numbers of parents was a high court priority. Other evidence-based parenting programs have been plagued by low participation rates when programs are offered under real-world conditions (i.e., typically only 1 to 17 percent of parents participate) (Fagan, Hanson, Hawkins, & Arthur, 2009; Matthey, Patterson, Mutton, & Kreutzfeldt, 2006; Spoth, Clair, Greenberg, Redmond, & Shin, 2007). Difficulties in engaging parents occur at multiple points: (1) most parents choose not to enroll in preventive parenting programs offered to them (e.g., Heinrichs, Bertram, Kuschel, & Hahlweg, 2005; Matthey et al., 2006); (2) many parents who enroll never attend a session (e.g., Garvey, Julion, Fogg, Kratovil, & Gross, 2006); and (3) half or more of parents who begin a parenting program do not complete it or attend irregularly (Heinrichs et al., 2005).

We developed a parent recruitment method for the effectiveness trial that involved showing a video to invite parents to the NBP in the brief parenting classes that are mandated for divorcing parents. This method has the advantage of reaching nearly all the target population inexpensively through a mechanism that is common in many family court systems, mandated parent information classes (Pollet & Lombreglia, 2008). We developed parent recruitment material based on social psychological principles of influence because many studies have shown that these principles are powerful motivators of compliance with requests to engage in specific behaviors (Cialdini, 2009). The principles targeted were: (1) reciprocation – desire to repay benefits and services one has received; (2) scarcity – perception that rare opportunities are more valuable than plentiful ones; (3) legitimate authority – trust in recommendations from sources perceived as credible; (4) social validation – tendency to mimic the behavior of similar others; (5) liking – inclination to concur with those we like; and (6) commitment/consistency – propensity to behave in ways that are consistent with our goals and commitments.

Prior to the NBP effectiveness trial, we conducted a randomized controlled trial with 1,123 attendees of a brief court-mandated parenting class to compare three versions of this video. The version of the video that was most effective for the overall sample incorporated techniques from five of the six principles of influence (all but commitment/consistency). Relative to an informational video, this video increased the percentage of parents who initially expressed an interest in attending (39 percent vs. 29 percent), the percentage of parents who signed up to attend (24 percent vs. 13 percent), and the actual initial attendance rate (15 percent vs. 7 percent) (Winslow et al., 2015). The rate of attendance in this condition was toward the upper end of rates found in large-scale effectiveness trials (Spoth et al., 2007). Although the motivational video provides a promising method for recruiting parents, the large gap between the percentage of parents who initially expressed interest in attending (39 percent) and those who attended at least one session (15 percent) prompted us to test a method to reduce this gap in the effectiveness trial, which we describe in the following section.

Effectiveness Trial: Testing the New Beginnings Program as a Collaborative Community Service

In this section, we discuss how the effectiveness trial of the NBP addresses the Society for Prevention Research (SPR) standards for establishing the effectiveness of a prevention program,[1] including testing the generalizability of program effects across variability in the population to whom it is delivered and variability in implementation of the program; describing the settings in which the program was implemented; and identifying the outcomes that are affected and the time frame within which effects occur (Gottfredson et al., in press). Consistent with our perspective on the role of effectiveness trials, we also discuss how information obtained by the trial will inform later approaches to sustain the program as a community service. At this time, we have completed the delivery phase and are now collecting the last cohort of follow-up data. Therefore, we only present descriptive information on program delivery and describe and discuss the specific aims of the trial.

1 www.preventionresearch.org/wp-content/uploads/2011/12/Standards-of-Evidence_2015.pdf.

Design of the Randomized Trial

The study was implemented as a two-arm randomized control trial with assessment at pretest, posttest and ten-month follow-up. Parents were recruited to be in the trial by the invitational video that was shown in the parent education class, referral from the courts, and self-referral from parents who learned about it through the media. Eligibility criteria were greatly reduced from the efficacy trials and included only having a child between three and eighteen years old; having contact with child at least three hours per week or an overnight visit every other week; and being separated or divorced or be relitigating the divorce agreement within the past two years. Recruitment occurred across four cohorts between 2012 and 2014. Eligible parents who consented to participate in the trial were randomly assigned to either a two-session version of the NBP or a ten-session NBP after the pretest. The two-session version consisted of didactic presentations and discussion of the skills that are taught in the ten-session program but did not involve skill modeling or practice. Both versions were implemented in groups of up to ten parents, with separate mother and father groups. Randomization was conducted separately by parent gender. If both parents participated, the parent who was recruited second was assigned to the same experimental condition as the first parent. At pretest, posttest, and ten-month follow-up, the participating parent and children age nine to eighteen were interviewed by phone and the teachers of all children in school were sent a questionnaire. Parent report data were collected on all children in the family between the ages of three and eighteen.

The final sample included 830 parents (two-session version: N = 385 families, 705 children; ten-session version: N = 445 families, 822 children) with 1,527 children. As shown in Table 5.2, we were successful in recruiting a sample that was heterogeneous on ethnicity, gender of parent, and age range of children. Furthermore, sufficiently large samples were recruited to provide adequate power to assess program effects within subgroups of fathers and Mexican Americans and across ages of children.

Collaborations with the Courts and Community Agencies to Deliver the NBP

Family courts in four counties in Arizona (United States) participated in the effectiveness trial. The presiding judges in these courts agreed to have the brief (twelve-minute) video shown in their mandated brief parent-education programs in order to invite parents into the trial. Community agencies were recruited to provide the NBP using the normal process by which the courts solicit the provision of other family services, a competitive request for services process. Selection of applicants was conducted jointly to ensure that the agencies had the capacity to deliver the program, as determined by the research team, and were positively viewed by the court. Two courts initially volunteered to participate in the trial, but dropped out before the trial began due to a change in priorities following a change in leadership and difficulty in obtaining a community agency to deliver the NBP.

Specific Aim 1: Test whether the NBP has positive effects when delivered through a collaboration of the family court and community agencies. This specific aim tests whether the adapted NBP delivered as a community service achieves similar outcomes as those in the efficacy trial. We will compare the two-session and ten-session versions on the targeted proximal outcomes of parenting and children's exposure to interparental conflict and effects on child mental health problems using valid and reliable parent, youth, and teacher report measures comparable to those used in our prior efficacy trials. We will also test whether program effects on youth outcomes at the ten-month follow-up are mediated by program-induced effects on positive parenting or by exposure to interparental conflict at posttest, thus testing the theoretical model on which the program is based. These analyses are currently in progress and will be written in 2016.

Specific Aim 2: Test moderation of program effects. We will test whether program effects differ across four potential moderators: the gender and ethnicity of the parent, the child's level of risk at program entry, and the child's age. Although research has consistently shown that the quality of parenting by nonresidential fathers is related to children's outcomes after divorce (e.g., Sandler et al., 2012), there is very limited evidence of the effectiveness of parenting programs for divorced fathers (for an exception, see Cookston et al., 2007). Also, despite the recent increase in the Hispanic population in the United States (an increase of 58 percent since 1990–2000) and data showing that divorce is an important risk factor for Hispanic children (e.g., Umana-Taylor & Alfaro, 2006), evaluations of prevention programs for divorced families have not assessed their effects on Hispanic youth. We focus on Hispanics because we could recruit a sufficient number of Hispanic families in Arizona to have adequate power to test program effects on this subpopulation. We focus on age as a moderator because there is a much broader age distribution in this trial versus the efficacy trials. Because of the modifications we made to the NBP and the finding that other parenting programs have been effective for both mothers and fathers (e.g., Lundahl, Tollefson, Risser, & Lovejoy, 2008) and across ethnicity (Barrera et al., 2002) and youth age (e.g., Taylor & Biglan, 1998), we are not predicting differences in program effects across these demographic subgroups. However, on the basis of our findings in the efficacy trials that those who were at higher risk benefited most from the NBP (Tein et al., 2004; Dawson-McClure et al., 2004), we are predicting subgroup differences on the basis of children's level of risk at baseline. Replication of this finding in the effectiveness trial would suggest that reaching high-risk families would be an important part of delivery of the NBP as a community service.

Specific Aim 3: Examine whether variability in implementation accounts for variability in parenting and youth outcomes. We conceptualized four dimensions of implementation (Berkel, Mauricio, Schoenfelder, & Sandler, 2011), each of which has been found to be associated with better program outcomes

(Durlak & DuPre, 2008). Three of these dimensions refer to behaviors of the provider: fidelity (i.e., number of the activities in the program manual that are covered by the provider); quality of program delivery (i.e., quality of the provider's teaching and support in using program skills); and additive adaptation (i.e., the provider's positive additions to program content or methods). The fourth dimension refers to participant responsiveness (i.e., attendance, active engagement in the program, completion of home practice). We developed multiple measures of each dimension based on the reports of group leaders, supervisors, and parents. These data were entered on a web-based system of program monitoring, and videos of each session were uploaded to a secure website to be coded by objective raters. In the following, we briefly elaborate on the assessment of these dimensions and provide some preliminary data on fidelity of implementation.

Fidelity was evaluated using items that assessed adherence to the leader manual. The manual includes directions for what is to be said and done (i.e., content) and specific process components. For example, at many points in the manual, leaders are instructed to validate and normalize participants' experiences to ensure they know they are not alone in the postdivorce struggles they face. The program manual includes an average of 7.8 activities per session, with an average of 20 directions per activity. As a preliminary assessment of fidelity, objective raters coded one activity per session that was selected to represent different program structures (i.e. didactic presentations, roleplay of skills, etc.). Activities were coded to assess leader performance of each direction in the manual. For 45 percent of the activities, the leaders implemented most or all directions (70–100 percent); for 48.8 percent of the activities, leaders implemented some to most of the directions (40–69 percent); and for 5.8 percent of the activities, the leaders implemented few or none of the directions. The quality measure was tailored to fit the theoretical model of the NBP. It includes three subscales: Positive Engagement, which assesses the degree to which there is a positive relationship between the leader and parents; Skillful Presentation, which addresses the degree to which the provider presents the didactic material in a clear, enthusiastic, and natural way; and Skillful Feedback, which assesses skill in providing positive and constructive feedback on participants' use of program skills during the roleplay and home practice review components of each session.

Adaptation is a complex construct because it is by nature unknown before it happens. For this reason, we asked group leaders and supervisors to decide whether any content or processes had been added to the activity and describe these additions. We are currently developing in-depth schemes for observers to code the adaptations based on the work of Hansen and Dusenbury (2011). This coding system will assess whether an adaptation was an addition to content (i.e., adding nonprescribed information, such as legal advice) or methods (i.e., adding nonprescribed presentation strategies, such as letting a discussion evolve into advice giving) and also estimate the magnitude and expected positive or negative direction of the adaptation.

Participant responsiveness has been measured in many different ways, including retention, active engagement in sessions, satisfaction, perceived supportiveness of the group, and use of skills in participants' daily lives (Dane & Schneider, 1998). Parents' use of program skills with their families is of primary theoretical importance in the NBP, as stated many times in the manual, *Home Practice Is the Program*. We created a multimeasure, multiinformant (i.e., parents, providers) measure of home practice (Schoenfelder et al., 2012). Parent reports are collected via weekly home practice worksheets that indicate whether they attempted the assigned skill, whether each component of the skill was implemented, and how successfully the skills were implemented (efficacy). Providers rate the parents' competence with the skill based on the worksheet and the "Home Practice Review" activity of the session. At the posttest, parents report on their satisfaction with and use of each program skill.

The comprehensive assessment of implementation will allow us to probe several questions with important implications for delivering the NBP as a community service. What is the level of implementation of the program when delivered as a community service? Does implementation differ across characteristics of participants (e.g., ethnicity, gender) or characteristics of providers (e.g., attitudes toward manualized programs)? Another critical question is whether there are particular activities (e.g., didactic, roleplay) that are most influential in predicting program effects and what are the most efficient methods of sampling these activities. Addressing these questions will provide a knowledge base to monitor implementation of the NBP when delivered as a community service and to support continual program improvement methods.

Specific Aim 4: Test whether an experimental engagement interview increases parental engagement in the NBP. The findings from our research on the DVD invitation to parents led us to examine whether we could develop an engagement strategy that would reduce the drop-off between initial interest and attendance, a phenomenon that is widely observed in health promotion research (e.g., Webb & Sheeran, 2006). We based our strategy on Winslow and colleagues' (2015) theory-based, motivational engagement call. This engagement call was made by program providers who prompted parents to identify their child-focused goals and showed how the parenting program could help with these goals. The engagement call also helped parents identify and problem-solve barriers to attendance. In a predominantly low-income MA sample of parents with elementary school children, a package of strategies that included this engagement call nearly doubled the initial attendance rate compared to a brochure plus attention-control condition (48 percent vs. 25 percent) (Winslow et al., 2015). In the effectiveness trial, we are using a "trial within a trial" design (Braver & Smith, 1996), in which we randomly assigned NBP providers to conduct either the experimental engagement call or a general relationship-building introductory call one or two weeks prior to the first session. We hypothesized that the experimental engagement call would reduce the gap between initial interest and attendance compared to the relationship-building call.

Cost analysis of providing the NBP. Cost analysis of prevention programs is an important aspect of testing the effectiveness of a preventive intervention (Gottfredson et al., in press) because it has clear implications for how well it can be sustained as a community service, and because it provides the foundation for cost effectiveness and benefit-cost analysis (Crowley, Hill, Kuklinshi, & Jones, 2014), which are particularly relevant to policy makers. In the effectiveness trial, we are assessing costs of delivering the NBP from an agency perspective using invoices from service providers. Data were collected on the upfront and ongoing costs to train, supervise, and deliver the NBP in the six community agencies that participated in the trial. Staff time excluded research-specific activities (e.g., data collection), focusing instead on those activities required to implement the NBP in a community setting in real-world conditions. Costs include expenses to train and supervise the providers, leader time to deliver the program, materials for leaders and participants, administrative overhead, space and equipment, and support staff required by agencies to deliver the program (e.g. child care staff, site coordinator).

After the trial: Exploratory steps toward a sustainable service. To help create a bridge from the effectiveness trial to a community-based sustainable service, we held a feedback meeting with our collaborators from the four participating courts and six community agencies. Eighteen collaborators attended the full-day meeting, including current and former presiding judges and court and agency administrators. The discussion focused on three questions: (1) what was the collaborators' experience of the effectiveness trial and their role in it; (2) what could be done to promote the NBP as a sustained service in their communities; and (3) what role could our team play in helping sustain NBP in their communities. Comments from the meeting were transcribed, grouped, and arranged into a hierarchy of the most salient factors for the court and agency collaborators.

For both the court and agency collaborators, a theme of the potential benefits of the NBP to their organization and the people they serve emerged. Court representatives perceived the NBP as a tool to help them meet the goal of promoting positive outcomes for children, particularly for those in families that have a serious need for strengthened parenting (Singer, 2009; Kierstead, 2011). They highlighted the evidenced-based approach of the NBP for promoting positive outcomes for children as an important justification for supporting their mission to help families in need and disseminating useful information to the divorcing public. It was clear that the court interest in adopting the program would be very high if evidence emerged that the NBP helped with efficiency of court proceedings by reducing relitigation or noncompliance with court orders. Whether there are program effects on these outcomes will be tested in the effectiveness trial. The agency collaborators focused on the benefits to their agencies of delivering the NBP. Like the court representatives, the agency representatives highlighted the evidenced that the NBP promotes positive outcomes for children as an important program characteristic supporting their mission.

Logistical issues in delivering the NBP were a second theme that emerged for both the court and agency representatives. There was consensus among the court representatives that the NBP would need to delivered through a partnership with community agencies rather than through the court. Key issues for the agencies included the costs to implement the NBP; both fiscal and personnel time demands; and logistical issues related to space, child care needs, and security. Representatives also focused on the logistical issues for parents in participating in the NBP. Coordination between the courts and the community agencies would be important in establishing services in order to deal with issues such as accessibility and timing of the program relative to the timing of divorce proceedings.

A third theme that emerged in the discussion among the agency representatives centered on strategies for sustaining the NBP. This discussion included topics such as coordinating efforts across agencies and state agencies to access funds and ways to market the NBP program to attract a broader range of parents and funders. At the end of the meeting, we offered our assistance to collaborators interested in seeking funds to continue the program after the trial. In a very hopeful sign for sustainability of the NBP, one of the courts, Maricopa Superior Court, found funding to continue the program following the trial in a continuing partnership with the community agency trained during the trial. It is notable that this continued implementation of the NBP primarily involves the court mandating that parents it perceived as high risk participate in the program

Summary

This chapter described a case study of the development of an effectiveness trial of the NBP, a U.S.-based program with extensive evidence of positive long-term benefits for children from divorcing families. We describe the systematic, iterative steps in the process of adapting an experimental prototype of the program, which was tested in two efficacy trials, into a community service. These steps involved identifying collaborating organizations to deliver the program, studying organizational preferences that might influence adoption of the program, identifying program design features that would enable high-quality implementation, adapting aspects of the program to meet the needs of the diverse population of divorcing families, modifying delivery features to ensure that the program could be delivered with high quality and fidelity by community providers and that it fit community organization needs that were consistent with theory of the intervention, and designing an effective mechanism for recruiting divorcing parents. An effectiveness trial to test the impact of the NBP is described and initial evidence of sustainable ability following the trial is presented. Although the process of adaptation and testing effectiveness is lengthy, we see it as part of an ongoing process of program adaptation and improvement to meet the needs of an ever-changing population and the community organizations that serve them. We see program adaptation to fit with the needs of organizations that deliver prevention programs as an important step in the dissemination of evidence-based prevention programs. Although the NBP was developed and tested in the United States, it can be considered a promising prevention approach internationally because of the high rate of divorce in many countries and because similar parenting programs that target different populations have been found to have positive impacts both in developed countries (Sandler et al., 2011) and in low- and middle-income countries (Knerr, Gardner, & Cluver, 2013).

References

Aarons, G. A., Hurlburt, M., & Horwitz, S. M. (2011). Advancing a conceptual model of evidence-based practice implementation in public service sectors. *Administrative Policy Mental Health* 38: 4–23. doi: 10.1007/s10488-010–0327-7

Akao, Y., & Mazur, G. H. (2003). The leading edge in QFD: Past, present and future. *International Journal of Quality and Reliability Management* 20 :20–35.

Amato, P. R. (2001). Children of divorce in the 1990s: an update of the Amato and Keith (1991) meta-analysis. *Journal of Family Psychology* 15: 355–70. doi: 10.1037/0893–3200.15.3.355

Barrera, M., Jr., Biglan, A., Taylor, T. K., Gunn, B. K., Smolkowski, K., Black, C., Ary, D. V., & Fowler, R. C. (2002). Early elementary school intervention to reduce conduct problems: a randomized trial with Hispanic and non-Hispanic children. *Prevention Science* 3(2): 83–94.

Berkel, C., Mauricio, A. M., Schoenfelder, E., & Sandler, I. N. (2011). Putting the pieces together: an integrated model of program implementation. *Prevention Science* 12(1): 23–33.

Braver, S., Salem, P., Pearson, J., & DeLuse, S. (1996). The content of divorce education programs: results of a survey. *Family and Conciliation Court Review* 34: 41–59.

Braver, S. L., & Smith, M. C. (1996). Maximizing both external and internal validity in longitudinal true experiments with voluntary treatments: the "combined modified" design. *Evaluation and Program Planning* 19: 287–300. doi: 10.1016/S0149-7189(96)00029–8

Cialdini, R. B. (2009). *Influence: Science and Practice*. New York: Pearson Education.

Cookston, J. T., Braver, S. L., Griffin, W. A., De Luse, S. R., & Miles, J. C. (2007). Effects of the Dads for Life Intervention on interparental conflict and coparenting in the two years after divorce. *Family Process* 46: 123–37. doi: 10.1111/j.1545–5300.2006.00196.x

Cookston, J. T., Braver, S. L., Sandler, I. N., & Genalo, M.T. (2002). Prospects for expanded court-based services for children of divorce. *Family Court Review* 40: 190–203.

Crowley, M., Hill, L., Kuklinski, M., & Jones, D. (2014) Research priorities for economic analyses of prevention: current issues and future directions. *Prevention Science* 15: 789–98. doi: 10.1007/s11121-013–0429-z

Dane, A. V., & Schneider, B. H. (1998). Program integrity in primary and early secondary prevention: are implementation effects out of control? *Clinical Psychology Review* 18(1): 23–45.

Dawson-McClure, S. R., Sandler, I. N., Wolchik, S. A., & Millsap, R. E. (2004). Risk as a moderator of the effects of prevention programs for children from divorced families: a six-year longitudinal study. *Journal of Abnormal Child Psychology* 32: 175–90.

Durlak, J., & DuPre, E. (2008). Implementation matters: a review of research on the influence of implementation on program outcomes and the factors affecting implementation. *American Journal of Community Psychology* 41(3–4): 327–50.

Eisner, M., Nagin, D., Ribeaud, D., & Malti, T. (2012). Effects of a universal parenting program for highly adherent parents: a propensity score matching approach. *Prevention Science* 13: 252–66. doi: 10.1007/sr11121-011–0266-x

Fagan, A., Hanson, K., Hawkins, J. D., & Arthur, M. (2009). Translational research in action: implementation of the communities that care prevention system in 12 communities. *Journal of Community Psychology* 37(7): 809–29. doi: 10.1002/jcop.20332

Garvey, C., Julion, W., Fogg, L., Kratovil, A., & Gross, D. (2006). Measuring participation in a prevention trial with parents of young children. *Research in Nursing & Health* 29(3): 212–22. doi: 10.1002/nur.20127

Gottfredson, D. C., Cook, T. D., Gardner, F. E. M., Gorman-Smith, D., Howe, G. W., Sandler, I. N., & Zafft, K. M. (in press). Standards of evidence for efficacy, effectiveness, and scale-up research in prevention science: new generation. *Prevention Science*. doi: 10.1007/s11121-015–0555-x

Gottfredson, D. C., Kumpfer, K., Polizzi-Fox, D., Wilson, D., Puryear, V., Beatty, P., & Vilmenay, M. (2006). The Strengthening Washington D.C. Families Project: a randomized effectiveness trial of family-based prevention. *Prevention Science* 7: 57–76.

Hansen, W. B., & Dusenbury, L. (2011). *User's Manual Evaluation Lizard Assessments of Quality of Delivery: A Manual for Observers*. Greensboro, NC: Tanglewood Research.

Heinrichs, N., Bertram, H., Kuschel, A., & Hahlweg, K. (2005). Parent recruitment and retention in a universal prevention program for child behavior and emotional problems: barriers to research and program participation. *Prevention Science* 6(4): 275–86. doi: 10.1007/s11121-005-0006-1

Herman, P. M., Mahrer, N. E., Wolchik, S. A., Jones, S., & Sandler, I. N. (2015). Cost-benefit analysis of a preventive intervention for divorced families: reduction in mental health and justice system service use costs 15 years later. *Prevention Science* 16: 586–96.

Kelly, J. B. (2012). Risk and protective factors associated with child and adolescent adjustment following separation and divorce: social science applications. In Kuehnle, K., & Drozd, L. (eds.), *Parenting Plan Evaluations: Applied Research for the Family Court*. New York: Oxford University Press, pp. 49–85.

Kierstead, S. (2011). Parent education programs in family courts: balancing autonomy and state intervention. *Family Court Review* 49: 140–54. doi: 10/1111/j.1744-1617.2010.01358.x

Knerr, W., Gardner, F., & Cluver, L. (2013). Improving positive parenting skills and reducing harsh and abusive parenting in low- and middle-income countries: a systematic review. *Prevention Science* 14: 352–63. doi: 10.1007/s11121-o12-0314-1

Lundahl, B. W., Tollefson, D., Risser, H., & Lovejoy, M. C. (2008). A meta-analysis of father involvement in parent training. *Research on Social Work Practice* 18: 97–106. doi: 10.1177/104973157309828

Matthey, S., Patterson, P., Mutton, N., & Kreutzfeldt, K. (2006). Enrolment rates into parenting programs using a clinically viable recruitment strategy. *International Journal of Mental Health Promotion* 8(3): 6–14. doi: 10.1080/14623730.2006.9721740

McClain, D. B., Wolchik, S. A., Winslow, E., Tein, J. Y., Sandler, I. N., & Millsap, R. E. (2010). Developmental cascade effects of the New Beginnings Program on adolescent adaptation outcomes. *Development and Psychopathology* 22: 771–84. doi: 10.1017/S0954475941000453

National Center for Health Statistics (2008). Marriage and divorce. Retrieved from www.cdc.gov/nchs/fastats/divorce.htm.

National Research Council and Institute of Medicine (2009). *Preventing Mental, Emotional, and Behavioral Disorders among Young People: Progress and Possibilities*. Committee on the Prevention of Mental Disorders and Substance Abuse among Children, Youth, and Young Adults: Research Advances and Promising Interventions. O'Connell, M. E., Boat, T., & Warner, K. E. (eds.). Washington DC: National Academy Press.

Parkinson, S. (2011). *Family Law and the Indissolubility of Parenthood*. New York: Cambridge University Press.

Pollet, S. L., & Lombregila, M. (2008). A nationwide survey of mandatory parent education. *Family Court Review* 46: 375–94. doi: 10.1111/j.1744-1617.2008.00207.x

Rogers, E. M. (1995). *Diffusion of Innovations*. New York: Free Press.

Salem, P., Sandler, I., & Wolchik, S. (2013). Taking stock of parent education in the family courts: envisioning a public health approach. *Family Court Review* 51: 131–48. doi: 10.1111/fcre.12014

Sandler, I., Knox, P., & Braver, S. L. (2012). Collaboration of prevention science and the family court. *Administration and Policy in Mental Health and Mental Health Services Research* 29: 291–300.

Sandler, I., Schoenfelder, E., Wolchik, S. A., & MacKinnon, D. P. (2011). Long-term impact of prevention programs to promote effective parenting: lasting effects but uncertain processes. *Annual Review of Psychology* 62: 299–329.

Sandler, I., Wolchik, S., Winslow, E., Mahrer, N., Moran, J., & Weinstock, D. (2012). Quality of maternal and paternal parenting following separation and divorce. In Kuehnle, K., & Drozd, L. (eds.), *Parenting Plan Evaluations: Applied Research for the Family Court*. New York: Oxford University Press, pp. 85–123.

Schoenfelder, E., Sandler, I. N., Millsap, R. E., Wolchik, S. A., Berkel, C., & Ayers, T. S. (2012). Responsiveness to the Family Bereavement Program: What predicts responsiveness? What does responsiveness predict? *Prevention Science* 14(6): 545–56.

Sigal, A., Sandler, I. N., Wolchik, S. A., & Braver, S. L. (2011). Do parent education programs promote healthy post-divorce parenting? Critical distinctions and a review of the evidence. *Family Court Review* 49: 120–39.

Sigal, A. B., Wolchik, S. A., Tein, J. Y., & Sandler, I. N. (2012). Enhancing youth outcomes following parental divorce: a longitudinal study of the effects of the New Beginnings Program on educational and occupational goals. *Journal of Clinical Child and Adolescent Psychology* 41: 150–65.

Singer, J. B. (2009). Dispute resolution and the postdivorce family: implications of a paradigm shift. *Family Court Review* 47: 363–71.

Smith-Daniels, V., Sandler, I., & Wolchik, S. A. (2008). Use of quality management methods in the transition from efficacious prevention programs to effective prevention services. *American Journal of Community Psychology* 41: 250–61.

Spoth, R., Clair, S., Greenberg, M., Redmond, C., & Shin, C. (2007). Toward dissemination of evidence-based family interventions: maintenance of community-based partnership recruitment results and associated factors. *Journal of Family Psychology* 21(2): 137–45. doi: 10.1037/0893–3200.21.2.137

Spoth, R., Rohrbach, L. A., Greenberg, M., Leaf, P., Brown, C. H., Fagan, A., Catalano, R. F., Pentz, M. A., Sloboda, Z., & Hawkins, J. D (2013). Addressing core challenges for the next generation of type 2 translation research and systems: the Translational Science to Population Impact (TSci Impact) Framework. *Prevention Science* 14: 319–51. doi: 10.1007/211121-012-0362–6

Taylor, T. K., & Biglan, A. (1998). Behavioral family interventions for improving child-rearing: a review of the literature for clinicians and policy makers. *Clinical Child and Family Psychology Review* 1(1): 41–60.

Tein, J.-Y., Sandler, I. N., MacKinnon, D. P., & Wolchik, S. A. (2004). How did it work? Who did it work for? Mediation and mediated moderation of a preventive intervention for children of divorce. *Journal of Consulting and Clinical Psychology* 72: 617–24.

Umana-Taylor, A. J., & Alfaro, E. C. (2006). Divorce and relationship dissolution among Latino populations in the United States. In Fine, M. A. & Harvey, J. H. (eds.), *Handbook of Divorce and Relationship Dissolution*. Mahwah, NJ: Lawrence Erlbaum, pp. 515–30.

United Nations Statistical Division (UNSTAT) (2012). *Demographic Yearbook*. Retrieved from unstats.un.org/unsd/demographic/products/dyb/dyb2012.htm.

Velez, C., Wolchik, S. A., Tein, J. Y., & Sandler, I. N. (2011). Protecting children from the consequences of divorce: A longitudinal study of the effects of parenting on children's coping efforts and coping efficacy. *Child Development* 82: 244–57.

Webb, T. L., & Sheeran, P. (2006). Does changing behavioral intentions engender behavior change? A meta-analysis of the experimental evidence. *Psychological Bulletin* 132(2): 249–68. doi: 10.1037/0033–2909.132.2.249

Winslow, E. B., Betkowski, J., Lopez, M., Wheeler, L., Sandler, I., Braver, S., & Cialdini, R. (2015). Video-based approach to engaging parents into a preventive intervention for divorcing families: results of a randomized controlled trial. Manuscript in progress.

Winslow, E. B., Poloskov, E., Begay, R., Tein, J-Y., Sandler, I., & Wolchik, S. (2014). Engagement of low-income, Mexican American parents into preventive parenting interventions: a randomized experimental study. Manuscript submitted for publication.

Wolchik, S. A., Sandler, I. N., Millsap, R. E., Plummer, B. A., Greene, S. M., Anderson, E. R., et al. (2002). Six-year follow-up of a randomized, controlled trial of preventive interventions for children of divorce. *Journal of the American Medical Association* 288: 1–8.

Wolchik, S. A., Sandler, I. N., Tein, J.-Y., Mahrer, N. E.,Millsap, R. E., Winslow, E., & Reed, A. (2013). Fifteen year follow-up of a randomized trial of a preventive intervention for divorced families: effects on mental health and substance use outcomes in young adulthood. *Journal of Clinical and Consulting Psychology* 81: 600–73. doi: 10.1037/a0033235

Wolchik, S. A., Sandler, I., Weiss, L., & Winslow, E. B. (2007). New Beginnings: an empirically-based program to help divorced mothers promote resilience in their children. In Briesmeister, J. M., & Schaefer, C. E. (eds.), *Handbook of Parent Training: Helping Parents Prevent and Solve Problem Behaviors*. New York: John Wiley & Sons, pp. 25–62.

Wolchik, S. A., West, S. G., Sandler, I. N., Tein, J.-Y., Coatsworth, D., Lengua, L., et al. (2000). The New Beginnings Program for divorced families: an experimental evaluation of theory-based single-component and dual-component programs. *Journal of Consulting and Clinical Psychology* 68: 843–56.

Wolchik, S. A., West, S., Westover, S., Sandler, I. N., Martin A., Lustig, J., et al. (1993). The children of divorce parenting project: outcome evaluation of an empirically based parenting program. *American Journal of Community Psychology* 21: 293–331.

Zhou, Q., Sandler, I., Millsap, R., Wolchik, S., & Dawson-McClure, S. (2008). Mother-child relationship quality and effective discipline as mediators of the six-year effects of the New Beginnings Program for children from divorced families. *Journal of Consulting and Clinical Psychology* 76: 579–95.

6 The Science and Practice of Prevention from Multicultural and Social Justice Perspectives

Y. Joel Wong, Ellen L. Vaughan, & Elyssa M. Klann

From the wearing of seat belts to the consumption of vitamins to the monitoring of weather forecasts, the practice of prevention is ubiquitous in everyday life. Although there is widespread consensus and a large corpus of research on the benefits of prevention (APA, 2014; Romano, 2015), not every social group benefits equally from the fruits of prevention work (e.g., Earnshaw, Bogart, Dovidio, & Williams, 2013). Across diverse societies, substantial health and educational disparities exist as a function of gender, race, socioeconomic status (SES), sexual orientation, and other social statuses (Shin & Kendall, 2013; World Health Organization, 2015; Yoshikawa, Aber, & Beardslee, 2012). Against this backdrop, the goal of this chapter is to present a conceptual framework, the Multicultural Social Justice Framework (MSJF), to interpret previous prevention scholarship, identify existing limitations in the literature, and inform future research and practice on prevention. The MSJF was adapted from the Racial-Cultural Framework, a recently developed framework used to address suicide-related outcomes in racial and ethnic minority communities (Wong, Maffini, & Shin, 2014b). Our main thesis in this chapter is that multiculturalism and social justice should permeate all forms of prevention research and practice, especially those pertaining to minority and marginalized groups in society.

Before proceeding, we clarify the meaning of "prevention" used in this chapter. In contrast to a remedial approach to addressing problems, prevention generally focuses on intervening before a problem fully develops. Following Hage et al. (2007), we adopt an inclusive definition of prevention that includes stopping or delaying the onset of a problem; lessening the impact of problems; promoting attitudes, knowledge, and skills that influence well-being; and strengthening institutions, communities, and policies that enhance well-being.

Overview of the Multicultural Social Justice Framework

As earlier alluded to, the MSJF emphasizes the role of multiculturalism and social justice in prevention work. Multiculturalism acknowledges the increasing diversity of societies across the globe; recognizes the pervasive influence of culture on individuals and institutions; and calls for the respect and appreciation of diverse cultural worldviews, values, and practices (APA, 2003, Sue, 2001). Moreover, multiculturalism denotes multiple forms of diversity, including race, ethnicity, national origin, gender, SES, sexual orientation, age, religion, and disability status. We contend that multiculturalism should be infused into all aspects of prevention theories, research, and practice. Guided by Sue's (2001) multidimensional model of cultural competence, we argue that multicultural competence in prevention work includes prevention professionals' (a) awareness of their own cultural worldviews and biases, (b) knowledge of multicultural concerns relevant to diverse groups, and (c) multicultural skills in research and practice.

Inasmuch as multiculturalism prescribes the content of prevention work, social justice clarifies the values that should guide prevention efforts. Social justice includes both procedural justice and distributive justice. Procedural justice can be conceptualized as "scholarship and professional action designed to change societal values, structures, policies and practices, such that disadvantaged or marginalized groups gain increased access to these tools of self-determination" (Goodman et al., 2004, p. 795). Distributive justice, on the other hand, focuses on addressing social inequities by conferring the greatest benefits to the least advantaged and ensuring the equitable distribution of resources (Rawls, 1971). Because social justice psychologists locate the causes of problems in social inequities and oppressive environments (e.g., poverty and racism), they emphasize macro-level interventions that focus on eliminating inequities and oppression rather than rely exclusively on individual-centered interventions (Kenny & Hage, 2009). Moreover, social justice advocates are committed to reducing power imbalances between professionals and social groups that are the focus of prevention work – this requires prevention professionals to acknowledge their power and privileges as well as engage in collaborative relationships with local communities (Prilleltensky & Nelson, 2013). Throughout this chapter, we emphasize that social justice and multiculturalism are complementary perspectives. That is, the values of social justice often require a focus on diverse communities' cultural worldviews, values, and practices (Romano, Koch, & Wong, 2012; Vera & Kenny, 2013).

Similar to Wong, Maffini, & Shin's (2014b) Racial-Cultural Framework, the MSJF consists of nine principles embedded within three interrelated components: constructs, populations, and interventions. As reflected in Table 6.1, we propose a key question that each component addresses. The first question, *What* (Component 1, Principles 1–3), identifies the constructs that should be emphasized in prevention theories, research, and practice. The second question, *Who* (Component 2, Principles 4 and 5), identifies the populations that should be given greater attention in prevention work. The third question, *How* (Component 3, Principles 6–9), addresses how preventive interventions should be conducted as well as the focus of such interventions. What follows is a discussion of the three components and nine principles. Although much of the research we cite in this chapter is from the Western hemisphere, whenever possible, we also include studies from non-Western countries.

Table 6.1 *The Multicultural Social Justice Framework for Prevention Research and Practice*

Component	Questions	Principles
Constructs	What constructs should theories and research highlight in addressing prevention outcomes in diverse communities?	1. Identify social inequities and oppression as targets for prevention. 2. Examine the ways in which cultural constructs can constitute risk and protective factors. 3. Recognize culturally specific beliefs and attitudes.
Populations	Who should be given more consideration in prevention theory, research, and practice?	4. Disaggregate data to determine diverse subgroups that have been underserved. 5. Address the intersectionality of social identities.
Interventions	How should prevention professionals develop interventions and what should these interventions focus on?	6. Create culturally relevant preventive interventions. 7. Collaborate with stakeholders from diverse communities to produce, implement, and evaluate interventions. 8. Improve access to prevention resources. 9. Engage in macro-level preventive interventions.

Note: This framework was adapted from Wong et al.'s (2014b) Racial-Cultural Framework.

Component 1: Relevant Constructs in Prevention Theories, Research, and Practice

The first component of the MSJF, *Who* (Principles 1–3), identifies three broad domains of constructs that should be emphasized in prevention theories, research, and practice: social inequities and oppression, cultural risk and protective factors, and culturally specific lay beliefs and attitudes.

Principle 1: Identify Social Inequities and Oppression as Targets for Prevention

Consistent with social justice principles, we encourage prevention professionals to conceptualize social inequities and oppression as preventable risk factors for deleterious outcomes as well as to work to prevent such inequities (Kenny & Hage, 2009). These social injustices include poverty, homelessness, racism, sexism, heterosexism, and ageism that adversely affect minority and marginalized social groups. Such injustices could be overt or covert (Sue, 2010) and include individual- and macro-level manifestations of oppression (Buhin & Vera, 2009; Schwartz & Lindley, 2009).

A preventive emphasis on oppression and social inequities reframes the nature of societal problems, reconceptualizes research questions, and transforms the foci of preventive interventions. Specifically, in the United States (U.S.), LGBT, low SES, and racial minority children and adolescents exhibit higher rates of school dropout relative to their heterosexual, high SES, and White counterparts, respectively (Shin & Kendall, 2013). Informed by a social justice perspective, Shin and Kendall argued that such disparities cannot be conceptualized solely as a problem associated with individual factors (e.g., poor academic performance). Instead, the authors argued for a greater acknowledgment of social inequities that result in disproportionately high rates of expulsion and suspension of Latino and African American students as salient causes of disparities in school dropout rates.

A growing body of research has identified various forms of social inequities and oppression as risk factors negatively associated with well-being. Meta-analyses have documented greater rates of victimization among LGBT individuals relative to heterosexuals across eight countries (Katz-Wise & Hyde, 2012) and a positive association between U.S. African Americans' experiences of racism and psychological distress (Pieterse, Todd, Neville, & Carter, 2012). Evidence from many studies across multiple countries shows that poverty is associated with a host of negative outcomes, including higher rates of mental disorders, lower educational attainment, and poorer physical health (Yoshikawa et al., 2012).

In addition, the prevention of social inequities and oppression is not just a means to removing obstacles to well-being but is an outcome worthy of pursuit in its own right because it contributes to the development of a socially just society (Prilleltensky & Nelson, 2013). Among diverse forms of oppression, racism and sexism have been the focus of most preventive intervention research (Buhin & Vera, 2009; Schwartz & Lindley, 2009). In a multicountry study, Navarro, Velasquez, Ryan, and Megias (2014) showed that a twenty-hour workshop that addressed topics such as the social construction of gender, gender stereotypes, gender-based power, and sexual violence as expressions of gender inequity reduced various forms of sexism among university students in Argentina, Spain, and El Salvador. With regard to racism, a comprehensive review of 985 studies across the globe identified a wide range of (mostly racial) prejudice reduction interventions, among which cooperative learning was assessed as the intervention that best illustrated theoretically grounded, rigorous laboratory and field research (Paluck & Green, 2009). Applied mostly in school settings, this approach involves developing opportunities in which students from diverse backgrounds learn from and teach one another (Slavin, 1995).

Several limitations in the literature on preventing social inequities and oppression are noteworthy. With a few exceptions (e.g., Buhin & Vera, 2009;

Schwartz & Lindley, 2009), the literature on anti-oppression interventions has not been well integrated with the prevention science literature. We therefore advocate for the cross-fertilization of ideas between both bodies of scholarship. For instance, theoretical frameworks from prevention science, such as the classification of interventions as universal, selected, and indicated (Mrazek & Haggerty, 1994), can enrich the conceptualization of anti-oppression interventions. Additionally, there is a paucity of theory, research, and interventions to address the prevention of forms of social injustice other than racism and sexism. Several scholars have documented the need for more research on the prevention of ageism (Bugental & Hehman, 2007) and homelessness (Montgomery, Metraux, & Culhane, 2013). Furthermore, most research on the prevention of social injustices has been conducted in the Western hemisphere. Given that manifestations of social inequities likely differ across cultures (e.g., Lee, Pratto, & Li, 2007), interventions to prevent social injustices in African and Asian countries might need to be modified to address unique, local cultural norms.

Principle 2: Examine the Ways in Which Cultural Constructs Can Constitute Risk and Protective Factors

What cultural constructs serve as risk and protective factors for adverse and positive outcomes? Principle 2 of the MSJF aims to identify these important cultural constructs. Consistent with the principles of multiculturalism (Sue, 2001), prevention professionals are tasked with identifying the most salient cultural constructs for their target population. Within prevention science and practice, cultural constructs have been at the center of risk and protective research. Such work has utilized several conceptual models to aid prevention professionals in identifying cultural constructs that serve as risk and protective factors.

Ecological theories highlight the important contexts in which humans develop (Bronfenbrenner, 1979), and have been widely applied in prevention science (e.g., Pantin, Schwartz, Sullivan, Prado, & Szapocznik, 2004). Macro-level cultural factors help define a community or culture and encompass demographic characteristics, attitudes, and values of a population, as well as broader political climates. Examples include the ethnic or religious density of a community (e.g., Hong, Zhang, & Walton, 2014), the stability of neighborhoods due to mobility or economic deprivation (e.g., Hanibuchi et al., 2015), and the climate of a receiving culture with respect to cultural adaptation (Schwartz, Unger, Zamboanga, & Szapocznik, 2010). Other individual and micro-level factors such as religiosity, specific cultural values, and processes of acculturation and enculturation may directly impact outcomes or interact with broader cultural factors such as community stability.

Prevention professionals have made strides in recognizing and incorporating cultural constructs into prevention practice and science across a variety of outcomes (e.g. Hecht & Kreiger, 2006). In the U.S., community indicators of poverty (i.e., income, proportion of the population below the poverty line, and proportion of the community with less than a high school education) have been associated with increased mortality among infants with congenital heart defects (Kucik et al., 2014). Other neighborhood factors have also been linked to health behaviors. Among middle-aged Japanese adults, neighborhood instability and fewer years of residence in the neighborhood were associated with greater risk for smoking behaviors (Hanibuchi et al., 2015).

Individual cultural factors are also critical for implementation of prevention efforts. Religiosity, defined broadly, represents one's engagement in religious activities and the importance that religious beliefs and the search for the sacred play in one's life. This individual cultural context has been connected to various positive outcomes. Specifically, Amit and colleagues (2014) found that greater religiosity was associated with lower risk of indicators of self-injury among Jewish adolescents in Israel. In South Africa, religiosity was linked to lower risk for sexual activity among college students (Blignaut, Vergnani, & Jacobs, 2014). Finally, in Brazil, participants reporting higher levels of religiosity showed greater endorsement of policies and laws to deter alcohol use, such as higher taxes or restrictions on selling alcohol (Lucchetti, Koenig, Pinsky, Laranjeira, & Vallada, 2014). Together, these studies suggest that religiosity may be an important cultural context for understanding engagement in behaviors that might be targets of prevention.

There has also been growth in prevention research attending to the individual processes of acculturation and enculturation in the United States. Acculturation involves the changes an individual experiences when in contact with a dominant culture (Schwartz et al., 2010). Enculturation refers to socialization into one's heritage culture. These processes may interact with macro-level variables, such as characteristics of the receiving culture, to exert influence on adverse outcomes. Among U.S. racial minority samples, greater acculturation has been linked with a number of negative health outcomes, including greater risk of substance use (Zemore, 2007) and risk for suicide (Wong et al., 2014b). In Germany, greater acculturation has been associated with smoking during pregnancy among Turkish immigrants (Reiss et al., 2014). Among adolescents in the Dominican Republic, those with contact and greater involvement with the United States were at increased risk for suicide attempts (Peña, Zayas, Cabrera-Nguyen, & Vega, 2012). But greater acculturation is also protective in other areas, such as increased vaccination of daughters for humanpapilloma virus (HPV) by Latina American mothers (Gerend, Zapata, & Reyes, 2013) and self-reported health among Asian Americans (Lee, Chen, He, Miller, & Juon, 2013). Taken together, these studies underscore the complex relationships between macro- and individual-level cultural factors and prevention-related outcomes.

In terms of future directions, a particular area of growth for prevention would include research and practice that attend to macro-level cultural constructs. How might prevention research address the stability of neighborhoods, including measuring the impact of changing stability on outcomes? Further, more research is needed to understand the role that receiving cultures play in prevention-related outcomes (Schwartz et al., 2010). For instance, the risk and protective factors associated with immigrant Asian Americans' mental health might differ depending on whether they live in immigrant gateway cities (e.g., San Francisco) or in monocultural White-majority areas within the United States.

Principle 3: Recognize Culturally Specific Lay Beliefs and Attitudes.

We encourage prevention professionals to identify culturally specific lay beliefs and attitudes that are relevant to prevention work. Such beliefs and attitudes include cultural worldviews (e.g., beliefs about the ubiquity of change) and beliefs about the causes, duration, appropriate coping strategies, and solutions to problems (Wong, Tran, Kim, Van Horn Kerne, & Calfa, 2010). Culturally specific lay beliefs and attitudes can help prevention professionals identify cultural barriers to accessing prevention resources; such cultural lay beliefs can also be incorporated into preventive interventions to enhance their cultural relevance within diverse communities (see Principle 6).

The majority of prevention-related research on culturally specific lay beliefs and attitudes has focused on health-related concerns – these studies tend to be based explicitly or implicitly on what we term the *medical discordance paradigm*. That is, discordance between lay and expert medical beliefs is assumed to reflect lay people's misconceptions, which should be corrected to advance the cause of prevention work. Examples of such research include investigations of lay beliefs about tuberculosis in Addis Ababa, Ethiopia (Gebremariam, Bjune, & Frich, 2011), and HIV and AIDS among Black South Africans (Bogart et al., 2011). To illustrate, Neiderdeppe and Levy (2007) found that U.S. adults' fatalistic beliefs about cancer (e.g., the idea that not much can be done to lower the odds of getting cancer) varied as a function of language, race, and level of education. Spanish-speaking Latino respondents were more likely to than White respondents to endorse fatalistic cancer beliefs. Given previous research demonstrating that fatalistic cancer beliefs were negatively associated with health-promotion behaviors, the authors recommended that cancer prevention work should include educational interventions to "dispel" such fatalistic beliefs.

In contrast to the medical discordance paradigm, some scholars have called for a greater emphasis on honoring individuals' culturally specific lay beliefs and subjective experiences of illness (Carroll, 2013), a perspective that we believe is more consistent with the principles of social justice and multiculturalism undergirding the MSJF. Lay beliefs that diverge from expert medical viewpoints are not necessarily misperceptions to be corrected; instead, professionals and consumers of health services should seek to understand each other's perspectives and come to a consensus on how best to understand the experience of illness (Carroll, 2013). In designing culturally relevant health preventive interventions, prevention practitioners are encouraged to use concepts and vocabulary from both medical and lay models of illness to enhance the social validity of the interventions. To illustrate, individuals who adhere to a traditional Asian cultural health worldview may believe that mental illness is caused by somatic concerns (e.g., an imbalance in one's diet). Therefore, preventive programs that address mental health concerns for such individuals could incorporate practical strategies that address somatic concerns (e.g., a change in one's diet) in addition to other psychological interventions (Maffini & Wong, 2014). In another example, Blocker et al. (2006) identified several strength-based cultural beliefs among church-attending African Americans, such as the sacredness of one's physical body, that can be incorporated into prostate cancer prevention programs.

Beyond physical and mental health, more research is needed on other culturally relevant lay beliefs and attitudes relevant to prevention work, such as lay beliefs about education, career, crime, violence, and race. For instance, research has shown that students from East Asian Confucian cultures tend to view effort as more central to academic success than Western students, who are more likely to value the role of inherent ability (Tweed & Lehman, 2002). Such attributional beliefs about academic success can be addressed in preventive interventions for academically at-risk students.

Component 2: Populations

Component 2 of the MSJF is designed to help prevention professionals identify the *Who* of prevention efforts. The two principles aim to identify subpopulations that might be targets of prevention efforts.

Principle 4: Disaggregate Data to Determine Underserved Subgroups

The MSJF advocates for disaggregating data to better understand subpopulation differences in outcomes. Often heterogeneous groups are lumped together in epidemiologic samples to study an outcome (e.g., Oh & DeVylder, 2014). While there are practical reasons for doing so, at times important targets of prevention are obscured. For example, men and women, rural and urban participants, or large racial and ethnic groups may be grouped together (e.g., Asian Americans, without respect to national origin). Disaggregation of data provides depth and allows for the identification of subgroups that may be at high risk for adverse outcomes and targets of prevention practice (Wong, Vaughan, Liu, & Chang, 2014). Given the vast dimensions by which data can be disaggregated, (e.g., race/ethnicity, SES, biological sex, sexual orientation, geographic location), professionals ought to focus on data that accurately and specifically reflects their target population. For example, a prevention professional may be tasked with developing prevention programs for immigrants in Australia from China. Thus, research that disaggregates data from Asian immigrant populations helps to define specific prevention needs. While this list is not exhaustive, it provides a starting point for thinking about ways data can be disaggregated to best meet a population's prevention needs and to identify subpopulations whose prevention needs might be obscured by aggregated data.

Among the most predominant forms of disaggregation are studies testing biological sex and racial/ethnic differences in behaviors and conditions that might be targets of prevention. Sex and racial/ethnic differences are readily reported in large epidemiologic studies, such as the Youth Risk Behavior Surveillance System (Kann et al., 2014), which measures adolescent risk behavior in the United States. The World Health Organization (WHO) collects and disaggregates international health and health behavior data, making it publicly available for prevention professionals.[1] Recently, the WHO (2014) released the 2014 Global Status Report on Violence Prevention, which provides disaggregated data on violence by age, biological sex, country income, and global region. These large-scale data sources are important places for access to disaggregated data. However, further disaggregation may shed light on populations with different prevention needs and may help when prevention professionals are doing prevention work with a more narrow population.

There are a growing number of studies that underscore the importance of disaggregation to better understand the nature of a target of prevention. Among physical and mental health behaviors in the United States, important subgroup differences have been shown within large racial and ethnic groups. For example, overall, Asian American adolescents use substances at lower rates than other racial and ethnic groups in the United States (SAMHSA, 2011). This assertion obscures subgroup data among Asian American subgroups; specifically, Lee, Han, and Gfroerer (2013) found that the rates of binge alcohol use in the preceding month ranged from a high of 24.6 percent among Korean Americans to a low of 8.1 percent among Chinese Americans. Likewise, U.S. Latino adolescents, whose substance use rates are often aggregated, show subgroup differences in alcohol use. In particular, Mexican American adolescents use alcohol at greater rates than other Latino groups (Siqueira & Crandall, 2008). In China, disaggregated data on rural and urban differences demonstrated that participants in rural areas had higher rates of chronic disease such as diabetes, hypertension, and heart disease (Wang et al., 2014). These aforementioned studies illustrate the need to narrow in to identify populations that might be important targets of prevention efforts.

However, there remain limitations in researchers' abilities to disaggregate data in all possible manners. One statistical limitation may be garnering enough participants from a particular population to make meaningful conclusions about findings. Again, this might obscure important differences or highlight differences that with larger numbers might not be as important. Finally, the myriad ways data can be disaggregated might hamper one's decisions about one's target population. One way to address this limitation is for prevention

1 www.who.int/healthinfo/en/.

professionals to get to know the communities they aim to target and then to identify the meaningful ways they might disaggregate data.

Principle 5: Address the Intersectionality of Social Identities

Principle 5 of the MSJF, which addresses intersectionality of identities, is an extension of our discussion on data disaggregation enumerated in Principle 4. Multicultural models for understanding human development acknowledge that people's multiple identities are important to understanding their well-being (Neville & Mobley, 2001). Further, risk or protective factors may operate differently depending upon the intersection of multiple identities. Indeed, prevention efforts often target populations with intersecting identities. Examples might include HIV prevention targeting gay men from a particular racial or ethnic background, suicide prevention for immigrant women, or heart disease prevention for men from a particular religious background. There is a growing literature applying the notion of intersectionality to understanding outcomes (e.g., Watkins-Hays, 2014). Empirically, this is most often seen in the form of moderator research questions. Such moderator questions may be related to the intersection of identities and a particular outcome or moderators of the relationships between risk and protective factors and the target of prevention efforts. Both strategies are important to developing culturally competent prevention.

Research on the intersection between identities has grown significantly with questions that are central to understanding a prevention professional's target population (e.g., Lipsicas et al., 2012). For example, if a prevention professional in the United States is interested in risky sexual behaviors among Asian American and Latino American adolescents, he or she might want to understand the intersectional identity of immigrant status. To illustrate, Hussey and colleagues (2007) found that, for both Asian and Latino Americans, being born outside the United States was associated with lower engagement in risky behaviors. Similarly, Lipsicas et al. (2012) tested gender and immigrant status differences in suicide attempts across several European countries. These authors found that not only did the gender ratios of suicide attempts vary by immigrant status, but there was also variation by national origin of the immigrant. Therefore, the authors conclude that, among immigrants, risk and protective factors for suicide attempts may be different for men and women. These studies underscore the salience of addressing intersecting identities when developing culturally competent prevention strategies.

Building upon the empirical literature that addresses questions of moderation with respect to outcomes, prevention programming should aim to address intersecting identities. For example, Harper (2007) calls for the inclusion of culture and context in HIV prevention efforts with gay men. Intersectionality might be addressed through programming that attends to racial and/or ethnic identity as well as the role that masculinity plays in sexual behavior. Overall, prevention professionals should incorporate aspects of salient intersecting identities in the communities they aim to serve.

Component 3: Interventions

The third component of the MSJF, *How* (Principles 6–9), provides four recommendations on preventive interventions that address cultural relevance, collaboration with community stakeholders, access to preventive resources, and macro-level interventions.

Principle 6: Create Culturally Relevant Preventive Interventions

Prevention professionals are encouraged to design, implement, and evaluate culturally relevant prevention programs (Vera & Kenny, 2013). Cultural relevance is defined as the degree to which a preventive intervention incorporates the cultural values, practices, and beliefs of a particular community (Kumpfer, Alvarado, Smith, & Bellamy, 2002). Although most prevention professionals agree that culture is a relevant factor in preventive interventions, there is a diversity of views concerning how and to what extent preventive interventions should be modified when applied to diverse cultural groups (Castro, Barrera, & Steiker, 2010). In addressing the cultural relevance of a preventive intervention, there also exists a dynamic tension between fidelity and modification (Castro et al., 2010). The principle of fidelity dictates that an intervention's effectiveness is enhanced when prevention professionals adhere to the intervention's main procedures (particularly when there is already a body of research supporting an intervention's effectiveness). In contrast, proponents of modification argue that preventive interventions are often developed and tested in environments that reflect the cultural values and practices of a dominant cultural group (e.g., European Americans), which may be less applicable to other cultural groups (Castro et al., 2010). Hence, the principle of modification favors altering an existing intervention to fit the preferences and needs of a particular cultural group. What follows is a review of five approaches (Castro et al., 2010; Okamoto, Kulis, Marsiglia, Holleran Steiker, & Dustman, 2014) to addressing cultural relevance in preventive interventions that differ in the extent to which they adhere to the principles of fidelity and modification: (a) culturally generic, (b) culturally attuned, (c) culturally adapted, (d) culturally informed, and (e) culturally grounded interventions.

Culturally generic preventive interventions are those that adhere strongly to fidelity and are not altered when applied to a new cultural group. For instance, Fang and Schinke (2014) demonstrated that a randomized controlled, culturally generic, Web-based substance use preventive intervention that involved Asian American adolescent daughters and their mothers improved the girls' family relationships and self-efficacy, which was in turn associated with the girls' reduced substance use two years later.

Culturally attuned interventions retain most of the original intervention procedures but make several minor modifications that help boost the recruitment and retention of participants from diverse backgrounds (Castro et al.,

2010; Okamoto et al., 2014). Examples include providing services in participants' native language or minor changes in the vocabulary of the intervention to be more consistent with participants' culture.

Culturally adapted interventions represent a middle ground between the principles of fidelity and modification in that most of the core components of the original intervention are retained, while modifications are made to the intervention to enhance its compatibility with a particular cultural group's values and practices (Castro et al., 2010). Grau and colleagues (2013) described the cultural adaptation of a U.S.-based psychoeducational intervention to reduce sexual risk behavior in St. Petersburg, Russia. These adaptations included introducing the notion of "latent infections" when chlamydia is untreated (to be congruent with Russian medical views) and a more gradual approach to using roleplays to practice health-promoting behaviors (given Russians' unfamiliarity with roleplay exercises).

Culturally informed interventions go a step further in conceptualizing culture not merely as an add-on component but as a core feature that is interwoven throughout the intervention protocol (Castro et al., 2010). To illustrate, Santisteban and Mena (2009) developed a culturally informed family-based intervention to address substance abuse among U.S. Latino youth. Although the intervention was based on structural family therapy, extensive modifications to the intervention protocol were made to address salient cultural issues such as acculturation and immigration stress (e.g., family conflicts arising from differences in parent–child acculturation levels).

Finally, culturally grounded interventions strongly favor the principle of modification in that the entire intervention is developed from the bottom up, often in close collaboration between researchers and community stakeholders, to fully reflect the values and practices of a cultural group (Okamoto et al., 2014). An example of a culturally grounded intervention is the People Awakening Project, a long-term prevention program aimed at reducing the rates of alcohol abuse among Yup'ik Alaskan Natives (Allen, Mohatt, Beehler, & Rowe, 2014). University researchers and members of the Yup'ik community collaborated on conducting research, developing a strength-based indigenous theoretical model of sobriety, and designing a preventive intervention based on this model.

Based on our literature review, we offer three principles that prevention professionals can use to determine which of these approaches to use when there is no prior evidence that the original intervention is effective for a particular cultural group.

First, time and resources (e.g., the number of available prevention practitioners) are pragmatic factors that can help determine how to address the cultural relevance of an intervention (Okamoto et al., 2014). For example, Helm and Okamoto's (2013) culturally grounded Ho'ouna Pono drug prevention program for Hawaiian youth took about six years to develop, a time frame that may be considered too resource-intensive for some communities. In this regard, the approaches that favor fidelity (e.g., culturally attuned interventions) tend to be easier to implement because prevention professionals can rely on preexisting intervention protocols.

Second, we encourage prevention professionals to assess the social validity of existing preventive interventions before deciding on their approach to cultural relevance (Reese & Vera, 2007). Adopting a wisdom-of-the-crowd approach, social validity refers to the acceptability and perceived utility of an intervention by intervention participants and community stakeholders (e.g., elders in the community). One potential indication that an intervention lacks social validity is when participants from a cultural group demonstrate a higher drop-out rate and poorer attendance in an intervention than members of another cultural group (Lau, 2006). A lack of social validity might signal the need to consider approaches that favor cultural modifications (e.g. culturally informed interventions).

Third, the need for cultural modifications of an existing intervention becomes more compelling when there is evidence that risk and protective factors associated with a targeted outcome differ across cultural groups (Lau, 2006). For example, several studies have found that interpersonal factors (e.g., family relationships) are a better predictor of suicide-related outcomes for certain African American and Asian American groups relative to their White American counterparts (Wong, Maffini, & Shin (2014b). Accordingly, suicide preventive interventions for these cultural groups might benefit from cultural modifications that emphasize interpersonal factors (Wong & Poon, 2010).

Principle 7: Collaborate with Stakeholders from Diverse Communities

To the extent that cultural relevance prescribes the content of preventive interventions, collaboration with community stakeholders is a key process through which an intervention attains cultural relevance (Wong et al., 2014b). There are several advantages afforded by such collaboration. From a multicultural standpoint, collaboration enhances the cultural relevance of preventive interventions because members of a local community can provide an insider's view of a community's cultural history, needs, preferences, and customs, which can be explicitly addressed in a preventive intervention. For instance, during the development of a suicide preventive intervention for U.S. Zuni tribal members, focus group feedback from tribal members resulted in a name change of the intervention from Zuni "suicide prevention" to "life skills development" (LaFromboise & Lewis, 2008). Collaboration also generates buy-in from community members, which increases an intervention's social validity, leading to greater participation and retention in preventive programs (Hage et al., 2007). Furthermore, collaboration dovetails with the social justice principle of establishing egalitarian partnerships with local communities. That is, community stakeholders must be given an active voice in prevention work for it to be considered socially just (Reese & Vera, 2007).

We therefore encourage prevention professionals to partner with community members and leaders (e.g., religious leaders) in the design, implementation, and evaluation of preventive interventions (Vera & Kenny, 2013). The nature and degree of collaboration likely differs across the aforementioned five approaches to attaining cultural relevance (refer to Principle 6), with culturally grounded interventions requiring a far greater degree of collaboration than approaches that emphasize the principle of fidelity. Other examples of collaboration, grounded in community-based participatory research, include strategies that foster community members' self-determination (e.g., training community members in research methods and program implementation) and opportunities for prevention professionals to increase their cultural competence by spending time with and learning from community members (Jason, Keys, Suarez-Balcazar, Taylor, & Davis, 2004).

Interorganizational collaborations can also contribute to the cultural relevance of preventive interventions. Flynn, Check, Eggerth, and Tonda (2013) described a collaborative effort between the U.S. National Institute for Occupational Safety and Health and the Mexican Ministry of Foreign Affairs to reduce incidences of fatal work injuries among immigrant Mexican workers. Because the ministry operated fifty consulates in the United States that provide millions of service contacts with Mexicans annually, the consulates were used to disseminate information on occupational safety and health as well as to gather information on unsafe working conditions provided by consumers of consulate services.

In terms of future directions, prevention researchers can assess whether the quality and extent of collaboration between prevention professionals and community members are associated with improved outcomes and greater social validity for preventive interventions (Wong et al., 2014b). We hypothesize that such collaborations would not only enhance the acceptability and effectiveness of preventive programs but also strengthen the quality of relationships between prevention professionals and community members as well as increase prevention professionals' cultural competence, factors that are crucial for the long-term success of culturally relevant preventive interventions.

Principle 8: Improve Access to Preventive Resources

Across diverse communities, members of minority and marginalized groups tend to consume prevention services at lower rates than those from majority cultures. For example, Wong and colleagues (2014a) found that among U.S. college students with suicide ideation, Asian Americans were less likely to seek professional psychological help relative to White Americans, and this disparity was explained by Asian Americans receiving advice to seek help at lower rates. Disparities in access to preventive resources are a social justice concern because they reflect the inequitable distribution of societal resources to the detriment of the least advantaged (Prilleltensky & Nelson, 2013).

Culturally relevant prevention services are of little value if they are not utilized by the communities for which they are intended. The reasons for disparities in the use of preventive services are multifaceted: they include structural barriers (e.g., the inability to pay for services), the lack of culturally relevant services, historic mistrust of services provided by members of a dominant cultural group, and minority groups' experiences of discrimination when accessing preventive services (Earnshaw et al., 2013; Ibaraki, Hall, & Sabin, 2014).

Given these concerns, we urge professionals who engage in preventive interventions to work toward the elimination of disparities in access to preventive resources. Such strategies include increasing the accessibility of prevention services and removing structural barriers to such services. For example, to address cultural mistrust of health professionals, prevention health services can be located in local community centers instead of in health care institutions (Earnshaw et al., 2013). In another example, Carpentier et al. (2007) described efforts to recruit Mexican American families for a school-based, family-focused preventive intervention to address academic engagement and mental health. The researchers devised strategies to reduce barriers to participation, such as offering services in either English or Spanish; personalized recruitment phone calls to all eligible families; home visits from prevention professionals; and the provision of child care, food, and transportation. These efforts resulted in a reasonably high recruitment rate: 62 percent of eligible families agreed to enroll in the intervention.

Principle 9: Engage in Macro-level Interventions

From a social justice standpoint, problems such as low academic achievement, crime, mental illness, and unemployment are often not just the result of individual weakness but also arise from macro-level social pathogens that unfairly disadvantage individuals from marginalized backgrounds (Prilleltensky & Nelson, 2013). Accordingly, the goals of socially just preventive interventions must include not only individual-level interventions but also macro-level interventions to alter the social conditions underlying individuals' experience of distress as well as to promote community wellness (Buhin & Vera, 2009; Schwartz & Lindley, 2009). In this regard, we define macro-level preventive interventions as those that address organizational, community-level, and societal outcomes or use environment-centered preventive strategies (e.g., social policies and the mass media). What follows are examples of three types of macro-level preventive interventions: media interventions, community interventions, and social policies.

Given that the media is a macro-level institution that plays an important role in shaping people's attitudes and behavior, prevention professionals are encouraged to engage such media (e.g., television, radio, newspaper, and the Internet) in their prevention efforts (Randolph and Viswanath, 2004). A recent meta-analysis of seventy-two mass-media HIV preventive interventions around the world found that overall these interventions were related to increased condom use and knowledge about HIV transmission and prevention (LaCroix, Snyder, Huedo-Medina, & Johnson, 2014). However, from a multicultural viewpoint, such efforts are ineffective if the type of media used for the transmission of prevention messages is not viewed or listened to by members of minority groups. Hence, it is important for prevention professionals to utilize the types of media outlets used by minority groups. To illustrate, Alexander, Kwon, Strecher, and Bartholomew (2013) described the recent efforts of the U.S. National Cancer Institute in developing a media outreach program to disseminate evidence-based cancer education tailored to racial/ethnic communities. These efforts include disseminating culturally relevant information in English and other languages through media interviews, articles in ethnic newspapers, and video vignettes in social media. In another example, messages about the prevention of group violence and reconciliation were embedded in a radio drama program broadcast in Rwanda, a country that experienced a devastating interracial genocide in 1994 (Staub, 2013). The story broadcast over radio described two villages that shifted from conflict to a collaborative effort to prevent group violence. An experimental study of this radio drama program found that participants who listened to it exhibited more positive attitudes, such as greater empathy for other Rwandans, compared to a control group (Paluck & Green, 2009).

Community-based interventions are another type of macro-level preventive intervention. In a study of a peer-outreach community violence prevention program that involved mediation of conflicts and outreach to youth who were at risk for gun violence, Webster, Whitehill, Vernick, and Curriero (2013) reported that three of the four intervention neighborhoods in Baltimore, Maryland (U.S.), experienced reductions in gun violence after the intervention. The authors estimated that the intervention may have prevented about thirty-five nonfatal shootings and at least five homicides.

Organizational and governmental policies are another crucial type of macro-level preventive interventions. To illustrate, the climate of an organization has been found to be one of the strongest predictors of workplace sexual harassment (Willness, Steel, & Lee, 2007). Therefore, Buchanan, Settles, Hall, and O'Connor (2014) argued that the problem of women's experiences of workplace sexual harassment must be addressed at the organizational level through changes in organizational policies. These include establishing procedures that protect complainants and initiate prompt disciplinary actions when complaints are validated, requiring training programs on sexual harassment policies, and increasing the number of female leaders in male-dominated workplaces. Prevention professionals are also encouraged to advocate for socially just government policies that address the roots of societal challenges. For instance, given evidence that poverty exerts a deleterious effect on children's mental and behavioral health, Yoshikawa et al. (2012) argued that social policies that reduce poverty can contribute to children's mental and behavioral health. In the United States., the Earned Income Tax Credit

(EITC) is an antipoverty policy that provides a tax credit for low-income individuals who work. An evaluation study of the EITC's effects on children's school performance estimated that an increase of $1,000 in income from the EITC was associated with higher math and reading test scores by 6 percent of a standard deviation in the short term (Dahl & Lochner, 2012).

Given that research on macro-level preventive interventions is relatively rare compared to individual-level prevention efforts (Prilleltensky & Nelson, 2013), we encourage greater research attention to such interventions. Additionally, a focus on macro-level interventions, especially those related to social policy, requires prevention professionals to move beyond their traditional responsibilities as clinicians and educators to embrace the roles of organizational consultants and social policy advocates (Hage et al., 2007). In sum, we commend the use of macro-level preventive interventions as a crucial means to achieving socially just societal outcomes.

Having discussed the nine principles of the MSJF, we now use the example of substance use prevention to illustrate how the MSJF can be applied to enhance the quality of prevention research and practice.

Applying the MSJF to Substance Abuse Prevention

In 2013, Latino eighth graders had higher rates of lifetime marijuana use and thirty-day alcohol use than White and Black U.S. eighth graders (Johnston, O'Malley, Bachman, Schulenberg, & Miech, 2014). In response to this challenge, there has been a growing body of prevention programs targeting Latino youth.

The Keepin' It R.E.A.L. substance abuse prevention program is an empirically supported, ten-session, school-based program for twelve-to-fourteen-year-olds based on a multicultural framework[2] (Gosin, Marsiglia, & Hecht, 2003; Hecht et al., 2003). The program addresses substance use norms and skills for resisting substance use in culturally specific ways. There are three versions of the program to meet different population needs: a Mexican American version, a version addressing aspects of White American and African American cultures, and a multicultural version that combines the two aforementioned versions (Hecht et al., 2003). It has been implemented across the United States, Canada, Mexico, and the United Kingdom. For our purposes here, we will describe the Mexican American version. Although the program was not designed using the MSJF, it includes many of the MSJF principles. While not all principles of the MSJF will be addressed, we will discuss each of the three components – the *What, Who,* and *How.*

What? With respect to the MSJF, Principles 2 and 3 are most evident in the development of this prevention program. The Curriculum was developed with

2 www.nrepp.samhsa.gov/ViewIntervention.aspx?id=133.

special attention to cultural values and narratives of Mexican American youth. Specifically, Keepin' It R.E.A.L aims to enhance values that promote drug resistance skills that are congruent with youths' cultural scripts. Examples of core Mexican American values included in the curriculum are *familismo* (a strong family orientation), *respeto* (respect), and *personalismo* (a strong preference for personable relationships) (Hecht et al., 2003).

Who? Principles 4 and 5 of the MSJF advocate for disaggregation of data and intersectionality to identify target populations. The Keepin' It R.E.A.L prevention program was developed based upon knowledge of substance use patterns among Mexican American youth in Phoenix, Arizona (U.S.) (Hecht et al., 2003). Further, Mexican American youth in this area may be born in the United States or in Mexico and have varying levels of English language usage. At the time of its development, Phoenix was experiencing incredible growth in the Latino population, including a growing immigrant population. To address the varying levels of language usage, the prevention program is available in English and in Spanish. However, the program does not explicitly have different versions developed for students of varying levels of acculturation or based upon nativity, which might be a limitation from an intersectionality perspective.

How? The final component of the MSJF enumerates principles for interventions. Specifically, Principle 6 advocates for the adoption of culturally relevant preventive interventions. Conceptually, the Keepin' It R.E.A.L program is a culturally grounded prevention program designed to meet the needs of Mexican heritage youth. When considering ecological risk and protective factors, the model explicitly considers broader cultural contexts and values, as well as local neighborhood effects (Gosin et al., 2003). Given the Latino values of *familismo*, *respeto,* and *personalismo*, one learning objective for the Latino youth was to understand the impact of their behaviors on others. Consistent with Principle 7, the development of the program's curriculum involved members of the community (Gosin et al., 2003). Initial dialogues between researchers and community members addressed the need for substance abuse prevention in the community (Marsiglia & Daley, 2002) and then included the target population in the design of the curriculum. For example, researchers used participatory action research (Jason et al., 2004) involving middle school youth to create narratives for drug resistance strategies. High school youth created videos of drug resistance strategies utilizing the middle school youths' narratives and cultural scripts (Hecht & Krieger, 2006).

With respect to Principle 8, the extent to which Keepin' It R.E.A.L. facilitates access to services for students with greater need has not been studied. However, the program developers recommend training to help teachers follow up on student self-disclosures of sensitive material with effective ways of responding and a list of resources for helping students (Harthun, Dustman, Reeves, Hecht, & Marsiglia, 2008). Finally, Principle 9 of the MSJF advocates for macro-level interventions. The Keepin' It R.E.A.L. program addresses psychosocial outcomes rather than macro-level problems, such as racism or economic factors that promote drug availability in communities. Immigration-related policy and legislation (e.g., laws that target undocumented immigrants) can impact the extent to which Latino populations retain protective cultural characteristics that buffer against substance abuse. Thus, macro-level interventions could include advocacy for policy and legislation that promotes multiculturalism and social justice.

Conclusions

In this chapter, we presented the MSJF, a framework to interpret previous prevention scholarship, assess limitations in the literature, and inform future research and practice on prevention. Guided by multicultural and social justice perspectives, the nine principles and three components in the MSJF identify the constructs, populations, and interventions that should be the foci of prevention science and practice. Several overarching implications of the MSJF should be noted. First, it is worth emphasizing that our framework is relevant to all types of prevention efforts and populations, not just to prevention work centered on minority and marginalized communities. Because no human experience is divorced from culture (i.e., the values and practices of a social group transmitted across generations; Sue, 2001), multicultural considerations are relevant to everyone, including individuals from dominant social groups (e.g., Han in China and Malays in Malaysia). Moreover, the pursuit of socially just ideals requires the participation of dominant social groups in preventive interventions. Because dominant social groups are often responsible for the perpetration of oppression (whether intentionally or unintentionally), preventive interventions must address the attitudes, behaviors, and institutional power of such groups (Buhin & Vera, 2009; Schwartz & Lindley, 2009). For example, a racism prevention strategy that focuses exclusively on helping minority groups cope with racism without any interventions that engage oppressive groups is arguably not socially just.

A second overarching implication is that the principles embedded in the MSJF require not just a set of foci in prevention efforts but ultimately a particular type of *prevention professional.* It is important for prevention professionals to reflect on their power, privileges, values, and biases when engaging in prevention work (Prilleltensky & Nelson, 2013). Moreover, the development of prevention professionals' cultural competence is as important as their implementation of culturally relevant preventive interventions (Castro et al., 2010). Cultural competence involves not just a collection of skills and knowledge but also a particular set of attitudes, especially cultural humility (Hook, Davis, Owen, Worthington, & Utsey, 2013). In conclusion, our hope is that prevention researchers and practitioners will use the MSJF to enrich their prevention efforts, and in so doing contribute to the development of culturally inclusive and social just societies across the globe.

References

Alexander, J., Kwon, H., Strecher, R., & Bartholomew, J. (2013). Multicultural media outreach: increasing cancer information coverage in minority communities. *Journal of Cancer Education* 28: 744–7. doi: 10.1007/s13187-013-0534-5

Allen, J., Mohatt, G. V., Beehler, S., & Rowe, H. (2014). People awakening: collaborative research with Alaska Native rural communities to address alcohol use disorders and suicide health disparities. *American Journal of Community Psychology* 54: 100–11. doi: 10.1007/s10464-014-9647-1

Amit, B., Krivoy, A., Mansbach-Kleinfeld, I., Zalsman, G., Ponizovsky, A., Hoshen, M., & Shoval, G. (2014). Religiosity is a protective factor against self-injurious thoughts and behaviors in Jewish adolescents: findings from a nationally representative survey. *European Psychiatry* 29: 509–13. doi: 10.1016/j.eurpsy.2014.04.005

APA (American Psychological Association) (2003). Guidelines on multicultural education, training, research, practice, and organizational change for psychologists. *American Psychologist* 58: 377–402. doi: 10.1037/e381582004-001

APA (American Psychological Association) (2014). Guidelines for prevention in psychology. *American Psychologist* 69: 285–96. doi: 10.1037/a0034569

Blignaut, R. J., Vergnani, T., & Jacobs, J. J. (2014). Correlates of sexual activity versus non-activity of incoming first-year students at a South African university. *African Journal of AIDS Research* 13: 81–91. doi: 10.2989/16085906.2014.901977

Blocker, D., Romocki, L., Jones, B., Jackson, E., Reid, L., Thomas, K., & Campbell, M. (2006). Knowledge, beliefs and barriers associated with prostate cancer prevention and screening behaviors among African-American men. *Journal of the National Medical Association* 98: 1286–95.

Bogart, L., Skinner, D., Weinhardt, L., Glasman, L., Sitzler, C., Toefy, Y., & Kalichman, S. (2011). HIV/AIDS misconceptions may be associated with condom use among black South Africans: an exploratory analysis. *African Journal of Aids Research* 10: 181–7. doi: 10.2989/16085906.2011.593384

Bronfenbrenner, U. (1979). *The Ecology of Human Development: Experiments by Nature and Design*. Cambridge, MA: Harvard University Press. doi: 10.1080/00131728109336000

Buchanan, N. T., Settles, I. H., Hall, A. T., & O'Connor, R. C. (2014), A review of organizational strategies for reducing sexual harassment: insights from the U. S. military. *Journal of Social Issues,* 70: 687–702. doi: 10.1111/josi.12086

Bugental, D. B. & Hehman, J. A. (2007). Ageism: a review of research and policy implications. *Social Issues and Policy Review* 1: 173–216. doi: 10.1111/j.1751-2409.2007.00007.x

Buhin, L., & Vera, E. M. (2009). Preventing racism and promoting social justice: person centered and environment-centered interventions. *Journal of Primary Prevention* 30: 43–59. doi: 10.1007/s10935-008-0161-9

Carpentier, F., Mauricio, A., Gonzales, N., Millsap, R., Meza, C., Dumka, L., & Genalo, M. (2007). Engaging Mexican origin families in a school-based preventive intervention. *Journal of Primary Prevention* 28: 521–46. doi: 10.1007/s10935-007-0110-z

Carroll, J. J. (2013). Key theories from critical medical anthropology for public health research. Part I: starting with Foucault: cultures of medicine and meanings of illness. *Tobacco Control and Public Health in Eastern Europe* 3: 39–46. doi: 10.6084/m9.figshare.729258

Castro, F. G., Barrera, M. J., & Steiker, L. H. (2010). Issues and challenges in the design of culturally adapted evidence-based interventions. *Annual Review of Clinical Psychology* 6: 213–39. doi: 10.1146/annurev-clinpsy-033109-132032

Dahl, G. B., & Lochner, L. (2012). The impact of family income on child achievement: evidence from the earned income tax credit. *American Economic Review* 102: 1927–56. doi: 10.3386/w14599

Earnshaw, V. A., Bogart, L. M., Dovidio, J. F., & Williams, D. R. (2013). Stigma and racial/ethnic HIV disparities: moving toward resilience. *American Psychologist* 68: 225–36. doi: 10.1037/a0032705

Fang, L., & Schinke, S. P. (2014). Mediation effects of a culturally generic substance use prevention program for Asian American adolescents. *Asian American Journal of Psychology* 5: 116–25. doi: 10.1037/a0035928

Flynn, M. A., Check, P., Eggerth, D. E., & Tonda, J. (2013). Improving occupational safety and health among Mexican immigrant workers: a binational collaboration. *Industrial Health* 48: 231–5. doi: 10.2486/indhealth.48.231

Gebremariam, M., Bjune, G., & Frich, J. (2011). Lay beliefs of TB and TB/HIV co-infection in Addis Ababa, Ethiopia: a qualitative study. *BMC Research Notes* 4: 277. doi: 10.1186/1756-0500-4-277

Gerend, M. A., Zapata, C., & Reyes, E. (2013). Predictors of human papillomavirus vaccination among daughters of low-income Latina mothers: the role of acculturation. *Journal of Adolescent Health* 53: 623–9. doi: 10.1016/j.jadohealth.2013.06.006

Goodman, L. A., Liang, B., Helms, J. E., Latta, R. E., Sparks, E., & Weintraub, S. (2004). Major contribution: training counseling psychologists as social justice agents: feminist and multicultural theories in action. *Counseling Psychologist* 32: 793–837. doi: 10.1177/0011000004268802

Gosin, M., Dustman, P., Drapeau, A., & Harthun, M. (2003). Participatory action research: creating an effective prevention curriculum for adolescents in the southwestern US. *Health Education Research* 18: 363–79. doi: 10.1093/her/cyf026

Gosin, M., Marsiglia, F. F., & Hecht, M. L. (2003). Keepin' it REAL: a drug resistance curriculum tailored to the strengths and needs of pre-adolescents of the Southwest. *Journal of Drug Education* 33: 119–42. doi: 10.2190/dxb9-1v2p-c27j-v69v

Grau, L. E., Krasnoselskikh, T. V., Shaboltas, A. V., Skochilov, R. V., Kozlov, A. P., & Abdala, N. (2013). Cultural adaptation of an intervention to reduce sexual risk behaviors among patients attending a STI clinic in St. Petersburg, Russia. *Prevention Science* 14: 400–10. doi: 10.1007_s11121-012-0301-6

Hage, S. M., Romano, J. L., Conyne, R. K., Kenny, M., Matthews, C., Schwartz, J. P., & Waldo, M. (2007). Best practice guidelines on prevention practice, research, training, and social advocacy for psychologists. *Counseling Psychologist* 35: 493–566. doi: 10.1177/0011000006291411

Hanibuchi, T., Nakaya, T., Honjo, K., Ikeda, A., Iso, H., Inoue, M., Sawada, N., & Tsugane, S. (2015). Neighborhood contextual factors for smoking among middle-aged Japanese: a multilevel analysis. *Health & Place* 31: 17–23. doi: 10.1016/j.healthplace.2014.10.010

Harper, G. W. (2007). Sex isn't that simple: culture and context in HIV prevention interventions for gay and bisexual male adolescents. *American Psychologist* 62: 803–19. doi: 10.1037/0003-066x.62.8.806

Harthun, M. L., Dustman, P. A., Reeves, L. J., Hecht, M. L., & Marsiglia, F. F. (2008). Culture in the classroom: developing teacher proficiency in delivering a culturally-grounded prevention curriculum. *Journal of Primary Prevention* 29: 435–54. doi: 10.1007/s10935-008-0150-z

Hecht, M., & Krieger, J. (2006). The principle of cultural grounding in school-based substance abuse prevention: the drug resistance strategies project. *Journal of Language and Social Psychology* 25: 301–19. doi: 10.1177/0261927X06289476

Hecht, M. L., Marsiglia, F. F., Elek, E., Wagstaff, D. A., Kulis, S., & Dustman, P. (2003). Culturally-grounded substance use prevention: an evaluation of the Keepin' It REAL curriculum. *Prevention Science* 4: 233–48. doi: 10.1023/A:1026016131401

Helm, S., & Okamoto, S. (2013). Developing the Ho'ouna Pono substance use prevention curriculum: collaborating with Hawaiian youth and communities. *Hawai'i Journal of Medicine & Public Health: A Journal of Asia Pacific Medicine & Public Health* 72: 66–9.

Hong, S., Zhang, W., & Walton, E. (2014). Neighborhoods and mental health: exploring ethnic density, poverty, and social cohesion among Asian Americans and Latinos. *Social Science & Medicine* 111: 117–24. doi: 10.1016/j.socscimed.2014.04.014

Hook, J. N., Davis, D. E., Owen, J., Worthington, Jr., E. L., & Utsey, S. O. (2013). Cultural humility: measuring openness to culturally diverse clients. *Journal of Counseling Psychology* 60: 353–66. doi: 10.1037/a0032595

Hussey, J. M., Hallfors, D. D., Waller, M. W., Iritani, B. J., Halpern, C. T., & Bauer, D. J. (2007). Sexual behavior and drug use among Asian and Latino adolescents: association with immigrant status. *Journal of Immigrant Minority Health* 9: 85–94. doi: 10.1007/s10903-006-9020-z

Ibaraki, A. Y., Hall, G. N. C., & Sabin, J. A. (2014) Asian American cancer disparities: the potential effects of model minority health stereotypes. *Asian American Journal of Psychology* 5: 75–81. doi: 10.1037/a0036114

Jason, L. A., Keys, C. B., Suarez-Balcazar, Y. E., Taylor, R. R., & Davis, M. I. (2004). *Participatory Community Research: Theories and Methods in Action*. Washington, DC: American Psychological Association. doi: dx.doi.org/10.1037/10726-000

Johnston, L. D., O'Malley, P. M., Bachman, J. G., Schulenberg, J. E., & Miech, R. A. (2014). Demographic subgroup trends among adolescents in the use of various licit and illicit drugs, 1975–2013. Monitoring the Future Occasional Paper 81. Ann Arbor: Institute for Social Research, University of Michigan.

Kann, L., Kinchen, S., Shanklin, S. L., Flint, K. H., Kawkins, J., Harris, W. A., & Zaza, S. (2014). Youth risk behavior surveillance – United States, 2013. *Morbidity and Mortality Weekly Report. Surveillance Summaries*. 63 (supplement 4): 1–168.

Katz-Wise, S. L., & Hyde, J. S. (2012). Victimization experiences of lesbian, gay, and bisexual individuals: a meta-analysis. *Journal of Sex Research* 49: 142–67. doi: 10.1080/00224499.2011.637247

Kenny, M. E., & Hage, S. M. (2009). The next frontier: prevention as an instrument of social justice. *Journal of Primary Prevention* 30: 1–10. doi: 10.1007/s10935-008-0163-7

Kucik, J. E., Nembhard, W. N., Donohue, P., Devine, O., Wang, Y., Minkovitz, C. S., & Burke, T. (2014). Community socioeconomic disadvantage and the survival of infants with congenital heart defects. *American Journal of Public Health* 104: 150–7. doi: 10.2105/AJPH.2014.302099

Kumpfer, K. L., Alvarado, R., Smith, P., & Bellamy, N. (2002). Cultural sensitivity and adaptation in family-based prevention interventions. *Prevention Science* 3: 241–6.

LaCroix, J. M., Snyder, L. B., Huedo-Medina, T. B., & Johnson, B. T. (2014). Effectiveness of mass media interventions for HIV prevention, 1986–2013: a meta-analysis. *Journal of Acquired Immune Deficiency Syndromes* 66: S329–S340. doi: 10.1097/qai.0000000000000230

Lafromboise, T., & Lewis, H. (2008). The Zuni Life Skills Development Program: a school/community-based suicide prevention intervention: advancing prevention research on the role of culture in suicide prevention. *Suicide & Life-Threatening Behavior* 38: 343–53. doi: 10.1521/suli.2008.38.3.343

Lau, A. S. (2006). Making the case for selective and directed cultural adaptations of evidence-based treatments: examples from parent training. *Clinical Psychology: Science and Practice* 13: 295–310. doi: 10.1111/j.14682850.2006.00042.x?journalCode=cpsp

Lee, S., Chen, L., He, X., Miller, M. J., & Juon, H. S. (2013). A cluster analytic examination of acculturation and health status among Asian Americans in the Washington DC metropolitan area, United States. *Social Science & Medicine* 96: 17–23. doi: 10.1016/j.socscimed.2013.07.007

Lee, H. K., Han, B., & Gfroerer, J. C. (2013). Differences in the prevalence rates and correlates of alcohol use and binge alcohol use among five Asian American subpopulations. *Addictive Behaviors* 38: 1816–23. doi: 10.1016/j.addbeh.2012.11.001

Lee, I., Pratto, F., & Li, M. (2007). Social relationships and sexism in the United States and Taiwan. *Journal of Cross-Cultural Psychology* 38: 595–612. doi: 10.1177/0022022107305241

Lemus, S., Navarro, L., Velásquez, M. J., Ryan, E., & Megías, J. L. (2014). From sex to gender: a university intervention to reduce sexism in Argentina, Spain, and El Salvador. *Journal of Social Issues* 70: 741–62. doi: 10.1111/josi.12089

Lipsicas, C. B., Mäkinen, I. H., Apter, A., Leo, D. D., Kerkhof, A., Lönnqvist, J., & Wasserman, D. (2012). Attempted suicide among immigrants in European countries: an international perspective. *Social Psychiatry and Psychiatric Epidemiology* 47: 241–51. doi: 10.1007/s00127-010-0336-6

Maffini, C. S., & Wong, Y. J. (2014). Assessing somatization with Asian American clients. In Benuto, L. T., Thaler, N., & Leany, B. (eds.), *Guide to Psychological Assessment with Asian Americans*. New York: Springer. doi: 10.1007/978-1-4939-0796-0_22

Marsiglia, F. F., & Daley, J. M. (2002). Latinos participating in multiethnic coalitions to prevent substance abuse: a case study. *Journal of Human Behavior in the Social Environment* 5: 97–121. doi: 10.1300/j137v05n03_06

Montgomery, A. E., Metraux, S., & Culhane, D. (2013). Rethinking homelessness prevention among persons with serious mental illness. *Social Issues and Policy Review* 7: 58–82. doi: 10.1111/j.1751-2409.2012.01043.x

Mrazek, P. J., & Haggerty, R. J. (eds.). (1994). *Reducing Risks for Mental Disorders: Frontiers for Preventive Intervention Research*. Washington, DC: National Academy Press. doi: 10.1002/hpm.4740100216

Neville, H., & Mobley, M. (2001). Social identities in contexts: an ecological model of multicultural counseling psychology processes. *Counseling Psychologist* 29: 471–86. doi: 10.1177/0011000001294001

Niederdeppe, J., & Levy, A. G. (2007). Fatalistic beliefs about cancer prevention and three prevention behaviors. *Cancer Epidemiology, Biomarkers & Prevention* 16: 998–1003. doi: 10.1158/1055-9965.epi-06–0608

Oh, H. Y., & DeVylder, J. E. (2014). Mental health correlates of past homelessness in Latinos and Asians. *Community Mental Health Journal* 50: 953–9. doi: dx.doi.org/10.1007/s10597-014-9721-z

Okamoto, S. K., Kulis, S., Marsiglia, F. F., Holleran Steiker, L. K., & Dustman, P. (2014). A continuum of approaches toward developing culturally focused prevention interventions: from adaptation to grounding. *Journal of Primary Prevention* 35: 103–12. doi: 10.1007/s10935-013-0334-z

Paluck, E. L., & Green, D. P. (2009). Prejudice reduction: what works? A critical look at evidence from the field and the laboratory. *Annual Review of Psychology* 60: 339–67.

Pantin, H., Schwartz, S. J., Sullivan, S., Prado, G., & Szapocznik, J. (2004). Ecodevelopmental HIV prevention programs for Hispanic adolescents. *American Journal of Orthopsychiatry* 74: 545–58. doi: 10.1037/0002-9432.74.4.545

Peña, J. B., Zayas, L. H., Cabrera-Nguyen, P., & Vega, W. A. (2012). U.S. cultural involvement and its association with suicidal behavior among youths in the Dominican Republic. *American Journal of Public Health* 102: 664–71. doi: 10.2105/ajph.2011.300344

Pieterse, A. L., Todd, N. R., Neville, H. A., & Carter, R. T. (2012). Perceived racism and mental health among black American adults: a meta-analytic review. *Journal of Counseling Psychology* 59: 1–9. doi: 10.1037/a0026208

Prilleltensky, I., & Nelson, G. (2013). Critical psychology, prevention, and social justice. In Vera, E. (ed.), *The Oxford Handbook of Prevention in Counseling Psychology*. New York: Oxford University Press, pp. 141–59. doi: 10.1093/oxfordhb/9780195396423.013.0010

Randolph, W., & Viswanath, K. (2004). Lessons learned from public health mass media campaigns: marketing health in a crowded media world. *Annual Review of Public Health* 25: 419–37. doi: 10.1146/annurev.publhealth.25.101802.123046

Rawls, J. (1971). *A Theory of Justice*. Cambridge, MA: Harvard University Press.

Reese, L. E., & Vera, E. M. (2007). Culturally relevant prevention programs: scientific and practical considerations. *Counseling Psychologist* 35: 763–78. doi: 10.1177/0011000007304588

Reiss, K., Breckenkamp, J., Borde, T., Brenne, S., David, M., & Razum, O. (2014). Smoking during pregnancy among Turkish immigrants in Germany: are there associations with acculturation? *Nicotine & Tobacco Research*. doi: 10.1093/ntr/ntu237

Romano, J. L. (2015). *Prevention Psychology: Enhancing Personal and Social Well-being*. Washington, DC: American Psychological Association. doi: 10.1037/14442-000

Romano, J. L., Koch, J., & Wong, Y. J. (2012). Prevention in counseling psychology: promoting education, health, and well-being across the life cycle. In Fouad, N., & Subich, L. (eds.), *Handbook of Counseling Psychology*. Washington, DC: APA Books, pp. 345–67. doi: 10.1037/13754-013

SAMHSA (Substance Abuse and Mental Health Services Administration), Center for Behavioral Health Statistics and Quality (2011). *The NSDUH Report: Substance Use among Asian Adolescents*. Rockville, MD: SAMHSA.

Santisteban, D., & Mena, M. (2009). Culturally informed and flexible family-based treatment for adolescents: a tailored and integrative treatment for Hispanic youth. *Family Process* 48: 253–68. doi: 10.1111/j.1545-5300.2009.01280.x

Schwartz, J. P., & Lindley, L. D. (2009). Impacting sexism through social justice prevention: implications at the person and environmental levels. *Journal of Primary Prevention* 30: 27–41. doi: 10.1007/s10935-008-0162-8

Schwartz, S. J., Unger, J. B., Zamboanga, B. L., & Szapocznik, J. (2010). Rethinking the concept of acculturation: Implications for theory and research. *American Psychologist* 65: 237–51. doi: 10.1037/a0019330

Shin, R. Q., & Kendall, M. A. (2013). Dropout prevention: a (re)conceptualization through the lens of social justice. In Vera, E. (ed.), *The Oxford Handbook of Prevention in Counseling Psychology*. New York: Oxford University Press, pp. 213–25.

Siqueira, L. M., & Crandall, L. A. J. (2008). Risk and protective factors for binge drinking among Hispanic subgroups in Florida. *Journal of Ethnicity in Substance Abuse* 7: 81–92. doi: 10.1080/15332640802083238

Slavin, R. E. (1995). *Cooperative Learning: Theory, Research, and Practice*. Boston: Allyn & Bacon.

Staub, E. (2013). Building a peaceful society: origins, prevention, and reconciliation after genocide and other group violence. *American Psychologist* 68: 576–89. doi: 10.1037/a0032045

Sue, D. W. (2001). Multidimensional facets of cultural competence. *Counseling Psychologist* 29: 790–821. doi: 10.1177/0011000001296002

Sue, D. W. (2010). Microaggressions, marginality and oppression. In Sue, D. W. (ed.) *Microaggressions and Marginality*. Hoboken, NJ: Wiley, pp. 3–22.

Tweed, R. G., & Lehman, D. R. (2002). Learning considered within a cultural context: Confucian and Socratic approaches. *American Psychologist* 57: 89–99. doi: 10.1037//0003-066x.57.2.89

Vera, E. M., & Kenny, M. E. (2013). *Social Justice and Culturally Relevant Prevention*. Thousand Oaks, CA: Sage. doi: 10.4135/9781452275598

Wang, S., Kou, C., Liu, Y., Li, B., Tao, Y., D'Arcy, C., & Yu, Y. (2014). Rural–urban differences in the prevalence of chronic disease in Northeast China. *Asia-Pacific Journal of Public Health*. doi: 1010539514551200

Watkins-Hayes, C. (2014). Intersectionality and the sociology of HIV/AIDS: past, present, and future research directions. *Annual Review of Sociology* 40: 431–57. doi: dx.doi.org/10.1146/annurev-soc-071312-145621

Webster, D. W., Whitehill, J. M., Vernick, J. S., & Curriero, F. C. (2013). Effects of Baltimore's Safe Streets program on gun violence: a replication of Chicago's CeaseFire program. *Journal of Urban Health* 90: 27–40. doi: 10.1007/s11524-012-9731-5

Willness, C. R., Steel, P., & Lee, K. (2007). A meta-analysis of the antecedents and consequences of workplace sexual harassment. *Personnel Psychology* 60: 127–62. doi: 10.1111/j.1744-6570.2007.00067.x

Wong, Y. J., Brownson, C., Rutkowski, L., Nguyen, C. P., & Becker, M. (2014a). A mediation model of professional psychological help seeking for suicide ideation among Asian American and white American college students. *Archives of Suicide Research* 18: 259–73. doi: 10.1080/13811118.2013.824831

Wong, Y. J., Maffini, C., & Shin, M. (2014b). The racial-cultural framework: a framework for addressing suicide-related outcomes in communities of color. *The Counseling Psychologist* 42: 13–54. doi: 10.1177/0011000012470568

Wong, Y. J., & Poon, M.-L. (2010). Counseling Asian American men who demonstrate suicidal behavior. In Liu, W. M., Iwamoto, D., & Chae, M. (eds.), *Culturally Responsive Counseling with Asian American Men*. New York: Routledge, pp. 279–98).

Wong, Y. J., Tran, K. K., Kim, S. H., Van Horn Kerne, V., & Calfa, N. A. (2010). Asian Americans' lay beliefs about depression and seeking professional help. *Journal of Clinical Psychology* 66: 317–32. doi: 10.1002/jclp.20653

Wong, Y. J., Vaughan, E. L., Liu, T., & Chang, T. K. (2014). Asian Americans' proportion of life in the United States and suicide ideation: the moderating effects of ethnicity. *Asian American Journal of Psychology* 5: 237–42. doi: 10.1037/a0033283

WHO (World Health Organization) (2014). Global status report on violence prevention. www.who.int/violence_injury_prevention/violence/status_report/2014/en/

Yoshikawa, H., Aber, J. L., & Beardslee, W. R. (2012). The effects of poverty on the mental, emotional, and behavioral health of children and youth: implications for prevention. *American Psychologist* 67: 272–84. doi: 10.1037/a0028015

Zemore, S. E. (2007) Acculturation and alcohol among Latinos in the United States: a comprehensive review. *Alcoholism: Clinical and Experimental Research* 31: 1968–90. doi: 10.1111/j.1530-0277.2007.00532.x

Methodology

7 International Standards on Drug Use Prevention

Tools to Support Policy Makers Globally to Implement an Evidence-Based Prevention Response

Giovanna Campello, Hanna Heikkila, & Wadih Maalouf

This chapter discusses the challenges faced by policy makers in applying evidence-based prevention responses, including (1) poor understanding of the etiology of the problem, (2) narrow-angled vision of the response both in terms of age groups and social settings that could be targeted, (3) multidisciplinary approach in designing an integrated system of evidence-based responses, and (4) value and cost effectiveness of prevention responses that are based on science. Moreover, this chapter contextualizes this discussion through describing the experience generated through two specific initiatives of United Nations Office on Drugs and Crime (UNODC). The first introduced initiative is "Prevention Strategy and Policy Makers," which focuses on disseminating the International Standards on Drug Use Prevention (later referred to as the Standards) and through it supporting policy makers to utilize evidence-based approaches in their prevention programming at the national level. The second initiative is "Global Piloting of Family Skills Training Programs," which operates at the program level focusing on helping national counterparts to adapt, train, pilot, and evaluate evidence-based family skills programs in different low- and middle-income countries across different geographical subregions. The lessons learned as well as implications for future action in the field of prevention are also discussed.

Introduction

Despite some remaining gaps, the science on prevention of drug use is quite established with a wealth of evidence on the effectiveness of some interventions and the lack of effectiveness of others (NIDA, 2003; UNODC, 2013). Applying this knowledge would make it possible to influence significantly the health and well-being of children, youth, and adults. Moreover, it would allow prevention of drug use to fulfill concretely its pivotal role in the context of a balanced, comprehensive, and health-centered response. Such a response would

The opinions expressed in this chapter represent those of the authors and not necessarily those of the United Nations Office on Drugs and Crime.

comprise and integrate prevention of drug use, treatment care, rehabilitation of drug dependence, and supply reduction while ensuring the access to controlled drugs for medical purposes (UNODC, 2014a).

Unfortunately, the relatively rudimentary data available as to the coverage and the quality of prevention activities implemented globally are not encouraging. UNODC collects annually data from all its 194 member states on the drug use situation in their countries, including on the prevention response. An average of 95 (close to 50 percent of all member states) respond on an annual basis to the call for data, which provide a general representation of the global response to reducing drug demand. Across the different waves of reports, evidence-based approaches are reported to be implemented in only a minority of cases. As an example, the most common prevention activity reported as having a high coverage by most member states continues to be information campaigns (UNODC, 2014b). This is despite the fact that the scientific literature regarding information campaigns indicates at best very limited effectiveness (UNODC, 2013). Furthermore, an average of 60 percent of the member states reporting annually to UNODC have never evaluated any of the prevention activities they implement. In addition, whenever applicable, most of these reported evaluations focused on assessing the process and the outcome of the intervention. The impact of prevention activities on actual substance use or on indicators predicting it has been evaluated only in 8 percent or less of cases.

This situation is of great concern on a number of accounts. Firstly, drug use remains a significant problem compromising the health, well-being, and productivity of people globally despite the availability of well-documented evidence-based prevention interventions. Moreover, prevention activities of poor coverage and quality rather than evidence-based ones mean that scarce resources are being wasted. Furthermore, prevention activities that are already known to carry iatrogenic effects or whose effectiveness or safety have not been assessed are still being implemented, which leads to a significant ethical concern.

There is a clear gap in bridging the science with practice and transferring the evidence into prevention practices worldwide, with a strong need for supporting the quality of evidence-based prevention, as well as its coverage. Member states of the United Nations have unanimously called for more evidence-based prevention on multiple occasions (Resolution 57/3) (United Nations, 2014). In this context, UNODC works to promote evidence-based prevention globally in a variety of ways, and this chapter presents and discusses the process and results of two initiatives of UNODC in this field.

The first initiative, labeled Prevention Strategy and Policy Makers, focused on systematically summarizing the globally existing evidence of what works in prevention and creating the UNODC International Standards of Drug Use Prevention (referred to later as the Standards). This initiative also works on disseminating the Standards to global policy makers facilitating evidence-based prevention planning in the different geographical regions of the world. The second initiative is the Global Piloting of Family-Skills Training Programs, UNODC's ongoing effort in systematically adapting and piloting evidence-based family skills training programs in a number of countries. Thus, while Prevention Strategy and Policy Makers disseminated basic knowledge about *all* drug prevention interventions and policy that work among *one* kind of stakeholder (policy makers), the Global Piloting of Family-Skills Training Programs focused on *one* kind of intervention (family skills training) involving *all* stakeholders (children, youth, families, facilitators, trainers, policy makers at the local and national level, local and international researchers, program developers).

These are not the only two initiatives of UNODC, nor is UNODC the only active institution either globally or regionally in this domain. However, they are the two initiatives most extensively undertaken by UNODC in drug prevention. It is hoped that the experience generated from these initiatives can provide lessons learned, and suggestions and recommendations for future actions with regard to improving the coverage and the quality of prevention, resulting in the healthy and safe development of children and youth and ultimately in improved health and well-being among entire population.

Other national and international governmental and nongovernmental institutions are contributing to the promotion of evidence-based prevention with initiatives of global relevance. These include the European Monitoring Centre on Drugs and Drug Addiction (EMCDDA); (see e.g. Burkhhart 2015), the Canadian Centre on Substance Abuse (CCSA); the Inter-American Drug Abuse Control Commission (CICAD) at the Organization of the American States; the Mentor Foundation (Mentor); the United States National Institute on Drug Abuse (NIDA); and the World Health Organization (WHO).

Prevention Strategy and Policy Makers

As mentioned previously, the specific aim of the Prevention Standards and Policy Makers initiative was to increase the capacity of national-level policy makers in planning and implementing effective and cost-effective prevention responses as recommended by the International Standards on Drug Use Prevention.

To a certain extent, policy makers represent the natural audience of focus for an organization such as UNODC that is at the service of member states. The targeted policy makers under this initiative are the ones making decisions on the types of prevention activities and implementation modalities that are supported at a national level in their respective countries. They also have a role in directing the allocation of financial resources for prevention, thus influencing the type of organizations and professional groups that are involved in prevention, as well as the contents of the prevention activities. Such policy makers have considerable influence on the prevention field via policies, guidelines, and recommendations and other support structures, such as capacity building, accreditation systems, national-level coordination structures, and support for evaluation (or lack thereof). Finally, they might be in a position to influence legislation regulating substance use prevention, for example on the marketing of legal substances (e.g., tobacco) or on prevention education implemented as part of national school curricula.

It should be noted that considerable variation exists in the way drug prevention policies and programs are planned and delivered worldwide. Many countries, but by no means all, have centralized decision-making processes, while a significant number of other countries decentralize such decisions. Moreover, there exist different levels of policy makers. While the ultimate decision is often in the hands of political appointees whose term in office might be relatively short, they are usually surrounded by, and rely on, cadres of civil servants whose term in office can often span into the long term. It is the latter group that was mostly targeted by the UNODC Prevention Strategy and Policy Makers initiative.

UNODC International Standards on Drug Use Prevention

The Standards is a document that was written on the basis of a systematic review of current scientific literature under the guidance of a globally representative group of prevention experts. The synthesis of the literature drew mainly on available systematic reviews. This was supplemented by primary studies, when additional evidence (or further geographical representative evidence) not covered by the systematic reviews was available. All studies were assessed as to their methodological soundness based on criteria developed with the support of a group of over eighty scientists and governmental experts representing the different subfields of prevention research as well as different geographical regions. The Standards also build on and recognize the work of many other organizations (e.g., EMCDDA, CCSA, CICAD, Mentor International, NIDA, WHO) that have previously developed standards and guidelines on various aspects of drug prevention, such as on quality of process (EMCDDA, 2011), or on specific subfields, such as school-based prevention (CCSA, 2010) (see also Burkhart, 2015).

The Standards encompass all interventions and policies aimed at delaying or avoiding the onset of substance use at early ages or preventing substance abuse or the transition to substance use disorders. This covers all psychoactive substances regardless of their legal or controlled status (nationally or internationally). The Standards emphasize the importance of targeting different age groups in an age-appropriate manner. They also present an overview covering all the important social settings where prevention interventions could be applied, by adopting a developmental perspective to prevention and framing prevention in support for the general developmental and socialization processes. The Standards outline the most important developmental goals for each developmental stage for contextualizing the rationale for prevention interventions and policies that are described age group by age group. Finally, the standards as well as the related capacity building processes highlight the positive effect of evidence-based substance use prevention as an investment in healthy and safe development, promoting a healthy lifestyle and also preventing many other risky behaviors across age groups and beyond substance use.

On the basis of the systematic review of the evidence, the Standards list and describe interventions and policies that have been found to be efficacious in preventing drug use and substance abuse. For each strategy, a short description of the main activities and theoretical basis is provided, together with the available evidence and the characteristics that appear to be linked to positive, negative, or no prevention outcomes. Prevention issues requiring further research are also briefly addressed, including interventions and policies for which no acceptable quality evidence was found, such as utilizing sport in prevention or strategies targeting particularly vulnerable children.

Finally, to support the planning and implementation of the evidence-based prevention strategies, the Standards also give an overview of the possible components for an effective national prevention system and of the supporting structures it requires. This is another area where further research is urgently needed. The investigations have traditionally focused more on the effectiveness of single interventions and policies. Therefore, besides the available evidence, this section of the Standards relied heavily on the consensus among the group of experts involved. The Standards describe effective national drug prevention systems as delivering an integrated range of interventions and policies based on scientific evidence in multiple settings, targeting relevant ages and levels of risk, and being sustained over time. The planning of such systems should respond to the complex interplay of factors that make children, youth, and adults alike vulnerable to substance abuse and other risky behaviors. This system should also correspond to the particular context, situation, and available resources where these vulnerabilities exist.

To deliver such an integrated range of prevention interventions and policies effectively, strong structural foundations are required. These include supportive policy and legal frameworks, scientific evidence, research and data-collection systems, coordination of multiple sectors and levels (national, subnational, and municipal/local), and training of policy makers and practitioners, as well as providing adequate resources and sustaining the system over the long term. In this context, the Prevention Strategy and Policy Makers initiative can be seen as an important contribution to building stronger drug prevention systems worldwide in the form of building the capacity of policy makers at the national level.

Implementation of Prevention Standards and Policy Makers

The initiative was implemented between mid-2013 and the end of 2014 via a series of regional three-day training seminars and some related follow-up communications. It trained over 250 national policy makers from 60 different countries in Central America, the Middle East, northern Africa, eastern Africa, southeastern Europe, Central Asia, and East Asia. The capacity-building process targeted policy makers and civil servants who are in charge of the planning and implementation of drug use prevention activities and policies in the different governmental sectors in their respective countries at the national level.

National governments were invited to nominate two to four policy makers from different sectors. The nominations normally included representation from the different governmental sectors in charge of drug use prevention in the given country, such as the ministries of health, education, social welfare, youth, or the interior. These cross-sectional delegations allowed for multidisciplinary perspectives for the discussions in the training and, most importantly, for networking not only between the countries but also within the countries (across the multiple sectors and organizations involved in prevention). This provided excellent opportunities for looking at the current and the potential prevention activities in the countries from a broader perspective (including different settings and target groups) as well as for planning improvement for the coordination, planning, and evaluation of the prevention activities at the national level. The seminars were all regional with the exception of the seminar in Nigeria, where UNODC had the opportunity to work with more than twenty policy makers and some nongovernmental organization (NGO) managers from a wide range of sectors all from one country.

The seminar was designed to be conducted within three days in an effort to balance the need to deliver all content deemed important to guide policy makers while ensuring that the duration of the training would not impede the attendance of the needed participants. In addition to these training seminars, UNODC had the possibility to deliver shorter (one-day) sessions introducing the Standards to various governmental stakeholders (in Brazil, Iran, Israel, and Russia). The following analysis only summarizes the information generated through the three-day regional meetings.

In addition to the Standards document, the training seminar relied on the following tools, which were also developed with the assistance of leading researchers:

1. Introduction to the etiology of drug use and substance abuse.
2. A series of participatory exercises focusing on the etiology of drug use and substance abuse, the methodology of development of the Standards, as well as what constitutes evidence-based practice and how to use media for drug use prevention in the most effective way possible.
3. A series of guiding PowerPoint presentations summarizing the same topics mentioned under point 2, as well as the effective intervention and policies included in the Standards, by age group, and the main component of an effective national drug prevention system.
4. Basic tools and participatory exercises to guide the discussion in the national groups, critically reflecting on the current coverage and quality of drug prevention and planning an improvement response.

These tools were translated when necessary to Arabic, Chinese, French, Russian, and Spanish and were provided to participants in an electronic format and used during the training.

The first day of the seminar was opened by a keynote speaker, who generally introduced prevention science, the Standards, and the Prevention Strategy and

Policy Makers initiative. Following that, the first day of the seminar comprised a series of sessions each including both a participatory component and a presentation on the following topics: the etiology of drug use and substance use, the methodology of developing the Standards, the definition of evidence-based practice, an overview of the effective drug prevention interventions and policies included in the Standards, and the use of media for drug use prevention in the most effective way possible. During the first day, the group work was conducted in mixed national groups, thus supporting wider regional networking among the participants.

During the second day of the seminar, sessions were organized within the context of a developmental framework, and each of the sessions focused on a specific age group. Each session described the interventions and policies found to be effective in preventing drug use and substance abuse targeting that age period. To better contextualize these interventions and policies and their rationale, a summary of the key developmental goals, and most common vulnerability factors for each of targeted age period, was also presented. In addition, the characteristics that have been associated with positive outcomes, or with no or iatrogenic outcomes, were highlighted under each strategy.

Following this, in each of the sessions, participants were divided into national groups, in which they discussed the coverage and quality of their existing national prevention systems and compared them to the ones that the Standards suggest. This was also contrasted in light of the resources, stakeholders, and most important factors of vulnerability present in their countries. As a result, they identified initiatives and activities that might be useful in improving the situation in their respective countries. Working within these national groups, the participants were able to combine their insights coming from the perspective of different fields and governmental sectors.

Finally, during the third day, the national delegations worked to combine the planned improvements for each specific age group into a coherent and comprehensive plan for improving the drug prevention system, aimed to cover the entire developmental span of children, youth, and adults. These plans also integrated improvements for the support structures of the national drug prevention systems, such as training, evaluation, data collection, and regulatory frameworks. The national delegations were encouraged to prioritize at least one short- or long-term goal per age in order to create more realistic and achievable "road maps." All delegations had the possibility to present the results of their work and receive feedback.

The seminar provided participants with an opportunity to share experiences on current national policies and best practices in drug use prevention with the other countries from the same region. Following the seminars, in some cases it was possible to arrange teleconferences among the national delegations, the UNODC field offices, and the UNODC headquarters to support further the development and realization of the national action plans developed during the seminar as well as networking between the national parties.

The seminar consisted of sessions that were regarded as core and mandatory for the full comprehension of the subject matter, and these were delivered in all training seminars. These were (in chronological order) the etiology presentation and workgroup; the evidence-based prevention presentation and workgroup; the media in prevention presentation; the early childhood interventions presentation and national workgroup; the middle childhood interventions presentation and national workgroup; the early adolescence interventions presentation and national workgroup; the adolescence and adulthood interventions presentation and national workgroup; and the presentation on national drug prevention system and related workgroup to build a comprehensive plan for improvement. In addition, the training had sessions that clarified the contents and allowed for more detailed and practical-level discussions, and these were delivered only whenever feasible, and so due to the local circumstances (such as translation or other time restraints), on average only half of the non-core sessions were delivered during the training seminars. This distinction between core and non-core sessions was maintained in order to ensure a fidelity in the delivery of the training.

Short-Term Outcomes of Prevention Strategy and Policy Makers

The short-term impact of the seminars was assessed through anonymous evaluation questionnaires completed by the participants before and after the three days of seminars, and out of the total of 250 participants 208 completed both the preseminar and the postseminar questionnaires.

The questionnaires included questions on the background and work responsibilities of the participants, on their understanding and opinions about substance use and substance use prevention, as well as on feedback about the training seminars. They were translated as necessary to facilitate accurate understanding of questions. The aim of the assessment was to analyze possible changes in participants' perceptions and opinions resulting from attending the seminars. This helped to draw conclusions about the short-term impact of the seminars. The main findings follow.

Only half of the participants (53 percent out of 208) reported through the preseminar questionnaire ever receiving any formal training on prevention of substance use. This was despite the fact that on average, the participants had seven years of service in their current position, where in the majority of cases substance use prevention was central to their role (see Figure 7.1). Practically all of the participants (97 percent) stated they would find such training useful. This further supported the view that there is a great demand for such capacity-building efforts targeting policy makers in the field of prevention.

The mean score change in perceptions on effectiveness of prevention of alcohol and drug prevention programs in different age groups was measured through a Likert scale ranging from 1 (very effective) to 3 (ineffective) pre- and postseminar and presented in Table 7.1.

It is interesting to note that both before and after the seminars, participants deemed prevention interventions and policies to be most effective when targeting

Table 7.1 *Mean Score of Perception of Effectiveness of Prevention Targeting Different Age Groups across the Regions (on Scale 1 = Very Effective, 2 = Somewhat Effective, 3 = Ineffective)*

Targeted age group	Pretest (N = 208) Mean (SD)	Posttest (N = 219) Mean (SD)
Infancy and early childhood	2.16 (0.59)	2.01 (0.78)
Middle childhood	1.81 (0.75)	1.69 (0.7)
Early adolescence	1.52 (0.65)	1.44 (0.67)
Late adolescence and adulthood	1.65 (0.69)	1.50 (0.62)

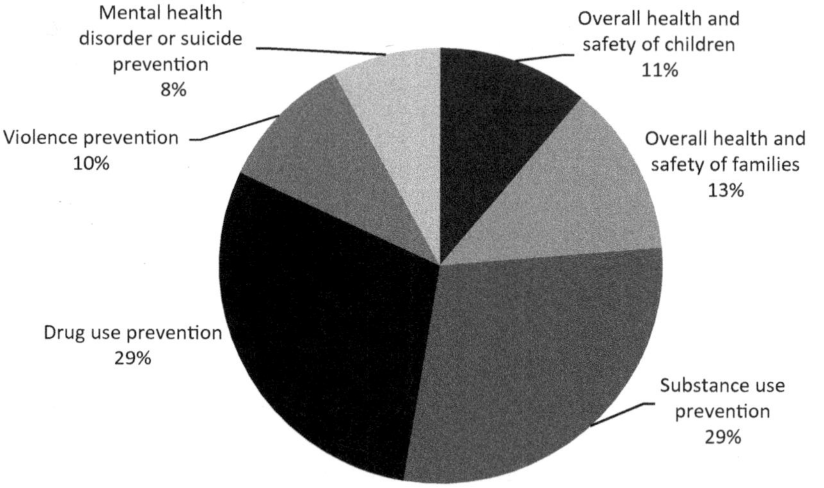

Figure 7.1. *Objectives of the current position held by Prevention Strategy and Policy Makers seminar participants (n = 208).*

early adolescents. This was true despite slight differences across regions with the mean of the perceived effectiveness of prevention targeting the age group of early adolescents ranging from 1.16 in Southeast Asia to 2.38 in Central America. The postseminar results indicated that the training appeared to influence the perceptions on the effectiveness of prevention favorably across age groups. In other words, the seminars increased participants' perceptions of the effectiveness of evidence-based prevention across the target age groups. As one of the main goals of the seminars was to encourage the national-level policy makers to support more evidence-based prevention and to increase its reach and coverage, these results seem encouraging and suggest a potential change in the right direction, as discussed in the conclusions of this chapter.

To further detail the change in perceptions of effectiveness, participants were also asked about their perceptions of the effectiveness of different types of prevention approaches within each age group. For each age group, a menu of different possible prevention interventions was provided in the pre- and post-questionnaires, out of which the participants were asked to rank the three most effective in their opinion. In the analysis, 3 points were assigned to the approach deemed most effective, 2 points for the one deemed second in effectiveness, and 1 point for the third most effective approach. Participants ranking more than three interventions per age group were excluded from the analysis. Accordingly, an average of twenty policy makers (11 percent) were excluded per age group of analysis for meeting this exclusion criteria. The scores were tallied for interventions having good or adequate quality of efficacy for preventing substance use according to the Standards and for interventions having only limited or no evidence on efficacy. In order to assess change in knowledge, such segregation of level of effectiveness was done during the analysis and naturally not available to the policy makers completing the questionnaires.

To assess the change in perceptions of effectiveness, the mean score for each group of interventions (group 1, interventions and policies with good evidence of effectiveness; and group 2, interventions and policies with no or limited evidence of effectiveness) was calculated in each age category. A chi square analysis indicated a significant change in mean scores from pretest to posttest and in each groups of interventions (evidence-based and nonevidence-based). This difference was significant at the level of 0.01. The analyses were additionally done separately for each targeted age group, as well as for the evidence-based and nonevidence-based interventions and policies.

After pooling the data of all policy makers receiving the seminar and regardless of the age group of the interventions, a significant ($p < 0.05$) increase in perceived effectiveness of evidence-based interventions was noted from pretest to posttest. Moreover, a statistically significant reduction ($p < 0.05$) in the perception of effectiveness of interventions with no or poor evidence of effectiveness was also recorded in the posttest. This change was true across the regions, despite minor fluctuations (see Figure 7.2 and Table 7.2).

Before the three-day training seminar participants ranked the approaches having no or only limited evidence on efficacy higher, perceiving them as more effective than the evidence-based approaches. This was consistent across the age groups and the regions. After the seminar, these perceptions on effective types of interventions had changed, and the participants were better able to recognize evidence-based approaches, rating the evidence-based approaches higher than the approaches with no or limited evidence on efficacy. This crossing over of the value score, reflecting perception of effectiveness across these two types of interventions, is a rewarding outcome of the seminar. These changes have potential for significant practical implications, as it is conceivable that in the future at least some of the targeted policy makers might shift their support from strategies with little or no evidence of efficacy to strategies with adequate or good evidence.

As an illustration detailing this change of perception, Figure 7.3 shows the perceived effectiveness score by individual interventions and policies for middle childhood. A significant shift has been noted for the score provided for each

Table 7.2 *Pre- and Posttest Change in Perceived Effectiveness* of Prevention Strategies across Ages, by Level of Scientific Evidence, as Classified in the Standards*

Age Group	Efficacy of Interventions	% of Maximum Score Preseminar (N = 170–183)	% of Maximum Score Postseminar (N = 187–196)	X^2 p-value
Middle Childhood	Interventions and policies with **good or adequate** evidence of efficacy[1]	55.0	75.0	< 0.01
	Interventions and policies with **limited or no** evidence on efficacy[1]	41.7	23.3	< 0.01
Early Adolescents	Interventions and policies with **good or adequate** evidence of efficacy[1]	41.6	61.6	< 0.01
	Interventions and policies with **limited or no** evidence on efficacy[1]	55.0	36.6	< 0.01
Late Adolescence and Adulthood	Interventions and policies with **good or adequate** evidence of efficacy[1]	30.0	46.6	< 0.01
	Interventions and policies with **limited or no** evidence on efficacy[1]	66.6	36.6	< 0.01
All Age Groups Combined	Interventions and policies with **good or adequate** evidence of efficacy[2]	42.2	61.1	< 0.01
	Interventions and policies with **limited or no** evidence on efficacy[2]	55.0	37.7	< 0.01

*% of maximum total score
[1]Maximum possible score 6.
[2]Maximum possible score 18.

intervention, reducing the perceived effectiveness of those having no or limited evidence of effectiveness (such as information in schools or raising awareness) and increasing the perceived effectiveness of interventions and policies with good evidence of effectiveness (particularly family-based programs). As some of the nonevidence-based programs bear a risk of iatrogenic outcomes, the potential practical implications are important.

Finally, as an elemental step in achieving a change in the commitment of the national policy makers to invest in evidence-based prevention, it was deemed necessary to increase their understanding not just in evidence-based prevention as such but also in the science upon which it is based. Accordingly, the training

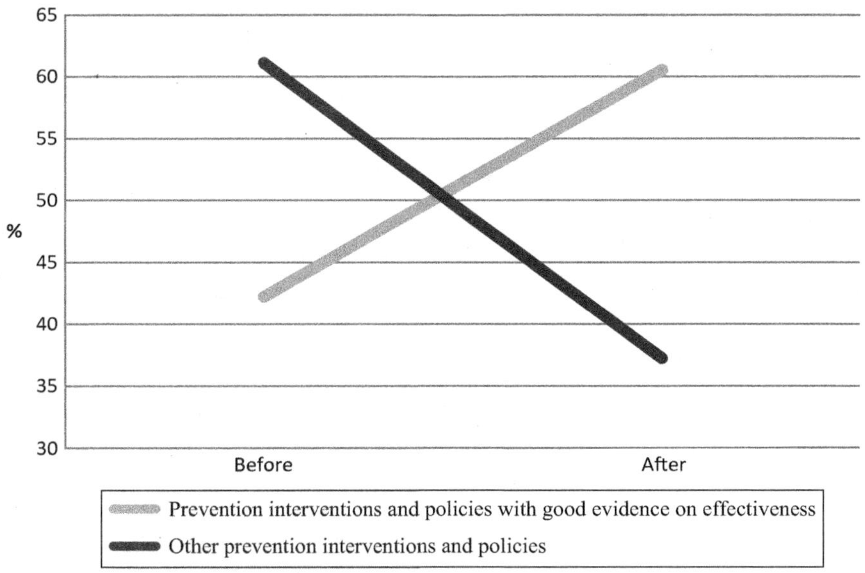

Figure 7.2. *Pre- and posttest change in perceived effectiveness* of prevention strategies across ages, by level of scientific evidence (n = 208).*

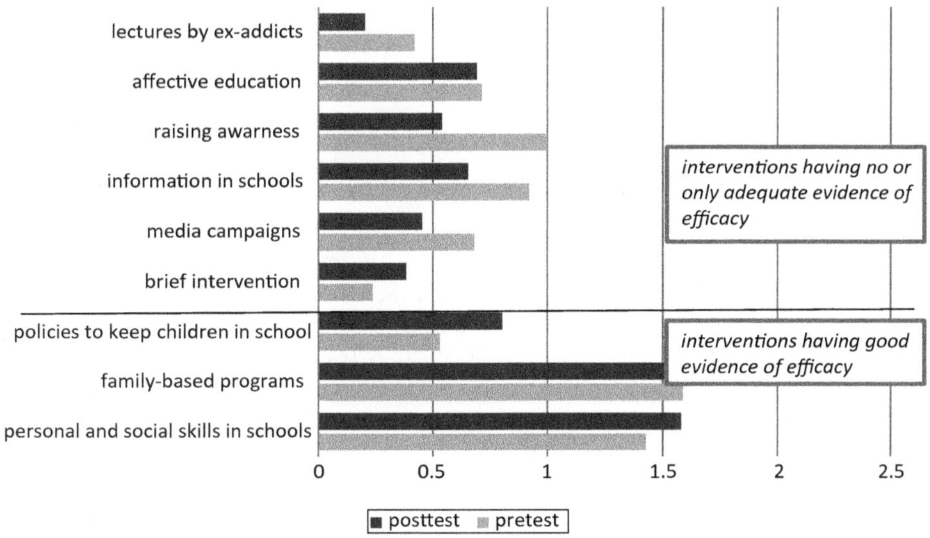

Figure 7.3. *Changes in perceived effectiveness of different prevention approaches targeting middle childhood*

included also in its first day introduction to the etiology of substance use and during the second day summaries of the most important developmental goals for each of the targeted age groups. For further insight, the participants were provided with a background paper (in most cases translated) on etiology. Despite the relatively limited content, as a result of these presentation, a shift in the participants' understanding of the causes of drug use was found at the end

Table 7.3 *Three Most Identified Causes of Drug Use as Identified by Participants before (n = 208) and after (n = 219) the Seminar*

	Causes of Drug Use	%
Before	Poor parenting (e.g., lack of supervision, teaching, role modeling, involvement, etc.)	49
	Lack of awareness and knowledge	48
	Bad parenting (e.g., mistreatment, abuse, neglect, parental substance addiction, etc.) and family dysfunction	45
After	Poor parenting (e.g., lack of supervision, teaching, role modeling, involvement, etc.)	68
	Bad parenting (e.g., mistreatment, abuse, neglect, parental substance addiction, etc.) and family dysfunction	52
	Accessibility and availability of illicit drug use	42

of the seminar (from pretest to posttest). Both pre- and postquestionnaire included a question that asked respondents to select the most significant causes of drug use in their countries out of a list of sixteen possible options. Table 7.3 presents the three most important factors for substance abuse, as identified by the policy makers before and after the seminar

As seen in Table 7.3, before the seminar the policy makers perceived poor or bad parenting and lack of awareness and knowledge as the reasons for substance abuse, while after the seminar they indicated accessibility – rather than lack of awareness and knowledge – as a significant risk factor and also perceived parenting, especially poor parenting, as an even more significant reason explaining substance abuse. This subtle shift in paradigm fits well with the changes observed in the types of prevention interventions and policies that the participants regarded as the most effective ones, before and after the seminar. As described previously, after the seminar participants tended to regard parenting and skills-based interventions as more effective and purely information-based approaches as less effective ones. These changes in the understanding of the underlying factors explaining substance use fit also well with the anecdotal information received via the follow-up communications, where some participants reported changes occurring in their national prevention systems toward more evidence-based practices after the seminar.

The participants valued very positively the participation in the training seminar as it carried practical impact on and applicability to their work. When provided with a scale of 1 (least useful) to 5 (most useful) to rate each of the training components, the average score per component was on average greater than 4. The recognition of the value of the training was further detailed in the qualitative feedback, where participants identified the essence of evidence-based prevention programming – that is, understanding of the etiology, the science behind and the contents of evidence-based prevention – as one of the most valuable components of training. The second most useful outcome of the training was making possible national-level discussions on priorities and supportive structures that could facilitate the adoption of a revised evidence-based prevention strategy inspired by the

Standards. Moreover, participants started to put further importance and value on the evaluation components of the prevention response. Guidance on how to monitor and evaluate prevention interventions and policies was the most common request for future follow-up training. The second most frequent request was guidance on how to implement specific interventions and policies in practice. Both requests are positive indications of a change in attitude and an affinity to quality implementation of prevention interventions.

The main concerns reported by the participants to implement higher-quality prevention were lack of resources, lack of cooperation between all key stakeholders, and cultural barriers. The experience of UNODC in providing technical assistance on how to directly pilot an evidence-based program as detailed in the following section for the second initiative, Global Piloting of Family Skills Training Program, provided an indirect response to these concerns.

Global Piloting of Family Skills Training Programs

One type of the interventions described in the International Standards of Drug Use Prevention with "very good" indication of efficacy is family-based programs. These programs in essence support caregivers in being better parents and strengthen positive age-specific and age-appropriate family functioning and interactions in general. They promote a warm child-rearing style, where parents set rules for acceptable behaviors, closely monitor free time and friendship patterns, and become good role models while helping their children to acquire skills to make informed decisions (UNODC, 2013). These programs have been found to be effective in preventing drug use and substance abuse as well as a range of other risky behaviors (UNODC, 2009).

One of the behaviors positively impacted by these family skills programs is reduction of violence (Maalouf & Campello, 2014; WHO, 2010), and WHO, in its series of briefings on the existing evidence for violence prevention, listed "increasing safe, stable and nurturing relationships between children and their parents and caregivers" as one of the seven main strategies for preventing interpersonal and self-directed violence (WHO, 2010). The physical and mental health of children is also directly impacted by the quality of parenting they receive (UNODC, 2010). Parenting skill programs have been shown to impact healthy parenting practice positively (Cooper et al., 2009; Knerr, Garder, & Cluver, 2013; Rahman, Iqbal, Roberts, & Hussain, 2009). Along these lines as well, parenting programs that focus on communication show promising results in the field of discussing risky sexual practices and protective measures (Wight & Fullerton, 2013). The UNODC compilation of evidence-based family skills programmed outlines also how these programs could carry a positive effect on the mental well-being of parents in the form of reduced parental stress, or reduced occupational stress, while supporting the development of children in terms of reducing behavioral and emotional problems (such as anxiety, internalizing behaviors, and social withdrawal) and raising self-esteem (UNODC, 2009, 2010).

From an educational outcome perspective, family and parenting skills training should be considered as one of the primary means by which positive student development and academic success can be fostered (Biglan et al., 1997; Zins, Weissberg, Wang, & Walberg, 2004). Voluminous research supports the important role of parents, family, and community in determining young people's academic success in schools (Coombes, Allen, & McCall, 2012). Parents generating positive social goals in children promote attachment to school, and studies show a direct link to academic success (Denham & Weissberg, 2004; Spoth, Randall, & Chin, 2008).

The majority of these evidence-based programs were predominantly designed and conceived in the United States. However, others with well-documented evidence have also been designed in other nations, such as Australia (Positive Parenting Programme, or Triple P [Sanders, 1999]; Parents under Pressure [Dawe & Harnett, 2007]; and Resilient Families [Shortt, Toumbourou, & Chapman, 2006]) and Canada (Stop Now and Plan, or SNAP; Koegl, Farrington, Augimeri, & Day, 2008). Moreover, most of these programs have been adapted, replicated, and piloted outside their country of origin with successful outcomes (UNODC, 2010). While most of these rigorously evaluated replications remain from high-income countries, other implementations (very few having strong methodological design) have also occurred in Africa, Asia, the Middle East, and Latin America (Meija, Ulph, & Calam, 2014). Nevertheless, such replications with positive results support the wider application of such rigorously designed programs when implemented with fidelity.

In November 2009, UNODC launched an initiative for Global Piloting of Evidence Based Family Skills Programs in low- and middle-income countries. The first building block of this initiative was the development of the "Guide to Implementing Family Skills Training Programs for Drug Abuse Prevention," which was translated to all six official United Nations languages (UNODC, 2009). The guide was developed in consultation with a global representation of experts. It summarized the evidence available at the time with regard to the effectiveness of family-based programs, as well as provided guidance on how to implement family-based programs from a practical point of view. The aforementioned conclusion of replicability of these results to other countries has been backed by the consultative process with this international panel of experts. This same guide also describes the main principles to follow to ensure greater success of such initiatives, including guidance on adaptation (UNODC, 2009).

A supplementary document published through this initiative was entitled "Compilation of Evidence-Based Family Skills Training Programed" (UNODC, 2010). This compilation provided policy makers, program managers, nongovernmental organizations, and others interested in implementing family skills training programs with a review of existing evidence-based family skills training programs, including descriptions of contents; groups targeted; and indications on the needed materials, training, and related costs. It aimed to assist users in selecting the program best suited to their needs and to offer guidance as to the kind of programs available (UNODC, 2010).

Despite the importance of these two building blocks (the guide and the compilation), the initiative went one additional step forward to further encourage policy makers to adopt evidence-based and family-centered interventions within their national prevention strategies. This was through initiating a technical capacity-building exercise to work directly with member states on jointly adapting, piloting, monitoring, and evaluating family skills programs as described later in this section. This was particularly helpful for policy makers from low- and middle-income countries, who were still reluctant and required further advocacy to dissipate the impression that such programs are foreign and not necessarily culturally suitable in their countries.

Since inception of this initiative in November 2009, a total of twenty-four low- and middle-income countries have become part of this initiative. These countries are scattered across four geographical regions. The first region is Central and South America (Panama, Nicaragua, Honduras, El Salvador, Guatemala, Dominican Republic, Mexico, and Brazil), and the second Southeast Europe (Serbia, Albania, Montenegro, Bosnia and Herzegovina, and Macedonia). Third region was Central and West Asia (Kazakhstan, Uzbekistan, Tajikistan, Kyrgyzstan, Turkmenistan, Iran, Pakistan, and Afghanistan), and the fourth East Africa (Kenya and Ethiopia). Of the aforementioned list of countries, by August 2015, Kenya, Ethiopia, Pakistan, and Afghanistan were still in early stages of implementation. The expansion of this initiative is hampered by financial resources, as the number of countries interested to join is even larger than those in which it is active.

Process of Implementation of Family Skills Training Programs

Since its launch, the technical capacity building component of this initiative has reached around 10,000 family members and trained 500 facilitators and 150 national trainers of facilitators in 19 active countries of Central Asia, Central America, South America, and Southeast Europe. The programs piloted so far by UNODC are the Strengthening the Family Programme 10-14 (SFP 10-14; Molgaard, Spoth, & Redmond, 2000) and Family and Schools Together (FAST; Kratchowill, McDonald, Levin, Scalia, & Coover, 2009). Both FAST and SFP 10-14 are composed by a series of interactive group sessions that aim to increase parental empowerment, family communication, cohesion, support and trust; build family unity and bonds; increase self-esteem; create a supportive network for parents; and build peer relations for children. To date, FAST has been piloted in Brazil and the five Central Asian countries, and SFP 10-14 has been piloted in Southeast Europe, Central America, and Brazil. These two programs were selected given the fact that (1) they target two important developmental age groups (pre- and early school years for FAST and early adolescence for SFP 10-14) (2) they require a relatively limited number of sessions (seven) and (3) the developers were available to participate in the process of adaptation and piloting in these low- and middle-income countries.

Despite the difference in the age group targeted by each of the two piloted family skills programs, the process of implementation was relatively similar for both programs. The process was formulated to ensure a higher likelihood of voluntary participation of member states to the pilots as well as higher odds of governmental endorsement and scale-up prospects once the pilots are over. That is why, as a first step, UNODC formally invited governmental counterparts to participate in the pilot. Depending on the country, the governmental counterpart was either the ministry of health or education or both, in addition to the national drug coordination body. Family skills interventions were presented to the government as components of social, community, and human development rather than just serving the purpose of preventing drug use. Moreover, following acceptance, national counterparts nominated both the schools that participated in the pilot and the facilitators to be trained. In very limited instances, such as Panama, the gathering of families in a few of the cycles happened in social settings outside the school, such as in churches.

To ensure that the programs are culturally fit and avoid them being perceived as foreign, the national counterpart was requested to assign a cultural adaptation team to review and assess appropriateness of the translated material to local cultures and norms. Any recommendations from these teams were accounted with the program developers to ensure adherence to the theories upon which the programs are designed. The first principle of adaptation as described in the UNODC guide to implement evidence-based family skills programs is "adapt minimally at first." This was a core message sent to participating member states. Accordingly, in the vast majority of cases, the adaptation was cosmetic, changing names, examples, and/or game content. There were no changes affecting the structure, content, or order of the sessions. The adaptation was not only at the level of the materials but also covered the process of implementation. The implementing partners (e.g., schools, NGOs), the timing and venue of the sessions, as well as the invitations to schools and parents to participate were also discussed in the cultural adaptation team. In most instances, the sessions were held on weekday evenings at a rate of one session per week.

To ensure quality and acceptability, facilitators were selected to be culturally representative from the communities where the families were to be served and were directly trained by the developers or a senior certified trainer of each of the programs. For both selected programs, the training of facilitators in the vast majority of cases was undertaken by the developers themselves over a period of five days. The number of facilitators per training was between fifteen and twenty-five. The national facilitators were then assigned in teams of two or three, each team serving a group of a maximum of ten to fifteen families. The teams were requested to implement all sessions of the programs. Facilitators were paid minor compensation for their time and efforts.

The facilitators were supervised nationally by an assigned trained quality assurance person. Conference calls were also undertaken with the developers/ senior personnel for troubleshooting purposes during the implementation.

For FAST, a program integrity checklist was also utilized by the facilitators in each session. For SFP 10-14, a process evaluation tool was administered during the second and fifth session of interaction with families. Customer satisfaction and family retention rates were further measured to reflect quality and fidelity. Furthermore, qualitative evaluations through expert opinion, provided by the developers of the programs, were also utilized to troubleshoot where and if necessary.

Participating schools were selected and approached by the governmental counterparts for consent. Minor incentives, in the form of investments in the infrastructure of the schools, were allotted to schools to encourage them to participate. The programs were implemented on a universal basis, and participation was strictly voluntary. Given the stigma associated with substance use in countries where pilots were undertaken, a common concern raised across all cultural adaptation teams was that families were not encouraged to participate in a program labeled as drug prevention. Accordingly, the invitation for families to attend promoted the core element that these programs target, which is family functioning improvement, without directly referring to the anticipated drug prevention outcomes. Families were invited to attend the first sessions, where they would learn firsthand of the content and benefit of such programs to their families. During further implementation cycles, families benefiting from the program also invited other families, after which they were typically encouraged to attend to the entire program. Informed consent was also sought from families on participation. Confidentiality of data was explained to participating families. No direct incentives were paid to the participating families.

The evaluation reports from the pilot programs provided feedback to their national counterparts. The evaluations were followed by structured national meetings that included all national stakeholders to document lessons learned and national needs to ensure a solid framework for endorsement and national scale-up. These national meetings prepared for regional ones where such results and experiences were shared with neighboring countries. A total of three regional meetings were held to date. The first was for Central and West Asia (involving eight countries: Tajikistan, Turkmenistan, Kazakhstan, Kyrgyzstan, Uzbekistan, Iran, Pakistan, and Afghanistan). The second was in Central America and the Caribbean (involving Panama, Honduras, Guatemala, El Salvador, the Dominican Republic, and Nicaragua). The third was for Southeast Europe (involving Albania Serbia, Montenegro, Croatia, Bosnia and Herzegovina, and the Former Yugoslav Republic of Macedonia). These regional meetings encourage exchange of expertise among countries involved in the pilot and stimulate the interest among those not yet fully involved.

Results of the Pilot Projects

Evaluation of the pilot projects was carefully designed, given that it is a key ingredient for scalability and sustainability. However, as the family-based programs were implemented for the very first time in some countries, a randomized clinical case control assessment of the pilot was avoided given that such family skills programs are completely new to these communities, which might bias the results for reasons related to the process and not necessarily related to the materials per se. Accordingly, the pilot process and related evaluation was regarded as "feasibility study" and "prototyping," and the evaluation was designed to be quasi-experimental, evaluating the process of implementation and the outcomes on a pretest-posttest basis only.

For SFP 10-14 (Molgaard et al., 2000), a retrospective pretest-posttest modality was implemented after the last session of each pilot. The measurement tools were modified from the original version focusing on indicators of immediate concern to the national counterparts by the national cultural adaptation teams and in consultation with the developers and lead consultants. These tools came in two complementary versions, one filled by parents and the other by the participating youth. For FAST (Kratchowill et al., 2009), the anonymous pretest questionnaires were filled by parents at the time of their contact with the FAST facilitator inviting them to the sessions and by the teachers, upon receipt of parental consent prior to the undertaking of the sessions. Within two weeks of the program's ending, the posttest questionnaires were distributed to the participating parents and teachers (McDonald & Doostgharin, 2013).

Both programs (i.e., FAST and SFP 10-14) showed significant positive effect on almost all indicators assessed. These indicators assessed several aspects of family functioning (such as family bonding, communication, respecting rules, conduct problems in child or adolescent, etc.), and these indicators are considered to be the main mediators to several health and social outcomes. Furthermore, a specific analysis was undertaken of indicators of violence, both relating to the violent behavior of parents and children attending the sessions. A statistically significant change in anger management indicators reported by parents, as well as in indicators relating to children's violent behavior reported both by children themselves and by their teachers, was noted between pre- and posttest in the vast majority of the parental groups assessed (Maalouf & Campello, 2014). This study combined data from the SFP 10-14 pilots undertaken in Panama, Honduras, Guatemala, and Serbia as well as the FAST pilots undertaken in Kazakhstan, Kyrgyzstan, Turkmenistan, Tajikistan, and Uzbekistan. Both programs indicated positive impact on the aforementioned indicators in all countries concerned. It is also worth noting that all results were cross-validated via more than one data source (parents, child, and teacher's assessments), further strengthening conclusions on changes noted across indicators (see Table 7.4 and Figure 7.4.). The results of the FAST pilots undertaken in Central Asia (Kazakhstan, Kyrgyzstan, Tajikistan, and Turkmenistan) generated comparable, and partly even stronger, positive pretest and posttest changes in parental functioning to those generated in the United States pilots – their original format and their country of design (McDonald & Doostgharin, 2013).

A qualitative study was undertaken in Panama following up families benefiting from the UNODC adapted version of SFP 10-14, twelve to thirty-six months post-implementation. This study documented that the changes in family functioning

Table 7.4 *Change Level (Mean Likert Scale Ranging from 1 to 4) from Pretest to Posttest of Indicators in SFP 10-14 in Serbia and Panama; Based on Parent and Youth Reports*

	Serbia			Panama		
	N	Mean pret-est SD	Mean postt-est SD	N	Mean pret-est SD	Mean postt-est SD
Parents' indicators						
1. Wait to deal with problems with my child until I have cooled down.	42	2.66	3.31**	47	1.77	3.10**
		1.00	0.75		0.86	0.81
2. Help my youth understand what the family and house rules are.	42	2.66	3.43**	47	2.28	2.51
		0.79	0.77		1.01	0.64
3. Take time to do something fun together as a family.	42	2.88	3.48**	51	2.43	3.15**
		1.01	0.80		1.02	0.86
4. Let my youth know what the consequences are for breaking rules.	42	3.00	3.48**	52	2.67	3.50**
		0.72	0.71		1.1	0.75
5. Follow through with consequences each time he or she breaks a rule.	42	2.94	3.00	51	2.24	2.98**
		1.05	0.88		1.11	0.96
6. Spend special time one-on-one with my youth.	42	2.75	3.07	53	2.32	3.00**
		0.95	0.87		1.05	0.85
7. Let my youth know the reason for the rules we have.	42	3.03	3.55*	53	2.57	2.40
		0.78	0.55		1.1	0.72
8. Listen to my youth when he or she is upset.	31	3.42	3.66*	49	2.73	3.40**
		0.67	0.57		1.06	0.88
9. Have regular times for homework.	41	2.91	3.10	53	2.70	3.20**
		0.97	0.99		1.03	0.75
10. Work together with my youth to solve problems that come up at home.	42	3.00	3.29	49	2.55	3.06**
		0.86	0.71		0.98	0.81
11. Try to see things from my youth's point of view.	42	2.90	3.19*	50	2.16	3.00**
		0.71	0.74		1.06	0.96

Table 7.4 (*cont.*)

	Serbia			Panama		
	N	Mean pretest SD	Mean posttest SD	N	Mean pretest SD	Mean posttest SD
Youths' indicators						
1. I know one step to take to reach one of my goals.	40	2.74 0.92	3.25** 0.93	58	2.16 10.9	3.79** 1.81
2. I do things to help me feel better when I am under stress.	38	2.63 1.00	3.00 0.99	57	1.96 0.98	2.58** 0.98
3. I appreciate the things my parent(s)/caregiver(s) do for me.	39	3.10 1.02	3.46* 0.72	58	2.53 0.98	3.18** 0.78
4. We have family meetings to discuss plans, schedules, and rules.	40	1.69 0.86	2.28 1.01	58	1.95 1.02	2.60** 0.99
5. I know how to tell when I am under stress.	40	2.88 0.95	3.43** 0.84	58	2.14 1.15	2.60** 0.79
6. I listen to my parent(s)/caregiver(s)' point of view.	39	2.85 0.89	3.44* 0.72	58	2.43 1.03	3.02** 0.98
7. I understand the values and beliefs my family has.	40	3.02 0.95	3.38* 0.84	58	2.95 0.94	3.21 0.86
8. I know there are consequences when I don't follow a given rule.	45	3.00 0.85	3.53** 0.79	57	2.77 1.00	3.23** 0.87
9. My parent(s)/caregiver(s) and I can sit down together to work on a problem without yelling or getting mad.	40	2.92 0.87	3.38* 0.79	55	2.13 0.98	2.67** 0.98
10. I know what my parent(s)/caregiver(s) think I should do about drugs and alcohol.	39	3.56 0.69	3.67 0.62	58	2.79 1.06	3.33** 0.79
11. My parent(s)/caregiver(s) are calm when they discipline me.	40	2.92 0.98	3.13 0.97	58	2.67 0.89	3.11** 0.89
12. I feel truly loved and respected by my parent(s)/caregiver(s).	40	3.57 0.77	3.63 0.71	57	2.88 1.12	3.52** 0.76

Note:
*$p < 0.10$;
**$p < 0.05$.

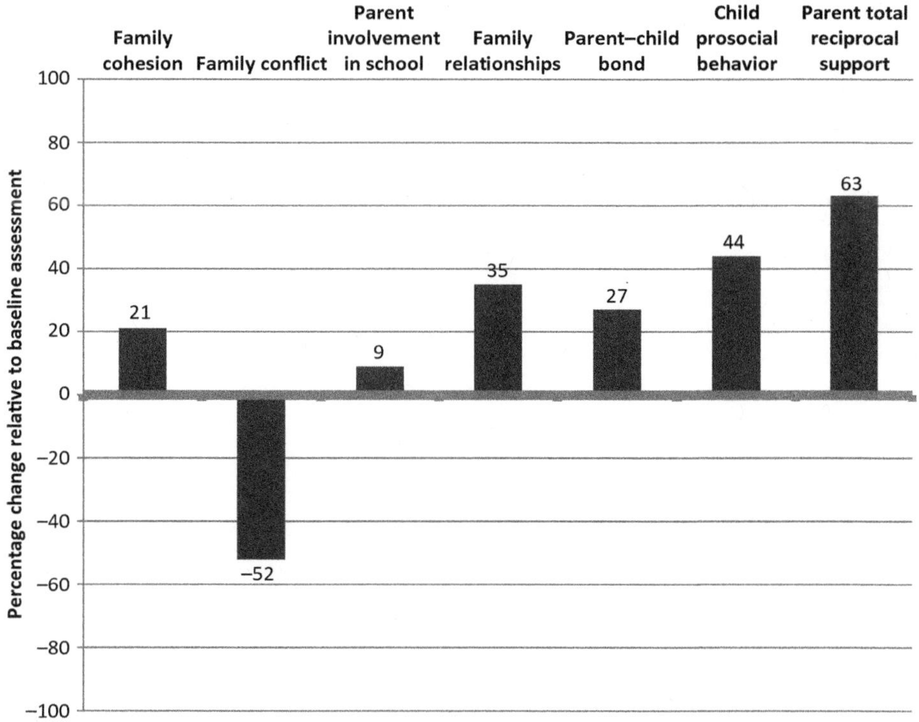

Figure 7.4. *Pretest and posttest change in the family functioning scores combined for all Central Asian countries piloting Families and Schools Together (FAST).*[a]
[a]*Adapted from McDonald & Doogstgharin, 2013.*

had a long-lasting effect among those attending the programs continuing up to three years after receiving the program (Meija et al., 2014).

Across all pilot countries, another level of evaluation was assessing the affinity of the tools developed and implemented. This was done through seeking information from the families, teachers, school principals, facilitators, trainers, and national counterparts. National meetings were organized to document this affinity and discuss further needs for scale-up.

The process through which both programs were implemented was designed in a way to carry an impact on improving relationships at the community level, bringing communities closer together to support each other in different aspects in their life, as well as on the broader social level, changing social and cultural norms and attitudes. Despite the original hesitation, at best, or lack of interest, at worse, of countries implementing such pilots, the process as implemented has generated a high level of affinity across countries to scale up such evidence-based programs. The level of affinity was documented at the level of families, teachers, and policy makers undertaking the pilots (Maalouf & Campello, 2014; McDonald & Doostgharin, 2013). For instance, the adapted piloted programs have been endorsed and received recognition at the level of the office of the presidency of Guatemala, Panama, and Honduras.

Discussion

While the limitations of the UNODC initiatives in terms of scope, coverage, and methodology of the evaluation studies are clear, the results were encouraging both from the point of view of their short-term impact and of their significance in the context of promoting evidence-based drug prevention in long-term perspective. There is a real demand for working with both policy makers in capacity building as well as with practitioners in the concrete programming in the field of prevention globally. This notion is true especially in low- and middle-income countries, where the prevention field is generally less developed and not as well resourced.

The demand for building the capacities of the national authorities in charge of planning and implementing the prevention is evident. Despite the fact that the engagement with policy makers was done in a relatively few number of days, the results achieved were encouraging and had a significant impact on the perception of the value of evidence-based prevention. This increased value to prevention in general and especially to evidence-based prevention interventions and policies among the policy makers could translate into improving the quality of prevention in participating countries. This would eventually be to the benefit of the health and well-being of children and youth in these countries.

Naturally, changes in the practical prevention programming in these countries would still need to be further supported to reap stronger and more concrete benefits. As UNODC seeks to continue the dialogue with the policy makers started during these trainings, it is hoped that more signs of these practical changes will become apparent. Already, positive examples of countries that are starting to adopt new evidence-based programs and readapt their national plans, bringing them closer to the scientific evidence, as summarized in the Standards, are starting to materialize following exposure to the trainings. As a concrete step to assist the countries further in supporting the implementation of evidence-based programs, the UNODC experience of implementing family skills programs in low- and middle-income countries has been instrumental. This has helped participating countries generate national evidence of the value of such intervention in preventing risky behaviors, including substance use and violence, and such evidence has also served as an important positive example to other countries not yet implementing such evidence-based programs. Moreover, it has given these countries an opportunity to experience firsthand the transferability, the ease of adaptability, the practicality in execution, and the high level of affinity to such programs. This is particularly relevant given the needs of the families from the countries concerned. The large spectrum of impacted outcomes and factors through the implemented pilots has given these countries a clearer sense of the positive spectrum of effective outcomes that can be generated through such investment. Further studies from these countries, particularly in the form of randomized clinical trials, could further substantiate these findings.

The future directions of this initiative and of UNODC actions in the field of prevention in general are focused around its pursuit to advance global understanding and recognition of evidence-based prevention, and especially its concrete implementation in low- and middle-income countries, via disseminating the International Standards on Drug Use Prevention. An encouraging sign in this direction is the recognition of the Standards at the highest political level of the UNODC member states, who have recently unanimously supported the implementation of evidence-based prevention, as described in the Standards (UNODC, 2013).

During the national and regional meetings with policy makers discussing the evidence-based prevention based on the Standards, policy makers repeatedly expressed the need of, and the interest in, guidance on evaluation of prevention. To respond to this need, and to further continue the ongoing dialogue with the national-level policy makers in charge of prevention, UNODC is producing a guidance initiative focusing on evaluation of prevention interventions and policies and delivering related training seminars to disseminate the guidance to relevant national policy makers. This guidance expands the preliminary indications that are already included in the Standards. It is hoped that this initiative will raise global awareness of the need for establishing prevention planning and implementation on a scientific basis and will encourage member states to invest in evaluation of their ongoing prevention programs.

UNODC, within its availed funding, continues to support the piloting and dissemination of specific evidence-based programs globally by assisting in scaling up activities in countries that have already piloted family skills initiatives; by increasing the number of low- and middle-income countries participating to such pilots; and by supplementing the family skills programs with school-centered life skills as well as classroom management programs in an effort to build models of comprehensive evidence-based prevention systems.

These efforts combine with the efforts of many other organizations and institutions that are all striving to promote safe, effective evidence-based prevention globally, addressing different aspects and stakeholders such as improving the quality standards of prevention initiatives, developing the capacity of practitioners, and identifying minimum competences of practitioners and institutions. It is hoped that the synergic effect of these complementary initiatives will contribute substantially to improve the coverage and quality of drug prevention, enabling healthy and safe development of children and youth worldwide.

References

Biglan, A., Duncan, T., Irvine, A., Ary, D., Smolkowski, K., & James, L. (1997). A drug abuse prevention strategy for rural America. *NIDA Research Monograms* 168: 364–97.

Burkhart, G. (2015). International standards in pervention: how to influence prevention systems by policy interventions? *International Journal of Prevention and Treatment of Substance Use Disorders* 1: 18–37. ijptsud.sljol.info/articles/abstract/10.4038/ijptsud.v1i3-4.7836/.

CCSA (Canadian Centre on Substance Abuse) (2010). *Building on Our Strengths: Canadian Standards for School-Based Youth.* Ottawa, ON: Canadian Centre. www.ccsa.ca/Resource%20Library/ccsa-011815-2010.pdf

Coombes, L., Allen, D., & McCall, D. (2012). The Strengthening Families Programme 10-14 (UK): engagement and academic success at school. *Community Practice* 85: 30–3.

Cooper, P., Tomlison, M., Swartz, L., Landman, M., Molteno, C., Stein, A., ... Murray, L. (2009). Improving quality of mother–infant relationship and infant attachment in socioeconomically deprived community in South Africa: randomised clinical trials. *BMJ* 14: 338.

Dawe, S., & Harnett, P. H. (2007). Reducing potential for child abuse among methadone-maintained parents: results from a randomised controlled trial. *Journal of Substance Abuse Treatment* 32: 381–90.

Denham, S., & Weissberg, R. (2004). Social-emotional learning in early childhood: what we know and where we go from here. In Chesebrough, E., King, P., Gullotta, T., & Bloom, M., *A Blueprint for the Promotion of Prosocial Behavior in Early Childhood.* New York: Kluwer/Plenum, pp. 13–50.

EMCDDA (European Monitoring Centre for Drugs and Drug Addiction) (2011). *European Drug Prevention Quality Standards.* Lisbon: European Monitoring Centre for Drugs and Drug Addiction.

Knerr, W., Garder, F., & Cluver, L. (2013). Improving positive parenting skills and reducing harsh and abusive parenting in low- and middle-income countries: a systematic review. *Prevention Science* 14: 352–63.

Koegl, C., Farrington, D., Augimeri, L., & Day, D. (2008). Evaluation of a targeted cognitive-behavioral program for children with conduct problems – the SNAP under 12 Outreach Project: service intensity, age and gender effects on short and long term outcomes. *Clinical Child Psychology & Psychiatry* 13: 419–34.

Kratchowill, T. R., McDonald, L., Levin, J. R., Scalia, P. A., & Coover, G. (2009). Families and Schools Together: an experimental study of multifamily support groups for children at risk. *Journal of School Psychology* 47: 245–65.

Maalouf, W., & Campello, G. (2014). The influence of family skills programmes on violence indicators: experience from a multi-site project of the United Nations Office on Drugs and Crime in low and middle income countries. *Aggression and Violent Behavior* 19: 616–24.

McDonald, L., & Doostgharin, T. (2013). UNODC Family Skills Initiative: outcome evaluation in Central Asia of Families and Schools Together (FAST) Multi-Family Groups. *Social Work and Social Sciences Review* 16: 51–75.

Mejia, A., Calam, R., & Sanders, M. R. (2012). A review of parenting programs in developing countries: opportunities and challenges for preventing emotional and behavioral difficulties in children. *Clinical Child & Family Psychology Review, 15* 163–75.

Meija, A., Ulph, F., & Calam, R. (2014). An exploration of parents' perceptions and beliefs about changes following participation in a family skill training program: a qualitative study in a developing country. *Prevention Science* 16: 674–84.

Molgaard, V. K., Spoth, R. L., & Redmond, C. (2000). Competency training: the Strengthening the Families Programme – for parents and youth 10–14. *Juvenile Justice Bulletin* (NCJ 182208), 1–11. Washington, DC: U.S. Department of Justice, Office of Juvenile Justice and Delinquency Prevention (OJJDP).

NIDA (National Institute on Drug Abuse) (2003). *Preventing Drug Use among Children and Adolescents: A Research-based Guide for Parents and Community Leaders*, 2nd ed. Bethesda, MD: NIH.

Rahman, A., Iqbal, Z., Roberts, C., & Hussain, N. (2009). Cluster randomized trial of a parent-based intervention to support early development of children in a low-income country. *Child Care & Health Development* 35: 56–62.

Sanders, M. R. (1999). Triple P–Positive Parenting Programme: towards an empirically validated multilevel parenting and family support strategy for the prevention of behavior and emotional problems in children. *Clinical Child and Family Psychology Review* 2: 71–90.

Shortt, A. L., Toumbourou, J. W., & Chapman, R. (2006). The Resilient Family Program: helping to prepare adolescents for success in school and life. *Youth Studies Australia* 25: 57–88.

Spoth, R., Randall, G., & Chin, C. (2008). Increasing school success through partnership-based family competency training: experimental study of long-term outcomes. *School Psychology Quarterly* 23: 70–89.

United Nations. (2014). Resolution 57/3: Promoting prevention of drug abuse based on scientific evidence as an investment in the well being of children, adolescents, youth, families and communities. In *Commission on Narcotic Drugs Report on the Fifty-Seventh Session*. New York: United Nations Economic and Social Council, p. 25.

UNODC (United Nations Office on Drugs and Crime) (2009). *Guide to Implement Evidence Family Programmes*. Vienna: United Nations Office on Drugs and Crime.

UNODC (United Nations Office on Drugs and Crime) (2010). *Compilation of Evidence-based Family Skills Training Programmes*. Vienna: United Nations Office on Drugs and Crime.

UNODC (United Nations Office on Drugs and Crime) (2013). *International Standards on Drug Use Prevention*. Vienna: UNODC. The standards are available at UNODC webpage: www.unodc.org/unodc/en/prevention/prevention-standards.html.

UNODC (United Nations Office on Drugs and Crime) (2014a). Joint ministerial statement. 2014 high level review by the Commission on Narcotic Drugs of the Implementation by member states of the Political Declaration and Plan of Action on International Cooperation towards Integrated and Balanced Strategy to Counter the World Drug Problem. Commission on Narcotic Drugs Fifty-seventh Session, Vienna. Official Records of the United Nations Economic and Social Council, Supplement No. 8A (E/2014/28/Add.1): 6–19.

UNODC (United Nations Office on Drugs and Crime) (2014b). Report of the Secretariat on the world situation with regard to drug abuse. Commission on Narcotic Drugs Fifty-eighth Session, Vienna. Official record of the United Nations Economic and Social Council (E/CN.7/2014/3).

Wight, D., & Fullerton, D. (2013). A review of interventions with parents to promote the sexual health of their children. *Journal of Adolescent Health* 52: 4-27.

WHO (World Health Organization) (2010). *Violence Prevention: The Evidence*. Geneva, Switzerland: World Health Organization.

Zins, J., Weissberg, R., Wang, M., & Walberg, H. (2004). *Building Academic Success on Social and Emotional Learning. What Does the Research Say?* New York: New York Teachers College Press.

8 Methodological Issues in Outcome Evaluation of Complex Interventions Aiming at Lifestyle Change

Maria Rosaria Galanti, Karin Engström, Yvonne Forsell, Anna Månsdotter, & Jette Möller

The aim of this chapter is to review some of the methodological challenges in the evaluation of public health interventions, addressing health-related behaviors, and to propose strategies to meet these challenges, albeit with no ambition to provide a comprehensive guide to the evaluation of these interventions.

Public health interventions aimed at disease prevention and health promotion through lifestyle modification – for example, smoking cessation, increase of physical activity, or changes in eating habits – are typically complex (Craig et al., 2008). Complexity may concern the following:

a. The *content* of the intervention itself, including the application of different components sustained over a long time
b. The *target*, often involving diverse population groups
c. The *outcome,* which may consist of modifications of multiple events/traits
d. The *provider*, represented by different professional categories and agencies
e. The *setting*, requiring the mobilization of different sectors in a community

All of these complexity features do not need to be present, but in most interventions they coexist. For instance, a literature search conducted by our research group, for an ongoing systematic review on randomized controlled studies of environmental school interventions for the promotion of physical activity, indicated that in most studies (forty-four out of sixty-five identified), the intervention involved at least two components out of the aforementioned. Most frequently, the complexity stems from a combination of educational activities and parents' and/or teachers' support. Also, in forty-two out of the sixty-five studies, at least one additional outcome besides physical activity was included in the evaluation.

But, what does complexity imply for intervention evaluation? Usually, the results of an evaluation translate into possibly two general implications: (a) inferring the causal effect of the intervention in modifying the natural history of the target health problem or health behavior (Miettinen, 2010); and (b) addressing the question whether the intervention or program is suitable for large-scale dissemination (Flay et al., 2005). Referring to these implications, intervention complexity might strongly challenge the causal inference step, thus introducing additional uncertainty in the decision-making process about dissemination. The challenges posed to causal inference are related to the following:

a. Incomplete knowledge of the causal association between intervention components (and their interaction) and behavioral modification, as well as between behavioral modification and the health outcome (often a prevented case of disease). This includes aspects such as induction time and dose.
b. The inter- and intraindividual variability of the processes involved in intervention adoption, delivery, and postintervention modifications in contextual variables, exposing the processes to multiple sources of systematic errors.
c. The imperfect measurement of most variables, above all the behavior itself.

Not surprisingly, these features have often deterred researchers from conducting a rigorous evaluation of behavioral and lifestyle interventions. As a consequence, many prevention programs that are in use lack sound evidence of effectiveness and even of no harm (Saltz, Biglan, Miller Brotman, Gonzalez Castro, & Gorman-Smith, 2015), leading to a vicious circle between lack of quality and paucity of resources devoted to public health intervention research. Therefore, in the past ten years there has been an increasing emphasis on the scientific evaluation of interventions of public health importance (Des Jarlais, Lyles, & Crepaz, 2004; Hawe, Di Ruggiero, & Cohen, 2012). Nevertheless, studies in the field do not consistently use a methodology adequate to sound inference. For instance, in a Cochrane review on the effectiveness of telephone counseling for smoking cessation (Stead, Hartmann-Boyce, Perera, & Lancaster, 2013) about 42 percent of the 113 excluded studies failed to meet appropriate standards for the evaluation of the intervention's effectiveness (Flay et al., 2005), most frequently because of lack of randomized comparison and/or short follow-up. Of the 77 included studies, 55 percent did not report sufficient information to judge on selection bias (33 percent among studies published in 2008 or later); 22 percent reported insufficient data on attrition among participants; 57 percent were judged to be at high risk of selection, attrition, or detection bias (65 percent among the studies published in 2008 or later).

The current chapter's goal is to present and discuss issues that are related to outcome evaluation of complex interventions. This would be achieved by further elaborations on the following issues: (1) the importance of background theories in intervention evaluation; (2) how to proceed beyond experiments: multiple study design and of multistage evaluation; (3) the importance of studying intermediary end-points and intervention implementation; and (4) how to proceed from scientific results to judgment of applicability and dissemination.

The Importance of Background Theories in Intervention Evaluation

While the use of theories or theoretical models is acknowledged in intervention development (APA, 2014), the theoretical background is less used to make predictions on the causal pathway for the anticipated effects (Shepperd et al., 2009), and therefore less used to inform evaluation practices. An illustration of these shortcomings was presented in a recent analysis (Molinar, Coppo, & Faggiano, 2014) of drug prevention interventions, where the authors investigated the correspondence between alleged theories, intervention components, and choice of the intermediate outcomes. The compared programs were the Health Belief Model; Problem Behavior Theory; Social Learning Theory; Social Norms Theory; Theory of Planned Behavior; Comprehensive Social Influence; Communication Competence Theory; Focus Theory of Norms; and Narrative Theory. This analysis showed a rather poor discriminative power of the theoretical base, as the same theory could be used as background to different intervention components and choice of putative mediators; conversely, similar mediators could be targeted by components referring to different theories (Molinar et al., 2014)

If a study hypothesis rests on a theoretical frame, rather than solely on empirical observation, the theory should inform both on the choice of the intervention components and on the specific causal pathway for the anticipated effects (Craig et al., 2008). Figure 8.1 illustrates this concept, while referring to Social Learning Theory (Bandura, 1977), in the context of smoking prevention. In this example, the theory has been used to hypothesize that smoking in adolescence is "learned" through exposure to role-modeling behavior by parents, older siblings, and peers (Bricker et al., 2006).

In the example in Figure 8.1, the hypothetical theory-based intervention is supposed to have an impact on the pathway linking (a) role-model identification, (b) norm appraisal, and (c) the wish to imitate or conform, in order to prevent smoking onset. For instance, the intervention may consist of interactive sessions, during which normative expectations are corrected with the help of objective statistics, or sessions in which social acceptance of a certain behavior is questioned by influential role models. However, this intervention might not affect the direct pathway (the thick arrow) leading from cigarette availability at

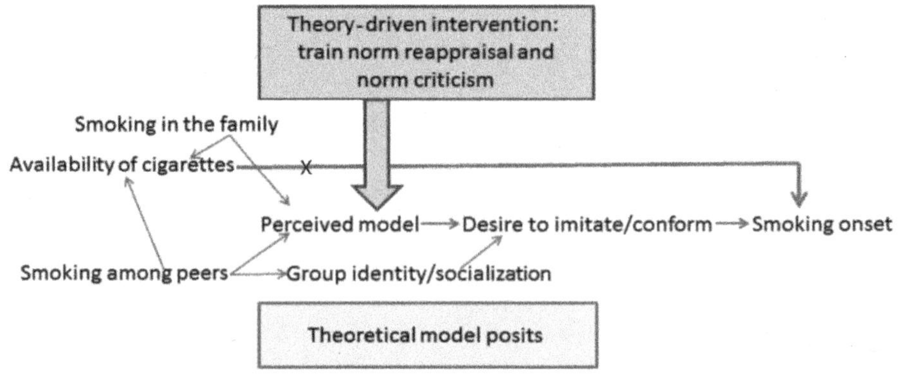

Figure 8.1. *Causal pathways to smoking uptake in adolescence and anchor points for a hypothetical intervention based on Social Learning Theory.*

home to smoking onset in the home environment. Since this latter pathway is likely to be a quite important one, an evaluation of the intervention that would ignore it might yield only a partial understanding of the phenomenon, once stating that the overall effect of the hypothetical intervention, if any, is small (Abar, Jackson, Colby, & Barnett, 2014).

In fact, the advantage of using a detailed visual frame, linking step-by step theory constructs to intervention components and to proposed behavioral modifications, is that in most cases it will allow both a reasoned and coherent choice of intermediary and distal outcomes, as well as a prediction of the direction, shape, and magnitude of the effects of the intervention.

How to Proceed Beyond Experiments

It is important to clarify that the outcome evaluation of a preventive or health-promoting intervention usually strives to answer questions of efficacy and/or effectiveness. The term "efficacy" refers to the ability of the intervention to modify the natural history of an event (either a disease or a behavior or equivalent risk factor for ill health), among those exposed to it, in strictly standardized conditions – that is, in conditions resembling as far as possible the laboratory setting – thus making it unlikely to attribute the revealed effects to other causes (Flay, 1986). The term "effectiveness" usually means the ability of the intervention to achieve the desired modifications in real-life settings, where one or more aspects of the intervention delivery, reach, use, and potential alternative explanatory factors are not thoroughly controlled by the investigators (Flay, 1986).

Irrespective of the question being posed, being able to draw a valid inference on an intervention's effects is largely a matter of study design, that is, of the way alternative interventions or no-intervention conditions are compared and the way relevant information on this comparison is collected. To start with, differences between study designs result in different potential for bias, that is, systematic errors driving the results away from the truth. These potential errors (bias) are usually classified into selection bias, information bias, and confounding (Sorensen, Lash, & Rothman, 2006). Although the distinction among these errors is not always straightforward (Schwartz, Campbell, Gatto, & Gordon, 2015) one can say that selection bias occurs when individuals are recruited and/ or followed up differentially in the groups to be compared, so that a distorted association between intervention and outcome will appear in the results. Information bias results from imperfect measurement of either exposure (e.g., intervention) or outcome (e.g., behavioral modification), so that again the comparison between exposed and nonexposed is impaired. Finally, confounding relates to unbalance of naturally occurring risk or protective factors for the outcome in question between the groups being compared: for instance, the level of smoking-related symptoms, and therefore the readiness to quit smoking, may differ between smokers signing up for a particular smoking cessation intervention and smokers who do not. Directly comparing these two groups would entail a great risk of biased conclusions.

Any of these systematic errors can spuriously obscure an effect when it actually exists (bias toward the null) as well as exaggerate an effect or even produce evidence of an effect when in reality none is present (bias away from the null). This latter occurrence is frequent in observational studies where participants choosing to take up an intervention based on behavioral modification are compared to people choosing to decline because of important – and often unmeasured – predictors of "success," for instance motivation to change. In general, the scientific community is more willing to accept the risk of falsely concluding that the intervention was ineffective rather than the risk of the opposite false conclusion. However, from a public health perspective, preventing a population from receiving a potential beneficial intervention because systematic errors obscure its effectiveness may also be detrimental. Indeed, this eventuality is rather frequent even in well-designed and well-conducted studies due to imperfect measurement of the actual exposure to the intervention, of the outcome, or of both (information bias) (Sorensen et al., 2006). For instance, in experimental studies with random assignment of participants to two or more interventions (randomized control trials, or RCTs), not all individuals will get the intervention to which they are assigned. Yet, they will be primarily analyzed as if they were exposed to the same one. These measurement errors, when not differential between groups to be compared (e.g., exposed or not exposed to a particular intervention), often lead to an underestimation of the effect of the intervention itself (Hofler, 2005b).

There is an accepted hierarchy of study designs in terms of bias minimization, with RCTs providing the highest possible level of evidence (Guyatt et al., 2011; Rickles, 2009). This is because RCTs represent the best approximation to an ideal counterfactual world,[1] where the outcome of interest would be simultaneously observed under exposure and nonexposure conditions in each and the same individual (Hofler, 2005a).

However, taking for granted RCT as gold standard in studies on prevention evaluation may lead to overlook some important issues:

1. There are inherent weaknesses of RCTs when applied to complex public health interventions. First of all, their feasibility may be limited by practical, ethical, or economic constraints. Also, randomized trials applied to behavioral modification or other nonmedical interventions often lack some methodological features of "pure" experiments such as a placebo component or participant and

1 Counterfactual theory is at the base of causal inference (see Höfler, 2005a). It posits that the only valid comparison to establish causality is to compare the disease risk (or the behavior occurrence) in the same individual under two theoretical conditions: with and without the intervention of interest. Since this situation never occurs in practice (the same individual cannot be at the same time exposed and nonexposed) it is called "counterfactual," that is, contrary to the facts. In order to approximate this condition, we compare groups of different individuals – some with and some without the intervention. How similar these groups are in the characteristics predicting the outcome marks their degree of approximation to the counterfactual world.

deliverer blindness, with consequent limitations in relation to the validity of the results (Campbell et al., 2000).

Bias can arise because of participants' postrandomization behavior or because of loss to follow-up if these are related to the outcome, an occurrence that is not unlikely (Hernan, Hernandez-Diaz, & Robins, 2013). For instance, if actual participation in an intensive smoking cessation program is determined by motivation to quit – in itself a predictor of "success" – nonmotivated individuals randomized to the intervention group may fail to comply with the intervention to a larger extent than nonmotivated individuals assigned to a brief counseling session in the comparison arm. This would lead to an underestimation of the program's effects, if any.

Finally, and perhaps most important in a public health context, unintended selection of participants in a trial, be it at the individual and/or at the group level (e.g., schools, medical practices), is in most cases unavoidable, because of efficiency or other feasibility reasons (eligibility criteria) and because of volunteer participation. This selection would bias the range of participant characteristics and thus make it difficult to estimate the potential impact of the intervention once going to scale (low external validity of the results) (Britton et al., 1999).

2. A second important consideration is the level of inference that the evaluation requires. As pinpointed by Habicht, Victora, and Vaughan (1999), sometimes decision makers are satisfied with knowing that a certain program is accompanied by changes in the desired direction, or even that it is being conducted with the desired standard of activity and resources. For instance, if the efficacy and/or the effectiveness of an intervention has been already evaluated based on previous well-conducted studies, population attendance or reach may convey enough information to judge whether the projected goal is being attained. In other cases, robust inference about intervention effectiveness coming from an RCT needs to be complemented with evidence about uptake and level of delivery in order to infer adequate population impact (Victora, Habicht, & Bryce, 2004).

3. In many cases where the effectiveness of a complex intervention still needs to be established, there has been a tendency among evaluators to immediately launch complex field experiments. It has been claimed that in many countries, preventive interventions still lack accreditation systems and processes comparable to those historically in use for drug development and marketing (Faggiano et al., 2014). No prescription drug would be evaluated in a large unselected patient population without prior assessment of efficacy and safety in smaller-scale, strictly monitored, trials. In this regard, an important question arising in the evaluation of complex interventions is how well established was the efficacy and safety of *each* intervention component *before* their assemblage into a complex package. Imagine a novel substance use prevention program consisting of (a) teacher-led, skill-enhancing sessions targeting students in schools; (b) parental support sessions; and (c) joint communication training sessions, involving both parents and their children. Before testing the effectiveness of

such a complex package on substance use outcomes, one would need to assess whether the student sessions achieved the expected skill modifications; whether the parent sessions actually have an impact on parenting style; whether the joint parent–student sessions are followed by the purported changes in communication style (if this was the goal); whether there are synergic effects among all these components (i.e., an effect that is greater than the sum of their individual effects, thus justifying this complex intervention); and finally whether there may be undesired side effects attributable to any of them, for instance increase in other risk-taking behaviors among students, or to a combination of them (e.g., moderating effects).

In line with the sequential approach proposed by Campbell et al. (2000), the Multiphase Optimization Strategy (MOST) model (Collins et al., 2011) has been proposed as a multistage procedure to identify promising components of an intervention and to test simultaneously for efficacy of these components and of their interactions in a series of factorial RCTs. At the end of the procedure, only the combination of components that has shown promising effects will be retained in a complex intervention, to be subsequently field-evaluated.

4. Quasi-experimental and observational studies should be considered as a complement or sometimes as an alternative to experimental studies (Sorensen et al., 2006). We refer to the numerous textbooks of epidemiology and public health for the description of classical study designs such as RCT, cohort, and case-control studies. In this chapter, we provide a brief description of the case-crossover study, infrequently used in evaluation, but an efficient alternative in some cases, especially in the upcoming field of e-health promotion interventions (Atherton, Huckvale, & Car, 2010).

We conclude this section with the description of a case recently managed by our group in order to illustrate the advantages of combining several study designs in the same evaluation task. In fact, to accommodate the frequently encountered time constraints in decision making, we suggest the possibility to collapse some steps in the sequential-circular model of intervention development and evaluation suggested, for instance, by Campbell et al. (2000) and Lich, Ginexi, Osgood, and Mabry (2013). In particular, pragmatic RCT and population-based cohort studies can be designed and conducted as part of the same evaluation plan.

The Case-Crossover Design

This design is particularly useful to identify short-term risk (triggers) and protective (deterrents) factors (Maclure & Mittleman, 2000). The case-crossover method can be understood as an extension of the matched case-control design, except that instead of comparing exposure information from different individuals (cases and controls), a sample of past time from each case is used as control information. Hence, only a sample of cases is needed and confounding from time-invariant factors, both measured and unmeasured, is inherently controlled for. Further, even when case-crossover studies have to rely on retrospectively self-reported data, the risk for differential misclassification is reduced, since within the same individual exposure information for both the case and control periods are nested. The magnitude of the problem with exchangeability is, as in most epidemiological studies, dependent on the exposure under study (Mittleman & Mostofsky, 2014). Such a design is most suitable for studying intermittent exposures, where the effect (outcome) is immediate and transient, such as the evaluation of the effects of mass media health messages on patients' contact with general practitioners (Eriksson, Maclure, & Kragstrup, 2005). The studies by Bleich and colleagues used the case-crossover approach to evaluate whether providing information on energy content of sugar-sweetened beverages (SSB) had any effect on adolescents' consumption. The intervention used four signs that represent caloric information: absolute calories, number of teaspoons of sugar, number of minutes of running, and number of miles of walking necessary to burn off a beverage; thus, each can was signed by one of these four caloric signs. Data at 6 points of sales were collected for 4,516 purchases by a sample of Black adolescents, including both baseline and postintervention periods, when signs were removed. In this way, sweetened beverage purchases were compared for each individual during a "sign-exposed period" and "sign-unexposed period."

Besides evaluating the direct effect of information on the purchases of SSB (Bleich, Herring, Flagg, & Gary-Webb, 2012) it was also possible to evaluate the effect of different types of information and whether the effect on behavior persisted after the messages were removed (Bleich, Barry, Gary-Webb, & Herring, 2014).

Combining Study Designs: A Case of Field Evaluation

A large municipality in the Stockholm region of Sweden, presenting several unfavorable indicators of health risks associated to lifestyle in the resident population (e.g. high prevalence rates of smoking and obesity), planned to launch an outpatient clinic in order to promote lifestyle changes among primary care patients. The whole intervention consisted of three components:

a. A prompt by general practitioners (GPs), consisting of the assessment of lifestyle risk and brief advice, followed by the offer to be referred to the "lifestyle clinic," that is, a facility offering organized programs to assist in behavior modification related to eating habits, tobacco and alcohol use, physical activity, and stress management.
b. An intensive lifestyle change individualized program led by an experienced counselor at the "clinic," complemented in the appropriate cases by the following.
c. Interventions managed outside the clinic (e.g., subsidized exercise program in a gym facility).

The municipality council wished to assess the effectiveness of this multicomponent program as a whole, compared to the usual praxis of brief advice only by the GP, the program's population reach, its impact, and associated costs.

The proposed evaluation plan included the combination of an RCT with an observational study, consisting of follow-up of a cohort of patients not willing to be randomized; a time series of population prevalence of cigarette smoking, overweight, and sedentary lifestyle; and a time series of incidence of hospital admissions for cardiovascular disease.

Figure 8.2 shows the approach combining RCT and cohort study in order to illustrate its informative advantages.

Patients seeking care at the clinic were screened for lifestyle risk factors (e.g. smoking, overweight). Eligible patients are then asked for consent to be randomized to be referred to the lifestyle clinic or just to receive brief advice. Consenting patients are then randomly allocated to one of the two interventions (squares labeled as 2 in Figure 8.2), while patients not willing to be randomized receive one of the two interventions according to preference (squares labeled as 1).

While the randomized cohort provides an estimate of the (unconfounded) effects of the intervention on behavioral modification, the total exposed cohort (i.e., composed of individuals undergoing the intervention either by randomization or spontaneously choosing to be referred) compared to the total unexposed cohort receiving only brief advice provides an estimation of the effects under nonexperimental conditions. As a second advantage, the comparison between randomized and nonrandomized individuals within each condition (exposed and nonexposed to the intervention) will inform about sociodemographic and clinical determinants of the choice of the intervention. Finally, studying cohort-wise the participants' compliance with the behavioral modification plan agreed upon during the intensive counseling ("as treated" analysis in the randomized

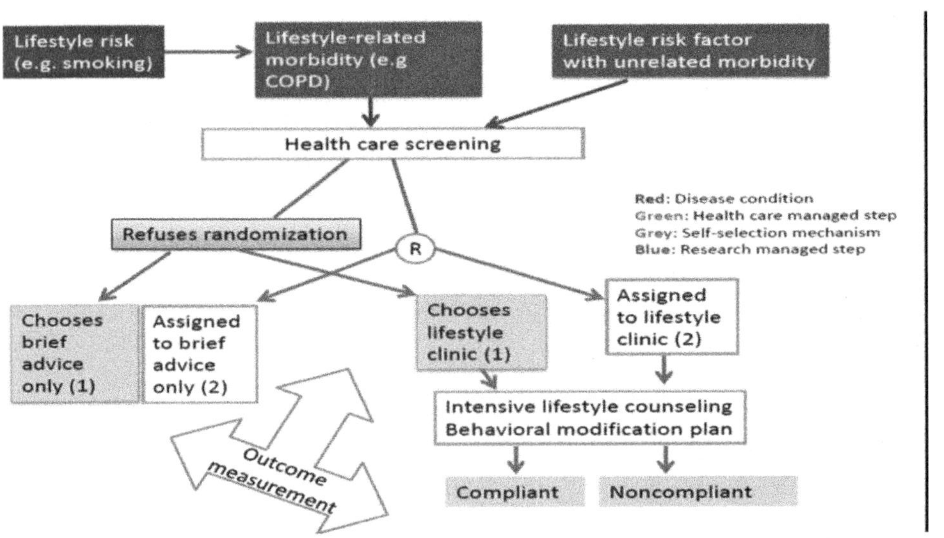

Figure 8.2. *Combining RCT and observational cohort design in the evaluation of a complex intervention.*

group) will provide insights on acceptance at the target level and on effective doses (see also the next paragraph).

The Importance of Studying Intermediary End-Points and Intervention Implementation

Evaluating the effects of an intervention is not only a question of "whether" the intervention has any impact but also of "why" and "how" the proposed actions work or do not work. The answer to this "why" is usually pursued through the analysis of intermediary end-points that should reflect the theoretical framework on which the intervention rests (Green, 2015). These can be represented by events or processes situated along the causal chain of the problem to be modified, proximally to the outcome of primary interest. For instance, in the example presented in Figure 8.1, one may want to know whether adolescents' exposure to the intervention would modify their normative perception of smokers as role models to a higher extent than adolescents who were not exposed to the same intervention. Or, in a comprehensive program aimed at reducing weight in an overweight/obese population, one may want to know whether the desired levels of physical activity and dietary modifications are actually attained. The interest in studying intermediary end-points becomes particularly evident in the following four occasions:

1. Some steps in the causal chain linking a particular behavior to a health problem are not well known. For instance, it may not be clear whether and how motivation to lose weight is associated to weight reduction practices and/or to actual weight loss (Teixeira, Silva, Mata, Palmeira, & Markland, 2012).
2. The intervention is based on a theoretical model the importance of which is to be assessed. For instance, if a "life-skills" based intervention (WHO, 1997) achieves the desired behavioral effects (e.g., refraining from smoking initiation) without modifying the skills postulated by the theory (e.g., resistance skills), then the relevance of the theoretical model to the targeted behavioral change should be revisited.
3. One is interested in estimating how much of the intervention's effect on a particular outcome (e.g., smoking cessation) is mediated by a change in a particular intermediary factor (e.g., change in motivation to quit) and how much is explained by other factors (direct effect) (Mascha, Dalton, Kurz, & Saager, 2013).
4. The success of the intervention requires that the target conforms to prespecified steps in the conduction of the intervention (e.g., attend counseling sessions or purchase the suggested nicotine replacement medications).

This compliance (adherence) constitutes a crucial step in the analysis of the possible effect of an intervention (Flay et al., 2005). Since adherence of the participants to a given program will differ, decisions on how to measure it are of great importance. For some interventions, adherence can be predefined based on optimal knowledge of what represents a possible threshold for the expected effects or a meaningful difference from the comparison group; for example, a certain number of sessions may need to be attended. In other interventions, this might prove difficult since the "minimal dosage" is unknown, and its assessment might actually constitute a research question per se.

Point 4 is illustrated in the following example. The Regassa study (Hallgren et al., 2015) is an RCT conducted in six health care regions of Sweden. The study goal was to compare the effects of physical exercise Internet-based Cognitive Behavioral Therapy and treatment as usual on mild to moderate depression among primary care patients. One of the secondary research questions was to assess the frequency of physical exercise needed to reach measurable effects on depression, since this aspect is still unclear (Cooney et al., 2013). Thus, adherence was analyzed as the number of sessions and percentage of total recommended sessions attended, according to patients' self-reports. Documenting adherence in an objective way may pose problems. In the Regassa study, pulse watches and accelerometers were used in order to measure physical exercise, with the additional advantage of an increase in the adherence among participants, because of regular feedback (Hysong, Best, & Pugh, 2006). Collecting data from the participants during an intervention will also be a "natural" way of reminding them of their participation. However, objective measurements, such as the one proposed in the Regassa study, often require staff participation as well (e.g., for the explanation of how to use the instrument, for the assessment of height and weight), which should be considered if high levels of implementation are required.

In fact, in complex interventions involving behavioral modification, adherence needs to be measured both at the participants' level and at the providers' level. Events that may impact implementation mostly occur at the organization level, for instance leadership, staff turnover, and local routines affecting the staff's behaviors such as task distribution (Aarons, 2005). At the individual level, the staff's expertise, attitudes, and belief in the effectiveness of the intervention and individual workload are the most prominent predictors of adherence to an intervention (Aarons, 2005). In order to increase provider's adherence, it is often necessary to adapt the intervention protocol to the local culture (Henderson et al., 2012). However, all deviations from the original protocol should be documented and considered in the analysis of the effects. To this end, we propose to appoint locally an independent group with the task of documenting the intervention's delivery, a strategy that may also be found useful in order to identify the implementation cues necessary to generalize the results to other settings. This documentation will also be valuable for the later implementation of the intervention on a larger scale.

Proceeding from Scientific Results to Judgment of Applicability and Dissemination

In order to "go to scale" with disease prevention and health promotion interventions, decision makers normally need information beyond that of established efficacy/effectiveness. Feasibility and acceptance at the broad target level, conditions for sustainability, costs, and potential interactions with existing programs/policies are examples of important information often not accrued during efficacy or effectiveness evaluation (Flay et al., 2005; Glasgow & Emmons, 2007; Glasgow, Klesges, Dzewaltowski, Bull, & Estabrooks, 2004).

Decreased differences in health within a population and wise use of limited resources represent two essential considerations. These ethical principles are embedded in the normative framework regarding social policy in general, which principally include the principle of autonomy (society's duty to respect individuals' right to decide for themselves), the utilitarian principle of caring (society's duty to do no harm, to prevent and diminish suffering, and to promote well-being), and the distributional principle of fairness (society's duty to benefit disadvantaged individuals and groups in the distribution of benefits and burdens).

We will address here these aspects under three perspectives: cost effectiveness; equality in health; and balancing cost-effectiveness and equality issues.

1. Health economic evaluation aims at offering decision makers information on how to allocate resources for maximum individual and population health benefit. There are two main normative foundations and evaluation methods. The traditional economic theory is welfarism, combined with the ethical principle of maximizing personal utility, which refers to subjective well-being (Sen, 1980). This is linked to the evaluation method known as cost-benefit analysis. In the case of disease prevention and health promotion, however, the welfarist approach is normally less useful, since people may gain immediate well-being from drinking alcohol or eating french fries. Hence, an extrawelfarist approach has been developed by health economists, according to which health should be the outcome of interest in health care and public health intervention. The evaluation method is cost-effectiveness analysis, combined with the ethical principle of maximizing health (Culyer, 1989).

The *first step* in establishing cost-effectiveness is to estimate costs for the interventions, such as time and wages for professionals and participants, information material, venues for meetings, travel and subsistence, and share of overhead. The *second step* is to estimate health gains from the intervention. Common outcomes are the prevented number of cigarettes or of daily smoking, promoted minutes of physical activity, or added life-years. The *third step* is to estimate savings from the interventions, such as prevented need of health care and medicine, social services, juridical system, and production loss. In practice, this normally means calculating various costs linked to the addressed outcome (e.g., mild depression) and risk of subsequent adverse outcomes (such as severe depression) through available data sources (questionnaires, municipality records, national registers, published literature, etc.), resulting in the average cost for one individual during one year. This quantity may then be used to estimate the savings (i.e., prevented costs) connected to the intervention, either restricting these estimates to the actual follow-up period or considering longer follow-up periods (five, ten, or twenty years) and eventually a lifetime perspective based on modeling techniques. Since cost-effectiveness is a relative measure, and hence is established by comparing the index intervention with others, these latter interventions should have been economically evaluated and available in reports or scientific articles with similar outcomes (i.e., it is not possible to compare reduced units of the body mass index [BMI] with reduced number of kilograms). This may not always be the case; therefore, it is recommended that health gains, such as from public health interventions, are measured in quality-adjusted life-years (QALY), an index combining effects on qualitative and quantitative aspects of health (Drummond, O'Brien, Stoddart, & Torrance, 2005). As an example, let us consider smoking-related outcomes. Smokers tend to have worse health-related quality of life (HRQoL) than nonsmokers due to ill health and sickness. They also have an increased risk of premature mortality (years lost). Hence, the health gains in QALYs from preventing smoking are the product of gained quality of life (which is normally anchored on a scale from 0, referring to death, and 1, referring to perfect health) times the number of gained life-years.

The result from a cost-effectiveness analysis is presented as the ratio of net costs per gained QALY, or as cost saving if savings exceed costs, resulting in the so-called incremental cost-effectiveness ratio (ICER). The willingness to pay (WTP) for a QALY is a societal measure and differs between contexts. In Sweden, for instance, the threshold is often set at fifty thousand euros (TEUR) (National Board of Health and Welfare), while in the United Kingdom it is set at thirty TEUR (National Institute for Health and Care Excellence [NICE]). This means that interventions demonstrating ratios below fifty TEUR or thirty TEUR per gained QALY, respectively, may be deemed as cost-effective and therefore considered for implementation.

This utility economics may be illustrated by a cost-effectiveness analysis of school-based prevention of cannabis in Sweden (Deogan et al., 2015). This analysis, based on the Swedish WTP threshold, demonstrated that these programs are not cost-effective (ICER 926 709 EUR per QALY) during a follow-up period of ten years, but cost-effective (ICER 14 981 EUR per QALY) considering the lifetime perspective. Further, if boys are targeted in socially disadvantaged areas, such programs are likely to be cost saving (ratio 1:3.2) after twenty years of follow-up.

2. The concept *equality* in health is here restricted to differences in health-related lifestyles, or their health consequences, that is, observable variation in a single outcome. This may be differentiated from equity in health, a normative concept considering values such as fairness, justice, right/wrong, and so on, based on ethical considerations such as freedom of choice and capability to achieve one's life goals. However, systematic and potentially avoidable differences (i.e., inequalities) in health, between individuals or groups, are often

identified as unfair (i.e., inequities) (Institute of Health Equity, 2010). Therefore, the distinction between equality and equity deserves further elaboration alongside intensive societal and political references.

The consideration of equality of health is orthogonal to the distinction between types of preventive public health interventions, principally divided into "selective" (targeting groups with a relatively high risk of a health-damaging lifestyle) and "universal" (targeting all individuals irrespective of their risk profile) (Mrazek & Haggerty, 1994). The first type of interventions (selective) is straightforward. If effective, they may also be assumed to decrease health inequalities in the society (holding constant all other circumstances). The second type of interventions (universal) is analytically more complex, because not only may the probability of a healthy/unhealthy lifestyle before the intervention differ between groups – for instance, by gender, education, ethnicity, living area, sexual identity, and disability – but also the efficacy/effectiveness of the intervention may differ. In this situation, absolute and/or relative inequality may occur, the former referring to subgroup difference in measures of morbidity or risk factor burden, the latter referring to the subgroup ratio of the corresponding measures (Charafeddine, Demarest, Van der Heyden, Tafforeau, & Van Oyen, 2013).

Therefore, when evaluating universal public health interventions aimed at disease prevention and health promotion, the following steps are needed (Oxman, Lavis, Lewin, & Fretheim, 2009):

a. Determine whether the studied health-related lifestyle is likely to differ between social groups based on theoretical and/or empirical knowledge (such as gender, education, ethnicity, residence area, sexual identity, disability, etc.). For instance, in Sweden as in many other high-income countries, cigarette smoking is disproportionately more frequent in subgroups with low education and low income.
b. Collect data on these relevant social characteristics.
c. Stratify the baseline and follow-up of the studied lifestyle for relevant social groups. It should be noted that if one launches a universal preventive intervention without caring for evaluation of a differential effectiveness, this may translate in the end to widening the gap between social groups. Incidentally, this has been the case for smoking cessation interventions, in which low-SES individuals not only make less use but also benefit less from smoking cessation interventions (e.g., Hiscock et al., 2013).
d. Estimate likely consequences on relative and absolute equality in health, based on efficacy/effectiveness of the intervention in relevant social groups.

On the same line, the Marmot Review (Institute of Health Equity, 2010) underpins the concept of "proportionate universalism," that is, scaling an intervention's intensity in relation to the level of health disadvantage (or need) in the population (Institute of Health Equity, 2010). Facilitated access to services and dedicated referral systems are examples of this approach, as illustrated by the case of smoking cessation services in the United Kingdom (Brown, Platt, & Amos, 2014).

The consideration of the ethical goals of equality of health and cost-effectiveness may harmonize as well as clash. The former situation does not present problems; on the contrary, the combination of decreased differences in health and wise use of society's resources is a strong argument for "going to full scale" with an intervention aimed at lifestyle modification. The cost-effectiveness analysis of cannabis prevention (Deogan et al., 2015) constitutes such an example where the two goals were perfectly in harmony (i.e., targeting boys in vulnerable areas would increase equality in health and at the same time be cost saving). The latter situation is more difficult, leaving evaluators/researchers to either restrict themselves to presenting the goal conflict or making some further analytic steps. For instance, some studies on preferences for trading off equality with effectiveness have shown that people are willing to sacrifice QALYs in groups with good health for the purpose of adding QALYs in groups with poor health (Lindholm & Rosen, 1998). An example of that is a Swedish study reporting that people are willing to sacrifice 1 QALY in a group of people with good health in order to give 0.45 QALY to a group of people with bad health (Johannesson & Gerdtham, 1996).

In fact, health as compared to (e.g.) income is particularly fundamental for human well-being: "a goal in itself and means for achieving other goals." This kind of information may be incorporated in cost-effectiveness analyses of universal[2] interventions by giving different QALY weights, or accepting different willingness-to-pay thresholds for a QALY, for different social groups (Bobinac, van Exel, Rutten, & Brouwer, 2012). However, the ultimate decision on how to balance equality in health and cost-effectiveness when "going to scale" pertains to the political rather than the scientific domain.

Summary

Complex interventions in public health, such as those aiming at lifestyle modification, entail challenges to the evaluation of their efficacy and effectiveness. These challenges regard all steps of the evaluation, in particular the choice of the outcome to be evaluated; the design of the evaluation and the relevant comparisons; the type of inference to be drawn; measurement issues; and the impact on the population at large, particularly the reduction or widening of social inequality in health.

In this chapter, we offer some reflections to address these challenges. In particular, we suggest to use theories not only to develop interventions, but also to identify the end-points for the evaluation, especially intermediate end-points along the chain of possible determinants of the behavior; to combine traditional and less traditional study types in order to enhance the strength of the evidence; to study the implementation of the intervention; and to give

2 Selective and indicated interventions do not need to be weighted, inasmuch as all outcomes are measured in the group with the highest need or risk profile.

careful consideration to the intervention's effects in population subgroups, especially those defined by socioeconomic circumstances.

References

Aarons, G. A. (2005). Measuring provider attitudes toward evidence-based practice: consideration of organizational context and individual differences. *Child and Adolescent Psychiatric Clinics of North America* 14: 255–71, viii. doi: 10.1016/j.chc.2004.04.008

Abar, C. C., Jackson, K. M., Colby, S. M., & Barnett, N. P. (2014). Common and unique parenting predictors of adolescent tobacco and alcohol use. *Addictive Behaviors* 39: 1528–32. doi: 10.1016/j.addbeh.2014.06.003

APA (American Psychological Association). (2014). Guidelines for prevention in psychology. *American Psychologist*, *69*, 285–296. doi: 10.1037/a0034569

Atherton, H., Huckvale, C., & Car, J. (2010). Communicating health promotion and disease prevention information to patients via email: a review. *Journal of Telemedicine and Telecare* 16: 172–5. doi: 10.1258/jtt.2010.004002

Bandura, A. (1977). *Social Learning Theory*. Englewood Cliffs, NJ: Prentice Hall.

Bleich, S. N., Barry, C. L., Gary-Webb, T. L., & Herring, B. J. (2014). Reducing sugar-sweetened beverage consumption by providing caloric information: how black adolescents alter their purchases and whether the effects persist. *American Journal of Public Health* 104: 2417–24. doi: 10.2105/AJPH.2014.302150

Bleich, S. N., Herring, B. J., Flagg, D. D., & Gary-Webb, T. L. (2012). Reduction in purchases of sugar-sweetened beverages among low-income black adolescents after exposure to caloric information. *American Journal of Public Health* 102: 329–35. doi: 10.2105/AJPH.2011.300350

Bobinac, A., van Exel, N. J., Rutten, F. F., & Brouwer, W. B. (2012). Inquiry into the relationship between equity weights and the value of the QALY. *Value in Health* 15: 1119–26. doi: 10.1016/j.jval.2012.07.002

Bricker, J. B., Peterson, A. V., Robyn Andersen, M., Leroux, B. G., Bharat Rajan, K., & Sarason, I. G. (2006). Close friends', parents', and older siblings' smoking: reevaluating their influence on children's smoking. *Nicotine & Tobacco Research* 8: 217–26.

Britton, A., McKee, M., Black, N., McPherson, K., Sanderson, C., & Bain, C. (1999). Threats to applicability of randomised trials: exclusions and selective participation. *Journal of Health Services Research & Policy* 4: 112–21.

Brown, T., Platt, S., & Amos, A. (2014). Equity impact of European individual-level smoking cessation interventions to reduce smoking in adults: a systematic review. *European Journal of Public Health* 24: 551–56. doi: 10.1093/eurpub/cku065

Campbell, M., Fitzpatrick, R., Haines, A., Kinmonth, A. L., Sandercock, P., Spiegelhalter, D., & Tyrer, P. (2000). Framework for design and evaluation of complex interventions to improve health. *British Medical Journal* 321: 694–6.

Charafeddine, R., Demarest, S., Van der Heyden, J., Tafforeau, J., & Van Oyen, H. (2013). Using multiple measures of inequalities to study the time trends in social inequalities in smoking. *European Journal of Public Health* 23: 546–51. doi: 10.1093/eurpub/cks083

Collins, L. M., Baker, T. B., Mermelstein, R. J., Piper, M. E., Jorenby, D. E., Smith, S. S., . . . Fiore, M. C. (2011). The multiphase optimization strategy for engineering effective tobacco use interventions. *Annals of Behavioral Medicine* 41: 208–26. doi: 10.1007/s12160-010-9253-x

Cooney, G. M., Dwan, K., Greig, C. A., Lawlor, D. A., Rimer, J., Waugh, F. R., . . . Mead, G. E. (2013). Exercise for depression. *Cochrane Database of Systematic Reviews* 9: CD004366. doi: 10.1002/14651858.CD004366.pub6

Craig, P., Dieppe, P., Macintyre, S., Michie, S., Nazareth, I., & Petticrew, M. (2008). Developing and evaluating complex interventions: the new Medical Research Council guidance. *British Medical Journal* 337: a1655. doi: 10.1136/bmj.a1655

Culyer, A. J. (1989). The normative economics of health care finance and provision. *Oxford Review of Economic Policy* 5: 34–58.

Deogan, C., Zarabi, N., Stenstrom, N., Hogberg, P., Skarstrand, E., Manrique-Garcia, E., . . . Mansdotter, A. (2015). Cost-effectiveness of school-based prevention of cannabis use. *Applied Health Economics and Health Policy* 13: 525–42. doi: 10.1007/s40258-015-0175-4

Des Jarlais, D. C., Lyles, C., & Crepaz, N. (2004). Improving the reporting quality of nonrandomized evaluations of behavioral and public health interventions: the TREND statement. *American Journal of Public Health* 94: 361–6.

Drummond, M. F., O'Brien, B., Stoddart, G. L., & Torrance, G. W. (2005). *Methods for Economic Evaluation of Health Care Programmes*, 3rd ed. Corby Northants, UK: Oxford University Press.

Eriksson, T., Maclure, M., & Kragstrup, J. (2005). To what extent do mass media health messages trigger patients' contacts with their GPs? *British Journal of General Practice* 55: 212–17.

Faggiano, F., Allara, E., Giannotta, F., Molinar, R., Sumnall, H., Wiers, R., . . . Conrod, P. (2014). Europe needs a central, transparent, and evidence-based approval process for behavioural prevention interventions. *PLoS Medicine* 11: e1001740. doi: 10.1371/journal.pmed.1001740

Flay, B. R. (1986). Efficacy and effectiveness trials (and other phases of research) in the development of health promotion programs. *Preventive Medicine*, *15*, 451–474.

Flay, B. R., Biglan, A., Boruch, R. F., Castro, F. G., Gottfredson, D., Kellam, S., . . . Ji, P. (2005). Standards of evidence: criteria for efficacy, effectiveness and dissemination. *Prevention Science* 6: 151–75.

Glasgow, R. E., & Emmons, K. M. (2007). How can we increase translation of research into practice? Types of evidence needed. *Annual Review of Public Health* 28: 413–33.

Glasgow, R. E., Klesges, L. M., Dzewaltowski, D. A., Bull, S. S., & Estabrooks, P. (2004). The future of health behavior change research: what is needed to improve translation of research into health promotion practice? *Annals of Behavioral Medicine* 27: 3–12. doi: 10.1207/s15324796abm2701_2.

Green, J. (2015). Editorial: process to progress? Investigative trials, mechanism and clinical science. *Journal of Child Psychology and Psychiatry and Allied Disciplines* 56: 1–3. doi: 10.1111/jcpp.12377

Guyatt, G., Oxman, A. D., Akl, E. A., Kunz, R., Vist, G., Brozek, J., . . . Schunemann, H. J. (2011). GRADE guidelines: 1. Introduction-GRADE evidence profiles and summary of findings tables. *Journal of Clinical Epidemiology* 64: 383–94. doi: 10.1016/j.jclinepi.2010.04.026

Habicht, J. P., Victora, C. G., & Vaughan, J. P. (1999). Evaluation designs for adequacy, plausibility and probability of public health programme performance and impact. *International Journal of Epidemiology* 28: 10–18.

Hallgren, M., Kraepelien, M., Ojehagen, A., Lindefors, N., Zeebari, Z., Kaldo, V., & Forsell, Y. (2015). Physical exercise and Internet-based cognitive behavioural therapy in the treatment of depression: randomised controlled trial. *British Journal of Psychiatry* 207: 227–34. doi: 10.1192/bjp.bp.114.160101

Hawe, P., Di Ruggiero, E., & Cohen, E. (2012). Frequently asked questions about population health intervention research. *Canadian Journal of Public Health* 103: e468–71.

Henderson, J., Milligan, K., Niccols, A., Thabane, L., Sword, W., Smith, A., & Rosenkranz, S. (2012). Reporting of feasibility factors in publications on integrated treatment programs for women with substance abuse issues and their children: a systematic review and analysis. *Health Research Policy and Systems* 10: 37. doi: 10.1186/1478-4505-10-37

Hernan, M. A., Hernandez-Diaz, S., & Robins, J. M. (2013). Randomized trials analyzed as observational studies. *Annals of Internal Medicine* 159: 560–2. doi: 1735165

Hiscock, R., Murray, S., Brose, L. S., McEwen, A., Bee, J. L., Dobbie, F., & Bauld, L. (2013). Behavioural therapy for smoking cessation: the effectiveness of different intervention types for disadvantaged and affluent smokers. *Addictive Behaviors* 38: 2787–96, doi: 10.1016/j.addbeh.2013.07.010

Hofler, M. (2005a). Causal inference based on counterfactuals. *BMC Medical Research Methodology* 5: 28. doi: 1471–2288-5-28

Hofler, M. (2005b). The effect of misclassification on the estimation of association: a review. *International Journal of Methods in Psychiatric Research* 14: 92–101.

Hysong, S. J., Best, R. G., & Pugh, J. A. (2006). Audit and feedback and clinical practice guideline adherence: making feedback actionable. *Implementation Science* 1: 9. doi: 1748–5908-1–9

Institute of Health Equity (2010). *Fair Society, Healthy Lives: The Marmot Review Executive Summary*. www.instituteofhealthequity.org/projects/fair-society-healthy-lives-the-marmot-review

Johannesson, M., & Gerdtham, U. (1996). A note on the estimation of the equity-efficiency trade-off for QALYs. *Journal of Health Economics* 15: 359–68.

Lich, K. H., Ginexi, E. M., Osgood, N. D., & Mabry, P. L. (2013). A call to address complexity in prevention science research. *Prevention Science* 14: 279–89. doi: 10.1007/s11121-012-0285-2

Lindholm, L., & Rosen, M. (1998). On the measurement of the nation's equity adjusted health. *Health Economics* 7: 621–8. doi: 10.1002/(SICI)1099-1050(1998110)

Maclure, M., & Mittleman, M. A. (2000). Should we use a case-crossover design? *Annual Review of Public Health* 21: 193–221. doi: 10.1146/annurev.publhealth.21.1.193

Mascha, E. J., Dalton, J. E., Kurz, A., & Saager, L. (2013). Statistical grand rounds: understanding the mechanism: mediation analysis in randomized and nonrandomized studies. *Anesthesia & Analgesia* 117: 980–94. doi: 10.1213/ANE.0b013e3182a44cb9

Miettinen, O. S. (2010). Etiologic study vis-a-vis intervention study. *European Journal of Epidemiology* 25: 671–5. doi: 10.1007/s10654-010-9486-9

Mittleman, M. A., & Mostofsky, E. (2014). Exchangeability in the case-crossover design. *International Journal of Epidemiology* 43: 1645–55. doi: 10.1093/ije/dyu081

Molinar, R., Coppo, A., & Faggiano, F. (2014). Effective interventions for prevention of alcohol abuse and illicit substance use in adolescence: reviewing theories and mediators. Paper presented at the European Society for Prevention Research, Palma de Mallorca. euspr.org/fifth-euspr-conference/

Mrazek, P. J., & Haggerty, R. J. (eds.). (1994). *Reducing Risks for Mental Disorders: Frontiers for Preventive Intervention Research*. Washington, DC: Institute of Medicine (US) Committee on Prevention of Mental Disorders.

Oxman, A. D., Lavis, J. N., Lewin, S., & Fretheim, A. (2009). SUPPORT Tools for evidence-informed health policymaking (STP) 10: taking equity into consideration when assessing the findings of a systematic review. *Health Research Policy and Systems* 7 (Suppl 1): S10. doi: 10.1186/1478-4505-7-S1-S10

Rickles, D. (2009). Causality in complex interventions. *Medicine, Health Care and Philosophy* 12: 77–90. doi: 10.1007/s11019-008-9140-4

Saltz, R., Biglan, A., Miller Brotman, L., Gonzalez Castro, F., & Gorman-Smith, D. *Advocacy for Prevention Science*. www.preventionresearch.org/Advocacy_principles_051205RFSa2.pdf

Schwartz, S., Campbell, U. B., Gatto, N. M., & Gordon, K. (2015). Toward a clarification of the taxonomy of "bias" in epidemiology textbooks. *Epidemiology* 26: 216–22. doi: 10.1097/EDE.0000000000000224

Sen, A. (1980). *Equality of What? The Tanner Lectures on Human Values*. Cambridge, UK: Cambridge University Press.

Shepperd, S., Lewin, S., Straus, S., Clarke, M., Eccles, M. P., Fitzpatrick, R., . . . Sheikh, A. (2009). Can we systematically review studies that evaluate complex interventions? *PLoS Medicine* 6: e1000086. doi: 10.1371/journal.pmed.1000086

Sorensen, H. T., Lash, T. L., & Rothman, K. J. (2006). Beyond randomized controlled trials: a critical comparison of trials with nonrandomized studies. *Hepatology* 44: 1075–82. doi: 10.1002/hep.21404

Stead, L. F., Hartmann-Boyce, J., Perera, R., & Lancaster, T. (2013). Telephone counselling for smoking cessation. *Cochrane Database of Systematic Reviews* 8: CD002850. doi: 10.1002/14651858.CD002850.pub3

Teixeira, P. J., Silva, M. N., Mata, J., Palmeira, A. L., & Markland, D. (2012). Motivation, self-determination, and long-term weight control. *International Journal of Behavioral Nutrition and Physical Activity* 9: 22. doi: 10.1186/1479-5868-9-22

Victora, C. G., Habicht, J. P., & Bryce, J. (2004). Evidence-based public health: moving beyond randomized trials. *American Journal of Public Health* 94: 400–5.

WHO (World Health Organization), Programme on Mental Health (1997). *Life Skills Education for Children and Adolescents in Schools*. Geneva, Switzerland: World Health Organization.

9 Methodology and Statistical Approaches for Conducting Valid and Reliable Longitudinal Prevention Science Research

Jenn-Yun Tein

Epidemiologically based prevention research, like most other sciences, includes an empirical study that starts with research questions and hypotheses generally derived from theory. Research methodologies are tools to address the questions and evaluate the hypotheses – such as assessing whether the intervention program works as intended, how it works, for whom and under which conditions it works, how large the effect is, and how long it works. It is imperative to maintain high standards of research methodology to best address these questions. Research questions and methodologies need to be considered hand in hand while conducting prevention studies. Research questions should be formulated in a way that can be addressed with sound methodology, sometimes involving new methodological developments. In reciprocal, the proposed methodological procedures should provide "analytical understanding" (Cázares & Beatty, 1994; p. 15) of the hypothesized theory.

Research methodologies for prevention studies include a whole spectrum of research processes. Substantial progress has been made in the development of methodologies and statistics in the last two decades. This chapter focuses on three methodological areas concerning prevention research: (1) sampling and participants, (2) measurement, and (3) evaluation of intervention effects, specifically under the framework of *randomized control trials (RCT)*. Note that each of the topics can be a chapter or a book by itself. The intention is to do an introductory overview of these areas and to outline statistical options, procedures, and techniques to handle potential methodological issues related to these areas. This chapter can be used as a starting point for planning a rigorous preventive intervention. Key references are provided so that prevention scientists can integrate state-of-the-art methodological and analytical approaches for conducting a well-designed study.

Samples and Participants

Preventive interventions are most effective when they are appropriately designed to address the intervention need of the target population.

The target may be the general public (i.e., *universal preventive interventions*); high-risk individuals whose risk of developing problem behaviors are higher than average (i.e., *selective preventive interventions*); or individuals who are having detectable signs of behavioral problems (i.e., *indicated preventive interventions*). A research sample should be selected that best represents the defined population. Evaluations of preventive interventions are done most often with randomized control trials (RCT; Brown & Liao, 1999; Brown, et al., 2008), where participants being studied are randomly allocated to different intervention groups. Analysis that appropriately compares outcomes for the participants in these groups leads to inferential statements about intervention effects for the target population (National Research Council & Institute of Medicine, 2009). However, the extrapolation of results from the trial groups to individuals in the larger population hinges upon the method of the selection of participants for the trial. Only if the participants were selected at random from the defined population can the results be generalized to members of the larger group, although randomization alone is not enough to allow a researcher to generalize the finding to the population. *Sample representativeness* and sample size are factors that must be considered. The degree to which the findings of a study can be generalized beyond the sample is referred to as *external validity*. More specifically, external validity is the extent to which the results can be generalized to the target population. Note that sampling selection affects not only external validity but also internal validity. *Internal validity* is the extent to which a researcher can be sure that the observed changes or differences are the result of the intervention. That is, the researcher can confidently conclude that the intervention caused the change in the outcomes and that the changes are not related to other extraneous factors, such as differences in participants in the intervention and control conditions that may exist outside of the intervention.

Ideally, a random sample should be drawn from every available individual who fulfills the criteria relevant for the trial. In reality, this is impractical and almost unattainable. A narrower defined sampling frame is deemed necessary (Elwood, 1982). For example, an intervention study promoting school performance for children of low-income families is done by sampling families from a particular city whose incomes are below the poverty threshold. Ideally, a series of replications may be necessary to ensure the validity of the findings. Precise information on every factor used to define the selection process should be documented so that the generalizability of the results from the trial can be clearly established. When feasible, testing of sample representativeness against the population from which the sample was drawn (e.g., the particular city) should be performed. One simple way of checking is to compare the demographic characteristics of the sample against those of the population, for example, how well the distribution of family incomes for the families in the sample reflects the distribution of incomes for all families from the city whose incomes are below the poverty threshold.

Statistical Power and Sample Size

Adequate sample size is needed to demonstrate an effect in a trial with a specific *statistical power* at a defined level of statistical significance (e.g., probability of *Type I error*, $\alpha \leq 0.05$). A true intervention effect is likely to be missed because not enough data are collected. As a result, calculations of statistical power and estimations of the optimal sample sizes are essential to demonstrate preventive intervention effects. Few researchers perform this calculation, and few journal articles ever mention the statistical power of their tests. Without information on statistical power, a conclusion such as "not statistically significant" might just be due to insufficient data to detect the real effect.

Depending on the nature of the sampling or the intervention, some interventions are more appropriate to be delivered on individual levels while others are more appropriate to be delivered on group levels (e.g., classroom level, small intervention group level). For example, for a school-based intervention, even though the outcome of interest is at the level of an individual student, the recruitment and random assignment typically occur at the classroom or school level. The individuals tend to be more similar within the same cluster than among clusters – a phenomenon called *intraclass correlation (ICC)*. The intraclass correlation among the individuals in clustered samples leads to an inflation in the variance of the outcome variables and consequently reduces *power*. As a result, a larger sample size is generally required in studies where cluster sampling (i.e., *multilevel data*) is applied compared to simple individual sampling. As a general rule, having more groups is more important than having more cases per group for getting sufficient statistical power (Hox, 2010; Snijders & Bosker, 2012).

There are books about *power analysis* (e.g., Cohen, 1988; Hedges & Rhoads, 2009), statistical software for calculating *power* (e.g., *G*Power*, Faul, Erdfelder, Buchner, & Lang, 2009; *Mplus Monte Carlo* simulations, Muthén & Muthén, 2002; *Optimal Design*, Raudenbush et al., 2011; *SAS PROC POWER* function, SAS Institute Inc., 2008), and published simulation work that provides guidelines of sample sizes for different effects (e.g., Demidenko, 2007 for *logistic regression*; Hsieh, Bloch, & Larsen, 1998 for *linear* and *logistic regression*; Fritz & MacKinnon, 2007, and Taylor, MacKinnon, & Tein, 2008, for *mediation analysis*). Some of these apply to multilevel data (Hedges & Rhoads, 2009; Raudenbush et al., 2011). Most power estimation methods and software cannot account for all design features (e.g., uneven sample size, multilevel data, blocking). It is better to compute power with various estimation methods to account for conditions such as different cell sizes (e.g., using lower and higher bounds, using *harmonic mean*), ICCs, and covariate effects. Reporting range or average of power estimates when they differ across methods and conditions is a good strategy.

Sample Maintenance and Retention

Intervention studies are longitudinal in nature, where participant data are collected at multiple follow-up times. Attrition is inevitable with longitudinal studies since it cannot be controlled by experimental design (Cronbach et al., 1980; Riecken & Boruch, 1974), such as participants having the right to refuse participation and, for various reasons, exiting the study prematurely. Nonrandom attrition, such as differential attrition rates across experimental conditions and attrition due to certain pretest sample characteristics, limit *internal validity* (i.e., the evidence of an intervention on the outcome is questionable and the causal conclusion of the finding is biased) as well as *external validity* (i.e., experimental results cannot be generalized to the population that was originally sampled) (Shadish, Cook, & Campbell, 2002). The best strategy of dealing with attrition is to minimize attrition. It is important to establish procedures that will be used to maintain participants' cooperation and to locate them throughout the study (Cotter, Burke, Loeber, & Navratil, 2002). Interviewers need to develop good rapport and utilize culturally sensitive skills that address barriers within families or environments that may interfere with the process of engagement (McKay & Bannon, 2004; Sullivan, Rumptz, Campbell, Eby, & Davidson, 1996). Using a token economy that rewards session attendance and completion of assessments also increases retention. Methods of maintaining contact with participants include obtaining and updating multiple contact information (e.g., phones and addresses of self and three relatives or friends), making regular contacts (e.g., sending birthday or holiday cards), and sending newsletters to share information about the study that will be of interest to the participants. In the case of losing contact with the participants, modern Internet search engines (e.g., Facebook, Google, PeopleSmart) and online directories are good sources of retrieving hard-to-locate participants. For example, using similar strategies, the New Beginnings Program for children of divorce was able to retain 80 percent of participants over fifteen years (Wolchik et al., 2013).

Attrition analyses provide methodology for testing the *internal* and *external threats*. Jurs and Glass (1971) and Hansen, Collins, Malotte, Johnson, and Fielding (1985) provide guidelines for testing these threats. Briefly, testing *external* or *internal validities* involves the following methods:

1. Testing whether the dropouts differ from the completers on pretest values of the studied variables and on demographic characteristics
2. Testing whether the rates of attrition differ among conditions
3. Testing whether there is a significant interaction between attrition status and intervention conditions on pretest values of the studied variables and on demographic characteristics

Test 1 addresses *external validity* issues – examining the generalizability to the larger population. Tests 2 and 3 address *internal validity* issues – examining selective attrition. Test 3 is an extension of Test 1. While Test 1 examines the main effect of attrition status, Test 3 examines the interaction effect of attrition by experimental condition. Attrition analyses can be easily done using the following statistical methods. Test 2 involves a *Chi-square test* of attrition status by condition crosstabs. For Test 1, examining differences between the completers and dropouts, *t-test* or *one-way analysis of variance (ANOVA)* can be used to examine differences of the continuous variables and *Chi-square tests* to examine differences of the categorical variables. For Test 3, two-way *ANOVA* (for continuous variables) or *logistic regression* (for categorical variables) can be used to examine the interaction of attrition status and intervention conditions.

Differential attrition and threats of *internal* and *external validities* compromise findings. Researchers often control for the variable that shows differences across attrition status or attrition by condition interaction. However, such procedures do not restore either *internal* or *external validity* (Cronbach et al., 1980; Hansen, Collin, Malotte, Johnson, & Fielding, 1985). Therefore, researchers should make every attempt to track and retain participants. Additionally, *attrition analyses* should be a common practice for prevention studies. The results of the attrition analysis can also inform the mechanisms of missing data as described in the following section.

Missing Data

Closely related to issues of attrition is the issue of missing data and methods of handling missing data. Other than that which is due to attrition, missing data occur because of nonresponse – such as participants refusing to answer certain items or the entire questionnaire. The modern missing data methodologies define mechanisms of missing data as the following based on Rubin's (1976) terminology:

1. *Missing completely at random (MCAR)* – missingness is independent of all observed and unobserved variables. When data are MCAR, the analyses performed on the data are unbiased; however, data are rarely missing completely at random.
2. *Missing at random (MAR)* – missingness is related to a particular variable, but it is not related to the value of the variable that has the missing data.
3. *Missing not at random (MNAR)* – missingness depends on the variable that has the missing data.

In a longitudinal study with missing data arising from attrition or nonresponse, these mechanisms can be interpreted as the following, as conceptualized by Hedeker and Gibbons (1997), Little (1995), and Schafer and Graham (2002). For MCAR, the missing data are independent of responses at every assessment – missing data are not related to any observable or nonobservable variables. For example, there is no specific reason why some participants provided information on drinking behaviors and the other did not. For MAR, the missingness depends on responses at any occasion prior to dropout – missing data are related to a particular variable or a set of variables collected from previous assessments. For example, participants who had high scores on risk-taking behaviors in previous assessments were less likely to disclose their drinking behaviors. For MNAR, missingness depends on unseen responses after participants drop out – missing data are related to current unobserved outcome variables. For example, participants who had drinking problems currently were less likely to report their drinking behaviors. MAR is also called ignorable nonresponse or noninformative missingness, and MNAR is also called nonignorable nonresponse, outcome-dependent dropout, or informative missingness (Diggle & Kenward, 1994). Attrition analysis provides some insight of the missing mechanism. *Little's MCAR test* (Little, 1988) also provides guidelines for detecting the missing data mechanism, which can be easily done with the statistical software programs, *SAS* (Statistical Analysis System; SAS Institute Inc., 2008) or *SPSS* (Statistical Package for the Social Sciences; IBM Corp, 2013) (see Enders, n.d).

Not handling missing data properly can have a significant effect on the conclusions that can be drawn from the sample data. The traditional *listwise deletion* method (i.e., deleting individuals who have missing data on any variables from an analysis), which conducts analysis only with the complete cases, has been shown to be biased if data are not MCAR (Little & Rubin, 2002; Schafer & Graham, 2002). Specifically, the complete cases are not a random sample of all of the cases; they are not representative of the full population. Using simulation studies, King, Honaker, Joseph, and Scheve (2001) and Schafer and Graham (2002) show that listwise deletion methods result in substantial biases in *parameter estimates* under the MAR or MNAR mechanism. Even with MCAR, the listwise deletion method does not produce optimal results because of loss of sample and loss of statistical power. Methodologies for handling missing data have been much advanced since Rubin, Little, and colleagues' work in this area (Dempster, Laird, & Rubin, 1977; Little & Rubin, 2002; Rubin, 1976, 1987), especially under the two modern methods – *multiple imputation (MI)* and *maximum likelihood (ML)*. Multiple imputation (Rubin, 1996; Schafer, 1997) replaces missing values with a set of simulated values based on the distribution and produces N plausible alternative sets of the complete data. The hypothesis model is then tested with each complete data set. The results of the N analysis are then pooled together to obtain overall estimates and *standard errors* (Schafer & Olsen, 1998). Maximum likelihood does not involve data imputation, but rather uses each case with available data to compute maximum likelihood estimates that are most likely to have resulted in the observed data. MI and ML make similar assumptions and have similar statistical properties. When implemented with models with comparable variables, the two approaches produce similar results (Schafer & Graham, 2002).

Only in the late 1990s, with the advancement of computer software, have ML and MI become popular (Schafer, 1997). In fact, ML and MI are now becoming standard procedures for handling missing data and are available in mainstream statistical software such as *SAS*, *SPSS*, *Stata* (StataCorp, 2013), *R* statistical package (R Development Core Team, 2007), and *Mplus* (Muthén & Muthén, 1998–2014). It is the default feature for most of the Mplus programs in handling missing data. MI and ML produce unbiased solutions for missing data under the assumption of MAR or MCAR. Methods of dealing with MNAR have also been developed, such as *pattern-mixed models*

(Hedeker & Gibbons, 1997; Little, 1993) and *Diggle-Kenward selection models* (Diggle & Kenward, 1994; see also Enders, 2011) and are incorporated into a couple of software packages (e.g., Mplus, SAS).

Measurement

Measurement is at the center of prevention research, enabling researchers to determine whether their findings had the intended effects. Well-founded prevention research relies on reliable and valid measurement; therefore, researchers must take steps to ensure the statistical test is reliable and valid, minimize error and biases, and use measures that contain the most precise and accurate values. This section summarizes various procedures for examining psychometric properties of measures, and methods of testing measurement equivalence across subpopulations or across times.

Measurement Psychometrics and Confirmatory Factor Analysis

Reliable and valid measures and methods are essential to minimize measurement errors and assess individual and environmentally relevant variables. Measures with low reliability attenuate the relations of these measures to other variables, including intervention effects. Researchers often rely on existing well-established psychological measures, with reasonable reliability, for hypothesis testing. Furthermore, taking a comprehensive approach that accounts for contextual variations (behaviors happen at school or at home) as well as avoids *common-method variance* and minimizes measurement errors, researchers often use multiple informants and multiple methods to assess and examine psychosocial constructs (De Los Reyes, Thomas, Goodman, & Kundey, 2013; Hunsley & Mash, 2007). For example, to assess child conduct problems, researchers collect reports from the child himself or herself, teachers, and parents as well as collect laboratory observation data from child–peer interaction tasks. Likewise, to assess parental warmth, researchers collect data from various sources that reflect acceptance, rejection, positive reinforcement, and family routine, for example.

Confirmatory factor analysis (CFA) is often the analytical tool that integrates the measures from the multiple sources and tests whether these measures are consistent with the underlying construct – for example, construct validity. More specifically, CFA is a multivariate statistical procedure that is used to investigate how well a set of observed or measured variables represent one or more latent constructs or factors. Figure 9.1 illustrates a one-factor CFA model with nine measured variables. For a one-factor model to be properly identified, more than three measured variables are necessary. Often, a straightforward one-factor model may be too simplistic to evaluate the underlying construct. Different forms of CFA are sometimes necessary, such as second-order CFA models and bifactor CFA models. *Second-order models* assess several related constructs

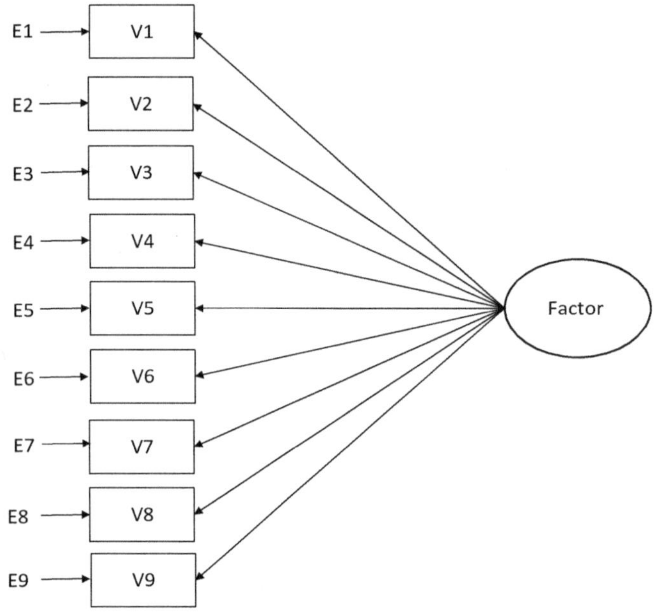

Figure 9.1. *A one-factor confirmatory factor model.*

that can be accounted for by one higher-order common underlying construct. For example, Kwok et al. (2005) applied a *second-order CFA* to examine the construct of positive parenting, which comprised lower-order constructs of child report of warmth, parent report of warmth, child report of discipline, and parent report of discipline, where each of the lower-order constructs were comprised of several psychological measures (e.g., warmth by acceptance, rejection, positive reinforcement). *Bi-factor models*, also known as *general-specific models*, comprise a general factor that accounts for the commonality of the constructs and domain-specific factors, each of which accounts for the unique influence of the specific domain over and above the general factor (Chen, West, & Sousa, 2006). For example, acceptance, rejection, talk with assurance, positive reinforcement, consistency of discipline, and monitoring are all measures of parenting (the general factor); however, acceptance, rejection, talk with assurance, and positive reinforcement reflect parent–child relationship quality while consistency of discipline and monitory reflect quality of discipline (two specific factors). Figures 9.2 and 9.3 illustrate a second-order model and a bifactor model. Testing the models as shown in Figures 9.1 through 9.3 can be done with any of the *structure equation modeling (SEM)* software programs, such as *Mplus, AMOS* (Arbuckle, 2006), *EQS* (Bentler, 2006), *Lavaan* (Rosseel, 2012), and *LISREL* (Jöreskog & Sörbom, 2006).

Conducting CFA and its various forms should be guided by hypotheses. The goodness-of-fit indices, such as *RMSEA* (root mean error of approximation; Steiger, 1990), *CFI* (comparative fit index; Bentler, 1990), and *SRMR*

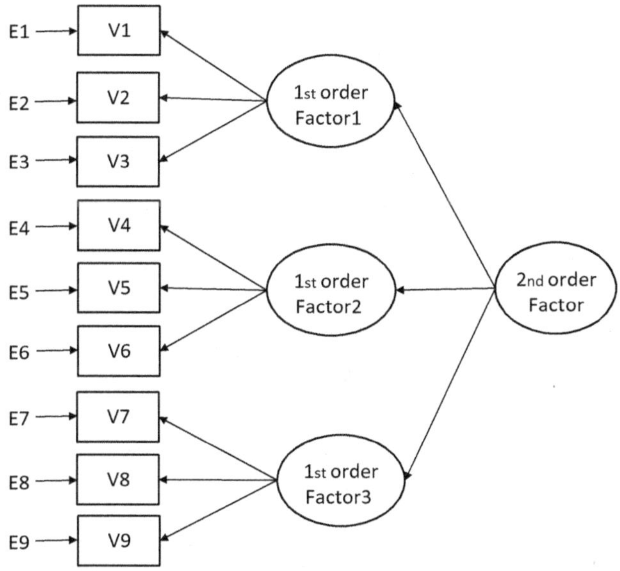

Figure 9.2. *A second-order measurement model.*

(standardized root mean square residual; Jöreskog & Sörbom, 1988), evaluate fit between the hypothesized model and the observed data. If the fit indices is poor, then the hypothesized measurement model will differ greatly from the actual values. It should be noted that for CFA with multiple informants' reports, discrepancies of reports among informants often exist and yield inconsistent findings (Achenbach, McConaughy, & Howell, 1987; Tein, Roosa, & Michaels, 1994). For example, in a study of parent–child agreement on parenting behaviors from a (United States) sample consisting of 134 fourth-, fifth-, and sixth-grade children and both of their parents, Tein et al. (1994) found that cross-generational convergent validity of the parenting measures was low. The correlations of parent and child reports concerning acceptance, rejection, firm control, hostile control, and inconsistent discipline, separately, ranged from 0.13 to 0.36 for mother–child agreement and from 0.19 to 0.31 for father–child agreement. Discrepancies might well reflect measurement errors or informants' reporting biases; they might, as well, reveal the unique perspectives held by each informant providing a report (Achenbach et al., 1987; De Los Reyes et al., 2013; Hunsley & Mash, 2007). Further investigation of discrepancies is necessary. Researchers accordingly incorporate the reasons for any discrepancy into hypothesis testing and data interpretation (see De Los Reyes et al., 2013).

Measurement Equivalence

The premise of conducting cross-cultural, cross-country, or other comparisons requires equivalent psychosocial measurements. Much cross-cultural prevention research involves adaptions or applications of intervention concepts and

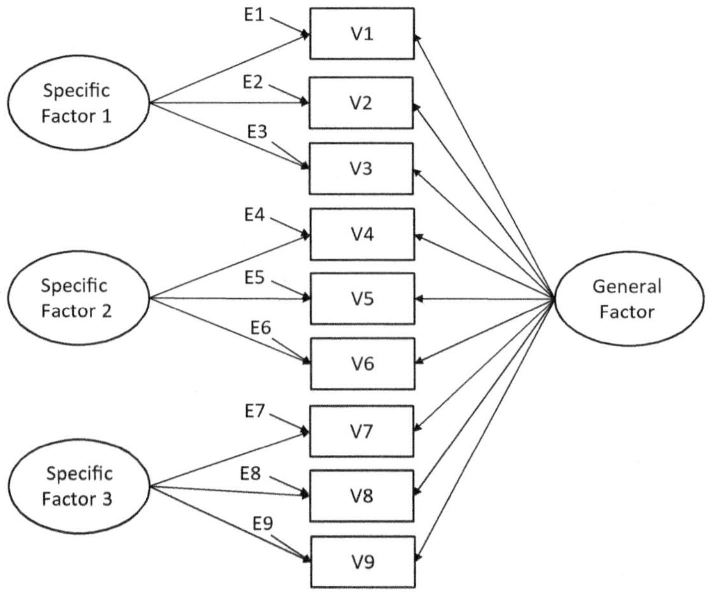

Figure 9.3. *A bifactor measurement model.*

measures developed in one cultural setting to another. Processes of adaptation or translation of existing questionnaires should consider (1) whether the construct is meaningful and recognized in the new culture, (2) whether the measure assesses the same construct in the new culture, (3) whether the meaning of each item remains the same after translation, and (4) whether the measure has the same relation with previously established criteria for the same phenomena (see Hui & Triandis, 1985; Prince, 2008). If a researcher wants to claim that a measure applies to individuals of all cultural backgrounds or subgroups or wants to make comparisons of the subgroups, *measurement invariance* across the subpopulation needs to be met first to ensure that the measures are interpreted in a conceptually similar fashion across the subgroups.

Prevention research aims at changes in behaviors or attitudes over time. Longitudinal developmental studies require balance in the use of measures that provide consistency across time yet recognize changes in the developmental contexts. The accuracy of gauging the changes hinges on the assumption of *measurement invariance* across assessment times.

Studies have demonstrated the procedures for using CFA models (see Figure 9.1) to test *measurement invariance* across subgroups (e.g., Widaman & Reise, 1997, for continuous indicators; Millsap & Tein, 2004, for categorical indicators) and across time (e.g., Widaman, Ferrer, & Conger, 2010, for continuous indicators; Coertjens, Donche, De Maeyer, Vanthournout, & Van Petegem, 2012, for ordinal categorical indicators). Basically, there are four levels of invariances, with one building upon the other, across group or time. Levels of measurement invariance are often tested by fitting and comparing the four hierarchical models with different equality constraints imposed on the estimated parameters. The first level is the *configure invariance model*, a baseline model that assumes that common factor structures are the same. That is, the general patterns of factor loadings need to be the same across group or time. The model implies that the same construct can be assessed by the same set of observed variables across subgroup or across time. This baseline model should provide a good fit of the data in order to proceed to the next level, the *metric or loading invariance model*, which assumes equivalence of *factor loadings* for all indicators. That is, the relations between the observed variables and the latent construct are the same across group or across time. If the *loading invariance* holds, the *intercept invariance model* for continuous indicators or the *threshold invariance model* for binary or ordinal-categorical variables can proceed. *Threshold invariance* assumes that for each observed variable, the threshold levels from one response to the next (e.g., from response 1 to 2, 2 to 3, etc.) are equivalent for either group or time. When loadings and intercepts/thresholds prove to be invariant, then the *unique variance invariance model* will be examined. This model requires variances that are not accounted for by the latent construct to be constrained as equal. If the unique variance invariance still holds, the models may be interpreted as full invariance (Millsap, 2011), indicating that group differences in the means, variances, and covariances are entirely attributable to the differences in the latent constructs. Only with both the loadings and intercepts/thresholds being invariant can researchers compare the means of the common factors across group or time. The *unique variance invariance model* is a highly constrained model and is often not likely to hold in practice. Empirical examples of using these steps to examine *measurement invariance* can be found in the studies by Blankson and McArdle (2013; across subgroup and time for continuous observed variables), Milfont and Fischer (2010; across subgroup for continuous observed variables), and Liu et al. (in press; across time for ordered-categorical observed variables).

Evaluation of Intervention Effects

Preventive interventions develop and implement programs or policies to prevent problem behaviors and their negative outcomes or to promote positive behaviors. Evaluation of the performance of the intervention is necessary; it provides the basis for decisions regarding whether the intervention should continue, improve, or expand. Evaluation of the intervention involves a series of analyses to investigate the program implementation and delivery (i.e., *process evaluation*) and the program impact or outcomes (i.e., *outcome analysis*). In addition, *mediation analysis* and *moderation analysis* enhance understanding of intervention effects. As intervention designs become increasingly sophisticated in their efforts to target program components for change, it is essential that researchers extract more detailed information from their studies regarding on which groups or under what conditions the intervention has effects (i.e., moderation analysis) and how the intervention achieves the effects (i.e., mediation analysis). This section reviews methodologies regarding process and outcome evaluations as well as moderation analysis to assess differential effects for subpopulations and mediation analysis to assess the mechanisms of the intervention on outcomes.

Process Evaluation

Meta-analytic studies have shown that quality of program implementation is a critical factor affecting participant outcomes (Durlak & DuPre, 2008; Wilson & Lipsey, 2007). Accurate interpretation of outcomes depends on knowing what aspects of the intervention were delivered and how well they were implemented (Durlak & DuPre, 2008). *Process evaluation* looks at how the intervention is implemented from start to finish. Durlak and DuPre (2008) identified several aspects that involve program implementation; the first four relate to how well providers deliver the program: (a) *fidelity* refers to the amount of curriculum delivered that corresponds to the originally intended program; (b) *dosage* refers to how much of the original program has been delivered; (c) *additive adaptations*, independent from a lack of fidelity, refer to quality of unscripted content added by providers during delivery of the program; and (d) *process quality* refers to the clinical and interactive skills providers use to convey the program information to participants. Another aspect, *participant responsiveness*, relates to behaviors of participants. Responsiveness refers to participants' active engagement in the program, which implies the degree to which the program stimulates the interest or holds their attention. Some of these aspects also overlap with Dane and Schneider's (1998) conceptualization of implementation integrity. However, Dane and Schneider (1998) define "dosage" as participant attendance. Other participant related aspects of process evaluation have also been proposed including completion of homework practice, perception of group cohesion, and levels of satisfaction of the intervention sessions (Tobler & Stratton, 1997).

Process evaluations are straightforward (mostly descriptive statistics) but often overlooked. Few studies conduct process evaluations. However, each of these aspects represents an important feature of program implementation and directly or indirectly affects intervention effects. A comprehensive process evaluation ensures implementation quality and integrity and enhances the interpretability of research on the outcomes of prevention programs. Deficiencies in any of the implementation processes can compromise the potential value of an intervention program (Dane & Schneider, 1998).

Outcome Evaluation

Outcome evaluation assesses the effectiveness of an intervention in producing changes as hypothesized. For a randomized control trial, researchers typically collect data at the pretest and posttest to test the hypothesis that intervention improves functioning on targeted outcomes in comparison to the control condition. Depending on the type of outcome variables, *multiple regression* or *analyses of covariance* (for continuous variables), *logistic regression* (for binary or categorical variables), *Poisson regression* (for count variables), and *survival analysis* (for time-to-event or survival time) are common statistical procedures to compare the posttest scores across the intervention and control conditions while controlling for the pretest scores.

Often researchers collect follow-up data after posttest for evaluation of short-term or long-term effects. Similar analytical procedures as the pre- and posttest evaluation are applied to evaluate findings of each of these follow-up assessment points. With pretest assessment, posttest assessment, and two or more follow-up assessments of the outcomes, researchers can examine the intervention effects on the developmental trajectories of the outcomes over time, using latent growth modeling (Muthén & Curran, 1997). *Latent growth modeling (LGM)* estimates whether individual growth trajectories of the outcome variable (i.e., within-person estimations) vary from person to person and whether the interindividual variation is systematically related to the intervention condition (i.e., between-person estimations). Performing latent growth curve models under the *finite-mixture random effects* modeling framework (i.e., *latent growth mixture modeling [LGMM]*, Muthén et al., 2002; *latent class growth analysis [LCGA]*, Nagin, 1999] is recommended to account for possible differential growth trajectory patterns across individuals. Conventional LGM assumes that all individuals have a uniform growth trajectory (e.g., linear, quadratic) whereas LGMM or LCGA assumes that not all of the individuals have the same patterns of trajectory and the model identifies multiple unobserved subpopulations within which individuals have similar patterns of trajectory that are different from the patterns of other subgroups. LGMM or LCGA allows researchers to identify distinct groups based on response patterns of growth trajectories and examine the impact of intervention within each group (see Muthén et al., 2002). LCGA is a special type of LGMM whereby the variance estimates for the growth factors within each class are assumed to be fixed to zero (i.e., all individuals growth trajectories within a class are assumed to be homogeneous). LGM, LGMM, and LCGA can be performed with Mplus and LCGA can be further performed with SAS procedure *PROC Traj* (Jones, Nagin, & Roeder, 2001).

As mentioned earlier, individuals assigned to intervention conditions may not be independent. For a group-based intervention, individuals assigned to the same group receive the program from the same interventionist. For a school-based intervention, the random assignment and delivery of the intervention most often occur at the classroom or the school level. Such data are referred to as nested data or clustered data (students nested within classrooms; individuals nested within groups), and data within the same cluster are likely to correlate to a certain extent. For example, Hedges and Hedberg (2007) provide a compilation of ICC values for academic achievement and related covariate effects on the basis of national representative samples in the United States and conclude that ICCs for mathematics or reading achievement are in the range of 0.15 to

0.25 for the national samples and for samples with low-SES schools. Even with an individual-based intervention, if individuals share some background, their data may not be independent. For example, for a large-scale universal intervention, individuals from the same geographic region (i.e., census tracks) may be more similar to each other with regard to socioeconomic status than individuals from other regions. With clustered data, random effects modeling or multilevel modeling are necessary (Raudenbush & Bryk, 2002; Snijders & Bosker, 2012). Most of the mainstream statistical software packages have the capacity to conduct multilevel analysis. HLM software (Raudenbush & Bryk, 2002; Raudenbush, Bryk, & Congdon, 2004) is also common software specifically for multilevel modeling.

As discussed earlier, RCT often suffers from noncompliance and missing data. The Consolidated Standards of Reporting Trials (CONSORT; Moher et al., 2010) guidelines recommend that participants in each group should be analyzed by the *intention-to-treat (ITT)* principle with full reporting of deviations from random allocation and missing responses. The ITT analysis includes all of the randomized participants, ignoring noncompliance, early withdrawal, and protocol deviations. As a result, the ITT analysis prevents bias caused by the loss of participants, which may disrupt the baseline equivalence established through random assignment.

The ITT analysis combines outcomes for individuals who comply with or adhere to the intervention and those who do not, although there should be little effect of intervention for those who do not comply with the intervention. As a result, the ITT estimates are conservative toward the null hypothesis. That is, ITT analysis minimizes Type I error but is more susceptible to Type II error. The ITT analysis underestimates the effects of intervention, especially when the number of individuals who are assigned to the intervention condition but do not actually comply with the intervention is not negligible (Ye, Beyene, Browne, & Thabane, 2014). However, excluding noncompliers from the analysis (i.e., per-protocol analysis) breaks randomization and has a potential for biasing the results (Connell, 2009).

A relatively novel statistical technique, *complier average causal effect (CACE)* analyses, defined as the average effect of intervention on those who complied with the intervention assignments (Angrist, Imbens, & Rubin, 1996; Jo, 2008), serves as an alternative in dealing with noncompliance. CACE analysis, originated from Rubin's causal modeling framework (Rubin, 1978), evaluates the causal effect of an intervention on the people who are intended to receive it based on original group assignment, and it accounts for potential selection bias associated with participation or compliance. Particularly, accounting for predictors of compliance with intervention in a randomized control trial, CACE evaluates the impact of the intervention by adjusting the ITT estimators for those in the intervention group who do not receive intervention services and for the crossovers in the control group who receive the intervention services. For example, Connell (2009) employed the CACE method to examine the effects of youth tobacco use from the Adolescent

Transition Program, a family-focused randomized encouragement trial, designed for delivery in the school setting. Participating families in the intervention condition engaged with intervention services as they saw fit. As a result, the degree of engagement varied. Connell compared the results between the ITT and CACE analyses and demonstrated that the ITT analysis had nonsignificant intervention effects while the CACE analysis, accounting for the engagement variable, showed significant intervention effects of reducing tobacco use for youth from families who were more likely to engage with the intervention services. CACE analysis is available in Mplus, SAS, and R and has been increasingly used for evaluating intervention effects in the last decade (Connell, 2009; Jo, 2002, 2008).

Moderation Analysis

Intervention programs often do not produce equal effects across participants (Brown & Liao, 1999). Often, interventions have bigger effects on the outcome for individuals who have more problems at baseline or for certain cultures, such as people from the Western culture in comparison with people from the Eastern culture. Moderation analysis investigates the condition under which or for whom the intervention works. If a moderated intervention exists, then the intervention does not produce a uniform effect across all individuals.

Statistically, a moderator is a variable that affects the direction or strength between a predictor and an outcome. There are two approaches for testing moderation effects – one applies to moderators, which can be a continuous variable (e.g., baseline problems) or a categorical variable (e.g., gender, nationality); another one applies to a moderator, which is only a categorical variable. The first is to test the moderation effect through the test of intervention condition × moderator interaction. Figure 9.4a illustrates the interaction model, with X being the intervention condition, Z being the moderator, and Y being the outcome. A significant product of X and Z (XZ; a_3) represents differences in the X to Y relation across levels of Z. Given a significant interaction, one needs to probe how exactly the moderator affects the direction and strength of the effect of the intervention on the outcome. The techniques for probing are plotting the interaction and conducting post hoc statistical testing of the simple effect at a specific level of the moderator (e.g., simple slope for males and for females). For a continuous moderator, it is not practical to probe the regression lines at each value of the moderator. Cohen, Cohen, West, and Aiken (2003) suggest that researchers probe three values of the moderator: one standard deviation above the mean (+1 SD; Z_{+1SD}), the mean (Z_{Mean}), and one standard deviation below the mean (–1 SD; Z_{-1SD}). Aiken and West (1991) also provide detailed instructions for probing simple effects.

Another approach is to use multiple-group structural equation modeling (SEM) to examine directly whether the coefficients of X to Y differ across discrete groups. Figure 9.4b illustrates the model for individual groups. If $c_1 \neq c_2$,

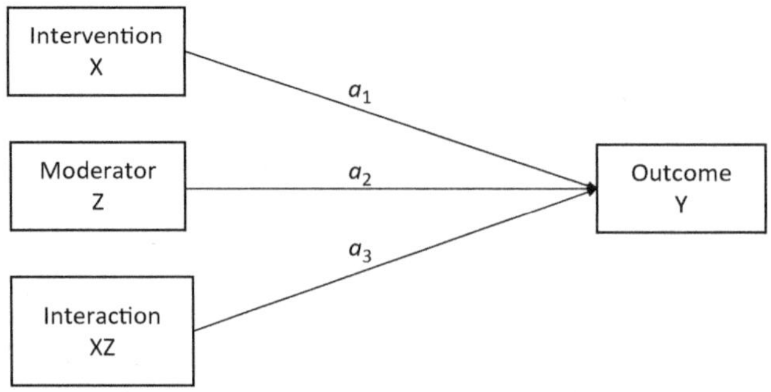

Figure 9.4a. *Testing moderation effect by XZ interaction* $Y = i_1 + a_1X + a_2Z + a_3XZ$.

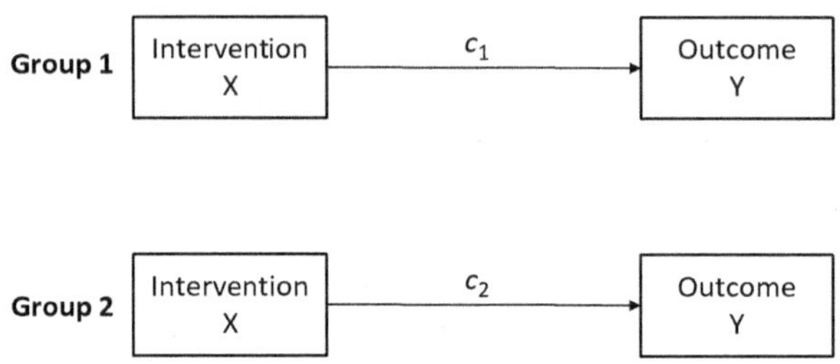

Figure 9.4b. *Testing a moderation using multiple-group SEM strategy, that is, testing* $c_1 = c_2$.

then there exists a moderation effect. It is not recommended to apply the multiple-group modeling approach to examine moderation effects when the moderator is a continuous variable. One common practice for conducting moderation analysis is to use a median split and dichotomize a continuous moderator to form high and low groups. Based on a simulation study, MacCallum, Zhang, Preacher, and Rucker (2002) demonstrate that dichotomization of a continuous predictor would result in loss of effect sizes and loss of power. Using all of the information available in the predictors, including the moderator, provides better power.

A couple of features should be noted for moderation analysis. First, Kraemer, Stice, Kazdin, Offord, and Kupfer (2001) argue that for a variable to influence the association between two other variables (e.g., $X \rightarrow Y$), that variable needs to precede both X and Y. Thus, by nature of the definition, a moderator should precede both the intervention condition and outcome variables such as a characteristic of the individual (e.g., gender, baseline behavioral problems) and a contextual factor (e.g., family environment). Second, *power* to detect moderation effects in intervention research can be challenging. Power of detecting interactions and moderation effects is often low because of the small effect sizes observed in social science studies (Aguinis et al., 2005; McClelland & Judd, 1993). Researchers should plan for an adequate sample size for moderation analysis.

Mediation Analysis

Mediation analysis is essential to investigate the mechanisms by which an intervention affects targeted mediating variables, which in turn affect outcome variables. For example, most parenting-focused intervention programs are designed to strengthen children's resilience or reduce children's behavioral problems through promoting effective parenting (see Sandler, Ingram, Wolchik, Winslow, & Tein, in press); namely, effective parenting mediates the impact of an intervention on the development of child's resilience. It can be argued that the underlying model in prevention research is the *mediation model* (MacKinnon, 2008). Prevention research builds upon etiologic or epidemiological research that studies behavioral, environmental, or biomedical risk or protective factors that may increase or decrease risks of the outcomes of interest (Cázares & Beatty, 1994; Lipsey, 1990). Theoretically based intervention integrates the etiological or epidemiological research and develops a program that aims at changing the risk or protective factors that are supposed to lead to changes in the outcome. That is, changes of the mediating factors represent the mechanisms by which the intervention affects the outcome (Sandler, Wolchik, MacKinnon, Ayers, & Roosa, 1997).

Methods for analyzing mediation effects of intervention effects have advanced rapidly. The traditional mediation analysis follows Baron and Kenny's (1986) paradigm. Figure 9.5a and 9.5b illustrate the paradigm under a simple one-mediation model, where the top diagram represents the total effect of X (independent variable; i.e., intervention condition) on Y (dependent variable; i.e., outcome), and the bottom diagram represents the mediated effect of X (intervention) on Y (outcome) through M (mediator); c' is the direct effect of X on Y adjusted for M; a is the effect of X on M; and b is the effect of M on Y adjusted for X. The indirect effect (i.e., mediated effect) is equal to the product of a and b, $a \times b$. The total effect is the sum of direct and indirect effects (i.e., $c = c' + a \times b$). In the evaluation of intervention, the a path is to test the action theory because X is directly manipulated by the intervention, whereas the b path is to test the conceptual theory because M is hypothesized to be related to Y (Chen, 1990; MacKinnon, Taborga, & Morgan-Lopez, 2002).

According to Baron and Kenny (1986), a mediation effect exists when the following conditions hold: (1) the intervention must affect the outcome, (2) the intervention must affect the mediator, and (3) the mediator must affect the outcome controlling for the intervention effect. It is debatable whether it is necessary to demonstrate that the total intervention effect on the outcome (i.e., c) needs to be significant for a mediation effect to exist. Most of the modern mediation methodologists agree that there may still be important mediation effects even if the overall intervention effect on the outcome is not significant (e.g., Kraemer, Wilson, Fairburn, & Agras, 2002; MacKinnon, 2008; Zhao, Lynch, & Chen, 2010). It is possible that the indirect effect and the direct effect have opposite signs because of a suppression effect (MacKinnon, Krull, & Lockwood, 2000) or the direct effect reflects the net effect of some omitted

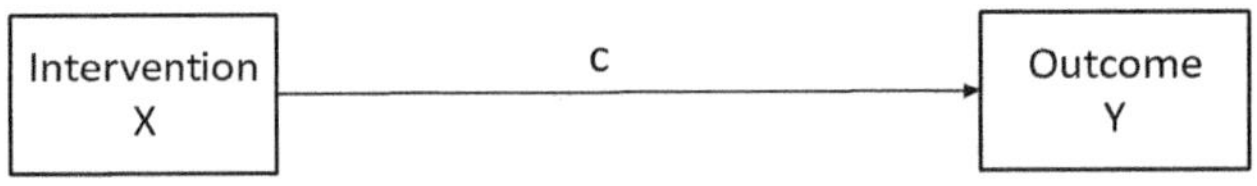

Figure 9.5a. *Total effect model from Intervention to outcome.*

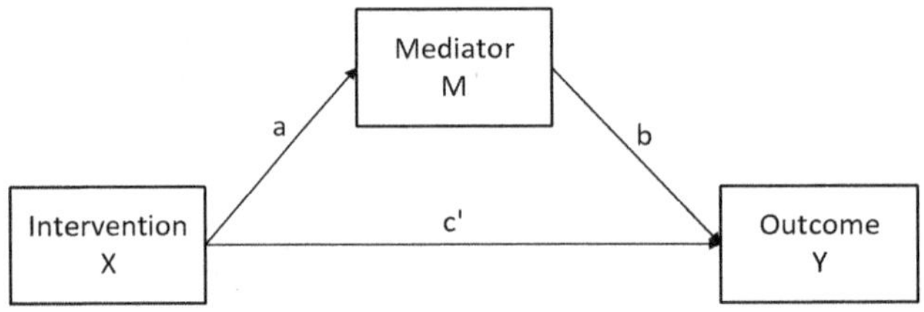

Figure 9.5b. *Mediation model where indirect effect is* $a \times b$ and direct effect is c'. The total effect is the sum of direct and indirect effects ($c = c' + a \times b$).

mediators that have different signs from the targeted mediator (Zhao et al., 2010), resulting in a nonsignificant total effect.

Most interventions are designed to change multiple mediators simultaneously or in sequence that is believed to relate to the outcome. Figures 9.6a and 9.6b illustrate extensions of Figure 9.5b. Figure 9.6a represents a multicomponent mediation model where an intervention is designed to change several mediating factors simultaneously. The multicomponent mediation analysis allows one to examine the unique mediation effect (e.g., $a_1 \times b_1$ controlling for $a_2 \times b_2$ and $a_3 \times b_3$) and the combined mediation effect (e.g., $a_1 \times b_1 + a_2 \times b_2 + a_3 \times b_3$). Figure 9.6b represents a multilink mediation model where, using a three-link model as an example (see Taylor et al., 2008), an intervention is designed to change two mediators in turn, such that the intervention affects the first mediating factor (a_1), which in turn affects the second mediating factor (b_1), which in turn leads to a change in the outcome (b_2). The mediation effect passing through both mediators is $a_1 \times b_1 \times b_2$. Note there are two other effects of X to Y, passing through only one of the mediators, $a_1 \times b_3$, and $a_2 \times b_2$.

Generally, SEM is applied to conduct mediation analysis. Several methods have been proposed for assessing significance of mediation effects. MacKinnon and his colleagues (Fritz & MacKinnon, 2007, MacKinnon, Lockwood, Hoffman, West, & Sheet, 2002; Taylor et al., 2008) have extensively evaluated these methods and concluded that joint significant tests and the bootstrap methods are better methods with smaller Type I error and/or better power. The joint significant test requires each of the path coefficients along the mediation pathway to be significant (e.g., a and b are both significant in Figure 9.5b; a_1, b_1, and b_2 are all significant in Figure 9.6b). The bootstrap method of testing mediation requires a random sample to be taken from the original data with replacement repeatedly. The values for a and b, in a two-link model as an example, are then found, and the indirect effect (e.g., $a \times b$) is computed for this bootstrap sample. This process of taking a bootstrap sample is then repeated a large number of times and the indirect effect is

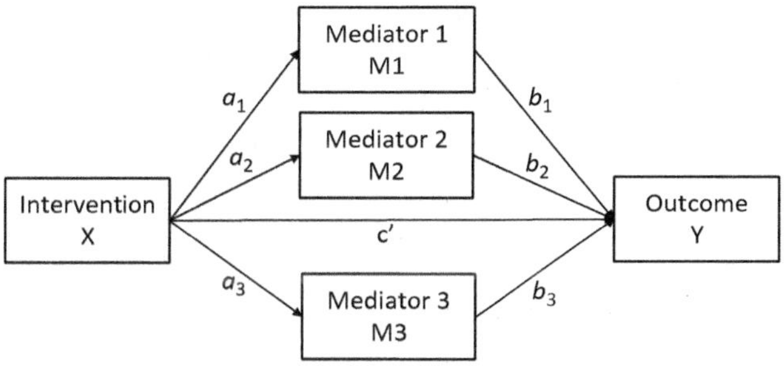

Figure 9.6a. *Multicomponent mediation model with three indirect effects,* $a_1 \times b_1$, $a_2 \times b_2$, and $a_3 \times b_3$, and where the direct effect is c'.

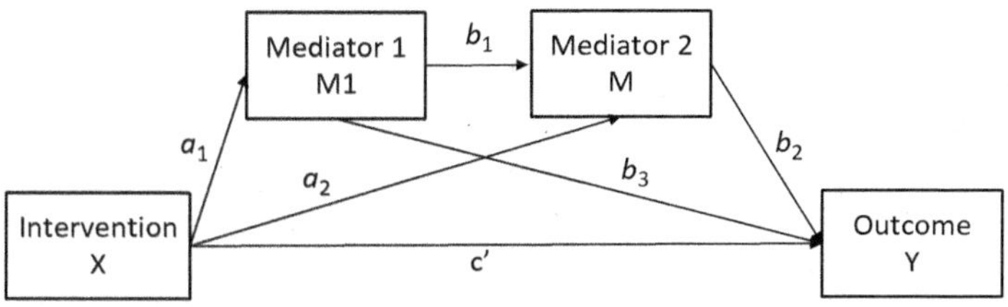

Figure 9.6b. *Multilink mediation model with three indirect effects,* $a_1 \times b_1 \times b_2$, $a_1 \times b_3$, and $a_2 \times b_2$, and where the direct effect is c'.

computed for each of the bootstrap samples. The large number of the estimates of the indirect effects from the repeated bootstrap samples then form a bootstrap distribution (e.g., probability distribution of $a \times b$ obtained from each of the two thousand bootstrap samples). The hypothesis of the mediation effect is supported if the confidence interval of the distribution (at the 95 percent or 99 percent level) does not contain zero.

Statistical relations alone cannot determine the causal relations that are essential for mediation models. Temporal precedence of intervention condition, mediator, and outcome, in this order, is necessary to define mediation effects (Kraemer et al., 2002; Maxwell & Cole, 2007). Having the outcomes being assessed at a later point in time than the mediators enables the researcher to clarify the temporal sequencing of causal processes and to rule out bidirectional pathways. However, some researchers argue that without randomizing both the intervention condition and the mediator, the causal inference of the mediation effect might be biased due to unmeasured confounders (e.g., the confounder explains the *M* to *Y* relation; see Imai, Keele, & Tingley, 2010; Lynch, Cary, Gallop, & Ten Have, 2008). Experimental approaches that directly manipulate the mediator are often impractical in prevention research because program components are interrelated and it is inefficient to separate them. Recently developed mediation analysis based on *Rubin's causal model* or the *potential outcomes* framework (Rubin, 2005; see also Albert, 2008; Imai et al., 2010; Pearl, 2014; Shpitser, 2013; VanderWeele & VanSteelandt, 2009) shows potential for more complete investigation of causal inference. By considering a participant's outcomes in the *counterfactual group* (i.e., counterfactual group membership is membership in a group that the participant *could* have been assigned, not the group in which the participant *was* assigned), the *potential outcomes model* gains insight into causal inference. Potential outcomes models for investigating mediation processes are complex and still relatively new, and software for potential outcomes analysis has just begun to appear in Mplus, SAS, R, and so on.

Summing Up

In the last two decades, there has been a rapid growth of applied statistical techniques in response to the increasing needs for more systematic and sophisticated research methodology in the field of preventive science. The advancement in research methodologies and statistical techniques has contributed to improved understanding of the etiological or epidemiological theories and theories of changes behind a preventive intervention (National Research Council and Institute of Medicine, 2009). Prevention research involves integrated processes – including conceptual specification, intervention design, and program evaluation. From the very first initiation of prevention study (research proposal, grant application), substantive researchers need to work closely with research methodologists in planning a rigorous research proposal and well-designed study, refining research design by considering new avenues for exploration, integrating state-of-the-art methodological and analytical approaches into the study, and identifying issues of concern in assessing effectiveness of the preventive intervention strategies (see also Cázares & Beatty, 1994).

This chapter provides a brief overview of research methodologies under three general areas that concern prevention research: (1) sampling and participants, (2) measurement, and (3) evaluation of intervention effects. The section on sampling and participants covers methods of recruiting samples, computing statistical power, steps of conducting attrition analysis, and modern methods of dealing with missing data. The measurement section reviews methods of testing psychological constructs under the confirmatory factor analysis framework and procedures of testing measurement invariance across subgroup and across time. In the last section of evaluating intervention effects, process and outcome evaluations as well as analyses to investigate further the mechanisms of intervention effects are discussed. In addition to explaining traditional analysis, this chapter provides more recently developed research methodologies as well as outlines statistical options, procedures, and techniques related to the methodology. Relevant references are also provided. Due to space limitation, only a few empirical examples are given. Nevertheless, preventive intervention researchers may use this chapter and listed references as resources to explore further new methodological and statistical approaches and integrate them into their intervention studies.

References

Achenbach, T. M., McConaughy, S. H., & Howell, C. T. (1987). Child/adolescent behavioral and emotional problems: implications of cross-informant correlations for situational specificity. *Psychological Bulletin* 101: 213–32. doi.org/ 10.1037/0033–2909.101.2.213

Aguinis, H., Beaty, J. C., Boik, R. J., & Pierce, C. A. (2005). Effect size and power in assessing moderating effects of categorical variables using multiple regression: a 30-year review. *Journal of Applied Psychology* 90: 94–107. doi: 10.1037/ 0021–9010.90.1.94

Aiken, L. S., & West, S. G. (1991). *Multiple Regression: Testing and Interpreting Interactions*. Newbury Park, CA: Sage.

Albert, J. M. (2008). Mediation analysis via potential outcomes models. *Statistics in Medicine* 27(8): 1282–1304. doi: 10.1002/sim.3016

Angrist, J., Imbens, G., & Rubin, D. (1996). Identification of causal effects using instrumental variables. *Journal of the American Statistical Association* 91: 444–72. doi: 10.1080/01621459.1996.10476902

Arbuckle, J. L. (2006). *Amos 7.0 User's Guide*. Chicago, IL: SPSS.

Baron, R. M., & Kenny, D. A. (1986). The moderator-mediator variable distinction in social psychological research: conceptual, strategic, and statistical considerations. *Journal of Personality and Social Psychology* 51: 1173–82. doi.org/ 10.1037/0022–3514.51.6.1173

Bentler, P. M. (1990). Comparative fit indexes in structural models. *Psychological Bulletin* 107: 238–46. doi.org/10.1037/0033–2909.107.2.238

Bentler, P. M. (2006). *EQS 6 Structural Equation Program Manual*. Encino, CA: Multivariate Software, Inc.

Blankson, A. N., & McArdle, J. J. (2013). Measurement invariance of cognitive abilities across ethnicity, gender, and time among older Americans. *Journals of Gerontology, Series B: Psychological Sciences and Social Sciences* 70: 386–97. doi: 10.1093/geronb/gbt106

Brown, C. H., & Liao, J. (1999). Principles for designing randomized preventive trials in mental health: an emerging developmental epidemiology paradigm. *American Journal of Community Psychology* 27: 673–710. doi.org/10.1023/A:1022142021441

Brown, C. H., Wang, W., Kellam, S. G., Muthén, M. O., Petras, H., Topinbo, P., ... et al., Prevention Science and Methodology Group (2008). Methods for testing theory and evaluating Impact in randomized field trials: intent-to-treat analyses for integrating the perspectives of person, place, and time. *Journal of Drug and Alcohol Dependence* 95(Supplement 1): s74–s104. doi.org/10.1016/ j.drugalcdep.2007.11.013

Cázares, A., & Beatty. L. A. (eds.) (1994). *Scientific Methods for Prevention Intervention Research*. Rockville, MD: National Institute on Drug Abuse Research Monograph.

Chen, F. F., West. S. G., & Sousa, K. H. (2006). A comparison of bifactor and second-order models of quality of life. *Multivariate Behavioral Research* 41: 189–225. doi.org/10.1207/s15327906mbr4102_5

Chen, H.-T. (1990). *Theory-Driven Evaluations*. Newbury Park, CA: Sage.

Coertjens, L., Donche, V., De Maeyer, S., Vanthournout, G., & Van Petegem, P. (2012). Longitudinal measurement invariance of Likert-type learning strategy scales:

are we using the same ruler at each wave? *Journal of Psychoeducational Assessment* 30: 577–87. doi.org/10.1177/0734282912438844

Cohen, J. (1988). *Statistical Power Analysis for the Behavioral Sciences*. Hillsdale, NJ: Lawrence Erlbaum.

Cohen, J., Cohen, P., West, S. G., & Aiken, L. S. (2003). *Applied Multiple Regression/Correlation Analysis for the Behavioral Sciences*, 3rd ed. Hillsdale, NJ: Lawrence Erlbaum.

Connell, A. (2009). Employing complier average causal effect analytic methods to examine effects of randomized encouragement trials. *American Journal of Drug and Alcohol Abuse* 35: 253–59. doi: 10.1080/00952990903005882

Cotter, R. B., Burke, J. D., Loeber, R,, & Navratil, J. L. (2002). Innovative retention methods in longitudinal research: a case study of the developmental trends study. *Journal of Child and Family Studies* 11: 485–98. doi: 10.1023/A:1020939626243

Cronbach, L. J., Ambron, S. R., Dornbursch, S. M., Hess, R. D., Hornik, R. C., Phillips, D. C., . . . Weiner, S. S. (1980). *Toward Reform of Program Evaluation*. San Francisco, CA: Jossey-Bass.

Dane, A. V., & Schneider, B. H. (1998). Program integrity in primary and early secondary prevention: are implementation effects out of control? *Clinical Psychology Review* 18: 23–45. doi.org/10.1016/S0272-7358(97)00043–3

De Los Reyes, A., Thomas, S. A., Goodman, K. L., & Kundey, S. M. A. (2013). Principles underlying the use of multiple informants' reports. *Annual Review of Clinical Psychology* 9: 123–49. doi: 10.1146/annurev-clinpsy-050212–185617

Demidenko, E. (2007). Sample size determination for logistic regression revisited. *Statistics in Medicine* 26: 3385–97. doi: 10.1002/sim.2771

Dempster, A. P., Laird, N. M., & Rubin, D. B. (1977). Maximum likelihood estimation from incomplete data via the EM algorithm (with discussion). *Journal of the Royal Statistical Society, Series B* 39: 1–38.

Diggle, P. J., & Kenward, M. G. (1994). Informative dropout in longitudinal data analysis (with discussion). *Applied Statistics* 43: 49–73. doi.org/10.2307/2986113

Durlak, J. A. & DuPre, E. P. (2008). Implementation matters: a review of research on the influence of implementation on program outcomes and the factors affecting implementation. *American Journal of Community Psychology* 41: 327–50. doi.org/10.1007/s10464-008–9165-0

Elwood, P. C. (1982). Randomised controlled trials: sampling, *British Journal of Clinical Pharmacology* 13: 631–6. doi: 10.1111/j.1365–2125.1982.tb01429.x

Enders, C. K. (n. d.). Applied missing data.com: companion website for applied missing data analysis. www.appliedmissingdata.com/macro-programs.html.

Enders, C. K. (2011). Missing not at random models for latent growth curve analyses. *Psychological Methods* 16: 1–16. doi.org/10.1037/a0022640

Faul, F., Erdfelder, E., Lang, A. G., & Buchner, A. (2009). Statistical power analyses using G * Power 3.1: tests for correlation and regression analyses. *Behavior Research Methods* 41: 1149–60. doi: 10.3758/BRM.41.4.1149

Fritz, M. S., & MacKinnon, D. P. (2007). Required sample size to detect the mediated effect. *Psychological Science* 18: 233–9. doi.org/10.1111/j.1467–9280.2007.01882.x

Hansen, W. B., Collin, L. M., Malotte, C. K., Johnson, C. A., & Fielding, J. E. (1985). Attrition in prevention research. *Journal of Behavioral Medicine* 8: 261–75. doi.org/10.1007/BF00870313

Hedeker, D., & Gibbons, R. D. (1997). Application of random-effects pattern-mixture models for missing data in longitudinal studies. *Psychological Methods* 2: 64–78. doi.org/10.1037/1082–989X.2.1.64

Hedges, L. V., & Hedberg, E. C. (2007). Intraclass correlations for planning group-randomized experiments in education. *Educational Evaluation and Policy Analysis* 29: 60–87.

Hedges, L. V., & Rhoads, C. (2009). *Statistical Power Analysis in Education Research (NCSER 2010–3006)*. Washington, DC: National Center for Special Education Research, Institute of Education Sciences, U.S. Department of Education.

Hox, J. (2010). *Multilevel Analysis: Techniques and Applications*, 2nd ed. New York: Routledge.

Hsieh, F. Y., Bloch, D. A., & Larsen, M. D. (1998). A simple method of sample size calculation for linear and logistic regression. *Statistics in Medicine* 17: 1623–34. doi.org/10.1002/(SICI)1097-0258(19980730)17:14%3C1623::AID-SIM871%3E3.0.CO;2-S

Hui, C. H., & Triandis, H. C. (1985). Measurement in cross-cultural psychology: a review and comparison of strategies. *Journal of Cross-Cultural Psychology* 16: 131–52. doi: 1177/0022002186017002006

Hunsley, J., & Mash, E. J. (2007). Evidence-based assessment. *Annual Review of Clinical Psychology* 3: 29–51. doi.org/10.1146/annurev.clinpsy.3.022806.091419

IBM Corp. (2013). *IBM SPSS Statistics for Windows, Version 22.0.* Armonk, NY: IBM Corp.

Imai, K., Keele, L., & Tingley, D. (2010). A general approach to causal mediation analysis. *Psychological Methods* 15: 309–34. doi.org/10.1037/a0020761

Jo, B. (2002). Estimating intervention effects with noncompliance: alternative model specifications. *Journal of Educational and Behavioral Statistics* 27: 385–420. doi.org/10.3102/10769986027004385

Jo, B. (2008). Causal inference in randomized experiments with mediational processes. *Psychological Methods* 13: 314–36. doi.org/10.1037/a0014207

Jones, B. L., Nagin, D. S., & Roeder, K. (2001). A SAS procedure based on mixture models for estimating developmental trajectories. *Sociological Methods & Research* 29: 374–93.

Jöreskog, K. G. & Sörbom, D. (1988). *LISREL 7 – a Guide to the Program and Applications*, 2nd ed. Chicago, IL: SPSS.

Jöreskog, K. G., & Sörbom, D. (2006). *LISREL 8.8 for Windows* [computer software]. Skokie, IL: Scientific Software International, Inc.

Jurs, S. G., & Glass, G.V. (1971). The effect of experimental mortality on the internal and external validity of the randomized comparative experiment. *Journal of Experimental Education* 40: 62–6. doi: 10.1080/00220973.1971.11011304

King, G., Honaker, J., Joseph, A., & Scheve, K. (2001). Analyzing incomplete political science data: an alternative algorithm for multiple imputation. *American Political Science Review* 95: 49–69.

Kraemer, H. C., Stice, E., Kazdin, A., Offord, D., & Kupfer, D. (2001). How do risk factors work together? Mediators, moderators, and independent, overlapping and proxy risk factors. *American Journal of Psychiatry* 158: 848–83. doi.org/10.1176/appi.ajp.158.6.848

Kraemer, H. C., Wilson, G. T., Fairburn, C. G., & Agras, W. S. (2002). Mediators and moderators of treatment effects in randomized clinical trials. *Archives of General Psychiatry* 59: 877–84. doi.org/10.1001/archpsyc.59.10.877

Kwok, O., Haine, R. A., Sandler, I. N., Ayers, T. S., Wolchik, S. A., & Tein, J.-Y. (2005). Positive parenting as a mediator of the relations between parental psychological distress and mental health problems of parentally bereaved children. *Journal of Clinical Child and Adolescent Psychology* 34: 260–71. doi: 10.1207/s15374424jccp3402_5

Lipsey, M. W. (1990). *Design Sensitivity: Statistical Power for Experimental Research.* Newbury Park, CA: Sage.

Little, R. J. A. (1988). A test of missing completely at random for multivariate data with missing values. *Journal of the American Statistical Association* 83: 1198–1202. doi.org/10.1080/01621459.1988.10478722

Little, R. J. A. (1993). Pattern-mixture models for multivariate incomplete data. *Journal of the American Statistical Association* 88: 125–34. doi.org/10.1080/01621459.1993.10594302

Little, R. J. A. (1995). Modeling the dropout mechanism in repeated-measures studies. *Journal of the American Statistical Association* 90: 1112–21. doi.org/10.1080/01621459.1995.10476615

Little, R. J. A., & Rubin, D. B. (2002). *Statistical Analysis with Missing Data*, 2nd ed. New York: John Wiley & Sons.

Liu, Y., Millsap, R., West, S. G., Tein, J.-Y., Tanaka, R., & Grimm, K. J. (in press). Testing measurement invariance in longitudinal data with ordered-categorical measures. *Psychological Methods.*

Lynch, K. G., Cary, M., Gallop, R., & Ten Have, T. (2008). Causal mediation analyses for randomized trials. *Health Services and Outcomes Research Methodology* 8: 57–76. doi: 10.1007/s10742-008-0028-9

MacCallum, R. C., Zhang, S., Preacher, K. J., & Rucker, D. D. (2002). On the practice of dichotomization of quantitative variables. *Psychological Methods* 7: 19–40. doi: 10.1037//1082–989X.7.1.19

MacKinnon, D. P. (2008). *Introduction to Statistical Mediation Analysis.* New York: Taylor & Francis Group.

MacKinnon, D. P., Krull, J. L., & Lockwood, C. M. (2000). Equivalence of the mediation, confounding, and suppression effect. *Prevention Science* 1: 173–81. doi.org/10.1023/A:1026595011371

MacKinnon, D. P., Lockwood, C. M., Hoffman, J. M., West, S. G., & Sheets, V. (2002). A comparison of methods to test the significance of the mediated effect. *Psychological Methods* 7: 83–104. doi.org/10.1037/1082–989X.7.1.83

MacKinnon, D. P., Taborga, M. P., & Morgan-Lopez, A. A. (2002). Mediation designs for tobacco prevention research. *Journal of Drug and Alcohol Dependence* 68 (Supplement 1): s74–s104. doi.org/10.1016/S0376-8716(02)00216–8

Maxwell, S. E., & Cole, D. A. (2007). Bias in cross-sectional analyses of longitudinal mediation. *Psychological Methods* 12: 23–44. doi.org/10.1037/1082–989X.12.1.23

McClelland, G. H., & Judd, C. M. (1993). Statistical difficulties of detecting interactions and moderator effects. *Psychological Bulletin* 114: 376–90. doi.org/10.1037/0033–2909.114.2.376

McKay, M. M., & Bannon, W. M. J. (2004). Engaging families in child mental health services. *Child and Adolescent Psychiatric Clinics of North America* 13: 905–21. doi: 10.1016/j.chc.2004.04.001

Milfont, T. L., & Fischer, R. (2010). Testing measurement invariance across groups: application in cross-cultural research. *International Journal of Psychological Research* 3: 111–21.

Millsap, R. E. (2011). *Statistical Approaches to Measurement Invariance*. New York: Routledge.

Millsap, R. E., & Tein, J.-Y. (2004). Assessing factorial invariance in ordered-categorical measures. *Multivariate Behavioral Research* 39: 479–515. doi: 10.1207/S15327906MBR3903_4

Moher, D., Hopewell, S., Schulz, K. F., Montori, V., Gøtzsche, P. C., Devereaux, P. J., Elbourne, D., Egger, M., & Altman, D. G. (2010). CONSORT 2010 explanation and elaboration: updated guidelines for reporting parallel group randomised trials. *Journal of Clinical Epidemiology* 63: e1–e37. doi: 10.1016/j.jclinepi.2010.03.004

Múthen, B. O., Brown, C. H., Masyn, K., Jo, B., Khoo, S., Yang, C.-C., Wang, C.-P, Kellam, S., Carlin, J. B., & Liao, J. (2002). General growth mixture modeling for randomized preventive interventions. *Biostatistics* 3: 459–75. doi.org/10.1093/biostatistics/3.4.459

Múthen, B. O., & Curran, P. J. (1997). General longitudinal modeling of individual differences in experimental designs: a latent variable framework for analysis and power estimation. *Psychological Methods* 2: 371–402. doi.org/10.1037/1082–989X.2.4.371

Muthén, L. K., & Muthén, B. O. (1998–2014). *Mplus User's Guide*, 7th ed. Los Angeles, CA: Muthén & Muthén.

Muthén, L. K., & Muthén, B. O. (2002). How to use a Monte Carlo study to decide on sample size and determine power. *Structural Equation Modeling* 9: 599–620. doi.org/10.1207/S15328007SEM0904_8

Nagin, D. S. (1999). Analyzing developmental trajectories: a semiparametric group-based approach. *Psychological Methods* 4: 139–57. doi.org/10.1037/1082–989X.4.2.139

National Research Council and Institute of Medicine (2009). *Preventing Mental, Emotional, and Behavioral Disorders among Young People: Progress and Possibilities. Committee on the Prevention of Mental Disorders and Substance Abuse among Children, Youth, and Young Adults: Research Advances and Promising Interventions*. O'Connell, M. E., Boat, T., & Warner, K. E. (eds.), Board on Children, Youth, and Families, Division of Behavioral and Social Sciences and Education. Washington, DC: National Academies Press.

Pearl, J. (2014). Interpretation and identification of causal mediation. *Psychological Methods* 19: 459–81. doi: 10.1037/a0036434

Prince, M. (2008). Measurement validity in cross-cultural comparative research. *Epidemiology and Psychiatric Science* 17: 211–20. doi: 10.1017/S1121189X00001305

R Development Core Team (2007). *R: A Language and Environment for Statistical Computing*. Vienna: R Foundation for Statistical Computing. www.R-project.org

Raudenbush, S. W., & Bryk, A. S. (2002). *Hierarchical Linear Models: Applications and Data Analysis Methods*. Thousand Oaks, CA: Sage.

Raudenbush, S. W., Bryk, A. S., & Congdon, R. (2004). *HLM 6 for Windows* [computer software]. Skokie, IL: Scientific Software International, Inc.

Raudenbush, S. W., Spybrook, J., Congdon, R., Liu, X., & Martinez, A., Bloom, H., & Hill, C. (2011). *Optimal Design Software Plus Empirical Evidence (Version 3.0)* [software]. www.wtgrantfoundation.org

Riecken, H. W., & Boruch, R. F. (1974). *Social Experimentation: A Method for Planning and Evaluating Social Intervention*. New York: Academic Press.

Rosseel, Y. (2012). lavaan: an R package for structural equation modeling. *Journal of Statistical Software* 48: 1–36. www.jstatsoft.org/v48/i02/

Rubin D. B. (1976). Inference and missing data. *Biometrika* 63: 581–92. doi.org/10.1093/biomet/63.3.581

Rubin, D. B. (1978). Bayesian inference for causal effects: the role of randomization. *Annals of Statistics* 6: 34–58. doi.org/10.1214/aos/1176344064

Rubin D. B. (1987). *Multiple Imputation for Nonresponse in Surveys*. New York: John Wiley & Sons.

Rubin, D. B. (1996). Multiple imputation after 18+ years. *Journal of the American Statistical Association* 91: 473–89. doi.org/10.1080/01621459.1996.10476908

Rubin, D. B. (2005). Causal inference using potential outcomes. *Journal of the American Statistical Association* 100: 322–31. doi: 10.1198/016214504000001880

SAS Institute Inc. (2008). SAS/STAT® 9.2 User's Guide. Cary, NC: SAS Institute Inc.

Sandler, I. N., Ingram, A., Wolchik, S. A., Winslow E. B., & Tein, J.-Y. (in press). Long-term effects of parenting preventive interventions to promote resilience of children and adolescents. *Child Development Perspectives*.

Sandler, I. N., Wolchik, S. A., MacKinnon, D., Ayers, T. S., & Roosa, M. W. (1997). Developing linkages between theory and intervention in stress and coping processes. In Wolchik, S. A., & Sandler, I. N. (eds.), *Handbook of Children's Coping: Linking Theory and Intervention*. New York: Plenum, pp. 3–40.

Schafer, J. L. (1997). *Analysis of Incomplete Multivariate Data*. London: Chapman & Hall.

Schafer, J. L., & Graham, J. W. (2002). Missing data: our view of the state of the art. *Psychological Methods* 7: 147–77. doi.org/10.1037/1082–989X.7.2.147

Schafer, J. L., & Olsen, M. K. (1998). Multiple imputation for multivariate missing-data problems: a data analyst's perspective. *Multivariate Behavioral Research* 33: 545–71. doi: 10.1207/s15327906mbr3304_5

Shadish, W. R., Cook, T. D., & Campbell, D. T. (2002). *Experimental and Quasi-Experimental Designs for Generalized Causal Inference*. Boston: Houghton-Mifflin.

Shpitser, I. (2013). Counterfactual graphical models for longitudinal mediation analysis with unobserved confounding. *Cognitive Science* 37: 1011–35. doi: 10.1111/cogs.12058

Snijders, T. A. B., & Bosker, R. J. (2012). *An Introduction to Basic and Advanced Multilevel Modeling*, 2nd ed. Thousand Oaks, CA: Sage.

StataCorp (2013). *Stata Statistical Software: Release 13*. College Station, TX: StataCorp LP.

Steiger, J.H. (1990). Structural model evaluation and modification: an interval estimation approach. *Multivariate Behavioral Research* 25: 173–80. doi.org/10.1207/s15327906mbr2502_4

Sullivan, C. M., Rumptz, M. H., Campbell, R., Eby, K. K., Davidson II, W. S. (1996). Retaining participants in longitudinal community research: a comprehensive protocol. *Journal of Applied Behavioral Science* 32: 262–76.

Taylor, A. B., MacKinnon, D., & Tein, J.-Y. (2008). Test of the three path mediated effect. *Organization Research Methods* 11: 241–69. doi: 10.1177/1094428107300344

Tein, J.-Y., Roosa, M.W., & Michaels, M. (1994). Agreement between parent and child reports on parental behaviors. *Journal of Marriage and the Family* 56: 341–55. doi.org/10.2307/353104

Tobler, N., & Stratton, H. (1997) Effectiveness of school-based drug prevention programs: a meta-analysis of the research. *Journal of Primary Prevention*, 18: 71–128. doi.org/10.1023/A:10246302059999

VanderWeele, T., & Vansteelandt, S. (2009). Conceptual issues concerning mediation, interventions and composition. *Statistics and Its Interface* 2: 457–68. doi.org/10.4310/SII.2009.v2.n4.a7

Widaman, K. F., & Reise, S. P. (1997). Exploring the measurement invariance of psychological instruments: Application in substance use domain. In Kendall, B. I., Windle, M. T., & West, S. G. (eds.), *The Science of Prevention: Methodological Advances from Alcohol and Substance Abuse Research*. Washington, DC: American Psychological Association, pp. 281–324.

Widaman, K. F., Ferrer, E., & Conger, R. D. (2010). Factorial invariance within longitudinal structural equation models: measuring the same construct across time. *Child Development Perspectives* 4: 10–18. doi.org/10.1111/j.1750–8606.2009.00110.x

Wilson, S. J., & Lipsey, M. J. (2007). Effectiveness of school-based intervention programs on aggressive behavior: update of a meta-analysis. *American Journal of Preventive Medicine* 33(Supplement 2): S130–S143. doi: 10.1016/j.amepre.2007.04.011

Wolchik, S. A., Sandler, I. N., Tein, J. Y., Mahrer, N., Millsap, R., Winslow, E. B., ... Reed, A. B. (2013). Fifteen-year follow-up of a randomized trial of preventive intervention for divorced families: effects on mental health and substance use outcomes in young adulthood. *Journal of Consulting and Clinical Psychology* 81: 660–73. doi: 0091–0627/04/0400-0175/0

Ye, C., Beyene, J., Browne, G., & Thabane, L. (2014). Estimating treatment effects in randomised controlled trials with non-compliance: a simulation study. *BMJ Open* 4: e005362. doi: 10.1136/bmjopen-2014-005362

Zhao, X., Lynch, J. G., Jr., & Chen, Q. (2010). Reconsidering Baron and Kenny: myths and truths about mediation analysis. *Journal of Consumer Research* 37: 197–206. doi: 10.1086/651257

Implementation

10 Prevention in Recreational Nightlife

Amador Calafat & Montse Juan

Relevance of the Recreational Use of Drugs: Cultural Implications

Traditionally, the use of alcohol and illegal drugs has been related to several risk factors such as poverty, exclusion, lack of network, personality problems, and so on. However, during the last decades the situation has changed. In certain locations and regions worldwide, the use and abuse of these substances is basically conducted by normative young people in nightlife recreational settings. This implies a quite radical change in the sort of people who consume legal or illegal drugs and the risk factors to be considered. In fact, what should be taken into consideration is that the socialization of these adolescents and young people is rapidly and drastically changing through the consolidation of these new social practices.

This takes us to the following issue. Behind these recreational contexts, so appealing for youngsters, there is an important industry as well as government interest (at local, regional, or national level) in fostering young people to participate in nightlife. A document produced by the Greater London Authority shows clearly that "consuming/drinking alcohol in the night-time economy (NTE) can have many benefits. For example, it generates economic activity and employment; it can bring people together to socialise; and it is an enjoyable pastime that many people value" (Wickham, 2012, p. 2).

This relatively recent development of the recreational use of drugs, as we currently understand the phenomena, has produced an impressive change in the way that people, including professionals and institutions, look at drugs and to the so called problematic drug use (PDU): In the official United Kingdom strategy on drugs, PDUs are related to "those using opiates (e.g. heroin, morphine, codeine) and/or crack cocaine" (HM Government, 2008, p. 50), and, according to this source, these drugs account for 99 percent of the costs to society. For the European Monitoring Centre on Drugs and Drug Addiction (EMCDDA), PDU is reduced to "injection drug use or long duration/regular use of opioids, cocaine and/or amphetamines..., but neither includes their rare nor irregular use, nor the use of ecstasy or cannabis" (EMCDDA, 2011). Of course, this restrictive view has been criticized because the use of other drugs, such as methamphetamines, cannabis, ecstasy, and psychotropics, have not been much studied. Just as an example, the estimated economic burden of methamphetamine use in the United States in 2005 was $23.4 billion, which amounts to approximately 20 percent of the estimated total cost for drug use in the country (Nicosia, Pacula, Kilmer, Lundberg, & Chiesa, 2009).

Drug use is very connected to the cultural context. We used to think of cannabis as linked to the hippie culture. In the same way, ecstasy or MDMA (methylenedioxymethamphetamine) has been, for many years, the paradigm of nightlife for many people. These drugs have even been baptized with a name that emphasizes their relationship with a specific environment, such as club drugs, dance drugs, recreational drugs, and so on. In addition, taking as an example the United Kingdom, one speaks of the ecstasy generation or the ecstasy culture (Fountain & Griffiths, 1997):

> The synthesis of house music and ecstasy has produced the largest youth cultural phenomenon that Britain has ever seen. Ecstasy culture had become the primary leisure activity for British youth, seamlessly integrated into the fabric of the weekend ritual. It was a highly lucrative business for operators on both sides of the law. The market place for the British dance scene had grown more than fivefold in a decade, while the gross financial proceeds had multiplied well over ten times (Collins, 1997, p. 267).

This paragraph has summarized the elements that work together to create this powerful new context: young people, use of certain drugs, culture, nightlife, and recreational industry. Through the synergy of these elements something that was reserved to certain social elite becomes, since the 1980s, open to many people.

Nightlife is now linked to a legitimate and well-considered industry that supplies postindustrial "lifestyle consumption" goods to cities and enhances cities' images as lively, cosmopolitan urban habitats (Hobbs, Winlow, Hadfield, & Lister, 2005). Nightlife has risen as a policy priority in some countries, such as Britain, Sweden, and Australia. Since the late 1980s, some deindustrializing cities adopted the mantra of the "twenty-four-hour" city, seeking to develop a "nighttime economy (NTE)" as part of efforts to develop a postindustrial economy (Heath, 1997).

All these issues have important prevention implications. Classical risk factors for drug and alcohol use considered up to now, such as underachievement at school, social exclusion, sensation seeking, lack of family control, and so on, become less important and/or play a different role in this new nightlife context. Most of the people participating in nightlife are studying or working, belong to a middle-class family, and have a good network of friends, and going out contributes to increase their social capital. Meanwhile, contextual factors become more relevant (e.g., intense involvement in recreational activity, selection of venues that are more permissive, special interest in certain types of music) as the new risk factors for drug and alcohol use and abuse (Calafat, Fernández, Juan, & Becoña, 2008a). From the age of fourteen or fifteen years onward, the majority of young people in certain countries go out to bars, nightclubs, and parties with their friends and mates. Attendance in these settings often goes hand in hand with alcohol and/or other drugs consumption.

These considerations force us to reconsider risk factors, prevention, and socials norms. Both individuals and society have difficulties identifying the potential harmful links to recreational nightlife, and therefore prevention is not considered important.

Depending on the city, young Europeans devote between four and seven hours to nightlife every weekend night that they go out (Calafat et al., 1999). For example, to ascertain going-out frequency among the general adolescent population in Spain, a survey was conducted in 2010 with 31,967 Spanish students (fourteen to eighteen years old) attending secondary schools (Delegación del Gobierno para el Plan Nacional sobre Drogas, 2010). Data showed that 49 percent of these students attended a nightlife setting at least once a week. Looking at the last time they went out during the weekend, 16.5 percent of them arrived home before midnight, 58.8 percent between 12:00 and 4:00 A.M., and the rest (24.7 percent) after 4.00 A.M.; percentages differed for each group by age. In this study, the frequency of alcohol (eighteen years is the legal age to consume alcohol in public venues in Spain) and drug use is firmly linked to the time they go home. Among seventeen-year-old adolescents, who return home before midnight, 37.7 percent had taken at least one drug, while among those who went home after 4.00 A.M. the percentage rises to 91.8 percent. Summing up, as this study showed, going out is a very frequent social practice in some countries, starting at a very young age, and the more time devoted to nightlife increases the chances of using legal and illegal alcohol and drugs. Frequencies vary from country to country depending on factors such as cultural traditions, widespread NTE, low prices, social permissiveness, and alcohol and drug accessibility, among others.

Given the globalization of youth cultures, it would be advisable to address the emerging problem in its early stages, by developing new approaches to prevent drug and alcohol abuse in recreational environments and by sharing experiences between countries with a sound record in dealing with the problem and those that are new to it (United Nations, 2002).

What Problems Are Related to Nightlife?

It is not a question here to discuss the multiple benefits that arise from a NTE. What we need to do is to call attention to certain problems that arise from this activity and that most of the time are not well identified and addressed. It is not easy to make people aware of the problems or to plan prevention activities in recreational contexts. Why should something as positive as having fun be problematic? Why should an activity practiced by so many "normal" youngsters be a problem? What are the risks, where, and to whom? These questions can be analyzed from different perspectives: according to the substances consumed or the type of problem, or in relation to the place where it takes place or the type of people who are more affected.

Problems to be considered are not only drunkenness and taking drugs. We should consider also health problems (e.g., involuntary injuries, hearing damage, heat stroke, etc.), violence, unsafe and involuntary sex, transport to and from recreational settings under the effects of alcohol and other substances, social nuisance (noise, street drinking, vandalism, etc.), underage drinking, and crime and law offences.

Violence

Research consistently shows that the peak time for violent offenses are weekend nights in and around pubs and clubs (Allen, Nicholas, Salisbury, & Wood, 2003). Nightlife settings are known to be common locations for alcohol-related harm, including physical and verbal aggression, drunkenness, and unintentional injury (Schnitzer et al., 2010). Research on alcohol-related harm in nightlife environments across Europe is rare, but there have been a few studies indicating the extent of such harm. A study of sixteen to thirty-five year olds in nine European cities found that the proportion of participants who reported involvement in violence in nightlife in the past twelve months ranged from 7.5 percent in Ljubljana (Slovenia) to 29.1 percent in Berlin (Schnitzer et al., 2010).

Research (Hughes et al., 2011a) involving 6,502 young British and German tourists who visited different Mediterranean tourist resorts gives some hints on how violence arises. As expected, males are the most involved in fights. Being involved in violence is more probable based on the destination and the tourists' interest in nightlife. Accordingly, the level of violence is higher in those destinations where nightlife is more prominent (Majorca, Cyprus, or Crete). Nationality is also important, but in the Hughes et al. (2011a) research, British and German tourists share nearly the same prevalence of violence in Majorca (around 6 percent have been involved in a fight), but not in Crete where violence involves mainly British tourists. As expected, most of the violence, regardless of nationality, occurs under the influence of alcohol (90 percent), and illegal drugs play a minor role. Probably this is because illegal drugs are less accessible to tourists during such short visits. Nevertheless, when people consume drugs, whether cannabis or others, they are frequently involved in fights. Half of the violence in this study took place in bars and clubs and 36 percent in the streets. About 62 percent of the fights resulted in injury.

Sexual Risk Behaviors and Sexual Harassment

Different matters are covered under the umbrella of sexual risk behaviors (e.g., sex against one's will, sex without control on birth or sexually transmitted disease, sexual harassment, sexuality under the effects of alcohol and drugs). Nightlife and the use of substances are central to the way many people experience sexuality nowadays. People go to bars and other nightlife venues for socialization, looking to meet potential partners, and so on. These encounters between people are not exempt from misunderstandings. Sometimes sexual contacts are positive and consensual, but aggression related to sexual advances is a common experience. In a qualitative research study (Graham et al., 2014) observing aggressive incidents in large-capacity nightlife venues involving sexual advances (e.g., invasiveness, persistence), 258 aggressions were analyzed. Ninety percent of incidents involved male initiators and female targets, with almost all incidents involving intentional or probable intentional aggression. Targets mostly responded nonaggressively, usually using evasion. Staff rarely intervened. The level of invasiveness was related to intoxication of the targets, but not of the initiators, suggesting intoxicated women were more often targeted.

Whether or not behaviors are perceived as sexual harassment is likely to vary according to culture, context, individuals, and time frames. For example, a cross-national study of college students found that those from Brazil were more likely to categorize as flattering behaviors that were considered harassment by their North American counterparts (Pryor et al., 1997).

During holiday periods, according to researchers, there is a behavioral inversion whereby meanings, morals, or norms of ordinary behavior are changed, held in abeyance, or even reversed (Graburn, 1983). Thus, research has shown that casual sexual encounters in youth holiday resorts are commonplace and often involve substance use (Downing et al., 2011). Men's alcohol use is cited as a factor in more than half of the reported sexual coercion incidents (Abbey, Zawacki, Buck, Clinton, & McAuslan, 2001). Equally, in some cultures, female alcohol use might suggest sexual availability (Bellis, Hughes, & Hughes, 2006), while intoxicated women appear to be easy targets for sexual activity or sexual assault (Calafat et al., 2008b).

Findings of a survey to 6,502 holidaymakers in the summer 2009, during a relatively short stay (on average less than nine days) in southern European resorts, showed that nearly one in ten British or German holidaymakers reported having been sexually harassed and 1.5 percent having had sex against their will (Calafat et al., 2013). In particular, sexual harassment was strongly associated with drunkenness and drug (cocaine) use, while gay and bisexual holidaymakers were at significantly increased risk of involvement in sex against their will.

Among people in nightlife, being a current drug user is associated with sexual risk taking. Thus in the last twelve months, regular cocaine users were 5.6 times more likely to have had multiple sexual partners, 2.7 times more likely to have had sex without using birth control, and 5.1 times more likely to have paid for sex (Bellis et al., 2008).

Transport to and from Recreational Areas

The role of transport as a cause of problems related to nightlife participation varies greatly from case to case (quality of public transport services, use of private cars, location of venues, etc.). In one study (Calafat et al., 2009a) undertaken in several European cities, private car was the most frequent form of transport when going out to nightlife settings (37.5 percent), which can be a serious problem when driving (or riding in car with a driver) under the influence of alcohol or other drugs. On the "last month" frequency, 18 percent of the respondents reported having driven a car after drinking too much, while 37 percent of the respondents reported having taken a lift from someone drunk or under the influence of drugs.

Alcohol is not the only substance that can affect driving safety. Other drugs affecting driving include cannabis, medicinal drugs, cocaine, and amphetamines (Appenzeller, Schneider, Yegles, Maul, & Wennig, 2005). A study of 10,748 drivers involved in fatal road traffic incidents in France found that at least 2.5 percent of fatal crashes were attributed to cannabis and 28.6 percent to alcohol (Laumon, Gadegbeku, Martin, & Biecheler, 2005). Simultaneous use of different drugs was confirmed in 28 percent of all cases (Appenzeller et al., 2005).

Social Nuisance and Crime

Nightlife has also become a focal point for the rallying cries of neighbourhood residents against the nuisance effects of nightlife businesses, such as excessive noise, heavy traffic, and vandalism.

In the neighborhood of some nightlife areas in Australia, almost 90 percent of residents were concerned about alcohol-related crime in their main entertainment precincts, and they had low perceptions of safety in such areas. Given the perceived safety problems, it is not surprising that most respondents reported feeling too unsafe to walk or wait for transport alone after dark (Miller et al., 2012).

Serving Alcohol to Drunk People

This is very common problem. In an investigation of seventy-three randomly selected pubs, bars, and nightclubs in a city in Northwest England using pseudodrunk actors, 83 percent of purchase attempts resulted in a sale of alcohol (Hughes et al., 2014). Similar results are found using also pseudointoxicated actors in other studies (Gosselt, Van Hoof, Goverde, & De Jong, 2013).

Underage Drinking

Underage drinking is a very frequent occurrence with very important consequences and should clearly be a priority for society to confront. In a Spanish national representative survey among secondary school students, 30.8 percent had been drunk during the previous month; and, 46.1 percent had been drinking in bars and pubs, although the legal drinking age in Spain is eighteen years of age (Punto Focal Nacional Reitox, 2013).

Use of Alcohol and Other Drugs

"Research studies targeted at young people in the European Union (EU) who attend dance music events consistently report much higher prevalence of drug use than that found in surveys of the general population. This appears to be the case in all of the countries where such surveys have been conducted" (EMCDDA, 2006, p. 56).

There is broad evidence of a high prevalence of recreational substance use. Epidemiological studies have shown that party people (clubbers, attendants to electronic music festivals and dance events) are more experienced with drug use, and the relationship between specific nightlife recreational environments and synthetic substance use has been well documented (Bellis, Hale, Bennett, Chaudry, & Kilfoyle, 2000; Calafat et al., 1999). Deehan and Saville (2003), in a study among clubbers in the Southeast of England, showed that most participants (people attending mainstream clubs) were aware of the risks inherent in their drug-taking lifestyle and of the legal and physical consequences, and pointed out that practices that could be seen as spontaneous where in fact calculated and ritualized. Many of these practices were based on harm reduction techniques (e.g., keeping hydrated through the event or not mixing drugs and alcohol), while others were nothing but urban myths (e.g., taking vitamins or exercising prior to a night out). The study also showed that users were using a wider range of illicit substances and increasingly using synthetic drugs; among users, 44 percent agreed with the statement "taking drugs is an integral part of my social life" (Deehan & Saville, 2003, p. 17).

Millions of young people holiday abroad at tourist resorts each year. Most of them choose their holidays depending on the nightlife. There is a link between drug use abroad and that in an individuals' country of origin. Furthermore, tourist resorts offer tourists the opportunity to increase levels of drug consumption and try different drugs in a context favorable to experimentation (Bellis, Hughes, Bennet, & Thompson, 2003).

Nightlife Prevention Interventions

NTE is essential for many cities and regions. On that basis, some of these locations strive to find the best balance between the benefits and the problems produced by NTE. As an example, the Council of the City of Sydney (Australia) is currently involved in the process of devising a "Night-time City Policy" (NTCP) that will provide a twenty-year vision for the future sustainable development of Sydney's NTE (Hadfield, 2011). Some research reviews, focusing on evidence in nightlife interventions, have been recently published, mainly regarding European countries (Akbar et al., 2011; Bolier, Voorham, Monshouwer, van Hasselt, & Bellis, 2011; Calafat, Duch, Juan, & Leckenby, 2012; Calafat, Juan, & Duch, 2009a; Hadfield, 2009, 2011; Ker & Chinnock, 2008; Hughes, K., Furness, Jones, & Bellis, 2010). These reviews acknowledge that this topic is underresearched, despite the fact that this is the context in many countries where young people experiment and use alcohol and other drugs. After a literature review, Hughes et al. (2010) pointed out that the majority of research on drinking environment interventions stemmed from non-European countries. More than two-thirds of the studies reviewed by Hughes at al. (2010) (n = 23), from a total of thirty-seven papers identified, had been conducted in the United States, Australia, or Canada. Of the twelve conducted in European countries, five of them had been conducted in the United Kingdom. However, the fact that most of the recent studies were conducted in Europe, which constitutes an important part of the nightlife activity worldwide, could signal an increase interest on the subject. In the meantime, Australia is currently making a big effort toward design and evaluation of NTE policies (Hadfield, 2011; Howard, Gordon, & Jones, 2014; Miller et al., 2012).

The biggest problems in nightlife are related to alcohol use. Although illegal drugs are a part of the equation, in most cases alcohol is present. Consequently, even though nightlife might have its own particularities, interventions and potential solutions should address chiefly alcohol. Concentrating on the alcohol problems, Babor et al. (2010) outlines seven broad areas of alcohol policy: (1) pricing and taxation; (2) regulation of physical availability; (3) modification of the drinking environment; (4) drink-and-driving countermeasures; (5) restrictions on marketing; (6) education and persuasion; and (7) treatment and early intervention.

Taxing and Alcohol Prices

Cheap drinks and alcohol promotions are related to increased alcohol consumption (Babor et al., 2010; Hughes et al., 2011b). It is frequent to find normative banning promotions (such as "happy hours," a period of time in which a bar or a disco offers a discount on alcoholic drinks) in different cities. In fact, this venue characteristic was most associated with alcohol-related aggression in research conducted in Melbourne (Australia) (McFadden, Young, & Markham, 2015). This is clearly an important venue characteristic, although politically sensitive since sometimes the general population does not support restrictions on alcohol pricing and availability.

A group of experts who participated in a qualitative study in Australia agreed that price is a key focal area for reducing alcohol problems (Fogarty & Chapman, 2013). According to their research, there is an opportunity for a united vision regarding minimum or floor pricing of alcohol to emerge in the public debate. Floor prices for alcohol (i.e., prices beneath which alcohol cannot be sold) are in place in Moldova, Russia, Ukraine, Uzbekistan, some U.S. states (e.g., Connecticut), and eight of the ten Canadian provinces. In 2012, Scotland legislated alcohol minimum unit pricing (i.e., the lowest price per unit of alcohol) the introduction of which is pending legal challenge.

In the United Kingdom, minimum unit pricing is the subject of substantial political and policy debate. U.K. alcohol prices in the off-trade, particularly supermarkets, have risen more slowly than have taxes on alcohol. A minimum alcohol price was withdrawn under pressure from the alcohol and trade industry, despite evidence that it would reduce premature mortality and antisocial behavior (Meng et al., 2013). The U.K. government dropped its plan to introduce a minimum unit price of £0·45 (approximately $0.67 U.S.), citing concerns that responsible drinkers on a low income might be disadvantaged. In fact, however, people from low socioeconomic backgrounds are the ones with fewer resources to protect themselves from the ill effects of drinking, and they also show higher levels of alcohol-related mortality and hospital admission at all levels of drinking compared with people from higher socioeconomic backgrounds. This is the same argument used in Australia when minimum pricing was contested by sectors of the drinks industry, who contended that a minimum price would adversely affect moderate drinkers and low-income households while having limited impact on heavy drinkers (Fogarty & Chapman, 2013).

Another approach would be to tax beverages according to their percentage of alcohol, instead of the current system based on product categories. Although among professionals there is a high degree of consensus on the benefits this measure would provide, its approval is highly improbable due again to the interests of the alcohol industry.

Venues: Physical Factors

A range of physical factors, including poor ventilation, poor cleanliness, crowding, noise, low lighting, high temperature, shabby décor, and low maintenance, have been associated with increased aggression in bars and nightclubs in various countries, either individually or combined (Hughes et al., 2011b). In Europe, music volume has been linked to alcohol consumption and faster drinking speed in the Netherlands and France, but to lower levels of overserving to individuals who are intoxicated in Sweden (Hughes et al., 2011b). Contradictory research results are frequent due to different factors. For example, getting drinks in a crowded venue can be harder and facilitates friction between customers themselves or with the staff, but at the same time people get fewer drinks and overserving is lower.

NTE premises should be designed in order to maximize health and minimize the risks of disorder and crime. Many issues can be addressed, such as the following:

- Regulate room temperature and ventilation to prevent smoky atmospheres and overheating.
- Make available chill-out areas with free or affordable water and calm music.
- Venues might provide harm reduction information about the use of drugs or counseling and crisis intervention. Venues can also provide water, condoms, ear plugs, and other aids.
- Glassware policy, such as clearing away empty and broken glasses and bottles, cleaning spills, and eliminating other hazards, can reduce risks.

- Reduce music volume to allow, at least in some areas, intimate conversation.
- Remove obstacles that might restrict and/or disturb people's flowing between bar, dance, and seating areas.
- Reduce queuing in bar areas.
- Provide good ratios of staff to patrons to avoid competition for service.
- Make random checks of toilets to monitor illegal and disruptive activities.
- Provide flat surfaces for drinks to reduce spillage and broken glass.
- Reduce dark areas inside premises and improve outside street lighting.

Closed-circuit television (CCTV) plays a major role in the governance of the NTE, especially in the prevention of crime and violence, sexual harassment, and other problems, and allows close collaboration with police. The use of CCTV is spreading quickly in nightlife and is very well accepted by the population. However, the impact of CCTV on the prevention of alcohol-related problems is not clear (Hadfield, 2011). The use of CCTV is well accepted in Britain, but not as much in Canada. Large discos in Ibiza (Spain) have all the areas of the club controlled through this system. Depending on local legislation, public areas, parking areas, public transports to the nightlife districts, and such can be also under CCTV surveillance in certain cities normally by the police station. Sometimes this technology has been used by club owners to select people to be admitted into the venues (Hadfield, 2008).

Venues: Managerial Approach

Alcohol-related harms tend to concentrate in some bars and nightclubs (Briscoe & Donnelly, 2001; Quigg et al., 2014), which seems to indicate that certain factors are present in those venues while not as much in others. Consequently, altering those factors could help reduce the risks of alcohol-related harms. Observation conducted in 118 large-capacity (> 300) bars and clubs in Toronto (Canada) has identified a wide range of staffing, customer, and environmental factors that are significantly associated with incidents of harm, such as a permissive environment, and high levels of intoxication among patrons (Graham, Bernards, Osgood, & Wells, 2006). Similar findings were found in European research involving bars in four cities in the Netherlands, Slovenia, Spain, and the United Kingdom (Quigg et al., 2014); however, when applying a final logistic regression model, only one factor remained significant: a permissive environment. In a U.K. study, poorly managed and problematic bars (PMP), according to ten established markers (Graham et al., 2014), are associated with increased sales of alcohol to drunken young customers (Hughes et al., 2014). Unfortunately, the cooperation of managers in prevention measures is frequently difficult to achieve unless the plan of action is mandatory or combined with enforcement. Interventions to raise and enforce venue managerial standards include (a) collaboration among various stakeholders (e. g. venue managers, local council representatives, etc.) involved in nightlife management; (b) collaboration of venue managers with police; and (c) adoption of codes of practice and other agreements.

An important question to address is whether harms are more likely to occur within or outside the venues. In a U.K. study of nightlife users (Anderson, Hughes, & Bellis, 2007), more participants reported having being involved in, or witnessing, a physical fight in the streets surrounding nightlife venues than inside (e.g., intoxicated patrons). Suggesting security staff might be moving problematic patrons outside to reduce the likelihood of the venue being associated with alcohol-related harms.

Venue: Staff Training

Several issues related to bar staff have been identified as factors that might cause problems, including the following:

- Low staff/patron ratio (Homel & Clark, 1994; Miller et al., 2012)
- Staff serving to intoxicated people (Homel & Clark, 1994; Hughes et al., 2014)
- Hostile and aggressive staff who are poorly trained and poorly coordinated by the manager and each other (Babor et al., 2010).
- High proportion of male staff, and "bouncers" behaving too aggressively or openly in a discriminatory way (Homel & Clark, 1994; Miller et al., 2012)
- Lack of monitoring of all entrances, allowing, for example, the entrance of people clearly intoxicated by alcohol or illegal drugs (Gripenberg, Wallin, & Andreasson, 2007) or not controlling the introduction of illegal drugs inside the venue
- Bar staff and security personnel being unfriendly to patrons

Training servers and sellers is very popular and widely implemented across Australia, Canada, Europe, and the United States. Server training is initiated by a manager as part of *responsible beverage service (RBS)* or *responsible service of alcohol.* However, RBS effectiveness is controversial (Babor et al., 2010; Hadfield, 2011). RBS is more effective when connected to venue policies and especially when it is systematically enforced. RBS should be adapted to each community and type of venue or event. The state of Oregon (the United States) introduced mandatory training of all alcohol servers in December 1986.

After conducting a qualitative evaluation of RBS in thirty-two U.S. states to establish minimum required components, Mosher, Toomey, Good, Harwood, and Wagenaar (2002) concluded that minimum RBS requirements should include the following:

- Comprehensive training with information about the social impact of alcohol as well as its physical effects on the body; local and state laws related to alcohol use; skills with role playing that includes techniques to prevent service or sales to underage persons; cutoff of service and refusal to sale to intoxicated patrons. Training should be for a minimum of four hours.
- Training that targets both managers *and* servers. Managers should be trained because they are responsible for supervising the servers.

- Policy development for management that includes skills such as writing house policies.
- Development of criteria and procedures for certifying training, trainers, and trainees
- Periodic refresher or booster training.
- Active monitoring of training programs, trainee, and manager compliance.

Research on aggression in bars shows that for training to be very effective, it needs to go beyond RBS training so that all staff are prepared to intervene effectively in any problem situation that might arise, including security staff, who are important to manage, control, and reduce problems. However, a study carried out among recreational industry representatives in fourteen European member-state countries evidenced that, with the exception of the United Kingdom, where it is a criminal offense to take a job as a door supervisor without a Security Industry Authority (SIA) license, no specific training was required in any other European country studied (Calafat et al., 2012). In Spain, training has become recently required by law in certain regions (e.g., Madrid, Catalonia, and the Balearic Islands) but not nationwide.

Opening Hours, Lockouts, and Density of Venues

One of the ways of decreasing alcohol availability is restricting the trading hours. A review (Stockwell & Chikritzhs, 2009) of forty-nine studies (fourteen included baseline and control measures) related to Australia, New Zealand, North America, and the United Kingdom suggests that extended late-night trading hours lead to increased consumption and related harm. One interesting experiment took place in Newcastle (Australia). In this study, trading hours ended at 3:30 A.M., and a lockout (restricting reentrance of patrons to venues after a set time), along with other elements, such as restricting drinks, not serving alcohol after a certain hour, or limiting the number of drinks served to patron at one time, was studied. The data showed that the restriction of trading hours had an immediate and long-term effect on alcohol-related harm and the culture of intoxication. The effects of other measures such as lockouts were less conclusive (Miller et al., 2012).

Lockouts aim to restrict the movement of patrons between establishments by setting a time (prior to closing) after which entry or reentry is no longer permitted. This measure has been implemented in different states or local jurisdictions in Australia. There is limited formal evidence of the effectiveness of lockouts due to a lack of comprehensive evaluation studies, and lockout polices are often only one component of a range of programs aimed at curbing late-night alcohol-related problems. In a follow-up to the Miller et al. (2012) intervention in Newcastle (Australia), there was no evidence that lockouts in isolation of reductions in opening hours were effective (Kypri, McElduff, & Miller, 2014).

Another variable, higher density of licensed venues and its association with higher levels of alcohol-related harms, has been studied. A review of the effectiveness of limiting alcohol venue density found that greater outlet density is associated with increased alcohol consumption and related harm, including medical harm, injury, crime, and violence. Primary evidence was supported by secondary evidence from correlational studies. The regulation of the density of alcohol outlets (places where alcohol can be sold) may be a useful public health tool for the reduction of excessive alcohol consumption and related harm, according to Campbell et al. (2009). In their review of five studies across three countries (Canada, the United Kingdom, and the United States), a positive association was found between density outlet and consumption of alcohol.

In research in Australia, the number of alcohol outlets per population of ten thousand was identified within geographic regions in Victoria. A state-representative student survey (N = 10,143) identified adolescent reports of alcohol purchasing. Each extra sales outlet per ten thousand population was associated with a significant increase in the risk of underage adolescent purchasing. The strongest effect was for club density (odds ratio = 1.22) and packaged takeaway outlet density (odds ratio = 1.12) (Rowland, Toumbourou, & Livingston, 2015).

Educational Interventions and Campaigns

Patron education (e.g., through pamphlets, peer-to-peer approaches) has been frequently implemented as a form of harm-reduction intervention in recreational contexts. In many places where NTE is a developed activity, this has been the most implemented and frequently the only intervention supported by municipalities. Delivery of information relies often on trained peers. However, there has been little assessment of its effect on patron's intoxication or harm reduction. Its effectiveness as an isolated measure will probably be reduced or nonexistent unless combined with enforcement and other types of interventions (Babor et al., 2010; Hadfield, 2011). Public education campaigns on safer drinking addressed to the general population or targeted at "high-risk" groups have a role to play as part of a package of measures within community-based programs (Hadfield, 2011).

We should consider that mass media interventions (brief and recurrent messages to inform and motivate individuals to abstain or reduce substance use) are sometimes very effective measures, especially when they are implemented together with community actions (Faggiano & Vigna-Taglianti, 2008).

The use of peer interventions in recreational settings has been quite popular, placing the accent on the importance of the information being delivered by peer educators of similar ages to those of the audience. However, there has been little assessment of their effect on patrons' intoxication or on harm reduction. Their effectiveness, as an isolated measure, is probably reduced or nonexistent unless combined with enforcement or other types of interventions (Graham, 2000; Hadfield, 2011).

Collaboration with Industry, Public Policy, and Codes of Practice

Relationships between public policies and the alcohol and entertainment industries are very complex and unavoidable. We have already mentioned that the NTE is an important issue to many municipalities and governments. For example, the British government enacted deregulatory measures for nightlife businesses, such as allowing for the extension of nightlife operating hours under the 2003 Licensing Act. North American cities have promoted nightlife to attract tourists as well as new residents to downtown areas of major cities. However, city governments have also realized the challenges of facilitating an NTE that balances "public well-being" and "quality of life" with integrating cultural amenities and leisure business, in order to position the city in the competitive regional/global market, while coping with the nuisances produced by nightlife businesses (Hae, 2011).

The nightlife industry is a powerful stakeholder, covering a very wide spectrum. Its collaboration is essential, but as we know, the industry has its own interests and a big capacity to adapt and to overcome new obstacles. The industry has responsibilities in alcohol beverages advertising and marketing, pricing, venue managing, alcohol promotion campaigns, underage selling, and so on. In the middle of so many interests, public health concerns are not normally the priority. Leaving the alcohol industry to self-regulate is unlikely to be effective, as a single bar in an area that is not compliant with voluntary controls would benefit from patrons rejected from compliant bars. There is also repeated evidence of code breaches when self-regulatory policies are implemented, funded, and administered by the alcohol industry on a voluntary basis (Howard et al., 2014).

To implement strategies and interventions in this area is a clear priority, but they depend on political priorities. For example, we have seen in the United Kingdom the difficulties in implementing an alcohol minimum price scheme. In a recent study on the willingness of the recreational industry to collaborate on several recognized prevention standards, no major differences were found between European countries in the assessment of the key components identified in the literature review (Calafat et al., 2012). Most of the industry representatives were familiar with the identified prevention components and aware of their effectiveness. Furthermore, many of the consulted venues reported having already adopted them. However, differences were found in the number of enforced legislative standards across countries studied (Calafat et al., 2012). The United Kingdom was clearly identified as the most regulated country and has enforced a number of legislative standards. Nevertheless, legislation and enforcement measures were difficult to compare in most explored countries due to the number and range of agencies and authorities involved. This study is especially interesting because we can identify the opinion of the recreational industry on the feasibility and readiness to accept a range of evidence-based preventive interventions. Indeed, in countries where NTE is not well developed or suffering the impact of the current economic crisis, nightlife industry representatives were not keen to adopt measures that they perceived may lower their incomes, while in countries where preventive practices were well implemented, such representatives were reluctant for the practices to be regulated or enforced since they would require a higher level of compliance.

Nevertheless, to have written house policies (e.g., house rules specifying acceptable and unacceptable behaviors for both staff and customers) and a code of practice can be a step in getting the recreational industry more involved in preventive strategies. At least it implies the acceptance that those in the industry have a role and a responsibility to address this issue.

There are other industry prevention initiatives that look promising, such as the Pubwatch scheme.[1] This initiative started in the United Kingdom (2003) as a partnership where NTE establishments unify as an independent group to preempt crime and antisocial behavior in licensed premises. They work closely with local authorities and intend to maintain a safe and secure social environment for customers and staff. Individual patrons caught with or taking drugs, being violent, or misbehaving in any of the venues enrolled in an existing Pubwatch can receive a six-month ban from all the network venues.

Award schemes are initiatives quite popular in certain countries such as the United Kingdom to promote good venue managing. A good example of this is the *Best Bar None* award scheme, initiated in 2003 by the Greater Manchester Police (U.K.), to reduce alcohol-related crime and irresponsible drinking practices through the promotion of responsible venue management operations. These initiatives have not been studied and their effectiveness is uncertain.

International Nightlife Resorts

International resorts play a trendsetting role spreading youth cultures and lifestyles (including substance use) among young travelers that visit them (Collins, 1997). These resorts that target young people are often oriented around nightlife with high concentrations of bars and nightclubs, offering opportunities for hedonistic partying every night of the week, and research has shown that substance use and sexual activity among young people increases during holiday periods (Hughes et al., 2011a). However, problems related to nightlife in tourist resorts are normally underreported because in most cases both the tourist industry and local authorities are afraid of possible economic problems if the issue is aired in the media. Consequently, there is often a lack of implementation of preventive measures. However, sometimes the problems created by NTE become an important media issue and there is a need to react. This is the case in the United States, where spring break venues often have adopted preventive measures.

International quality standards should be promoted and implemented to ensure visitors' health and safety when traveling to recreational nightlife resorts.

1 www.nationalpubwatch.org.uk/.

The implementation of standards should depend on the establishment of a robust and long-lasting network of representatives from tourist-provider and tourist-recipient countries, including those working at local and national levels (industry representatives, police, local authorities, health services) as well as internationally (consulates, tour operators and travel agencies, and youth tourist and other international organizations) to ensure distribution of responsibilities and tasks in the implementation and maintenance of safety procedures for international resorts (Calafat, 2010).

Licensing Legislation, Law Enforcement, and Policing

All the interventions reviewed in this section of the chapter, to be effective, depend on a great deal of regulation and enforcement, as their application dramatically improves when regulated and enforced. While regulations vary from country to country and from city to city, more important than regulation is the level of enforcement in each location.

Accordingly, interventions to reduce alcohol-related harm in the recreational context often use targeted policing and enforcement of licensing legislation to improve practices in drinking environments; however, findings from studies on the effectiveness of policing and enforcement activity are mixed. Some studies show higher levels of alcohol-related problems following policing and enforcement activity even though it might be due to better detection and reporting of such problems (Hughes, Furness, Jones, & Bellis, 2010).

Licensing requirements for venues vary greatly across Europe (Hughes et al., 2010) and elsewhere, sometimes even within different cities/regions in the same country. In certain locations, such as in the United Kingdom, specific conditions can be imposed on individual premises on a case-by-case basis. There are also additional laws, acts, and regulations that are not specifically designed for improving nightlife standards, but they are related to health and safety of staff and patrons. This makes legislation and enforcement measures difficult to compare. Whereas in some countries, as in Sweden, licensing is an essential tool in the management of alcohol policy, in other countries regulation is less strict or venues can even operate without a proper license, at least for a while.

Another issue to be considered is that regulations when voluntary or not enforced create differences between those who comply and those who do not. Mandatory implementation of measures creates a level playing field for all venue operators (Miller et al., 2012). Our experience working with the recreational industry in the Balearic Islands indicates that unless there are clear conditions established, good operators are penalized while bad operators avoid penalties.

Level of enforcement is also related to circumstantial issues, such as media coverage of alcohol-related violence, because this forces authorities to be stricter. It is clear that enforcement requires political commitment and financial resources. In practice, enforcement might be affected due to limited resources, the working relationship between police and venue owners, poor understanding of the benefits of enforcement, and concerns about the effects on the NTE. Finally, effectiveness of the enforcement measures depends on their application for long periods. In any case, leaving the alcohol industry to self-regulate is unlikely to be effective. Effectiveness of most initiatives depends on the NTE and venue enforcement, yet research suggests that police target individuals more than establishments (Howard et al., 2014).

Underage Drinking

This is very central issue. Legal drinking age varies widely. In Europe, minimum age is sixteen years in countries such as Belgium and Austria, and in the United States twenty-one years. In addition, even when countries prevent the sale or consumption of alcohol to minors, and not always with the same enforcement, underage people gain access to alcohol in various ways. Still, prosecutions to establishments infringing the law are rare in some countries or areas. While the health consequences of extreme intoxication are unambiguous, local authorities may be concerned that actions intended to reduce nightlife alcohol use will damage local nighttime economies.

Checks for proof of age identification should be carried out routinely as in many parts of the United States and other countries. Alcohol industry representatives are well aware in theory of the need to implement this action. In a European survey involving venue managers, 81 percent of them agreed that age check is a key regulation to ensure health and safety of patrons, and it is a practice easily implementable at low cost (Calafat et al., 2012). Nevertheless, just 66 percent of all industry representatives interviewed in this study reported carrying out age checks at entrance, and in most cases they are not done routinely but at discretion of door staff. Independently of the control system used, what is needed is industry collaboration together with enforcement. ID scanners are a very useful technology to respond not only to underage identification but also to respond to security and safety within licensed venues. In some countries (e.g., Australia, the United States), ID scanners are used to check for age at venue establishments. ID scanners also serve a role as deterrents to antisocial or violent behaviors, and they can detect fake ID documents (Miller et al., 2012). Scanning technology is quite developed, and Clubscan has been installed in more than thirty countries and is capable of reading 233 different IDs and 162 different passports.

Transport: Drinking and Driving Programs

People do not become involved with problems solely based on their consumption. The existence of effective transport to and from recreational areas is a key issue when addressing alcohol- and drug-related problems. Lack of availability of public transport (Homel, Carvolth, Hauritz, McIlwain, & Teague, 2004) or queuing for taxis or buses can trigger arguments and fights (Allen & Goody,

2002). The fact is that many clubbers use private cars because of a lack of public transport or due to cultural issues. Males are more prone to use private cars in Mediterranean countries (Calafat et al., 2009a).

Different actions can be effective to correct these environmental influences, such as (a) routing late-night crowds away from residential areas; (b) improving clients' dispersal from venues; (c) providing easy and free night transportation (e.g., NightRider buses) or extending the working hours of public transports; (d) ensuring the provision of taxis; and (e) allowing staff to call taxis for patrons.

In the "European action plan to reduce the harmful use of alcohol 2012–2020" (WHO, 2012), strategies to reduce motor vehicle crashes and fatalities include enforcing blood alcohol content limits through intelligent random breath-testing and sobriety checkpoints and introducing punishments with severe personal consequences (such as on-the-spot fines, driving license penalty points, and, as appropriate, driving license suspension, court-mandated interventions, and the use of alcohol ignition locks for specified periods).

"Designated drivers" programs are very popular, but their outcomes are not always as good as expected. According to data from the "2007 National Roadside Survey" in the United States (Lacey et al., 2009), almost one-third (30 percent) of nighttime drivers reported being designated drivers, with 84 percent of them having a blood alcohol concentration of zero. However, one-fifth of passengers riding with the designated drivers reported having consumed five or more drinks that day. But because designated driving separates drinking from driving, it may encourage passengers in a group traveling together to binge drink, which is associated with many adverse health consequences in addition to those arising from alcohol-impaired driving. Besides the impact that the initiative might have on encouraging higher alcohol consumption rates of passengers, research shows that it had no impact on rates of alcohol-related road accidents (Howard et al., 2014). Nevertheless, designated driving programs and campaigns, although not proven to be effective when used alone, can complement proven effective interventions to help reduce excessive drinking and alcohol-impaired driving (Bergen, Yao, Shultus, Romano, & Lacey, 2014).

Placing an interlock in the ignition to avert an impaired driver from driving is in theory a good approach to the problem. However, the problem for now is to keep breathalyzer devices in good working order since they are still very expensive to replace. Studies in the United States and Canada since the 1980s have shown that alcohol interlocks can be highly effective in preventing recidivism among penalized drivers (Voas, Fell, McKnight, & Sweedeler, 2004).

Hospital Emergency Departments and First-Aid Services

Emergency departments (ED) provide a measure of the number of serious violence and other harm related to alcohol and drug use that is independent from the one measured by police. They can be useful as indicators (e.g., the number of ED services administered) on the impact of prevention or policy initiatives,

An ED visit may also represent an important "teachable moment," and different interventions have been developed. Nevertheless, the evidence remains inconclusive as to whether their implementation has clear benefits as might be expected (Wojnar & Jakubczyk, 2014). According to Wojnar and Jakubczyk, the usefulness of brief interventions (BIs) may depend significantly on the target population. BIs have proved to be beneficial for male individuals and those patients who do not abuse other psychoactive substances. In contrast, evidence indicates that BIs in health settings are not effective when dealing with men admitted as a consequence of a violence-related event. In addition, Wojnar and Jakubczyk were unable to confirm the effectiveness of BI with females in hospital emergency room settings.

A proportion of big clubs (e.g., in Spain, the U.K.) have "club medic" rooms for managing individuals in need of medical assistance, but there have been no evaluations of such interventions, and they do not follow clear protocols. One club in London (U.K.) has implemented a medic room and developed a pilot set of guidelines, including implementing appropriate staff training (Wood et al., 2008).

Community-Based and Multicomponent Programs

The governance of nightlife involves many agencies, industries, and stakeholders, and cooperation among them is essential in order to broaden the scope and increase the results of interventions. Multi-agency partnerships working in collaboration to prevent alcohol- and drug-related harms at the community level are increasing in Europe, but with the exception of the STAD (STockholm combats Alcohol and Drug problems) project carried out in Sweden (Gripenberg et al., 2007; Wallin & Andreáson, 2004), not many initiatives have been evaluated to demonstrate their effectiveness. STAD involved community mobilization, training in responsible beverage service, and enforcement. At the baseline (in 1996), the rate for refusal to serve someone who was drunk was 5 percent, and at follow-up (after the STAD program implementation) the refusal rate was 70 percent (with a statistically significant difference between the intervention and the area of the town where the program was not implemented).

Although there is general consensus that a multicomponent approach is the most promising, in practice, partnerships are difficult to establish and it takes some time to succeed in creating synergies among the different agencies and components involved. Leadership of the coalition, community involvement, and funding are some of the potential problems faced in establishing these partnerships. Other problems faced by community-based multicomponent programs are the difficulties posed evaluating such approaches. However, community-evaluated projects such as STAD and the Club against Drugs project (Gripenberg et al., 2011), also implemented in Sweden, and studies on interventions in Geelong and Newcastle (Australia) permit comparison of different initiatives using a wide range of research methods (Miller et al., 2012).

Effective integral or multicomponent prevention programs combine some of the following components:

- Community mobilization by increasing the awareness of alcohol-related problems and gaining multi-agency support for action
- Training programs for staff working in drinking environments and raising awareness among other stakeholders
- Increased enforcement of existing laws and alcohol legislation
- Regular partnership meetings to develop and coordinate strategies
- Interventions in drinking environments
- School and family programs

Conclusions

Recreational use of alcohol and drugs is a very common occurrence in many cities. Among adolescents and young adults participating in nightlife activities, it is a much appreciated way of socializing. The profile of this group of people, even when they abuse alcohol and take illegal drugs, is perceived by many as socially normative. Traditional risk factors, previously linked to marginalized or problematic people, are not so applicable to these young consumers. Risk and protective factors are more linked to the context itself. Accordingly, prevention interventions need to be specific to this particular context. We must take into account that the alcohol and recreational industries along with municipalities are supporting the NTE. These facts and awareness of the complexity of the interrelationship between industry and authorities are key elements that determine the development of any prevention policy. Despite all this, we have to acknowledge that the topic of this chapter is an underresearched area in the field of addiction and prevention. The situation needs immediate attention, because nightlife contexts are very important for the socialization of young people. The socialization is related to the use and abuse of alcohol and illegal drugs and has important consequences for the health, safety, and future development of people.

Both individuals and society often have difficulty acknowledging the problems in nightlife settings. People tend to look at the advantages (e.g., having fun, economic benefits) and overlook problems of the NTE. Nevertheless, problems exist and they are not only the problem of alcohol or drug use, but also those of crime, violence, and risky sexual behaviors associated with substance abuse that may be prevalent within the NTE. Developing understanding of the impact of environmental factors in modern bars and nightclubs requires a multicomponent study that incorporates intelligence on both the micro level (i.e., environmental factors in bars and nightclubs) and macro level (e.g., national legislation) aspects of drinking environments.

Different types of interventions have been developed to address nightlife problems. However, as happens in some other contexts, most of the interventions implemented in recreational settings have not been well supported by research. For example, providing information about alcohol and drug use to patrons and conducting more complex interventions such as "responsible beverage serving" or "designated driver" programs have limited impact (Babor et al., 2010; Bergen et al., 2014; Hadfield, 2011; Howard et al., 2014). Other initiatives that have not been discussed in this review (such as onsite drug checking and alternative leisure activities) are often used, but there is little evidence of their effectiveness. Multicomponent approaches where enforcement occupies a relevant place are likely to be more successful, and political and social support are essential ingredients to ensure sustainability and institutionalization. Mobilizing communities, especially with a community intervention approach, is an essential tool for success. Communities can be mobilized through promoting partnerships and building coalitions, defined as interorganizational, cooperative, and synergistic working alliances (Butterfoss, Goodman, & Wandersman, 1993).

Recreational nightlife industry, implicitly or explicitly, shows a reasonable consensus on what should be done in order to promote health and safety in nightlife venues, but there is a concurrent fear surrounding the regulation and enforcement of such procedures. Furthermore, some administrations/governments are not proactive in developing and enforcing new or old regulations (Calafat et al., 2012). But, as it has been demonstrated in the Newcastle (Australia) experience (Miller et al., 2012), when such measures are introduced and given adequate notice, many will welcome the measures and negative consequences to businesses can be reduced if not eliminated.

The success of NTE prevention initiatives will depend on maintaining a balance between differing needs of and support from stakeholders and evaluating and adopting evidence-based practices and policies. Preventing unwanted nightlife behaviors and problems will take time, but setting realistically high goals is important for all concerned within a community context.

References

Abbey, A., Zawacki, T., Buck, P. O., Clinton, A., & McAuslan, P. (2001). Alcohol and sexual assault. *Alcohol Health and Research World* 25: 43–51.

Akbar, T., Baldacchino, A., Cecil, J., Riglietta, M., Sommer, B., & Humphris, G. (2011). Polysubstance use and related harms: a systematic review of harm reduction strategies implemented in recreational settings. *Neuroscience Biobehavior Review* 35: 1186–1202. doi: 10.1016/j.neubiorev.2010.12.002

Allen, C., & Goody, H. (2002). *All Day and All of the Night: An LGA Discussion Paper.* London: LGA Publications, the Local Government Association.

Allen, J., Nicholas, S., Salisbury, H., & Wood, M. (2003). Nature of burglary, vehicle and violent crime. In Flood-Page, C., & Taylor, J. (eds.), *Crime in England and Wales 2001/2002: Supplementary Volume. Home Office Statistical Bulletin 01/03*. London: Home Office.

Anderson, Z., Hughes, K., & Bellis, M. A. (2007). *Exploration of Young People's Experience and Perceptions of Violence in Liverpool's Nightlife*. Liverpool: Centre for Public Health, Liverpool John Moores University. www.cph.org.uk/wp-content/uploads/2012/08/exploration-of-young-peoples-experience-and-perceptions-of-violence-in-liverpools-nightlife.pdf

Appenzeller, B. M. R., Schneider, S., Yegles, M., Maul, A., & Wennig, R. (2005). Drugs and chronic alcohol abuse in drivers. *Forensic Science International* 155: 83–90.

Babor, T., Caetano, R., Casswell, S., Edwards, G., Giesbrecht, N., ... Rossow, I. (2010). *Alcohol: No Ordinary Commodity: Research and Public Policy* (2nd ed.). Oxford: Oxford University Press.

Bellis, M. A., Hale, G., Bennett, A., Chaudry, M., & Kilfoyle, M. (2000). Ibiza uncovered: changes in substance use and sexual behaviour amongst young people visiting an international night-life resort. *International Journal on Drug Policy* 11: 235–44.

Bellis, M. A., Hughes, K., Bennet, A., & Thomson, R. (2003). The role of an international nightlife resort in the proliferation of recreational drugs. *Addiction* 98: 1713–21.

Bellis, M., Hughes, K., Calafat, A., Juan, M., Ramon, A., Rodriguez, J. A., ... Phillips-Howard, P. (2008). Sexual uses of alcohol and drugs and the associated health risks: a cross sectional study of young people in nine European cities. *BMC Public Health* 8: 155. doi: 10.1186/1471–2458-8-155

Bellis, M. A., Hughes, K., & Hughes, S. (2006). *Intimate Partner Violence and Alcohol*. Geneva, Switzerland: World Health Organization.

Bergen, G., Yao, J., Shultus, R. A., Romano, E., & Lacey, J. H. (2014). Characteristics of designated drivers and their passengers from the 2007 National Roadside Survey in the United States. *Traffic Injury Prevention* 15: 273–7. doi: 10.1080/15389588.2013.810334

Bolier, L., Voorham, L., Monshouwer, K., van Hasselt, N., & Bellis, M. (2011). Alcohol and drug prevention in nightlife settings: a review of experimental studies. *Substance Use & Misuse* 46: 1569–91. doi: 10.3109/10826084.2011.606868

Briscoe, S., & Donnelly, N. (2001). *Assaults on Licensed Premises in Inner-Urban Areas. Alcohol Studies Bulletin 2*. Perth, Australia: Curtin University of Technology (Western Australia National Drug Research Institute).

Butterfoss, F. D., Goodman, R. M., & Wandersman, A. (1993). Community coalitions for prevention and health promotion. *Health Education Research* 8: 315–30.

Calafat, A. (2010). *Prevention Interventions in Recreational Settings*. Strasbourg: Council of Europe. Pompidou Group. wcd.coe.int/wcd/com.instranet.InstraServlet?Index=no&command=com.instranet.CmdBlobGet&InstranetImage=1717657&SecMode=1&DocId=1638156&Usage=2

Calafat, A., Blay, N., Juan, M., Adrover, D., Bellis, M. A., Hughes, K., ... Bohrn, K. (2009a). Traffic risk behaviours at nightlife: drinking, taking drugs, driving and use of public transport by young people. *Traffic Injury Prevention* 10: 162–9.

Calafat, A., Bohrn, K., Juan, M., Kokkevi, A., Maalsté, N., Mendes, F., ... Zavatti, P. (1999). *Night Life in Europe and Recreative Drug Use*. Palma de Mallorca: Irefrea. Retrieved from www.irefrea.eu.

Calafat, A., Duch, M., Juan, M., & Leckenby, N. (2012). Health and safety European standards for nightlife venues. *Adicciones* 24: 355–64.

Calafat, A., Fernández, C., Juan, M., & Becoña, E. (2008a). Recreational nightlife: risk and protective factors for drug misuse among young Europeans in recreational environments. *Drugs: Education, Prevention and Policy* 15: 189–200.

Calafat, A., Hughes, K., Blay, N., Bellis, M. A., Mendes, F., Juan, M., Lazarov, P. Cibin, B., & Duch, M. (2013). Sexual harassment among young tourists visiting Mediterranean resorts. *Archives of Sexual Behavior* 42: 603–13. doi: 10.1007/s10508-012-9979-6

Calafat, A., Juan, M., Becoña, E., & Mantecón, A. (2008b). Que drogas se prefieren para las relaciones sexuales en contextos recreativos. *Adicciones* 20: 37–48.

Calafat, C., Juan, M., & Duch, M. (2009a). Preventive interventions in nightlife: a review. *Adicciones* 21: 387–414.

Campbell, C. A., Hahn, R. A., Elder, R., Brewer, R., Chattopadhyay, S., Fielding, J., ...Task Force on Community Preventive Services (2009). The effectiveness of limiting alcohol outlet density as a means of reducing excessive alcohol consumption and alcohol-related harms. *American Journal of Preventive Medicine* 37: 556–69. doi: 10.1016/j.amepre.2009.09.028

Collins, M. (1997) *Altered State*. London: Serpent's Tail.

Deehan, A., & Saville, E. (2003). *Calculating the Risk: Recreational Drug Use among Clubbers in the South East of England*. London: Home Office.

Delegación del Gobierno para el Plan Nacional sobre Drogas (2010). *Encuesta estatal sobre uso de drogas en enseñanzas secundarias*. Madrid: Ministerio de Sanidad y Consumo. www.pnsd.msc.es/Categoria2/observa/pdf/ESTUDES_2010.pdf.

Downing, J., Hughes, K., Bellis, M. A., Calafat, A., Juan, M., & Blay, N. (2011). Factors associated with risky sexual behaviour: a comparison of British, Spanish and German holidaymakers to the Balearics. *European Journal of Public Health* 21: 275–81. doi: 10.1093/eurpub/ckq021

EMCDDA (European Monitoring Centre on Drugs and Drug Addiction) (2011). Problematic drug use population: an overview of the methods and definitions used. Retrieved from www.emcdda.europa.eu/stats11/pdu/methods

EMCDDA (European Monitoring Centre on Drugs and Drug Addiction) (2006). *Annual Report 2006*. Lisbon: EMCDDA. Downloadable from www.emcdda.europa.eu

Faggiano, F., & Vigna-Taglianti, F. (2008). Drugs, illicit – primary prevention strategies. In Heggenhougen, K., & Quah, S. (eds.), *International Encyclopaedia of Public Health*, vol. 2. San Diego: Academic Press.

Fogarty, A. S., & Chapman, S. (2013). What should be done about policy on alcohol pricing and promotions? Australian experts' views of policy priorities: a qualitative interview study. *BMC Public Health* 13: 610. www.biomedcentral.com/1471-2458/13/610.

Fountain, J., & Griffiths, P. (1997). *Inventory, Bibliography and Synthesis of Qualitative Research in the European Union (Rep. No. 1)*. London: National Addiction Centre.

Gosselt, J. F., Van Hoof, J. J., Goverde, M. M., & De Jong, M. D. (2013). One more beer? Serving alcohol to pseudo-intoxicated guests in bars. *Alcohol Clinical and Experimental Research* 37: 1213–19. doi: 10.1111/acer.12074

Graburn, N. H. H. (1983). The anthropology of tourism. *Annals of Tourism Research* 10: 9–33.

Graham, K. (2000). Preventive interventions for on-premise drinking: a promising but underresearched area of prevention. *Contemporary Drug Problems* 27: 593–668.

Graham, K., Bernards, S., Osgood, D. W., Abbey, A., Parks, M., Flynn, A., … Wells, S. (2014). "Blurred lines?" Sexual aggression and barroom culture. *Alcohol Clinical and Experimental Research* 38: 1416–24. doi: 10.1111/acer.12356

Graham, K., Bernards, S., Osgood, D. W., & Wells, S. (2006). Bad nights or bad bars? Multi-level analysis of environmental predictors of aggression in late-night large-capacity bars and clubs. *Addiction* 101, 1569–80.

Gripenberg, J., Wallin, E., & Andréasson, S. (2007). Effects of a community-based drug use program targeting licensed premises. *Prevention. Substance Use & Misuse* 42: 1883–98. doi: 10.1080/10826080701532916

Gripenberg, J., Wallin, E., & Andréasson, S. (2011). The "Clubs against Drugs" program in Stockholm, Sweden: two cross-sectional surveys examining drug use among staff at licensed premises. *Substance Abuse Treatment and Prevention Policy* 6: 2. doi: 10.1186/1747–597X-6-2

Hadfield, P. (2008). From threat to promise: Nightclub "security", governance and consumer elites. *British Journal of Criminology* 48: 429–47.

Hadfield, P. (2009). Nightlife and crime in international perspective. In Hadfield, P. (ed.), *Nightlife and Crime: Social Order and Governance in International Perspective*. Oxford, UK: Oxford University Press.

Hadfield, P. (2011) *Night-Time Economy Management: International Research and Practice*. Retrieved from www.philhadfield.co.uk

Hae, L. (2011). Gentrification and politicization of nightlife in New York City. *ACME: An International E-Journal for Critical Geographies* 11: 564–84. www.acme-journal.org/vol10/Hae2011.pdf

Heath, T. (1997). The twenty-four hour city concept: a review of initiatives in British cities. *Journal of Urban Design*, *2*, 193–204.

HM Government (2008). *Drugs: Protecting Families and Communities – the 2008 Drugs Strategy*. drugs.homeoffice.gov.uk/publication-search/drugstrategy/drug-strategy-2008?view=Binary

Hobbs, D., Winlow, S., Hadfield, P., & Lister, S. (2005). Violent hypocrisy. *European Journal of Criminology* 2: 161–83.

Homel, R., Carvolth, R., Hauritz, M., McIlwain, G., & Teague, R. (2004). Making licensed venues safer for patrons: what environmental factors should be the focus of interventions? *Drug and Alcohol Review* 23: 19–29.

Homel, R.. & Clark, J. (1994). The prediction and prevention of violence in pubs and clubs. *Crime Prevention Studies* 3: 1–46.

Howard, S. J., Gordon, R., & Jones, S. C. (2014). Australian alcohol policy 2001–2013 and implications for public health. *BMC Public Health* 14: 848. www.biomedcentral.com/1471–2458/14/848

Hughes, K., Bellis, M. A., Calafat, A., Blay, N., Kokkevi, A., Boyiadji, G., … Bajcàrova, L. (2011a). Substance use, violence and unintentional injury in young holidaymakers visiting Mediterranean destinations. *Journal of Travel Medicine* 18: 80–9. doi: 10.1111/j.1708–8305.2010.00489.x

Hughes, K., Bellis, M. A., Leckenby, N., Quigg, Z., Hardcastle, K., Sharples, O., & Llewellyn, D. J. (2014). Does legislation to prevent alcohol sales to drunk individuals work? Measuring the propensity for night-time sales to drunks in a UK city. *Journal of Epidemiology Community and Health* 68: 453–6. doi: 10.1136/jech-2013–203287

Hughes, K., Furness, L., Jones, L., & Bellis, M. A. (2010). *Reducing Harm in Drinking Environments. Evidence and Practice in Europe*. Liverpool: Centre for Public Health. Liverpool John Moores University. Retrieved from www.cph.org.uk/showPublication.aspx?pubid=692.

Hughes, K., Quigg, Z., Eckley, L., Bellis, M., Jones, L., Calafat, A., … van Hassel, N. (2011b). Environmental factors in drinking venues and alcohol-related harm: the evidence base for European intervention. *Addiction* 106(Supplement 1): 37–46. doi: 10.1111/j.1360-0443.2010.03316.x

Ker, K., & Chinnock, P. (2008). Interventions in the alcohol server setting for preventing injuries. *Cochrane Database of Systematic Reviews* 3: Art No. D005244

Kypri, K., McElduff, P., & Miller, P. (2014). Restrictions in pub closing times and lockouts in Newcastle, Australia five years on. *Drug and Alcohol Review* 33: 323–6. doi: 10.1111/dar.12123

Lacey, J. H., Kelley-Baker, T., Furr-Holden, D., Voas, R. B., Romano, E., Torres, P, … Berning, A. (2009). *2007 National Roadside Survey of Alcohol and Drug Use by Drivers*. Washington, DC: National Highway Traffic Safety Administration (NHTSA). www.nhtsa.gov/Driving+Safety/Research+&+Evaluation/2007+National+Roadside+Survey+of+Alcohol+and+Drug+Use+by+Drivers

Laumon, B., Gadegbeku, B., Martin, J. L., Biecheler, M. B., & SAM Group. (2005). Cannabis intoxication and fatal road crashes in France: population based case-control study. *British Medical Journal* 331: 1371–4.

McFadden, A. J., Young, M., & Markham, F. (2015). Venue-level predictors of alcohol-related violence: an exploratory study in Melbourne, Australia. *International Mental Health and Addiction*, forthcoming. doi: 10.1007/s11469-015–9552-3

Meng, Y., Brennan, A., Holmes, J., Hill-McManus, D., Angus, C.,. . ., Meier, P. (2013). *Modelled Income Group-Specific Impacts of Alcohol Minimum Unit Pricing in England in 2014/15: Policy Appraisals Using New Developments to the Sheffield Alcohol Policy Model (v2.5)*. Sheffield: University of Sheffield. www.sheffield.ac.uk/polopoly_fs/1.291621!/file/julyreport.pdf

Miller, P., Tindall, J., Sønderlund, A., Groombridge, D., Lecathelinais, C., . . ., Wiggers, J. (2012). *Dealing with Alcohol-Related Harm and the Night-Time Economy (DANTE). Final Report. Monograph Series No. 43*. Canberra, Australia: National Drug Law Enforcement Research Fund. www.ndlerf.gov.au/sites/default/files/. . ./mono43execsummary.pdf

Mosher, J. F., Toomey, T. L., Good, C., Harwood, E., & Wagenaar, A. C. (2002). State laws mandating or promoting training programs for alcohol servers and establishment managers: an assessment of statutory and administrative procedures. *Journal of Public Health Policy* 23: 90–113.

Nicosia, N. Pacula, R. L., Kilmer, B., Lundberg, R., & Chiesa, J. (2009). *The Economic Cost of Methamphetamine Use in the United States, 2005*. Santa Monica, CA: RAND. Corporation. www.rand.org/pubs/monographs/MG829.html

Pryor, J. B., DeSouza, E. R., Fitness, J., Hutz, C., Kumpf, M., Lubbert, K., …, Erber, M. W. (1997). Gender differences in the interpretation of social-sexual behavior: a cross-cultural perspective on sexual harassment. *Journal of Cross Cultural Psychology* 28: 509–34.

Punto Focal Nacional Reitox (2013). *Informe Nacional 2013 (datos del 2012) al OEDT*. Madrid: Delegación del Gobierno PNSD. www.pnsd.msssi.gob.es/Categoria2/publica/pdf/2013INFORMENACIONAL.pdf

Quigg, Z., Hughes, K., Bellis, M. A., van Hasselt, N., Calafat, A., . . ., Goossens, F. X. (2014). Incidents of harm in European drinking environments and relationships with venue and customer characteristics. *International Journal of Alcohol and Drug Research* 3: 269–75. doi.org/10.7895/ijadr.vXiY.180

Rowland, B., Toumbourou, J. W., & Livingston, M. (2015). The association of alcohol outlet density with illegal underage adolescent purchasing of alcohol. *Journal of Adolescent Health* 56: 146–52. doi: 10.1016/j.jadohealth.2014.08.005

Schnitzer, S., Bellis, M. A., Anderson, Z., Hughes, K., Calafat, A., Juan, M., & Kokkevi, A. (2010). Nightlife violence – a gender specific view on risk factors for violence in nightlife settings; a cross sectional study in nine European countries. *Journal of Interpersonal Violence* 25: 1094–1112. doi: 10.1177/0886260509340549

Stockwell, T., & Chikritzhs, T. (2009). Do relaxed trading hours for bars and clubs mean more relaxed drinking? A review of international research on the impacts of changes to permitted hours of drinking. *Crime Prevention and Community Safety* 11: 153–70.

United Nations. (2002). *Commission on Narcotic Drugs Report of the Executive Director, Forty-Fifth Session Vienna, 11–15 March 2002*. www.unodc.org/documents/commissions/CND/CND_Sessions/CND_45/E-CN-7-2002-9/E-CN7-2002-9_E.pdf

Voas, R. B., Fell, J. C., McKnight, A. S., & Sweedler, B. M. (2004). Controlling impaired driving through vehicle programs: an overview. *Traffic Injury Prevention* 5: 292–8.

Wallin, E., & Andreásson, S. (2004) Can I have a beer, please? A study of alcohol service to young adults on licensed premises in Stockholm. *Prevention Science* 5: 221–9.

WHO (World Health Organization). (2012). *European Action Plan to Reduce the Harmful Use of Alcohol 2012–2020*. Copenhagen: WHO Regional Office for Europe. Retrieved from www.euro.who.int/__data/assets/pdf_file/0008/178163/E96726.pdf?ua=1

Wickham, M. (2012). *Alcohol Consumption in the Night-Time Economy: Policy Interventions. Working Paper 55*. London: Greater London Authority.

Wood, D. W., Greene, S. L., Alldus, G., Huggett, D., Nicolaou, M., Chapman, K., . . .Dargan, P. I. (2008). Improvement in the pre-hospital care of recreational drug users through the development of club specific ambulance referral guidelines. *Substance Abuse Treatment, Prevention and Policy* 3: 14. doi: 10.1186/1747–597X-3-14 www.substanceabusepolicy.com/content/3/1/14

Wojnar, M., & Jakubczyk, A. (2014). Brief interventions for hazardous and harmful alcohol consumption in accident and emergency departments. *Front Psychiatry* 3(5):152. doi: 10.3389/fpsyt.2014.00152. eCollection 2014.

11 Preventing Distress and Promoting Psychological Well-Being in Uncertain Times through Career Management Intervention

Annamaria Di Fabio, Maureen E. Kenny, & Milena Claudius

The relationship of work to psychological well-being (PWB) and life satisfaction across the life course has been well documented across many fields (Blustein, 2008; Fouad & Bynner, 2008). Whereas one's work life may contribute positively to well-being, well-being can be threatened by problematic features of the work environment, risks associated with unemployment, and job instability. Given the contribution of work to well-being and the challenges many people now face in deriving at least part of their lifelong well-being from work activity (Blustein, 2008), attention to the types and scope of career preventive interventions that can serve to promote well-being is warranted.

This chapter is a response to what we see as a growing need for preventive and growth enhancing interventions to promote the capacity of individuals to access the benefits of work that contribute to well-being. Our sense of urgency is derived in part from the complexities of the contemporary workplace, including the economic and social factors that are changing the structure of the world of work. The combination of rapid technological change, globalization, and economic crises means that individuals are increasingly faced with the need to change jobs, interspersed with periods of unemployment. Frequent job change has become more normative among larger segments of the world population, as employers seek to outsource work with short-term contracts. Automation has eliminated many jobs that can be programmed by a computer or completed by a robot or by persons thousands of miles away who will work for less money (Jerald, 2009). In postindustrial nations, declines in the numbers of unskilled and manufacturing jobs and growth in positions requiring technological training have led to worker dislocation and unemployment for those without advanced skills.

While older workers have been displaced by globalization and technological change, young people are often unclear on how to best prepare for a productive and satisfying work future. Labor market opportunities continue to shift rapidly, such that the types of jobs that are in demand today might be obsolete by the time today's youth graduate from college or even high school (Peck, 2010).

The changing global marketplace and recent global recession have thus generated high levels of uncertainty and anxiety for many young people, who are no longer confident that they will secure work offering opportunities for growth, or even any work at all, despite good academic preparation (Peiró, Sora, & Caballer, 2012).

In this chapter, we take an international perspective on prevention and PWB with a focus on preparing individuals, particularly young people, to adapt effectively to the currently unpredictable and somewhat chaotic world of work. We devote particular attention to recent research and intervention carried out in Italy through the International Research and Intervention Laboratory in "Psychology for Vocational Guidance, Career Counseling and Talents (*LabOProCCareer&T*)" and the newly founded International Research and Intervention Laboratory in "Positive Psychology, Prevention and Sustainability" (PosPsycP&S)" at the University of Florence. Italy, along with other nations across Europe and the world, has experienced ongoing global and regional economic and policy change. While persons with advanced education and training continue to be most advantaged in job entry and advancement, pathways to secure, meaningful, and stable work have diminished across many segments of society (Stiglitz, 2012). In response to the challenges posed by the twenty-first-century workplace, we propose that promoting competencies for career management is an important focus for prevention psychologists. Career management is an ongoing process by which individuals develop, implement, and monitor career goals and engage in adaptive strategies that increase the probability that their career goals will be achieved (Greenhaus, Callanan, & Godshalk, 2010).

While this chapter focuses on North America and Europe, we are cognizant that many workers in the least developed and least affluent nations of the globe outside of Europe and North America have never enjoyed job security or choice in seeking meaningful work (Blustein, Kenny, & Kozan, 2014). Efforts to enhance PWB globally must consider the individual needs and life contexts of those who enjoy choice in managing their careers and those who lack choice and are focused on meeting survival needs. Prevention efforts ultimately entail a broad range of economic, psychological, health, and social factors (e.g., Seedat, Niekerk, Suffla, & Ratele, 2014). In this chapter, we focus specifically on preventive interventions designed to promote well-being by preparing individuals to navigate the instability and uncertainty presented by the changing global workplace

Work and Well-Being

A number of psychological frameworks are helpful in understanding how work is related to the well-being of individuals and communities (Blustein, 2008; Fouad & Bynner, 2008). For those who experience unemployment, threats to well-being are clear. Persons who are unemployed typically have less money for purchasing products that contribute to physical and mental well-being and experience high levels of stress (Blustein, 2008). At a community level, economic downturns and high levels of unemployment can also have negative effects, contributing to increases in crime, substance abuse, violence, and overall diminished access to resources that improve the quality of life (Blustein, 2008).

The psychology of working framework (Blustein, 2006) describes how work contributes to PWB and life satisfaction by offering a means to meet human needs for power, social connection, and self-determination. For individuals, unemployment thus presents risks to well-being by undermining financial security and by diminishing access to the social and psychological benefits that can be derived from work, including opportunities to create, contribute, and collaborate with others (Blustein et al., 2014). It thus follows that merely having a job is not enough to ensure PWB, but that many characteristics of the work itself and the work environment influence the capacity for work to meet the array of human needs associated with well-being. Preventive interventions intended to promote well-being, thus, need to help individuals to consider ways to meet their relational, power, and self-determination needs through their work and life choices.

Social-cognitive theory (Lent, 2004) explicates the importance of satisfaction in the specific life domains of school and work as contributors to overall life satisfaction and well-being. This model posits that an individual's satisfaction at school or work is influenced by the interaction of personal and environmental factors. Personal factors include malleable social-cognitive skills (e.g., self-efficacy expectations, outcome expectations, progress in goal-directed activities) and traitlike personality characteristics (e.g., positive affect, extraversion, optimism). Environmental barriers and supports are conceptualized as contextual factors, whose impact is influenced by social-cognitive and personality factors at the individual level. The model has been supported in U.S. research (Lent & Brown, 2006, 2008) and in a growing number of international studies (e.g., Lent, Taveira, & Lobo, 2012; Lent et al., 2014).

The critical importance of work can also be understood according to hedonic and eudaimonic models of well-being. Hedonic well-being refers to an absence of distress, depression, or unhappiness. In empirical investigations, the hedonic perspective is generally operationalized as subjective well-being (SWB), marked by positive affect (PA), the absence of negative affect (NA), and satisfaction with life (SWL) (Diener & Lucas, 1999). The eudaimonic perspective focuses on the attainment of PWB as related to personal growth, life purpose, mastery, and autonomy (Ryff & Singer, 2008). Although PWB is often accompanied by a sense of SWB, PWB goes beyond the attainment of SWB and is derived from a sense of achievement and the realization of one's potential. PWB has been broadly associated with indices of physical and mental health and is recognizably relevant to the understanding of work as a means for satisfying human needs for autonomy, competence, and relatedness (Ryan & Deci, 2001).

The field of positive organizational behavior (POB; Bakker & Schaufeli, 2008), a branch of organizational psychology derived from positive psychology, focuses on identifying the individual psychological and job resources, including opportunities to exercise autonomy and enjoy positive relationships, that enable employees to perform optimally, attain meaning, and experience PWB in the workplace (Xanthopoulou, Bakker, Demerouti, & Schaufeli, 2012). Whereas SWB emphasizes an affective state that has been conceptualized in traitlike terms, PWB focuses on agentic aspects of individuals' thinking and behavior in ways that may be modified through prevention efforts (Sheu & Lent, 2009). POB has also sought to identify the personal resources (e.g., resilience, self-efficacy, hope, self-regulation, meaning-making) and organizational factors that enable employees to be engaged and productive in the new and ever-changing workplace (Heuvel, Denerouti, Schaufeli, & Bakker, 2010).

Constructs central to Blustein's (2006) psychology of working, social-cognitive theory (Lent & Brown, 2004), PWB, and POB (Bakker & Schaufeli, 2008) have stimulated research that informs our understanding of career management as prevention.

Prevention and Career Management

Although vocational psychology has a longstanding prevention and social justice orientation (Blustein, McWhirter, & Perry, 2005), career education and vocational guidance have not typically been central in the prevention agenda (Brown, Lamp, Telander, & Hacker, 2012; Kenny & Di Fabio, 2009). Given the well-established relationship between work and well-being over the life course (Blustein, 2008), efforts to prepare young people for developing satisfying work lives and for managing career transitions that might otherwise threaten their well-being can, however, clearly be understood as prevention activities. Our discussion of career management focuses largely on the promotion of assets and protective factors that may help individuals to maintain well-being in times of work uncertainty. Interventions that seek to enhance the capacity of individuals, particularly young people, to prepare for life and career transitions that may otherwise undermine social and PWB are aligned with primary prevention. Interventions that seek to work with the unemployed or others who are already disconnected from the world of work and experiencing distress are aligned with the goals for secondary prevention.

Career guidance has traditionally assisted individuals in choosing a career that yields a good vocational fit (Blustein et al., 2005; Lent, 2013). Given today's unstable and rapidly changing world of work (Kenny & Minor, 2015), new models of intervention have emerged to augment the traditional approaches that focus on a single vocational choice and a linear process of career development. Vocational psychologists now refer to the need for career management (Savickas, 2011) involving proactive adaptation to a constantly changing work environment. As large corporations and governmental organizations can no longer be counted on as sites for long-term employment and career advancement, individuals need to assume greater responsibility for creating their own career possibilities, maintaining their employability, and managing their career transitions (Savickas, 2011). Di Fabio (2014c) suggests that self-management is an integral component of career management, since a constant process of self-assessment is needed for individuals to integrate new experiences and evolve new understandings of possible career roles and opportunities. Lent and Brown (2013) have proposed the concept of career self-management with a focus on the processes and factors that influence individuals' use of agentic and purposeful behaviors to navigate normative career developmental tasks and to cope with the less predictable events and crises that are presented by the changing work context. Given the level of uncertainty and anxiety experienced by many young people who feel unprepared to meet the demands of a shifting global workplace (Peiró et al., 2012), career management emerges as promising direction for prevention efforts focused on promoting well-being.

Psychological Factors Associated with Career Management

In order to cope adaptively with recurring career transitions and to manage their lives to yield PWB, individuals need to be equipped with advanced academic and technical skills and psychological competencies (Kenny & Minor, 2015). Research drawing from career and self-construction theories (Guichard, 2005; Savickas, 2005), relational theory (Blustein, 2011), the psychology of working (Blustein, 2006), positive youth development (Lerner, Almerigi, Theokas, & Lerner, 2005), social-cognitive theory (Brown & Lent, 2013), and positive psychology (Snyder & Lopez, 2002) has identified a range of psychological competencies pertinent to career management. We will turn now to discuss the psychological factors related to proactive career management and well-being with an interest in those competencies that may serve as foci for future prevention intervention.

The career construction model of Savickas and colleagues (Savickas, 2011; Savickas & Porfeli, 2012) focuses on the importance of career adaptability, or the personal capacity for change to cope with undefined, unfamiliar, and uncertain life demands, and the processes by which persons strive to bring their inner needs into harmony with external realities. In addition to a secure and coherent sense of self and identity, Savickas and Porfeli (2012) suggest that capacities for self-reflection and self-regulation are important for youth to maintain direction, purpose, and continuity. Career construction theory specifies four sets of career adaptability skills that contribute to the personal capacity for change, including concern about the future; control or the application of self-discipline, effort, and persistence to shape and prepare for the future; curiosity or the capacity to think about oneself in a variety of future roles; and confidence that one can pursue hoped-for choices and aspirations (Savickas, 2013).

Research emerging from the positive youth development perspective (PYD: Lerner et al., 2005) has also identified individual assets that promote positive adaptation in school and work and enable youth to develop resilience despite adversity. In U.S. research, Lerner and colleagues (2005) identified three individual assets (self-control or regulation, school engagement, and hopeful future expectations) that are consistently associated with positive youth development. Taken together, career construction and PYD research reveal an overlapping array of psychological attributes, ranging from a positive and secure sense of self, self-control, hopeful future expectations, curiosity, and engagement in school, associated with positive development. Education and training are thus challenged to equip individuals with these competencies in preparation for lives of agency, productivity, and engaged citizenship.

The value of these psychological attributes and their potential value as a focus for prevention are evident from a broad base of research, which we briefly and selectively discuss here (see Kenny & Minor, 2015, for a review). Research derived from the perspective of positive psychology (Juntunen & Wettersten, 2006; Snyder & Lopez, 2002), for example, suggests that hope has a central role in fostering motivation and preventing disengagement from school and work. Hopeful future expectations are aligned with well-being and adaptive career management from the PYD and self and career construction perspectives (Brown et al., 2012). Juntunen and Wettersen (2006) describe the relevance of hope in the vocational domain and suggest that identifying attainable career goals and the means for achieving them may foster motivation, while a lack of goals and unclear future possibilities may undermine motivation. Kenny, Walsh-Blair, Blustein, Bempechat, and Seltzer (2010) found that work hope was positively associated with achievement motivation among students attending an urban high school in the United States.

Consistent with the notion that PWB is derived from work and life activity that is meaningful, the construct of calling has received recent attention in vocational psychology (Dik & Duffy, 2009; Duffy, Allan, & Dik, 2011). Persons who describe themselves as having a calling, view work as having personal or social purpose and meaning beyond income or social status. Having a calling has been associated in a series of studies with positive work and well-being indicators including confidence in one's career choice, commitment and satisfaction with school, higher educational attainment, commitment to work, work and life satisfaction, and low levels of stress and depression (Duffy, Allan, & Bott, 2012). Work hope has been identified as one mediator between calling and academic satisfaction among college students (Duffy et al., 2011). Furthermore, having a calling appears to buffer the potentially negative impact of low core self-evaluation, characterized by low self-esteem, low self-efficacy, and pessimism, for the attainment of life satisfaction among college students (Duffy et al., 2012).

Blustein's (2011) relational theory of working and social-cognitive theory (Brown & Lent, 2013) underscore the importance of relational support for prevention and career management, which has been affirmed across a large body of research (see Kenny & Medvide, 2013). A series of studies with urban high school youth in the United States documented the contributions of relational support from teachers, family, peers, and work supervisors to positive academic and career development across the adolescent years (Kenny & Bledsoe, 2005; Kenny, Blustein, Chaves, Grossman, & Gallagher, 2003; Kenny et al., 2007a). Research with Italian high school and university students has also documented the association of perceived relational support from family, teachers, and friends with positive developmental outcomes, including resilience, self-perceived employability, and adaptive decision making (Di Fabio & Kenny, 2015).

Research on Career Management and Well-being in Italy

The International Research and Intervention Laboratory in "Psychology for Vocational Guidance, Career Counseling and Talents (LabOProCCareer&T)" and the newly founded International Research and Intervention Laboratory in "Positive Psychology, Prevention and Sustainability" (PosPsycP&S)" at the University of Florence have built upon career construction (Savickas, 2005), self and life construction (Guichard, 2005, 2013), relational theory of working (Blustein, 2011), and positive psychology (Snyder & Lopez, 2002) frameworks to further examine the range of protective psychological assets aligned with prevention, career management, and well-being across the life course. Italy is one of the European Union nations that was harshly impacted by the economic crisis of the past decade, with overall unemployment continuing at a high level of over 12 percent and youth unemployment above 40 percent (Harris, 2013). Given the severity and persistence of the social and economic crisis experienced in Italy and the resulting despair, especially among young people (Nadeau, 2014), the Laboratories at the University of Florence set out to study factors that enable individuals to take an agentic role in navigating career and life uncertainty. The Laboratories strive to identify factors and test theoretical models that can inform the development of preventive interventions to promote well-being in the context of social and economic turbulence.

Di Fabio & Kenny (2016) recently proposed the framework of Positive Self and Relational Management (PS&RM) to integrate psychological constructs derived from each of the preceding theoretical perspectives to guide the development of prevention and positive development interventions. PS&RM focuses on building individual strengths to promote effective lifelong self and relational management across numerous personal and professional challenges. Consistent with a lifelong focus, the researchers have carried out a systematic program of inquiry encompassing high school students, young adults in vocational training, college students, and adults employed in a variety of fields.

Emotional intelligence has been a principal focus of research as one mechanism for fostering positive development and resilience (see Di Fabio, Kenny, & Minor, 2014, for a review). Di Fabio and colleagues have studied the relationship of three distinct models (Bar-On, 1997; Mayer, Salovey, & Caruso, 2002; Petrides & Furnham, 2000) of emotional intelligence (EI) with a range of social (perceived social support), psychological (core self-evaluation, resilience, decisional styles), academic (grade point average), and career outcomes (career decision-making self-efficacy, career decision-making difficulties, perceived employability). Although there have been some variations across EI models and measures, the findings of Di Fabio and colleagues show EI to be a robust construct associated with adaptive social, psychological, and career outcomes, after accounting for the effects of cognitive abilities and stable dimensions of personality (e.g., Di Fabio, 2015a; Di Fabio & Kenny, 2012; Di Fabio & Saklofske, 2014). When dependent variables are self-reported, trait emotional intelligence seems to have a somewhat greater contribution, whereas when the dependent variable is performance-based (e.g., academic grade point average [GPA]), ability-based emotional intelligence has the greater role (Di Fabio & Kenny, 2012). The findings with regard to EI in the Italian context largely replicated findings in the United States, Spain, and other Western nations (Di Fabio, Bernaud, & Loarer, 2014).

The Laboratories have also studied emotional intelligence among employed adults with a focus on employee workplace' behaviors and characteristics of the work environment. Attention to the role of the work environment for well-being is emphasized in the psychology of working (Blustein, 2006), social-cognitive theory (Lent, 2004), POB (Bakker & Schaufeli, 2008), and prevention (Kenny, Horne, Orpinas, & Reese, 2009) frameworks. Among Italian nurses and physicians, trait emotional intelligence (Bar-On, 1997) has been positively associated with organizational resilience (Di Fabio, 2011a), organizational justice (Di Fabio & Palazzeschi, 2012), acceptance of change (Di Fabio, in press c) and inversely associated with workplace incivility (Di Fabio, in press b) and resistance to change (Di Fabio et al., 2014). These findings suggest that when workers have higher levels of EI, a healthier work environment may ensue.

Di Fabio (2014a, 2014e) introduced the construct of purposeful identitarian awareness as a preventive self-management competency that draws upon the constructs of adaptability (Savickas, 2011) and identity (Guichard, 2010). Purposeful identitarian awareness includes attention to the authentic self and self-attunement. Awareness of the authentic self (Di Fabio, 2014a, 2014e) includes knowledge of one's intrinsic interests (Sheldon & Houser-Marko, 2001) and goals that matter both personally and socially (Di Fabio, 2014d). Self-attunement (Di Fabio, 2014e) involves attention to one's objective (what I am able to do) and subjective (what energizes me, what motivates me to do) talents, and the attainment of balance between individual and collective needs and care for oneself and for others.

Di Fabio (2014c) has also proposed the construct of intrapreneurial self-capital (ISC) to account for a set of personal resources for use in innovative and effective problem solving in the context of uncertainty and change. Building upon prior research (Di Fabio, 2104c), nine individual-level factors were hypothesized to contribute to the ISC metaconstruct, including core self-evaluation, or positive self-concept (Judge, Erez, Bono, & Thorensen, 2003); the commitment, control, and challenge dimensions of hardiness (Maddi, 1990);

creative self-efficacy, or the perceived ability to generate new ideas and to solve problems creatively (Tierney & Farmer, 2002); resilience, the perceived ability to cope with adversity in an adaptive way (Luthar, Cicchetti, & Becker, 2000); goal mastery, motivation to develop and to learn new skills (Midgley et al., 2000); decisiveness, the perceived ability to make decisions in a timely manner (Frost & Shows, 1993); and vigilance, an adaptive decision-making style that includes the search for relevant information and careful evaluation of options before making a decision (Mann, Burnett, Radford, & Ford, 1997). Among Italian high school and university students, research to date has found core self-evaluation, creative self-efficacy, hardiness, and goal mastery to be associated with career decision-making self-efficacy (Di Fabio, 2014b, in press a) and inversely associated with career decision-making difficulties (Di Fabio, 2014b; Di Fabio, in press a; Di Fabio & Palazzeschi, 2014; Di Fabio, Palazzeschi, & Bar-On, 2012). Core self-evaluation (Di Fabio, 2014b), hardiness (Di Fabio, in press a) and goal mastery (Di Fabio, in press a) were associated with perceived employability. Core self-evaluation, creativity, self-efficacy, and trait emotional intelligence have been associated with eudaimonic indices of well-being (Di Fabio, 2014b).

Di Fabio (2014c) has confirmed the factor structure of the ISC metaconstruct as derived from the seven underlying constructs. The correlations of ISC were positive with career decision self-efficacy, negative with career decision-making difficulties, and positive with perceived employability and GPA. With regard to construct validity, ISC was also found to be positively associated with career adaptability and purposeful identity, after accounting for the variance explained by fluid intelligence and personality (Di Fabio, 2014b). To the extent that ISC is associated with career management and well-being and can be developed through intervention, it represents a promising construct for prevention and the promotion of well-being.

Examples of Preventive Interventions for Career Management

Preventive interventions can be designed to reduce risks or to buffer the potential negative effects of environmental risks by enhancing personal assets or protective factors (Kenny & Romano, 2009). The preceding summarized research identified a number of personal assets that can serve as targets for career management prevention in efforts intended to foster well-being and prevent distress. We now discuss some of these individual- and group-focused career education and development interventions designed to equip individuals with a range of strength-oriented career resources.

Based upon the identification of the reflective self as central in career management, the Career Construction Interview (CCI; Savickas, 2005) and Counseling for Self-Construction Interview (Guichard, 2005) were designed to engage individuals in dialogue and self-reflection to envision new ways of being that transcend static and narrow conceptions of career choice. The CCI, for example, begins by asking clients to tell stories about how they construct their self, identity, and career. Reflection on those narratives leads to a process of deconstruction, reconstruction, co-construction, and action to create a new narrative and plan for action in relation to shifting work opportunities.

A number of online-accessible tools have been developed to assist individuals in planning and clarifying their life priorities as related to career management. Framed around Savickas' (2005) research emphasizing adaptability, *My Career Story Workbook for Life Career Success* (Savickas & Hartung, 2012) engages individuals in a developmental process of self-construction as actors, agents, and eventually authors of their career and life narratives. The workbook, which poses questions designed to provoke individuals to enact their life story and vocational choices (e.g., "telling, hearing, and enacting my story"), can be used by individuals alone, in groups, or with educators.

Psycho-educational programs in school and community settings in the United States incorporate research from career construction (Savickas, 2005) and positive youth development (Lerner et al., 2005) models in efforts to foster academic, social, and vocational development and other positive outcomes (Lapan, 2004). Such programs promote individual characteristics that are needed to manage uncertain futures, such as having a hopeful outlook, positive identity, school engagement, and the ability to challenge barriers to self-confidence. Several psycho-educational programs also aim to foster critical consciousness and an understanding of the ways that systems of oppression may act as barriers to vocational success. Research has demonstrated that youth who adopt a critical lens to systemic injustice hold more optimistic vocational expectations and perceive work as a critical component in their lives (e.g., Watts, Williams, & Jagers, 2003; Diemer et al., 2010).

Tools for Tomorrow (TFT: Kenny, Sparks, & Jackson, 2007b) is an example of a psychoeducational intervention built on PYD principles (Lerner et al., 2005) and emancipatorian communitarian values (Prilleltensky & Nelson, 2012) and designed to help U.S. students develop self-awareness and personal and vocational identities within a broader sociocultural context. Urban U.S. high school students are guided in drawing connections between their academic participation and vocational futures, thereby enhancing school engagement and decreasing risk of early dropout. The year-long curriculum, implemented once per week, is composed of three primary modules: In the *Who am I* module, students explore issues related to personal, cultural backgrounds and ethnic identity. The *Connecting School and Career* module allows students to draw connections between their educational and vocational aspirations. Students learn about the academic and training requirements related to their careers of interest and how they can apply their strengths and talents to realize their career aspirations. The *Identifying Resources and Barriers* module guides students in identifying external and internal resources that can be accessed to reduce barriers that may impede pursuit of their chosen vocational path. Program assessment suggests that engagement in TFT activities is associated with increases in U.S. student school engagement over the academic year (Kenny, Blustein, Haase, Jackson, & Perry, 2006).

Making My Future Work, a college and career readiness program for urban middle and high school students developed in the United States by Perry and colleagues (2014), consists of four modules: (a) *Exploring Self and Identity*; (b) *Career Exploration*, *Planning*, and *Post-secondary Pathways*; (c) *My 21st Century Skills Toolkit* (e.g., including skills in communications, stress management and coping, multiculturalism, and growth mindsets); and (d) *College Entry, Survival, and Success*. The program includes eighty lessons that are aligned with academic standards, allowing teachers choice in selecting the most relevant lessons for their classroom. The intervention is being evaluated using a mixed-methods quasi-experimental design with preliminary findings revealing a positive impact on academic grade point average and gains on measures of school engagement, career planning, and career decision making.

Related to the recent recession in the United States and the adverse impact of unemployment for well-being (Fouad & Bynner, 2008), interventions have also been developed to minimize psychological risks and to equip individuals with new skill sets for employment. Programs grounded in community and social justice seek to address the complex needs of unemployed adults, with attention to internal and external systemic barriers. For example, Bhat (2010) developed an intensive fifteen-day group intervention that focused on fostering personal awareness, self-efficacy, and empowerment among unemployed adults. The program taught group members employment search skills and engaged members with a community employer liaison to provide ongoing case management and advocacy. Notably, through the support of the group, employment seekers began to feel empowered and reconnected to their respective community. Similarly, Creed, Bloxsome, and Johnston (2001) found that unemployed adults who participated in a community-based vocational skills development program demonstrated greater self-efficacy, a central construct in social-cognitive models of career self-management (Brown & Lent, 2013). Along this vein, Juntunen and colleagues (2006) developed a program to increase self-efficacy and address common vocational barriers for welfare recipients, including lack of transportation and child care. Participants who completed the program reported decreased symptoms of depression and greater self-efficacy.

Promising Preventive Interventions for Career Management in Italy

Prevention efforts carried out through the International Research and Intervention Laboratory in "Psychology for Vocational Guidance, Career Counseling and Talents (*LabOProCCareer&T*)" and the International Research and Intervention Laboratory in "Positive Psychology, Prevention and Sustainability" (*PosPsycP&S*)" at the University of Florence to promote career management include school- and workplace-based interventions focused on the narrative assessment of career competencies, life design, and the promotion of specific career management competencies, such as emotional intelligence and intrapreneurial self-capital.

The narrative assessment of career competencies, for example, is an individual or group guidance intervention focused on the development of an adaptable self. The group version of the intervention utilizes the power of the audience method (Di Fabio & Maree, 2012), developed in the Laboratories to expand the number of clients served through a single intervention. This method includes written exercises completed individually by all group members and exercises in which participants interact individually with a counselor while other group members listen without intervening. Over a four-day period (eight hours each), group members are guided in examining their personal strengths and limitations to construct a new narrative of their competencies and employability (Di Fabio, 2014a, 2014e). The effectiveness of the assessment of career competencies has been evaluated with Italian female entrepreneurs, showing an increase in career decision-making self-efficacy and a decrease in career decision-making difficulties for the intervention group in comparison with a control group (Di Fabio, 2011b).

The Laboratories have also evaluated an application of the Career Construction Interview (CCI; Savickas, 2005) with university students and adults in Italy. This intervention is intended to increase self-awareness and promote agency and flexibility in designing one's career and life path and has face validity for use given the current economic context in Italy. The Laboratories adapted the CCI for delivery in a group format, employing the power of the audience approach (Di Fabio & Maree, 2012). The validity of the adapted CCI in the Italian context was assessed through mixed-method evaluation, including quantitative measures to assess expected intervention outcomes and qualitative measures to capture changes in individuals' self-narratives (Di Fabio, 2012a, 2014f; Rehfuss & Di Fabio, 2012). Qualitative evaluation, using the Future Career Autobiography (Rehfuss, 2009), revealed more specific life and occupational goals after the CCI for the intervention group in comparison with the control group (Di Fabio, 2012a). Another qualitative study found that the narratives of the intervention group reflected personal and professional change and increased career adaptability (Savickas & Porfeli, 2012), which were not evident for the control group (Di Fabio, 2012b, 2015b, 2016b). Expected changes were also found for relevant quantitative measures, including gains in career decision-making self-efficacy and decreases in self-reported career decision-making difficulties (Di Fabio, 2013; Di Fabio & Maree, 2012), lending further support for the validity of the adapted CCI for use in Italy.

The Life Design Genogram (Di Fabio, 2015c, 2016a) was developed by the Laboratories in Italy to help individuals experiencing a shifting life and work context to connect and give meaning to their past, present, and future life experiences and to inform the further development of their authentic self (Di Fabio, 2014a, 2014e). The Life Design Genogram engages participants in the development of two genograms focusing on personal and career dimensions of their lives (Di Fabio, 2015c). Validation of the intervention is limited to date, but promising with evaluation revealing positive narrative change assessed through the Future Career Autobiography (FCA; Rehfuss, 2009; Rehfuss & Di Fabio, 2012) and gains on a quantitative measure of authenticity (Wood, Linley, Maltby, Baliousis, & Joseph, 2008).

Constructing My Future Purposeful Life is a recently developed intervention (Di Fabio, 2014g) based on the PS&RM framework (Di Fabio & Kenny, 2016). This intervention was designed to develop a purposeful identitarian awareness and authentic self (Di Fabio, 2014a, 2014e). The first module focuses on fostering adaptability through the Life Design Genogram and the *Me and the Future* exercise. The second module, *Self-Advising the Future Self*, adopts Guichard's (2005, 2013) self-advising technique to foster self-reflection. The third module, *Constructing the Purposeful Self*, builds on Guichard's (2004) process *To Make Oneself Self* by assisting individuals in integrating their life experiences on the basis of their authentic intentions. Evaluation of this intervention found positive changes on the Future Career Autobiography (FCA; Rehfuss, 2009) and the Career Counseling Innovative Outcomes (CCIO) measure, an open-ended narrative assessment of counseling outcomes developed by Di Fabio (2014b, 2016b) and by increases on the quantitative measures of core self-evaluation (Judge et al., 2003) and authenticity (Wood et al., 2008).

The Laboratories have also sought to promote prevention and career management through interventions designed to foster emotional intelligence and intrapreneurial self-capital (Di Fabio, 2014c; Di Fabio & Kenny, 2011). Each of the four sessions (two and a half hours each) of the emotional intelligence intervention focus on one component of the Mayer and Salovey (1997) model, with the first session focusing on perceiving emotions in oneself and others, in objects, art, stories, music, and other similar stimuli; the second session focusing on facilitating thought or the ability to generate, use, and feel emotion to communicate feelings and use them in other cognitive processes; the third session focusing on understanding emotions; and the fourth session focusing on managing emotions or the capacity to modulate emotions in oneself and others so as to promote personal understanding and growth. Evaluation revealed that the intervention group of Italian high school students demonstrated higher ability-based and self-reported emotional intelligence and reduced career indecision and indecisiveness in comparison with the student control group (Di Fabio & Kenny, 2011).

A recently designed intervention to enhance ISC offers short and long versions. The short version (five sessions of four hours each) includes reflection on the chapters of one's life story in the first session; a focus on positive self-concept and hardiness in the second session; specific exercises to stimulate reflection on creative self-efficacy and resilience in the third session; reflection on goal mastery, decisiveness, and vigilance in the fourth session; and integrative reflection to achieve a new voice of authorship in building the next chapter in one's own life-story in the fifth session. The long version (five sessions of eight hours each) augments the short version with exercises designed to foster greater self-evaluation; to recognize and focus on positive components of ISC;

to deepen analysis from the past through the present to the future; and to integrate positive components of ISC in one's own life story. Research to date with Italian university students indicates that the intervention is effective in fostering individual intrapreneurial resources (i.e., as aligned with the nine ISC constructs) hypothesized as integral for effective and creative adaptation to change and for overcoming environmental constraints (Di Fabio & Van Esbroeck, 2016).

Career Management and the Ecology of People's Lives

The research and interventions described in this chapter that are derived from self and career construction theories, PYD, social-cognitive theory, and life design models of career intervention focus on building personal assets for prevention and career management but give minimal attention to altering ecological factors that limit individual choice and success. Systemic barriers related to social class, race, gender, age, and disability status influence career opportunities and the experience of power, connection, and autonomy in the workplace and opportunities for career management and PWB (Blustein et al., 2014). Prilleltensky (Prilleltensky & Nelson, 2012) posits an ecological model of well-being, derived from the balanced and simultaneous satisfaction of individual, relational, organizational, communal, and environmental needs and from the enactment of just policies and practices in each of these contexts. According to this model, well-being cannot be achieved only by empowering individuals but requires attention to the satisfaction of objective and subjective needs across multiple contexts, including the work context.

The contemporary challenge, exacerbated by the recent recession and technological change, extends beyond individual adaptability and resilience to a concern for the availability of work that affords dignity and a livable wage for all. The psychology of working perspective (Blustein, 2006) and best practices in prevention (APA, 2014) acknowledge the need to modify factors external to the person that limit access to educational and work opportunities and other resources associated with well-being. Vocational psychologists are now emphasizing the importance of providing universal access to decent work (Guichard, 2013).

To date, most prevention and positive development interventions focusing on ecological change have targeted the proximal contexts. Prilleltensky and colleagues (Myers et al., 2014) have designed interventions to promote social justice and well-being in the community and workplace by simultaneously attending to survival (money, shelter, food) and self-determination needs (autonomy, freedom, power). These interventions, described by the acronym SPECS (strengths, prevention, empowerment, and community change), seek to guide processes of internal organizational change focused on building a healthy organizational climate that gives voice and choice to employees and fosters feelings of safety, respect, belonging, and trust (Evans et al., 2010).

Conclusions

Economic and technological changes worldwide are transforming the world of work encountered by young people today and for the future. We argue that new models of career intervention that are aligned with prevention and positive development frameworks can help to equip young people with a range of competencies that will allow them not only to cope adaptively with contemporary challenges but to proactively imagine and create better futures. Many scholars, including researchers at the Laboratories in Florence, are developing and evaluating promising interventions that have the potential for preventive impact in other national contexts.

While we are energized by the emergent research on relevant psychological constructs and interventions, we are also humbled by an awareness of the prevalence of systemic social and economic barriers and inequities that limit access to opportunity for all people. With this awareness, the effectiveness of preventive interventions that emphasize awareness, empowerment, and the construction of choice will inevitably be circumscribed in impact. At a basic level, more work opportunities need to be developed worldwide that offer stable employment, that affirm the dignity of the worker, and that provide a living wage. Emerging efforts to design and deliver interventions that reduce systemic barriers and create more just work environments offer additional promise, but this work remains in an early phase. Despite our awareness of the inevitable limitation of individually focused prevention in a world where decent work opportunities are constricted by systemic inequities and injustice, we maintain that the development of individual skills and empowerment is an essential component of any prevention strategy to foster career management and well-being for all. We hope that the international audience of this book will advance both the individual and ecological prevention efforts documented in this chapter.

References

APA (American Psychological Association) (2014). Guidelines for prevention in psychology. *American Psychologist* 69: 285–96.

Bakker, A. B., & Schaufeli, W. B. (2008). Positive organizational behavior: engaged employees in flourishing organizations. *Journal of Organizational Behavior,*29: 147–54. doi: 10.1002/job.515

Bar-On, R. (1997). *The Emotional Intelligence Inventory (EQ-I): Technical Manual.* Toronto, Canada: Multi-Health Systems.

Bhat, C. S. (2010). Assisting unemployed adults find suitable work: a group intervention embedded in community and grounded in social action. *Journal for Specialists in Group Work* 35: 246–54.

Blustein, D. L. (2006). *The Psychology of Working: A New Perspective for Career Development, Counseling, and Public Policy.* Mahwah, NJ: Lawrence Erlbaum.

Blustein, D. L. (2008). The role of work in psychological health and well-being: a conceptual, historical, and public policy perspective. *American Psychologist* 63(4): 228–40.

Blustein, D. L. (2011). A relational theory of working. *Journal of Vocational Behavior* 79: 1–17. doi: 10.1016/j.jvb.2010.10.004

Blustein, D. L., Kenny, M. E., & Kozan, S. (2014). Education and work as human birthrights: eradicating poverty through knowledge, innovation, and collaboration. In United Nations Development Program (ed.), *Barriers to and Opportunities for Poverty Reduction: Prospects for Private Sector–Led Interventions*. Istanbul: UNDP Istanbul International Center for Private Sector in Development.

Blustein, D. L., McWhirter, E. H., & Perry, J. C. (2005). An emancipatory communitarian approach to vocational development theory, research, and practice. *Counseling Psychologist* 33: 141–79.

Brown, S. D., Lamp, K., Telander, K. J., & Hacker, J. (2012). Career development as prevention: toward a social cognitive model of vocational hope. In Vera, E. (ed.), *The Oxford Handbook of Prevention in Counseling Psychology*. New York: Oxford University Press, pp. 374–92.

Brown, S. D., & Lent, R. W.. (eds.) (2013). *Career Development and Counseling: Putting Theory and Research to Work*, 2nd ed. Hoboken, NJ: Wiley & Sons.

Creed, P. A., Bloxsome, T. D., & Johnston, K. (2001). Self-esteem and self-efficacy outcomes for unemployed individuals attending occupational skills training programs. *Community, Work and Family* 4: 285–303.

Di Fabio, A. (2011a). L'intelligenza emotiva: nuove ricerche, nuove frontiere e nuovi strumenti per gli interventi in Italia [Emotional intelligence: new research, new frontiers and new instruments for intervention in Italy]. Keynote address presented at the 1st International Conference in Italy on Emotional Intelligence, Florence, Italy, June.

Di Fabio, A. (2011b). Bilancio per l'intraprendenza professionale: Valorizzazione del Sé professionale e della capacità di fare rete [Assessment for professional enterprise: valuing professional self and the ability to networking]. Paper presented at the CNR Ibimet conference "Creative enterprise networks: results of a path for the development of female entrepreneurship in crafts textile," Parma, Italy, May.

Di Fabio, A. (2012a). Narratabililty and career construction: empirical evidence of intervention effectiveness. State-of-the-Science Invited Lecture in the Field of Psychology of Counseling presented at the International Congress of Psychology (ICP) 2012, Cape Town, South Africa, July.

Di Fabio, A. (2012b). The effectiveness of the Career Story Interview from the perspective of Life Designing. *South African Journal of Higher Education* 26(4).

Di Fabio, A. (2013). Applying career construction in group-based contexts with adults. In Di Fabio, A., & Maree, J. G. (eds.), *Psychology of Career Counseling: New Challenges for a New Era. Festschrift in Honour of Prof. Mark Savickas*. New York: Nova Science, pp. 83–99.

Di Fabio, A. (2014a). Due meta-competenze chiave narrative per la nuova consapevolezza identitaria purposeful nel XXI secolo [Two key narrative meta-competences for the new, purposeful identitarian awareness in the twenty-first century]. *Counseling. Giornale Italiano di Ricerca e Applicazioni* 7: 133–41.

Di Fabio, A. (2014b). In light of the changing work scene: new challenges for research and intervention. Invited keynote address at the symposium "Career Development and the Psychology of Working," February, sponsored by Lynch School of Education of Boston College, D. L. Blustein, chair.

Di Fabio, A. (2014c). Intrapreneurial self-capital: a new construct for the 21st century. *Journal of Employment Counseling* 51: 98–111.

Di Fabio, A. (2014d). Positive preventive perspective for a positive lifelong self and relational management (PLS&RM): new challenges and opportunities for research and intervention. Invited keynote address at the Conference on Psychology and Health (PHC 2014), Beijing, China, November.

Di Fabio, A. (2014e). The new purposeful identitarian awareness for the twenty-first century: valorize themselves in the life construction from youth to adulthood and late adulthood. In Di Fabio, A., & Bernaud, J.-L. (eds.), *The Construction of the Identity in 21st Century: A Festschrift for Jean Guichard*. New York: Nova Science, pp. 157–68.

Di Fabio, A. (2014f). Career counseling and positive psychology in the 21st century: new constructs and measures for evaluating the effectiveness of intervention. *Journal of Counsellogy* 1: 193–213.

Di Fabio, A. (2014g). "Constructing my future purposeful life": a new Life Construction intervention. In Di Fabio, A., & Bernaud, J.-L. (eds.), *The Construction of the Identity in 21st Century: A Festschrift for Jean Guichard.* New York: Nova Science, pp. 219–39.

Di Fabio, A. (2015a). Beyond fluid intelligence and personality traits in social support: The role of ability-based emotional intelligence. *Frontiers in Psychology* 6: 395. doi: 10.3389/fpsyg.2015.00395

Di Fabio, A. (2015b). Life Adaptability Qualitative Assessment (LAQuA): a narrative instrument for evaluating counseling intervention effectiveness. In Maree, J. G., & Di Fabio, A. (eds.), *Exploring New Horizons in Career Counselling: Turning Challenges into Opportunities*. Rotterdam: Sense, pp. 43–62.

Di Fabio, A. (2015c). The Life Design genogram. In McMahon, M., & Watson, M. (eds.), *Career Assessment: Qualitative Approaches.* Rotterdam: Sense, pp. 97–103.

Di Fabio, A. (2016a). The Life Design genogram: a case study of an Italian female graduated student. In Busacca, L., & Rehfuss, M. (eds.), *Postmodern Career Counseling: A Handbook of Culture, Contexts, and Cases* (pp. 229–244). American Counseling Association.

Di Fabio, A. (2016b). Life Design and Career Counseling Innovative Outcomes (CCIO): a case study. *Career Development Quarterly* 64: 35–48.

Di Fabio, A. (in press a). Hardiness and goal mastery per promuovere adaptive career outcomes [Hardiness and goal mastery to promote adaptive career outcomes]. *Counseling. Giornale Italiano di Ricerca e Applicazioni.*

Di Fabio, A. (in press b). Intrapreneurial self-capital training. Counseling. Giornale Italiano di Ricerca e Applicazioni.

Di Fabio, A. (in press b). Personality traits and self-reported emotional intelligence: Which role in workplace incivility? *Counseling. Giornale Italiano di Ricerca e Applicazioni.*

Di Fabio, A. (in press c). The role of personality traits and self-reported emotional intelligence in relation to acceptance of change. *Counseling. Giornale Italiano di Ricerca e Applicazioni.*

Di Fabio, A., Bernaud, J.-L., & Loarer, E. (2014). Emotional intelligence or personality in resistance to change? Empirical results in an Italian health context. *Journal of Employment Counseling* 51: 146–57.

Di Fabio, A., & Kenny, M. E. (2011). Promoting emotional intelligence and career decision making among Italian high school students. *Journal of Career Assessment* 19: 21–34.

Di Fabio, A., & Kenny, M. E. (2012). Emotional intelligence and perceived social support among Italian high school students. *Journal of Career Development* 39: 461–75.

Di Fabio, A., & Kenny, M. E. (2015). The contributions of emotional intelligence and social support for adaptive career progress among Italian youth. *Journal of Career Development* 42: 48–59.

Di Fabio, A., & Kenny, M. E. (2016). From decent work to decent lives: positive Self and Relational Management (PS&RM) in the twenty-first century. *Frontiers in Psychology* 7(361). doi: 10.3389/fpsyg.2016.00361

Di Fabio, A., Kenny, M., & Minor, K. (2014). Emotional intelligence: school-based research and practice in Italy. In Furlong, M. J., Gilman, R., & Huebner, E. S. (eds.), *Handbook of Positive Psychology in the Schools,* 2nd ed. New York: Routledge, Taylor and Francis, pp. 450–64.

Di Fabio, A., & Maree, J. G. (2012). Group-based life design counseling in an Italian context. *Journal of Vocational Behavior* 80: 100–7.

Di Fabio, A., & Palazzeschi, L. (2012). Organizational justice: personality traits or emotional intelligence? An empirical study in an Italian hospital context. *Journal of Employment Counseling* 49: 31–42.

Di Fabio, A., & Palazzeschi, L. (2014). Creative self-efficacy e career decision-making difficulties in studenti italiani di scuola secondaria di secondo grado [Creative self-efficacy and career decision-making difficulties in Italian high school students]. *Counseling. Giornale Italiano di Ricerca e Applicazioni* 7: 171–81.

Di Fabio, A., Palazzeschi, L., & Bar-On, R. (2012). The role of personality traits, core self-evaluation and emotional intelligence in career decision-making difficulties. *Journal of Employment Counseling* 49: 118–29.

Di Fabio, A., & Saklofske, D. H. (2014). Promoting individual resources: the challenge of trait emotional intelligence. *Personality and Individual Differences* 65: 19–23.

Di Fabio, A. & Van Esbroeck, R. (2016). Intrapreneurial Self-Capital: A concept fitting a life-designing intervention. *Giornale Italiano di Ricerca e Applicazioni* 9(2).

Diemer, M. A., Wang, Q., Moore, T., Gregory, S., Hatcher, K. & Voight, A. M. (2010). Sociopolitical development, work salience, and vocational expectations among low-SES African American, Latin American, and Asian American youth. *Developmental Psychology* 46(3): 619–35.

Diener, E., & Lucas, R.E. (1999). Personality and subjective well-being. In Kahneman, D., & Diener, E. *The Foundations of Hedonic Psychology*. New York: Russel Sage Foundation, pp. 213–29.

Dik, B., & Duffy, R. D. (2009). Calling and vocation at work. *Counseling Psychologist* 37(3): 424–50.

Duffy, R., Allan, B., Bott, E. (2012). Calling and life satisfaction among undergraduate students: investigating mediators and moderators. *Journal of Happiness Studies* 13(3): 469–79.

Duffy, R. D., Allan, B. A., & Dik, B. J. (2011). The presence of a calling and academic satisfaction: examining potential mediators. *Journal of Vocational Behavior* 79(1): 74–80.

Evans, S., Prilleltensky, O., McKenzie, A., Prilleltensky, I., Nogueras, D., Huggins, C., & Mescia, N. (2010). Promoting strengths, prevention, empowerment, and community change through organizational development: lessons for research, theory, and practice. *Journal of Prevention and Intervention in the Community* 39(1): 50–64.

Fouad, N. A., & Bynner, J. (2008). Work transitions. *American Psychologist* 63(4): 241–51.

Frost, R. O., & Shows, D. L. (1993). The nature and measurement of compulsive indecisiveness. *Behavior Research Therapy* 31: 683–92.

Greenhaus, J. H., Callanan, G., & Godshalk, V. (2010). *Career Management,* 4th ed. Thousand Oaks, CA: Sage.

Guichard, J. (2004). Se faire soi [To make oneself Self]. *L'Orientation Scolaire et Professionnelle* 33: 499–534.

Guichard, J. (2005). Life-long self-construction. *International Journal for Educational and Vocational Guidance* 5: 111–24.

Guichard, J. (2010). Les théories de la construction des parcours professionnels et de la construction de soi: Deux approches de la construction de la vie individuelle. Paper presented at Colloque International, L'Institut national d'étude du travail et d'orientation professionnelle (INETOP), Paris, March.

Guichard, J. (2013). Career guidance, education, and dialogues. Presentation at the Congress of the International Association for Educational and Vocational Guidance. Montpellier, France, September.

Harris, K. (2013). Italy's youth unemployment reaches new all time high. *Time.* world.time.com/2013/10/01/italys-youth-unemployment-reaches-new-all-time-high/

Heuvel, M., Demerouti, E., Schaufeli, W., & Bakker, A. B. (2010). Personal resources and work engagement in the face of change. In Houdmont, J., & Leka, S. (eds.), *Contemporary Occupational Health Psychology: Global perspectives on research and practice.* Chichester, UK: John Wiley & Sons, pp. 124–50.

Jerald, C.D. (2009). Defining a 21st Century Education. Alexandria, VA: Center for Public Education. www.centerforpubliceducation.org/Main-Menu/Policies/21st-Century/Defining-a-21st-Century-Education-Full-report-PDF.pdf

Judge, T. A., Erez, A., Bono, J. E., & Thoresen, C. J. (2003). The core self-evaluations scale: development of a measure. *Personnel Psychology* 56: 303–31.

Juntunen, C. L., Cavett, A. M., Clow, R. B., Rempel, V., Darrow, R. E., & Guilmino, A. (2006). Social justice through self-sufficiency: vocational psychology and the transition from welfare to work. In Toporek, R. L., Gerstein, L. H., Fouad, N. A., Roysircar, G., & Israel, T. (eds.), *Handbook for Social Justice in Counseling Psychology.* Thousand Oaks, CA: Sage, pp. 294–309.

Juntunen, C. L., & Wettersen, K. B. (2006). Work hope: development and initial validation of a measure. *Journal of Counseling Psychology,*53: 94–106.

Kenny, M. E., & Bledsoe, M. (2005). Contributions of the relational context to career adaptability among urban adolescents. *Journal of Vocational Behavior* 66: 257–72

Kenny, M. E., Blustein, D., Chaves, A., Grossman, J., & Gallagher, L. A. (2003). The role of perceived barriers and relational support in the educational and vocational lives of urban high school students. *Journal of Counseling Psychology* 20: 142–55.

Kenny, M. E., Blustein, D. L., Haase, R. F., Jackson, J., & Perry, J. (2006). Setting the stage: career development and the school engagement process. *Journal of Counseling Psychology* 53: 272–9.

Kenny, M., & Di Fabio, A. (2009). Prevention and career development. *Risorsa Uomo. Rivista di Psicologia del Lavoro e dell'Organizzazione* 15: 361–74.

Kenny, M. E., Gualdron, L., Scanlon, D., Sparks, E., Blustein, D., & Jernigan, M. (2007a). Urban adolescents' construction of supports and barriers to their educational and career attainment. *Journal of Counseling Psychology* 54: 336–43.

Kenny, M. E., Horne, A. M., Orpinas, P., & Reese, L. E. (2009). Social justice and the challenge of preventive interventions: an introduction. In Kenny, M. E., Horne, A. M., Orpinas, P., & Reese, L. E. (eds.), *Realizing Social Justice: The Challenge of Preventive Interventions*. Washington, DC: American Psychological Association, pp. 3–14.

Kenny, M. E., & Medvide, M. B. (2013). Relational influences. In Brown, S. D., & Lent, R. W. (eds.), *Career Development and Counseling: Putting Theory and Research to Work,* 2nd ed. Hoboken, NJ: John Wiley, pp. 329–56.

Kenny, M., & Minor, K. (2015). Developing self and resilience for an uncertain future: positive youth development. In Di Fabio, A., & Bernaud, J.-L. (eds.), *The Construction of the Identity in 21st Century: A Festschrift for Jean Guichard.* New York: Nova Science, pp. 87–102.

Kenny, M. E., & Romano, J. (2009). Promoting positive development and social justice through prevention: a legacy for the future. In Kenny, M. E., Horne, A. M., Orpinas, P., & Reese, L. E. (eds.), *Realizing Social Justice: The Challenge of Preventive Interventions.* Washington, DC: American Psychological Association, pp. 17–30.

Kenny, M. E., Sparks, E., & Jackson, J. (2007b). Striving for social justice through interprofessional university school collaboration. In Aldarondo, E. (ed). *Advancing Social Justice through Clinical Practice*. Mahwah, NJ: Lawrence Erlbaum, pp. 313–35.

Kenny, M. E., Walsh-Blair, L., Blustein, L., Bempechat, J., & Seltzer, J. (2010). Achievement motivation among urban adolescents: work hope, autonomy support, and achievement-related beliefs. *Journal of Vocational Behavior* 77: 205–12.

Lapan, R. T. (2004). *Career Development across the K-16 Years: Bridging the Present to Satisfying and Successful Futures*. Alexandria, VA: American Counseling Association.

Lent, R. W. (2004). Toward a unifying theoretical and practical perspective on well-being and psychosocial adjustment. *Journal of Counseling Psychology* 51(4): 482–509.

Lent, R. W. (2013). Career-life-preparedness: revisiting career planning and adjustment in the new workplace. *Career Development Quarterly* 61: 2–14. doi: 10.1002/j.2161-0045.2013.00031.x

Lent, R. W. & Brown, S. D. (2006). Integrating person and situation perspectives on work satisfaction: a social-cognitive view. *Journal of Vocational Behavior* 69: 236–47.

Lent, R. W., & Brown, S. D. (2008). Social cognitive career theory and subjective well-being in the context of work. *Journal of Career Assessment* 16: 6–21.

Lent, R. W., & Brown, S. D. (2013). Promoting work satisfaction and performance. In S. D. Brown & R. W. Lent (Eds.), *Career Choice and Development: Putting Theory and Research* (pp. 621–652). New York, NY: Wiley.

Lent, R. W., Taveira, M., & Lobo, C. (2012). Two tests of the social cognitive model of well-being in Portuguese college students. *Journal of Vocational Behavior* 80: 362–71. doi: 10.1016/j.jvb.2011.08.009

Lent, R. W., Taveira, M., Pinto, J. C., Silva, A. D., Blanco, Á, Faria, S., & Gonçalves, A. M. (2014). Social cognitive predictors of well-being in African college students. *Journal of Vocational Behavior* 84(3): 266–72.

Lerner, R. M., Almerigi, J. B., Theokas, C., & Lerner, J. V. (2005). Positive youth development: a view of the issues. *Journal of Early Adolescence* 25(1): 10–16.

Luthar, S. S., Cicchetti, D., & Becker, B. (2000). The construct of resilience: a critical evaluation and guidelines for future work. *Child Development* 71: 543–62.

Maddi, S. R. (1990). Issues and interventions in stress mastery. In Friedman, H. S. (ed.), *Personality and Disease*. New York: Wiley, pp. 121–54.

Mann, L., Burnett, P., Radford, M., & Ford, S. (1997). The Melbourne Decision Making Questionnaire: an instrument for measuring patterns for coping with decisional conflict. *Journal of Behavioral Decision Making* 10: 1–19.

Mayer, J. D., & Salovey, P. (1997). What is emotional intelligence? In Salovey, P., & Sluyter, D. (eds.), *Emotional Development and Emotional Intelligence: Educational Implications*. New York: Basic Books, pp. 3–31.

Mayer, J. D., Salovey, P., & Caruso, D. R. (2002). *Mayer–Salovey–Caruso Emotional Intelligence Test (MSCEIT): User's Manual.* Toronto, Canada: Multi-Health Systems.

Midgley, C., Maehr, M. L., Hruda, L., Anderman, E. M., Anderman, L., Freeman, K. E., Gheen, M., Kaplan, A., Kumar, R., Middleton, M. J., Nelson, J., Roeser, R., & Urdan, T. (2000). *Manual for the Patterns of Adaptive Learning Scales (PALS)*. Ann Arbor: University of Michigan.

Myers, N. D. Prilleltensky, I, Jin, Y., Dietz, S., Rubenstein, C. Prilleltensky, O., & McMahon, A. (2014). Empirical contributions of the past in assessing multidimensional well-being. *Journal of Community Psychology,*42:,789–98.

Nadeau, B.L. (2014). Italy's lost generation: youth unemployment hits nearly 50 percent. *Daily Beast*. www.thedailybeast.com/articles/2014/06/07/italy-s-lost-generation-youth-unemployment-hits-nearly-50-percent.html

Peck, D. (2010). How a new jobless era will transform America [electronic version]. *Atlantic*. www.theatlantic.com/magazine/archive/2010/03/how- a-new-jobless-era-will-transform-america/7919/

Peiró, J. M., Sora, B., & Caballer, A. (2012). Job insecurity in the younger Spanish workforce: causes and consequences. *Journal of Vocational Behavior* 80: 444–53.

Perry, J. C., President, M. A., Harmon, J. A., Mizen, A. S., Calhoun-Butts, C., Riley, S. A. . . ., & Arendt, C. (2014). *Making My Future Work: A College and Career Readiness Program* (manual). Cleveland, OH: Cleveland State University. www.csuohio.edu/cehs/mmfw/making-my-future-work-0

Petrides, K. V., & Furnham, A. (2000). On the dimensional structure of emotional intelligence. *Personality and Individual Differences* 29: 313–20.

Prilleltensky, I., & Nelson, G. (2012). Critical psychology, prevention, and social justice. In Vera, E., ed., *The Oxford Handbook of Prevention in Counseling Psychology*. New York: Oxford University Press, pp. 141–59.

Rehfuss, M. C. (2009). The *Future Career Autobiography*: a narrative measure of career intervention effectiveness. *Career Development Quarterly* 58(1): 82–90.

Rehfuss, M., & Di Fabio, A. (2012). Validating the *Future Career Autobiography* as a measure of narrative change. *Journal of Career Assessment* 20: 452–62.

Ryff, C. D., & Singer, B. H. (2008). Know thyself and become what you are: a eudaimonic approach to psychological well-being. *Journal of Happiness Studies* 9: 13–39.

Ryan, R. M., & Deci, E. L. (2001). On happiness and human potentials: a review of research on hedonic and eudaimonic well-being. *Annual Review in Psychology* 52: 141–66.

Savickas, M. L. (2005). The theory and practice of career construction. In Brown, S. D., & Lent, R. W. (eds.), *Career Development and Counseling: Putting Theory and Research to Work*. Hoboken, NJ: John Wiley & Sons, pp. 42–70.

Savickas, M. L. (2011). *Career Counseling*. Washington, DC: American Psychological Association.

Savickas, M. L. (2013). Career construction theory and practice. In Lent, R. W., & Brown, S. D. (eds.), *Career Development and Counseling: Putting Theory and Research to Work,* 2nd ed. Hoboken, NJ: John Wiley, pp. 144–80.

Savickas, M. L., & Hartung, P. J. (2012). My career story: an autobiographical workbook for life-career success. www.vocopher.com/CSI/CCI_workbook.pdf.

Savickas, M. L., & Porfeli, E. J. (2012). Career adapt-abilities scale: construction, reliability, and measurement equivalence across 13 countries. *Journal of Vocational Behavior* 80: 661–73.

Seedat, M., Niekerk, A., Suffla, S., & Ratele, K. (2014). Psychological research and South Africa's violence prevention responses. *South African Journal of Psychology* 44: 136–44.

Sheldon, K. M., & Houser-Marko, L. (2001). Self-concordance, goal attainment, and the pursuit of happiness: can there be an upward spiral? *Journal of Personality and Social Psychology* 80: 152–65.

Sheu, H. B., & Lent, R. W. (2009). A social cognitive perspective on well-being in educational and work settings: cross-cultural considerations. *International Journal for Educational and Vocational Guidance* 9: 45–60. doi: 10.1007/a10775-008-9147-7

Snyder, C. R., & Lopez, S. J. (eds.) (2002). *The Handbook of Positive Psychology*. New York: Oxford University Press.

Stiglitz, J. E. (2012). *The Price of Inequality: How Today's Divided Society Endangers Our Future*. New York: Norton.

Tierney, P., & Farmer, S. M. (2002). Creative self-efficacy: its potential antecedents and relationship to creative performance. *Academy of Management Journal* 45: 1137–48.

Watts, R., Williams, N. C., & Jagers, R. J. (2003). Sociopolitical development. *American Journal of Community Psychology* 31(1/2): 185–94.

Wood, A. M., Linley, P. A., Maltby, J., Baliousis, M., & Joseph, S. (2008). The authentic personality: a theoretical and empirical conceptualization and the development of the Authenticity Scale. *Journal of Counseling Psychology* 55: 385–99.

Xanthopoulou, D., Bakker, A. B., Demerouti, E., & Schaufeli, W. B. (2012). A diary study on the happy worker: how job resources relate to positive emotions and personal resources. *European Journal of Work and Organizational Psychology* 21(4): 489–517. doi: 10.1080/1359432X.2011.584386

12 Family-Based Prevention

Efficacy, Effectiveness, and Widespread Implementation of Parenting Programs to Reduce Child Behavior Problems

Abigail H. Gewirtz & Adriana M. Youssef

Introduction

Early onset aggressive behavior and conduct problems are costly for children and for society. Psychological costs to children include social exclusion, impaired school performance, higher rates of psychopathology, and subsequently child welfare and juvenile justice system involvement, which incur high financial costs. The prevention and amelioration of conduct problems are of high priority to governments and health systems alike (e.g., Ogden, Forgatch, Askeland, Patterson, & Bullock, 2005). Moreover, effective prevention interventions to reduce child behavior problems have been developed and validated over the past four decades. The current challenge is to implement these programs effectively on a large scale in order to reduce the prevalence of conduct and behavior problems among children. In this chapter, we review evidence regarding effective prevention interventions to reduce child behavior problems by promoting positive parenting. We discuss key prevention programs and address efforts and challenges to bring these programs to large-scale implementation.

Developmental theories of the emergence, maintenance, and growth of conduct problems focus on negative and coercive social interactions occurring between parents and children as key predictors of subsequent child antisocial behavior. Gerald Patterson's (1982) coercion theory (later termed *social interaction learning theory*) provides a developmental approach to account for how parenting is associated with later child antisocial behavior. Patterson suggested that children learn antisocial behavior through multiple negative and coercive interactions with parents. Coercive interactions may be initiated either by children or by parents, but are characterized by escalating negative interactions, known as *conflict bouts* (Patterson, Reid, & Eddy, 2002). These bouts are typically terminated through positive or negative reinforcement of the aversive behaviors. For example, a parent whose child has refused to complete a task may escalate into shouting, which results in the child withdrawing from the conflict bout and completing the parent's bidding. Empirical data demonstrate that frequency, intensity, and length of coercive parent–child interactions are associated with multiple poor outcomes related to child antisocial behavior, including arrests, substance use, delinquency, and poor school performance (Reid, Patterson, & Snyder, 2002).

Coercive parenting is more likely when parents are stressed (e.g., undergoing family transitions such as divorce and repartnering, living in poverty) or are experiencing depression, antisocial behavior, and/or other psychopathology. Family stress models (e.g., Conger et al., 2002) document how stress impairs parenting, which, in turn, impairs child adjustment. Both social interaction learning (SIL) theory and family stress models propose that parenting *mediates* the impact of stressful environmental circumstances on children's externalizing behavior (Conger et al., 2002; Patterson, 2005). While family stress models provide a macro perspective, SIL documents the microsocial (moment-by-moment) parent–child interactions that influence child risk for psychopathology, as specified previously – that is, through conflict bouts.

A variety of parent training prevention interventions based on SIL theory and family stress models have been developed. These range from universal (for all) to selective (risk) to indicated (high-risk) prevention programs, and they have been tested with diverse family populations primarily across America, Europe, and Australia. Parent training models share the same theoretical premise but vary in the details of their approach. All models focus on the reduction of coercive parenting through the teaching of positive parenting strategies. These strategies typically include the use of positive reinforcement to teach children prosocial behaviors, mild contingent discipline to curb negative behaviors, monitoring and supervision of children's behaviors, problem solving, and positive engagement. Parent training prevention interventions have been widely tested in efficacy and effectiveness trials over the last thirty years, and some data also are available from large-scale implementation trials (Forgatch & DeGarmo, 2011; Shapiro, Prinz, & Sanders, 2012).

With randomized trial data that clearly demonstrate the effectiveness of parent training programs in improving parenting and reducing children's antisocial behavior, federal, state, and local governments are calling for the broad utilization of empirically validated, effective models of intervention for children and families (National Institute of Mental Health, 2008; Prinz & Sanders, 2007). Further, initiatives such as the Grand Challenges in Global Mental Health (Collins et al., 2011) have called for scaling up the delivery of evidence-based mental health interventions worldwide.

Although a growing number of child-serving systems (mental health, child welfare, schools) recognize the importance of serving families with evidence-based programs, few of these programs are actually adopted into routine care (United States Department of Health and Human Services, 2006). More frequently, community-based agencies delivering parenting programs provide "homegrown" programs without attention to their evaluation or claim that they are providing an evidence-based parent training program when, in fact, little attention is paid to fidelity. Without large-scale implementation of evidence-based programs, there will be little public health benefit from the billions of tax dollars spent to support stressed parents and their children.

Without doubt, deploying an evidence-based program on a large scale is challenging, in large part due to the lack of research focused on effective and efficient ways to *implement* evidence-based practices. Implementation research, as defined by Eccles and Mittman (2006, p. 2), is the "scientific study of methods to promote the systematic uptake of research findings and other evidence-based practices into routine practice, and, hence, to improve the quality and effectiveness of health services and care." In this chapter, we review a conceptual framework for implementation and then discuss the development, testing, and large-scale implementation outcomes from three well-validated parent training programs: the Parent Management Training-Oregon Model (PMTO); Positive Parenting Program (Triple P), and the Incredible Years (IY). Although a much larger number of parent training prevention programs are well validated, few other than these also have been implemented on a large-scale basis (in large numbers of municipalities, states, and countries beyond the development location). We review implementation data in an effort to highlight what is known, as well as the research that remains to be done in order for parent training programs to effectively reach large swathes of families.

A Conceptual Model for Implementation Research

This review is guided by the conceptual model of implementation research put forth by Proctor and colleagues (2009; see Figure 12.1). This model suggests that implementation efforts require input from both intervention and implementation strategies. Intervention strategies are those evidence-based practices that support the intervention's effectiveness. Implementation strategies are purposeful, specified, and systematic processes to adopt and integrate evidence-based practices into routine care (Fixsen, Naoom, Blasé, Friedman, & Wallace, 2005; Powell, Proctor, & Glass, 2014; Proctor et al., 2011). The model also draws attention to the various contextual levels at which implementation strategies can take place, including systems environment, organizational, group/learning, supervision, and individual providers/consumers.

Figure 12.1 shows three hierarchical and interrelated types of outcomes. The first, implementation outcomes (adoption, appropriateness, cost, feasibility, fidelity, penetration, and sustainability) result from a combination of intervention and implementation strategies. The second set of outcomes occurs at the service level and refer to efficiency, safety, and timeliness (Institute of Medicine, 2001). The third level, client outcomes, focuses on reduction in symptoms and improved functioning and quality of life. While intervention strategies are important for establishing efficacy and effectiveness, these alone will not provide a complete picture of how large-scale interventions are carried out successfully. Implementation strategies may impact all three types of outcomes.

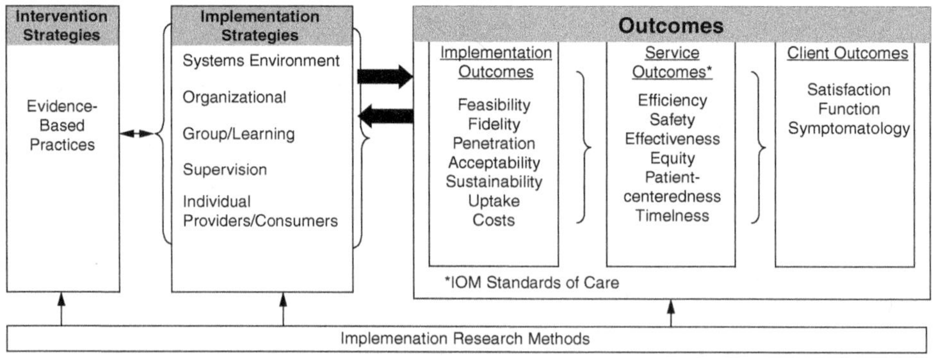

Figure 12.1. *Conceptual model of implementation research (Proctor et al., 2009; reprinted with permission).*

Thus, it becomes critical to better understand how implementation strategies impact implementation outcomes, as they may indicate intervention success, inform us on the process of implementation, and serve as key intermediate outcomes in relation to service- and client-level outcomes (Powell et al., 2014). We begin our review of parent training programs by reviewing intervention strategies and client outcomes from efficacy and effectiveness trials.

Empirically Supported Parent Training Models – Efficacy and Effectiveness Trials

Parent Management Training – Oregon Model (PMTO)

Developed by Marion Forgatch, Gerald Patterson, and their colleagues, PMTO is a principle-based intervention that provides parents with practice and support to implement five positive parenting practices, the putative mechanisms for improvement in child adjustment. PMTO can be delivered as treatment or prevention, in individual family or group format, in homes, clinics, schools, or community settings, for children from preschool through adolescence. The length of the intervention varies from fourteen weekly sessions in parent groups designed for prevention to four to nine months in individual family therapy.

Reflecting the SIL model upon which PMTO is based (Patterson, 1982, 2005), modification of the social environment is core to the intervention, and is reflected at multiple levels both in delivery and in broad implementation (e.g., training and coaching; Forgatch & Ogden, 2006). For example, foundational parenting skills include using contingent positive reinforcement to reward children for prosocial behaviors. Discipline is taught only after parents have mastered and are predominantly using skill encouragement. In parallel, facilitators teach parents encouragement skills by punctuating and reinforcing the positive actions parents accomplish. In implementation, a coach begins debriefing a trainee's videotaped therapy session by highlighting specifically what the facilitator has accomplished. Roleplay is used both to teach parents and to teach facilitators to strengthen delivery skills.

Efficacy trials. Experimental tests (i.e., randomized controlled trials) are excellent ways to test a theory of change. Replication of findings across populations and contexts provides evidence for generalizability. To test the SIL model, multiple randomized controlled trials of PMTO interventions have been executed. These studies have been conducted with a range of populations, aimed at children across developmental stages, and family contexts; for example, those in divorced and step-families, those exposed to a parent's military deployment, and those at risk for, or displaying conduct problems. (Dishion & Andrews, 1995; Forgatch & DeGarmo, 1999; Forgatch, DeGarmo, & Beldavs, 2005; Reid, Eddy, Fetrow, & Stoolmiller, 1999; Gewirtz, DeGarmo, & Zamir, 2016). (Bank, Marlowe, Reid, Patterson, & Weinrott, 1991; Chamberlain, 1999; Patterson, 1982; Patterson, Chamberlain, & Reid, 1982, Reid & Kavanagh, 1985). Chamberlain and colleagues developed an extension of PMTO known as Treatment Foster Care targeting youth removed from their homes, in which foster parents serving as the intervention agents. (Chamberlain, 2003). The intensity of intervention provided varies dependent on levels of indication or risk, but the core principles of the interventions remain the same.

Beyond testing the efficacy and effectiveness of prevention programs, randomized controlled trials (RCT) also can allow for an understanding of unfolding developmental processes within a theoretical model, demonstrating how the mechanisms result in positive outcomes. In such instances, it is crucial to assess processes and outcomes repeatedly with valid instruments and appropriate analytic procedures. An example of this is provided in a study conducted by Forgatch and colleagues with the Oregon Divorce Study, in which random assignment to PMTO or a no-treatment control was carried out with a sample of 238 recently separated mothers and their sons in grades K through 3 (e.g., Forgatch, Patterson, DeGarmo, & Beldavs, 2009; Patterson, Forgatch, & DeGarmo, 2010). Mothers participated in PMTO parent training groups; no intervention was provided to the youngsters. Assessments were conducted at six-month and then yearly intervals, with data available up to nine years following baseline.

Results of the RCT demonstrated prevention effects on both mother's parenting and child behavior, with some cascading effects on family outcomes. At thirty months after baseline, mothers in the intervention group reported reductions in their depression and increases in per capita annual income, as well as a rise out of poverty relative to the control group. Nine-year follow-up data using intent-to-treat (ITT) analyses revealed direct effects for children whose mothers were assigned to the PMTO group for both behavior and emotional adjustment: teacher-reported youth delinquency, deviant peer association, police arrest data, and youth-reported depression and substance use. At nine years, mothers in the intervention group had higher standard of living (i.e., education, occupation, income) and fewer police arrests.

The study also provided an understanding of the *processes* through which change takes place. The theoretical model – SIL – postulated that PMTO would yield positive distal outcomes by altering proximal mechanisms (i.e., the specified parenting practices). In turn, it was hypothesized that the parenting practices would mediate intervention effects on the outcomes. The findings did indeed support the model. In one study, reduced coercive and increased positive parenting – that is, less inept discipline and improved skill encouragement, problem solving, monitoring, and positive involvement – each explained significant variance in reduced child noncompliance. The surprise was that positive parenting was a more powerful predictor of change in child noncompliance than was coercive parenting (Martinez & Forgatch, 2001). Additional analysis using latent growth curve modeling, and longitudinal sequencing showed that both coercive parenting and positive parenting served as mediators for reduction in delinquency over the course of nine years. The first change was a reduction in coercive parenting from baseline to twelve months, which was followed by an increase in positive parenting from twelve to thirty months. Within the same analysis, the contribution of deviant peer association was evaluated as a mediator. The analysis examined intervention effects on reduction in deviant peer association from baseline to eight years. That reduction had a significant and independent effect on delinquency growth (Forgatch et al., 2009).

As noted earlier, data gathered in PMTO trials are multiple-method and multi-informant. Key measures of parenting are gathered using observational data (videotaped family interaction tasks) that include standardized problem solving and teaching tasks, coded by trained and reliable observational coders (e.g., see Gewirtz, DeGarmo, Plowman, August, & Realmuto, 2009). Informants typically include parents, teachers, and youth themselves, with latent growth curve modeling allowing for the creation of latent factors that combine parent, teacher, and child report of adjustment or deviant peer behavior, for example. Broadband measures of child adjustment are used to assess child outcome (for example, the Behavior Assessment Scale for Children (BASC-2; Reynolds & Kamphaus, 2006).

Positive Parenting Program (Triple P)

The Positive Parenting Program, most commonly referred to as Triple P (Sanders, 1999), provides a tiered system of behavioral parent training, using a population-based public health approach to improving parenting and reducing child behavior problems. In contrast to PMTO, which is based on SIL and coercion theory (i.e., a combination of social learning and social interactional perspectives; see Patterson, 2005), Triple P's theoretical basis is in social learning theory. In addition, PMTO data rely on multimethod, multi-informant data, and in particular observational data to examine parent–child interactions, while Triple P typically relies on parent-report data. Triple P programs are provided at five levels of intensity, from universal (Level 1) to indicated (Level 5). Level 1 uses mass media, print, and electronic media to disseminate positive parenting messages to entire communities. Levels 2 and 3 provide brief selected prevention programs with one to four sessions of twenty to ninety minutes in a group or individual format, in a variety of settings including primary care (Level 3; Sanders, 2012). Level 4 (originally known as Standard Triple P) provides programming for parents of children with behavior problems in eight to ten sessions in various formats, including individual, group (plus individual phone sessions), and online.

Empirical evidence for Triple P has been gathered via multiple studies of different programs and levels of the system (Sanders, 1999, 2012; Sanders, Dittman, Farrugia, Keown, 2014a; Sanders, Kirby, Tellegen, & Day, 2014b). Triple P's Level 4 has the most empirical support via randomized trials comparing different levels of intensity of the intervention (Sanders, Markie-Dadds, Tully, & Bor, 2000), as well as different formats of the program (Sanders et al., 2014a). Triple P also is quite unique among parent training programs in that it has data demonstrating effectiveness of the program in producing population-level reductions in child maltreatment (Prinz, Sanders, Shapiro, Whitaker, & Lutzker, 2009). The U.S. Triple P Population Trial assigned eighteen counties in South Carolina to Triple P or services as usual. All counties had comparable rates of child maltreatment reports prior to the trial. Counties assigned to the Triple P program received mass media messages directed to parents, training for child welfare workers, and group-based Triple P. At posttest (two years later), counties assigned to Triple P demonstrated significantly lower rates of substantiated child maltreatment reports, out-of-home placements, and emergency-room visits for child abuse injuries than counties randomly assigned to the control group. Effect sizes were in the large to very large range (Prinz et al., 2009).

Several meta-analyses have evaluated data on the Triple P system. Four papers published between 2007 and 2008 concluded that Triple P produced reductions in child behavior problems, especially in younger children (de Graaf Speetjens, Smit, de Wolff, & Tavecchio, 2008; Nowak & Heinrichs, 2008; Thomas & Zimmer-Gembeck, 2007). More recently, Wilson et al. (2012) conducted a meta-analysis of thirty-three randomized controlled trials of Triple P, reporting medium effect sizes for differences between experimental and control groups in mothers' reports of reductions in child behavior problems from baseline to posttreatment, but no differences in fathers' reports. Methodological concerns were raised, including the dearth of evidence for longer-term effects of the Triple P program. Coyne and Kwakkenbos (2013), in a related article, raised concerns regarding evaluations of Triple P that rely on small and underpowered sample sizes.

In response, Sanders et al. (2014a) reported meta-analytic findings from all 101 published Triple P studies (both experimental and nonexperimental) from 1980 to 2013. The authors reported significantly reduced child social, emotional, and behavior problems with a medium effect size at posttest and up to thirty-six months post baseline.

The Incredible Years (IY)

Developed by Carolyn Webster-Stratton, the Incredible Years Parent Training (IY) program was originally developed as a universal prevention program to improve parenting in mothers of two- to seven-year-old children (Webster-Stratton, 1981). Based on social learning theory (e.g. Bandura, 1971) and using videotape modeling, the program aims to improve parent–child bonding, decrease coercive discipline, and improve problem-solving capacity (Webster-Stratton & Reid, 2003). Since its inception, the program has expanded to four programs targeting infants, toddlers, preschoolers, and school-aged children from six to thirteen years of age. The program currently includes both BASIC and ADVANCE components for parents, and teachers; ADVANCE is completed after BASIC and is a targeted program aimed at parents whose behaviors may place their children at risk for poor adjustment outcomes (Webster-Stratton & Reid, 2003).

The IY BASIC program, for which the most efficacy and effectiveness data are available, is a group-based, 9 to 20-week long, two hours per week program. The shorter groups target parents of infants; longer groups target parents of toddlers and preschoolers. Groups center around the use of video clips that model effective parenting skills such as setting up routines, using praise and incentives, and problem-solving. The video clips are designed to foster discussion, and facilitators use role play and rehearsal to help parents master and consolidate skills (Webster-Stratton & Reid, 2003).

Randomized trials of IY have demonstrated the program to result in improved parenting practices and decreased children's problem behaviors among a range of populations, including maltreating and foster families (Linares, Montalto, Li, & Oza, 2006), those enrolled in Head Start (Hurlburt, Nguyen, Reid, Webster-Stratton, & Zhang, 2013; Webster-Stratton, 1998), and parents of children with developmental delays (McIntyre, 2008) and ADHD (Webster-Stratton, Reid, & Beauchaine, 2013). As with Triple P, and unlike PMTO, which uses observational measures, IY studies have typically used the Eyberg Child Behavior Inventory (ECBI; Eyberg, 1999), a parent-report measure of child behavior outcomes.

A recent meta-analysis of IY that included fifty outcome studies published over a thirty-year period showed that IY was effective in preventing and treating child behavior problems (i.e., disruptive, aggressive, and/or noncompliant behaviors; Menting, Orobio de Castro, & Matthys, 2013). Overall, small effect sizes were evident for prevention programs, and medium effect sizes for treatment studies, using parent report of child problems as the outcome. Children reported as having more severe problems showed greater improvements. Longer-term follow up studies of IY have demonstrated program gains maintained for as long as three years after BASIC (Jones, Daley, Hutchings, Bywater, & Eames, 2008) and twelve years after ADVANCE programs (Webster-Stratton, Rinaldi, & Reid, 2011). Data from a recent randomized trial in the Netherlands with 144 families demonstrated improvements favoring the intervention group in observed and parent reports of parenting practices, and reductions in observed children's problem behavior (Posthumus, Raaijmakers, Maassen, Van Engeland, & Matthys, 2012).

In sum, robust evaluation data from a wide range of randomized trials suggest that PMTO, Triple P, and IY have strong evidence for improving client outcomes in intervention studies. We now review research on five specific *implementation* outcomes of these parent training programs: adoption, penetration, acceptability, fidelity, and cost.

Adoption

Adoption is defined by Proctor and colleagues (2011, p. 89) as "the intention, initial decision, or action to try and employ an intervention." Research in this area of implementation science may examine the approach used to adopt an intervention or those factors that influence adoption such as cost or perceptions of acceptability. In the following section, we focus on the process of how parent training programs are adopted, as this may influence how staff perceives the program and how often and well they implement it.

Research on intervention approaches to adoption has been examined in Triple P. In a study done in Ontario, Canada, of sixty-nine different agencies using Triple P, it was explored whether adoption of the program was initiated via "top-down" (e.g., government funders decide whether an agency will deliver an evidence-based program) or "bottom-up" (e.g., an agency identifies a problem and adopts a program of its choice) approaches (Asgary-Eden & Lee, 2011). It was found that the majority of agencies (67 percent) adopted Triple P from the bottom up, whereas only 25 percent reported a top-down initiative where a government funder selected Triple P. Whether the agency utilized a top-down or bottom-up approach was unrelated to other factors associated with decisions to adopt an evidence-based practice, such as the agencies' readiness for implementation, openness to new ideas, resistance to adoption, and program usage once trained (Asgary-Eden & Lee, 2011).

Although empirical data on adoption initiatives are lacking in PMTO and IY, it has been reported that several wide-scale implementation efforts have utilized top-down approaches. In PMTO, for example, top-down approaches have been reported for implementation efforts in Norway (Ogden et al., 2005), Mexico (Baumann, Domenech Rodríguez, Amador, Forgatch, & Parra-Cardona, 2014), and Michigan and Kansas in the United States (Forgatch, Patterson, & Gewirtz, 2013). In IY, top-down approaches have also been described for efforts in Portugal (Webster-Stratton, Gaspar, & Seabra-Santos, 2012), the United Kingdom (eg,. Hutchings et al., 2007), and Wales (Department for Training and Education in Wales, 2005).

The process of adoption has the potential not only to impact practitioners and other stakeholders, but perhaps also to influence client outcomes. For example, Romney, Israel, and Zlatevski (2014) examined how community-based agencies' use of a structured site readiness process affected parent graduation rates in Triple P levels 4 and 5. This process involved using a worksheet to educate agencies about Triple P and the requirements necessary for implementation so that thoughtful consideration about feasibility could take place before adoption. Agencies then met with implementation staff to ask questions, problem-solve concerns, and discuss budget. Results suggest that agencies who used the readiness process had parents who were 12.2 times more likely to graduate from the program than parents from agencies who did not use the process. This finding persisted even after accounting for parent-level factors that could impact graduation, such as socioeconomic status, history of child protective services involvement, and parental stress. Additionally, the readiness process proved to save money: the cost-per-graduate was seven times higher in the agencies that did not use the readiness process compared to those that did (Romney et al., 2014). Agencies in this study were not randomized, thus future RCT studies with larger sample sizes are needed to replicate these findings. Nonetheless, this study highlights how implementation strategies for adoption employed at the agency level can impact implementation outcomes (cost) and client outcomes (retention).

In summary, adoption approaches for single-agency implementation are likely to involve both bottom-up and top-down approaches to initiate the process. Though not studied empirically, large-scale implementation efforts of PMTO, IY, and Triple P have been described in the literature using more top-down approaches. Top-level leaders must engage and generate support from all levels of a community in order to create "buy-in" for an evidence-based intervention to be adopted; how this is achieved and sustained is a question for future research (Forgatch et al. 2013). Additionally, although we have qualitative accounts of how parent training programs are adopted on a large scale, there is no empirical evidence that examines the factors associated with adoption such as stakeholders' attitudes on the acceptability, appropriateness, feasibility, and fidelity monitoring process of an evidence-based practice (Aarons, Cafri, Lugo, & Sawitzky, 2012).

Penetration

Penetration has been defined as the integration of an intervention into a service system and its subsystems (Proctor et al., 2011) and is similar to the concept of "reach." Research on Triple P has examined the concept of penetration as it relates to the number of practitioners trained relative to the number of practitioners who then go on to use Triple P with families. This line of investigation is critical to understanding how large numbers of families are exposed to an intervention. By better understanding those factors impacting the percentage of practitioners who complete training and subsequently go on to deliver an intervention, we can learn how to best support the cost-effective goals of implementation efforts.

In the United States and other countries, practitioners who start the training process in PMTO, Triple P, and IY often complete it. For example, across three PMTO "generations," 73 percent of Icelandic and 92 percent of Norwegian providers completed the training and certification process (Sigmarsdóttir & Gudmundsdóttir, 2013). In the previously mentioned population-level study of Triple P in the United States, about 83 percent of providers trained became accredited in Triple P (Sanders, Prinz, & Shapiro, 2009; Seng, Prinz, & Sanders, 2006). Seng and colleagues (2006) reported that practitioners from diverse backgrounds and settings, with varying levels of previous training, experience, self-efficacy, and confidence, were equally likely to complete Triple P training. Practitioners who did not complete training reported significantly more barriers to program use than practitioners who were completers. The barriers identified were associated with workplace characteristics (e.g., difficulty integrating Triple P into caseload, lack of recognition of Triple P work, and insufficient provision of supervision), issues of program/provider fit (e.g., perceptions of training as being inadequate and materials being unavailable), and problems in practitioners' program management (e.g., difficulty in coordinating with other practitioners involved with the family, difficulty covering scheduled material in the scheduled amount of time). Taken together, the research suggests that despite some barriers, high numbers of trainees complete training, which may contribute to better implementation fidelity and increase the chance that the population will see a return on training investment.

Though the completion of training is important, once trained to certification, a practitioner's program use is not assured. Other factors may impact practitioners' initiating and sustaining program use (Aarons & Palinkas, 2007; Glisson et al., 2008; Seng et al, 2006). Research on Triple P has examined factors at the organizational, practitioner, and client level that may impact penetration in terms of how often practitioners utilize Triple P with families once they are trained to accreditation. In the Triple P U.S. population study, practitioners could select the level of Triple P at which they wished to be trained. Six months after training, their usage of Triple P with families was examined. Approximately 63 percent had implemented the program with at least one family, 58 percent had used it with two or more families, and 37 percent had not used the intervention at all. Immediately after training, provider knowledge, skill, and self-confidence were associated with Triple P usage (Shapiro et al., 2012). Six months following training, high program delivery was associated with being trained in Level 4 Group Triple P (compared to practitioners trained at other levels), incorporating Triple P knowledge and skills into general workflow, and consulting with other Triple P practitioners (Sanders et al., 2009). Practitioner-level factors associated with low program use 6 months following training included having a different theoretical orientation or approach which clashed with Triple P principles, having low confidence in parent consultation work, experiencing difficulty incorporating Triple P into everyday job activities, and lacking knowledge in behavioral family intervention (Sanders et al., 2009). Sustained use of Triple P two to three years following training has been related to practitioners' perceived self-efficacy (Shapiro et al., 2014).

In terms of client characteristics, practitioners were more likely to use Triple P six months following training when they encountered clients whose presenting problems were appropriate for the intervention that they were trained to deliver and when they received positive parent feedback regarding the program, (Sanders et al., 2009). Qualitative data suggest that sustained use of Triple P two to three years following training may be related to practitioners' early experiences of success with the program and the positive impact it has on families (Shapiro et al., 2014). Practitioners who continue using the program for long periods experience success with a wide range of clients who are typically perceived as being difficult to reach, such as teen parents, parents with cognitive delays, and parents in the social service system (Shapiro et al., 2014). Using qualitative data on practitioners' perspectives of implementation of Triple P in Canada, Breitkreuz, McConnell, Savage, and Hamilton (2011) found that impact of Triple P on families was a theme related to program usage. Thus, these "wins" with clients and positive impact with parents appear to be important factors influencing practitioners' initial and sustained use of Triple P.

At the organizational level, factors associated with low program use six months following training were practitioner-reported lack of access to consultation or supervision, lack of overtime for after-hours appointments, clash with after-hours appointments, lack of recognition by colleagues for Triple P work, and difficulty coordinating with other service providers working with the family (Sanders et al., 2009). Additionally, across practitioner and organization levels, Turner, Nicholson, and Sanders (2011) found that for primary care practitioners, workplace barriers and supports were significantly associated with practitioner self-efficacy; self-efficacy, in turn, predicted Triple P usage with parents six months following training. One workplace support that may be particularly important is the provision of peer support. In a study of Triple P practitioners from fifteen different countries, those that found peer support (e.g., to rehearse skills and for supervision) to be particularly helpful were more likely to deliver Triple P to families a month after training (Turner, Sanders, & Hodge, 2014).

In summary, the completion of Triple P training seems to have less to do with individual provider characteristics and more to do with larger agency-level barriers and support systems. Research is needed investigating whether these same associations are present in PMTO and IY contexts. Once trained, predictors of practitioner intervention usage are complex, likely involving multiple factors at various levels (e.g., client/provider/organization; Beidas & Kendall, 2010). Research is needed to examine how these factors interact to predict initial and sustained usage. Future research also is needed to investigate how penetration outcomes moderate client outcomes.

Acceptability and Appropriateness

Acceptability is the perception that a given intervention is satisfactory or agreeable. Features of an intervention that may be acceptable include, but are not limited to, its content, complexity, format, and modes of delivery. A conceptually similar implementation outcome is that of appropriateness, which refers to the perceived relevance, fit, or compatibility of an intervention for a targeted setting, provider, or consumer. Because these constructs often overlap and are not consistently used in research, the term *acceptability* will be used to refer to studies that have looked at aspects of both acceptability and appropriateness.

Acceptability in parent programs has been most commonly studied at the level of clients. This has allowed researchers a better understanding of how to adapt interventions for new target populations. In general, parents from diverse ethnic backgrounds, cultures, and contexts have found these parent training programs to be acceptable, as measured by self-report satisfaction ratings looking at variables such as program usefulness, cultural appropriateness, and satisfaction with staff. For example, Triple P has been found to be acceptable to Japanese parents living in Australia (Matsumoto, Sofronoff, & Sanders, 2007) as well as Japanese parents living in Tokyo (Matsumoto, Sofronoff, & Sanders, 2010). Panamanian parents have found Triple P to be relevant and culturally acceptable (Mejia, Calam, & Sanders, 2014b). Parents utilizing IY in Portugal have found the program to be satisfactory (Seabra-Santos, Gaspar, Azevedo, Homem, & Pimentel, 2011), as well as Maori and non-Maori parents in New Zealand (Fergusson, Stanley, & Horwood, 2009). Low-income Hispanic, Asian, African American, and Caucasian parents alike have found the IY program to be acceptable (Reid, Webster-Stratton, & Beauchaine, 2001), as well as economically disadvantaged parents in New York's child welfare system, with room for improvement in group leaders' cultural competence (Marcynyszyn, Maher, & Corwin, 2011). Cultural adaptations made to PMTO for use with Spanish-speaking Latino families living within the United States and for Muslim immigrants from Pakistan and Somalia living in Norway have been found to be acceptable (Bjørknes & Manger, 2013; Martinez & Eddy, 2005; Parra-Cardona et al., 2012). PMTO also was found to be highly acceptable to women residing in a battered women's shelter (Gewirtz & Taylor, 2009). Additionally, a modified version of PMTO for use with families in the U.S. military was found to be highly satisfactory by parents in the National Guard and Reserve (Gewirtz, Pinna, Hanson, & Brockberg, 2014).

Compared to available data on parents' satisfaction of these programs, relatively less is known regarding perceptions of acceptability of other stakeholders who are involved in the implementation process. How practitioners perceive programs may be particularly relevant as they are often regarded as "gatekeepers" of an intervention and have influence on the adoption, penetration, and sustainability of programs. However, little is known regarding how practitioners, particularly those from various cultures, perceive parenting training programs. In a low resource setting in Panama (Mejia et al., 2014a), 97 percent of school-based practitioners responded that they would encourage a family to participate in a program like Triple P and 100 percent felt that a parenting program was needed in their community. Practitioners rated the program as being acceptable and useful, with some specific strategies being more acceptable than others. For example, strategies for developing a positive relationship were rated higher in acceptability than strategies for encouraging positive behavior and managing difficult behavior (Mejia et al., 2014a). Health care practitioners in Australia also rated Triple P as being highly acceptable and useful for a culturally diverse population, with higher preference for individual sessions with a therapist and less preference for online self-directed formats of Triple P (Morawska, Sanders, O'Brien, McAuliffe, & Anderson, 2012). Although these studies illustrate how therapists from different cultures view these programs, we still need a better understanding of how cultural views of mental health, parenting, and child behavior influence how practitioners perceive these parent training programs.

The wide-scale implementation of parent training programs necessitates an examination of how parents from diverse cultures and contexts perceive these programs in terms of acceptability and appropriateness. These data will help inform the development of adaptations of these programs for targeted populations. However, the research must move beyond the client level and examine acceptability at the practitioner, supervisor, agency, and government-stakeholder level, because top-down support for an intervention has the potential to influence how resources are allocated and the overall penetration and sustainability of an intervention. Additionally, as stakeholders gain more experience with an intervention over time, this may impact their perceptions of the acceptability of the program; thus, longitudinal studies are needed that measure the factors that are related to sustained satisfaction with an intervention. As parent training programs gear up for wide-scale implementation, agencies will be encouraged to engage in novel implementation strategies, such as fidelity monitoring, peer and group consultation, outcome measurement, as well a new technologies (e.g., online tools) to support implementation and program delivery. Thus, it will be critical to examine stakeholders' perceptions of acceptability and appropriateness of these methods to better understand how interventions are implemented successfully.

Implementation Fidelity

Much attention in implementation research has focused on the development of clear and feasible strategies for measuring implementation fidelity (Lee et al., 2008; Mihalic, Fagan, & Argamaso, 2008) – the degree to which an intervention is delivered as intended by the developers. The assessment of fidelity is critical in understanding how and why an intervention works. Fidelity can act as a potential moderator of the relationship between interventions and their intended outcomes (Mihalic, 2004) and can also contribute to the internal and external validity of an intervention, as well as the statistical power of a study. Fidelity may be operationalized as adherence to the intervention protocol, coverage of core components, dose (frequency and duration), and/or quality of delivery (Dane & Schneider, 1998; Mihalic, 2004; Waltz, Addis, Koerner, & Jacobson, 1993). Research on implementation fidelity in PMTO, Triple P, and IY is beginning to uncover how these programs use implementation strategies to facilitate high fidelity and its maintenance over time in various settings and cultures, and the clinical implications of high fidelity in terms of improvements in parenting and reductions in child problem behaviors. The following section will first review the fidelity measurement tools that have been developed for use in PMTO, IY, and Triple P. Next, implementation strategies to enhance fidelity in these parent programs will be discussed.

PMTO utilizes an observer-rated Fidelity of Implementation Rating Scale (FIMP; Knutson, Forgatch, Rains, & Sigmarsdóttir, 2009) to measure fidelity in the areas of adherence to the intervention protocol and competence of program delivery. Because PMTO is strongly theory-based, the guiding principle of the FIMP is that fidelity can be achieved if the core components are skillfully taught with competent clinical and teaching processes in a manner that brings about change. Employing observational methodology to assess fidelity, the FIMP manual details procedures for scoring five skill dimensions: *knowledge* – demonstrated understanding of PMTO content and theoretical principles; *structure* – demonstrated skill in balancing several activities at once including leading without dominating, following an agenda, and using sensitive timing and pacing; *teaching* – how information is imparted to promote parents' mastery and independent use of PMTO skills; *process skills* – demonstrated skill in providing support to create a safe and supportive context; and *overall development* – the family's apparent satisfaction with the intervention and growth in knowledge of PMTO components and the likelihood that parents will continue participating in the intervention and will use the skills at home. The predictive validity of the FIMP establishes the relationship between fidelity and program outcomes. In an RCT evaluating a PMTO program for stepfamilies, high FIMP ratings predicted change in observed parenting practices for mothers and stepfathers at twelve months. Fidelity accounted for 30 percent of the variance in mother and stepfather parenting (Forgatch, Patterson, & DeGarmo, 2005). In a larger-scale setting – a nationwide implementation of PMTO conducted in Norway – FIMP ratings predicted improvements in observed effective parenting practices for mothers and fathers from pre- to posttreatment (Forgatch & DeGarmo, 2011). Thus, higher fidelity as measured by the FIMP is predictive of improvements in parenting.

Fidelity in IY has been assessed in various ways. The developer of IY created the Leader Session Checklist, a practitioner-report measure of adherence, and the Leader Rating Scale, a measure of quality of delivery in the areas of *group process skills* (e.g., creating a safe, accepting atmosphere), *leadership skills* (e.g., structuring an agenda), *relationship-building skills* (e.g., normalizing problems), *leader's knowledge* (e.g., developmentally appropriate behavior) and *teaching methods* (e.g., using videotape modeling and roleplay), and *parents' responses* (Webster-Stratton, 2004). The Leader Rating Scale may be completed by a peer, supervisor, or IY consultant or mentor. Research is needed examining the validity of these two fidelity measures. Another measure called the Leader Observation Tool (LOT) has been developed to assess implementation fidelity in IY using observational methodology (Eames et al., 2008). The LOT measures clinical process skills used in delivering the program, in the domains of *listening, empathy, physical encouragement*, and *positive behavior,* as well as negative behaviors. An IY study of fidelity conducted in Wales with parents of preschool-age children at risk for developing conduct disorder (Eames et al., 2008, 2009; Hutchings et al., 2007) demonstrated that LOT scores for each process domain were associated with greater changes in observed positive parenting, with effects sizes ranging from 0.29 to 0.35 (Eames et al., 2009). In turn, changes in both observed positive parenting and parent-reported change in parenting style predicted positive child outcomes (Eames et al., 2009). Two key LOT process skills – praising parents and using reflective behaviors (e.g., comments and questions) – predicted observed changes in parents use of praise and reflective behaviors with their children (Eames et al., 2010). Other tools to measure fidelity in IY include Scott, Carby, and Rendu's (2008) measure of therapist skill (e.g., in teaching, encouraging parent participation, and highlighting the positives) and level of organization (e.g., having materials ready, making practical arrangements for smooth flow of content delivery). Scott and colleagues reported that group therapist skill significantly predicted posttreatment antisocial behavior, controlling for pretreatment behavior, therapist organization, and quality of alliance with the parents. Thus, fidelity measurement tools for IY suggest that therapist competence and quality of delivery are associated with improvements in parenting.

There are currently no validated fidelity measures for Triple P. To measure adherence, researchers have used session-specific checklists provided by Triple P manuals and completed by practitioners (Asgary-Eden & Lee, 2011; Taylor, Asgary-Eden, Lee, & LaRoche, 2015). To further explore adherence, Taylor and colleagues (2015) coded the checklists into the following activities: *process* – activities to set the organization or flow of the session; *homework* – activities to promote practicing the skills outside of sessions; *Triple P therapeutic interventions* – activities that form the curriculum of positive parenting; and *exercises* – activities to engage parents in relating the material to their own family. The relationship between these adherence categories and program outcomes has yet to be explored; therefore, the predictive validity of this fidelity measurement tool is unknown. Taylor and colleagues examined fidelity at the practitioner level and found that 63 percent of practitioners reported less than 100 percent adherence to the checklist. Adherence was highest for process activities and exercises and relatively lower for homework and therapeutic interventions. Practitioners' years of experience providing parenting training interventions was related to greater adherence in the areas of process activities and exercises

(Taylor et al., 2015). The most common reasons for general nonadherence were time constraints, perceived inappropriateness for particular parents, and forgetting content (Asgary-Eden & Lee, 2011).

Applying Proctor and colleagues' (2009; Figure 12.1) model of implementation research, several studies have examined implementation strategies at the supervision and group/learning levels in investigating the impact of training on fidelity. The training process for PMTO, Triple P, and IY employs implementation strategies that aim to improve practitioner fidelity. For example, training processes for these programs involve multiple days of intensive workshop training, modeling of key components, video and trainer roleplays, simulation practice with peers, and expert feedback and consultation. Trainees complete an accreditation or certification process and are evaluated on competency of delivery, with expert feedback provided. Details on the training process for Triple P (Sanders, Cann, & Markie-Dadds, 2003a; Shapiro et al., 2008; Turner & Sanders, 2006), PMTO (Knutson et al., 2009), and IY (Webster-Stratton & Herman, 2010) can be found elsewhere. Because training for these programs is intensive and costly (some training-to-certification processes can last up to eighteen months or more), it is important to examine the association of training and fidelity. Research on Triple P has suggested that practitioners who complete the training series report an increase in self-efficacy in consultation tasks such as conducting behavioural rehearsals with parents (Sanders, 2008; Sanders, Tully, Turner, Maher, & McAuliffe, 2003c; Sanders, Murphy-Brennan, & McAuliffe, 2003b). Behavioral observation data also suggest that training is associated with improved parent consultation skills (Sanders et al., 2003c). Forgatch and DeGarmo (2011) assessed fidelity to PMTO using FIMP scores at three time points in the training process (early, mid, and end), finding improvements as well as less variability in skills by the completion of the training program. Moreover, an examination of fidelity over three generations of practitioners in Norway (the first trained by the developers, the second and third trained by the first generation) found no decay in fidelity as training continued across generations (Forgatch & DeGarmo, 2011; Sigmarsdóttir & Guðmundsdóttir, 2013).

Qualitative research on IY suggests that effective supervision and training are critical aspects of achieving and maintaining fidelity (Stern, Alaggia, Watson, & Morton, 2008). More recently, quantitative IY research has examined components of training associated with changes in fidelity. In an RCT with practitioners in a community mental health setting, practitioners received either a three-day workshop or an enhanced training model (the workshop plus weekly coaching phone calls) and consultation for practitioners and agency supervisors. The enhanced model was associated with improved fidelity in the domains of offering practical support, having a collaborative approach, showing knowledge of content, and using skills in mediating discussions on vignettes (Webster-Stratton, Reid, & Marsenich, 2014). This is promising considering that therapists may have difficulty adhering to the use of vignettes when they perceive them to be inappropriate for parents' needs (Stern et al., 2008).

The RCT also revealed no differences in leadership, the building of positive relationships with parents, home activities review, and the use of roleplays (Webster-Stratton et al., 2014). This last finding is significant because the use of roleplay may greatly contribute to a parent's learning of a skill (e.g., Forgatch, Bullock, Patterson, & Steiner, 2004); however, practitioners may not adhere to using roleplay due to their own discomfort with this method (Stern et al., 2008; Webster-Stratton, 2004).

It becomes difficult to draw conclusions on the factors that promote fidelity in parent training programs because Triple P, IY, and PMTO each measure different components of fidelity. Even when they examine similar themes, such as therapists' skill and quality of delivery, each measurement system has a different way of defining these variables. Research on Triple P suggests that practitioner experience with parent interventions is related to adherence. PMTO and IY have provided evidence that training is positively associated with improvements in fidelity (we could find no published data regarding Triple P); however, little is known about what constitutes "core components" of training to ensure high adherence and quality. Quality supervision and ongoing organizational support appear to be critical to establishing high fidelity, though research is still needed to understand how much and how often. Furthermore, research is needed investigating those factors that support and maintain high fidelity after certification within a setting over time.

Other than supervision and training, there is little research on agency- and policy-level factors impacting fidelity in parent training programs. One example of this is research done by Asgary-Eden and Lee (2011), who examined how the adoption of Triple P (a government-funded top-down approach or practitioner-led bottom-up approach) was related to practitioner adherence to session protocol. More research such as this is needed to examine how contextual factors impact how practitioners implement interventions.

Research also is needed into how to make fidelity assessment feasible for implementation in "real-world" settings. Observational assessment remains the "gold standard" for measuring fidelity (Dusenbury, Brannigan, Falco, & Hansen, 2003; Mihalic et al., 2008) and is most often used in clinical trials. However, the training to become reliable to assess fidelity and the process of collecting, scoring, and reviewing therapy sessions can be costly and labor intensive. There are recommendations for strategies available to help administrators promote and maintain fidelity (e.g., Mazzucchelli & Sanders, 2010) and even low-cost questionnaires that administrators can use to assess program delivery (e.g., Webster-Stratton, 2006). Though these strategies use research to inform their use, quantitative data are needed to support specific recommendations for use with certain parent training programs, populations, and contexts. Cost-benefit data are needed to inform budget- and time-efficient ways to assess fidelity (Schoenwald et al., 2011). It has also been argued that videotaping sessions and coding practitioner–client interactions may promote adherence at the cost of increasing therapists' perceptions that the intervention requires rigid delivery without the flexibility to respond to individual clients' needs (Sanders & Kirby, 2014). This may stifle practitioners' sense of work autonomy, though the research has shown that fidelity monitoring may benefit agencies, such as by contributing to greater staff retention (Aarons, Sommerfeld, Hecht, Silovsky, & Chaffin, 2009). Future research is needed examining how fidelity monitoring may change the organizational climate and impact various stakeholders.

Cost of Implementation

The analysis of implementation cost is crucial for decisions about intervention adoption and allocating scarce resources to prevention programs. The published research on implementation cost for IY and Triple P is scant, and none is available on PMTO other than general cost information on sites such as Blueprints for Healthy Youth Development (Mihalic, n.d.). Currently, cost studies for parent training programs focus more on calculating cost-effectiveness and cost-benefit analysis on intervention strategies with little emphasis on the cost of implementation strategies.

Cost-effectiveness studies compare intervention delivery costs with parent and child outcomes. Studies done in various countries have found that parenting training programs are typically cost-effective. For example, the IY parenting program implemented in Ireland and the United Kingdom has been found to be cost-effective in reducing child conduct problems (Edwards, O'Ceilleachair, Bywater, Hughes, & Hutchings, 2007; Furlong et al., 2012; O'Neill, McGilloway, Donnelly, Bywater, & Kelly, 2013).

There is growing interest from government policy makers to invest in high-quality early interventions that will produce short- and long-term economic returns. Cost-benefit analysis can be calculated by estimating the costs of a problem on society and comparing this value to intervention costs. The IY program implemented in community programs in Ireland was found to have an estimated rate of return of 11 percent when considering the long-term cost of child conduct problems on key outcomes (crime, unemployment, and education) in adulthood (O'Neill et al., 2013). When considering similar long-term outcomes of conduct disorder until age twenty-eight in Australia, the delivery of Triple P on a large scale would need to avert less than 1.5 percent of cases of conduct disorder to pay for itself. Delivering the intervention on a population-wide basis was considered cost-effective until the prevalence rate of conduct disorder reductions fell below 7 percent, in which case there would be a positive cost associated with the intervention (Mihalopoulos, Sanders, Turner, Murphy-Brennan, & Carter, 2007). It has also been estimated that the cost associated with the delivery of Triple P on a populationwide level in the United States could be recovered in one year by a 10 percent reduction in rates of child abuse and neglect (Aos et al., 2011; Foster, Prinz, Sanders, & Shapiro, 2008). Though these studies are based on estimates and further research is needed to confirm these findings, they suggest that these parent training programs have the potential to save more than they cost and may provide a favorable rate of return in the long run.

There are fewer published studies examining the cost of implementation strategies. The cost-effectiveness of providing a site readiness process during the exploration phase of Triple P implementation has been explored (Romney et al., 2014). Research on Triple P has also estimated the cost of training practitioners to provide the program on a population level (Foster et al., 2008). This research may aid stakeholders as they consider adopting a program. IY research has elucidated how implementation costs can differ based on having newly trained leaders versus the recurrent cost of delivery with trained leaders and materials already paid for (Charles, Edwards, Bywater, & Hutchings, 2013). This line of research may help agencies estimate the costs of sustaining programs over the long term.

Parent Training Prevention Programs in the Twenty-first Century: Challenges and Opportunities for Implementation Research

Despite the burgeoning of an evidence base for parent training programs over the past three decades, the promise of their widespread implementation and corresponding decreases in the prevalence of childhood behavior problems remains elusive. Implementation is costly both in time and money, and implementation research is in its infancy. Nonetheless, the preceding data reviewed provide important clues regarding cost, penetration, and fidelity as implementation outcomes for parent training programs. As implementation science advances, its research and methodology will become more sophisticated (e.g., Crowley, Coffman, Greenberg, Feinberg, & Spoth, 2014). For example, longitudinal studies that concurrently examine fidelity, cost, and penetration at multiple time points are needed in order to help implementing organizations plan, forecast, and sustain evidence-based parent training programs.

While this review focused on the associations of implementation strategies and implementation outcomes, there is a growing literature on – and need to understand – the association of *intervention* strategies and implementation outcomes. For example, what components, sequence, or formats of parent training prevention programs result in the greatest acceptability or penetration? Does the personalization of interventions for families' needs or preferences (e.g., He, Gewirtz, Lee, August, & Morrell, 2015) lead to their greater penetration?

While randomized trials are now the sine qua non of intervention testing, there are very few data from RCTs examining implementation strategies (e.g. Glisson, Hemmelgarn, Green, & Williams, 2013). Implementation strategies are typically "homegrown" by intervention developers – evidence-informed, but rarely evidence-based. Far more research is needed to validate theory-driven implementation models and strategies. Studies that meet standards of rigor set forth by the Cochrane EPOC group (EPOC, 2015) should use designs capable of testing the impact of implementation strategies both on implementation and intervention outcomes (Landsverk, Brown, Rolls Reutz, Palinkas, & Horwitz, 2011).

Cost data examining how parent training programs benefit society in terms of factors other than crime rates, educational attainment, and unemployment are also needed. For example, far more research is needed to examine cost-benefits associated with reductions in maltreatment rates, out-of-home placements, and parental mental illness. More research also is needed examining the costs of sustaining parenting programs over time, particularly as agencies incorporate into routine practice systems to maintain fidelity to the program. Finally, comparative studies examining detailed economic analyses associated with varying implementation efforts and in varying contexts (e.g., private versus public sector) are needed to inform decision and policy makers as they consider adopting, implementing, and sustaining effective interventions.

Finally, very little is known about whether and to what extent widespread implementation efforts are sustained in communities and systems. Despite the extensive implementation and testing of the three programs, we could find little published data on their long-term *sustainability* in diverse communities (see Gewirtz & Forgatch, 2016, for data on sustainability of PMTO). Indeed, there is a dearth of data on sustainability of evidence-based practices in general, with recent calls to increase this research (Chambers, Glasgow, & Stange, 2013). Reducing the prevalence of child behavior problems through the widespread, efficient, and sustained implementation of evidence-based parenting programs is a feasible challenge for the twenty-first century. Implementation science can provide the tools for effectively addressing this challenge.

In sum, a large body of empirical evidence exists for the utility of parent training programs for reducing child behavior problems and promoting youth adjustment. These programs have been validated in primarily Western, developed countries around the world and with diverse populations. The promise of widespread implementation of these programs is their potential to decrease the prevalence of child behavior problems across entire communities. However, far less research exists on the widespread implementation and in particular on the sustainability of these programs than on their effectiveness. Expanding the implementation of these programs across cultures and countries – particularly in the developing world – and developing a research agenda to examine sustainability are the next challenges for the field.

Acknowledgments

The first author gratefully acknowledges Marion Forgatch for her mentorship and inspiration, and Kate Gliske for her diligent research on IY and Triple P efficacy. The authors are supported with funding from the Division of

Epidemiology, Services, and Prevention Branch, the National Institute on Drug Abuse (NIDA), via R01DA030114 to Abigail Gewirtz, and a NIDA Research Supplement to Promote Diversity in Health-Related Research to Adriana Youssef.

References

Aarons, G. A., Cafri, G., Lugo, L., & Sawitzky, A. (2012). Expanding the domains of attitudes towards evidence-based practice: The Evidence Based Practice Attitude Scale-50. *Administration and Policy in Mental Health,* 39(5), 331–340.

Aarons, G. A., & Palinkas, L. A. (2007). Implementation of evidence-based practice in child welfare: service provider perspectives. *Administration and Policy in Mental Health and Mental Health Services Research* 34(4): 411–19.

Aarons, G. A., Sommerfeld, D. H., Hecht, D. B., Silovsky, J. F., & Chaffin, M. J. (2009). The impact of evidence-based practice implementation and fidelity monitoring on staff turnover: evidence for a protective effect. *Journal of Consulting and Clinical Psychology* 77(2): 270–80.

Aos, S., Cook, T. D., Elliott, D. S., Gottfredson, D. C., Hawkins, J. D., Lipsey, M. W., & Tolan, P. (2011). Commentary on Valentine, Jeffrey, et al.: replication in prevention science. The Advisory Board of Blueprints for Violence Prevention. *Prevention Science* 12(2): 121–2.

Asgary-Eden, V., & Lee, C. M. (2011). So now we've picked an evidence-based program, what's next? Perspectives of service providers and administrators. *Professional Psychology: Research and Practices* 42(2): 169–75.

Bandura, A. (1971). *Social Learning Theory*. New York: General Learning Press.

Bank, L., Marlowe, J. H., Reid, J. B., Patterson, G. R., & Weinrott, M. R. (1991). A comparative evaluation of parent-training interventions for families of chronic delinquents. *Journal of Abnormal Child Psychology* 19(1): 15–33.

Baumann, A. A., Domenech Rodríguez, M. M., Amador, N. G., Forgatch, M. S., & Parra-Cardona, J. R. (2014). Parent Management Training-Oregon Model (PMTOTM) in Mexico City: integrating cultural adaptation activities in an implementation model. *Clinical Psychology* 21(1): 32–47.

Beidas, R. S., & Kendall, P. C. (2010). Training therapists in evidence-based practice: a critical review of studies from a systems-contextual perspective. *Clinical Psychology: Science and Practice* 17(1): 1–30.

Bjørknes, R., & Manger, T. (2013). Can parent training alter parent practice and reduce conduct problems in ethnic minority children? A randomized controlled trial. *Prevention Science* 14(1): 52–63.

Breitkreuz, R., McConnell, D., Savage, A., & Hamilton, A. (2011). Integrating Triple P into existing family support services: a case study on program implementation. *Prevention Science* 12(4): 411–22.

Chamberlain, P. (1999). *Residential Care for Children and Adolescents with Oppositional Defiant Disorder and Conduct Disorder*. Dordrecht, Netherlands: Kluwer Academic.

Chamberlain, P. (2003). *Treating Chronic Juvenile Offenders: Advances Made through the Oregon Multidimensional Treatment Foster Care Model.* Washington, DC: American Psychological Association.

Chambers, D. A., Glasgow, R. E., & Stange, K. C. (2013). The dynamic sustainability framework addressing the paradox of sustainment amid ongoing change. *Implementation Science* 8(1): 117.

Charles, J. M., Edwards, R. T., Bywater, T., & Hutchings, J. (2013). Micro-costing in public health economics: steps towards a standardized framework, using the Incredible Years toddler parenting program as a worked example. *Prevention Science* 14(4): 377–89.

Collins, P. Y., Patel, V., Joestl, S. S., March, D., Insel, T. R., Daar, A. S., . . . Fairburn, C. (2011). Grand challenges in global mental health. *Nature* 475(7354): 27–30.

Conger, R. D., Wallace, L. E., Sun, Y., Simons, R. L., McLoyd, V. C., & Brody, G. H. (2002). Economic pressure in African American families: a replication and extension of the family stress model. *Developmental Psychology* 38(2): 179–93.

Coyne, J. C., & Kwakkenbos, L. (2013). Triple P-Positive Parenting programs: the folly of basing social policy on underpowered flawed studies. *BMC Medicine* 11(1): 11.

Crowley, D. M., Coffman, D. L., Feinberg, M. E., Greenberg, M. T., & Spoth, R. L. (2014). Evaluating the impact of implementation factors on family-based prevention programming: methods for strengthening causal inference. *Prevention Science* 15(2): 246–55.

Dane, A. V., & Schneider, B. H. (1998). Program integrity in primary and early secondary prevention: are implementation effects out of control? *Clinical Psychology Review* 18(1): 23–45.

de Graaf, I., Speetjens, P., Smit, F., de Wolff, M., & Tavecchio, L. (2008). Effectiveness of the Triple P – Positive Parenting Program on behavioral problems in children: a meta-analysis. *Behavior Modification* 32(5): 714–35.

DeGarmo, D. S., Patterson, G. R., & Forgatch, M. S. (2004). How do outcomes in a specified parent training intervention maintain or wane over time? *Prevention Science* 5: 73–89.

Department for Training and Education in Wales (DfTE) (2005). *Parenting Action Plan: Supporting Mothers, Fathers, and Careers with Raising Children in Wales.* Welsh Assembly Government. Information Document No: 054–05. Cardiff: DfTE.

Dishion, T. J., & Andrews, D. W. (1995). Preventing escalation in problem behaviors with high-risk young adolescents: immediate and 1-year outcomes. *Journal of Consulting and Clinical Psychology* 63(4): 538–48.

Dusenbury, L., Brannigan, R., Falco, M., & Hansen, W. B. (2003). A review of research on fidelity of implementation: implications for drug abuse prevention in school settings. *Health Education Research* 18(2): 237–56.

Eames, C., Daley, D., Hutchings, J., Hughes, J. C., Jones, K., Martin, P., & Bywater, T. (2008). The Leader Observation Tool: a process skills treatment fidelity measure for the Incredible Years parenting program. *Child: Care, Health and Development* 34(3): 391–400.

Eames, C., Daley, D., Hutchings, J., Whitaker, C. J., Bywater, T., Jones, K., & Hughes, J. C. (2010). The impact of group leaders' behaviour on parents' acquisition of key parenting skills during parent training. *Behaviour Research and Therapy* 48(12): 1221–6.

Eames, C., Daley, D., Hutchings, J., Whitaker, C. J., Jones, K., Hughes, J. C., & Bywater, T. (2009). Treatment fidelity as a predictor of behaviour change in parents attending group-based parent training. *Child: Care, Health and Development* 35(5): 603–12.

Eccles, M. P., & Mittman, B. S. (2006). Welcome to implementation science. *Implementation Science* 1(1): 1.

Edwards, R. T., O'Ceilleachair, A., Bywater, T., Hughes, D. A., Hutchings, J. (2007). Parenting program for parents of children at risk of developing conduct disorder: cost effectiveness analysis. *BMJ* 334(7595): 683–8.

EPOC (Effective Practice and Organisation of Care) (2015). EPOC taxonomy. epoc.cochrane.org/epoc-taxonomy

Eyberg, S. (1999). *Eyberg Child Behavior Inventory*. Odessa, FL: Psychological Assessment Resources.

Fergusson, D., Stanley, L., & Horwood, L. J. (2009). Preliminary data on the efficacy of the Incredible Years Basic Parent Program in New Zealand. *Australian and New Zealand Journal of Psychiatry* 43: 76–9.

Fixsen, D. L., Naoom, S. F., Blase, K. A., Friedman, R. M., & Wallace, F. (2005). *Implementation Research: A Synthesis of the Literature*. Tampa, FL: University of South Florida, Louis de la Parte Florida Mental Health Institute, National Implementation Research Network (FMHI Publication #231).

Forgatch, M. S., Beldavs, Z. G., Patterson, G. R., & DeGarmo, D. S. (2008). From coercion to positive parenting: putting divorced mothers in charge of change. In Kerr, M., Stattin, H., & Engels, R. (eds.), *What Can Parents Do? New Insights into the Role of Parents in Adolescent Problem Behavior*. London: Wiley, pp. 191–209.

Forgatch, M. S., Bullock, B. M., Patterson, G. R., & Steiner, H. (2004). From theory to practice: increasing effective parenting through role-play. In Steiner, H. (ed.), *Handbook of Mental Health Interventions in Children and Adolescents: An Integrated Developmental Approach*. San Francisco, CA: Jossey-Bass, pp.782–812.

Forgatch, M. S., & DeGarmo, D. S. (1999). Parenting through change: an effective prevention program for single mothers. *Journal of Consulting and Clinical Psychology* 67(5): 711–24.

Forgatch, M. S., & DeGarmo, D. S. (2002). Extending and testing the social interaction learning model with divorce samples. In Reid, J. B., Patterson, G. R., & Snyder, J. (eds.), *Antisocial Behavior in Children and Adolescents: A Developmental Analysis and Model for Intervention*. Washington, DC: American Psychological Association, pp. 235–56.

Forgatch, M. S., & DeGarmo, D. S. (2007). Accelerating recovery from poverty: prevention effects for recently separated mothers. *Journal of Early and Intensive Behavioral Intervention* 4(4): 681–702.

Forgatch, M. S., & DeGarmo, D. S. (2011). Sustaining fidelity following the nationwide PMTO implementation in Norway. *Prevention Science* 12(3): 235–46.

Forgatch, M. S., DeGarmo, D. S., & Beldavs, Z. G. (2005). An efficacious theory-based intervention for stepfamilies. *Behavior Therapy* 36(4): 357–65.

Forgatch, M., & Ogden, T. (2006). Enhancing resilience in a nationwide system of care for children with behavior disorders. Paper presented at the Fourth World Conferences on the Promotion of Mental Health and Prevention of Mental and Behavioural Disorders, Enhancing Resilience, Oslo, Norway.

Forgatch, M. S., Patterson, G. R., & DeGarmo, D. S. (2005). Evaluating fidelity: predictive validity for a measure of competent adherence to the Oregon model of parent management training (PMTO). *Behavior Therapy* 36(1): 3–13.

Forgatch, M. S., Patterson, G. R., DeGarmo, D. S., & Beldavs, Z. G. (2009). Testing the Oregon delinquency model with nine-year follow-up of the Oregon Divorce Study. *Development and Psychopathology* 21(2): 637–60.

Forgatch, M. S., Patterson, G. R., & Gewirtz, A. H. (2013). Looking forward: the promise of widespread implementation of parent training programs. *Perspectives on Psychological Science* 8: 682–94.

Forgatch, M. S., & Toobert, D. J. (1979). A cost-effective parent training program for use with normal preschool children. *Journal of Pediatric Psychology* 4: 129–45.

Foster, E. M., Prinz, R. J., Sanders, M. R., & Shapiro, C. J. (2008). The costs of a public health infrastructure for delivering parenting and family support. *Children and Youth Services Review* 30: 493–501.

Furlong, M., McGilloway, S., Bywater, T., Hutchings, J., Smith, S. M., & Donnelly, M. (2012). Behavioural and cognitive-behavioural group-based parenting programmes for early-onset conduct problems in children aged 3 to 12 years. *Cochrane Database of Systematic Reviews* 2. onlinelibrary.wiley.com/doi/10.1002/14651858.CD00 8225.pub2/pdf/standard

Gewirtz AH, DeGarmo DS, Plowman EJ, August G, Realmuto G. Parenting, parental mental health, and child functioning in families residing in supportive housing. American Journal of Orthopsychiatry. 2009;79:336–347.

Gewirtz, A. H., & Forgatch, M. S. (2016). Creating and sustaining science-based delivery systems for psychological interventions: The widespread implementation of a parent training intervention. Manuscript in preparation.

Gewirtz, A. H., Pinna, K. L. M., Hanson, S. K., & Brockberg, D. (2014). Promoting parenting to support reintegrating military families: after deployment, adaptive parenting tools. *Psychological Services* 11(1): 31–40.

Gewirtz, A., & Taylor, T. (2009). Participation of homeless and abused women in a parent training program: science and practice converge in a battered women's shelter. In Hindsworth, M. F., & Lang, T. B. (eds.). *Community Participation and Empowerment*. Hauppage, NY: Nova Science, pp. 97–114.

Glisson, C., Hemmelgarn, A., Green, P., & Williams, N. J. (2013). Randomized trial of the availability, responsiveness and continuity (ARC) organizational intervention for improving youth outcomes in community mental health programs. *Journal of the American Academy of Child & Adolescent Psychiatry* 52(5): 493–500.

Glisson, C., Landsverk, J., Schoenwald, S., Kelleher, K., Hoagwood, K. E., Mayberg, S., … & Research Network on Youth Mental Health. (2008). Assessing the organizational social context (OSC) of mental health services: Implications for research and practice. *Administration and Policy in Mental Health and Mental Health Services Research* 25(1–2): 98–113.

He, Y., Gewirtz, A., Lee, S., Morrell, N., & August, G. (2015). A randomized preference trial to inform personalization of a parent training program implemented in community mental health clinics. *Translational Behavioral Medicine*, under review.

Hurlburt, M. S., Nguyen, K., Reid, J., Webster-Stratton, C., & Zhang, J. (2013). Efficacy of the Incredible Years group parent program with families in Head Start who self-reported a history of child maltreatment. *Child Abuse & Neglect* 37(8): 531–43.

Hutchings, J., Bywater, T., Daley, D., Gardner, F., Whitaker, C., Jones, K., … Edwards, R. T. (2007). Parenting intervention in Sure Start services for children at risk of developing conduct disorder: pragmatic randomised controlled trial. *BMJ* 334(7595): 678.

Institute of Medicine (2001). *Crossing the Quality Chasm: A New Health System for the 21st Century*. Washington, DC: National Academy Press.

Jones, K., Daley, D., Hutchings, J., Bywater, T., & Eames, C. (2008). Efficacy of the Incredible Years Program as an early intervention for children with conduct problems and ADHD: long-term follow-up. *Child: Care, Health and Development* 34(3): 380–90.

Knutson, N., Forgatch, M., Rains, L., & Sigmarsdóttir, M. (2009). *Fidelity of Implementation Rating System (FIMP): The Manual for PMTO™*, revised ed. Eugene, OR: Implementation Sciences International.

Landsverk, J., Brown, C. H., Reutz, J. R., Palinkas, L., & Horwitz, S. M. (2011). Design elements in implementation research: a structured review of child welfare and child mental health studies. *Administration and Policy in Mental Health and Mental Health Services Research* 38(1): 54–63.

Lee, C.-Y. S., August, G. J., Realmuto, G. M., Horowitz, J. L., Bloomquist, M. L., & Klimes-Dougan, B. (2008). Fidelity at a distance: assessing implementation fidelity of the Early Risers Prevention Program in a going-to-scale intervention trial. *Prevention Science* 9(3): 215–29.

Linares, L. O., Montalto, D., Li, M., & Oza, V. S. (2006). A promising parenting intervention in foster care. *Journal of Consulting and Clinical Psychology* 74(1): 32.

Marcynyszyn, L. A., Maher, E. J., & Corwin, T. W. (2011). Getting with the (evidence-based) program: an evaluation of the Incredible Years parenting training program in child welfare. *Children and Youth Services Review* 33: 747–57.

Martinez, C. R. Jr., & Eddy, J. M. (2005). Effects of culturally adapted parent management training on Latino youth behavioral health outcomes. *Journal of Consulting and Clinical Psychology* 73(4): 841–51.

Martinez, C. R., Jr., & Forgatch, M. S. (2001). Preventing problems with boys' noncompliance: effects of a parent training intervention for divorcing mothers. *Journal of Consulting and Clinical Psychology* 69: 416–28.

Matsumoto, Y., Sofronoff, K., & Sanders, M. R. (2007). The efficacy and acceptability of the Triple P – Positive Parenting Program with Japanese parents. *Behavioral Change* 24: 205–18.

Matsumoto, Y., Sofronoff, K., Sanders, M. R. (2010). Investigation of the effectiveness and social validity of the Triple P – Positive Parenting Program in Japanese Society. *Journal of Family Psychology* 24(1): 87–91.

Mazzucchelli, T. G., & Sanders, M. R. (2010). Facilitating practitioner flexibility within an empirically supported intervention: lessons from a system of parenting support. *Clinical Psychology Science and Practice* 17: 238–52.

Mejia, A., Calam, R., & Sanders, M. R. (2014a). Examining the fit of evidence-based parenting programs in low-resource settings: a survey of practitioners in Panama. *Journal of Child and Family Studies*. doi: 10.1007/s10826-014-0028-z

Mejia, A., Calam, R., & Sanders, M. R. (2014b). Examining delivery preferences and cultural relevance of an evidence-based parenting program in a low-resource setting of Central America: approaching parents as consumers. *Journal of Child and Family Studies*. doi: 10.1007/s10826-014–9911-x

McIntyre, L. L. (2008). Adapting Webster-Stratton's Incredible Years parent training for children with developmental delay: findings from a treatment group only study. *Journal of Intellectual Disability Research* 52(12): 1176–92.

Menting, A. T., Orobio de Castro, B., & Matthys, W. (2013). Effectiveness of the Incredible Years parent training to modify disruptive and prosocial child behavior: a meta-analytic review. *Clinical Psychology Review* 33(8): 901–13.

Mihalic, S. F. (n.d.). Blueprints for Healthy Youth Development | Blueprints Programs. Retrieved from www.blueprintsprograms.com

Mihalic, S. F. (2004). The importance of implementation fidelity. *Emotional & Behavioral Disorders in Youth* 4(4): 83–6, 99-101, 105.

Mihalic, S. F., Fagan, A. A., & Argamaso, S. (2008). Implementing the LifeSkills Training drug prevention program: factors related to implementation fidelity. *Implementation Science* 3(5): 1–16.

Mihalopoulos, C., Sanders, M. R., Turner, K. M., Murphy-Brennan, M., & Carter, R. (2007). Does the Triple P–Positive Parenting Program provide value for money? *Australian and New Zealand Journal of Psychiatry* 41(3): 239–46.

Morawska, A., Sanders, M. R., O'Brien, J., McAuliffe, C., & Anderson, E. (2012). Practitioner perceptions of the use of parenting programs with culturally diverse families. *Australian Journal of Primary Health* 18: 313–20.

National Institute of Mental Health (2008). Child and adolescent effectiveness research in clinical practice and community settings: needs, challenges, and opportunities. Retrieved from www.nimh.nih.gov/research-priorities/scientific-meetings/2008/

Nowak, C., & Heinrichs, N. (2008). A comprehensive meta-analysis of Triple P-Positive Parenting Program using hierarchical linear modeling: effectiveness and moderating variables. *Clinical Child and Family Psychology Review* 11(3): 114–44.

Ogden, T., Forgatch, M. S., Askeland, E., Patterson, G. R., & Bullock, B. M. (2005). Implementation of parent management training at the national level: the case of Norway. *Journal of Social Work Practice* 19(3): 317–29.

O'Neill, D., McGilloway, S., Donnelly, M., Bywater, T., & Kelly, P. (2013). A cost-effectiveness analysis of the Incredible Years parenting program in reducing childhood health inequalities. *European Journal of Health Economics* 14(1): 85–94.

Parra-Cardona, J. R., Domenech-Rodriguez, M., Forgatch, M., Sullivan, C., Bybee, D., … Bernal, G. (2012). Culturally adapting an evidence-based parenting intervention for Latino immigrants: the need to integrate fidelity and cultural relevance. *Family Process* 51(1): 56–72.

Patterson, G. R. (1982). *Coercive Family Process*. Eugene, OR: Castalia.

Patterson, G. R. (2005). The next generation of PMTO models. *Behavior Therapist* 28(2): 25–32.

Patterson, G. R., Chamberlain, P., & Reid, J. B. (1982). A comparative evaluation of a parent-training program. *Behavior Therapy* 13(5): 638–50.

Patterson, G. R., Forgatch, M. S., & DeGarmo, D. S. (2010). Cascading effects following intervention. *Development & Psychopathology* 22 (Special Issue 04), 949–70.

Patterson, G. R., Reid, J. B., & Eddy, J. M. (2002). A brief history of the Oregon model. In Reid, J. B., Patterson, G. R., & Snyder, J. J. (eds.), *Antisocial Behavior in Children and Adolescents: A Developmental Analysis and Model for Intervention*. Washington, DC: American Psychological Association, pp. 3–21.

Posthumus, J. A., Raaijmakers, M. A., Maassen, G. H., Van Engeland, H., & Matthys, W. (2012). Sustained effects of Incredible Years as a preventive intervention in preschool children with conduct problems. *Journal of Abnormal Child Psychology* 40(4): 487–500.

Powell, B. J., Proctor, E. K., & Glass, J. E. (2014). A systematic review of strategies for implementing empirically supported mental health interventions. *Research on Social Work Practice* 24(2): 192–212.

Prinz, R. J., & Sanders, M. R. (2007). Adopting a population-level approach to parenting and family support interventions. *Clinical Psychology Review* 27(6): 739–49.

Prinz, R. J., Sanders, M. R., Shapiro, C. J., Whitaker, D. J., & Lutzker, J. R. (2009). Population-based prevention of child maltreatment: the US Triple P system population trial. *Prevention Science* 10(1): 1–12.

Proctor, E. K., Landsverk, J., Aarons, G., Chambers, D., Glisson, C., & Mittman, B. (2009). Implementation research in mental health services: an emerging science with conceptual, methodological, and training challenges. *Administration and Policy in Mental Health and Mental Health Services Research* 36(1): 24–34.

Proctor, E., Silmere, H., Raghavan, R., Hovmand, P., Aarons, G., Bunger, A., … Hensley, M. (2011). Outcomes for implementation research: conceptual distinctions, measurement challenges, and research agenda. *Administration and Policy in Mental Health and Mental Health Services Research* 38(2): 65–76.

Reid, J. B., Eddy, J. M., Fetrow, R. A., & Stoolmiller, M. (1999). Description and immediate impacts of a preventive intervention for conduct problems. *American Journal of Community Psychology* 27(4): 483–517.

Reid, J. B., & Kavanagh, K. (1985). A social interactional approach to child abuse: risk, prevention, and treatment. In Chesney, M., & Rosenman, R. (ed.), *Anger and Hostility in Behavioral and Cardiovascular Disorders* New York: Hempisphere/ McGraw-Hill, pp. 113–34.

Reid, J. B., Patterson, G. R., & Snyder, J. (2002). *Antisocial Behavior in Children and Adolescents: A Developmental Analysis and Model for Intervention*. Washington, DC: American Psychological Association.

Reid, M. J., Webster-Stratton, C., & Beauchaine, T. P. (2001). Parent training in Head Start: a comparison of program response among African American, Asian American, Caucasian, and Hispanic mothers. *Prevention Science* 2(4): 209–27.

Reynolds, C. R., and Kamphaus, R. W. (2006). *BASC-2: Behavior Assessment System for Children*, 2nd ed. Upper Saddle River, NJ: Pearson Education.

Romney, S., Israel, N., & Zlatevski, D. (2014). Exploration-stage implementation variation: its effect on the cost-effectiveness of an evidence-based parenting program. *Zeitschrift fur Psychologie* 222: 37–48.

Sanders, M. R. (1999). Triple P-Positive Parenting Program: Towards an empirically validated multilevel parenting and family support strategy for the prevention of behavior and emotional problems in children. *Clinical Child and Family Psychology Review* 2(2): 71–90.

Sanders, M. R. (2008). Triple P-Positive Parenting Program as a public health approach to strengthening parenting. *Journal of Family Psychology* 22(4): 506–17.

Sanders, M. R. (2012). Development, evaluation, and multinational dissemination of the Triple P-Positive Parenting Program. *Annual Review of Clinical Psychology* 8: 345–79.

Sanders, M. R., Cann, W., & Markie-Dadds, C. (2003a). The Triple P-Positive Parenting Program: a universal population-level approach to the prevention of child abuse. *Child Abuse Review* 12(3): 155–71.

Sanders, M. R., Dittman, C. K., Farruggia, S. P., & Keown, L. J. (2014a). A comparison of online versus workbook delivery of a self-help positive parenting program. *Journal of Primary Prevention* 35(3): 125–33.

Sanders, M. R., & Kirby, J. N. (2014). Surviving or thriving: quality assurance mechanisms to promote innovation in the development of evidence-based parenting interventions. *Prevention Science*. doi: 10.1007/s11121-014-0475-1

Sanders, M. R., Kirby, J. N., Tellegen, C. L., & Day, J. J. (2014b). The Triple P-Positive Parenting Program: a systematic review and meta-analysis of a multi-level system of parenting support. *Clinical Psychology Review* 34(4): 337–57.

Sanders, M. R., Markie-Dadds, C., Tully, L. A., & Bor, W. (2000). The Triple P-Positive Parenting Program: a comparison of enhanced, standard, and self-directed behavioral family intervention for parents of children with early onset conduct problems. *Journal of Consulting and Clinical Psychology* 68(4): 624.

Sanders, M. R., Murphy-Brennan, M. & McAuliffe, C. (2003b). The development, evaluation, and dissemination of a training programme for general practitioners in evidence-based parent consultation skills. *International Journal of Mental Health Promotion* 5(4): 13–20.

Sanders, M. R., Prinz, R. J., & Shapiro, C. J. (2009). Predicting utilization of evidence-based parenting interventions with organizational, service-provider and client variables. *Administration and Policy in Mental Health and Mental Health Services Research* 36(2): 133–43.

Sanders, M. R., Tully, L. A., Turner, K. M. T., Maher, C., & McAuliffe, C. (2003c). Training GPs in parent consultation skills: an evaluation of training for the Triple P-Positive Parenting Program. *Australian Family Physician* 32(9): 763–8.

Schoenwald, S. K., Garland, A. F., Chapman, J. E., Frazier, S. L., Sheidow, A. J., & Southam-Gerow, M. A. (2011). Toward the effective and efficient measurement of implementation fidelity. *Administration and Policy in Mental Health and Mental Health Services Research* 38(1): 32–43.

Scott, S., Carby, A., & Rendu, A. (2008). *Impact of Therapists' Skill on Effectiveness of Parenting Groups for Child Antisocial Behavior*. London: King's College, Institute of Psychiatry, University College London.

Seabra-Santos, M. J., Gaspar, M. F., Azevedo, A., Homem, T. C., & Pimentel, M. (2011). Incredible Years Parent Training Program in ADHD: parents attendence and satisfaction. *ADHD Attention Deficit Hyperactivity Disorder* 3: 168–9.

Seng, A. C., Prinz, R. J., & Sanders, M. R. (2006). The role of training variables in effective dissemination of evidence-based parenting interventions. *International Journal of Mental Health Promotion* 8(4): 20–8.

Shapiro, C. J., Prinz, R. J., & Sanders, M. R. (2008). Population-wide parenting intervention training: initial feasibility. *Journal of Child and Family Studies* 17(4): 457–66.

Shapiro, C. J., Prinz, R. J., & Sanders, M. R. (2012). Facilitators and barriers to implementation of an evidence-based parenting intervention to prevent child maltreatment: the Triple P-Positive Parenting Program. *Child Maltreatment* 17(1): 86–95.

Shapiro, C. J., Prinz, R. J., & Sanders, M. R. (2014). Sustaining use of an evidence-based parenting intervention: practitioner perspectives. *Journal of Child and Family Studies*. dx.doi.org/10.1007/s10826-014-9965-9

Sigmarsdóttir, M., & Guðmundsdóttir, E. V. (2013). Implementation of parent management training–oregon model (PMTO™) in Iceland: building sustained fidelity. *Family Process* 52(2): 216–27.

Stern, S. B., Alaggia, R., Watson, K., & Morton, T. R. (2008). Implementing an evidence-based parenting program with adherence in the real world of community practice. *Research on Social Work Practice* 18(6): 543–54.

Taylor, W. D., Asgary-Eden, V., Lee, C. M., & LaRoche, K. J. (2015). Service providers' adherence to an evidence-based parenting program: what are they missing and why? *Journal of Child and Family Studies* 24: 50–6.

Thomas, R., & Zimmer-Gembeck, M. J. (2007). Behavioral outcomes of parent–child interaction therapy and Triple P–Positive Parenting Program: a review and meta-analysis. *Journal of Abnormal Child Psychology* 35(3): 475–95.

Turner, K. M., Nicholson, J. M., & Sanders, M. R. (2011). The role of practitioner self-efficacy, training, program and workplace factors on the implementation of an evidence-based parenting intervention in primary care. *Journal of Primary Prevention* 32(2): 95–112.

Turner, K. M., & Sanders, M. R. (2006). Dissemination of evidence-based parenting and family support strategies: learning from the Triple P–Positive Parenting Program system approach. *Aggression and Violent Behavior* 11(2): 176–93.

Turner, K. M., Sanders, M. R., & Hodge, L. (2014). Issues in professional training to implement evidence-based parenting programs: the preferences of indigenous practitioners. *Australian Psychologist* 49: 384–94.

United States Department of Health and Human Services (2006). *The Road Ahead: Research Partnerships to Transform Services: A Report by the National Advisory Mental Health Council's Workgroup on Services and Clinical Epidemiology Research*. Bethesda, MD: National Institutes of Health, National Institute of Mental Health.

Waltz, J., Addis, M. E., Koerner, K., & Jacobson, N. S. (1993). Testing the integrity of a psychotherapy protocol: assessment of adherence and competence. *Journal of Consulting and Clinical Psychology* 61(4): 620.

Webster-Stratton, C. (1981). Modification of mothers' behaviors and attitudes through a videotape modeling group discussion program. *Behavior Therapy* 12(5): 634–42.

Webster-Stratton, C. (1998). Preventing conduct problems in Head Start children: strengthening parenting competencies. *Journal of Consulting and Clinical Psychology* 66(5): 715.

Webster-Stratton, C. (2004). Quality training, supervision, ongoing monitoring, and agency support: key ingredients to implementing the Incredible Years programs with fidelity. Retrieved from http://incredibleyears.com/research-library/.

Webster-Stratton, C. (2006). Treating children with early-onset conduct problems: Key ingredients to implementing the Incredible Years programs with fidelity. In Neill, T. K. (ed.), *Helping Other Help Children: Clinical Supervision of Child Psychotherapy*. Washington, DC: American Psychological Association, pp. 161–75.

Webster-Stratton, C., Gaspar, M. F., & Seabra-Santos, M. J. (2012). Incredible Years parent, teachers, and children's series: transportability to Portugal of early intervention programs for preventing conduct problems and promoting social and emotional competence. *Psychosocial Intervention* 21(2): 157–69.

Webster-Stratton, C., & Herman, K. C. (2010). Disseminating Incredible Years series early-intervention programs: integrating and sustaining services between school and home. *Psychology in the Schools* 47(1): 36–54.

Webster-Stratton, C., & Reid, M. J. (2003). The Incredible Years parents, teachers, and children training series: a multifaceted treatment approach for young children with conduct problems. In Kazdin, A. E., & Weisz, J. R. (eds.), *Evidenced-Based Psychotherapies for Children and Adolescents*. New York: Guilford Press, pp. 194–210.

Webster-Stratton, C., Reid, M. J., & Beauchaine, T. P. (2013). One-year follow-up of combined parent and child intervention for young children with ADHD. *Journal of Clinical Child & Adolescent Psychology* 42(2): 251–61.

Webster-Stratton, C., Reid, M. J., & Marsenich, L. (2014). Improving therapist fidelity during implementation of evidence-based practices: incredible years program. *Psychiatric Services* 65(6): 789–95.

Webster-Stratton, C., Rinaldi, J., & Reid, J. M. (2011). Long-term outcomes of Incredible Years parenting program: predictors of adolescent adjustment. *Child and Adolescent Mental Health* 16(1): 38–46.

Wilson, P., Rush, R., Hussey, S., Puckering, C., Sim, F., Allely, C. S., ... Gillberg, C. (2012). How evidence-based is an "evidence-based parenting program"? A PRISMA systematic review and meta-analysis of Triple P. *BMC Medicine* 10(1): 130.

13 Preventing Violence and Victimization among Racial/Ethnic Minority and Immigrant Youth in the United States

Looking beyond the Individual Factors

Jun Sung Hong, Anthony A. Peguero,
Dorothy L. Espelage, & Paula Allen-Meares

Introduction

Violence and victimization involving children and adolescents are pressing social and public health concerns in the United States. Studies have consistently revealed that children and adolescents who experience violence and victimization at home, at school, and in the neighborhood are at a heightened risk of physical and psychosocial health problems, such as depression, anxiety, aggressive behaviors, sexual risk behaviors, and suicidal thoughts and behaviors (Flannery, Singer, & Wester, 2001; Voisin, Jenkins, & Takahashi, 2011). Children exposed to violence and victimization are also likely to perform poorly in school, engage in illicit drug use, develop interpersonal conflicts, and perpetrate violence against romantic partners (e.g., Low & Espelage, 2014). Although the rate of delinquent activities has decreased since the mid-1990s in the United States (Puzzanchera, 2013), significant number of students had reported experiencing violent victimization. To illustrate, in 2013 the National Center for Educational Statistics of the U.S. Department of Justice reported violent victimization among 749,200 youth, ages twelve to eighteen (Robers, Kemp, Rathbun, & Morgan, 2014).

Certain children and adolescent populations are at higher risk for violence than others. Those youth not only are at risk for perpetrating violence but are also at higher risk for being victims of violence (Centers for Disease Control and Prevention, 2006; Reed et al., 2014). More specifically, the growing number of racial and ethnic minorities and immigrant youth in the United States are confronted with violence and victimization. Bullying involvement and peer conflicts appear to be serious concerns for African American and Hispanic/Latino children (Peguero, 2009; Peguero & Popp, 2012). The higher rates of violence and victimization experienced by African American youth and youth originally from immigrant families reflect major differences in vulnerability, marginalization, and victimization, as well as privilege and power, that are inherent in the U.S. school districts.

Violence and Victimization of African American Youth

Past research evidence suggests that African American children and adolescents are exposed to significantly higher rates of violence compared to youth of other races. To illustrate, studies report that African American youth are significantly more likely to be victims and perpetrators of violence in the home, school, and community (Black et al., 2013; Patton, Hong, Williams, & Allen-Meares, 2013). Bullying perpetration and physical fighting in schools and in neighborhoods appear to be more frequent among African American youth than among White youth (Wang, Ianotti, & Nansel, 2009). A more recent study conducted by Elsaesser and Voisin (2014), also found high prevalence of multiple forms of violence exposure among urban African American youth. These youth typically reside in low-income areas where risk of exposure to violence is probable (see Black et al., 2013). Violence victimization can also significantly reduce the average lifespan of African American men. Homicide is the leading cause of death among African Americans, and African American males eighteen to twenty-five years of age have the highest homicide victimization rates (Harrell, 2007).

Violence and Victimization of Immigrant Youth in the United States

The rate of immigrant youth populations has also been increasing due to globalization, technology transfer, and migrant labor force. In the United States, one in every four children identifies as Hispanic/Latino or non-White (Appleby, Colon, & Hamilton, 2011), and it is estimated that within thirty years, non-White youth originally from immigrant families are expected to increase by 30 percent (United States Census Bureau, 2012). Many immigrant children and adolescents, particularly those who recently immigrated to the United States, are also confronted with violence exposure, assault, and related psychological distress resulting from experiences before, during, and after the immigration (Decker, Raj, & Silverman, 2007). Until recently, studies on victimization of children and adolescents originally from immigrant families have been relatively scant. However, in recent years, there has been a growing interest in examining violence and victimization of youth originally from immigrant families because they are representative of the future of the United States (Peguero, 2009). Indeed, Hispanic/Latino, Asian, and Arab American children and adolescents are at a heightened risk of violence victimization and are subjected to negative treatment such as discrimination, ridicule, threats, and harassments from other students, teachers, and school administrators, which are attributed to language and cultural barriers, social isolation, and anti-immigrant policies that reinforce discriminatory treatment. For instance, Abdelkarim (2003) found that U.S. school districts have witnessed a dramatic increase in physical and verbal bullying directed at Arab American and Middle Eastern students. The U.S. Department of Justice (2009) also revealed that youth originally from immigrant families, particularly Hispanic/Latino and Asian families, are more likely to be victimized by their mainstream classmates and peers in school than their non-Hispanic, White peers (United States Department of Justice, 2009).

The Importance of Culturally Relevant Violence Prevention

As previously mentioned, in the United States the rate of youth crime and violence fell since the mid-1990s (Puzzanchera, 2013). However, as evidenced by several empirical findings, disparities in violence persist among racial and ethnic minority and immigrant youth. According to the Centers for Disease Control and Prevention (2013), the homicide rate is highest among African American youth and second highest among Hispanic/Latino youth in the United States. The U.S. Department of Justice also reported that homicide rate among African American male youth (ages ten to twenty-four) between 1980 and 2008 was significantly higher than among non-Hispanic White males in the same group (Cooper & Smith, 2011). Further, Hispanic/Latino, Asian/Pacific Islander, and American Indian adolescents are also reported to engage in high levels of violent behaviors and have high rates of self-inflicted violence, which causes problems for themselves, their families, and their communities (e.g., Perry, 2004). Despite these findings, development of culturally relevant youth violence prevention programs in racial and ethnic minority communities is rare, although researchers have attempted to examine culturally specific antecedents, mediators, and moderators of violence (e.g., Reese, Vera, & Hasbrouck, 2003; Wright & Fagan, 2013). However, cultural factors are difficult to examine, as studies have shown that violence is influenced by a confluence of risk factors occurring in various levels (Reese et al., 2003). Racial and ethnic minority and immigrant children and adolescents are confronted with a wide array of adversities (Jensen & Fraser, 2006) in their communities. Examples include unemployment and/or underemployment, access to illicit drugs, and dilapidated housing, all of which can increase their likelihood of being involved in violence and criminal activities (Compton, Gfroerer, Conway, & Finger, 2014) in their neighborhood and in their school. Thus, racial and ethnic minorities residing in such neighborhoods are disproportionately affected by violence occurring in their home and school (Reese et al., 2003) and are subsequently likely to be overrepresented in the juvenile justice system as a result (Duran & Posadas, 2013).

Theoretical Frameworks for Violence Prevention

Youth violence prevention can be found at various school levels (i.e., primary, secondary, and tertiary) and in various contexts, such as individual, family, school, peer groups, community, and policy (Swearer et al., 2006). The types of extant prevention studies, however, have followed similar patterns found among youth violence research in general (Wong, 2008). In other words, applying the tradition of the medical model, prevention studies for the most part have been developed by adults and have focused on the individual levels and, more specifically, individual pathology (Swearer et al., 2006; Wong, 2008). Scholars and educators are understandably interested in why an individual engages in certain behavior. Given that focusing solely on individual-level determinants is incomplete, researchers have begun to consider prevention in the broader social-ecological context (Swearer et al., 2006). The social-ecological framework is particularly important in developing comprehensive and sustainable violence prevention initiatives that target racial/ethnic minority and immigrant children and adolescents (Umemoto et al., 2009). However, in order to achieve this, it is imperative that researchers develop and tailor prevention by considering contexts that are germane to racial/ethnic minority and immigrant youth, such as family, neighborhood, and culture.

Social-Ecological Framework

The social-ecological framework has a long history, and it emerged from developments in various disciplines, such as public health, psychology, sociology, and biology, all of which formed the foundations of health promotion (Green, Richard, & Potvin, 1996). Organizations, such as the World Health Organization, the Centers for Disease Control, the National Institute of Health and Prevention, and the Institute of Medicine have called for incorporating the social-ecological framework in prevention and intervention program development (Golden & Earp, 2012). The social-ecological framework provides guidance for understanding the constellation of risk and protective factors that may promote or inhibit violence and victimization (Bograd, 1999). This framework identifies both proximal and distal factors that are related to violence and victimization at the individual, interpersonal, community, and societal levels (Bronfenbrenner, 1979). Although numerous theories (e.g., social learning theory) from multiple disciplines (e.g., sociology, criminology) have illuminated our understanding of why some youth are predisposed to violence and victimization, such theories have primarily focused on individual level factors as means of sustaining behavioral changes. As a result, stigmatization, condemnation, retribution, and segregations have been the hallmarks of youth violence prevention in the past (see, e.g., Hillyard & McDermott, 2014). On the contrary, the social-ecological framework is based on the premise that no single factor can explain why certain youth are at higher risk of violence and victimization than others (Richardson, 2008). Individual behavior is influenced by factors within social environments, such as home, school, and community. Moreover, the social, physical, and cultural aspects of the social environments have a cumulative effect on individual behavior (Stokols, 1996), which is not simply additive but rather complex (Espelage, Rao, & De La Rue, 2013). This framework has been widely employed by researchers to better understand and prevent violence (e.g., Dahlberg & Krug, 2002).

Individual. The first level of the social-ecological framework, the individual level, consists of personal and biological determinants of violence and victimization. Examples of factors at the individual level are psychological problems, personality disorders, aggressive behavior, and alcohol and drug use. Studies have documented that youth with a history of psychiatric problems, such as conduct disorder, are predisposed to aggressive behaviors (e.g., Singh et al., 2007). Moreover, research has also found that youth who use illicit substances are also prone to violence and victimization (e.g., Herrenkohl et al., 2000).

Interpersonal. Youths' relationships with their family, friends, peers, and romantic partners can also influence or inhibit the likelihood of violence. Youths' social circles, such as parents, siblings, peers, teachers, and romantic partners can shape their behavior and their relationships with others. Indeed, studies have shown that youths' abusive relationships with their parents, negative peer influence and deviant peer affiliation, and conflicts with teachers have been positively related to violence perpetration and victimization (for review, see Hong & Espelage, 2012).

Community. A community environment in which the individual operates, attitudes of the community residents, and relationships among various institutions within communities can all shape youths' psychosocial well-being (Fielding, Teutsch, & Breslow, 2010). Community environment is important in that youth spend considerable time in their home and school, both of which are nested in their community (Elder et al., 2007). Further, previous research has also reported on community influence as a moderator on the association between parenting practices and youth behaviors (Beyers, Bates, Pettit, & Dodge, 2003). Institutions within community settings, such as schools, and community-level characteristics, such as poverty, low socioeconomic status, unemployment, and criminal activities, have all been implicated in research on violence and victimization (Kramer, 2000).

Societal. Intrinsic to our social environment are societal factors, such as policies and norms, which provide social infrastructure (Fielding et al., 2010). Social norm theory purports that individual behavior is shaped by the pervasive social norms surrounding a behavior (Perkins & Berkowitz, 1986). Cultural norms that shape youth behaviors can also be influenced by the media (Thornburgh & Lin, 2002), which play a pivotal role in youths' socialization (DiClemente, Salazar, & Crosby, 2007). Although less frequently examined in comparison to individual, interpersonal, and community factors, researchers have found that societal factors, such as beliefs that are supportive of aggressive behaviors, are salient factors that are correlated with youths' risk of violence (Simon, Miller, Gorman-Smith, Orpinas, & Sullivan, 2010).

Resilience Framework

The idea of identifying risk factors to illuminate our understanding of experiences in violence of children and adolescents has gained widespread acceptance (Jenson & Fraser, 2006; Fergus & Zimmerman, 2005). Over the past several decades, we have learned about the causes and development of problem behaviors in youth (Jenson & Fraser, 2006). Research on youth violence has informed us about the risks and impact of children and adolescents' experiences in violence and victimization. Studies have long reported that risk factors function directly and indirectly to render youth vulnerable to poor developmental outcomes (e.g., Narayan, Englund, Carlson, & Egeland, 2014), and the association between risk factors and outcomes may be influenced by specific aspects of the youths' social environment, such as home, school, and neighborhood. However, a framework for prevention and intervention should focus on not only identifying the risk factors, but also understanding how resilience as a protective factor can explain positive outcomes for some children and adolescents. Resilience research in behavioral sciences emerged around 1970 from studies conducted by scholars seeking to understand and prevent the development of psychopathology (Masten, 2007). Scholars were inspired by several cases of resilience and also by the variability of outcomes of individuals who were at a heightened risk for problems (Rutter, 1985). Resilience scholars had predicted that it was important to utilize strengths and positive adaptation of individuals to prevent or ameliorate extreme adversity (Masten, 2007). *Resilience* can be defined most broadly as "[t]he capacity of a dynamic system to withstand or recover from significant challenges that threaten its stability, viability, or development" (Masten, 2011, p. 494). Research on resilience represents a significant paradigm shift in health-related fields, from focusing exclusively on risk factors to emphasizing the strengths and competencies of individuals (Michaud, 2006). Also inherent to a developmental psychopathology perspective is the manner in which the individual responds to and interacts with risk and protective factors at various levels of the social ecology, which results in diversity in developmental outcomes (Cicchetti & Rogosch, 1996). Although individual youth, such as racial/ethnic and immigrant youth in adverse situations, may begin on the same or similar developmental trajectory, many display different patterns of maladaptation or positive adaptation (Cicchetti, 2013; Cicchetti & Rogosch, 2012). An enhanced understanding of resilience has a strong potential for informing the development of prevention and interventions that focus on how racial and ethnic minority and immigrant youth might be protected from adversities that place them at risk of experiencing violence.

Violence Prevention Targeting Risk and Resilience in Multiple Social Environments

It is essential that youth violence prevention target risk and resilient factors in multiple social environments, given that the individual youth is directly and indirectly embedded in such environments as culture/society, policy/laws, parents/families, peers/friends, classroom/school, and community/neighborhood. Widely disseminated prevention programs have been developed, such as the Olweus Bullying Prevention Program (OBPP; Olweus, 2004), a universal program that was first developed in Norway; the components of the program target individual, classroom, school, and community levels. OBPP has been found to reduce youths' behavior problems, such as bullying and increase their prosocial behaviors (Olweus & Limber, 2010). Indeed, a recent review of evaluations using quasi-experimental or experimental research design to assess violence prevention found that effective interventions across settings and development are likely to reduce youth violence substantially (Fagan & Catalano, 2013).

Culture/Society

At the societal level, there are sociocultural mechanisms and factors that may marginalize racial and ethnic minority and immigrant youth, which in turn can contribute to making these populations vulnerable to violence and victimization (Peguero, 2012; Peguero, Popp, & Koo, 2011). Societal level is the departure point for better understanding of the historical, structural, systemic, and overarching racial/ethnic stratification in the United States in relationship to violence and victimization. Namely, the growing populations of racial/ethnic minorities and immigrants are exacerbating tensions and conflict often imposed on racial/ethnic minorities and immigrants as well as their children. The "threat hypothesis" suggests dominant groups protect their advantageous position in society by targeting and identifying subordinate groups as threatening whereas, individual-level threat occurs when a specific competitive individual is perceived as a threat to limited resources and opportunities (Jacobs, Malone, & Iles, 2012). Some researchers demonstrate that violence and victimization also derail competitive racial/ethnic minorities and immigrants from economic access and success. Racial riots, lynching, hate crimes, and interpersonal violence have been partially explained by an increasing number of competitive racial and ethnic minorities and immigrants seeking economic access and success (Alexander, 2010; Stacey, Carbone-López, & Rosenfeld, 2011). The threat of racial/ethnic minority and immigrant youth is finding its way within schools. The increasing population of racial and ethnic minority and immigrant youth within schools can be perceived as a threat, particularly in schools where there are limited educational resources and opportunities available to all students (Bankston & Caldas, 2002; Renzulli & Evans, 2005). Because of the perception that education is a zero-sum game with educational resources and opportunities, the increasing racial/ethnic and immigrant youth population is considered to be a threat, which can result in increased hostility, aggression, and violence and victimization.

Policy/Laws

As noted in the prior section, the threat of the increasing immigrant population can contribute to violence against and victimization of immigrants because they are perceived as threat to the dominant class's interests. There is a significant increase in creating, implementing, and enforcing stringent justice policies that are punitive and marginalizing immigrants and their children (Filindra, Blanding, & García Coll, 2011; Kubrin, Zatz, & Martínez, 2012). The growing population of immigrants, especially in a "post-9/11 society," has been a social, political, economic, and justice "war" on immigration and immigrants (Kubrin et al., 2012). At the federal level, there are unprecedented enforcement policies that target immigrants and their children with increased employment raids, detentions, deportations, and a public discourse establishing phenomena of "illegal immigrants" (Kubrin et al., 2012). At the state level, Florida, Texas, California, Alabama, and Arizona create, implement, and enforce policies that deny basic health and social services to immigrants and their children (Provine & Chavez, 2009). It also appears that policies the address the threat on immigration and immigrant families are also extending into the U.S. school system. Filindra et al. (2011) argue that the effects of political ideology and policies that are marginalizing immigrants have detrimental consequences for their children's overall well-being, development, school experiences, and educational progress. For instance, there is a positive relationship between access to the welfare system and graduation rates of children of immigrants, and these children and their families have limited access to social programs that could adversely affect their educational progress (Filindra et al., 2011). Thus, as result of these policies and laws, immigrants and their children are more likely to be victims of violence, because they are less likely to report their victimization to authorities due to fear of deportation, and also more likely to face discrimination, peer aggression and harassment, and unwelcoming communities and schools (Filindra et al., 2011; Hong et al., 2014; Kubrin et al., 2012).

Parents/Family

Relationships between youth and parents in the home can affect youths' attitudes and behaviors in their school (Espelage, Low, Rao, Hong, & Little, 2014b), and youth development occurs in the context of their caregivers (Dishion & Stormshak, 2007; Eddy, Reid, & Fetrow, 2000; Reese, Vera, Simon, & Ikeda, 2000). For this reason, a number of interventions have focused on parents and adult caregivers in the home. Studies reveal that family-focused parenting skills training interventions can reduce adolescents' aggressive, hostile, and violent behaviors (see Eddy et al., 2000; Serketich & Dumas, 1996). A recent systematic review of the effectiveness of parenting intervention for reducing harsh/abusive parenting and increasing positive parenting in low-income and developing countries also found that such intervention holds some promise for improving parenting practices and reducing maltreatment and violence against children in developing countries (Knerr, Gardner, & Cluver, 2013). Parent skills training is effective when the following components are included: increasing positive parent–child interactions and emotional communication skills, teaching parents how to use time-out and the importance of parenting consistency, and requiring parents to practice new skills with their children during the training session (Kaminski, Valle,

Filene, & Boyle, 2008). Targeting parents and family in prevention and intervention efforts appears to be promising for racial and ethnic minority and immigrant youth, as studies have shown that Latino and Asian children tend to be family-oriented (e.g., Garcia-Reid, Reid, & Peterson, 2005). However, barriers to family-focused youth violence prevention and intervention among racial and ethnic minority and immigrant youth, such as an acculturation gap between parents and children and difficulty in parental involvement in children's education and social competence, also need to be addressed in prevention efforts (Leidy, Guerra, & Toro, 2010).

Peers/Friends

Friends and peers play an increasingly important role in youth development, and friendships and peer support are critical components of overall functioning of youth. Friends and peers provide opportunities for youth to explore their identities, to feel a sense of belonging, and to develop social skills. Similarly, peer relationships also influence the development of youths' behavior problems (Deutsch, Crockett, Wolff, & Russell, 2012; Wang & Dishion, 2012). As expected, a bulk of violence prevention programs have targeted youths' peer ecologies. Conducting interventions with groups of youth with similar or the same clinical issues has been a major focus of youth violence prevention. However, studies also point out that youth with similar levels of antisocial and violent tendencies are likely to affiliate with one another (Espelage, Holt, & Henkel, 2003; Salmivalli, Huttunen, & Lagerspetz, 1997), and there is also potential harm in interventions involving peer groups with similar tendencies (Dishion & Stormshak, 2007).

Healthy peer relationships and friendships are essential for racial and ethnic minority and immigrant youth in achieving successful educational and psychosocial outcomes and in fostering a sense of belonging. Peer-level youth violence programs that are specifically geared toward racial and ethnic minority and immigrant youth need to have two specific goals. First, given that victimization commonly experienced by racial and ethnic minority and immigrant youth is due to language spoken, immigration status, and acculturation (Yu, Huang, Schwalberg, Overpeck, & Kogan, 2003), practitioners may need to be particularly sensitive to the peer experiences of these groups of youth. Likewise, practitioners need to also conduct a thorough assessment of youths' experiences in racially and ethnically motivated violence (McKenney, Pepler, Craig, & Connolly, 2006).

Classroom/School

Classroom and school environments are important consideration in youth violence prevention (Ozer, 2006), given that they play a major role in shaping the attitudes and behaviors of children and adolescents. Schools provide opportunities for youth to develop not only academic skills but also social and interpersonal skills. Researchers have focused on classroom and school context variables (e.g., lack of teacher support) that are positively associated with youth violence (Espelage, Low, & Jimerson, 2014a; Astor, Benbenishty, Zeira, & Vinokur, 2002). However, certain classroom and school variables have been identified as protective elements in youth violence prevention. For instance, opportunities for classroom discussions and learning have been recognized as an essential component of bullying prevention programs (see, e.g., Beale & Scott, 2001). Moreover, due to frequent interactions between youth and teachers in school, teachers' attitudes and involvement in particular are important. Youths' perceptions of their teachers as supportive and involved has been found to be an important component of reducing behavior problems, such as bullying (Flaspohler, Elfstrom, Vanderzee, Sink, & Birchmeier, 2009; Frey, Ruchkin, Martin, & Schwab-Stone, 2009). Findings from Verkuyten and Thijs' (2002) study also revealed that fewer children reported experiencing racially motivated bullying when they perceived their teachers as being involved. Teachers need to be trained to take a stand effectively to protect racial and ethnic minority and immigrant youth who are victimized.

Community/Neighborhood

Community-level patterns of racial inequality and discrimination and how they contribute to racial and ethnic minority and immigrant youths' involvement in violence have been researched extensively (Desmond & Kubrin, 2009; Sampson, Morenoff, & Raudenbush, 2005). Study findings have revealed that for racial minorities, residence in neighborhoods that are characterized as violent are significantly associated with violence and delinquent behavior (Chen, Voisin, & Jacobson, 2013; McMahon et al., 2013). Interestingly, Desmond and Kubrin (2009) also found that immigrant concentration is negatively associated with youth violence. Prevention programs are embedded within community and neighborhood contexts (Dishion & Stormshak, 2007), and community leaders and residents' involvement can foster prosocial youth development (McWhirter, McWhirter, McWhirter, & McWhirter, 2007). Also considering that family, peers, and schools are embedded in the community, school officials and professionals (e.g., social workers) need to work with the community leaders and residents in monitoring youth activities and providing needed resources that promote positive youth behaviors. Salcido, Ornelas, and Garcia's (2002) examination of a university community–based neighborhood watch program called Kid Watch found that youth participants perceived a sense of community, given their collaborations with school officials, researchers, and law enforcement, which decreased their fears and victimization. Kid Watch is a community-based program developed in 1995 and designed to keep "at-risk" children in school and to reduce youth crime and violence (Salcido et al., 2002). Collaborative work for organizing neighborhood watch programs or other community-based programs requires expanded roles for school practitioners.

A Call to Prevention Science

Relative to the voluminous research literature in the area of youth violence in the United States, studies that examine risk and protective factors among racial/ethnic minority and immigrant youth are sparse. Thus, it is imperative that more prevention scientists conduct basic research with diverse populations of youth in order to engage in culturally relevant violence prevention (Neville, Tynes, & Utsey, 2009). For example, findings from research on African American children and adolescents highlight an urgent need for additional research, particularly related to the strengths (individual, cultural, and contextual) that youth possess that may buffer against the negative outcomes that are associated with violence and victimization (American Educational Research Association, 2013). These studies need to move beyond crude measures of race and ethnicity and tap culturally relevant constructs, such as racial/ethnic identity, cultural capital, acculturation stress, and collective efficacy, to name a few (see, for example, Oyserman & Yoon, 2009). This call is also consistent with the importance of conceptualizing violence and victimization outcomes from a positive psychology framework, which emphasizes moving away from a risk-only or "pathologizing" focus and identifying strength and resilience of youth. In addition to identifying culturally relevant protective and resilience factors associated with violence and victimization experiences, prevention science scholars need to design studies that consider the intersection of the various structures of the social ecology (Espelage et al., 2014b).

Further, prevention science researchers also need to consider how efficacy of programs vary or are moderated by race, ethnicity, immigrant status, gender, and the intersections of these sociodemographic variables. This is most important for groups of youth who were not part of the development of programs. Perhaps the most striking example of this problem is the widely implemented OBPP, which has been found to be effective in decreasing bullying behavior and increasing prosocial behaviors, as indicated in several international study findings (Olweus & Limber, 2010). However, little to no adaptation is made when it is transported to the United States. The one and only U.S.-based randomized controlled trial study of the OBPP that has been published included an RCT of ten schools, where reductions of bullying were reported only for non-Hispanic White students (Bauer, Lozano, & Rivara, 2007), not racial and ethnic minority students. This points to the importance of developing programs with the input from the target populations, such as racial and ethnic minority and immigrant youth, which is particularly important when applying U.S.-based research in other countries.

Conclusion

This chapter makes a substantive contribution to the literature on youths' experiences in violence and victimization in relation to race/ethnicity and immigrant status. We are reminded of the importance of sociocultural factors that may act to marginalize and oppress racial/ethnic and immigrant youth, which can contribute to their experiences in violence victimization and perpetration. The other unique contribution of this chapter is that it is not limited to individual/sociodemographic characteristics; instead, it draws upon social-ecological (i.e., individual, family, school, and neighborhood environments) and resilience frameworks to understand more deeply both risk and protective factors that may foster or inhibit involvement in violence. The next logical step is to make recommendations to policy makers, school administrators, counselors, psychologists, and social workers on ways to address inequities that are inherent in the existing laws and improve the quality of services for racial and ethnic minority and immigrant children and adolescents who are both victims and perhaps even perpetrators of violence. To achieve this, it is imperative that we have an understanding of how to develop evidence-based remedial and preventative interventions that are culturally relevant for the growing number of racial and ethnic minority and immigrant youth in the United States.

References

Abdelkarim, R.Z. (2003). Arab and Muslim Americans: collateral damage in the wars on terrorism, Iraq. *Washington Report on Middle East Affairs* 22: 55–6.

Alexander, M. 2010. *The New Jim Crow: Mass Incarceration in the Age of Colorblindness.* New York: New Press.

American Educational Research Association (2013). *Prevention of Bullying in Schools, Colleges, and Universities: Research Report and Recommendations.* Washington, DC: American Educational Research Association.

Appleby, G. A., Colon, E., & Hamilton, J. (2011). *Diversity, Oppression, and Social Functioning: Person-in-Environment Assessment and Intervention* (3rd ed. Boston: Allyn & Bacon.

Astor, R. A., Benbenishty, R., Zeira, A., & Vinokur, A. (2002). School climate, observed risky behaviors, and victimization as predictors of high school students' fear and judgments of school violence as a problem. *Health Education & Behavior* 29: 716–36. doi: 10.1177/109019802237940

Bankston, C. L., & Caldas, S. J. (2002). *A Troubled Dream: The Promise and Failure of School Desegregation in Louisiana.* Nashville, TN: Vanderbilt University Press.

Bauer, N. S., Lozano, P., & Rivara, F. P. (2007). The effectiveness of the Olweus Bullying Prevention Program in public middle schools: a controlled trial. *Journal of Adolescent Health* 40: 266–74. doi: dx.doi.org/10.1016/j.jadohealth.2006.10.005

Beale, A. V., & Scott, P. C. (2001). "Bullybusters": using drama to empower students to take a stand against bullying behavior. *Professional School Counseling* 44: 300–5.

Beyers, J. M., Bates, J. E., Pettit, G. S., & Dodge, K. A. (2003). Neighborhood structure, parenting processes, and the development of youths' externalizing behaviors: a multilevel analysis. *American Journal of Community Psychology* 31: 35–53. doi: 10.1023/A:1023018502759

Black, B. M., Chido, L. M., Preble, K. M., Weisz, A. N., Yoon, J. S., Delaney-Black, V., Kernsmith, P., & Lewandowski, L. (2013). Violence exposure and teen dating violence among African American youth. *Journal of Interpersonal Violence*. doi: 10.1177/0886260514552271

Bograd, M. (1999). Strengthening domestic violence theories: intersections of race, class, sexual orientation, and gender. *Journal of Marriage and Family Therapy* 25: 275–89. doi: 10.1111/j.1752-0606.1999.tb00248.x

Bronfenbrenner, U. (1979). *Ecology of Human Development: Experiments by Nature and Design*. Cambridge, MA: Harvard University Press.

Centers for Disease Control and Prevention (2006). *Youth Violence: Fact Sheet*. www.cdc.gov.proxy.lib.umich.edu/ncipc/factsheets/yvfacts.htm

Centers for Disease Control and Prevention (2013). Homicide rates among persons aged 10–24 years – United States, 1981–2010. *MMWR* 62: 545–8.

Chen, P., Voisin, D. R., & Jacobson, K. C. (2013). Community violence exposure and adolescent delinquency: examining a spectrum of promotive factors. *Youth & Society*. doi: 10.1177/0044118X13475827

Cicchetti, D. (2013). Annual research review: resilient functioning in maltreated children: past, present, and future perspectives. *Journal of Child Psychology and Psychiatry* 54: 402–22. doi: 10.1111/j.1469-7610.2012.02608.s

Cicchetti, D., & Rogosch, F. A. (1996). Equifinality and multifinality in developmental psychopathology. *Development and Psychopathology* 8: 597–600. dx.doi.org/10.1017/S0954579400007318

Cicchetti, D., & Rogosch, F. A. (2012). Gene by environment interaction and resilience: effects of child maltreatment and serotonin, corticotropin releasing hormone, dopamine, and oxytocin genes. *Development and Psychopathology* 24: 411–27. doi: 10.1017/S0954579412000077

Compton, W. M., Gfroerer, J., Conway, K. P., & Finger, M. S. (2014). Unemployment and substance outcomes in the United States 2002–2010. *Drug and Alcohol Dependence*. Advance online publication. dx.doi.org/10.1016/j.drugalcdep.2014.06.012

Cooper, A., & Smith, E. L. (2011). *Homicide Trends in the United States, 1980–2008: Annual Rates for 2009 and 2010*. Washington, DC: U.S. Department of Justice, Office of Justice Programs, Bureau of Justice Statistics. www.bjs.gov/content/pub/pdf/htus8008.pdf

Dahlberg, L. L., & Krug, E. G. (2002). Violence: a global public health problem. In Krug, E., Dahlberg, L. L., Mercy, J. A., Zwi, A. B., & Lozano, R. (eds.), *World Report on Violence and Health*. Geneva, Switzerland: World Health Organization, pp. 1–56.

Decker, M., Raj, A., & Silverman, J. G. (2007). Sexual violence against adolescent girls: influence of immigration and acculturation. *Violence against Women* 13: 498–513. doi: 10.1177/1077801207300654

Desmond, S. A., & Kubrin, C. E. (2009). The power of place: immigrant communities and adolescent violence. *Sociological Quarterly* 50: 581–607. doi: 10.1111/j.1533-8525.2009.01153.x

Deutsch, A. R., Crockett, L. J., Wolff, J. M., & Russell, S. T. (2012). Parent and peer pathways to adolescent delinquency: variations by ethnicity and neighborhood context. *Journal of Youth and Adolescence* 41: 1078–94. doi: 10.1007/s10964-012-9754-y

DiClemente, R. J., Salazar, L. F., & Crosby, R. A. (2007). A review of STD/HIV preventive interventions for adolescents: sustaining effects using an ecological approach. *Journal of Pediatric Psychology* 32: 888–906. doi: 10.1093/jpepsy/jsm056

Dishion, T. J., & Stormshak, E. A. (2007). *Intervening in Children's Lives: An Ecological, Family-Centered Approach to Mental Health Care*. Washington, DC: American Psychological Association.

Duran, R., & Posadas, C. E. (2013). Disproportionate minority contact in the land of enchantment: juvenile justice disparities as a reflection of white-over-color ascendancy. *Journal of Ethnicity in Criminal Justice* 11: 93-111. doi: 10.1080/15377938.2013.739430

Eddy, J. M., Reid, J. B., & Fetrow, R. A. (2000). An elementary school-based prevention program targeting modifiable antecedents of youth delinquency and violence: linking the interests of families and teachers (LIFT). *Journal of Emotional and Behavioral Disorders* 8: 165–76. doi: 10.1177/106342660000800304

Elder, J. P., Lytle, L., Sallis, J. F., Young, D. R., Steckler A., Simons-Morton, D., . . . & Ribisl, K. (2007). A description of the social-ecological framework used in the trial of activity for adolescent girls (TAAG). *Health Education Research* 22: 155–65. doi: 10.1093/her/cyl059

Elsaesser, C. M., & Voisin, D. R. (2014). Correlates of polyvictimization among African American youth: an exploratory study. *Journal of Interpersonal Violence*. doi: 10.1177/0886260514554424

Espelage, D. L., Holt, M. K., & Henkel, R. R. (2003). Examination of peer-group contextual effects on aggression during early adolescence. *Child Development* 74: 205–20. doi: 10.1111/1467-8624.00531

Espelage, D. L., Low, S., & Jimerson, S. (2014a). Understanding school climate, aggression, peer victimization, and bully perpetration: contemporary science, practice, and policy. *School Psychology Quarterly* 29: 233–7. doi: dx.doi.org/10.1037/spq0000090

Espelage, D. L., Low, S., Rao, M. A., Hong, J. S., & Little, T. D. (2014b). Family violence, bullying, fighting, and substance use among adolescents: a longitudinal mediational model. *Journal of Research on Adolescence* 24: 337–49. doi: 10.1111/jora.12060

Espelage, D. L., Rao, M. A., & De La Rue, L. (2013). Current research on school-based bullying: a social-ecological perspective. *Journal of Social Distress and the Homeless* 22: 21–7. doi: dx.doi.org/10.1179/1053078913Z.0000000002

Fagan, A. A., & Catalano, R. F. (2013). What works in youth violence prevention: a review of the literature. *Research on Social Work Practice* 23: 141–56. doi: 10.1177/104973151245899

Fergus, S., & Zimmerman, M. A. (2005). Adolescent resilience: a framework for understanding healthy development in the face of risk. *Annual Review of Public Health* 26: 399–419. doi: 10.1146/annurev.publhealth.26.021304.144357

Fielding, J. E., Teutsch, S., & Breslow, L. (2010). A framework for public health in the United States. *Public Health Reviews* 32: 174–89.

Filindra, A., Blanding, D., & García Coll, C. (2011). The power of context: state-level policies and politics and the educational performance of the children of immigrants in the United States. *Harvard Educational Review* 81: 407–37.

Flannery, D. J., Singer, M. I., & Wester, K. (2001). Violence exposure, psychological trauma, and suicide risk in a community sample of dangerously violent adolescents. *Journal of the American Academy of Child & Adolescent Psychiatry* 40: 435–42. doi: dx.doi.org.10.1097/00004583-200104000-00012

Flaspohler, P. D., Elfstrom, J. L., Vanderzee, K. L., Sink, H. E., & Birchmeier, Z. (2009). Stand by me: the effects of peer and teacher support in mitigating the impact of bullying on quality of life. *Psychology in the School* 46: 636–49. doi: 10.1002/pits.20404

Frey, A., Ruchkin, V., Martin, A., & Schawb-Stone, M. (2009). Adolescents in transition: school and family characteristics in the development of violent behaviors entering high school. *Child Psychiatry & Human Development* 40: 1–13. doi: 10.1007/s10578-008-0105-x

Garcia-Reid, P., Reid, R. J., & Peterson, N. A. (2005). School engagement among Latino youth in an urban middle school context. *Education and Urban Society* 37: 257–75. doi: 10.1177/0013124505275534

Golden, S. D., & Earp, J. A. L. (2012). Social ecological approaches to individuals and their contexts: Twenty years of Health Education & Behavior Health promotion interventions. *Health Education & Behavior, 39*, 364–372. doi: 10.1177/1090198111418634

Green, L. W., Richard, L., & Potvin, L. (1996). Ecological foundations of health promotion. *American Journal of Health Promotion, 10*, 270–281. doi: http://dx.doi.org/10.4278/0890-1171-10.4.270

Harrell, E. (2007). *Black Victims of Violent Crime: Bureau of Justice Statistics Special Report*. Washington, DC: Department of Justice. Bureau of Statistics. www.ojp.usdoj.gov/bjs/pub/pdf/bvvc.pd

Herrenkohl, T. I., Maquin, E., Hill, K. G., Hawkins, J. D., Abbott, R. D., & Catalano, R. F. (2000). Developmental risk factors for youth violence. *Journal of Adolescent Health* 26: 176–86. doi: 10.1016/S1054-139X(99)00065-8

Hillyard, D., & McDermott, M. J. (2014). Ecological, peacemaking, and feminist considerations. In Muschert, G. W., Henry, S., Bracy, N. L., & Peguero, A. A. (eds.), *Responding to School Violence: Confronting the Columbine Effect*. Boulder, CO: Lynne Rienner, pp. 173–88.

Hong, J. S., & Espelage, D. L. (2012). A review of research on bullying and peer victimization in school: an ecological system analysis. *Aggression and Violent Behavior* 17: 311–22. doi: 10.1016/j.avb.2012.03.003

Hong, J. S., Peguero, A. A., Choi, S., Lanesskog, D., Espelage, D., & Lee, N. Y. (2014). School bullying and peer victimization of Latino and Asian American youth: a social-ecological framework. *Journal of School Violence* 13: 315–38. doi: 10.1080/15388220.2013.856013

Jacobs, D., Malone, C., & Iles, G. (2012). Race and imprisonment: vigilante violence, minority threat, and racial politics. *Sociological Quarterly* 53: 166–87. doi: 10.1111/j.1533-8525.2012.01230.x

Jenson, J. M., & Fraser, M. W. (2006). A risk and resilience framework for child, youth, and family policy. In J. M. Jenson & M. W. Fraser (Eds.), *Social policy for children and families: A risk and resilience perspective* (pp. 1–18). Thousand Oaks, CA: Sage.

Kaminski, J. W., Valle, L. A., Filene, J. H., & Boyle, C. L. (2008). A meta-analytic review of components associated with parent training program effectiveness.

Journal of Abnormal Child Psychology 36: 567–89. doi: 10.1007/s10802-007-9201-9

Knerr, W., Gardner, F., & Cluver, L. (2013). Improving positive parenting skills and reducing harsh and abusive parenting in low- and middle-income countries: a systematic review. *Prevention Science* 14: 352–63. doi: 10.1007/s11121-012-0314-1

Kramer, R. C. (2000). Poverty, inequality, and youth violence. *Annals of the American Academy of Political and Social Science* 567: 123–39. doi: 10.1177/000271620056700109

Kubrin, C., Zatz, M., & Martínez, R. (2012). *Punishing Immigrants: Policy, Politics, and Injustice*. New York: NYU Press.

Leidy, M. S., Guerra, N. G., & Toro, R. I. (2010). Positive parenting, family cohesion, and child social competence among immigrant Latino families. *Journal of Family Psychology* 24: 252–60. doi: dx.doi.org/10.1037/2168-1678.1.S.3

Low, S., & Espelage, D.L. (2014). Conduits from community violence exposure to bullying and victimization: contributions of parental monitoring, impulsivity and deviancy. *Journal of Counseling Psychology* 61: 221–31. doi: dx.doi.org/10.1037/a0035207

Masten, A. S. (2007). Resilience in developing systems: progress and promise as the fourth wave rises. *Development and Psychopathology* 19: 921–30. doi: dx.doi.org/10.1017/S0954579407000442

Masten, A. S. (2011). Resilience in children threatened by extreme adversity: frameworks for research, practice, and translational synergy. *Development and Psychopathology* 23: 493–506. doi: dx.doi.org/10.1017/S0954579411000198

McKenney, K. S., Pepler, D., Craig, W., & Connolly, J. (2006). Peer victimization and psychosocial adjustment: the experiences of Canadian immigrant youth. *Electronic Journal of Research in Educational Psychology* 9: 239–64.

McMahon, S. D., Todd, N. R., Martinez, A., Coker, C., Sheu, C. F., Washburn, J., & Shaw, S. (2013). Aggressive and prosocial behavior: community violence, cognitive, and behavioral predictors among urban African American youth. *American Journal of Community Psychology* 51: 407–21. doi: 10.1007/s10464-012-9560-4

McWhirter, J. J., McWhirter, B. T., McWhirter, E. H., & McWhirter, R. J. (2007). *At Risk Youth: A Comprehensive Response for Counselors, Teachers, Psychologists, and Human Service Professionals*, 4th ed. Belmont, CA: Thomson Brooks/Cole.

Michaud, P. A. (2006). Adolescents and risks: why not change our paradigm? *Journal of Adolescent Health* 38: 481–3. doi: 10.1016/j.jadohealth.2006.03.003

Narayan, A. J., Englund, M. M., Carlson, E. A., & Egeland, B. (2014). Adolescent conflict as a developmental process in the prospective pathway from exposure to interparental violence to dating violence. *Journal of Abnormal Child Psychology* 42: 239–50. doi: 10.1007/s10802-013-9782-4

Neville, H. A., Tynes, B. M., & Utsey, S. O. (2009). *African American Psychology: Trends and Future Directions*. Thousand Oaks, CA: Sage. search.proquest.com/docview/621807131?accountid=14553

Olweus, D. (2004). The Olweus Bullying Prevention Programme: design and implementation issues and a new national initiative in Norway. In Smith, P. K., Pepler, D., & Rigby, K. (eds.), *Bullying in Schools: How Successful Can Interventions*

Be? Cambridge, UK: Cambridge University Press, pp. 13–36. dx.doi.org/10.1017/CBO9780511584466.003

Olweus, D., & Limber, S. P. (2010). The Olweus Bullying Prevention Program: Implementation and evaluation over two decades. In Jimerson, S.R., Swearer, S.M., & Espelage, D.L. (eds.), *Handbook of Bullying in Schools: An International Perspective*. New York: Routledge, pp. 377–402.

Oyserman, D., & Yoon, K.-I. (2009). Neighborhood effects on racial–ethnic identity: the undermining role of segregation. *Race and Social Problems,* 1(2), 67–76. dx.doi.org/10.1007/s12552-009-9007-1

Ozer, E. J. (2006). Contextual effects in school-based violence prevention programs: a conceptual framework and empirical review. *Journal of Primary Prevention* 27: 315–40. doi: 10.1007/s10935-006-0036-x

Patton, D. U., Hong, J. S., Williams, A. B., & Allen-Meares, P. (2013). A review of research on school bullying among African American youth: an ecological systems analysis. *Educational Psychology Review* 25: 245–60. doi: 10.1007/s10648-013-9221-7

Peguero, A. A. (2009). Victimizing the children of immigrants: Latino and Asian American student victimization. *Youth & Society* 41: 186–208. doi: 10.1177/0044118X09333646

Peguero, A. A. (2012). Schools, bullying, and inequality: intersecting factors and complexities within the stratification of youth victimization at school. *Sociology Compass* 6: 402–12. doi: 10.1111/j.1751-9020.2012.00459.x

Peguero, A. A., & Popp, A. M. (2012). Youth violence at school and the intersection of gender, race, and ethnicity. *Journal of Criminal Justice* 40: 1–9. doi:10.1016/j.jcrimjus.2011.11.005

Peguero, A. A., Popp, A. M., & Koo, D. J. (2011). Race, ethnicity, and school-based adolescent victimization. *Crime & Delinquency* 61: 323–49. doi: 10.1177/0011128711398021

Perkins, H. W., & Berkowitz, A. D. (1986). Perceiving the community norms of alcohol use among students: some research implications for campus alcohol education programming. *International Journal of the Addictions* 21: 961–76. doi: 10.3109/10826088609077249

Perry, S. W. (2004). *American Indians and Crime: A BJS Statistical Profile, 1992–2002*. Washington, DC: U.S. Department of Justice, Office of Justice Programs, Bureau of Justice Statistics.

Provine, M. D., & Chavez, J. M. (2009). Race and the response of state legislatures to unauthorized immigrants. *Annals of the American Academy of Political and Social Science* 623: 78–92. doi: 10.1177/0002716208331014

Puzzanchera, C. (2013). *Juvenile Arrests 2011*. Washington, DC: Office of Juvenile Justice and Delinquency Prevention.

Reed, E., Lawrence, D. A., Santana, M. C., Seth, C., Welles, L., Horsburgh, C. R., ... Raj, A. (2014). Adolescent experiences of violence and relation to violence perpetration beyond young adulthood among an urban sample of black and African American males. *Journal of Urban Health* 91: 96–106.

Reese, L., Vera, E. M., & Hasbrouck, L. M. (2003). Examining the impact of violence on ethnic minority youth, their families, and communities: issues for prevention practice and resilience. In Bernai, G., Trimble, J. E., Burlew, K., & Leong, F. T. L. (eds.), *Handbook of Racial & Ethnic Minority Psychology*. Thousand Oaks, CA: Sage, pp. 465–85.

Reese, L. E., Vera, E. M., Simon, T. R., & Ikeda, R. M. (2000). The role of families and caregivers as risk and protective factors in preventing youth violence. *Clinical Child and Family Psychology Review* 3: 61–77. doi: 10.1023/A: 1009519503260

Renzulli, L., & Evans, L. (2005). School choice, charter schools, and white flight. *Social Problems* 52(3): 398–418. doi: dx.doi.org/10.1525/sp.2005.52.3.398

Richardson, J. W. (2008). From risk to resilience: promoting school-health partnerships for children. *International Journal of Educational Reform* 17: 19–36.

Robers, S., Kemp, J., Rathbun, A., & Morgan, R. E. (2014). *Indicators of School Crime and Safety: 2013* (NCES 2014-042/NCJ 243299). Washington, DC: National Center for Education Statistics, U.S. Department of Education, and Bureau of Justice Statistics, Office of Justice Programs, U.S. Department of Justice.

Rutter, M. (1985). Resilience in the face of adversity: protective factors and resistance to psychiatric disorders. *British Journal of Psychiatry* 147: 598–611. doi: 10.1192/bjp.147.6.598

Salcido, R. M., Ornelas, V., & Garcia, J. A. (2002). A neighborhood watch program for inner city school children. *Children & Schools* 24: 175–87. doi: 10.1093/cs/24.3.175

Salmivalli, C., Huttunen, A., & Lagerspetz, K. M. J. (1997). Peer networks and bullying in schools. *Scandinavian Journal of Psychology* 38: 305–12. doi: 10.1111/1467-9450.00040

Sampson, R. J., Morenoff, J. D., & Raudenbush, S. (2005). Social anatomy of racial and ethnic disparities in violence. *American Journal of Public Health* 95: 224–32. doi: 10.2105/AJPH.2004.037705

Serketich, W. J., & Dumas, J. E. (1996). The effectiveness of behavioral parent training to modify antisocial behavior in children: a meta-analysis. *Behavioral Therapy* 27: 171–86. doi: 10.1016/S0005-7894(96)80013-X

Simon, T. R., Miller, S., Gorman-Smith, D., Orpinas, P., & Sullivan, T. (2010). Physical dating violence norms and behavior among sixth-grade students from four U.S. sites. *Journal of Early Adolescence* 30: 395–409. doi: 10.1177/0272431609333301

Singh, N. N., Lancioni, G. E., Joy, S. D. S., Winton, A. S. W., Sabaawi, M., Wahler, R. G., & Singh, J. (2007). Adolescents with conduct disorder can be mindful of their aggressive behavior. *Journal of Emotional and Behavioral Disorders* 15: 56–63. doi: 10.1177/10634266070150010601

Stacey, M., Carbone-López, K., & Rosenfeld, R. (2011). Demographic change and ethnically motivated crime: the impact of immigration on anti-Hispanic hate crime in the United States. *Journal of Contemporary Criminal Justice* 27: 278–98. doi: 10.1177/1043986211412560

Stokols, D. (1996). Translating social ecological theory into guidelines for community health promotion. *American Journal of Health Promotion* 10: 282–98. doi: dx.doi.org/10.4278/0890-1171-10.4.282

Swearer, S. M., Peugh, J., Espelage, D. L., Siebecker, A. B., Kingsbury, W. L., & Bevins, K. S. (2006). A socioecological model for bullying prevention and intervention in early adolescence: an exploratory examination. In Jimerson, S. R., & Furlong, M. J. (eds.), *The Handbook of School Violence and School Safety: From Research to Practice*. Mahwah, NJ: Erlbaum, pp. 257–73.

Thornburgh, D., & Lin, H. (eds.) (2002). *Youth, Pornography, and the Internet*. Washington, DC: National Academy Press.

Umemoto, K., Baker, C. K., Helm, S., Miao, T. A., Goebert, D. A., & Hishinuma, E. S. (2009). Moving toward comprehensiveness and sustainability in a social ecological approach to youth violence prevention: lessons from the Asian/Pacific Islander Youth Violence Prevention Center. *American Journal of Community Psychology* 44: 221–32. doi: 10.1007/s10464-009-9271-7

United States Census Bureau (2012). *Current Population Survey*. Washington, DC: U.S. Census Bureau, Population Division.

United States Department of Justice (2009). *FBI Uniform Crime Reports*. Retrieved from www.fbi.gov/about-us/cjis/ucr.

Verkuyten, M., & Thijs, J. (2002). Racist victimization among children in the Netherlands: the effect of ethnic group and school. *Ethnic and Racial Studies* 25: 310–31. doi: 10.1080/01419870120109502

Voisin, D. R., Jenkins, E. J., & Takahashi, L. (2011). Toward a conceptual model linking community violence exposure to HIV-related risk behaviors among adolescents: directions for research. *Journal of Adolescent Health* 49: 230–6. doi: 10.1016/j.jadohealth.2011.01.002

Wang, J., Iannotti, R. J., & Nansel, T. R. (2009). School bullying among adolescents in the United States: physical, verbal, relational, and cyber. *Journal of Adolescent Health* 45: 368–75. doi : 10.1016/j.jadohealth.2009.03.021

Wang, M. T., & Dishion, T. J. (2012). The trajectories of adolescents' perceptions of school climate, deviant peer affiliation, and behavioral problems during the middle school years. *Journal of Research on Adolescence* 22: 40–53. doi: 10.1111/j.1532-7795.2011.00763.x

Wong, N. T. (2008). A participatory youth empowerment model and qualitative analysis of student voices on power and violence prevention. (Unpublished doctoral dissertation). University of Michigan, Ann Arbor.

Wright, E. M., & Fagan, A. A. (2013). The cycle of violence in context: exploring the moderating roles of neighborhood disadvantage and cultural norms. *Criminology* 51: 217–49. doi: 10.1111/1745-9125.12003

Yu, S. M., Huang, Z. H., Schwalberg, R. H., Overpeck, M., & Kogan, M. D. (2003). Acculturation and the health and well-being of U.S. immigrant adolescents. *Journal of Adolescent Health* 33: 479–88. doi: 10.1016/S1054-139X(03)00210-6

14 Early Intervention to Prevent Lifelong Consequences of Childhood Antisocial Behavior and Social Exclusion

Sajid Humayun & Stephen Scott

Introduction

Persistent childhood antisocial behavior (ASB) is remarkably common. Even when using relatively conservative criteria, diagnosable disorders affect 5 percent of the population (Scott, 2015). The diagnostic term Oppositional-Defiant Disorder (ODD), generally applied with younger children, requires the presence of symptoms such as arguing, tantrums, refusal to carry out instructions, spitefulness and blaming others. The term Conduct Disorder (CD) requires the presence of more serious violations such as fighting, using a weapon, physical cruelty to people or animals, running away from home, and stealing with force (American Psychiatric Association, 2013).

Whether they have ODD, CD, or serious conduct problems that do not meet a clinical threshold, these children are seriously impaired: at home, they evoke criticism and have few friends, and at school they are disruptive. There is high comorbidity with other childhood mental health problems; for example, they are ten times more likely to have ADHD (Barker, Oliver, & Maughan, 2010). Long-term prognosis is poor: there is high continuity to adult criminality and Antisocial Personality Disorder (ASPD; Zoccolillo, Pickles, Quinton, & Rutter, 1992), and these children are more likely to leave school without qualifications, end up unemployed, misuse drugs, and become a teenage parent (Beecham, 2014; Fergusson, Horwood, & Ridder, 2005). In fact, CD is the most reliable precursor to diverse adult mental illness (Kim-Cohen et al., 2003). The lifetime cost to the public of such high-risk children has been estimated to be up to $2.3 million in the United States (U.S.; Cohen & Piquero, 2009) and in England individuals with CD aged ten cost society ten times as much as controls by age twenty-eight (Scott, Knapp, Henderson, & Maughan, 2001), with a large burden of the cost falling to education services (Snell et al., 2013).

To be worth attempting prevention, CD needs to (a) be detectable early (b) be amenable to preventive or early intervention strategies that are potentially available and effective; and (c) proceed to a more seriously damaging condition later in a substantial proportion of cases. How do conduct disorders measure up to these criteria? (a) Early signs are relatively easy to detect at the individual level – parents and nursery workers or teachers can spot disruptive disorders fairly reliably, and screening instruments such as the Strengths and Difficulties Questionnaire (Goodman, 2001) detect it with good sensitivity and specificity. At a group level, identifiable demographic characteristics are available that increase the odds of conduct disorders severalfold, for example parents who are long-term unemployed, teenage mothers, and parents with mental health disorders. (b) As will be discussed in more detail later in this chapter, there are interventions that can work and that can potentially be made available, for example teaching children socioemotional skills in schools and training parents to encourage child prosocial behavior and use effective strategies to handle misbehavior. (c) A substantial proportion of young children continue into teenage and adulthood to serious outcomes. In summary, conduct disorders are a good candidate for attempting prevention on all three criteria. This is not the case to the same degree for all childhood disorders – thus, for example, depression is hard to detect reliably under age eight, has a waxing and waning course, and has modestly successful treatments when fully established later.

Yet only about a quarter of children in the United Kingdom (U.K.) meeting criteria for ODD/CD receive specialist help (Ford, Hamilton, Goodman, & Meltzer, 2005). Furthermore, many children and families receive treatment only in late childhood or adolescence, when outcomes are poorer (Office of the Surgeon General, 2001). There are also a large number of intervention and prevention approaches being used that are not grounded in empirically based theory but rather on general beliefs about psychotherapeutic counseling or medication and have little or no evidence of effectiveness (Bickman, Noser, & Summerfelt, 1999). This is despite the fact that there are a number of different prevention approaches that have been shown to work.

In this chapter, we first review different levels of prevention and then summarize what is known about the risk factors for ASB that prevention approaches should target. We then describe the different types of prevention programs for ASB and review the evidence for their effectiveness. We conclude by discussing some of the barriers that currently exist to implementation of these approaches and widespread prevention of childhood and adolescent ASB.

Levels and Modes of Delivery

The U.S. Institute of Medicine (1994) has proposed a classification of levels of prevention in accordance with the population served. *Universal prevention* is offered to the entire population of a particular area. *Targeted prevention* is offered to particular groups. *Targeted selective prevention* is aimed at children at increased risk by virtue of their membership of a vulnerable subgroup (e.g., the children of highly stressed, economically disadvantaged, single mothers) or because they are about to experience a life transition or stressful event (e.g., leaving school, divorce).

Targeted indicated prevention is directed at groups that are identified as being at risk by virtue of symptom patterns (e.g., aggressive behavior at home or at school).

Prevention can also be classified in accordance with the *modality* and *timing* of intervention. The modality refers to whether the intervention is delivered directly to the individual or via the parent, the teacher, school, or a combination. Examples of prevention programs that address ASB, at each of the levels and modalities, are given in Table 14.1.

Table 14.1 *Levels of Prevention* of Conduct Disorder and Modes of Delivery*

	Mode of Delivery			
Level	*Young Person*	*Parent*	*Teacher/School*	*Multimodal*
Universal (for all children in a particular area/ community)	Information and media campaigns addressing child and young person risk behaviors, e.g., drinking, carrying knives; self-help manuals, e.g., *I Can Problem Solve*[1]	Information and media campaigns addressing parenting behavior e.g., *Triple P level 1*[3]	*Socioemotional Learning* (SEL) programs as part of normal classes; whole-school antibullying programs	Community-wide prevention, e.g., after-school clubs and youth activity programs; surveillance, including police, closed circuit TV cameras, etc.
Targeted - Selective (for populations with a general risk factor, such as poverty or a teenage parent)	Campaigns directed at particular groups of children and young people, e.g., emotional self-awareness and control, self-esteem, positive social skills, conflict resolution	Programs addressing populations at risk, e.g., *Nurse–Family Partnership*[4] home-visiting program for young, unsupported, or poor mothers	Emotional processing or behavioral programs, e.g., *Promoting Alternative Thinking Strategies (PATHS)*[6] *the Good Behaviour Game*[7] *(GBG)*	Multiple services for at risk groups, e.g., *SureStart Centres*[9] in high-need areas with a range of helping professionals
Targeted - Indicated (for individuals already showing behaviors or signs indicative of the problem)	Anger management programs, e.g., *Coping Power*[2]	Group parenting programs, e.g., *Incredible Years*[5]	Problem-solving therapies for small groups of children with disruptive behavior, e.g., *Dinosaur School*[8]	Programs with several elements covering home and school, e.g., *Families and Schools Together (Fast Track)*[10]

* Using the Institute of Medicine (1994) classification.
Please note that the preceding interventions are examples of such programs.
[1] Aberson, Albury, Gutting, Mann, & Trushin (1987); [2] Larson & Lochman (2010); [3] Bor, Sanders, & Markie-Dadds (2002); [4] Olds (2007); [5] Webster-Stratton (2003); [6] Greenberg et al. (1998); [7] Barrish, Saunders, & Wolf (1969); [8] Webster-Stratton, Reid, & Stoolmiller. (2008); [9] Melhuish et al. (2008); [10] Conduct Problems Prevention Research Group (1999).

Timing refers to the developmental period when the intervention occurs: antenatal, infancy, preschool, middle childhood, or adolescence. While the aim of a prevention program will be to set a child off on a favorable life trajectory from the outset, just because an approach is effective early, for example by promoting secure attachment, this does not mean that the problem is solved. There may be new risk factors later in development, when a different approach to prevention may be needed, for example drug avoidance campaigns. Conversely, the fact that CD was not prevented early does not mean all hope of improvement is lost later – there are many interventions that are effective in adolescence (Lipsey, 2009).

Risk Factors

There is a great deal of research describing factors influencing ASB (Lahey, Moffitt, & Caspi, 2003; Loeber et al., 2005; Rutter, Giller, & Hagell, 1998), so a sensible starting point when deciding on intervention and prevention approaches is to consider the main causal factors and processes and then design approaches around them.

Parenting and Family Risk Factors

The relationship between parenting and family factors and the development of ASB is a particularly important one in informing prevention approaches. Specifically, the relationship between parent–child relationship quality and ASB is one of the most widely reported in the literature, repeatedly found in large-scale epidemiological investigations, intensive clinical investigations, and naturalistic studies of diverse samples using a mixture of methods (e.g. Denham et al., 2000). In particular, parenting styles characterized by low warmth and involvement, high hostility, inconsistent and harsh discipline, and poor supervision have been found to be associated with ASB (Stouthamer-Loeber, Loeber, Wei, Farrington, & Wikström, 2002). These are not just a reaction to child behavior; they have a causal role too (Patterson, 2002) and are modifiable (as discussed in the following).

Patterson (1982) proposed a specific mechanism to explain the relationship between poor parenting and the development of oppositional and aggressive behaviors in children. In this reinforcement model, a parent responds to mild oppositional behavior by a child with a prohibition to which the child responds by escalating his or her behavior, and mutual escalation continues until the parent backs off, thus negatively reinforcing the child's behavior. The parent's inconsistent behavior increases the likelihood of the child showing further oppositional or aggressive behavior. In addition to specific tests of Patterson's reinforcement model (Snyder & Patterson, 1995), there is ample evidence that conduct problems are associated with hostile, critical, punitive, and coercive parenting (Rutter et al., 1998).

In *44 Juvenile Thieves,* John Bowlby (1944) argued that a key factor in the development of criminal personality was early caregiving experiences and a resulting insecure attachment security status. Although attachment security is thought to be a lifelong organizer of personality development (Allen, Porter, McFarland, McElhaney, & Marsh, 2007), it has yet to be clearly established whether attachment difficulties have an independent causal role in the development of ASB. However, some evidence for this causal relationship is emerging. For example, Futh, O'Connor, Matias, Green, and Scott (2008) showed an independent association between insecure attachment and conduct problems using a doll play task with six year olds, and a recent metareview has shown that a secure attachment is protective against the development of ASB in childhood (Fearon, Bakermans-Kranenburg, van IJzendoorn, Lapsley, & Roisman, 2010). Less is known about attachment and ASB in adolescence. However, Scott, Briskman, Woolgar, Humayun, & O'Connor (2011) found that in adolescence insecure attachment predicted conduct problems, even after taking into account current parenting quality, suggesting it may have at least a maintaining role.

While research suggests a strong relationship between parenting styles and ASB, the role of different family characteristics is not as clear. On the one hand, there is some evidence to suggest that growing up in a chaotic and disorganized home acts as a causal risk factor for childhood ASB and juvenile delinquency, both by exacerbating the effect of bad parenting, but it also increases the risk of ASB independently of parenting, and this relationship is not due to household income or social class (Coldwell, Pike, & Dunn, 2006; Deater-Deckard et al., 2009; Humayun, Oliver, Malpass, Chesnokov, & Scott, 2015). In fact, while there is an association between severe poverty and early-childhood conduct problems (Murray & Farrington, 2010), research has indicated that the association is indirect, mediated via family processes such as marital discord and parenting deficits (Costello, Compton, Keeler, & Angold, 2003; Hill & Maughan, 2001).

Similarly, the relationship between growing up in a single-parent family and ASB is not a straightforward one. While the presence of a prosocial father appears to reduce the risk of ASB, the presence of an antisocial father increases the risk of ASB (Jaffee, Moffitt, & Caspi, 2003), and therefore in some cases children may have better outcomes in a single-parent family. Experiencing a broken home is predictive of ASB and of having a violent criminal conviction by age fifty (Theobald, Farrington, & Piquero, 2013). However, it is important to note that the relationship between ASB and divorce is at least partly mediated by the experience of family conflict leading up to divorce (Amato & Keith, 1991; Krishnakumar & Buehler, 2000). Longitudinal studies have shown that behavior problems are present before divorce (e.g. Block, Block, & Gjerde, 1988) and in some cases reduce after divorce (Johnston, Kline, & Tschann, 1989). Many studies have shown that children exposed to domestic violence between adults are subsequently more likely to themselves become aggressive (Moffitt & Caspi, 1998), possibly because of the effect of conflict on children's regulation of emotion (Cummings & Davies, 2002; Davies & Cummings, 1994) and because they may imitate the aggression they witness (Bandura, 1977; Osofsky, 1995).

The relationship between children's own experience of maltreatment and ASB are well established (Fergusson, Horwood, & Lynskey, 1996; Fergusson, Lynskey, & Horwood, 1996). However, little is known about the possible mechanisms linking maltreatment to conduct problems, although threats to security of attachment, difficulties in affect regulation, distortions of information processing, and self-concept are likely to be relevant. One study found that physical punishment was clearly associated with behavior problems in White American children, but not in African American children (Deater-Deckard, Dodge, Bates, & Pettit, 1996), although a more recent American study found that the association was present across different ethnic groups (Wang & Kenny, 2014).

Risks outside the Family: Neighborhood and Peers

Beyond the family, peers play an important role through two mechanisms, peer rejection and association with delinquent peers (Gifford-Smith, Dodge, Dishion, & McCord, 2005). Again, both of these are potentially modifiable. A particularly harmful aspect of the latter is membership of a gang (Gatti, Tremblay, Vitaro, & McDuff, 2005). The neighborhood a child lives in can also exacerbate delinquent tendencies, with low ties to the neighborhood, poor social control of behavior, and exposure to risky activities such as drug taking all contributing (Murray & Farrington, 2010). However, individual differences can determine the extent to which the child's neighborhood can affect his or her ASB (Lynam et al., 2000), and the combination of a violent neighborhood and the experience of childhood maltreatment has been shown to be particularly detrimental (Cecil, Viding, Barker, Guiney, & McCrory, 2014b).

Individual and Cognitive Risk Factors

Several prospective studies have shown associations between temperament and conduct problems (Keenan & Shaw, 2003), and that temperament also predicted ASPD and criminal offending into adulthood (Caspi, Moffitt, Newman, & Silva, 1996). Conduct disordered children, delinquent adolescents, and adult antisocial individuals also show poor performance on standardized tests of verbal ability, and in tests of IQ, poor verbal and performance scores (Lynam & Henry, 2001; Nigg & Huang-Pollock, 2003). Longitudinal studies show that persistence in ASB over periods of years is predicted by low verbal IQ in childhood (Lahey et al., 1995; Lynam & Henry, 2001). Several possible ways in which poor verbal ability might influence behavior can be drawn from Luria's theory of the role of verbal memory and verbal abstract reasoning in the development of self-control (Luria, 1961). The abilities to recall oral instructions and to use language to think through the consequences of actions contribute to the effective control of actions. Children who cannot reason or assert themselves verbally may attempt to gain control of social exchanges using aggression (Dodge, 1993). It is likely that there are also indirect effects in which low verbal IQ contributes to academic difficulties that in turn mean that the child's experience of school becomes unrewarding rather than a source of self-esteem and support.

Children and adolescents with conduct problems have been shown consistently to have poor tested executive functions (Hobson, Scott, & Rubia, 2011; Lynam & Henry, 2001; Moffitt, 1993b; Nigg & Huang-Pollock, 2003). Executive functions comprise those abilities implicated in successfully achieving goals through appropriate, effective actions and inhibiting inappropriate responses. These mental functions are largely, although not exclusively, associated with frontal lobes (Pennington & Ozonoff, 1996). Important data come from a Montreal cohort studied from the age of six years (Seguin, Pihl, Harden, Tremblay, & Boulerice, 1995). Chronic aggression was associated with lower scores on tests tapping executive functions of the frontal brain region, and the findings held after controlling for general memory, IQ, and ADHD. Although most studies of executive deficit involve adolescents, such deficits have also been linked with disruptive behaviors in very young preschool children (Hughes, Dunn, & White, 1998; Speltz, DeKlyen, Calderon, Greenberg, & Fisher, 1999).

Dodge (1993) proposed the leading information-processing model for the genesis of aggressive behaviors within social interactions. The model hypothesizes that children who are prone to aggression focus on threatening aspects of others' actions, interpret hostile intent in the neutral actions of others, and are more likely to select and to favor aggressive solutions to social challenges. Several studies have demonstrated that aggressive children make such errors of social cognition (Dodge, Coie, & Lynam, 2007). Dodge (1993) hypothesized that these tendencies are the result of repeated exposure to physical maltreatment, and there is some limited evidence to support this claim (Dodge, Pettit, Bates, & Valente, 1995).

Genetic Mechanisms

Genetic Liability

There is now solid evidence from twin and adoption studies that conduct problems assessed both dimensionally and categorically are substantially heritable (Moffitt, 2005; Rhee & Waldman, 2002). However, genetic risk will typically lead to adverse outcomes in interaction with circumstances in the child's environment. Adoption studies have reported an interaction between ASB in the biological parent and adverse conditions in the adoptive home that predicted the adopted child's antisocial outcome (Bohman, 2007; Cadoret, Yates, Woodworth, & Stewart, 1995). A twin study also yielded evidence that family genetic liability and the experience of maltreatment interact (Jaffee et al., 2005), and there is some limited evidence suggesting that the effect of universal school-based prevention programs can be modified by genetic factors (Musci et al., 2014).

An emerging area of research demonstrating the complexity of gene-environment interactions is the study of epigenetics. In a seminal series of studies on rats, Meaney and his colleagues have shown that experimentally induced poor parenting (a paradigm in which the young pups are removed from their cages for three hours a day, so their mothers fail to lick and groom them and thereby neglect their care) leads the offspring to behave in a disturbed way. However, it also affects the way their genes function (Bagot & Meaney, 2010). The result is methylation and acetylation of neurotransmitter promoting genes, which has the effect of dampening the expression of the genes without changes in the nucleotide sequence (Zhang et al., 2010). The research on the epigenetics of ASB in humans is in its infancy, but studies showing the role of epigenetic mechanisms are beginning to emerge (e.g. Cecil et al., 2014a).

The result of epigenetic effects may not be all bad. Thus, there is some evidence that under stressful conditions, rats that are raised harshly perform better than ones that are raised benignly (Bagot & Meaney, 2010). This suggests that epigenetics may be one of nature's mechanisms for adapting mammals to their environments, through which genetic and cellular mechanisms may confer evolutionary advantages (van IJzendoorn, Bakermans-Kranenburg, & Ebstein, 2011). It has been proposed that prenatal stress in humans may make male offspring better fitted to threatening environments by increasing their aggressiveness and may make female offspring better fitted for an adverse world by making them more anxious of threatening stimuli, so they become more protective mothers (Glover & Hill, 2012).

The genetic mechanisms described above are among a series of research findings that are beginning to alter the way in which the effects of an adverse environment on the development of ASB are conceptualized. There is increasing evidence that the traditional view that some children are at heightened risk for the development of ASB while others are resilient (Thomas & Chess, 1977) is too simplistic. Instead, the emerging view is that children differ in their susceptibility to the environment, for better or for worse (Belsky & Pluess, 2013; Ellis, Boyce, Belsky, Bakermans-Kranenburg, & van IJzendoorn, 2011). This has important implications for prevention approaches as some children may be more amenable to the effects of intervention than others.

Subtypes

As described previously, while risk factors are present in multiple domains (see Murray & Farrington, 2010, for a more thorough review), recent research indicates that there are likely to be three distinct pathways to antisocial and violent behavior, each with its own cluster of risk factors (Pardini & Frick, 2013).

First, the timing of onset of ASB has been shown to delineate groups of individuals, such that those with early onset of ASB (before age ten) appear to constitute a separate and more severe group than those whose ASB begins in adolescence (Moffitt, 1993a). Individuals with early onset ASB are more likely to exhibit early hyperactivity and oppositional behavior (Moffitt, 2006), tend to come from families who use harsh and inconsistent parenting practices (Odgers et al., 2008), and are at higher risk of lifetime criminality (Farrington, 2005; Odgers et al., 2008) and life failure (Piquero, Farrington, Nagin, & Moffitt, 2010). They are at substantially greater risk of delinquent acts in adolescence and continued violence and offending into adulthood, and many develop ASPD, a disorder synonymous with psychopathic traits and violence (Loeber et al., 2005; Soderstrom, Sjodin, Carlstedt, & Forsman, 2004; Sourander, Elonheimo, & Niemela, 2006). However, recent studies are beginning to challenge the view that the ASB that emerges in adolescence is likely to be limited to the teenage years (e.g. Farrington, Ttofi, & Coid, 2009).

Second, children with callous-unemotional (CU) traits appear to be an etiologically distinct group with low empathy and high fearlessness. These are children who are cruel to animals, have difficulty making friends, and engage in acts of premeditated violence. CU traits have higher genetic heritability than CD (Viding, Blair, Moffitt, & Plomin, 2005) and are associated with a different pattern of neurocognitive deficits such as reduced amygdala function (Kiehl et al., 2001). They are also strongly associated with the development of ASPD and psychopathy (Feilhauer & Cima, 2013; Frick & White, 2008) and are predictive of criminal offending in early adulthood (Kahn, Byrd, & Pardini, 2013). The presence of CU traits in antisocial children has important treatment implications. Studies have shown that these children are more resistant to punishment and are more difficult to treat (Hawes & Dadds, 2005). However, it is not the case that they cannot benefit from treatment (as discussed later in this chapter), and a key target for intervention may be empathy and the quality of the parent–child relationship (Dadds et al., 2011).

Third, a number of studies have begun to support a causal pathway associated with poor regulation of anger. These are children who misinterpret ambiguous social cues as threatening, which may lead them to respond in an aggressive and violent manner (De Castro, Veerman, Koops, Bosch, & Monshouwer, 2002). There is often a history of harsh discipline in this group (Pasalich, Dadds, Hawes, & Brennan, 2011). However, the association between harsh discipline and ASB seems to be most pronounced among those with a genetic susceptibility (Taylor & Kim-Cohen, 2007).

Implications for Prevention and Intervention Approaches

Social learning theory proponents (e.g., Patterson, 1982) suggest that the immediate environment is crucial in engendering ASB, with the responses to ASB provided by parents and then later peers, shaping delinquency. By ignoring prosocial behavior and inadvertently rewarding aggression (e.g., by giving in to threats or tantrums), parents reinforce ASB. This has formed the basis of parenting programs for ASB that try to change these contingent responses. The quality of the parent–child relationship may also be important, although care should be taken not to focus entirely on the attachment relationship (Woolgar & Scott, 2014).

Within the individual at a psychological level, different theories lead to different intervention approaches. For example, cognitive theory has led to cognitive therapies that concentrate on the way the youth perceives threats and cues (e.g. Kazdin, Bass, Siegel, & Thomas 1989). On the other hand, if the causal theory postulates that the fundamental problem is one of emotional overreactivity, then teaching youth to become more aware of their own emotions and develop strategies to control these emotions may be tried, as in anger management programs (e.g., Lochman & Wells, 2002). While evidence is accruing for neurobiological and genetic risks, rather few findings on these mechanisms have led to treatment approaches so far. On the other hand, the large body of evidence on the relationship between early onset of conduct problems and juvenile delinquency suggests that early prevention may be sensible (Loeber & Farrington, 2000).

It is important to note that prevention is not only about the removal of risks for ASB but also about enhancing protective factors. For example, this could involve encouraging children to engage in an activity or hobby in which they can take pride and that would therefore improve their self-esteem. Further, risk factors do not appear to operate in a purely additive way, with a linear increase in risk of conduct problems or delinquency per each additional risk factor. Instead, a larger number of risk factors appear to confer a disproportionately higher risk (Appleyard, Egeland, Dulmen, & Sroufe, 2005). The implications of this for prevention approaches would appear to be that several risk factors need to be tackled in order for interventions to be successful. It follows then that children should be assessed for these risk and protective factors and prevention approaches tailored accordingly.

Prevention and Intervention Approaches

Family-Based Approaches

Prevention Starting in Pregnancy

As noted previously, the effects of parenting start early, therefore prevention approaches that start equally early are likely to be particularly effective. There are two main types of very early intervention. Firstly, some interventions aim to strengthen the couple relationship in order to improve the quality of parenting in the early years. One of these programs, Family Foundations, has shown some initial evidence of improved child behavior at three to four years after birth (Feinberg, Jones, Kan, & Goslin, 2010) due to improved co-parenting (Solmeyer, Feinberg, Coffman, & Jones, 2014). Second, and more commonly, home visiting by trained nurses and health visitors has been used as a form of early prevention of child behavior problems. The results of evaluations of the majority of these programs have been mixed (Bernazzani & Tremblay, 2006; Bilukha et al., 2005). The exception is the *Nurse–Family Partnership* (NFP; disseminated in England under the name Family–Nurse Partnership), devised by David Olds and colleagues (2007).

In NFP, at-risk mothers (determined by, for example, being a poor teenaged parent) are visited at home before their child is born and then regularly for the next two years. A thorough evaluation is made and a range of evidence-based, manualized interventions is implemented by a nurse who has built up a trusting relationship with the mother. The nurses have three major goals: (1) improve the outcomes of pregnancy by helping women improve their prenatal health, for example, by smoking and drinking cessation where indicated; (2) improve the child's health and development by helping parents provide more competent care; and (3) improve parents' life course by helping them develop visions for their futures, make good choices about planning future pregnancies, complete their education, and find work. Toward these goals, the nurses help women build supportive relationships with family members and friends, especially boyfriends, fathers, and grandmothers, and link families with other services. There have been three major randomized controlled trials, and results show reduced abuse and neglect in mothers and lower levels of offending in the NFP group when the children were fifteen (Olds et al., 1998), although effects at age nineteen were significant only for girls (Eckenrode et al., 2010). While NFP is relatively expensive, cost-benefit analyses have shown a three- to four-times rate of return for every dollar spent on the program (Welsh & Farrington, 2011). However, evidence up to the present comes almost entirely from the United States, and results from a U.K. randomized controlled trial (RCT) are yet to be reported, although the initial pilot results have been promising (Barnes et al., 2011).

Programs Based on Social Learning Theory

These programs have evolved for more than forty years, and there is a large evidence base. Most are aimed at ASB as their proximal target outcome and take the form of parent management training. The content and delivery of a typical program are described in this section. There have been several adaptations for low- and middle-income countries (LMICs) (see the section "Parenting Programs in Low- and Middle-Income Countries" later in this chapter). Most basic programs take 8 to 12 sessions, lasting 1.5 to 2 hours each. Full accounts of programs are given by the developers (e.g. Markie-Dadds & Sanders, 2006; Webster-Stratton & Reid, 2003).

Format of Typical Social Learning Parenting Programs

Teaching a Child-Centered Approach

The first session covers play. Parents are asked to follow the child's lead rather than impose their own ideas. Instead of giving directions, teaching, and asking questions during play, parents are instructed simply to give a running commentary on their child's actions. As soon as the parent complies, the practitioner gives feedback. After ten to fifteen minutes, this directly supervised play ends and the parent is "debriefed" for half an hour or more alone with the clinician.

The second session involves elaboration of play skills. The previous week's "homework" of playing at home is discussed with the parent in considerable detail. Often there are practical reasons for not doing it ("I have to look after the other children, I've got no help"), and parents are then encouraged to solve the problem and find ways around the difficulty. For some parents, there may be emotional blocks ("it feels wrong – no one ever played with me as a child") that need to be overcome before they feel able to practice the homework.

After this discussion, live practice with the child is carried out. This time, the parent is encouraged to go beyond describing the child's behavior and to make comments describing the child's likely mood state (e.g., "you're really trying hard making that tower," or, "that puzzle is making you really fed up"). This process has benefits for both the parent and the child. The parent gets better at observing the fine details of the child's behavior, which makes the parent more sensitive to the child's mood. The child gradually gets better at understanding and labeling his or her own emotional states.

Increasing Desirable Child Behavior

Praise and rewards are covered here. The parent is required to praise the child for lots of simple everyday behaviors, such as playing quietly on his or her own, eating nicely, and so on. In this way the frequency of desired behavior increases. However, many parents find this difficult. Usually, with directly coached practice, praise becomes easier. Later sessions go through the use of reward charts.

Imposing Clear Commands

A hallmark of ineffective parenting is a continuing stream of ineffectual, nagging demands for the child to do something. Parents need to be taught to reduce the number of demands, but make them much more authoritative. This is done through altering both the manner in which they are given and what is said. The manner should be forceful (standing over the child, fixing him or her in the eye, and in a clear firm voice giving the instruction). The emotional tone should be calm, without shouting and criticism. The content should be phrased directly ("I want you to . . ."). It should be specific ("keep the sand in the box"' rather than vague ("do be tidy"). It should be simple (one action at a time, not a chain of orders) and performable immediately. Commands should be phrased as what the parent does want the child to do, not as what the child should stop doing ("please speak quietly" rather than "stop shouting"). Instead of threatening the child with vague, dire consequences ("you're going to be sorry you did that"), "when–then" commands should be given ("when you've laid the table, then you can watch television").

Reducing Undesirable Child Behavior

Consequences for disobedience should be applied as soon as possible. They must always be followed through: children quickly learn to calculate the probability that consequences will be applied, and if a sanction is given only every third occasion, a child is being taught he or she can misbehave the rest of the time. Simple logical consequences should be devised and enforced for everyday situations (e.g., if a child refuses to eat dinner, there will be no pudding). The consequences should "fit the crime," should not be punitive, and should not be long term (e.g., no bike riding for a month), as this will lead to a sense of hopelessness in the child, who may see no point in behaving well if it seems there is nothing to gain. Consistency of enforcement is central.

Time-out from positive reinforcement remains the final "big one" as a sanction for unacceptable behavior. The point here is to put the child in a place away from a reasonably pleasant context. Parents must resist responding to taunts and cries from the child during time-out, as this will reinforce the child by giving attention. Time-out provides a break for the adult to calm down also.

Effectiveness of Social Learning Parenting Programs

Behavioral parent training is the most extensively studied treatment for children's conduct problems, and there is considerable empirical support for its effectiveness (Furlong et al., 2012; Piquero et al. 2009; Weisz, Jensen-Doss, & Hawley, 2006) Several programs are considered well-established according to American Psychological Association criteria, after multiple randomized trials (e.g. Patterson, 1982; Webster-Stratton, Reid, & Hammond, 2001) and replications by independent research groups (e.g. Scott et al., 2001). Evaluations of the Incredible Years program show consistent reductions in conduct problems and disorder in a preventive context (Menting, Orobio de Castro, & Matthys, 2013; Scott et al., 2010b; Webster-Stratton & Reid, 2010) and improvements in aspects of parenting beyond those conceptualized in social learning theory, such as attachment-based measures of sensitive responding (O'Connor, Matias, Futh, Tantam, & Scott, 2013). Effects are bigger for more severe conduct problems and can be small in universal preventive approaches (Scott et al., 2010a). Randomized trials have shown the effectiveness of Triple P (e.g., Bor et al. 2002; Sanders, Kirby, Tellegen, & Day, 2014; Sanders, Markie-Dadds, Tully, & Bor, 2000; Wilson et al., 2012), and there is at least one independent replication supporting the Parent–Child Interaction Therapy model (Nixon, Sweeney, Erickson, & Touyz, 2003).

These studies suggest that behavioral parent training leads to short-term reductions in ASB, and there is evidence of positive effects in middle- as well as high-income countries (Baker-Henningham, 2011). Follow-up studies suggest enduring effects at up to six years after treatment (Hood & Eyberg, 2003; Reid, Webster-Stratton, & Hammond, 2003). Furthermore, a recent study found fewer elements of antisocial personality when children were followed up in adolescence (Scott, Briskman, & O'Connor, 2014). These effects were found in a sample of children screened in childhood for ASB but not in a sample of more severe clinic-referred children. Modeling analyses suggest that these reductions are likely to result in long-term savings to public expenditure (Bonin, Stevens, Beecham, Byford, & Parsonage, 2011). It should be noted that the wider terms "parenting support" and "parenting programs" cover a broad range of approaches, many of which are not evidence-based and therefore cannot be advocated.

Parenting Programs in Low- and Middle-Income Countries

The main technology used in parenting programs is human skill, so in principle, parenting programs should be capable of being used in LMICs with no loss of effectiveness, providing cultural issues are appropriately addressed and staff are suitably trained. The systematic review by Knerr, Gardner, and Cluver (2013) found twelve published trials of parenting programs in LMICs. These took place in a wide range of locations, including China, Pakistan, Ethiopia, South Africa, Brazil, Jamaica, and Iran. All studies reported significant ($p < 0.05$), positive effects of the intervention on parent–child interaction at all time points, which ranged from one month to six years. Effect sizes were provided or could be calculated for four of the seven parent–child interaction outcomes, and ranged from 0.24 (small) in the study with the largest sample to 1.59 (large) in the smallest study and thus were of similar magnitude to the effect sizes found in developed countries.

Given the differences between high-income countries and LMICs in cultural beliefs about families, and about what are desirable parenting practices, the interventions were adapted to suit the countries in which they were carried out. For example, the "Learning through Play" program, adapted for use in Pakistan, utilizes a pictorial calendar featuring information about child development, thus avoiding the need for parent literacy (Rahman, Iqbal, Roberts, & Husain, 2009, p. 57). In China, Jin et al. (2007) similarly used a program that had picture aids, including materials to encourage parents to play with their children using locally available materials.

Because ASB is also manifest in the school setting, Baker-Henningham, Scott, Jones, and Walker (2012) tested an adaptation of the Incredible Years program for teachers in large nursery classes (with thirty-five to forty children per teacher, whether teacher was unqualified) in Jamaica. Careful attention was given to training the staff to become adequately skilled in the program, and the study was notable for using direct observation rather than just teacher report to evaluate outcomes. The program was effective and significantly reduced ASB in the classroom and improved child friendliness.

Self-Help Programs

There will never be sufficient professional and volunteer practitioners to assist everyone who could benefit from help with parenting, and some parents may not have the time or inclination to seek help from other people. Therefore, there is a need for accessible, acceptable, and effective means for parents to learn by themselves. A trial comparing a typical eleven-session parenting group versus one session followed by instruction to use a book showed that both were superior to being on a waiting list, although the more intensive approach produced better results (Kling, Forster, Sundell, & Melin, 2010). A review of seven other RCTs of self-help concluded they were effective (O'Brien & Daley, 2011), and trials of Internet-based programs are on their way.

Family Therapy

As described in the preceding, parenting programs are one of the best researched interventions for behavior problems in children and are recommended by the U.K. National Institute for Clinical Excellence as the intervention of choice for CD (NICE, 2013). However, there is less evidence for their effectiveness in adolescents, and family-based interventions for delinquent youth have typically added additional elements to parent management techniques attempting to alter the structure and functioning of the family unit, being based on systemic family therapy theories. The best known in the context of delinquency is Functional Family Therapy (FFT), brought into being in 1969 by James Alexander and colleagues (Alexander, Pugh, Parsons, & Sexton, 2000). It is designed to be practicable and relatively inexpensive; eight to twelve one-hour sessions are given in the family home, to overcome attendance problems common in this client group; for more intractable cases, twenty-six to thirty hours are offered, usually over three months. The target age range is eleven to eighteen.

Following assessment, there are four phases to treatment. The first two are the *engagement* and *motivation* phases. Here the therapist works hard to enhance the perception that change is possible. The aim is to keep the family in treatment and then to move on to find what precisely the family wants. Techniques include reframing, whereby positive attributes are enhanced, such as a youth who offends often but does not get caught being labeled as bright, and the emotional motivation is brought out, such as a mother who continually nags being labeled as caring, upset, and hurt.

The third phase of FFT targets *behavior change*. There are two main elements to this: communication training and parent training. The success of this stage is dependent on the first two having been achieved, and it has not commenced unless they have been. This stage is applied flexibly according to family needs. Thus if there are two parents who continually argue and this is impinging on the adolescent, the "marital subsystem" will be addressed, using standard techniques. Parent training techniques are similar to those found in standard approaches, and include praise, rewards (called contracting in FFT – e.g., if you come home by 6 P.M. each night, I will take you to the cinema on Saturday), limit setting, consequences and response cost (e.g., losing TV time for swearing).

The fourth and final phase of FFT is *generalization*. Here the goal is to get the improvements made in a few specific situations to generalize to other similar family situations and to help the youth and family negotiate positively with community agencies, such as the school, and help them get the resources they need. Sometimes this latter goal may require the therapist to be a case manager for the family. To do this therefore requires that the therapist knows the community agencies and how the system works and is prepared to spend time engaging it – these characteristics are specified in the model. This is a very different approach from traditional therapies in which the therapist stays neutral with regard to outside agencies.

The effectiveness of FFT is fairly well established; there have been over ten replication studies (Alexander et al., 2000), of which over half have been independent of the developers. The trials published to date all have been positive, with typical recidivism rates being 20 to 30 percent lower than in controls, and cost-benefit analyses show a return of up to $14 per $1 invested (Lee et al., 2012). Like many evidence-based interventions, the importance of high fidelity to the model in order to achieve change has often been highlighted (Graham, Carr, Rooney, Sexton, & Wilson Satterfield, 2014; Sexton & Turner, 2010). However, most studies have been in the United States (although see Graham et al., 2014; Hartnett, Carr, & Sexton, 2015), and the methodological quality of evaluations has not always been high. Importantly, the first non-U.S. trial written in English and comparing FFT to an active, therapeutic control intervention (Youth Offending casework) found that it was no more effective at reducing ASB than the control intervention (Pearse & Humayun, 2015). Further research on this program is needed in order to establish its effectiveness when compared to the more substantial usual services in the United Kingdom and Europe.

Interventions with Individual Children and Youth

Prevention programs that have focused on the individual child rather than the family have typically either aimed to provide intellectual enrichment and social skills training or focused on helping children manage their emotions, usually using CBT approaches. These are sometimes delivered at an individual level and sometimes through schools.

Intellectual Enrichment Approaches

These preschool prevention approaches, such as the Perry Preschool project (Schweinhart, Barnes, Weikart, Barnett, & Epstein, 1993; Schweinhart et al., 2005), target risk factors of low intelligence and educational attainment. The aims are improved cognitive skills, school readiness, and better social and emotional development (Currie, 2001). Children who received the Perry Preschool intervention had lower arrest rates at ages nineteen and twenty-seven (Schweinhart et al., 1993) and at age forty (Schweinhart et al., 2005), and cost-benefit analyses indicate a $7 return for each $1 invested (Barnett, 1996), rising to a $17 return by age forty (Schweinhart et al., 2005). One of the other largest enrichment programs, Head Start, had similar but smaller effects, with lower arrest rates between ages eighteen and thirty (Garces, Thomas, & Currie, 2002; note that this is not a randomized study) and a $2 to $3 dollar for each $1 spent (Aos, Lieb, Mayfield, Miller, & Pennucci, 2004). More generally, a meta-analysis of preschool and daycare programs found a small but significant effect on reduced ASB (Farrington & Welsh, 2002).

School-Based Approaches

At a universal level, social and emotional learning (SEL) programs aim to enable children to acquire core competencies to recognize and manage emotions, set and achieve positive goals, appreciate the perspectives of others, establish and maintain positive relationships, make responsible decisions, and handle interpersonal situations constructively. The proximal goals of SEL programs are to foster the development of five interrelated sets of cognitive, affective, and behavioral competencies: self-awareness, self-management, social awareness, relationship skills, and responsible decision making (Durlak, Weissberg, Dymnicki, Taylor, & Schellinger, 2011). These competencies, in turn, should provide a foundation for better adjustment and academic performance as reflected in more positive social behaviors, fewer conduct problems, less emotional distress, and improved test scores and grades. Over time, mastering SEL competencies should result in a developmental progression that leads to a shift from being predominantly controlled by external factors to acting increasingly in accord with internalized beliefs and values, caring and having concern for others, making good decisions, and taking responsibility for one's choices and behaviors.

Probably the best researched and most widely implemented formal SEL program is Promoting Alternative Thinking Strategies (PATHS; Greenberg, Kusche, Mihalic, & Elliott, 1998). This is a program where children are encouraged through stories and roleplay to identify their emotions and how to cope with difficult situations in a problem-solving way. It is taught by the children's regular teachers in weekly lessons throughout the school year. Results of trials suggest that after exposure to PATHS, intervention children had greater skills in recognizing their own emotions and those of others and were rated by parents and teachers as more socially competent compared to peers. Further, teachers rated intervention children as less socially withdrawn at the end of the school year compared to controls (Domitrovich, Cortes, & Greenberg, 2007; Greenberg, Kusche, Cook, & Quamma, 1995; Kelly, Longbottom, Potts, & Williamson, 2004).

There have been many RCTs of a range of SEL programs, almost all in the United States. A meta-analysis of 213 school-based, universal SEL programs involving 270,034 primary and secondary school pupils found that compared to controls, SEL participants demonstrated significantly improved social and emotional skills, attitudes, behavior, and academic performance that reflected an 11-percentile-point gain in achievement (Durlak et al., 2011). Such findings are encouraging, but the huge problem is whether such demonstration projects can be translated into everyday life. There was widespread adoption in schools in England of Social and Emotional Aspects of Learning (SEAL) programs. The evaluation in primary schools of the small-group, selective-targeted aspect showed small effect sizes in some of the measured outcomes, with increases in pupil-rated overall emotional literacy; increases in staff-rated self-regulation; decreases in staff-rated peer problems; and increases in pupil-rated empathy, self-regulation, social skills, and overall emotional literacy (Humphrey et al., 2008). However, in secondary schools SEAL showed no overall effects on pupils (Humphrey, Lendrum, & Wigelsworth, 2010). Thus while these approaches appear to be promising, further evaluations are needed, including in LMICs.

Cognitive-Behavioral and Anger Management Programs

Anger management programs build on the evidence that aggressive children have poor recognition of their emotions, have overvalued beliefs about the effectiveness of aggression, and are quick to become emotionally aroused in situations they perceive as threatening. A number of programs exist, broadly based on cognitive behavioral principles. Elements include (1) attributional retraining, (2) anger management, (3) social problem solving, (4) social skills training, and (5) help for youth in setting targets for desirable behavior and negotiating rewards for achieving them. While each of these elements can be separated out on its own, most modern programs incorporate a number of these themes blended together. These programs are best delivered by skilled clinicians, either to children individually or in groups. Although groups offer several advantages (e.g., opportunities to practice peer interactions) and appear to be more effective when delivered to higher-risk children (Mytton, DiGuiseppi, Gough, Taylor, & Logan, 2002; Wilson & Lipsey, 2005), they may have potentially harmful effects (Dishion, McCord, & Poulin, 1999). These appear to be particularly common in larger groups and those with inadequate therapist supervision, where children learn deviant behavior from their peers and encourage each other to act antisocially.

Early therapeutic sessions involve assisting the children to recognize their anger in difficult interpersonal encounters, identify the triggers, and take the perspective of the other person, including recognizing whether their intentions are truly hostile. Attributional retraining helps correct the cognitive distortions identified by Dodge (1993) whereby the youth tends to perceive threat and hostile intent even in neutral scenarios, and work is done to help understand others' points of view. Realizing that the other person may have made a mistake, be bored, or be unable to communicate more effectively can reduce feelings of anger. The next stage is to practice coping techniques to reduce anger arousal and avoid impulsive, rage-filled responses. Techniques include the use of distraction, relaxation, and self-talk. These need to be repeatedly practiced, under conditions of increasing threat, for example initially with puppets but then by roleplay with other young people. The children are reinforced for creating a repertoire of coping self-statements that are meaningful and useful for them and encouraged to practice them in real-life situations.

In two RCTs, Kazdin and colleagues (Kazdin, Bass, Siegel, & Thomas, 1989; Kazdin, Esveldt-Dawson, French, & Unis, 1987) found that Problem-Solving Skills Training results in a significant decrease in deviant behavior and an increase in prosocial behavior. Outcomes were superior to a client-centered, relationship-based treatment and were maintained at a one-year follow-up. The addition of both real-life practice and a parent training component enhanced outcomes. Evaluations of the Coping Power Program found reductions in aggression and substance use and improved social competence (e.g., Lochman & Wells, 2002). Treatment effects were maintained at a one-year follow-up, particularly for those whose parents also received parent training (Lochman & Wells, 2004), and there is evidence of reduced substance misuse four years later (Larson & Lochman, 2010). A recent follow-up of a brief version found effects were maintained at a three-year follow-up, but that booster sessions did not improve intervention effects (Lochman et al., 2014). More generally, a meta-analysis of RCTs of social skills training confirmed its usefulness, although studies with larger samples led to smaller effect sizes (Losel & Beelmann, 2003). Limitations of anger management programs include the fact that quite a few young people with conduct disorders will not engage in them; there are few practitioners with the necessary skills available; and some young people can demonstrate the necessary steps in the clinic situation but in real-life provocations still cannot control their angry outbursts.

Multicomponent Approaches

A number of recent high-quality prevention trials have combined several evidence-based approaches. For example, Webster-Stratton et al., (2008) combined parent training with child social skills training to good effect. Some have added literacy or school behavior components led by teachers (Tolan, Gorman-Smith, & Henry, 2004). On the other hand, some multicomponent approaches have not been successful. Fast Track was a model efficacy trial, with six separate types of intervention, but as with many multimodal trials, the program had modest effects: the mean effect size on ASB was 0.11 (Conduct Problems Prevention Research Group, 1999). Another multicomponent program, the Syracuse University Family Development Research Program (U.S.), found significant differences between treatment groups on delinquency at age fifteen and lower costs to the justice system (Lally, Mangione, & Honig, 1988) but Aos, Phipps, Barnoski, and Lieb (2001) found that the costs of running the program outweighed the benefits by three to one. One recent meta-analysis of early prevention approaches which reported significant effects for delinquency (d = 0.48) found that while program duration and intensity were associated with effect sizes, whether programs were multicomponent was not (Manning, Homel, & Smith, 2010). However, the most recent and comprehensive meta-analysis of prevention programs for delinquency found that multimodal approaches carried out in the family context were the most effective (De Vries, Hoeve, Assink, Stams, & Asscher, 2015).

Multisystemic Therapy (MST) is one of the best developed multicomponent treatments and was developed by Henggeler et al. (1999) in the United States. There are nine treatment principles:

1. An assessment should be made to determine the fit between the problems and the wider environment: difficulties are understood as a reaction to a specific context, not seen as necessarily intrinsic deficits.
2. Therapeutic contacts emphasize the positive and use systemic strengths as levers for change. Already the assessment will have identified strengths (such as being good at sports, getting on well with grandmother, having prosocial peers in grandmother's neighborhood); the implementation of this principle means that each contact should acknowledge and work on these.
3. Interventions are designed to promote responsible behavior and decrease irresponsible behavior.
4. Interventions are focused in the present are action-oriented and have specific, well-defined goals. The approach is what can be done in the here and now, in contrast to some therapies that emphasize the need to understand the family and the youth's past.
5. Interventions target sequences of behavior in multiple systems that maintain problems.
6. Interventions are developmentally appropriate. They should fit the life stage and personal level of the family members
7. Interventions require daily or weekly effort by family members. This enables frequent practice of new skills and frequent positive feedback for efforts made; nonadherence to treatment agreements rapidly becomes apparent.
8. Intervention effectiveness is evaluated continuously from multiple perspectives, with the intervention team assuming responsibility for overcoming barriers to successful outcomes.
9. Interventions are designed to promote treatment generalization by empowering parents to address youth needs across multiple contexts.

The way the therapy is delivered is closely controlled. Due to the weekly monitoring of progress, if there are barriers to improvement these should be rapidly addressed, and the hypotheses of what is going on in the family and systems around the youth should be revised in the light of progress. Clinicians take on only four to six cases since the work is intensive; there is close attention to quality control by weekly supervision along prescribed lines, and parents and youth themselves fill in weekly questionnaires on whether they have been receiving therapy as planned. Therapy is given for three months and then stopped.

The first set of outcome studies by the program's developers was positive. Thus the meta-analysis of papers up to 2003, including one authored by of the program's developers, Charles Borduin, found that in seven outcome studies comparing MST to treatment as usual or an alternative treatment, with 708 youth by 35 therapists, the mean overall effect size across several domains was 0.55 (Curtis, Ronan, & Borduin, 2004). However, the three studies using the developers' own graduate students as therapists got noticeably larger effect sizes (mean 0.81) than when the developers were supervising local community therapists, where the effect size mean was down to 0.26. Long-term follow-up fourteen years later (when the individuals' mean age was twenty-nine years old) by the developers of one of the first trials gave recidivism rates of 50 percent versus 81 percent respectively.

There have also been at least twenty-seven published reviews of MST (Littell, 2005) and the sorts of findings previously discussed have led MST to be cited as an effective, evidence-based treatment by a number of U.S. government agencies. However, in the process of evaluation, the next test of any therapy is its effectiveness when evaluated independently. The first independent evaluation was also the first one to use proper intention to treat analyses (rather than exclude treatment refusers), and it found, with a large sample (N = 409) in Ontario, Canada, that MST yielded no improvement on treatment as usual on any outcome, either immediately or by three-year follow-up (Leschied & Cunningham, 2002). A smaller independent study in Norway (N = 75; Ogden & Hagen, 2006) was more positive, though here there was 40 percent missing data. Likewise, a totally independent trial by Timmons-Mitchell, Bender, Kishna, & Mitchell (2006) in the United States randomized ninety-three delinquents and also got substantial beneficial effects also. The Canadian study (not published in a peer-reviewed journal but of high quality) was included in the Cochrane Library's review of MST (Littell, 2005), but the other two independent Norwegian and U.S. studies were not. The Cochrane conclusion that "evidence suggests that MST is not consistently more effective than other alternatives" is thus in our view unduly harsh.

Furthermore, there have been a number of subsequent evaluations of MST in the last few years, one conducted by the program developers (Letourneau et al., 2009), and three independent evaluations. One of these was in the United States (Weiss et al., 2013) and found small but significant positive effects for MST on two out of four primary outcomes. A U.K. trial found greater reductions in offending in the MST group but only at the long-term follow-up and only for nonviolent offences (Butler, Baruch, Hickey, & Fonagy, 2011). Similarly, a Dutch trial found small effects but not for violence (Asscher, Deković, Manders, van der Laan, & Prins, 2013) with a two-year follow-up finding that effect sizes were bigger, but there were no differences between groups on official records of offending (Asscher et al., 2014). One recent cost-benefit analysis (which included one of the developers as a coauthor) found a $5 return per $1 invested when youth were followed-up twenty-five years after the intervention (Dopp, Borduin, Wagner, & Sawyer, 2014), with reductions in cost and offending in siblings of targeted youth also (Wagner, Borduin, Sawyer, & Dopp, 2014). However, cost-benefit analysis of the U.K. study found no significant differences in costs of criminal activity between groups at an eighteen-month follow-up (Cary, Butler, Baruch, Hickey, & Byford, 2013). While the MST group was less expensive in its use of youth offending services, this difference disappeared when the cost of MST was included.

Finally, a recent independent meta-analysis consisting of twenty-two studies and over four thousand youth concluded that MST has small but significant effects on delinquency and some secondary outcomes and is most effective with more severe youth (van der Stouwe, Asscher, Stams, Deković, & van der Laan, 2014). This conclusion is more cautious than the previously established view. A number of reasons are possible. First, some of the developers' own studies did not do full intention to treat analyses, and may have been more favorable since some cases with the worse outcomes (the dropouts) were excluded. Secondly, the degree of skill with which the intervention was delivered may have been higher in the developers' sites. Third, the comparison treatment may have been different in Canada, the Netherlands, and the United Kingdom, where the justice system may be better organized.

Interventions for Specific Groups

As described previously, there is increasing evidence to show that some children are more susceptible to their environments and that markers of this differential susceptibility may indicate differential susceptibility to interventions. Scott and O'Connor (2012) found that emotionally labile, reactive children benefited from improved parenting after parent training while headstrong children did not. However, Gatzke-Kopp, Greenberg, & Bierman (2015) found that low reactivity was associated with greater improvement over time. Clearly, research exploring this issue is in its infancy and further intervention studies testing moderation of treatment effect by these child characteristics are necessary.

Abusive Families and Fostered Children

While it has been known for some years that interventions in early infancy with a practical slant work with families that have mild to moderate difficulties, recent studies show that these approaches can work with children whose parents are frankly abusive (Cicchetti, Rogosch, Toth, & Sturge-Apple, 2011). Moreover, these interventions do not only improve infants' psychosocial functioning, but a range of biological changes can be detected as a result of parent training treatment that indicate improved functioning (Cicchetti et al., 2011; Woltering, Granic, Lamm, & Lewis, 2011). Parent–Child Interaction Therapy and the Incredible Years have both been shown to be effective with abusive parents (Chaffin, Funderburk, Bard, Valle, & Gurwitch, 2011; Letarte, Normandeau, & Allard, 2010), as has MST (Swenson, Schaeffer, Henggeler, Faldowski, & Mayhew, 2010). The effectiveness of these interventions with abusing families poses the question of why more social services departments do not train their staff to deliver them.

Children who have been abused or neglected so severely that they require removal from their birth parents do particularly poorly. However, recovery is possible when children are placed in a foster care family (Dozier et al., 2014), as high-quality foster care can result in improved psychosocial functioning, such as secure attachment relationships (Joseph, O'Connor, Briskman, Maughan, & Scott, 2014). Furthermore, effective interventions are emerging (see van IJzendoorn et al., 2015, for a review). For example, a recent U.K. RCT of parent training for foster carers showed large improvements in child behavior (Briskman et al., 2012).

Probably the best-known example of an intervention with this group is Multidimensional Treatment Foster Care (MTFC). MTFC evolved at the Oregon Social Learning Center (U.S.), beginning in 1983 (Chamberlain, 2003), where parent training with families of delinquents proved extremely difficult (although reasonably effective – Bank, Marlowe, Reid, & Patterson, 1991), due to the inability of the family to cope with the extreme demands of having a delinquent youth. This led to the idea of placing such youth in a specially trained foster family. It has a number of similarities with MST. The moment-to-moment interactions are seen as the key to change and part of the regime is based on the youth earning points for good behavior and losing them for bad behavior, while at school points are awarded for good behavior in class. The youth has to earn one hundred points a day; then he or she can get privileges, such as going to bed later, having time on the computer, getting extra time to phone friends, and so on.

For the youth, the immediacy of experiencing a contingent response to their behavior is often a stark contrast to being left alone or having long coercive interchanges with their parents. In addition to close liaison with the school, close supervision is key – the young person loses fully a point a minute for all time where he or she cannot verify his or her whereabouts, incurring a sizable fine. MTFC lasts for around six months, and then the young person returns to his or her birth family. However, crucial to the model is the birth family therapist, who while the youth is in the foster family, works with the birth family to inculcate the same regime to be used.

There have been two main trials completed with MTFC for delinquency, one in boys and one in girls, both by the program's developers. With boys ($N = 79$), MTFC compared to group care led to a reduction in the number of arrests at two-year follow-up (for two or more arrests 5 percent versus 24 percent), and reduced self-reports of aggression and fighting (Eddy, Bridges Whaley, & Chamberlain, 2004). With girls at one-year follow-up ($n = 81$), criminal referrals showed a trend (mean 0.76 referrals in MTFC, 1.3 for group care, $p = 0.10$), days locked up twenty-two versus fifty-six ($p < 0.05$), and a reduction on some measures of delinquency but not others (Leve, Chamberlain, & Reid, 2005). A Cochrane review of the intervention (Macdonald & Turner, 2008) concluded that it was a promising intervention and that there was some evidence for reductions in aggressive and violent behavior, but that the evidence base is less robust than usually reported. One recent trial has shown reductions in violent behavior in girls (Rhoades, Chamberlain, Roberts, & Leve, 2013), but a subsequent U.K. RCT showed no overall effect (Green et al., 2014).

Callous-Unemotional Traits

As discussed previously, CU traits are becoming recognized as a marker of a specific developmental path to violence and ASB. Youth with these traits are commonly seen in justice systems due to a combination of deceptiveness, violence, and ASB. Delinquent offenders with these psychopathic traits have an earlier onset of offending, commit more crimes, and reoffend more often (Forth & Burke, 1998) and more violently (Spain, Douglas, Poythress, & Epstein, 2004) than nonpsychopathic criminal youth. In addition, they exhibit insensitivity to punishment cues irrespective of whether or not they have conduct problems, making them especially hard to treat (O'Brien & Frick, 1996).

However, overconfident predictions about poor outcomes for youth with these traits should be avoided, as recent findings are challenging the previous view that children with CU traits do not respond to treatment for ASB. First, some recent studies have shown that children and adolescents with CU traits are more sensitive to parenting than previously thought (O'Connor, Humayun, Briskman, & Scott, 2016; Waller, Gardner, & Hyde, 2013). Second, some recent trials have shown improvements in conduct problems in children with CU traits when treatment models have focused on emotion recognition skills (Dadds, Cauchi, Wimalaweera, Hawes, & Brennan, 2012) and improving the parent–child bond (Somech & Elizur, 2012), and one recent study has shown that FFT can be equally effective with violent youth with CU traits (White, Frick, Lawing, & Bauer, 2012). While this is a promising finding, it should be noted that there was no control group in this study. Third, there have also been a handful of studies showing reductions in CU traits (rather than ASB) following treatment (Hawes & Dadds, 2007; Kolko et al., 2009; McDonald, Dodson, Rosenfield, & Jouriles, 2011; Somech & Elizur, 2012), and three recent reviews have concluded that parent training has some potential for producing improvements in this group (Frick, Ray, Thornton, & Kahn, 2014; Hawes, Price, & Dadds, 2014; Waller et al., 2013).

Ineffective Approaches

Unfortunately, evidence of effectiveness is not the only consideration to have shaped the choice of interventions for ASB. Other motivations, from the desire to punish violent youth, to making use of what is currently available at relatively low cost, have often driven policy making and commissioning in prevention services. These different motives may conflict with what is effective for children and young people and what works in reducing the damage they cause to society. One of the best examples of this is shock incarceration in military-style boot camps, which although recommended in the 1990s by the U.S. Office of Juvenile Justice and Delinquency Prevention, and satisfying the desire for retribution and somewhat lower running costs, have repeatedly proven at least ineffective and often positively harmful (Bottcher, 2005; Cullen, Blevins, Trager, & Gendreau, 2005; Meade & Steiner, 2010; Stinchcomb, 2005).

Another approach is to attempt to frighten delinquents with visits to prisons in an attempt to deter them, as for example in the "Scared Straight" program. However, a meta-analysis of nine controlled trials found that the intervention on average is more harmful than doing nothing, as it led to worse outcomes in participants (Petrosino, Turpin-Petrosino, & Buehler, 2003). Peer-group work can also be harmful. In an evaluation of the Adolescent Transitions Programs, Dishion and Andrews (1995) studied 120 families with an antisocial youth and found that at one- and three-year follow-up, adolescents allocated to a youth group intervention fared significantly worse on a number of outcomes. The famous Cambridge-Somerville delinquency project studied four hundred youth, half of whom were offered a range of interventions for four years that were state of the art at the time in the early 1940s, but a thirty-year follow-up showed increased criminal activity, drug, cigarette, and alcohol use by the intervention group compared to controls (McCord, 1978). Subsequent reanalysis or examination of videotapes has led authors to hypothesize that these poor outcomes are due to "deviancy training" among youth (Dishion et al., 1999; Granic & Dishion, 2003; McCord, 1997).

Another intervention is the use of medication. However, no pharmacological intervention is currently approved specifically for CD or ASB. Nevertheless, medication is used relatively frequently and increasingly for this behavior in the United States (Steiner, Saxena, & Chang, 2003). In the United Kingdom, medication would not generally be supported as good practice because there is very little evidence of effectiveness, particularly for children without comorbid ADHD.

Barriers to Implementation and Dissemination

While it is crucial to have well-designed trials, concern has been expressed that they do not reflect everyday practice, and that the effects in the real world are usually smaller. There may be several reasons for this. First, clinically referred cases have multiple comorbid problems; second, therapists have to deliver several different therapies in the course of a day, not just the one used by trial therapists; and third, the training, supervision, and motivation of the therapists may be less. Thus there is an increasing need for so-called effectiveness, rather than efficacy, trials that test interventions as they would be used in everyday service delivery.

Handling Treatment Failure

The great increase in the number of families who attend services for parenting interventions has resulted in (a) more families presenting who have relapsed after initial improvement and (b) more failing to improve with initial treatment.

For the former, studies are needed to see whether, some months after initial treatment, booster sessions should routinely be offered to prevent relapse. For the latter, systematic procedures are needed to address the difficulties of families for whom parenting programs didn't work. One helpful approach draws on four different theories to explain and treat failure to progress, which are applied according to the particular problems that families present (Scott & Dadds, 2009). It proposes motivational interviewing for parents who lack the drive to attend, attachment-theory informed interventions for parents who are failing to bond with their children, a family-systems approach if wider issues are interfering with progress, and cognitive restructuring therapy for parents whose beliefs stop them from making the necessary behavioral changes. Such an approach is attractive as it blends clear strategic thinking with clinical wisdom; it now needs to be tested in trials.

National Initiatives

If prevention of conduct disorders is to be anything more than a theoretical possibility or a rare activity occasionally undertaken in limited demonstration projects, it requires recognition of the problem and possible solutions at the governmental level. There have been a number of relevant European and American reports and initiatives in the last decade or so. For example, the U.S. Surgeon General's report (Office of the Surgeon General, 2001) on youth violence described it as an epidemic and called for rigorous evaluation of prevention programs. Subsequently, a number of prevention and intervention research centers (PIRCs) were funded. The National Resource Council's (2009) report on the prevention of mental, emotional, and behavioral (MEB) disorders stated that "Research on the prevention of MEB disorders should focus on interventions that occur before the onset of disorder but should broaden the range of outcomes to include accomplishment of age-appropriate developmental tasks (e.g., school, social, and work outcomes)." In Europe, in Norway, Sweden, and England there have been national initiatives rolling out evidence-based parenting programs on a large scale (Scott, 2009). The Allen review on early interventions in England (Allen, 2011) recommended the widespread implementation of a range of evidence-based approaches, but was not supported by any substantial new funding. However, to reduce the impact of poverty on poor outcomes more generally (not just ASB/conduct disorders), the government in England has continued to fund SureStart early intervention programs, which cost £500 million to set up and whose evaluation suggested improved parenting and child outcomes (Melhuish, Belsky, Leyland, & Barnes, 2008). Most recently, the U.K. Home Office has funded the Early Intervention Foundation as a What Works Centre to collate an evidence base on prevention of ASB and youth and gang violence.[1]

1 www.eif.org.uk.

Conclusion

Many of the risk factors for the development of ASB are well understood, and this has allowed for the identification of specific targets for prevention approaches. Over the last forty years, a number of interventions based on these principles have been developed and tested. Those based on social learning theory and incorporating parent management training have been shown to be highly effective in children. There is also some evidence for programs based on cognitive-behavioral approaches. Thus there are a number of effective prevention approaches available for ASB that, if implemented on a large scale, are likely to result in large medium- to long-term cost savings. At the same time, there are a number of approaches that have been shown to be ineffective and, in some cases, positively harmful. However, many interventions have been tested predominantly in the United States and against U.S. usual services. It is important to test these against the often more substantive existing services in Europe. Finally, the individual characteristics of the child or adolescent should be taken into account when selecting prevention approaches, with particular focus on identifying CU traits.

References

Aberson, B., Albury, C., Gutting, S., Mann, F., & Trushin, B. (1987). *I Can Problem Solve (ICPS): A Cognitive Training Program for Kindergarten Children.* Dade County, FL: Bureau of Education.

Alexander, J. F., Pugh, C., Parsons, B., & Sexton, T. L. (2000). *Blueprints for Violence Prevention, Book Three: Functional Family Therapy.* Boulder, CO: Center for the Study and Prevention of Violence.

Allen, G. (2011). *Early Intervention, The Next Steps: An Independent Report to Her Majesty's Government.* London: The Stationery Office.

Allen, J. P., Porter, M., McFarland, C., McElhaney, K. B., & Marsh, P. (2007). The relation of attachment security to adolescents' paternal and peer relationships, depression, and externalizing behavior. *Child Development* 78(4): 1222–39.

Amato, P. R., & Keith, B. (1991). Parental divorce and the well-being of children: a meta-analysis. *Psychological Bulletin* 110(1): 26.

American Psychiatric Association. (2013). *The Diagnostic and Statistical Manual of Mental Disorders: DSM 5.* Arlington, VA: bookpointUS. books.google.com/books?hl=en&lr=&id=_VzzAgAAQBAJ&oi=fnd&pg=PT2&dq=Diagnostic+and+statistical+manual+fifth+edition&ots=oTYnsdJ_3n&sig=s-L1kked6ZX3d0qnIu6ueDcIP8Q

Aos, S., Lieb, R., Mayfield, J., Miller, M., & Pennucci, A. (2004). *Benefits and Costs of Prevention and Early Intervention Programs for Youth.* Olympia, WA: Washington State Institute for Public Policy. courses.washington.edu/pbaf513m/prevention%20tech%20appendix.pdf

Aos, S., Phipps, P., Barnoski, R., & Lieb, R. (2001). *The Comparative Costs and Benefits of Programs to Reduce Crime. Version 4.0.* Olympia, WA: Washington State Institute for Public Policy. eric.ed.gov/?id=ED453340

Appleyard, K., Egeland, B., Dulmen, M. H. M., & Sroufe, A.L. (2005). When more is not better: the role of cumulative risk in child behavior outcomes. *Journal of Child Psychology and Psychiatry* 46(3): 235–45. doi.org/10.1111/j.1469-7610.2004.00351.x

Asscher, J. J., Deković, M., Manders, W. A., van der Laan, P. H., & Prins, P. J. (2013). A randomized controlled trial of the effectiveness of multisystemic therapy in the Netherlands: post-treatment changes and moderator effects. *Journal of Experimental Criminology* 9(2): 169–87.

Asscher, J. J., Deković, M., Manders, W., van der Laan, P. H., Prins, P. J., & van Arum, S. (2014). Sustainability of the effects of multisystemic therapy for juvenile delinquents in The Netherlands: effects on delinquency and recidivism. *Journal of Experimental Criminology* 10(2): 227–43.

Bagot, R. C., & Meaney, M. J. (2010). Epigenetics and the biological basis of gene X environment interactions. *Journal of the American Academy of Child & Adolescent Psychiatry* 49(8): 752–71.

Baker-Henningham, H. (2011). Transporting evidence-based interventions across cultures: using focus groups with teachers and parents of pre-school children to inform the implementation of the Incredible Years Teacher Training Programme in Jamaica: focus groups with pre-school teachers and parents in Jamaica. *Child: Care, Health and Development* 37(5): 649–61. doi.org/10.1111/j.1365-2214.2011.01208.x

Baker-Henningham, H., Scott, S., Jones, K., & Walker, S. (2012). Reducing child conduct problems and promoting social skills in a middle-income country: cluster randomised controlled trial. *British Journal of Psychiatry* 201(2): 101–8. doi.org/10.1192/bjp.bp.111.096834

Bandura, A. (1977). Self-efficacy: toward a unifying theory of behavioral change. *Psychological Review* 84(2): 191.

Bank, L., Marlowe, J. H., Reid, J. B., Patterson, G. R., & Weinrott, M. R. (1991). A comparative evaluation of parent-training interventions for families of chronic delinquents. *Journal of Abnormal Child Psychology* 19(1): 15–33.

Barker, E. D., Oliver, B. R., & Maughan, B. (2010). Co-occurring problems of early onset persistent, childhood limited, and adolescent onset conduct problem youth. *Journal of Child Psychology and Psychiatry* 51(11): 1217–26. doi.org/10.1111/j.1469-7610.2010.02240.x

Barnes, J., Ball, M., Meadows, P., Howden, B., Jackson, A., Henderson, J., & Niven, L. (2011). The Family-Nurse Partnership programme in England: Wave 1 implementation in toddlerhood and a comparison between Waves 1 and 2a of implementation in pregnancy and infancy. dera.ioe.ac.uk/1973/1/dh_123273.pdf

Barnett, W. S. (1996). *Lives in the Balance: Age-27 Benefit-Cost Analysis of the High/Scope Perry Preschool Program,* vol. 11. Ypsilanti, MI: High/Scope Press. eric.ed.gov/?id=ED410024

Barrish, H. H., Saunders, M., & Wolf, M. M. (1969). Good behavior game: effects of individual contingencies for group consequences on disruptive behavior in a classroom. *Journal of Applied Behavior Analysis* 2(2): 119.

Beecham, J. (2014). Annual research review: child and adolescent mental health interventions: a review of progress in economic studies across different disorders. *Journal of Child Psychology and Psychiatry* 55(6): 714–32.

Belsky, J., & Pluess, M. (2013). Beyond risk, resilience, and dysregulation: phenotypic plasticity and human development. *Development and Psychopathology* 25 (4pt2): 1243–61. doi.org/10.1017/S095457941300059X

Bernazzani, O., & Tremblay, R. E. (2006). Early parent training. In Welsh, B. C., & Farrington, D. P. (eds.), *Preventing Crime*. Netherlands: Springer, pp. 21–32. link.springer.com/chapter/10.1007/1–4020-4244-2_2

Bickman, L., Noser, K., & Summerfelt, W. T. (1999). Long-term effects of a system of care on children and adolescents. *Journal of Behavioral Health Services & Research* 26(2): 185–202.

Bilukha, O., Hahn, R. A., Crosby, A., Fullilove, M. T., Liberman, A., Moscicki, E., ... Briss, P. A. (2005). The effectiveness of early childhood home visitation in preventing violence. *American Journal of Preventive Medicine* 28(2): 11–39. doi.org/10.1016/j.amepre.2004.10.004

Block, J., Block, J. H., & Gjerde, P. F. (1988). Parental functioning and the home environment in families of divorce: prospective and concurrent analyses. *Journal of the American Academy of Child & Adolescent Psychiatry* 27(2): 207–13.

Bohman, M. (2007). Predisposition to criminality: Swedish adoption studies in retrospect. In Organizer, G. R. B., & Goode, J. A. (eds.), *Ciba Foundation Symposium 194 – Genetics of Criminal and Antisocial Behaviour*. Chicester, UK: John Wiley & Sons, pp. 99–114. onlinelibrary.wiley.com/doi/10.1002/9780470514825.ch6/summary

Bonin, E.-M., Stevens, M., Beecham, J., Byford, S., & Parsonage, M. (2011). Costs and longer-term savings of parenting programmes for the prevention of persistent conduct disorder: a modelling study. *BMC Public Health* 11(1): 803.

Bor, W., Sanders, M. R., & Markie-Dadds, C. (2002). The effects of the Triple P-Positive Parenting Program on preschool children with co-occurring disruptive behavior and attentional/hyperactive difficulties. *Journal of Abnormal Child Psychology* 30(6): 571–87.

Bottcher, J. (2005). Examining the effectiveness of boot camps: a randomized experiment with a long-term follow up. *Journal of Research in Crime and Delinquency* 42(3): 309–32. doi.org/10.1177/0022427804271918

Bowlby, J. (1944). Forty-four juvenile thieves: their characters and home life. *International Journal of Psychoanalysis* 25(19–52): 107–27.

Briskman, J., Castle, J., Blackeby, K., Bengo, C., Slack, K., Stebbens, C., ... Scott, S. (2012). *Randomised Controlled Trial of the Fostering Changes Programme* (No. DFE-RR237). London: Department for Education. www.education.gov.uk/publications/eOrderingDownload/DFE-RR237.pdf

Butler, S., Baruch, G., Hickey, N., & Fonagy, P. (2011). A randomized controlled trial of multisystemic therapy and a statutory therapeutic intervention for young offenders. *Journal of the American Academy of Child & Adolescent Psychiatry* 50(12): 1220–35.

Cadoret, R. J., Yates, W. R., Woodworth, G., & Stewart, M. A. (1995). Genetic-environmental interaction in the genesis of aggressivity and conduct disorders. *Archives of General Psychiatry* 52(11): 916–24.

Cary, M., Butler, S., Baruch, G., Hickey, N., & Byford, S. (2013). Economic evaluation of multisystemic therapy for young people at risk for continuing criminal activity in the UK. *PloS One* 8(4): e61070.

Caspi, A., Moffitt, T. E., Newman, D. L., & Silva, P. A. (1996). Behavioral observations at age 3 years predict adult psychiatric disorders: longitudinal evidence from a birth cohort. *Archives of General Psychiatry* 53(11): 1033–9.

Cecil, C. A. M., Lysenko, L. J., Jaffee, S. R., Pingault, J. B., Smith, R. G., Relton, C. L., … Barker, E. D. (2014a). Environmental risk, Oxytocin Receptor Gene (OXTR) methylation and youth callous-unemotional traits: a 13-year longitudinal study. *Molecular Psychiatry*. www.nature.com/mp/journal/vaop/ncurrent/full/mp201495a.html

Cecil, C. A., Viding, E., Barker, E. D., Guiney, J., & McCrory, E. J. (2014b). Double disadvantage: the influence of childhood maltreatment and community violence exposure on adolescent mental health. *Journal of Child Psychology and Psychiatry*. onlinelibrary.wiley.com/doi/10.1111/jcpp.12213/full

Chaffin, M., Funderburk, B., Bard, D., Valle, L. A., & Gurwitch, R. (2011). A combined motivation and parent–child interaction therapy package reduces child welfare recidivism in a randomized dismantling field trial. *Journal of Consulting and Clinical Psychology* 79(1): 84–95. doi.org/10.1037/a0021227

Chamberlain, P. (2003). The Oregon multidimensional treatment foster care model: features, outcomes, and progress in dissemination. *Cognitive and Behavioral Practice* 10(4): 303–12.

Cicchetti, D., Rogosch, F. A., Toth, S. L., & Sturge-Apple, M. L. (2011). Normalizing the development of cortisol regulation in maltreated infants through preventive interventions. *Development and Psychopathology* 23(03): 789–800. doi.org/10.1017/S0954579411000307

Cohen, M. A., & Piquero, A. R. (2009). New evidence on the monetary value of saving a high risk youth. *Journal of Quantitative Criminology* 25(1): 25–49.

Coldwell, J., Pike, A., & Dunn, J. (2006). Household chaos–links with parenting and child behaviour. *Journal of Child Psychology and Psychiatry* 47(11): 1116–22.

Conduct Problems Prevention Research Group. (1999). Initial impact of the Fast Track prevention trial for conduct problems: II. Classroom effects. *Journal of Consulting and Clinical Psychology* 67(5): 648.

Costello, E. J., Compton, S. N., Keeler, G., & Angold, A. (2003). Relationships between poverty and psychopathology: a natural experiment. *JAMA* 290(15): 2023–9.

Cullen, F. T., Blevins, K. R., Trager, J. S., & Gendreau, P. (2005). The rise and fall of boot camps: a case study in common-sense corrections. *Journal of Offender Rehabilitation* 40(3–4): 53–70. doi.org/10.1300/J076v40n03_03

Cummings, E. M., & Davies, P. T. (2002). Effects of marital conflict on children: recent advances and emerging themes in process-oriented research. *Journal of Child Psychology and Psychiatry* 43(1): 31–63.

Currie, J. (2001). Early childhood education programs. *Journal of Economic Perspectives* 15(2): 213–38.

Curtis, N. M., Ronan, K. R., & Borduin, C. M. (2004). Multisystemic treatment: a meta-analysis of outcome studies. *Journal of Family Psychology* 18(3): 411.

Dadds, M. R., Allen, J. L., Oliver, B. R., Faulkner, N., Legge, K., Moul, C., … Scott, S. (2011). Love, eye contact and the developmental origins of empathy v. psychopathy. *British Journal of Psychiatry* 200(3): 191–6. doi.org/10.1192/bjp.bp.110.085720

Dadds, M. R., Cauchi, A. J., Wimalaweera, S., Hawes, D. J., & Brennan, J. (2012). Outcomes, moderators, and mediators of empathic-emotion recognition training for complex conduct problems in childhood. *Psychiatry Research* 199(3): 201–7. doi.org/10.1016/j.psychres.2012.04.033

Davies, P. T., & Cummings, E. M. (1994). Marital conflict and child adjustment: an emotional security hypothesis. *Psychological Bulletin* 116(3): 387.

Deater-Deckard, K., Dodge, K. A., Bates, J. E., & Pettit, G. S. (1996). Physical discipline among African American and European American mothers: links to children's externalizing behaviors. *Developmental Psychology* 32(6): 1065–72. doi.org/10.1037/0012–1649.32.6.1065

Deater-Deckard, K., Mullineaux, P. Y., Beekman, C., Petrill, S. A., Schatschneider, C., & Thompson, L. A. (2009). Conduct problems, IQ, and household chaos: a longitudinal multi-informant study. *Journal of Child Psychology and Psychiatry* 50(10): 1301–8.

De Castro, B. O., Veerman, J. W., Koops, W., Bosch, J. D., & Monshouwer, H. J. (2002). Hostile attribution of intent and aggressive behavior: a meta-analysis. *Child Development* 73(3): 916–34.

Denham, S. A., Workman, E., Cole, P. M., Weissbrod, C., Kendziora, K. T., & Zahn-Waxler, C. (2000). Prediction of externalizing behavior problems from early to middle childhood: the role of parental socialization and emotion expression. *Development and Psychopathology* 12(1): 23–45.

De Vries, S. L. A., Hoeve, M., Assink, M., Stams, G. J. J. M., & Asscher, J. J. (2015). Practitioner review: effective ingredients of prevention programs for youth at risk of persistent juvenile delinquency - recommendations for clinical practice. *Journal of Child Psychology and Psychiatry* 56(2): 108–21. doi.org/10.1111/jcpp.12320

Dishion, T. J., & Andrews, D. W. (1995). Preventing escalation in problem behaviors with high-risk young adolescents: immediate and 1-year outcomes. *Journal of Consulting and Clinical Psychology* 63(4): 538.

Dishion, T. J., McCord, J., & Poulin, F. (1999). When interventions harm: peer groups and problem behavior. *American Psychologist* 54(9): 755.

Dodge, K. A. (1993). Social-cognitive mechanisms in the development of conduct disorder and depression. *Annual Review of Psychology* 44(1): 559–84.

Dodge, K. A., Coie, J. D., & Lynam, D. (2007). Aggression and antisocial behavior in youth. In Eisenberg, N. (ed.), *Handbook of Child Psychology*, vol. III. New York: John Wiley & Sons, p. 12. onlinelibrary.wiley.com/ doi/10.1002/9780470147658.chpsy0312/abstract

Dodge, K. A., Pettit, G. S., Bates, J. E., & Valente, E. (1995). Social information-processing patterns partially mediate the effect of early physical abuse on later conduct problems. *Journal of Abnormal Psychology* 104(4): 632.

Domitrovich, C. E., Cortes, R. C., & Greenberg, M. T. (2007). Improving young children's social and emotional competence: a randomized trial of the preschool "PATHS" curriculum. *Journal of Primary Prevention* 28(2): 67–91. doi.org/10.1007/s10935-007–0081-0

Dopp, A. R., Borduin, C. M., Wagner, D. V., & Sawyer, A. M. (2014). The economic impact of multisystemic therapy through midlife: a cost–benefit analysis with serious juvenile offenders and their siblings. psycnet.apa.org/psycinfo/2014-11068-001/

Dozier, M., Kaufman, J., Kobak, R., O'Connor, T. G., Sagi-Schwartz, A., Scott, S., . . . Zeanah, C. H. (2014). Consensus statement on group care for children and adolescents: a statement of policy of the American Orthopsychiatric Association. *American Journal of Orthopsychiatry* 84(3): 219–25. doi.org/10.1037/ort0000005

Durlak, J. A., Weissberg, R. P., Dymnicki, A. B., Taylor, R. D., & Schellinger, K. B. (2011). The impact of enhancing students' social and emotional learning: a meta-analysis of school-based universal interventions. *Child Development* 82 (1): 405–32. doi.org/10.1111/j.1467–8624.2010.01564.x

Eckenrode, J., Campa, M., Luckey, D. W., Henderson, C. R., Cole, R., Kitzman, H., . . . Olds, D. (2010). Long-term effects of prenatal and infancy nurse home visitation on the life course of youths: 19-year follow-up of a randomized trial. *Archives of Pediatrics & Adolescent Medicine* 164(1): 9–15.

Eddy, J. M., Bridges Whaley, R., & Chamberlain, P. (2004). The prevention of violent behavior by chronic and serious male juvenile offenders: a 2-year follow-up of a randomized clinical trial. *Journal of Emotional and Behavioral Disorders* 12(1): 2–8. doi.org/10.1177/10634266040120010101

Ellis, B. J., Boyce, W. T., Belsky, J., Bakermans-Kranenburg, M. J., & van IJzendoorn, M. H. (2011). Differential susceptibility to the environment: an evolutionary–neurodevelopmental theory. *Development and Psychopathology* 23(01): 7–28. doi.org/10.1017/S0954579410000611

Farrington, D. P. (2005). Childhood origins of antisocial behavior. *Clinical Psychology & Psychotherapy* 12(3): 177–90.

Farrington, D. P., Ttofi, M. M., & Coid, J. W. (2009). Development of adolescence-limited, late-onset, and persistent offenders from age 8 to age 48. *Aggressive Behavior* 35(2): 150–63.

Farrington, D. P., & Welsh, B. C. (2002). Family-based crime prevention. In Sherman, L. W., Farrington, D. P., Welsh, B. C., & MacKenzie, D. L. (eds.), *Evidence-Based Crime Prevention.* New York: Routledge, p. 22. books.google.com/books?hl=en&lr=&id=p-aCAgAAQBAJ&oi=fnd&pg=PA22&dq=farrington+welsh+2002+family-based+crime+prevention&ots=5PntOJtJR5&sig=fDE1jbrks0fuDvjhOThnIkEAoac

Fearon, R. P., Bakermans-Kranenburg, M. J., van IJzendoorn, M. H., Lapsley, A., & Roisman, G. I. (2010). The significance of insecure attachment and disorganization in the development of children's externalizing behavior: a meta-analytic study. *Child Development* 81(2): 435–56.

Feilhauer, J., & Cima, M. (2013). Youth psychopathy: differential correlates of callous-unemotional traits, narcissism, and impulsivity. *Forensic Science International* 224(1–3): 1–7. doi.org/10.1016/j.forsciint.2012.10.016

Feinberg, M. E., Jones, D. E., Kan, M. L., & Goslin, M. C. (2010). Effects of family foundations on parents and children: 3.5 years after baseline. *Journal of Family Psychology* 24(5): 532–42. doi.org/10.1037/a0020837

Fergusson, D. M., Horwood, L. J., & Lynskey, M. T. (1996). Childhood sexual abuse and psychiatric disorder in young adulthood: II. Psychiatric outcomes of childhood sexual abuse. *Journal of the American Academy of Child & Adolescent Psychiatry* 35(10): 1365–74.

Fergusson, D. M., Horwood, L. J., & Ridder, E. M. (2005). Show me the child at seven: the consequences of conduct problems in childhood for psychosocial functioning in adulthood. *Journal of Child Psychology and Psychiatry* 46(8): 837–49. doi.org/10.1111/j.1469–7610.2004.00387.x

Fergusson, D. M., Lynskey, M. T., & Horwood, L. J. (1996). Childhood sexual abuse and psychiatric disorder in young adulthood: I. Prevalence of sexual abuse and factors associated with sexual abuse. *Journal of the American Academy of Child & Adolescent Psychiatry* 35(10): 1355–64.

Ford, T., Hamilton, H., Goodman, R., & Meltzer, H. (2005). Service contacts among the children participating in the British child and adolescent mental health surveys. *Child and Adolescent Mental Health* 10(1): 2–9.

Forth, A. E., & Burke, H. C. (1998). Psychopathy in adolescence: Assessment, violence, and developmental precursors. In Cooke, D. J., Forth, A. E., & Hare, R. D. (eds.), *Psychopathy: Theory, Research and Implications for Society*. Dordrecht: Kluwer, pp. 205–29.

Frick, P. J., Ray, J. V., Thornton, L. C., & Kahn, R. E. (2014). Can callous-unemotional traits enhance the understanding, diagnosis, and treatment of serious conduct problems in children and adolescents? A comprehensive review. *Psychological Bulletin* 140(1): 1–57. doi.org/10.1037/a0033076

Frick, P. J., & White, S. F. (2008). Research review: the importance of callous-unemotional traits for developmental models of aggressive and antisocial behavior. *Journal of Child Psychology and Psychiatry* 49(4): 359–75. doi.org/10.1111/j.1469-7610.2007.01862.x

Furlong, M., McGilloway, S., Bywater, T., Hutchings, J., Smith, S. M., & Donnelly, M. (2012). Behavioural and cognitive-behavioural group-based parenting programmes for early-onset conduct problems in children aged 3 to 12 years. *Cochrane Database of Systematic Reviews*. onlinelibrary.wiley.com/doi/10.1002/14651858.CD008225.pub2/abstract

Futh, A., O'Connor, T. G., Matias, C., Green, J., & Scott, S. (2008). Attachment narratives and behavioral and emotional symptoms in an ethnically diverse, at-risk sample. *Journal of the American Academy of Child & Adolescent Psychiatry* 47(6): 709–18. doi.org/10.1097/CHI.0b013e31816bff65

Garces, E., Thomas, D., & Currie, J. (2002). Longer-term effects of head start. *American Economic Review* 92(4): 999–1012.

Gatti, U., Tremblay, R. E., Vitaro, F., & McDuff, P. (2005). Youth gangs, delinquency and drug use: a test of the selection, facilitation, and enhancement hypotheses. *Journal of Child Psychology and Psychiatry* 46(11): 1178–90.

Gatzke-Kopp, L. M., Greenberg, M., & Bierman, K. (2015). Children's parasympathetic reactivity to specific emotions moderates response to intervention for early-onset aggression. *Journal of Clinical Child & Adolescent Psychology* 44(2): 1–14.

Gifford-Smith, M., Dodge, K. A., Dishion, T. J., & McCord, J. (2005). Peer influence in children and adolescents: crossing the bridge from developmental to intervention science. *Journal of Abnormal Child Psychology* 33(3): 255–65. doi.org/10.1007/s10802-005-3563-7

Glover, V., & Hill, J. (2012). Sex differences in the programming effects of prenatal stress on psychopathology and stress responses: An evolutionary perspective. *Physiology & Behavior* 106(5): 736–40. doi.org/10.1016/j.physbeh.2012.02.011

Goodman, R. (2001). Psychometric properties of the strengths and difficulties questionnaire. *Journal of the American Academy of Child & Adolescent Psychiatry* 40(11): 1337–45.

Graham, C., Carr, A., Rooney, B., Sexton, T., & Wilson Satterfield, L. R. (2014). Evaluation of functional family therapy in an Irish context. *Journal of Family Therapy* 36(1): 20–38.

Granic, I., & Dishion, T. J. (2003). Deviant talk in adolescent friendships: a step toward measuring a pathogenic attractor process. *Social Development* 12(3): 314–34.

Green, J. M., Biehal, N., Roberts, C., Dixon, J., Kay, C., Parry, E., ... Sinclair, I. (2014). Multidimensional treatment foster care for adolescents in English care: randomised trial and observational cohort evaluation. *British Journal of Psychiatry* 204(3): 214–21. doi.org/10.1192/bjp.bp.113.131466

Greenberg, M. T., Kusche, C. A., Cook, E. T., & Quamma, J. P. (1995). Promoting emotional competence in school-aged children: the effects of the PATHS curriculum. *Development and Psychopathology* 7(01): 117–36.

Greenberg, M. T., Kusche, C. A., Mihalic, S. F., & Elliott, D. S. (1998). *Blueprints for Violence Prevention: Book Ten: Promoting Alternative Thinking Strategies.* Boulder, CO: Center for the Prevention of Violence. www.ncjrs.gov/App/abstractdb/AbstractDBDetails.aspx?id=174203

Hartnett, D., Carr, A., & Sexton, T. (2015). The effectiveness of functional family therapy in reducing adolescent mental health risk and family adjustment difficulties in an Irish context. *Family Process*. doi.org/10.1111/famp.1219

Hawes, D. J., & Dadds, M. R. (2005). The treatment of conduct problems in children with callous-unemotional traits. *Journal of Consulting and Clinical Psychology* 73(4): 737–41. doi.org/10.1037/0022–006X.73.4.737

Hawes, D. J., & Dadds, M. R. (2007). Stability and malleability of callous-unemotional traits during treatment for childhood conduct problems. *Journal of Clinical Child and Adolescent Psychology* 36(3): 347–55.

Hawes, D. J., Price, M. J., & Dadds, M. R. (2014). Callous-unemotional traits and the treatment of conduct problems in childhood and adolescence: a comprehensive review. *Clinical Child and Family Psychology Review*. doi.org/10.1007/s10567-014–0167-1

Henggeler, S. W., Rowland, M. D., Randall, J., Ward, D. M., Pickrel, S. G., Cunningham, P. B., ... Hand, L. D. (1999). Home-based multisystemic therapy as an alternative to the hospitalization of youths in psychiatric crisis: clinical outcomes. *Journal of the American Academy of Child & Adolescent Psychiatry* 38(11): 1331–9.

Hill, J., & Maughan, B. (2001). *Conduct Disorders in Childhood and Adolescence.* Cambridge: Cambridge University Press. books.google.co.uk/books?hl=en&lr=&id=QctzbWps7IQC&oi=fnd&pg=PP1&dq=Maughan,+B.+(2001)+Conduct+disorder+in+context.++&ots=5aJC9w6DST&sig=JdtnQbxVSGgI-lI5BfVBvivJNgs

Hobson, C. W., Scott, S., & Rubia, K. (2011). Investigation of cool and hot executive function in ODD/CD independently of ADHD. *Journal of Child Psychology and Psychiatry* 52(10): 1035–43. doi.org/10.1111/j.1469–7610.2011.02454.x

Hood, K. K., & Eyberg, S. M. (2003). Outcomes of parent–child interaction therapy: mothers' reports of maintenance three to six years after treatment. *Journal of Clinical Child & Adolescent Psychology* 32(3): 419–29. doi.org/10.1207/S15374424JCCP3203_10

Hughes, C., Dunn, J., & White, A. (1998). Trick or treat? Uneven understanding of mind and emotion and executive dysfunction in "hard-to-manage" preschoolers. *Journal of Child Psychology and Psychiatry* 39(07): 981–94.

Humayun, S., Oliver, B. R., Malpass, E., Chesnokov, M., & Scott, S. (2015). Drowned out? Household chaos negates the impact of positive parenting on non-violent antisocial behavior in juvenile delinquents. Paper presented at the Society for Research in Child Development Biennial Meeting, Philadelphia, PA.

Humphrey, N., Lendrum, A., & Wigelsworth, M. (2010). *Social and Emotional Aspects of Learning (SEAL) Programme in Secondary Schools: National Evaluation*. London: Department for Education. dera.ioe.ac.uk/11567/1/DFE-RR049.pdf

Humphrey, N., Kalambouka, A., Bolton, J., Lendrum, A., Wigelsworth, M., Lennie, C., & Farrell, P. (2008). *Primary Social and Emotional Aspects of Learning (SEAL): Evaluation of Small Group Work*. London: Department for Children, Schools and Families.

Institute of Medicine (1994). *Reducing Risks for Mental Disorders: Frontiers for Preventive Intervention Research*. Washington, DC: National Academy Press.

Jaffee, S. R., Caspi, A., Moffitt, T. E., Dodge, K. A., Rutter, M., Taylor, A., & Tully, L. A. (2005). Naturexnurture: genetic vulnerabilities interact with physical maltreatment to promote conduct problems. *Development and Psychopathology* 17(01): 67–84.

Jaffee, S. R., Moffitt, T. E., & Caspi, A. (2003). Life with (or without) father: the benefits of living with two biological parents depend on the father's antisocial behavior. *Child Development* 74(1): 109–26.

Jin, X., Sun, Y., Jiang, F., Ma, J., Morgan, C., & Shen, X. (2007). "Care for Development" intervention in rural China: a prospective follow-up study. *Journal of Developmental & Behavioral Pediatrics* 28(3): 213–18.

Johnston, J. R., Kline, M., & Tschann, J. M. (1989). Ongoing postdivorce conflict: effects on children of joint custody and frequent access. *American Journal of Orthopsychiatry* 59(4): 576.

Joseph, M. A., O'Connor, T. G., Briskman, J. A., Maughan, B., & Scott, S. (2014). The formation of secure new attachments by children who were maltreated: an observational study of adolescents in foster care. *Development and Psychopathology* 26(1): 1–14.

Kahn, R. E., Byrd, A. L., & Pardini, D. A. (2013). Callous-unemotional traits robustly predict future criminal offending in young men. *Law and Human Behavior* 37 (2): 87–97. doi.org/10.1037/b0000003

Kazdin, A. E., Bass, D., Siegel, T., & Thomas, C. (1989). Cognitive-behavioral therapy and relationship therapy in the treatment of children referred for antisocial behavior. *Journal of Consulting and Clinical Psychology* 57(4): 522.

Kazdin, A. E., Esveldt-Dawson, K., French, N. H., & Unis, A. S. (1987). Problem-solving skills training and relationship therapy in the treatment of antisocial child behavior. *Journal of Consulting and Clinical Psychology* 55(1): 76.

Keenan, K., & Shaw, D. (2003). Exploring the etiology of antisocial behaviour. In Lahey, B. B., Moffit, T. E., & Caspi, A. (eds.), *Causes of Conduct Disorder and Delinquency*. New York: Guilford Press, pp. 153–81.

Kelly, B., Longbottom, J., Potts, F., & Williamson, J. (2004). Applying emotional intelligence: exploring the promoting alternative thinking strategies curriculum. *Educational Psychology in Practice* 20(3): 221–40. doi.org/10.1080/0266736042000251808

Kiehl, K. A., Smith, A. M., Hare, R. D., Mendrek, A., Forster, B. B., Brink, J., & Liddle, P. F. (2001). Limbic abnormalities in affective processing by criminal psychopaths as revealed by functional magnetic resonance imaging. *Biological Psychiatry* 50(9): 677–84.

Kim-Cohen, J., Caspi, A., Moffit, T. E., Harrington, H., Milne, B. J., & Poulton, R. (2003). Prior juvenile diagnoses in adults with mental disorder: developmental follow-back of a prospective-longitudinal cohort. *Archives of General Psychiatry* 60(7): 709–17. doi.org/10.1001/archpsyc.60.7.709

Kling, A., Forster, M., Sundell, K., & Melin, L. (2010). A randomized controlled effectiveness trial of parent management training with varying degrees of therapist support. *Behavior Therapy* 41(4): 530–42.

Knerr, W., Gardner, F., & Cluver, L. (2013). Improving positive parenting skills and reducing harsh and abusive parenting in low- and middle-income countries: a systematic review. *Prevention Science* 14(4): 352–63. doi.org/10.1007/s11121-012–0314-1

Kolko, D. J., Dorn, L. D., Bukstein, O. G., Pardini, D., Holden, E. A., & Hart, J. (2009). Community vs. clinic-based modular treatment of children with early-onset ODD or CD: a clinical trial with 3-year follow-up. *Journal of Abnormal Child Psychology*, 37(5): 591–609. doi.org/10.1007/s10802-009–9303-7

Krishnakumar, A., & Buehler, C. (2000). Interparental conflict and parenting behaviors: a meta-analytic review. *Family Relations* 49(1): 25–44.

Lahey, B. B., Loeber, R., Hart, E. L., Frick, P. J., Applegate, B., Zhang, Q., ... Russo, M. F. (1995). Four-year longitudinal study of conduct disorder in boys: patterns and predictors of persistence. *Journal of Abnormal Psychology* 104(1): 83.

Lally, J. R., Mangione, P. L., & Honig, A. S. (1988). The Syracuse University Family Development Research Program: long-range impact on an early intervention with low-income children and their families. In Honig, A. S., & Powell, D. R. (eds.), *Parent Education as Early Childhood Intervention: Emerging Directions in Theory, Research and Practice,* vol. 3. Westport, CT: Ablex, pp. 79–104. psycnet.apa.org/psycinfo/1989–97054-005

Larson, J., & Lochman, J. E. (2010). *Helping Schoolchildren Cope with Anger: A Cognitive-Behavioral Intervention.* New York: Guilford Press. books.google.co.uk/books?hl=en&lr=&id=XlwGv5YCViwC&oi=fnd&pg=PP2&dq=Helping+Schoolchildren+Cope+with+Anger&ots=z-EaBs5GFf&sig=n32f2R5U9x-2HzVnmaJEMW9X7Bc

Lee, S., Aos, S., Drake, E., Pennucci, A., Miller, M., & Anderson, L. (2012). *Return on Investment: Evidence-Based Options to Improve Statewide Outcomes, April 2012* (Document No. 12-04-1201). Olympia: Washington State Institute for Public Policy.

Leschied, A. W., & Cunningham, A. (2002). Seeking effective interventions for serious young offenders: interim results of a four-year randomized study of multi-systemic therapy in Ontario, Canada. www.lfcc.on.ca/seeking.html

Letarte, M.-J., Normandeau, S., & Allard, J. (2010). Effectiveness of a parent training program "Incredible Years" in a child protection service. *Child Abuse & Neglect* 34(4): 253–61. doi.org/10.1016/j.chiabu.2009.06.003

Letourneau, E. J., Henggeler, S. W., Borduin, C. M., Schewe, P. A., McCart, M. R., Chapman, J. E., & Saldana, L. (2009). Multisystemic therapy for juvenile sexual offenders: 1-year results from a randomized effectiveness trial. *Journal of Family Psychology* 23(1): 89–102. doi.org/10.1037/a0014352

Leve, L. D., Chamberlain, P., & Reid, J. B. (2005). Intervention outcomes for girls referred from juvenile justice: effects on delinquency. *Journal of Consulting and Clinical Psychology* 73(6): 1181.

Lipsey, M. W. (2009). The primary factors that characterize effective interventions with juvenile offenders: a meta-analytic overview. *Victims & Offenders* 4(2): 124–47. doi.org/10.1080/15564880802612573

Littell, J. H. (2005). Lessons from a systematic review of effects of multisystemic therapy. *Children and Youth Services Review* 27(4): 445–63. doi.org/10.1016/j.childyouth.2004.11.009

Lochman, J. E., Baden, R. E., Boxmeyer, C. L., Powell, N. P., Qu, L., Salekin, K. L., & Windle, M. (2014). Does a booster intervention augment the preventive effects of an abbreviated version of the coping power program for aggressive children? *Journal of Abnormal Child Psychology* 42(3): 367–81. doi.org/10.1007/s10802-013-9727-y

Lochman, J. E., & Wells, K. C. (2002). Contextual social-cognitive mediators and child outcome: a test of the theoretical model in the Coping Power program. *Development and Psychopathology* 14(4): 945–67.

Lochman, J. E., & Wells, K. C. (2004). The coping power program for preadolescent aggressive boys and their parents: outcome effects at the 1-year follow-up. *Journal of Consulting and Clinical Psychology* 72(4): 571.

Loeber, R., & Farrington, D. P. (2000). Young children who commit crime: epidemiology, developmental origins, risk factors, early interventions, and policy implications. *Development and Psychopathology* 12(04): 737–62.

Loeber, R., Pardini, D., Homish, D. L., Wei, E. H., Crawford, A. M., Farrington, D. P., ... Rosenfeld, R. (2005). The prediction of violence and homicide in young men. *Journal of Consulting and Clinical Psychology* 73(6): 1074–88. doi.org/10.1037/0022-006X.73.6.1074

Losel, F., & Beelmann, A. (2003). Effects of child skills training in preventing antisocial behavior: a systematic review of randomized evaluations. *ANNALS of the American Academy of Political and Social Science* 587(1): 84–109. doi.org/10.1177/0002716202250793

Luria, A. R. (1961). *The Role of Speech in the Regulation of Normal and Abnormal Behavior*. New York: Pergamon Press. books.google.co.uk/books?hl=en&lr=&

id=5iqoBQAAQBAJ&oi=fnd&pg=PP1&dq=The+role+of+speech+and+the+regulation+of+normal+and+abnormal+behaviour.&ots=20odQCA3Ks&sig=kz0_f43XdbXAV_r3Ikhig3iigFY

Lynam, D. R., Caspi, A., Moffit, T. E., Wikström, P.-O., Loeber, R., & Novak, S. (2000). The interaction between impulsivity and neighborhood context on offending: the effects of impulsivity are stronger in poorer neighborhoods. *Journal of Abnormal Psychology* 109(4): 563.

Lynam, D. R., & Henry, W. (2001). The role of neuropsychological deficits in conduct disorders. In Hill, J., & Maughan, B. (eds.), *Causes of Conduct Disorder and Delinquency*. Cambridge, UK: Cambridge University Press.

Manning, M., Homel, R., & Smith, C. (2010). A meta-analysis of the effects of early developmental prevention programs in at-risk populations on non-health outcomes in adolescence. *Children and Youth Services Review* 32(4): 506–19. doi.org/10.1016/j.childyouth.2009.11.003

Macdonald, G., & Turner, W. (2008). Treatment foster care for improving outcomes in children and young people. *Cochrane Database of Systematic Reviews.* doi.wiley.com/10.1002/14651858.CD005649.pub2

Markie-Dadds, C., & Sanders, M. R. (2006). Self-Directed Triple P (Positive Parenting Program) for mothers with children at-risk of developing conduct problems. *Behavioural and Cognitive Psychotherapy* 34(03): 259. doi.org/10.1017/S1352465806002797

McCord, J. (1978). A thirty-year follow-up of treatment effects. *American Psychologist* 33(3): 284.

McCord, J. (1997). On discipline. *Psychological Inquiry* 8(3): 215–17. doi.org/10.1207/s15327965pli0803_10

McDonald, R., Dodson, M. C., Rosenfield, D., & Jouriles, E. N. (2011). Effects of a parenting intervention on features of psychopathy in children. *Journal of Abnormal Child Psychology* 39(7): 1013–23. doi.org/10.1007/s10802-011-9512-8

Meade, B., & Steiner, B. (2010). The total effects of boot camps that house juveniles: a systematic review of the evidence. *Journal of Criminal Justice* 38(5): 841–53. doi.org/10.1016/j.jcrimjus.2010.06.007

Melhuish, E., Belsky, J., Leyland, A. H., & Barnes, J. (2008). Effects of fully-established Sure Start Local Programmes on 3-year-old children and their families living in England: a quasi-experimental observational study. *Lancet* 372(9650): 1641–7.

Menting, A. T. A., Orobio de Castro, B., & Matthys, W. (2013). Effectiveness of the Incredible Years parent training to modify disruptive and prosocial child behavior: a meta-analytic review. *Clinical Psychology Review* 33(8): 901–13. doi.org/10.1016/j.cpr.2013.07.006

Moffitt, T. E. (1993a). Adolescence-limited and life-course-persistent antisocial behavior: a developmental taxonomy. *Psychological Review* 100(4): 674.

Moffitt, T. E. (1993b). The neuropsychology of conduct disorder. *Development and Psychopathology* 5(1–2): 135–51.

Moffitt, T. E. (2005). The new look of behavioral genetics in developmental psychopathology: gene-environment interplay in antisocial behaviors. *Psychological Bulletin* 131(4): 533.

Moffitt, T. E. (2006). A review of research on the taxonomy of life-course persistent versus adolescence-limited antisocial behavior. In Cullen, F. T., Wright, J. & Coleman, M. (eds.), *Advances in Criminological Theory: Taking Stock: The Status of Criminological Theory*, vol. 15. New Brunswick, NJ: Transaction, pp. 277–312. books.google.com/books?hl=en&lr=&id=4Apx0EeqCJEC&oi=fnd&pg=PA277&dq=moffitt+2006&ots=iGZJa3D2JB&sig=4vGiqPtb9NiYtw6OHsieWmWF_lM

Moffitt, T. E., & Caspi, A. (1998). Annotation: implications of violence between intimate partners for child psychologists and psychiatrists. *Journal of Child Psychology and Psychiatry* 39(02): 137–44.

Murray, J., & Farrington, D. P. (2010). Risk factors for conduct disorder and delinquency: key findings from longitudinal studies. *Canadian Journal of Psychiatry* 55(10): 633–42.

Musci, R. J., Bradshaw, C. P., Maher, B., Uhl, G. R., Kellam, S. G., & Ialongo, N. S. (2014). Reducing aggression and impulsivity through school-based prevention programs: a gene by intervention interaction. *Prevention Science* 15(6): 831–40. doi.org/10.1007/s11121-013–0441-3

Mytton, J. A., DiGuiseppi, C., Gough, D. A., Taylor, R. S., & Logan, S. (2002). School-based violence prevention programs: systematic review of secondary prevention trials. *Archives of Pediatrics & Adolescent Medicine* 156(8): 752–62.

National Research Council (U.S.) (2009). *Preventing Mental, Emotional and Behavioral Disorders among Young People,* O'Connell, M. E., Boat, T., & Warner, K. E. (eds.). Washington, DC: National Academies Press. www.ncbi.nlm.nih.gov/books/NBK32789/

NICE (National Collaborating Centre for Mental Health) (2013). CG158 conduct disorders in children and young people: NICE guideline [Guidance/Clinical Guidelines]. publications.nice.org.uk/antisocial-behaviour-and-conduct-disorders-in-children-and-young-people-recognition-intervention-cg158

Nigg, J. T., & Huang-Pollock, C. L. (2003). An early onset model of the role of executive functions and intelligence in conduct disorder/delinquency. In B. B. Lahey, T. E. Moffit, & A. Caspi (eds.), *Causes of Conduct Disorder and Delinquency*. New York: Guilford Press, pp. 227–53.

Nixon, R. D. V., Sweeney, L., Erickson, D. B., & Touyz, S. W. (2003). Parent–child interaction therapy: a comparison of standard and abbreviated treatments for oppositional defiant preschoolers. *Journal of Consulting and Clinical Psychology* 71(2): 251–60. doi.org/10.1037/0022-006X.71.2.251

O'Brien, M., & Daley, D. (2011). Self-help parenting interventions for childhood behaviour disorders: a review of the evidence: self-help intervention for childhood behaviour problems. *Child: Care, Health and Development* 37(5): 623–37. doi.org/10.1111/j.1365–2214.2011.01231.x

O'Brien, B. S., & Frick, P. J. (1996). Reward dominance: associations with anxiety, conduct problems, and psychopathy in children. *Journal of Abnormal Child Psychology* 24(2): 223–40.

O'Connor, T. G., Humayun, S., Briskman, J. A., & Scott, S. (2016). Sensitivity to parenting in adolescents with callous/unemotional traits: observational and experimental findings. *Journal of Abnormal Psychology* 125(4): 502–13. doi.org/10.1037/abn0000155

O'Connor, T. G., Matias, C., Futh, A., Tantam, G., & Scott, S. (2013). Social learning theory parenting intervention promotes attachment-based caregiving in young children: randomized clinical trial. *Journal of Clinical Child & Adolescent Psychology* 42(3): 358–70. doi.org/10.1080/15374416.2012.723262

Odgers, C. L., Moffitt, T. E., Broadbent, J. M., Dickson, N., Hancox, R. J., Harrington, H., ... Caspi, A. (2008). Female and male antisocial trajectories: from childhood origins to adult outcomes. *Development and Psychopathology* 20(02). doi.org/10.1017/S0954579408000333

Office of the Surgeon General. (2001). *Youth Violence: A Report of the Surgeon General.* Rockville, MD: U.S. Department of Health and Public Services.

Ogden, T., & Hagen, K. A. (2006). Multisystemic treatment of serious behaviour problems in youth: sustainability of effectiveness two years after intake. *Child and Adolescent Mental Health* 11(3): 142–9. doi.org/10.1111/j.1475-3588.2006.00396.x

Olds, D. L. (2007). Preventing crime with prenatal and infancy support of parents: the nurse-family partnership. *Victims & Offenders* 2(2): 205–25. doi.org/10.1080/15564880701263569

Olds, D., Henderson Jr, C. R., Cole, R., Eckenrode, J., Kitzman, H., Luckey, D., ... Powers, J. (1998). Long-term effects of nurse home visitation on children's criminal and antisocial behavior: 15-year follow-up of a randomized controlled trial. *JAMA* 280(14): 1238–44.

Osofsky, J. D. (1995). The effect of exposure to violence on young children. *American Psychologist* 50(9): 782.

Pardini, D., & Frick, P. J. (2013). Multiple developmental pathways to conduct disorder: current conceptualizations and clinical implications. *Journal of the Canadian Academy of Child and Adolescent Psychiatry* 22(1): 20.

Pasalich, D. S., Dadds, M. R., Hawes, D. J., & Brennan, J. (2011). Do callous-unemotional traits moderate the relative importance of parental coercion versus warmth in child conduct problems? An observational study. *Journal of Child Psychology and Psychiatry* 52(12): 1308–15. doi.org/10.1111/j.1469–7610.2011.02435.x

Patterson, G. R. (1982). *Coercive Family Process.* Eugene, OR: Castalia.

Patterson, G. R. (2002). Future extensions of the model. In Reid, J. B., Patterson, G. R., & Snyder, J. (eds.), *Antisocial Behavior in Children and Adolescents: A Developmental Analysis and Model for Intervention.* Washington, DC: APA, pp. 273–83.

Pearse, J., & Humayun, S. (2015). Functional family therapy in the UK: clinical practice, implementation and evaluation. Paper presented at the conference Aggression, Violence and Conduct Disorders: Bringing Together Basic Science, Prevention and Treatment. Association for Child and Adolescent Mental Health, London. www.acamh.org/events/2015/03/aggression-violence-and-conduct-disorders-bringing-together-basic-science-prevention

Pennington, B. F., & Ozonoff, S. (1996). Executive functions and developmental psychopathology. *Journal of Child Psychology and Psychiatry* 37(1): 51–87.

Petrosino, A., Turpin-Petrosino, C., & Buehler, J. (2003). Scared straight and other juvenile awareness programs for preventing juvenile delinquency: a systematic review of the randomized experimental evidence. *Annals of the American Academy of Political and Social Science* 589(1): 41–62. doi.org/10.1177/0002716203254693

Piquero, A. R., Farrington, D. P., Nagin, D. S., & Moffitt, T. E. (2010). Trajectories of offending and their relation to life failure in late middle age: findings from the Cambridge Study in Delinquent Development. *Journal of Research in Crime and Delinquency* 47(2): 151–73. doi.org/10.1177/0022427809357713

Piquero, A. R., Farrington, D. P., Welsh, B. C., Tremblay, R., & Jennings, W. G. (2009). Effects of early family/parent training programs on antisocial behavior and delinquency. *Journal of Experimental Criminology* 5(2): 83–120. doi.org/10.1007/s11292-009-9072-x

Rahman, A., Iqbal, Z., Roberts, C., & Husain, N. (2009). Cluster randomized trial of a parent-based intervention to support early development of children in a low-income country. *Child: Care, Health and Development* 35(1): 56–62. doi.org/10.1111/j.1365-2214.2008.00897.x

Reid, M. J., Webster-Stratton, C., & Hammond, M. (2003). Follow-up of children who received the Incredible Years intervention for oppositional-defiant disorder: maintenance and prediction of 2-year outcome. *Behavior Therapy* 34(4): 471–91.

Rhee, S. H., & Waldman, I. D. (2002). Genetic and environmental influences on antisocial behavior: a meta-analysis of twin and adoption studies. *Psychological Bulletin* 128(3): 490–529. doi.org/10.1037//0033-2909.128.3.490

Rhoades, K. A., Chamberlain, P., Roberts, R., & Leve, L. D. (2013). MTFC for high-risk adolescent girls: a comparison of outcomes in England and the United States. *Journal of Child & Adolescent Substance Abuse* 22(5): 435–49. doi.org/10.1080/1067828X.2013.788887

Rutter, M., Giller, H., & Hagell, A. (1998). *Antisocial Behavior by Young People*. Cambridge, UK; New York: Cambridge University Press.

Sanders, M. R., Kirby, J. N., Tellegen, C. L., & Day, J. J. (2014). The Triple P-Positive Parenting Program: a systematic review and meta-analysis of a multi-level system of parenting support. *Clinical Psychology Review* 34(4): 337–57. doi.org/10.1016/j.cpr.2014.04.003

Sanders, M. R., Markie-Dadds, C., Tully, L. A., & Bor, W. (2000). The Triple P-Positive Parenting Program: a comparison of enhanced, standard, and self-directed behavioral family intervention for parents of children with early onset conduct problems. *Journal of Consulting and Clinical Psychology* 68(4): 624–40. doi.org/10.1037//0022-006X.68.4.624

Schweinhart, L. J., Barnes, H. V., Weikart, D. P., Barnett, W., & Epstein, A. (1993). *Significant Benefits: The High/Scope Perry Preschool Study through Age 27*, vol. 27. Ypsilanti, MI.: High/Scope Press.

Schweinhart, L. J., Montie, J., Xiang, Z., Barnett, W. S., Belfield, C. R., & Nores, M. (2005). *Lifetime Effects: The High/Scope Perry Preschool Study through Age 40*. Ypsilanti, MI: High/Scope Press. works.bepress.com/william_barnett/3/

Scott, S. (2009). National dissemination of effective parenting programmes to improve child outcomes. *British Journal of Psychiatry* 196(1): 1–3. doi.org/10.1192/bjp.bp.109.067728

Scott, S., Briskman, J., & O'Connor, T. G. (2014). Early prevention of antisocial personality: long-term follow-up of two randomized controlled trials comparing indicated and selective approaches. *American Journal of Psychiatry* 171(6): 649. doi.org/10.1176/appi.ajp.2014.13050697

Scott, S., Briskman, J., Woolgar, M., Humayun, S., & O'Connor, T. G. (2011). Attachment in adolescence: overlap with parenting and unique prediction of behavioural adjustment. *Journal of Child Psychology and Psychiatry* 52(10): 1052–62. doi.org/10.1111/j.1469–7610.2011.02453.x.

Scott, S., & Dadds, M. R. (2009). Practitioner review: when parent training doesn't work: theory-driven clinical strategies. *Journal of Child Psychology and Psychiatry* 50(12): 1441–50.

Scott, S., Knapp, M., Henderson, J., & Maughan, B. (2001). Financial cost of social exclusion: follow up study of antisocial children into adulthood. *BMJ: British Medical Journal* 323(7306): 191.

Scott, S., & O'Connor, T. G. (2012). An experimental test of differential susceptibility to parenting among emotionally-dysregulated children in a randomized controlled trial for oppositional behavior. *Journal of Child Psychology and Psychiatry* 53(11): 1184–93. doi.org/10.1111/j.1469–7610.2012.02586.x.

Scott, S., O'Connor, T. G., Futh, A., Matias, C., Price, J., & Doolan, M. (2010a). Impact of a parenting program in a high-risk, multi-ethnic community: the PALS trial. *Journal of Child Psychology and Psychiatry* 51(12): 1331–41.

Scott, S., Sylva, K., Doolan, M., Price, J., Jacobs, B., Crook, C., & Landau, S. (2010b). Randomised controlled trial of parent groups for child antisocial behaviour targeting multiple risk factors: the SPOKES project. *Journal of Child Psychology and Psychiatry* 51(1): 48–57.

Seguin, J., Pihl, R. O., Harden, P. W., Tremblay, R. E., & Boulerice, B. (1995). Cognitive and neuropsychological characteristics of physically aggressive boys. *Journal of Abnormal Psychology* 104: 614–624.

Sexton, T., & Turner, C. W. (2010). The effectiveness of functional family therapy for youth with behavioral problems in a community practice setting. *Journal of Family Psychology* 24(3): 339.

Snell, T., Knapp, M., Healey, A., Guglani, S., Evans-Lacko, S., Fernandez, J.-L., … Ford, T. (2013). Economic impact of childhood psychiatric disorder on public sector services in Britain: estimates from national survey data. *Journal of Child Psychology and Psychiatry* 54(9): 977–85.

Snyder, J. J., & Patterson, G. R. (1995). Individual differences in social aggression: a test of a reinforcement model of socialization in the natural environment. *Behavior Therapy* 26(2): 371–91.

Soderstrom, H., Sjodin, A.-K., Carlstedt, A., & Forsman, A. (2004). Adult psychopathic personality with childhood-onset hyperactivity and conduct disorder: a central problem constellation in forensic psychiatry. *Psychiatry Research* 121(3): 271–80. doi.org/10.1016/S0165-1781(03)00270-1

Solmeyer, A. R., Feinberg, M. E., Coffman, D. L., & Jones, D. E. (2014). The effects of the family foundations prevention program on coparenting and child adjustment: a mediation analysis. *Prevention Science* 15(2): 213–23.

Somech, L. Y., & Elizur, Y. (2012). Promoting self-regulation and cooperation in prekindergarten children with conduct problems: a randomized controlled trial. *Journal of the American Academy of Child & Adolescent Psychiatry* 51(4): 412–22.

Sourander, A., Elonheimo, H., Niemela, S., Nuutila, A., Helenius, H., Sillanmaki, L., … Moilanen, I. (2006). Childhood predictors of male criminality: a prospective population-based follow-up study from age 8 to late adolescence. *Journal of the American Academy of Child & Adolescent Psychiatry* 45(5): 578–86.

Spain, S. E., Douglas, K. S., Poythress, N. G., & Epstein, M. (2004). The relationship between psychopathic features, violence and treatment outcome: the comparison of three youth measures of psychopathic features. *Behavioral Sciences & the Law* 22(1): 85–102. doi.org/10.1002/bsl.576

Speltz, M. L., DeKlyen, M., Calderon, R., Greenberg, M. T., & Fisher, P. A. (1999). Neuropsychological characteristics and test behaviors of boys with early onset conduct problems. *Journal of Abnormal Psychology* 108(2): 315.

Steiner, H., Saxena, K., & Chang, K. (2003). Psychopharmacologic strategies for the treatment of aggression in juveniles. *CNS Spectrums* 8(4): 298.

Stinchcomb, J. B. (2005). From optimistic policies to pessimistic outcomes: why won't boot camps either succeed pragmatically or succumb politically? *Journal of Offender Rehabilitation* 40(3–4): 27–52. doi.org/10.1300/J076v40n03_02

Stouthamer-Loeber, M., Loeber, R., Wei, E., Farrington, D. P., & Wikström, P.-O. H. (2002). Risk and promotive effects in the explanation of persistent serious delinquency in boys. *Journal of Consulting and Clinical Psychology* 70(1): 111–23. doi.org/10.1037//0022-006X.70.1.111

Swenson, C. C., Schaeffer, C. M., Henggeler, S. W., Faldowski, R., & Mayhew, A. M. (2010). Multisystemic therapy for child abuse and neglect: a randomized effectiveness trial. *Journal of Family Psychology* 24(4): 497–507. doi.org/10.1037/a0020324

Taylor, A., & Kim-Cohen, J. (2007). Meta-analysis of gene–environment interactions in developmental psychopathology. *Development and Psychopathology* 19(04). doi.org/10.1017/S095457940700051X

Theobald, D., Farrington, D. P., & Piquero, A. R. (2013). Childhood broken homes and adult violence: an analysis of moderators and mediators. *Journal of Criminal Justice* 41(1): 44–52.

Thomas, A., & Chess, S. (1977). *Temperament and Development*. New York: Brunner/Mazel. psycnet.apa.org/psycinfo/1978-03178-000

Timmons-Mitchell, J., Bender, M. B., Kishna, M. A., & Mitchell, C. C. (2006). An independent effectiveness trial of multisystemic therapy with juvenile justice youth. *Journal of Clinical Child & Adolescent Psychology* 35(2): 227–36. doi.org/10.1207/s15374424jccp3502_6

Tolan, P., Gorman-Smith, D., & Henry, D. (2004). Supporting families in a high-risk setting: proximal effects of the SAFEChildren preventive intervention. *Journal of Consulting and Clinical Psychology* 72(5): 855–69. doi.org/10.1037/0022–006X.72.5.855.

van der Stouwe, T., Asscher, J. J., Stams, G. J. J., Deković, M., & van der Laan, P. H. (2014). The effectiveness of Multisystemic Therapy (MST): a meta-analysis. *Clinical Psychology Review* 34(6): 468–81.

van IJzendoorn, M. H., Bakermans-Kranenburg, M. J., & Ebstein, R. P. (2011). Methylation matters in child development: toward developmental behavioral epigenetics. *Child Development Perspectives* 5(4): 305–10.

van IJzendoorn, M. H., Bakermans-Kranenburg, M. J., & Scott, S. (2015). Residential and Foster Care. In Thapar, A., Pine, D. S., Leckman, J. F., Snowling, M. J.,

& Taylor, E. (eds.), *Rutter's Child and Adolescent Psychiatry*. New York: Wiley-Blackwell, pp. 261–72. onlinelibrary.wiley.com/doi/10.1002/9781118381953.ch21/summary

Viding, E., Blair, R. J. R., Moffitt, T. E., & Plomin, R. (2005). Evidence for substantial genetic risk for psychopathy in 7-year-olds. *Journal of Child Psychology and Psychiatry* 46(6): 592–7. doi.org/10.1111/j.1469-7610.2004.00393.x

Wagner, D. V., Borduin, C. M., Sawyer, A. M., & Dopp, A. R. (2014). Long-term prevention of criminality in siblings of serious and violent juvenile offenders: a 25-year follow-up to a randomized clinical trial of multisystemic therapy. *Journal of Consulting and Clinical Psychology* 82(3): 492–99. doi.org/10.1037/a0035624

Waller, R., Gardner, F., & Hyde, L. W. (2013). What are the associations between parenting, callous–unemotional traits, and antisocial behavior in youth? A systematic review of evidence. *Clinical Psychology Review* 33(4): 593–608. doi.org/10.1016/j.cpr.2013.03.001

Wang, M.-T., & Kenny, S. (2014). Parental physical punishment and adolescent adjustment: bidirectionality and the moderation effects of child ethnicity and parental warmth. *Journal of Abnormal Child Psychology* 42(5): 717–30.

Webster-Stratton, C. (2003). The Incredible Years: parent, teacher, and child training series (IYS). In *Preventing Violence and Related Health-Risking Social Behaviors in Adolescents: An NIH State-of-the-Science Conference,* p. 73.

Webster-Stratton, C., Reid, M. J., & Hammond, M. (2001). Preventing conduct problems, promoting social competence: a parent and teacher training partnership in Head Start. *Journal of Clinical Child & Adolescent Psychology* 30(3): 283–302. doi.org/10.1207/S15374424JCCP3003_2

Webster-Stratton, C., Reid, M. J., & Stoolmiller, M. (2008). Preventing conduct problems and improving school readiness: evaluation of the incredible years teacher and child training programs in high-risk schools. *Journal of Child Psychology and Psychiatry* 49(5): 471–88.

Webster-Stratton, C., & Reid, M. (2010). Adapting the Incredible Years, an evidence-based parenting programme, for families involved in the child welfare system. *Journal of Children's Services* 5(1): 25–42. doi.org/10.5042/jcs.2010.0115

Weiss, B., Han, S., Harris, V., Catron, T., Ngo, V. K., Caron, A., . . . Guth, C. (2013). An independent randomized clinical trial of multisystemic therapy with non-court-referred adolescents with serious conduct problems. *Journal of Consulting and Clinical Psychology* 81(6): 1027.

Weisz, J. R., Jensen-Doss, A., & Hawley, K. M. (2006). Evidence-based youth psychotherapies versus usual clinical care: a meta-analysis of direct comparisons. *American Psychologist* 61(7): 671–89. doi.org/10.1037/0003-066X.61.7.671

Welsh, B. C., & Farrington, D. P. (2011). The benefits and costs of early prevention compared with imprisonment toward evidence-based policy. *Prison Journal* 91 (3 supplement): 120S–137S.

White, S. F., Frick, P. J., Lawing, K., & Bauer, D. (2013). Callous-unemotional traits and response to functional family therapy in adolescent offenders. *Behavioral Sciences & the Law* 31(2): 271–85. doi.org/10.1002/bsl.2041

Wilson, P., Rush, R., Hussey, S., Puckering, C., Sim, F., Allely, C. S., . . . Gillberg, C. (2012). How evidence-based is an "evidence-based parenting program"? A PRISMA systematic review and meta-analysis of Triple P. *BMC Medicine* 10(1): 130.

Wilson, S. J., & Lipsey, M. W. (2005). *The Effectiveness of School-Based Violence Prevention Programs for Reducing Disruptive and Aggressive Behavior*. Washington, DC: United States Department of Justice. www.ncjrs.gov/App/abstractdb/AbstractDBDetails.aspx?id=232642

Woltering, S., Granic, I., Lamm, C., & Lewis, M. D. (2011). Neural changes associated with treatment outcome in children with externalizing problems. *Biological Psychiatry* 70(9): 873–9. doi.org/10.1016/j.biopsych.2011.05.029

Woolgar, M., & Scott, S. (2014). The negative consequences of over-diagnosing attachment disorders in adopted children: the importance of comprehensive formulations. *Clinical Child Psychology and Psychiatry* 19(3): 355–66.

Zhang, T.-Y., Hellstrom, I. C., Bagot, R. C., Wen, X., Diorio, J., & Meaney, M. J. (2010). Maternal care and DNA methylation of a glutamic acid decarboxylase 1 promoter in rat hippocampus. *Journal of Neuroscience* 30(39): 13130–7. doi.org/10.1523/JNEUROSCI.1039-10.2010

Zoccolillo, M., Pickles, A., Quinton, D., & Rutter, M. (1992). The outcome of childhood conduct disorder: implications for defining adult personality disorder and conduct disorder. *Psychological Medicine–London* 22: 971–87.

15 Comprehensive School Counseling Programs

International Potential for Prevention

Julie M. Koch & Douglas Knutson

Introduction

In this chapter, we introduce readers to comprehensive school counseling programs as one means for prevention in school settings. Through comprehensive school counseling programs, professional school counselors are able to tailor prevention programs to their schools' needs, which may include prevention of dropout, substance abuse, bullying, and violence as well as promotion of career readiness, prosocial behaviors, and safe learning environments. Comprehensive school counseling programs as implemented in the United States are inherently preventive in nature. They are designed to target all children in a school system, in the areas of academic, career, and personal/social development. We summarize some of the similar challenges and opportunities faced by similar programs around the globe and provide examples of what elements of school counseling and school-based prevention programs look like internationally. Finally, we provide the reader with tools to implement and evaluate culturally relevant, needs-based comprehensive school counseling programs in schools in their home countries.

One challenge in the discussion of prevention programs offered in schools is that they look different around the globe. Even within countries, they may vary greatly. In the case of the United States, prevention efforts in schools are typically implemented in one of two ways. First, they may be provided by agencies outside of the school, but in collaboration with the school. An example of this would be a school district inviting an expert on suicide prevention to come and train faculty and staff. Another example would be a local counseling agency implementing a substance abuse prevention program for seventh and eighth graders at a school. The other method is when prevention efforts are an integral part of the school system, offered through school counselors, school social workers, school nurses, school psychologists, or administrators. Likewise, around the world, efforts focused on prevention in schools may be an integral part of the school system itself or may include outside agencies that work in collaboration with schools. In this chapter, we try to focus on school counselors, but occasionally that role carries a different label in another country, in which case we will point that out to the reader.

The main difference between *school-based prevention programs* and *comprehensive school counseling programs* is that school-based prevention programs can be any type of programming that occurs in a school setting, regardless of the provider. Comprehensive school counseling programs, on the other hand, are an integral part of the school system and are programmed by school counseling personnel who work with students, parents, and faculty on a daily basis. In function, the two can be closely related and are not mutually exclusive. In this chapter, however, we argue that comprehensive school counseling programs can be a highly effective and efficient means of prevention and health promotion with youth. Evidence shows that comprehensive school counseling programs have positive effects on academic achievement, prosocial behavior, and career development of school-age children and adolescents (Kim & Alamilla, 2008; McGannon, Carey, & Dimmitt, 2005; Whiston, Tai, Rahardja, & Eder, et al. 2011).

Although several definitions of prevention have been offered historically, in this chapter we apply Romano and Hage's (2000) definition of prevention to school settings. This includes school-based counseling programs that (a) stop (prevent) a problem from ever occurring; (b) delay the onset of an age-related problem or intervene with those at risk for a problem; (c) reduce the impact of an existing problem; (d) strengthen knowledge, attitudes, behaviors, and skills of individuals or groups to enhance protections against problems and disorders; and (e) support and advocate for institutional, community, and government policies that promote physical and emotional health and well-being (APA, 2014; Romano, 2015). We also use Gordon's (1987) classification system of universal, selective, and indicated prevention, as it seems to fit well with school structure. Universal prevention in this case would be a schoolwide effort, while selective and indicated prevention would be efforts at the small-group or individual level, targeted at children who have been identified to be at risk for some kind of problem.

Prevention is developmental in nature. In other words, some prevention efforts are best targeted at different age groups. In many cases, it is important that prevention programming focus on children at younger ages (Romano & Hage, 2000). There is evidence that prevention efforts beginning as early as prekindergarten programs such as Head Start are highly effective (Davis et al., 2013; Forness et al., 2000). With children being a primary focus of prevention efforts, school settings are a natural, logical environment in which prevention programs may be implemented (Romano, 2015). For many children and adolescents in the United States and elsewhere, schools are the major providers of mental health and social services (Adelman & Taylor, 2010; Burns et al., 1995). Schools have served as partners to prevent various problems, such as HIV/STD (Centers for Disease Control and Prevention, 2013); to promote the well-being of sexual orientation minority and gender identity minority children (Greytak & Kosciw, 2010); and to prevent bullying (Espelage & Swearer, 2004).

Prevention scholars have emphasized that school-based prevention programs should be comprehensive and integrated, as problems and issues are often interconnected, and there are too many issues seen in schools to address separately (Adelman & Taylor, 2000; Romano, 2015). These programs should be *comprehensive*, meaning that rather than having many discrete, fragmented efforts, they should be broad in range, include all levels of prevention, and include the whole school as well as communities (Adelman & Taylor, 2000). Programs should be *integrated* in that they should be integrated into the school system and should be coordinated with other prevention efforts in the school in a systematic manner (Adelman & Taylor, 2000).

In the United States, comprehensive school counseling programs based on the American School Counselor Association (ASCA) National Model (ASCA, 2003; 2012) are one means through which schools can make comprehensive and integrated prevention efforts. Comprehensive school counseling programs are directed by school counselors employed by schools. They include schoolwide prevention curriculum, small groups, and work with other school personnel and community members. Comprehensive school counseling programs are inherently preventive in nature. These programs are designed to target all children in a school system, in the areas of academic, career, and social/emotional development. They are flexible enough to allow individual schools or school systems to determine the areas of prevention that are most imperative for their needs. We provide an in-depth examination of comprehensive school counseling programs in the next section.

While historically there has been a dearth of empirical research examining the effectiveness of comprehensive school counseling programs (Whiston, 2002), this is gradually changing (Whiston et al., 2011). In addition to the longstanding journal *Professional School Counseling*, newer journals such as the *Journal of School Counseling* and *School Counseling Research and Practice* provide outlets for the dissemination of school counseling scholarship. The Center for School Counseling Outcome Research tracks the effectiveness of school counseling programs and produces monographs on recent positive outcomes (McGannon et al., 2005). Whiston et al. (2011) conducted a meta-analysis of 117 published and unpublished outcome studies on the effectiveness of school counseling programs. They examined both treatment-control and pretest/posttest comparisons, and found an overall weighted effect size of 0.30 for school counseling interventions, although many of these were not comprehensive in nature. One of the largest-scale studies of comprehensive school counseling programs was a statewide longitudinal study on academic achievement (Sink & Stroh, 2003). Findings indicated that elementary school children who attended schools with comprehensive school counseling programs had higher academic achievement test scores than students in schools without comprehensive school counseling programs. This effect increased the longer a child was enrolled in the same school with a comprehensive school counseling program (Sink & Stroh, 2003).

School counseling programs have great potential for prevention efforts geared toward children, adolescents, and their families. Being spearheaded by the schools themselves, they are able to address children in their natural environment, so to speak. School counselors who work with children on a daily basis may be highly aware of their needs and the needs of communities. They can be economically efficient as they use school personnel, facilities, and materials. With this in mind, it is crucial that scholars around the world continue to engage in conversations and collaborate on the development of school counseling programs (Romano, Goh, & Wahl, 2005). Around the world, school counseling and guidance programs have been well established in such countries as the United States, Taiwan, and Israel (Guo, Wang, Combs, Lin, & Johnson, 2013; Karayanni, 1996; Whiston et al., 2011). Educators in other countries, such as Kenya and Belize, have begun to recognize the utility of school-based counseling or comprehensive school counseling programs (Ajowi & Simatwa, 2010; Smith-Augustine & Wagner, 2012), and some countries such as Turkey (Aliyev, Erguner-Tekinalp, Ulker, & Shine-Edizer, 2012) and Israel (Israelashvili & Wegman-Rozi, 2012) have begun to institute these programs at even the early education level (ages three through four).

Comprehensive School Counseling Program Model in the United States

School counseling programs, historically often termed *guidance programs*, have a fairly long history in the United States, beginning with the rise of vocational guidance that developed in the Industrial Revolution of the late 1800s through the work of persons such as George Merrill and Frank Parsons (Schmidt, 2008). In the late 1890s, Merrill worked with a school in California to develop job training and job placement services for students. Beginning around 1908, Parsons put forth the notion that if people understood their own abilities and interests, and knew about the world of work and different types of employment, they could put that information together to make effective vocational decisions. The vocational guidance movement spread throughout U.S. schools (Schmidt, 2008). Eventually, in the 1950s, the ASCA was developed to standardize training of school counselors and the provision of services in schools (Myrick, 1997). Government funds were allotted to support school counseling programs (Schmidt, 2008), but no one seemed to agree exactly on the focus of school counseling programs (Myrick, 1997; Schmidt, 2008). Through the 1970s and 1980s, school counselors focused on academic and career development of students and a number of societal issues that were emerging – the need to advocate for special needs students, the need for gifted and talented education, racial and ethnic issues, and so on (Schmidt, 2008).

As school reform efforts became widespread in the United States in the 1980s and 1990s, it became apparent that school counseling programs were not always considered a crucial component to students' academic success. There was limited research linking the support services that school counselors provided to academic, personal, and career success (Stone & Dahir, 2006). In fact, some people perceived school counselors as only working with White, college-bound students, thereby maintaining the status quo of socioracial divides and inequities in the United States. The ASCA worked to develop and establish a system of delivery for all students that would be structured and systematic and promote academic achievement and career success, while preventing barriers to success (such as school dropout and substance abuse) (Stone & Dahir, 2006).

More recently, in 2003 with updates in 2012, ASCA developed the ASCA National Model of comprehensive school counseling programs to standardize provision of school counseling services in schools (ASCA, 2003; 2012). School counselors continue to face societal issues that affect students' lives, such as controversy over sexual orientation or gender identity; poverty and lack of resources in schools; domestic violence; suicide and major mental health issues; school violence; substance use and abuse; divorce; "parenting" by grandparents and extended family members; transitions and moves; and more. For example, on a daily basis, children in schools experience bullying from peers that affects their academic and personal development. In response to these challenges, with the ASCA National Model, school counselors have a stronger structure than ever before to guide them through their work. The ASCA National Model (2012) clearly puts preventive efforts at the forefront and delineates the roles of school counselors as personnel responsible for implementation of comprehensive school counseling programs. Furthermore, it requires school counselors to implement data-driven programs that are both based on evidence and gather further evidence, thereby linking school counseling programs to student success (Stone & Dahir, 2006). In the ASCA National Model, a comprehensive school counseling program consists of four components: foundation, delivery system, management, and accountability. Here, we summarize and offer examples of the components of the ASCA National Model as a backdrop against which we will analyze prevention efforts worldwide.

Foundation

The foundation of a comprehensive school counseling program consists of *program focus*, *student standards*, and *professional competencies* of the counselor.

Program focus. One key component of a comprehensive school counseling program is the belief that *all* students should benefit from such programs rather than a select few. Historically, United States school guidance counselors tended to give more attention to students with the highest grades and achievement or, conversely, the "problem" students who consistently were referred for disciplinary matters (Schmidt, 2008). Under a comprehensive school counseling program, all students' needs are addressed. To determine what the program focus will be, a school counselor will outline a vision for the school and student outcomes. This may be constructed in collaboration with other administrators, teachers, parents, and community members. The school counselor will also outline the mission, or specific goals, of the program. The mission may also include how goals are to be measured. Overall, school counseling programs are comprehensive and preventive (ASCA, 2012). Additionally, they are developmental in nature (ASCA, 2012), meaning, for example, that a substance abuse prevention program for sixth graders will look different from one aimed at twelfth graders.

Student competencies. Comprehensive school counseling programs focus on three main student competency domains: academic, career, and social/emotional development. In the academic realm, the school counseling program assists students with their academic development. This may mean that students are taught skills such as time management, test-taking skills, study skills, and so on. In the career realm, school counselors expose students to a wide range of career options and opportunities and administer appropriate career assessments to help students identify their interests and skills. In the social/emotional development domain, school counselors promote prosocial behaviors and positive interpersonal development (ASCA, 2012).

Professional competencies. According to ASCA (2012), professional school counselors should have the knowledge, attitudes, and skills required to provide competent services to students and to meet the high demands of being a school counselor. School counselors should be aware of ethical guidelines and laws that govern educational systems in their jurisdictions. The ASCA Ethical Standards for School Counselors outline standards for ethical behavior of school counselors (ASCA, 2010).

Delivery System

Comprehensive school counseling programs are delivered through four means: core curriculum, individual student planning, responsive services, and system support. These services are provided not only to students and school staff, but also to parents and to community members (ASCA, 2012). This delivery system fits with Romano and Hage's (2000) definition of prevention: first, prevention efforts are directed at the entire school (core curriculum, individual planning); next, prevention efforts are targeted at groups of students or individuals whose needs may not be met by the core curriculum (responsive services). This system is also compatible with the law of parsimony and allows for maximum use of school counselor time and resources in an efficient manner. For example, most students will respond positively to a schoolwide antibullying curriculum while there may be some students who are particularly vulnerable and may need additional support through group counseling. In their meta-analysis of comprehensive school counseling programs outcome research, Whiston et al. (2011) found that core curriculum and responsive services had the largest effects on cognitive, behavioral, and affective outcomes, with effect sizes of 0.35 and 0.35, respectively. Individual planning had an overall effect size of 0.26, and management had an effect size of 0.19. The findings of Whiston et al. provide evidence for the effectiveness of the delivery system of comprehensive school counseling programs, which is described in more detail later in this chapter.

School counseling core curriculum. The core curriculum is comprised of the guidance lessons or activities that counselors use to provide students with tools for positive development as well as prevention of things such as substance abuse and bullying. First, a school counselor conducts a needs assessment to determine the current high-priority needs of the children, parents, and community. For example, an elementary school principal might be concerned about the number of discipline referrals for fighting on a playground. The school administrators and school counselor might then determine that conflict resolution skills are an area of need at the school. School counselors seek out evidence-based curricula, if possible, to address those needs on a schoolwide basis. In this case, the school counselor looks for curricula, or guidance lessons, to use in the classroom with students. The curriculum is delivered systematically to all students in the classroom (universal prevention), schoolwide, in collaboration with school faculty (ASCA, 2012). For example, ten lessons teaching students conflict resolution skills may be taught over a course of ten weeks. Some examples of evidence-based curricula are *Peace Builders*, a violence prevention program;[1] Second Step, a program to build social skills;[2] and Bully Busters, a bullying prevention program.[3] The text, *Evidence-Based School Counseling* (Dimmitt, Carey, & Hatch, 2007), is an excellent resource and guide for school counselors who wish to implement core curriculum in their schools.

Responsive services. Individual and group counseling may also be done, when necessary, to serve students at risk or in a crisis (selective and indicated prevention) (ASCA, 2012). For example, the school counselor may have individual counseling sessions with a student who is being bullied at school, or the counselor might lead a small group focused on children whose parents are going through a divorce or other family transition (Omizo & Omizo, 1988). Group counseling also allows for response to a crisis such as the suicide of a student or an act of violence at school (Poland & McCormick, 1999).

Individual student planning. School counselors working within the ASCA model will also have a system in place to help students determine their own personal goals and future plans (ASCA, 2012). This does not necessarily mean one-on-one meetings, but rather a systemic effort to help all students (universal prevention) with these considerations. For example, all students in a school might be given a career assessment such as the Kuder Galaxy or Kuder Navigator.[4] These assessments are designed to help students as young as prekindergarten children learn about their own interests, skills, and values to make informed career decisions. Students will receive individual results in consultation with the school counselor to help them determine their future career and educational plans.

Indirect student services. School counselors also provide indirect services, which may not be as visible as other services. These may include referrals to

1 www.peacebuilders.com.
2 www.cfchildren.org/second-step.
3 www.researchpress.com.
4 Available at www.kuder.com.

other agencies outside of the school such as community mental health agencies for further assistance. School counselors may collaborate with parents or teachers or consult with community mental health providers or social workers (ASCA, 2012). For example, a school counselor may reach out to a local domestic violence agency to see whether there is shelter space available for a student's family.

Management

The management of a comprehensive school counseling program refers to the organization, structure, and assessment of the program. First, management involves assessment of the school counselors' performance and the strengths and weaknesses of the school's program. Management may include an assessment of how much time school counselors are spending on different activities. The ASCA National Model states that 80 percent of a school counselor's time should be spent on direct and indirect services to students as described previously (ASCA, 2012). The other 20 percent of the school counselor's time may be spent doing other school-related activities such as engaging in professional development or attending administrative meetings. Management also includes annual agreements between school counselor leaders in the school and school administrators about the focus of the program, the roles and responsibilities of the counselors, and the school counseling program goals. Often, advisory councils are used to guide the direction of the comprehensive school counseling program. Advisory councils may be made up of administrators, faculty, staff, parents, students, and community members, and their purpose, in addition to setting goals, is to assist the school counselors to manage and implement the comprehensive school counseling program. In managing the program, school counselors also must use data they have collected on the outcomes of their programs. Data may include student attendance rates, behavior/discipline referrals to the school counselors, student graduation rates, or other information. These data can be helpful to understand the effectiveness of comprehensive school counseling programs and may be presented to school boards, ministries of education, and so on to provide evidence and justification for comprehensive school counseling programs.

Management also includes action plans, their intended goals, and calendars for organization (ASCA, 2012). In this way, school counselors can organize and coordinate their programs. School counselors can use these tools to prioritize and track how they spend their time. A school may establish an action plan with goals to reduce dropout rates, for example. A calendar is used to establish, across a school year, the activities, lessons, meetings, and data collections to achieve that goal. The plan and calendar might include a schedule of all guidance lessons to be offered (where and when); parent–teacher association talks on the benefits of staying in school; small group meetings with students who are at higher risk of dropping out; and so on.

Accountability

School counselors are expected to evaluate the effectiveness of their comprehensive school counseling program, show its impact on school goals such as increased attendance or improved behavior, and determine what the needs are for future programming (ASCA, 2012). In this way, they are accountable for the delivery and outcomes of their comprehensive school counseling programs. Accountability remains one of the most important aspects of the success of comprehensive school counseling programs (ASCA, 2012; Whiston & Sexton, 1998). The notion of accountability answers the question, "How are students different as a result of the school counseling program?" (ASCA, 2003; Stone & Dahir, 2006). Stone and Dahir tell future school counselors: "Your school counseling program will be aligned with the educational enterprise, will be data-driven, proactive, and preventive in focus, and will assist students in acquiring and applying lifelong learning skills" (Stone & Dahir, 2006, p. 237). The ASCA national model requires school counselors to consider results that take into account local demographic needs and the climate of the community (ASCA, 2003; 2012).

One accountability process method proposed by Stone and Dahir (2004) is called *MEASURE.* It involves (a) establishing the mission and goals of the program; (b) identifying the critical data elements needed; (c) analyzing the critical data elements to establish a baseline; (d) including stakeholders and members of the community; (e) reanalyzing the data and comparing them to the baseline; and (f) educating the public and disseminating the data to show the positive impact of the school counseling program. Component (f) may be the most crucial piece: sharing support with stakeholders, administrators, and the community is essential for continued support of school counseling programs (Duarte & Hatch, 2014). Bemak, Williams, and Chi-Ying Chung (2015) assert that the most critical domains for accountability and promoting student success are grades, attendance, disciplinary referrals, and suspension.

An exemplar of the use of accountability comes from a school district in California that wrote a grant to fund comprehensive school counseling programs at three elementary schools (Duarte & Hatch, 2014). This program was extremely broad in scope, but here we will focus on the area of academic achievement and discipline issues to provide a clear example. Using the aforementioned *MEASURE* process, the program was designed as follows:

a. The mission and goals of the program were to implement a comprehensive school counselor program that would increase the academic achievement of all students and reduce barriers and increase resilience for students at risk of school failure.
b. The data elements were academic achievement test scores, the number of discipline referrals and suspensions, and the number of unexcused absences/ truancies.
c. Baseline data showed that there were 808 discipline referrals at all three schools combined the year of baseline and 2,140 unexcused absences at all schools combined.

d. Stakeholders included the school administration, teachers, the parent–teacher organization, and leadership teams.
e. After three years of the comprehensive school counseling program, data analysis showed increase in academic achievement and decrease in discipline issues. Standardized test scores in math and English increased by over 9 percent. The number of discipline referrals decreased by 64 percent, and unexcused absences decreased by 40 percent. Duarte and Hatch (2014) estimate that this saved approximately $40,000 (USD) for the school district that year.
f. Data from the program were shared in an intentional and purposive manner. Data were shared with principals, teachers, school board members, members of the community, and families. Presentations were made to the school superintendent and other school district administrators, emphasizing the improvements in attendance, improvements in academic achievement scores, and reduction of discipline problems. Based on this evidence, the school district agreed to not only continue to fund the program (as the grant funding ended), but to also expand the program to a middle school in the district (Duarte & Hatch, 2014).

Barriers

Unfortunately, there are many barriers to starting and implementing comprehensive school counseling programs. Even with evidence showing that comprehensive school counseling programs can result in positive outcomes, school systems with limited funding may have to prioritize. The result of this oftentimes is extremely high student-to-counselor ratios. For example, the state of California has over 6 million students and has struggled to fund education in recent years (Duarte & Hatch, 2014). In California, the student-to-counselor ratio was 1,016 to 1 in the 2010–2011 academic year (Keaton, 2012). When school systems do implement comprehensive school counseling programs, the actual quality of implementation can be compromised by differences of opinion between principals and school counselors about counselor responsibilities (Lapan & Harrington, 2010). If administrators do not fully understand or support comprehensive school counseling programs, school counselors may spend much of their time doing nonguidance work such as substitute teaching, enforcing disciplinary actions, or other tasks (Lapan & Harrington, 2010). In the first author's experience collecting data for a study on the implementation of comprehensive school counseling programs in elementary schools, there were issues with school counselor turnover; lack of principal support; lack of teacher support; and the training of school counselors on the guidance curriculum (Koch, 2008). In the first author's personal experience as a professional school counselor at the elementary and high school levels, comprehensive school counseling programs can be difficult to implement because teachers do not want to take away from instructional time; there is a lack of understanding overall about school counseling, and there may be differing opinions on the highest needs in the community. For example, one year the first author conducted a needs assessment at a high school with four groups: the student body, administration, teachers, and parents. The students requested more curricula to focus on race, diversity, and LGBT issues, while the administration wanted to focus on improving attendance rates, the teachers felt the highest priority should be study skills and student motivation, and the parents' organization wanted to focus on preparation for tests required for college admission. All of these obstacles can be challenges to the professional school counselor. At the same time, these barriers may be overcome with strong leadership and advocacy from professional school counselors to increase administrative support and understanding and educate the community and school personnel about the importance of comprehensive school counseling programs.

International School-Based Programs

Around the world, children and adults are affected by societal, geographical, political, and other issues that interfere with their personal and career development. The United Nations International Children Educational Fund (UNICEF, 2015) offers some statistics that are daunting. The UNICEF 2015 State of the World's Children Report provides statistics on children's well-being, including issues such as underweight children, access to water and sanitation, child labor, female genital mutilation, school attendance rates, and children orphaned by diseases such as AIDS. In 2013, the under-five mortality rate for children was over 10 percent in West and Central Africa. In that same year, the total worldwide deaths of children under five numbered 6.3 million. The United Nations (UN) Education First initiative reports that worldwide, 171 million children's growth is stunted by age five (UN, 2015). Yet, the UN and UNICEF both show that prevention and education efforts across the past forty years have produced large improvements in health and well-being. For example, the UN states that "the global increase in women's education has prevented more than four million child deaths" in the past four decades (UN, 2015, p. 1). Both organizations have prevention- and education-oriented plans to continue to target these needs. The UN predicts that if all children had basic reading skills, over 170 million people could be lifted out of poverty (UN, 2015). These statistics highlight the need worldwide for education and prevention efforts.

In response to these and other health-related issues, individual countries have developed preventive systems and networks of services that target developing young people as a way to reduce morbidity later in life. Terminology used to refer to school mental health practitioners can vary significantly between countries, as can training levels, education, roles, and expectations (Jimerson, Oakland, & Farrell, 2007b). Many authors note that counseling providers carry a variety of titles across the world, including social psychological help in Russia (Currie, Kuzmina, & Nadyuk, 2012); various types of guidance teachers in

Hong Kong (Yuen, 2003), Turkey (Stockton & Güneri, 2011), and South Africa (Berard, Pringle, & Ahmed, 1997); guidance counselors in Ireland (O'Leary, 1990); as well as psychopedagogues, or some subcategory of psychologist in other areas of the world (Hutz-Midgett & Hutz, 2012; Jimerson, Graydon, Curtis, & Staskal, 2007a),

The terminology used largely depends on the cultural, historical, educational, and legislative factors in a given country that give rise to the discipline of school counseling. For example, in Turkey, the Ministry of National Education (MONE) has regularly shaped the roles of school counselors (Stockton & Güneri, 2011). Similarly, Russian ministries have begun to fund and endorse various prevention programs and initiatives roughly parallel to Turkish school counseling (Currie et al., 2012; Stothard, Romanova, & Ivanova, 2007). Still, the core responsibility and function of these professionals, to provide guidance and support for students, families, and school personnel, remain fairly constant between nations regardless of title (Farrell, Jimerson, & Oakland, 2007). According to Farrell et al., (2007) newer dimensions of school interventions, such as developing and implementing prevention programs and activities, may require a level of training that is not yet offered in academic training programs worldwide and, therefore, may not be offered as consistently by school counselors throughout the world.

Here, we want to note that in discussing international school counseling programs, we are not including "overseas" or "international schools" that serve U.S. citizens or other international students in international settings. Rather, we are focusing exclusively on programs that serve the national students of their own countries. There has been no international assessment of the needs and function of school counselors similar to the International School Psychology Survey (Jimerson et al., 2007a), which assessed school psychology services in a variety of countries. Thus, collective analyses of comprehensive services worldwide are largely based on comparisons of reports and research from individual nations and globally informed understandings of the school counseling profession.

Some countries (such as the United States, Taiwan, and Israel) feature longer-standing, more regulated school guidance and/or counseling organizations, training programs, and services (Cunningham, 2007; Guo et al., 2013; Israelashvili & Wegman-Rozi, 2012; Karayanni, 1996). The length and visibility of counseling services may actually hinder the development and implementation of more comprehensive, especially preventive, services since national programs may become more resistant to change and may require demonstrated competence in a given area before practice can be allowed (Farrell et al., 2007). In places like Brazil and Israel, there has been some resistance among practitioners in related fields to forming separate legal and professional definitions for counselors as a group, although school counselors have existed for some time in Israel without legal codification (Hutz-Midgett & Hutz, 2012; Israelashvili & Wegman-Rozi, 2012). Therefore, it is possible that countries currently developing school counseling programs (e.g., Belize) are uniquely poised in the future to offer more comprehensive services. In the case of Belize, poverty and access to education are of urgent and primary importance (Smith-Augustine & Wagner, 2012). School counselors and related professionals in Belize have worked to increase access to education through fundraising, helping connect students to scholarships, and through the provision of mental health services that facilitate learning and self-efficacy. As indicated by the UN, this increased access to education may reduce poverty (UN, 2015).

Just as the titles assigned to school counselors may vary between countries, so do the types of services offered in schools (Jimerson et al., 2004). While some countries have instituted school counseling programs that implement a variety of the comprehensive school counseling tenets forwarded by the ASCA National Model, some function uniquely in each country and are shaped by historical, political, and situational concerns (Pokhrel, Masagutov, Kniazev, & Sussman, 2012). Here, we highlight some of these unique challenges, strengths, and similarities among programs in countries such as Israel, Taiwan, Brazil, Belize, Ireland, South Africa, and Turkey. We selected these countries in order to give readers a broader view of prevention efforts across the globe. While some Western nations have a history of longstanding, well-established preventive services, focusing only on Western programs would overlook efforts in a variety of countries to prevent and address a myriad of issues in innovative and effective ways (Perkins, 1971).

Challenges

School counselor availability. Some of the major issues facing school counselors are shared worldwide. One of the larger challenges is the wide gap in student-to–school counselor ratios and general lack of adequate numbers of counselors reported in countries such as Taiwan (much higher than 250-to-1), Belize (approximately 85,430-to-40), and Turkey (1,367-to-1) (Guo et al., 2013; Smith-Augustine & Wagner, 2012; Stockton & Güneri, 2011). This reduced availability of counselors may result in fewer interventions with students since counselors may be able to meet with each student only very briefly during the year (Berard et al., 1997; Guo et al., 2013). Additionally, confusion about what school counselors are supposed to do may result in a focus on teaching or teacher guidance roles that may preclude school counselors' ability to perform more counseling, prevention-oriented interventions (Guo et al., 2013; Stockton & Güneri, 2011).

Role confusion. In many countries, the delineation of counselor roles and responsibilities may be unclear due to a variety of factors. There may be a general confusion about differences in meaning between *counseling* and *guidance,* which may conflate support and guidance roles (Guo et al., 2013). This issue can be further complicated when guidelines and counselor roles are not nationally standardized in school counseling legislation, if it exists (Mandt, 2008; Stockton & Güneri, 2011). The title given to school counselors in legislation and/or the expectations placed on them by consumers can strongly influence the variety and availability of services provided (Cunningham, 2007; O'Leary, 1990; Stockton & Güneri, 2011). This lack of clarity about counselor roles, combined with a lack of funding, may increase pressure on counselors to shape services in accordance with pressure from parents, teachers, and or governments, which has been reported in places such as Turkey (Nazli, 2014) and Israel (Karayanni, 1996). These challenges are exacerbated when counselors face having their positions cut due to lack of funding and/or priority placed on school counseling among administrators and/or legislators (Guo et al., 2013; Stockton, & Güneri, 2011; Whiston & Sexton, 1998). As a result, the comprehensiveness of a school counseling program may be limited when a school counselor is regularly called upon to teach classes, provide testing services to large number of students, or perform administrative duties (Jimerson et al., 2007a; Mandt, 2008; Stockton & Güneri, 2011; Thomason & Qiong, 2008; Whiston & Sexton, 1998).

For example, in Turkey, the initial passage of the Ministry of National Education legislation 2001 served to increase school counseling services, but referred to school counselors as "guidance teachers" (Stockton & Güneri 2011). According to Stockton and Güneri (2011), this has led to utilization of school counselors for a variety of jobs and has, in some places, limited their role to addressing emotionally, socially, and/or academically challenged students through remediation rather than all students in a school with preventive services (universal prevention). These school counselors, who are already reportedly insufficient in number, may more often be called upon to perform teaching and/or administrative duties (Tekin, 2012). Similarly, in Ireland, a study indicated that school counselors worked longer hours than teachers because they were expected to both teach and provide support and guidance for students (O'Leary, 1990). The demands placed on school counselors, who are required by law to be present in schools, may be increased by a variety of factors, such as high student-to-counselor ratios, requirements to carry a teaching load, and poorly defined roles (Guo et al., 2013; Karayanni, 1996). Low numbers of school counselors, combined with role confusion, has resulted in the overworking of counselors worldwide. This is exacerbated by the serious and complex types of student concerns presented in schools.

Student concerns. School-based professionals must address issues such as increased presence of immigrant and refugee children in schools; natural disasters; and societal issues such as poverty, domestic violence, substance use, and war. Immigration can pose unique challenges for school counselors who wish to provide effective preventive services that meet students' unique needs (Goh, Wahl, McDonald, Brissett, & Yoon, 2007; Williams & Butler, 2003). For example, Israel has seen an increase in immigration of Jewish people from Ethiopia since 1973 and researchers such as Isralowitz, Shpiegel, Reznik, and Laytin (2009) have identified a variety of unique needs and challenges faced by this population (e.g., discrimination, elevated substance abuse). In an effort to address the needs of immigrant children in schools, the European Commission Directorate-General for Education and Culture (Eurydice, 2009) coordinated comparative studies of the integration of immigrant children and language proficiency in European schools, with reports provided for each European nation. Eurydice found that language barriers and communication with families were major concerns for schools.

Large natural disasters, war, and societal issues can also interrupt services and/or create an increased demand on school counselors to provide comprehensive preventive services. For example, one year after the devastating 2004 tsunami hit Thailand, scholars found that adolescents' behavior problems were closely tied to their experiences of the tsunami (Tuicomepee & Romano, 2008). In a study of adolescents eighteen months after Hurricane Katrina hit the Gulf Coast of the United States, researchers found ties to posttraumatic stress disorder (PTSD) and substance abuse (Overstreet, Salloum, & Badour, 2010). In Belize, the issue of poverty works in conjunction with other societal issues so that school counselors focus on helping students find funds for school uniforms and tuition costs so that they can continue their education beyond the compulsory level (approximately the eighth grade in the United States) (Smith-Augustine & Wagner, 2012).

Historical impact. Professional school counseling as a recognized discipline (e.g., offered in universities, subject to government oversight, utilized by communities) is relatively new in some countries, may operate under a variety of monikers (e.g., school psychologist, school counselor, guidance teacher, guidance counselor), and may fill a variety of preventive and preemptive roles (e.g., diagnosis, case management, psychoeducation). This wide variance in terminology, role, and function has led to a near indistinguishable blending of the disciplines of teaching, school counseling, and school psychology in some countries. The existence of a variety of professionals with various titles does not herald difficulties or conflict by default. For example, in Singapore, various professionals collaborate to provide more integrated, comprehensive preventive services (Yeo, Tan, & Neihart, 2012). In Singapore, teacher counselors, educational psychologists, allied educators, guidance specialists, and counselors work together to provide care for students and, as a team, may be better equipped to address more acute and/or complex concerns.

In some cultural contexts, counseling and psychological services carry longstanding stigma resulting from a troubled past. In some countries, psychological services were once used by governments and others to maintain power and control over the general public by diagnosing mental health concerns and thereby stigmatizing and in some cases discrediting citizens (Currie et al., 2012; Thomason, & Qiong, 2008). Initially, this may have contributed to a resistance in the general population to utilization of mental health services. However, in the last fifty years, school psychological and counseling services have been developed and offered by many countries and have garnered a presence in schools, especially in countries with public education systems due to increasing awareness of the need for mental health services and due to intercultural contact between countries (Jimerson et al., 2007a).

These programs and services have been significantly shaped by the historical and political contexts in which they are offered. In some countries, services may be more content-driven and psychoeducational while others may emphasize academic performance and focus on testing and assessment (Currie et al., 2012; Thomason, & Qiong, 2008). Romano et al. (2005) state that the role of school counselors in the Asia-Pacific region often focuses on high academic achievement and improving the reputation of the school. For example, China's guidance counseling services were shaped by its national history. Western psychology, with the exception of behaviorism, was largely absent from Chinese culture beginning with World War II through about 1976 (Lim, Lim, Michael, Cai, & Schock, 2010). To this day, many favor traditional Eastern healing approaches such as herbs and deep breathing exercises designed to treat metaphysical ailments (Lim et al., 2010), as opposed to Western psychological approaches to mental health. Furthermore, a historical and lasting emphasis on academic performance may contribute to greater attention to students' cognitive and academic functioning and may reinforce a more disciplinary role among "guidance teachers" in China (Hui, 1999; Lim et al., 2010). While this high emphasis on performance and discipline may dominate guidance counseling services in China, students may also receive support and resources from guidance teachers (Hui, 1999).

Strengths

Legislative oversight. Over time, changes have been created at a legislative level in such places as Turkey and Ireland, resulting in sweeping changes to countrywide education standards. These standards are implemented by school-based professionals such as guidance teachers and guidance counselors, as they are referred to in Turkey and Ireland respectively (O'Leary, 1990; Stockton & Güneri, 2011). For example, the minister for education in Ireland initiated a School Psychological Service in 1966 to provide prevention and intervention support for students (O'Leary, 1990). While such moves may result in the sorts of high student-to-counselor (or other school mental health professional) ratios addressed earlier, they also serve to institutionalize, standardize, and bolster services offered (Jimerson et al., 2007a; Stockton & Güneri, 2011). Over time, countries may move to more structured and organized standards, legislation, and professional organizations for school counselors. Countries such as the United States, New Zealand, and England currently feature such frameworks, although in the United States standards of conduct and requirements for licensure vary by state (Cunningham, 2007).

Needs-based services. Since the unique political climates and social expectations of a given country shape the availability of counseling services, school counselors are poised to identify and meet needs as they arise. In order to identify the gaps in care, some scholars have used the International School Psychology Survey (ISPS) to evaluate the availability and topography of school-based psychological services in a variety of countries. For example, the questionnaire was used in Egypt to assess, among other things, the amount of time allotted to student support among school-based mental health providers.

Based on the results, Jimerson, Alghorani, Darweish, and Abdelaziz (2010) pointed out that Egyptian school psychologists spend 17 percent of their time focused on primary prevention programs and 44 percent providing direct services, though these traditionally counseling-related tasks are usually carried out by school counseling staff in other countries. In Turkey, a study examined counseling and guidance services in early childhood education at select public schools in Malatya (Tekin, 2012) and identified a greater need for increased coordination among counselors, parents, children, and teachers. In South Africa, Berard et al. (1997) examined available counseling resources in high schools on the cape peninsula and identified a need for more counselors in schools.

Movements toward social justice. School counselors may meet student needs and challenges with cultural sensitivity, which is crucial to the success of counseling programs (Sue, Arredondo, & McDavis, 1992). For example, in Brazil a commitment to multiculturalism is a strength among school counselors, who are not yet a distinct presence but are distinguishing themselves by demonstrating cultural sensitivity in a diverse society by raising awareness about and advocating for individuals who are not members of the dominant socioracial population (Hutz-Midgett & Hutz, 2012). In Israel, results from a survey of 200 school counselors indicated that participants perceived their role to be that of a social advocate and as a leader on behalf of disadvantaged students (Erhard & Sinai, 2012) Outreach and advocacy efforts include culturally informed and culturally sensitive services that address the needs of immigrant students (Israelashvili & Wegman-Rozi, 2012). Respondents also reported a high sense of justice that informed their provision of services for all students (Erhard & Sinai, 2012). Egalitarian beliefs about the provision of counseling may be foundational for the dissemination of services for all students throughout culturally diverse schools.

School-Based Preventive Initiatives Worldwide

Based on the wide variety of literature available, it appears that components of the comprehensive school counseling model are being implemented effectively, although differently, across the globe. Regardless of cultural, political, and other challenges, many countries equal or surpass well-established programs such as those in the United States in provision of services to students. School counseling programs across the world range from those that are well-established (e.g., England, Israel, and the United States) to those that are in their formative stages (e.g., Belize, Brazil, and Russia). In this section, we will provide an in-depth look at the school counseling systems in Israel, Belize, Taiwan, Brazil, and Russia. Here, we illustrate the wide range of school counseling programs, from those that are well established and supported, to newer programs. We do so in order to provide illustrations of programs in countries across the globe, rather than focusing on Western nations.

Israel. In Israel, at least six research universities offer master's and/or doctoral programs in school counseling (Israelashivili & Wegman-Rozi, 2012).

School-based services have been offered for several decades in Israel since school counseling was introduced in Israeli schools during 1960 in response to an urgent need for vocational guidance and to manage learning difficulties among students (Karayanni, 1985). Later, in an updated review of the development of school counseling and guidance in Israel, Karayanni (1996) predicted that multicultural counseling would likely continue to be a major issue. He indicated that ideological and historical divisions between diverse populations in Israel would necessitate cultural sensitivity and awareness on the part of school counselors in the nation (Karayanni, 1996). His projections were later confirmed by Israelashvili and Wegman-Rozi (2012) in their discussion of formal and applied counseling in Israel. Fifteen years after Karyanni's work, Israelashvili and Wegman-Rozi (2012) advocate the primary concerns for counselors as being multiculturalism and terror management, which they extended to school-based professionals by pointing out the presence of security threats and large waves of immigration. Israeli school-based professionals have been called upon to address the needs of students who have been exposed to trauma and situations involving terror (Abel & Friedman, 2009; Gelkopf & Berger, 2008). These students may come from a variety of nations (Israelashvili & Wegman-Rozi, 2012). For example, Isralowitz et al. (2009) cite the recent influx of Ethiopian youth and identify specific stressors, including low socioeconomic status and prejudice, which may result in elevated rates of adolescent alcohol use among members of this subpopulation in Israel. Proactively addressing the culture-related challenges faced by all students may be a way to prevent prejudice-based violence and substance abuse among these minority populations and may reduce tensions with the majority population in Israel.

School counselors in Israel appear to have taken up the challenge put forth by Karayanni in 1996 by developing a professional identity that includes a value for social justice (Erhard & Sinai, 2012). In addition to their standard guidance and support work, school counselors have begun to institute psychoeducational programs for stress management and safety planning and have begun to focus on early identification of student needs (Abel & Friedman, 2009; Gelkopf & Berger, 2008). This identification with a social justice orientation and advocacy for student health and well-being is in alignment with Romano and Hage's (2000) definition of prevention.

Belize. In this description, we draw heavily from the experiences of the first author of this chapter consulting and collaborating with the Belize Ministry of Education in 2010–2011 as well as from Smith-Augustine and Wagner's (2012) description of school counseling in Belize. School counseling in Belize is a fairly recent practice (Smith-Augustine & Wagner, 2012). The Belize Ministry of Education recently passed and began implementing new legislation for school reform, including the requirement that teachers hold teaching licenses (Belize Ministry of Education, 2012). Teachers in Belize are not required to complete training beyond high school aside from some tertiary training and instruction. There are no current licensing or training requirements for school counselors above and beyond the requirements for teachers, and there are no training programs for school counseling in Belize. However, the new formation (beginning around 2010) of the Belize Association of School Counsellors and the Belize Catholic Association of School Counsellors (Smith-Augustine & Wagner, 2012) indicates that standards and training programs will likely be forthcoming.

In 2012, there were approximately 40 counselors in Belize, while there were 349 schools and approximately 85,000 students (Smith-Augustine & Wagner, 2012). Most counselors, who are designated as teachers within their schools, focus on secondary school needs (approximately ages fifteen through eighteen). Counselors in Belize face a variety of challenges when attempting to provide services for students. One primary issue is the fact that 40 percent of Belize's population is considered to be below the poverty line and school attendance comes with unavoidable costs (Smith-Augustine & Wagner, 2012; U.S. Department of Labor, 2013). Children in Belize often do not have adequate access to health care, are exposed to domestic violence, and are victims of abuse and neglect, and most do not complete education beyond the required primary level (approximately age fourteen) as they do not have the funds for private school. In Belize, primary school is compulsory and is mostly funded by the government, with some funding coming from religious organizations. Secondary schools, however, are all private. About 75 percent of students who complete primary school continue on to secondary school, but only about half of students who begin secondary school complete it (Belize Ministry of Education, 2013). According to Smith-Augustine and Wagner (2012), it is not uncommon for school counselors to become fundraisers in order to help pay for school fees and uniforms to keep students in school. School counselors may travel long distances to serve students at different schools. They often include parents and families in their work with children. Most school counseling work in Belize fits within Romano and Hage's (2000) component (c) of their definition of prevention: reducing the impact of existing problems. While school counseling is new to Belize, however, the passion that school counselors have for working with children was evident to the first author in her travels to Belize and visits with school counselors there. With little resources and materials, the school counselors have been determined to begin two national organizations and to further their training through workshops and travel to the United States for ASCA conferences.

Taiwan. According to Guo et al. (2013), guidance and counseling were initially cultivated in Taiwan in order to meet the needs of foreign students (mostly Westerners including individuals from the United States) during the mid-twentieth century, and it was not until around 1968 that services for Taiwan nationals were sanctioned by the Ministry of Education in schools. In 2011, a revision to the Citizen's Education Law was passed requiring that an increased number of school counselors be recruited in five years following the mandate to address increases in school bullying (Taiwan Ministry of Education, 2011). This may pose a unique challenge since the rapid growth in need of school counselors in recent years has not been met with an attenuating growth in financial resources to support school counselors (Guo et al., 2013).

In Taiwan, school-based service providers face a variety of challenges, such as limited funding, high student-to-counselor ratios, and the need to serve in dual roles (Guo et al., 2013). Though school counselors and guidance teachers are not required to be licensed, they may be expected to meet the criteria necessary for licensure (e.g., to obtain a master's degree and to pass the national licensing exam). Still, counselors continue to be engaged, whenever possible, in providing individual support and guidance for students in both primary and secondary schools in keeping with the three-tiered prevention system instituted by the government that splits the responsibility for student guidance among teachers, counselors, and the broader society (Guo et al., 2013). To guide and augment the work of school counselors, a variety of prevention-oriented literature is being produced in Taiwan to avert student tobacco use (Chen, Huang, & Chao, 2011), substance use (Huang, Chien, Cheng, & Guo, 2012), and Internet addiction behaviors that may lead to cyberbullying (Lan & Lee, 2013). For example, at least one group of researchers used the online curriculum platform provided by WebQuest[5] to provide anticyberbullying curriculum online (Lee, Zi-Pei, Svanström, & Dalal, 2013). School counselors in Taiwan may be able to cultivate optimally effective preventive services that will enable them to stop these problems from occurring (Romano & Hage, 2000).

Brazil. Brazil is somewhat of a unique case when it comes to school guidance and counseling since helping professionals (e.g., psychologists, social workers, and teachers) have provided counseling services in schools since the 1950s, but no distinct discipline or licensure has taken shape for school counselors as a separate group (Hutz-Midgett & Hutz, 2012). Thus, school counselors as separate, credentialed professionals are absent from Brazilian schools (Hutz-Midgett & Hutz, 2012). This absence is reflected in the research literature, which focuses on the involvement of teachers as guides and providers of support and education for students (Kashima et al., 2008). Licensure is only granted to psychology majors who complete a five-year undergraduate program that includes a two-year internship (Hutz, Gomes, & McCarthy, 2006).

The role of teacher-as-counselor is utilized in other countries such as Turkey and Belize, but these countries have distinct classifications for teachers who assume a counseling or guidance role (Smith-Augustine & Wagner, 2012; Tekin, 2012). While such an arrangement is not ideal, in the absence of visible school counselors, Brazilian teachers play a large role in the cultivation of positive school climates for LGBT students and others (Alexander, Santo, Cunha, Weber, & Russell, 2011) and in providing HIV/AIDS education and prevention (Kashima et al., 2008). Some researchers laud the accomplishments of guidance-focused teachers who create school climates that are more supportive for students facing a variety of challenges (Alexander et al., 2011; Kashima

5 webquest.org.

et al. 2008). As the demand for sex-education, multicultural competence, and vocational counseling grow, some argue, so will the demand for licensed school counselors (Hutz-Midgett & Hutz, 2012).

Implementation of Comprehensive School Counseling Programs

Comprehensive school counseling programs may be implemented in ways that are flexible, efficient, and time- and cost-effective, regardless of national, cultural, social, economic, or religious contexts or environments. In this section, we will discuss ways in which counselors, prevention-focused educators, and school personnel can implement comprehensive school counseling programs in their own countries and provide issues for consideration when developing such programs. As Romano et al. (2005) remind us, and as we have described in this chapter, there are significant international differences in educational systems, their philosophies, and their values that influence the role of school counseling programs and their implementation.

According to Adelman and Taylor (2000), educational systems that are organized effectively and have properly trained personnel are in a strong situation to (a) make decisions about allocation of resources; (b) plan, implement, maintain, and evaluate prevention activities; (c) engage in outreach to community and other partners; and (d) utilize best practices in prevention interventions and in modern technology. However, these efforts may require new philosophies about the roles of educators and restructuring of current systems (Adelman & Taylor, 2000). We encourage counselors and educators around the world to develop organized systems of school counseling, if not already in place, to address the needs of their communities and nations. As in Belize, these initiatives can start with simple conversations with other like-minded individuals, which may grow to a group of like-minded individuals, which with leadership can develop into a professional organization to provide leadership and advocacy for school counseling programs. If school counseling systems already are in place, we encourage educators to evaluate their current utility and determine whether reforms should be made.

Romano et al. (2005) developed suggestions for school counseling programs in the Asia-Pacific region, which we stretch to apply internationally. First, they encourage educators to keep in mind the importance of cultural context. They note Leong's (2002) model of cultural accommodation when applying Western theories to Asian countries, which includes looking for gaps in cultural norms; selecting culturally appropriate concepts to fill in the gaps; and testing the new model's effectiveness. We suggest that while applying a United States model to international settings may be helpful or appropriate for some, it may also be useful for countries to develop their own systems "from scratch" or through learning what not to do from mistakes other countries have made. We hope that by reviewing a broad range of existing and developing systems throughout the world, and with our suggestions in Table 15.1, we have provided some information that will be helpful in that regard. Second, Romano et al. (2005) note the importance of the sociopolitical climate of the countries in which school counseling programs exist. School counselors should understand how the role of preventive school counseling programs fits within their larger nation's goals for education and development of children. In planning school counseling programs, educators should evaluate how they match societal values as well. For example, a pressing need might be HIV/STD prevention, but if the district or country in which school counselors work has a taboo on sex-related education or discussions, it will be important to consider how this will be handled. Third, Romano et al. (2005) discuss the nature of education systems in Asia, specifically related to how school counseling programs may be used specifically to promote high educational achievement, a school's or a nation's reputation, or national labor needs. This will differ around the world based on different countries' perceptions of the role of education and whether school counseling programs are to focus on personal, career, or academic development of the child or on some other area. Is there a national emphasis on academic performance? Or perhaps on the need for more skilled workers in health professions? Fourth, Romano et al. (2005) state that it is important to consider what school counselors' roles are and how they are outlined. With role confusion being an issue worldwide, nations should standardize and clearly delineate the responsibilities and tasks of school counselors. Finally, they emphasize the need for school counselors to work with a team to address students' educational needs (Romano et al, 2005). Educators will need to determine whether this is most appropriate in their cultural context and who the members of the "team" would be.

Romano et al. (2005) developed excellent questions for educators in the Asia-Pacific region to keep in mind when developing or improving their school counseling programs and for training of school counselors. While we recognize that other scholars have provided recommendations of standards and guidelines regarding preventive school-based and/or comprehensive school counseling programs (e.g., Sink & Moore, 2013; Wright & Gray, 2007), we think that the questions offered by Romano et al. (2005) provide the most useful and helpful framework for consideration. Their questions include issues regarding training; skills; school administration understanding of school counseling programs; the need for program evaluation and research on efficacy; systemic change; the integral nature of school counseling programs; the need for school counseling programs at all levels (K–12); a need to focus on prevention; multicultural competencies; and collaboration with partners. Keeping the ASCA National Model (2012) and the current diverse nature of international school counseling approaches in mind, we expand on these questions. In Table 15.1, we provide issues for consideration when developing, implementing, or reforming comprehensive school counseling programs at the national, regional/district, and school levels. It is important for school counselors to keep in mind that administrative and policy support of comprehensive prevention programs can be crucial to their success (Adelman & Taylor, 2000).

Table 15.1 *Issues for Consideration When Developing, Implementing, or Reforming Comprehensive School Counseling Programs*

Issues for consideration at the national level

1. Governmental issues: What are the roles of the national government and national departments of education, if any, in standardizing school counseling programs?
2. Professional organizations: Are there national professional school counseling organizations in place?
3. Credentialing: Will there be a certification or license required to practice as a school counselor? Will this be determined at the national or local level (see also the next section of this table)?
4. Training needs: What educational systems are in place to train school counselors? Who decides what the training requirements will be and at what level? Is there funding available for this training? Are there nearby countries or partner countries or educational institutions where school counselors may acquire training? What areas, such as cultural competence, might be most important for school counselors to have?
5. Ethical issues: Who will determine the school counselor standards for ethics and behavior? Professional organizations? Government entities?

Issues for consideration at the local, regional, state, or district level

6. Support: Is there support at the local level for school counseling programs? How can local entities gain "buy in" from their communities for school counseling programs?
7. Financial resources: What kind of funds are available for the hiring of school counselors? How will school counseling programs be prioritized? What kind of job or financial security can be offered to school counselors?
8. Credentialing: Will the need for certain training, licensure, or certification be dictated at the local level? Who will make these determinations?
9. Hiring needs: How will school counselors be hired? What will their titles be? Will their pay or benefits be different from teachers?

Issues for consideration at the school level

10. Facility needs: Is separate space needed for the school counseling? For storage or for individual or group counseling? Will the school counselor(s) have an office to meet with parents?
11. Technology needs: What are the technology needs? Should the school counseling program have a website? What software is needed to manage data collection and evaluation?
12. Personnel needs: Are support staff needed (for filing, answering phones, scheduling, etc.)?
13. Relationships with school administrators, teachers, and staff: Do administrators understand the role of school counselors? Is there teacher "buy in" to the school counseling program? Will the school counseling program take away from instructional time (and how will this be presented to teachers)?
14. Materials: What school counseling materials are needed? At the secondary level, is there access to career assessments? At the primary level, does the school counseling program need books? Puppets?
15. Budget: What will be the costs of the school counseling program to the school? How will these be supported at the local or national level?
16. Roles: What roles will the school counselor have? How much power does the school counselor have within the school? Are they expected to coach sports, or act in an administrative role if the principal is unavailable? Do they manage testing or focus on classroom-based lessons?

Table 15.1 (*cont.*)

17.	Ethical issues: How is the school counselor expected to handle issues that are sensitive in the community (such as sexual education/HIV/STD prevention)? What are the expectations for student confidentiality? What are a student's rights? What are parents' rights?
18.	Accountability: How will school counselors show that their work is effective and meeting the needs of their school? How will school counselors measure any changes they have made (attendance records, number of students attending college, etc.)?
19.	Relationships with community: How will the school counseling program collaborate with community organizations and members? Are there parent volunteers who can be utilized for help? Are there community organizations willing to donate materials or funds? Will the school work with local nurses, dentists, physicians, social workers, and so on? How?
20.	Comprehensive School Counseling Program: What will the school counseling program look like? Will it have a curriculum that is preventive in nature? Will it focus on academic, career, or social development, or all of these? How and when will needs assessments be conducted?

Conclusion

Comprehensive school counseling programs have been shown to be effective as a preventive intervention throughout the world. We encourage readers to utilize such programs to promote the well-being of children and their families worldwide. While the model used in the United States makes strong recommendations about things such as professional school counselor preparation and student-to-counselor ratios, these are ideals based on U.S. cultural values and norms and may not be appropriate for school systems or contexts in other parts of the world. We have shown that many countries have instituted their own unique, school-based prevention programs or comprehensive school counseling programs in highly effective ways. We suggest that school administrators, teachers, and counselors continue to collaborate to develop comprehensive school counseling programs that are culturally appropriate and relevant while keeping the aspirational, preventive nature of these programs at the forefront.

References

Abel, R. M., & Friedman, H. A. (2009). Israeli school and community response to war trauma: a review of selected literature. *School Psychology International* 30: 265–81.

Adelman, H. S., & Taylor, L. (2000). Moving prevention from the fringes into the fabric of school improvement. *Journal of Educational and Psychological Consultation* 11: 7–36.

Adelman, H. S., & Taylor, L. (2010). *Mental Health in Schools.* Thousand Oaks, CA: Corwin.

Ajowi, J. O., & Simatwa, E. M. W. (2010). The role of guidance and counseling in promoting student discipline in secondary schools in Kenya: a case study of Kisumu District. *Educational Research and Reviews* 5: 263–72.

Alexander, M. M., Santo, J. B., Da Cunha, J., Weber, L., & Russell, S. T. (2011). Effects of homophobic versus non-homophobic victimization on school commitment and the moderating effect of teacher attitudes in Brazilian public schools. *Journal of LGBT Youth* 8: 289–308.

Aliyev, R., Erguner-Tekinalp, B., Ulker, R., & Shinde-Edizer, F. (2012). The perceptions of school counselors and principals towards new psychological counseling and guidance services in early childhood education in Turkey. *Educational Sciences: Theory and Practice* (Autumn, Special Issue): 3083–98.

APA (American Psychological Association) (2014). Guidelines for prevention in psychology. *American Psychologist* 69: 285–96. doi: 10.1037/a0034569

ASCA (American School Counselor Association) (2003). *The ASCA National Model: A Framework for School Counseling Programs*, 1st ed. Herndon, VA: Author.

ASCA (American School Counselor Association) (2010). Ethical standards for school counselors. www.schoolcounselor.org/school-counselors-members/legal-ethical

ASCA (American School Counselor Association) (2012). *The ASCA National Model: A Framework for School Counseling Programs*, 3rd ed. Herndon, VA: Author.

Belize Ministry of Education (2012). Belize Teaching Service Commission Public Announcement. Retrieved from www.moe.gov.bz

Belize Ministry of Education (2013). Abstract of Education Statistics 2012–13. Retrieved from www.moe.gov.bz

Bemak, F., Williams, J. M., & Chi-Ying Chung, R. (2015). Four critical domains of accountability for school counselors. *Professional School Counseling* 18: 100–10.

Berard, R. M., Pringle, E. F., & Ahmed, N. (1997). A preliminary investigation of high-school counseling resources on the Cape Peninsula. *Adolescence* 32: 373–9.

Burns, B. J., Costello, E. J., Angold, A., Tweed, D., Stangl, D., Farmer, E., & Erkanli, A. (1995). Children's mental health service use across service sectors. *Health Affairs* 14: 147–59.

Centers for Disease Control and Prevention (2013). *Schools Play Key Role in HIV/STD Prevention.* Atlanta, GA: Author. Retrieved from www.cdc.gov/features/HIVSTDPrevention/

Chen, P. L., Huang, W. G., & Chao, K. Y. (2011). Factors associated with Taiwanese junior high school personnel advising students to quit smoking. *Journal of School Health* 81(2): 91–9.

Cunningham, J. L. (2007). Centripetal and centrifugal trends influencing school psychology's international development. In Jimerson, S. R., Oakland, T., & Farrell, P. T. (eds.), *The Handbook of International School Psychology*. Thousand Oaks: Sage, pp. 463–74.

Currie, C. L., Kuzmina, M. V., & Nadyuk, R. I. (2012). The counseling profession in Russia: historical roots, current trends, and future perspectives. *Journal of Counseling & Development* 90: 488–93.

Davis, S. M., Sanders, S. G., FitzGerald, C. A., Keane, P. C., Canaca, G. F., & Volker-Rector, R. (2013). Chile: an evidence-based preschool intervention for obesity prevention in Head Start. *Journal of School Health* 83: 223–9. doi: 10.1111/josh.12018

Dimmitt, C., Carey, J. C., & Hatch, T. (2007). *Evidence-Based School Counseling.* Thousand Oaks, CA: Corwin.

Duarte, D. & Hatch, T. Successful implementation of a federally funded violence prevention elementary school counseling program: results bring sustainability. *Professional School Counseling* 18: 71–81.

Erhard, R. L., & Sinai, M. (2012). The school counselor in Israel: an agent of social justice? *International Journal for the Advancement of Counselling* 34(2): 159–73.

Espelage, D. L., & Swearer, S. M. (2004). *Bullying in American Schools: A Social-Ecological Perspective on Prevention and Intervention.* Mahwah, NJ: Lawrence Erlbaum.

Eurydice (2009). *Integrating Immigrant Children into Schools in Europe: Measures to Foster Communication with Immigrant Families and Heritage Language Teaching for Immigrant Children.* Brussels, Belgium: Author. eacea.ec.europa.eu/education/eurydice/documents/thematic_reports/101EN.pdf

Farrell, P. T., Jimerson, S. R., & Oakland, T. D. (2007). School psychology internationally: a synthesis of findings. In Jimerson, S. R., Oakland, T., & Farrell, P. T. (eds.), *The Handbook of International School Psychology.* Thousand Oaks: Sage, pp. 501–9.

Forness, S. R., Serna, L. A., Nielsen, E., Lambros, K., Hale, M. J., & Kavale, K. A. (2000). A model for early detection and primary prevention of emotional or behavioral disorders. *Education and Treatment of Children* 23: 325–45.

Gelkopf, M., & Berger, R. (2008). A school-based, teacher-mediated prevention program (ERASE-Stress) for reducing terror-related traumatic reactions in Israeli youth: a quasi-randomized controlled trial. *Journal of Child Psychology and Psychiatry* 50: 962–71.

Goh, M., Wahl, K. H., McDonald, J. K., Brissett, A. A., & Yoon, E. (2007). Working with immigrant students in schools: the role of school counselors in building cross-cultural bridges. *Journal of Multicultural Counseling and Development* 35: 66–79. doi: 10.1002/j.2161-1912.2007.tb00050.x

Gordon, R. (1987). An operational classification of disease prevention. In Sternberg, J. A., & Silverman, M. M. (eds.), *Preventing Mental Disorders.* Rockville, MD: U.S. Department of Health and Human Services, pp. 20–6.

Guo, Y. J., Wang, S. C., Combs, D. C., Lin, Y. C., & Johnson, V. (2013). Professional counseling in Taiwan: past to future. *Journal of Counseling & Development* 91: 331–5.

Greytak, E. A., & Kosciw, J. G. (2010). *Year One Evaluation of the New York City Department of Education Respect for All Training Program.* New York: GLSEN.

Huang, C. M., Chien, L. Y., Cheng, C. F., & Guo, J. L. (2012). Integrating life skills into a theory-based drug-use prevention program: effectiveness among junior high students in Taiwan. *Journal of School Health* 82: 328–35.

Hui, E. K. (1999). Building an effective guidance service in Hong Kong: a qualitative study. *Asia Pacific Journal of Education* 19: 78–88.

Hutz, C. S., Gomes, W., & McCarthy, S. (2006). Teaching of psychology in Brazil. *International Journal of Psychology* 41: 10–16.

Hutz-Midgett, A., & Hutz, C. S. (2012). Counseling in Brazil: past, present, and future. *Journal of Counseling & Development* 90: 238–42.

Israelashvili, M., & Wegman-Rozi, O. (2012). Formal and applied counseling in Israel. *Journal of Counseling & Development* 90: 227–32.

Isralowitz, R., Shpiegel, S., Reznik, A., & Laytin, A. (2009). Ethiopian youth in Israel: gender-related alcohol use and related problem behaviour. *Drugs: Education, Prevention, and Policy* 16: 273–8.

Jimerson, S. R., Alghorani, M. A., Darweish, A. H., & Abdelaziz, M. (2010). School psychology in Egypt results of the 2008 International School Psychology Survey. *School Psychology International* 31: 219–28.

Jimerson, S. R., Graydon, K., Curtis, M. J., & Staskal, R. (2007a). The international school psychology survey: insights from school psychologists around the world. In Jimerson, S. R., Oakland, T., & Farrell, P. T. (eds.), *The Handbook of International School Psychology*. Thousand Oaks: Sage, pp. 481–500.

Jimerson, S. R., Graydon, K., Farrell, P., Kikas, E., Hatzichristou, C., Boce, E., & Bashi, G. (2004). The International School Psychology Survey development and data from Albania, Cyprus, Estonia, Greece and northern England. *School Psychology International* 25: 259–86.

Jimerson, S. R., Oakland, T., & Farrell, P. T. (eds.). (2007b). *The Handbook of International School Psychology*. Thousand Oaks: Sage.

Karayanni, M. (1985). School counseling in Israel: issues and development. *International Journal for the Advancement of Counselling* 8: 297–307.

Karayanni, M. (1996). The emergence of school counseling and guidance in Israel. *Journal of Counseling & Development* 74: 582–7.

Kashima, S., de Castro, F. A., de Castro Amarante, M. F., ProSeguir, G., Barbieri, M. R., & Covas, D. T. (2008). HIV/AIDS researchers interaction with schoolteachers: a key to combat AIDS among Brazilian adolescents. *Journal of HIV/AIDS Prevention in Children & Youth* 9: 115–31.

Keaton, P. (2012). *Public Elementary and Secondary School Student Enrollment and Staff Counts from the Common Core of Data: School Year 2010–2011, First Look*. Washington, DC: U.S. Department of Education.

Kim, B. S. K., & Alamilla, S. G. (2008.) Research in and on school counseling. In Coleman, H. L. K., & Yeh, C. (eds.), *Handbook of School Counseling*. New York: Taylor & Francis, pp. 751–64.

Koch, J. M. (2008). An early elementary school counseling outcome study: academic achievement, discipline and pro-social behavior, and school climate (Doctoral dissertation). Retrieved from ProQuest Information & Learning (AAI3328318)

Lan, C. M., & Lee, Y. H. (2013). The predictors of addiction behaviours for Taiwanese elementary school students. *School Psychology International* 34: 648–57.

Lapan, R., & Harrington, K. (2010). *Paving the Road to College: How School Counselors Help Students Succeed.* Amherst, MA: Center for School Counseling Outcome Research.

Lee, M-S., Zi-Pei, W., Svanström, L., & Dalal, K. (2013). Cyber bullying prevention: intervention in Taiwan. *PLoS ONE* 8(5): 1–6.

Leong, F. T. L. (2002). Challenges for career counseling in Asia: variations in cultural accommodation. *Career Development Quarterly* 50: 277–84.

Lim, S. L., Lim, B. K. H., Michael, R., Cai, R., & Schock, C. K. (2010). The trajectory of counseling in China: past, present, and future trends. *Journal of Counseling & Development* 88: 4–8.

Mandt, G. (2008). The quality framework in Norway. *Intercultural Education*,19(2): 177–82.

McGannon, W., Carey, J., & Dimmitt, C. (2005). *The Current Status of School Counseling Outcome Research.* Amherst, MA: Center for School Counseling Outcome Research.

Myrick, R. D. (1997). *Developmental Guidance and Counseling*, 3rd ed. Minneapolis, MN: Educational Media Corporation.

Nazli, S. (2014). Career development of upper primary school students in Turkey. *Australian Journal of Guidance and Counselling* 24: 49–61.

O'Leary, E. (1990). Research on school counseling: an Irish perspective. *School Counselor* 37: 261–9.

Omizo, M. M., & Omizo, S. A. (1988). The effects of participation in group counseling sessions on self-esteem and locus of control among adolescents from divorced families. *School Counselor* 36: 54–60.

Overstreet, S., Salloum, A., & Badour, C. (2010). A school-based assessment of secondary stressors and adolescent mental health 18 months post Katrina. *Journal of School Psychology* 48: 413–31. doi: 10.1016/j.jsp.2010.06.002

Perkins, S. A. (1971). Secondary school counseling in England and Canada: a mini comparison. *Canadian Counsellor* 5: 219–23.

Pokhrel, P., Masagutov, R., Kniazev, V., & Sussman, S. (2012). Health-as-a-value, spirituality, and cigarette and alcohol use among Russian high school students. *Journal of Primary Prevention* 33: 239–48.

Poland, S., & McCormick, J. S. (1999). *Coping with Crisis: Lessons Learned.* Longmont, CO: Sopris West.

Romano, J. L. (2015). *Prevention Psychology: Enhancing Personal and Social Well-being.* Washington, DC: American Psychological Association.

Romano, J. L., Goh, M., & Wahl, K. H. (2005). School counseling in the United States: implications for the Asia-Pacific region. *Asia Pacific Education Review* 6: 113–23.

Romano, J. L., & Hage, S. M. (2000). Prevention and counseling psychology: revitalizing commitments in the 21st century. *Counseling Psychologist* 28: 733–63. doi: 10.1177/0011000000286001

Schmidt, J. J. (2008). History of school counseling. In Coleman, H. L. K., & Yeh, C. (eds.), *Handbook of School Counseling*. New York: Taylor & Francis, pp. 3–13.

Sink, C. A., & Moore, L. D. (2013). Sustaining professional school counseling through viable accountability practices. *Educational Research Journal* 28: 103–24.

Sink, C. A., & Stroh, H. R. (2003). Raising achievement test scores of early elementary school students through comprehensive school counseling programs. *Professional School Counseling* 6: 350–65.

Smith-Augustine, S., & Wagner, M. (2012). School counseling in Belize: poised for great development. *International Journal for the Advancement of Counselling* 34: 320–30.

Stockton, R., & Güneri, O. Y. (2011). Counseling in Turkey: an evolving field. *Journal of Counseling & Development* 89: 98–104.

Stone, C. B., & Dahir, C. A. (2004). *School Counselor Accountability: A Measure of Student Success.* Upper Saddle River, NJ: Pearson Education.

Stone, C. B., & Dahir, C. A. (2006). *The Transformed School Counselor*. Boston, MA: Houghton Mifflin.

Stothard, B., Romanova, O., & Ivanova, L. (2007). Recent developments in HIV/AIDS prevention for Russian adolescents. *Sex Education* 7: 175–89.

Sue, D. W., Arredondo, P., & McDavis, R. J. (1992). Multicultural counseling competencies and standards: a call to the profession. *Journal of Counseling & Development* 70: 477–86.

Taiwan Ministry of Education (2011). Guidelines for classroom sizes and employee numbers in public elementary and middle schools. Retrieved from english.moe.gov.tw

Tekin, G. (2012). Counseling and guidance services in early childhood education: the case of public preschools in Malatya, Turkey. *US–China Education Review* 10: 875–80.

Thomason, T., & Qiong, X. (2008). School counseling in China today. *Journal of School Counseling* 6: 213–19.

Tuicomepee, A., & Romano, J. L. (2008). Thai adolescent survivors 1 year after the 2004 tsunami: a mixed-methods study. *Journal of Counseling Psychology* 55: 308–20. doi: 10.1037/0022–0167.55.3.308

UN (United Nations) 2015. *Education First: Facts and Figures.* New York: Author. www.un.org/en/globalissues/children/index.shtml

UNICEF (United Nations International Children Education Fund) (2015). *The State of the World's Children 2015: Executive Summary.* New York: Author. Retrieved from www.data.unicef.org/resources/the-state-of-the-world-s-children-report-2015-statistical-tables

U.S. Department of Labor. (2013). *2013 Findings on the Worst Forms of Child Labor: Belize.* Washington, DC: Author. Retrieved from www.dol.gov/ilab/reports/child-labor/findings/2013TDA/belize.pdf

Whiston, S. C. (2002). Response to the past, present and future of school counseling: raising some issues. *Professional School Counseling* 5: 148–55.

Whiston, S. C., & Sexton, T. L. (1998). A review of school counseling outcome research: implications for practice. *Journal of Counseling & Development* 76: 412–26.

Whiston, S. C., Tai, W. L., Rahardja, D., & Eder, K. (2011). School counseling outcome: a meta-analytic examination of interventions. *Journal of Counseling and Development* 89: 37–55.

Williams, F. C., & Butler, K. S. (2003). Concerns of newly arrived immigrant students: implications for school counselors. *Professional School Counseling* 7: 9–14.

Wright, G., & Gray, N. D. (2007). The ISLLC standards: a unifying force in school administrator and counselor preparation. Paper based on a program presented at the Association for Counselor Education and Supervision Conference, Columbus, OH, October.

Yeo, L. S., Tan, S. Y., & Neihart, M. F. (2012). Counseling in Singapore. *Journal of Counseling & Development* 90: 243–8.

Yuen, M. (2003). Exploring Hong Kong Chinese guidance teachers' positive beliefs: a focus group study. *International Journal for the Advancement of Counselling* 24: 169–82.

16 Prevention in Early Childhood

Models of Parenting Interventions among Immigrants

Neha Navsaria & Ji Su Hong

> Investing in the healthy development of all our nation's children, including children of immigrants, is to invest into a brighter future – not just for these children themselves, but for our entire nation
>
> (Shields & Behrman, 2004, p. 4).

Introduction

Advances in the field of early childhood development have increased our awareness of the crucial importance of early experiences on health, development, and prevention of disorders. Central to early childhood is the notion of parenting. Based on this belief, the primary goal of early childhood mental health is fostering relationships between young children and their caregivers as the predominant focus of intervention. In this chapter on prevention in early childhood, we will examine mental health prevention efforts that target the parent–child dyad, with an emphasis on immigrant families. The chapter will begin by providing a conceptualization of early childhood mental health from a dyadic perspective. We will describe the specific ways in which the early years are scaffolded by a caregiver and the idea that strengthening parenting and thus positively influencing parent–child relationships can serve to optimize individual functioning and achievement.

Next, we will address the need to examine parenting from a cultural lens. In particular, we will highlight parenting in the context of immigrants, a population with rapidly increasing numbers across the globe. According to the International Organization for Migration (IOM, 2015), approximately 200 million people worldwide are currently living outside their country of origin. The Americas contain approximately 27 percent of the world's migrants (IOM, 2015). Specific to the United States (U.S.), the nation's immigrant population hit a record 41.3 million in July 2013, an increase of 10.2 million from 2000 (Zeigler & Camarota, 2014). Within the European Union (EU), there was an estimated 1.7 million immigrants to the EU from countries outside the EU (Eurostat, 2014).The number of international migrants in Asia in 2010 was estimated at 27.5 million, and the Oceanic region (Australia, New Zealand, and the Pacific Islands) hosts more than 6 million international migrants

(IOM, 2015). This marked global increase in the immigrant population demonstrates a need to focus prevention and intervention efforts on this population.

Our final objective for this chapter is to describe firmly established as well as newly emerging evidence-based parenting interventions as prevention models. We will first present general knowledge about each parenting intervention and summarize the global evidence base on the effectiveness of these programs in promoting child and family resilience. Research implementing these interventions to reach immigrant families in need will then be described with an emphasis on how the programs have been adapted for use with various immigrant populations. While the scope of this chapter is focused on immigrant families, we will also present some relevant studies of other ethnic groups. This information can be important in modifying intervention programs with immigrant groups in the future given the commonalities of cultural influences and hardships faced. Given the lack of cross-cultural information available on parenting interventions, any information within a cultural context can be beneficial for future implementation of parenting interventions within diverse populations.

Conceptualization of Early Childhood Mental Health from a Dyadic Perspective

A body of empirical studies across the globe has suggested that development in the early years may represent a window of opportunity during which experiences may either promote or hinder a child's optimal development (Anderson, 2002; Perry, 2002; Shonkoff & Phillips, 2000; Sroufe, Egeland, & Kreutzer, 1990; Zigler & Berman, 1983). In early childhood, the most fundamental principle is that the young child does not function as a psychologically autonomous individual and remains inextricably tied to the primary caregiver for adaptive and emotional functioning (Navsaria & Luby, 2015). While the caregiver–child relationship is important throughout a child's developmental trajectory, the interactions between a primary caregiver and child are central to the child's development at this early stage for multiple reasons. The parent–child relationship serves as a regulatory mechanism by which a child develops adaptive emotional regulation patterns and problem-solving skills and facilitates autonomy development, exploration, and self-control (Dallaire & Weinraub, 2005; Deater-Deckard, Ivy, & Smith, 2005; Hartup, 1989). This role of a parent supports the notion that some aspects of resilience may be systematically learned or internalized through this relationship experience (Merrel, Whitcomb, & Parisi, 2009), with parents playing an important role in shaping a child's inherent skills for adaptive coping.

The framework provided by a parent is often termed *parental scaffolding* (Carter, Briggs-Gowan, & Davis, 2004; Sclafani, 2004). In the academic and cognitive domain, Vygotsky (1978), when referring to scaffolding, states that until a child becomes a proficient problem solver, a child relies heavily on parents for assistance when confronted with tasks beyond the child's own abilities. A dyadic process emerges between primary caregiver and child where the caregiver scaffolds their children's problem-solving skills until the child gains mastery and self-initiates those skills, culminating in more independent functioning. When considering the importance of the parent–child relationship on a child's functioning, it can be concluded that parenting styles and techniques contribute to the prevention of emotional and behavioral problems in children. Appropriate intervention during the early years can also potentially offset negative social and economic outcomes for children and families. For example, early childhood intervention programs in the United States have been shown to have benefits for reducing crime (Aos & Drake, 2013), raising earnings, and promoting education (Heckman, 2011), as well as improved adult health (Campbell et al., 2014). The potential for greater efficacy for early intervention may prove that these techniques are cost-effective from a societal point of view.

Given the crucial importance of parenting in a child's developmental trajectory, prevention programs focusing on early childhood must target parenting skills and the caregiver–child relationship. There is substantial evidence (mostly in North America and Europe) that parenting interventions can improve parent–child relationships, reduce child problem behaviors, and prevent maltreatment (Barlow, Johnston, Kendrick, Polnay, & Stewart-Brown, 2006; Gardner, Montgomery, & Knerr, 2015; Piquero, Farrington, Welsh, Tremblay, & Jennings, 2008). When considering global contexts, an understanding of the impact of culture-specific norms and values on parenting is necessary in order to inform parenting interventions accurately. Gardner et al. (2015) asserts a need for careful consideration of not only the cultural and contextual variation when implementing parenting programs globally, but also the potential for commonalities across settings that may facilitate transportation of interventions across countries. There is evidence that parenting programs appear to transport well across cultures. A systematic review of evidenced-based programs developed in the United States and Australia found comparable effect sizes in ten recipient countries in five global regions (Gardner et al., 2015). While this significant review focused on the cultural transportability of interventions, it did not emphasize immigrant populations, a highly vulnerable, yet understudied, group. In planning these interventions in diverse societies, one must consider how these interventional programs can impact vulnerable populations, such as immigrant groups, which requires an understanding of the acculturation process.

Immigrants, Parenting, and Acculturation

Recent numbers from the United States indicate that children of immigrants represented more than one-fifth of all children under eighteen (Dettlaff & Earner, 2012), emphasizing the substantial presence of parenting scenarios in the context of migration. Immigrant children and families can frequently struggle in their new communities. Their hardships are often due to past traumas (i.e., persecution, conflicts, natural disasters), limited education, non-transferable job skills, and difficulties with immigration status (National Center for Mental Health Promotion and Youth Violence Prevention, 2011). Moreover, a significant hardship for these families centers on the stressful experience of current adjustment to a new environment and culture, termed *acculturative stress* (Williams & Berry, 1991). They can face the challenge of learning new rules and roles, lacking English-speaking ability, and being victimized by racism and discrimination (Berry, 2005) without the support of familiar social networks (Bornstein & Bohr, 2011). Compared to their parents, immigrant children are more exposed to socialization agents beyond their family members and therefore adapt more rapidly to the customs and language of the mainstream culture (Borstein, 2011). This dissonance in acculturation has been shown to complicate communication and mutual understanding between the two generations, in turn increasing tension and family conflict (McQueen, Getz, & Bray, 2003; Ying, 1999).

In the context of these difficulties, immigrant parents are navigating the process of raising their children in a new country. Many immigrants bring with them attitudes and beliefs about parenting that are embedded in their previous social and cultural environment. These beliefs may or may not contrast with parenting practices of their current environment. Research shows that immigrants do not always readily adopt cognitions of the receiving culture, and culturally significant parenting beliefs and norms tend to resist change (LeVine, Miller, & West, 1988). Additionally, different immigrants groups retain and adopt culture-specific practices differently (Lin & Fu, 1990), with a varied emphasis on what is practiced in the public versus private domain (Bornstein & Bohr, 2011). This simultaneous management of two cultures engenders complex transformations of parenting and a parent's own cultural identity.

One such example, relevant to childhood, of a culturally mitigated parenting belief is in the context of play. Play is an action that occurs across cultures; however, there are cultural differences in the frequency and content of play as well as caregiver–child interactions (Jent, Niec, & Baker 2011). Some families may value academic components of play over pretend play (Farver & Shinn 1997). Other families, depending on their values and life experiences, may emphasize individualism and self-reliance, preferring more child-directed play. For collectivistic families, early choice making may be discouraged due to the emphasis on child obedience and respect (Johnston & Wong, 2002). These dynamics could lead to seemingly restrained play that is more parent-driven. Furthermore, collectivistic societies often rely on the extended family or community to engage children in play activity. These parents may appear to place less importance on one-to-one playtime, when in reality, they expect the child has other adults and children involved in their play.

The contextual factors and risk trajectories as described in the preceding create a number of vulnerabilities for immigrant families in various countries. The complex and ongoing process of straddling two cultures and increased family conflict can lead to a greater risk of mental health problems for many parents and children (Berry, 2005). There is evidence that immigrant and ethnic minority communities display lower levels of sensitive parenting behaviors and a higher prevalence of child behavior problems (e.g., Yagmur, Mesman, Malda, Bakermans-Kranenburg, & Ekmekci, 2014). There are also concerns about elevated risks for child maltreatment. Children living with a foreign-born parent comprise 8.6 percent of all children who come to the attention of the child welfare system in the United States (Dettlaff & Earner, 2012). It has also been shown that parental beliefs about sensitive parenting in early childhood are similar across cultures, but attitudes toward discipline practices vary by culture (Yagmur et al., 2014). It has been hypothesized that cultural differences or misunderstandings play a role in the increased risk for child maltreatment in these families. These risk factors and resulting vulnerabilities suggest the need for parenting interventions in this population is paramount.

Often, based on immigrant parents' minimal response to traditional school and community engagement strategies (Falicov, 2007), it is assumed that these parents are not interested in learning about parenting their children. However, the reality is that most immigrant families care deeply about their children's education and health and often keep their distance from school and community agencies out of respect for educators, limited English proficiency, work schedules, and decreased comfort in interactions (National Center for Mental Health Promotion and Youth Violence Prevention, 2011; Kugler, 2009). To meet these challenges, researchers and community educators have implemented parenting interventions and education programs with various ethnic groups with the goal of making them more culturally adaptive and engaging.

Considerations in Cultural Adaptions of Parenting Interventions

While the use of evidenced-based parenting interventions with immigrant communities has been identified as a much needed resource, there are also concerns about forging ahead with culturally focused adaptations of these treatments. Developing a culturally modified model rests on the assumption that standard protocols are not helpful to ethnic minority communities. Although there is limited evidence supporting the effectiveness of evidenced-based treatments with minorities, evidence that they are less effective with minorities is likewise limited (Lau, 2006). Within this chapter, there are studies presented where the standard treatment model is just as effective as the culturally based model (McCabe & Yeh, 2009). There is also research presented where multiethnic populations are studied and there were no significant differences among minority or majority groups when receiving standard parenting interventions (Lieberman, Van Horn, & Ippen, 2005; Scott et al., 2010). Another concern with developing culturally relevant evidenced-based treatments is that adapting these treatments to be culturally responsive may prompt haphazard or inappropriate adaptations that may actually compromise the fidelity of the interventions and their effectiveness (Lau, 2006).

Overall, there is a dearth of research on parenting programs in countries outside of North America, Europe, and Australia. For the research that does exist in Western countries, there is minimal emphasis on immigrant communities within the study population. In this chapter, we will present a summary of findings from international studies on parenting interventions that include immigrant communities as well as those that focus on ethnic populations within their country of origin. Across these populations, information learned on cultural adaptations (or lack thereof) can be relevant to the implementation of global parenting interventions in order to prevent negative developmental trajectories for children.

Review of Parenting Interventions

Parenting Education Programs

Nurturing Parenting Program (NPP; www.nurturingparenting.com). NPP was developed as a treatment program for child abuse and neglect in the United States (Bavolek, Comstock, & McLaughlin, 1983; Bavolek, 2000). NPP is currently implemented in more than twenty-four countries in multiple regions of the world, such as North America, South America, Europe, Asia, and Australia. NPP is a group or home-based program lasting from twelve to twenty-three sessions totaling no more than forty-five sessions. At each session, parents learn age-specific parenting skills and self-nurturing skills for themselves. The goals of NPP include (1) developing a positive family self-concept, (2) building an empathic awareness of the developmental needs of others, (3) helping parents substitute nurturing behaviors for abusive ones, and (4) increasing healthy family communication.

The efficacy of NPP has been researched numerous times (Maher, Marcynyszyn, Corwin, & Hodnett, 2011; Palusci, Crum, Bliss, & Bavolek, 2008; Veso, Cooper, & Behforooz, 2006; Cowen, 2001). After the course of treatment, parents developed more appropriate expectations of child development, more empathic awareness of children's needs, and more positive attitudes toward children's independence and became less supportive of corporal punishment and attitudes reflecting parent–child role reversal. Recidivism decreased in groups who completed the program. There was improvement in family cohesion, expressiveness, independence, organization, and decreased family conflict.

Bavolek, Keene, Miranda, and Radcliff (2013) developed and implemented the "Crianza con Cariño Parenting Program," which is the Spanish version of NPP. This program was evaluated for Spanish-speaking families in Arizona, Colorado, Texas, Wisconsin, Mexico, and Venezuela. It has been field-tested in and disseminated in Mexico and Central and South America. The program was edited and reviewed by Hispanic human services professionals to improve cultural sensitivity and accuracy. In addition to the group program, home-based sessions were provided if the family needed additional support or needed to make up sessions. After treatment, there were gains made in empathy, alternatives to physical punishment, and a better understanding of the child's independence. This study showed that NPP can be successfully implemented in the Hispanic population as a preventive program. The authors believed that the findings challenged the common cultural myth that parents would not participate in parenting programs due to stigma.

Montañez, Devall, and Van Leeuwen (2010) implemented NPP for Mexican American families in New Mexico (U.S.). NPP was provided to Mexican American parents of preschool children. Parenting programs were delivered by parenting educators in English or Spanish. Montañez et al. considered three important cultural factors for Mexican families: sociocentrism (interdependence; social relationships; behaviors relying on others' thoughts, feelings, and actions), *familismo* (strong family orientation), and *compadrazgo* (honorary parents play an important role in parenting). The authors applied these cultural constructs into their adaptation of NPP in a number of ways. Parenting educators mailed postcards each week, called families before each class, and provided a special graduation ceremony with certificates and gifts. Results indicated that parents who completed the program had greater knowledge of positive discipline techniques, increased awareness of children's needs, decreased beliefs about physical punishment, decrease in role reversal, and decrease in inappropriate expectations of the child.

Anecdotal evidence of NPP with the Somali population is provided by the Lewiston School System in Maine (Northeast U.S.) (National Center for Mental Health Promotion and Youth Violence Prevention, 2011). The school district invited small groups of Somali women to participate in NPP using trusted cultural brokers and Somali interpreters. The parent educators used visuals to communicate concepts such as the importance of expressing bottled-up feelings (a demonstration of a volcano erupting) and how parent self-care allows mothers to take care of their families (the analogy of putting your oxygen mask on first before helping your child). Through the NPP, Somali mothers learned about developmentally appropriate expectations for children, appropriate discipline practices in the United States, the importance of communicating feelings, and ways to empower parents and children. A valued support system for Somali women was created, and women were also introduced to literacy volunteers to help them acquire English language skills. The Lewiston district identified the following strategies to be effective in their implementation of NPP with Somali immigrants: (1) working with Somali cultural brokers and interpreters to develop trust within the community, (2) collaboration with an extended network of trusted professionals to provide services and education to families, and (3) helping parents understand that participation in the program will help children succeed in school.

The Incredible Years (IY; www.incredibleyears.com). Webster-Stratton and her colleagues (1984) developed IY to treat externalizing disorders in children. The IY parenting program provides skills for improving parent–child relationships, reducing harsh discipline, increasing positive parenting practices, and fostering parents' ability to promote children's social-emotional development. Parenting skills are taught via video vignettes and roleplays. The topics include positive parenting behaviors, such as listening, following a child's lead, praising, and descriptive commenting. Parents of preschoolers and school-age children also learn how to promote school readiness skills and how to create good partnerships with teachers. In numerous countries (mostly North America and Europe), IY has been proven to be effective in improving children's self-regulation and social competence and parents' positive parenting skills while reducing coercive/harsh parenting practices (Gardner, Burton & Klimes, 2006; Larsson et al., 2009; Little et al., 2012; Posthumus, Raajimakers, Maassen, van Engeland & Matthys, 2012; Reid, Webster-Stratton, & Hammond, 2007; Webster-Stratton, 1984, 1990, 1994, 1998; Webster-Stratton & Hammond, 1997; Webster-Stratton, Hollinsworth, & Kolpacoff, 1989; Webster-Stratton, Reid, & Hammond, 2004). Positive outcomes from early interventions were mostly maintained eight to ten years later.

The existing research on IY provides rich information from numerous studies on immigrant communities in multiple countries. In the United States, Barrera et al. (2002) used IY as part of a comprehensive intervention to reduce conduct problems in children. European American and Hispanic children were selected for aggressiveness or reading difficulties and were randomly assigned to an intervention or no-intervention control condition. Intervention families received IY and their children received social behavior interventions and supplementary reading instruction over a two-year period. Groups were conducted in Spanish by bilingual/bicultural staff or English, depending on the parents' language preferences. At the end of the intervention, treated children displayed less negative social behavior. At the one-year follow-up, treated children showed less teacher-rated internalizing and parent-rated coercive and antisocial behaviors. The authors found that the intervention was as successful in decreasing conduct problems for Hispanic children as it was for European American children.

The IY program was implemented with a low-income sample of Caucasian, African American, Hispanic, and Asian mothers whose children were enrolled in the U.S. Head Start program (Reid, Webster-Stratton, & Beauchaine, 2001). Families were randomly assigned to an intervention group or a control group (Head Start only). When a sufficient number of families was present who spoke Spanish or Vietnamese, the group was led by trained native speakers. When there were fewer non-English speaking families in attendance, they participated in an English group with a translator. Families were assessed and then were reassessed one year later via observations of parent–child interactions and parent reports of parenting style, discipline strategies, and child behavior problems. After treatment, mothers in the intervention group were observed to be more positive, less critical, more consistent, and more competent in their parenting than mothers in the control group. Children in the intervention group were observed to exhibit fewer behavioral problems than children in the control group. Differences in treatment responses across ethnic groups were few.

Hispanic parents rated group leaders more highly than Caucasian parents. Asian parents displayed preferences for classes on parenting topics over group participation. The observations from this study suggest that considering the context of language may have important implications in how parent educators are received by immigrant families. The lack of differences between ethnic groups indicates an intervention design that could be used across a number of ethnic groups versus a program tailored to a specific group; however, it should be noted that different groups gravitated to various features of IY.

U.S. American Indian (AI) parents have also been studied using the IY model. While the AI population does not meet the formal definition of an "immigrant" group, there are many commonalities in the challenges faced by both of these groups. The high level of difficulty plaguing the AI community today, including mental stress, substance use, and economic difficulties, is likely a direct result of historical trauma passed through the generations, as well as ongoing prejudice and discrimination (Duran & Duran, 1995; Evans-Campbell, 2008; La Fromboise, 1998). These challenges have resulted in the rise of ineffective parenting practices and insensitivity to children's needs by some AI parents (Brasfield, 2001; Brave Heart, 1999). For these reasons, Dionne, Davis, Sheeber, and Madrigal (2009) studied a culturally adapted IY model for AI families. All families participated in a motivational phase and were subsequently randomized to the culturally based IY program or a control condition. The motivational phase consisted of the Indian Family Wellness Assessment motivational interview procedure (Dionne & Dishion, 1998) designed to motivate AI parents to participate in family interventions. Family coaches were trained and supervised by the lead investigator, an AI psychologist who completed the IY training program. The staff also participated in a cultural competency training focused on best practices for working with AI families.

In addition to the standard IY protocol, at the beginning of each session, coaches drew connections between the skills to be taught and traditional AI values, traditions, and beliefs. For example, given the importance of respect in the AI community, when discussing relationship-building play skills, coaches emphasized that parents are teaching the child respect by parents modeling respect for them. There was significant improvement in parenting effectiveness and children's externalizing problems in the intervention group when compared to those in the control group. The design of this study highlights the importance of motivating parents before engaging them in parenting training as well as grounding parenting topics in values emphasized in the ethnic minority community.

Regarding the Asian immigrant community, the IY program was provided to Korean American mothers (Kim, Cain, & Webster-Stratton, 2008). First-generation Korean American mothers of young children were randomly assigned to IY intervention and control groups. Each IY parenting video vignette was shown in English, and group leaders translated the content into Korean. All other components of the program were delivered in Korean. After completing the program, intervention group mothers significantly increased their use of positive discipline, and these results were maintained after a one-year follow-up. Interestingly enough, low-acculturated mothers were more receptive to decreasing harsh discipline while high-acculturated mothers were more open to adopting Westernized discipline strategies. These findings suggest the importance of providing parenting training in appropriate lingual contexts and conducting an acculturation assessment to understand the various ways immigrant parents could respond to new information on parenting.

In the context of immigrant communities in the United Kingdom (U.K.), Scott et al., (2010) conducted clinical trials with parents of young children living in a high-risk, ethnically diverse (British, Black African, African Caribbean), inner-city area. The intervention group received the IY program, and the remainder of parents received as-usual community services. There were no cultural adaptations to the protocol reported by the authors. At one-year follow-up, those allocated to the intervention group demonstrated significant improvements in the parent–child relationship, and these effects were similar across all ethnic groups (Scott et al., 2010). Given that the researchers did not apply cultural adaptations to the standard IY protocol, the positive findings speak to the generalizability of IY on a multiethnic parent sample. However, it should be noted that child behavioral problems did not improve; the authors suggested that low attendance rates may have contributed to these findings. These outcomes raise the question of whether or not cultural adaptations addressing rapport and motivation could have impacted attendance levels in this study.

Outside of immigrant communities, but relevant to the efficacy of cultural adaptions, the transferability of IY to Swedish parents and their children with oppositional symptoms was studied (Axberg & Broberg, 2012). Materials were translated into Swedish and sessions were delivered in Swedish. There was a significant reduction of symptoms in children, and this improvement was sustained at the one-year follow-up. In the United Kingdom, Scott et al. (2001), studied the impact of IY and found that there was a large reduction in antisocial behavior compared to the waiting list control group. While language translation was not needed, the IY video vignettes were dubbed over with English accents to make the information more relevant to the parents' cultural context.

Triple P-Positive Parenting Program (www.triplep.net). The Triple P-Positive Parenting Program (Sanders, 2012) was developed in Australia to prevent and treat behavioral, emotional, and developmental problems in children and adolescents by helping parents obtain parenting knowledge, skills, and confidence. Triple P has multiple levels of intervention based on the severity of children's problems and family dysfunction. The lower levels range from providing information about parenting through mass media (Level 1) to brief interventions for low- to moderate-intensity problems (Levels 2 and 3). Most studies on Triple P use Levels 4 and 5, which provide individual or group parenting programs for moderate- to high-intensity problems and additional sessions for high-intensity problems that provide training on coping skills for complex family problems.

Providers determine the level of service by what is observed to be the minimally sufficient effective intervention to serve the needs of parents.

Several studies and meta-analyses have shown that the Triple-P model produces positive outcomes in children's behavior and parents' parenting skills across the globe (de Graaf, Speetjens, Smit, De Wolff, & Tavecchio, 2008; Jalali, Shaeeri, Tahmasian, & Pourahmadi, 2009; Nowak & Heinrichs, 2008; Thomas & Zimmer-Gembeck, 2007). Sumargi, Sofronoff, and Morawska (2014a) implemented a pilot study of Triple P with Indonesian immigrant parents of children residing in Australia. Minor adaptations and cultural modifications were applied. These included translating materials and delivering the program in Indonesian, using culturally relevant examples, and using pictures of Indonesian families. Participants reported less frequent use of dysfunctional parenting and a reduction of children's emotional and behavioral problems three weeks after the seminar and at three-month follow-up. Most parents reported that the content of the seminar was culturally acceptable. Sumargi et al. (2014b) conducted a randomized-controlled trial of the Triple P program in Indonesia. Parents were assigned to an intervention group and to a waitlist control group. Parents in the intervention group reported a greater decrease in child behavioral problems, dysfunctional parenting, and parental stress and an increase in parenting confidence in comparison to the control group. The intervention effects were maintained at a six-month follow-up.

In another study, Matsumoto, Sofronoff, and Sanders (2007) examined the efficacy of Triple P with Japanese immigrant parents living in Australia. The program was delivered in Japanese by a Japanese Triple P trainer. At the sessions, the trainer made efforts to clarify Japanese parents' understanding and specific concerns, and considered cultural and language differences in the material. A randomized group comparison was conducted between the Triple P group and a waitlist control group. The intervention group had significant reductions in child behavior problems, parental overreactivity and laxness, and parental conflict as well as increases in parental competence. Matsumoto et al. (2010) then implemented the Triple-P program (with similar cultural modifications) in community settings in Japan. Japanese families were randomly assigned to intervention groups and a waitlist control group. The intervention group had significant improvements in children's behaviors, parenting practices, parental competence, family functioning, and parental adjustment. These findings (Matsumoto et al., 2010; Sumargi et al., 2014b) suggest the effectiveness of parenting programs with cultural modifications for Indonesian and Japanese immigrant parents as well as parents in their country of origin.

In working with the Chinese immigrant community, Crisante and Ng (2003) implemented the Triple P for Cantonese-speaking Chinese parents living in Australia. The intervention was delivered by appropriately trained bilingual facilitators in the Chinese community. The intervention consisted of four group sessions followed by four optional weekly telephone consultation sessions. The investigators observed that most parents were reluctant to complete questionnaires and had concerns that providing information about their child might result in them being disadvantaged in some way or their answers would somehow be linked to government bureaucracies. These observations highlight the crucial importance of trust between immigrants and those who deliver parent programs.

Leung, Sanders, Leung, Mak, and Lau (2003) implemented Triple P for Chinese parents of three- to six-year-old children with early onset conduct-related problems living in Hong Kong. Materials were translated into Chinese by a bilingual psychologist. Participants in the intervention group reported significantly lower levels of child behavior problems, lower dysfunctional parenting styles, and higher parent sense of competence. In further analysis of their data (Leung, Sanders, Ip, & Lau, 2006), they found that greater change in child behavior problems was related to low family income, new immigrant family status, and high preintervention levels of parenting stress. The engagement of new immigrant families and the maintenance of their involvement are important, as new immigrant families who completed the program reported greater changes in child behavior than nonimmigrant families. Furthermore, the authors described that new immigrant families had lower retention rates, suggesting the need to develop specific engagement procedures customized to parental need. This finding suggests that the parents who respond best to the intervention are also the most vulnerable.

Parent–Child Dyadic Interventions

Parent–Child Interaction Therapy (PCIT; www.pcit.org). PCIT was developed in the United States to treat preschool disruptive behaviors. In addition to the United States, it has been researched in Europe, Asia, and Australia (McNeil & Hembree-Kigin, 2010; Brinkmeyer & Eyberg, 2003; Bell & Eyberg, 2002). PCIT targets the improvement of parental nurturance and building firm limits, with an emphasis on child-directed interaction (CDI) and parent-directed interaction (PDI). In CDI, parents learn to follow their child's play with positive attention (behavioral descriptions, reflection, labeled praise) for appropriate behaviors and ignoring for inappropriate behaviors. In PDI, parents learn how to use commands when compliance is needed and how to use time-out for disruptive behaviors.

In clinical applications with the Spanish-speaking immigrant community, McCabe, Yeh, Garland, Lau, and Chavez (2005) developed a culturally modified version of PCIT for Mexican Americans. The developers stressed that Mexican Americans have a stronger emphasis on family relationships, affiliation and cooperation, avoidance of confrontation and competition, relationship hierarchies, and respect for authority and traditional gender roles. Extended family members are important in decision making, and there is a strong stigma regarding mental health. The investigators reflected these cultural characteristics in their adaptation of PCIT, naming their program Guiding Active Children (Guiando a Ninos Activos; GANA) rather than using the terms "therapy" or "treatment." Therapists were referred to as GANA teachers or child behavior experts. CDI was renamed as a "communication exercise," and PDI was reframed as "consistent discipline." Initial engagement phone calls lasted from thirty minutes to one hour. GANA teachers were encouraged to contact the family before the first session and could have unlimited phone calls and up to three visits with the family during the intervention. GANA teachers contacted fathers and/or grandparents in an attempt to engage them in the program. Time was spent in each session to encourage parents to voice their concerns rather than waiting for parents to report their concerns. All materials were provided in Spanish.

McCabe and Yeh (2009) conducted a clinical trial with Mexican American families who were randomized to the GANA group, standard PCIT, or treatment as usual (TAU). All therapists were bilingual. All three approaches produced significant improvements in disruptive behaviors. Both the GANA and PCIT groups had significant improvements compared to the TAU group. There was no significant difference between the GANA and PCIT groups, and families reported being more satisfied with both GANA and PCIT than TAU. The similar results for both GANA and PCIT suggest that conducting a parent–child therapy in Spanish (i.e., GANA and PCIT) may be more beneficial to families than the tailored family engagement strategies used in GANA.

Matos, Bauermeister, and Bernal (2009) implemented a culturally adapted version of PCIT with Puerto Rican families (in Puerto Rico) with preschoolers with ADHD and disruptive behaviors. Their cultural adaption (Matos, Torres, Santiago, Jurado, & Rodríguez, 2006) was similar to that of McCabe et al. (2005). All materials were provided in Spanish. Additional time was added to sessions to discuss contextual issues that could affect treatment with parents. Extra time was also spent to increase rapport. Special attention was given to help participating parents discuss the treatment process with their spouses and extended family members. This was done in order for parents to receive support and to prevent disruptions in treatment by nonparticipating family members. The time-out procedure was modified for children who refused to go to the time-out chair or demanded use of excessive force by parents, and as an alternative, loss of privileges was used. Families were randomized to a PCIT group and waitlist group. There was a significant reduction in hyperactivity, inattention, aggressive behaviors, oppositional-defiant behaviors, conduct problems, and parenting stress as well as significant increase in the use of adequate parenting practices in the intervention group. Treatment effects lasted at a 3.5-month follow-up assessment.

Leung, Tsang, Heung, and Yiu (2008) conducted a PCIT efficacy study for Chinese children with behavioral problems and their families in Hong Kong. The intervention group reported decreased child behavior problems and parenting stress after treatment than the comparison group. Parents in the intervention group showed less inappropriate child-management behaviors, such as criticisms, commands, questions, and corporal punishment as well as more positive parenting behaviors. The treatment effect was maintained at a three- to six-month follow-up. During the study, the authors made some relevant observations related to the cultural nuances at play when engaging Chinese families in the process of PCIT. First, many Chinese parents were hesitant to use praise as positive reinforcement for appropriate behaviors, resulting in PCIT therapists working more with parents to help them use praise. Second, most families had difficulty following their child's play and tended to be overdirective and interrupt play interactions. Third, Chinese families had difficulty using ignoring techniques for negative child behaviors. Lastly, a few participants faced difficulties in convincing their spouses and extended family members to share their views. These important observations indicate possible cultural factors that could impact the efficacy of PCIT with these families and inform future planning of interventions with this population.

Child-Parent Psychotherapy (CPP). CPP was developed and researched by Lieberman and her colleagues in the United States (Lieberman, 2008; Lieberman, Ippen, & Van Horn, 2006; Lieberman & Van Horn, 2004, 2009; Lieberman, Weston, & Pawl, 1991; Lieberman et al., 2005). CPP is a manually based dyadic therapeutic intervention for infants, toddlers, and preschoolers who experienced traumatic events and subsequently experience attachment, emotional, or behavioral problems (Lieberman, 2008; Lieberman & Van Horn, 2004). CPP aims to support and strengthen the parent–child relationship, which will restore and protect a child's sense of security and emotional-behavioral-physiological regulation. Intervention includes the correction of parents' and children's maladaptive representations of themselves and each other and their interactions. Therapists help parents to understand how their past experiences influence their perception of themselves and their children. CPP also helps parents to attune to their children's emotional state and inner experiences. The intervention encourages clinicians to tailor engagement strategies depending on the needs and background of the family and consider contextual factors that affect the parent–child relationship, such as cultural factors, socioeconomic factors, and immigration-related stressors.

Due to their contextual approach, studies in the United States on CPP have included ethnic minorities, immigrants, and disadvantaged populations: Mexican, Central and South Americans, recent immigrant Cambodians, and multigenerational African Americans. CPP has been implemented with careful consideration of the cultural factors present in each ethnic group. There have been several randomized CPP studies, and in most CPP research the Caucasian population comprises a small portion of study samples (Cicchetti, Rogosh & Toth, 2006; Lieberman et al., 1991; Lieberman et al., 2005).

Lieberman et al. (1991) implemented CPP with Spanish-speaking Latina immigrant mothers and their infants. Mothers were from Mexico or Central America and living in the United States for less than five years. Anxiously attached parent–infant dyads were randomly assigned to the CPP intervention group or a comparison group. Securely attached dyads formed a second control group. CPP was delivered by four bicultural/bilingual female therapists. CPP toddlers had significant improvements on avoidance, resistance, and anger toward their mothers and displayed increased partnerships with their mothers. CPP mothers had significant improvements on empathy and interactiveness with their children.

Lieberman et al. (2005) implemented CPP for preschoolers who were exposed to domestic violence in the United States. Ethnic groups represented were of mixed ethnicity: Latino, African American, white, and Asian. Parent–child dyads were randomly assigned to CPP, while a comparison group received services in the community and monthly case management for one year. CPP children were found to have greater reductions in total behavior problems and traumatic stress symptoms. CPP mothers had significantly greater reductions in avoidant symptomatology. At a six-month follow-up (Lieberman et al., 2006), CPP children showed greater reductions in total behavior problems, and CPP mothers showed significant reductions in general distress.

Toth, Maughan, Manly, Spagnola, and Cicchetti (2002) studied the treatment efficacy of CPP for maltreated preschoolers and their mothers in the United States. Parent–child dyads were randomly assigned to CPP, a psychoeducation home visitation (PHV), community standard treatment (CS), and a low-income normative comparison group (NC). The majority of study participants were ethnic minorities, predominantly African American. Children in the CPP group had significantly greater reductions in negative self-representations compared to children in the other three groups.

Parent–Child Interventions Using Video Feedback

Emerging research has shown the effectiveness of video feedback interventions in enhancing parental sensitivity and attunement as well as reducing child problem behaviors (Steele et al., 2014). However, there is limited evidence on the use of these short-term interventions with immigrant and ethnic minority communities. Despite the minimal research, video feedback has the potential to be a useful tool with these families. The viewing of parent–child interactions on video may provide the parent with more pertinent information that would otherwise be compromised by possible language and cultural barriers.

Video Feedback Intervention to Promote Positive Parenting and Sensitive Discipline (VIPP-SD; http://www.marinusvanijzendoorn.com/video-feedback-intervention-vipp). VIPP-SD was developed and researched by Juffer, Bakermans-Kranenburg, and Van IJzendoorn (2013) in the Netherlands. VIPP-SD is a brief, focused, and structured parent–child intervention using video feedback with a component of sensitive discipline to address signs of externalizing behaviors. The goal of VIPP-SD is to improve parents' sensitivity and discipline strategies to improve parent–child interaction and prevent or reduce the child's behavioral problems. While reviewing videotape, the therapist reviews specific video segments and discusses targeted themes with parents over four sessions. Booster sessions are included to consolidate intervention effects. There has been research of VIPP-SD and its extensions in Netherland, Lithuania, and United Kingdom (Kalinauskiene et al., 2009; Klein Velderman et al., 2006; Stein et al., 2006). Research findings indicate improvements in maternal sensitivity and more sensitive disciplinary attitudes and behaviors.

Yagmur et al. (2014) implemented a culturally modified version of VIPP-SD for Turkish immigrant families in the Netherlands called VIPP-TM (VIPP-Turkish Minorities). Participants were Turkish mothers of children with high levels of externalizing problems. Changes for cultural adaptation included the use of culturally appropriate toys and play activities, having only female therapists with Turkish backgrounds and following the language use of the mothers (Turkish/Dutch). Each home visit, in the context of Turkish culture, started with social conversation. Results indicated that the intervention group had significant benefits in the areas of maternal sensitivity and nonintrusiveness.

Interaction Guidance Intervention (IG). IG intervention was developed in the United States by McDonough (1995) and has been researched in the United States and Switzerland (McDonough, 2000; McDonough, 2004; Rusconi-Serpa, Sancho Rossignol, & McDonough, 2009). In the treatment sessions, the infant and family are video-recorded in play with developmentally appropriate toys. Video feedback is immediately provided highlighting positive play interactions between the infant and family and pointing out the family's strengths, positive parenting behavior, and sensitivity. Therapists may comment on parental attitudes and behaviors that need to change only when it is critically important. IG has been proven to be effective to help families caring for infants with growth failure, sleep disorder, feeding disorder, and substance exposure.

Parent–Child Interaction Assessment-II/Modifying Attributions of Parents (PCIA-II/MAP). Another method that utilizes the video feedback approach is the Parent–Child Interaction Assessment/Mapping Attributions of Parents (PCIA-II/MAP; Holigrocki, Kaminski, & Frieswyk, 2002). PCIA-II/MAP was developed in the United States and researched by Bohr, Holigrocki, and colleagues (Bohr & Holigrocki, 2005; Bohr et al., 2008) in the United States and Canada. This protocol relies on a set of videotaped parent–child dyadic interactions in the context of a structured story stem play activity. The therapist reviews video segments with parent(s), highlighting parental strengths and helping the parent(s) to explore their thoughts and feelings and how they perceived the child's thoughts, feelings, and intentions during the play tasks. The parent is also encouraged to develop an alternative narrative regarding what child was thinking, feeling, and intending. Through this intervention, the therapist helps parents to modify their attributions to a child and develop age-appropriate expectations and parental sensitivity.

Conclusions

The early years of childhood have proven importance in preventing and reducing risk, strengthening inherent abilities, promoting competence, and building a strong foundation for social and emotional development (Masten,

Gewirtz, & Sapienza, 2013). The aim of this chapter was to use this vital understanding to support the utilization of parenting programs as a preventive endeavor that can offset the risk factors that face today's immigrant families. Given the summary of findings presented in this chapter, it can be concluded that to have a significant impact on improving the health and well-being of children in immigrant families it is important to work with these families within their context in a collaborative manner. Experts in the area of cultural psychology and migration in America emphasize how "the future character of American society and economy will be intimately related to the adaptation of the children of today's immigrants" (Suárez-Orozco & Suárez-Orozco, 2001, p. 3). Therefore, investigations on parenting programs as factors of resilience and prevention for immigrant and ethnic minority children will benefit society as a whole. There is a clear lack of evidence of these programs in non-Western countries; however, the transportability of parenting interventions across countries shows promise, and the information gained on cultural adaptions in this review can easily facilitate planning of these programs in non-Western countries.

Table 16.1 provides a summary of the effective cultural adaptations and modifications made within the studies presented in this chapter. Overall, in the review of the existing literature on parent training programs and parent–child therapies, it was found that the following strategies for engaging and treating immigrant families and ethnic groups in their country of origin were commonly used:

- Translate written materials into the native language.
- Use bilingual and bicultural staff and clinicians.
- Use translators when content is presented in English.
- Give staff and clinicians cultural competency training specific to ethnicity.
- Introduce a motivational/supportive phase to increase potential for engagement before evidenced-based intervention begins.
- Ground key components of intervention in cultural values, beliefs, and constructs by using culture-specific examples, vignettes, and visuals.
- Build trust among the families, schools, and community through involvement of respected community agencies and trusted cultural brokers.
- Provide extra booster sessions, phone consultations, and home visits to provide support, reinforce information learned, and clarify any misunderstandings.

This summary of modifications can be beneficial in the planning of parenting interventions with immigrant and ethnic minority communities.

Future Directions

The effectiveness of culturally adapted parenting interventions as a preventive mechanism for the well-being of immigrant children remains an emerging area of clinical investigation. While evidence on how specific

Table 16.1 *Summary of Cultural Adaptations and Modifications*

Study Authors	Intervention	Group studied (host country)	Translation of written materials	Bilingual and/or bicultural staff	Translator present when content presented in English	Cultural competency training for staff	Motivational/ support phase	Cultural values, beliefs, constructs woven into content	Community agencies and/or trusted cultural brokers involved	Extra booster sessions, phone consultation or home visits provided
Bavolek et al. (2013)	Nurturing Parenting Program	Hispanic (U.S.)	X	X					X	X
Montañez et al. (2010)	Nurturing Parenting Program	Mexican (U.S.)		X				X		
National Center for Mental Health Promotion and Youth Violence Prevention, (2011).	Nurturing Parenting Program	Somali (U.S.)			X		X		X	
Axberg & Broberg (2012)	Incredible Years	Swedish (Sweden)	X	X						
Barrera et al. (2002)	Incredible Years	Hispanic (U.S.)		X						
Reid et al. (2001)	Incredible Years	Hispanic Asian Afr American (U.S.)	X		X					
Dionne et al. (2009)	Incredible Years	American Indian (U.S.)				X	X	X		
Kim et al. (2008)	Incredible Years	Korean (U.S.)		X	X					
Scott et al. (2001)	Incredible Years	British (U.K.)						X		
Sumargi et al. (2014a, b)	Triple P	Indonesian (Australia)	X	X				X		
Matsumoto et al. (2007, 2010)	Triple P	Japanese (Australia)	X	X				X		X

Table 16.1 (*cont.*)

Study Authors	Intervention	Group studied (host country)	Translation of written materials	Bilingual and/or bicultural staff	Translator present when content presented in English	Cultural competency training for staff	Motivational/ support phase	Cultural values, beliefs, constructs woven into content	Community agencies and/or trusted cultural brokers involved	Extra booster sessions, phone consultation or home visits provided
Leung et al., (2003)	Triple P	Chinese (Hong Kong)	X	X						
Crisante & Ng (2003)	Triple P	Chinese (Australia)		X						X
McCabe et al. (2005)	PCIT	Mexican (U.S.)	X	X			X	X		X
Matos et al. (2006)	PCIT	Puerto Rican (Puerto Rican)	X	X			X	X		
Leung et al. (2008)	PCIT	Chinese (Hong Kong)	X	X			X	X		
Lieberman et al. (1991)	CPP	Latina (U.S.)		X				X		
Yagmur et al. (2014)	VIPP-TM	Turkish (Netherlands)		X				X		

adaptations impact treatment outcomes is limited, the summary of information provided in this chapter can be utilized in a number of ways. The array of culturally adapted interventions presented can inform the design of future studies and recruitment and rapport building when conducting outreach with immigrant communities. While the studies presented show positive short-term results for culturally relevant interventions for immigrant parents, further investigation on the long-term effectiveness of these types of interventions is necessary. An understanding of the longer-term effects is especially important in the conceptualization of these types of interventions as prevention models. Finally, an examination of Table 16.1 tells us that researchers have used a variety of cultural adaptations to produce positive results. It does not appear there is one set way in which to treat these communities. What remains unknown is the effectiveness of one cultural adaptation over another. An explorative comparison of culturally adapted delivery formats and treatment features would be highly informative to the field.

The present chapter provides valuable insights about parenting interventions in the context of cultural adaptations. There is minimal literature that explores the use of these interventions as a protective mechanism in the well-being of children of immigrants. The present review of literature is unique in that it summarizes studies with immigrant communities and outlines the specific cultural adaptations that researchers found to be effective with the ethnic minority and immigrant communities. The information sets a foundation for developing culturally relevant parenting programs. This chapter also informs policy makers and professionals working with this population about the need to have accessible and relevant evidenced-based parenting interventions.

References

Anderson, P. (2002). Assessment and development of executive function (EF) during childhood. *Child Neuropsychology* 8(2): 71–82.

Aos, S. & Drake, E. (2013). *Prison, Police and Programs: Evidence-Based Options That Reduce Crime and Save Money*. Olympia, WA: Washington State Institute for Public Policy.

Axberg, U., & Broberg, A. G. (2012). Evaluation of "the Incredible Years" in Sweden: the transferability of an American parent training program to Sweden. *Scandinavian Journal of Psychology* 53(3): 224–32.

Barlow, J., Johnston, I., Kendrick, D., Polnay, L., & Stewart-Brown, S. (2006). Individual and group-based parenting programmes for the treatment of physical child abuse and neglect. *Cochrane Database of Systematic Reviews* 3. doi: 10.1002/14651858.CD005463.pub2

Barrera, M., Biglan, A., Taylor, T. K., Gunn, B. K., Smolkowski, K., Black, C., & Fowler, R. C. (2002). Early elementary school intervention to reduce conduct problems: a randomized trial with Hispanic and non-Hispanic children. *Prevention Science* 3(2): 83–94.

Bavolek, S. J. (2000). The Nurturing Parenting Program. *Juvenile Justice Bulletin* (November): 1–12.

Bavolek, S. J., Comstock, C. C., & McLaughlin, J. A. (1983). *The Nurturing Program: A Validated Approach for Reducing Dysfunctional Family Interactions*. Rockville, MD: National Institute of Mental Health.

Bavolek, S. J., Keene, R., Miranda, G., & Radcliff, J. (2013). *Implementation of the Nurturing Parenting Programs with Latino Families in Imperial County, California*. El Centro, CA: Imperial County Office of Education.

Bell, S., & Eyberg, S. M. (2002). Parent–Child Interaction Therapy. In VandeCreek, L., Knapp, S., & Jackson, T. L. (eds.), *Innovations in Clinical Practice: A Source Book*. Sarasota, FL: Professional Resource Press, pp. 57–74.

Berry, J. W. (2005). Acculturation: living successfully in two cultures. *International Journal of Intercultural Relations* 29(6): 697–712.

Bohr, Y., Dhayanandhan, B., Armour, L., Sockett DiMarco, N., Holigrocki, R. & Baumgartner, E. (2008). Mapping parent-infant interactions: a brief cognitive approach to the prevention of relationship ruptures and infant maltreatment (the MAP method). *Infant Mental Health Promotion* 51: 2–7.

Bohr, Y., & Holigrocki, R. J. (2005). PCIA-II/MAP treatment manual: modifying attributions of parents' intervention. Unpublished manuscript, York University, Toronto, Canada; and University of Indianapolis, Indianapolis, IN.

Borstein, M. (2011). *Immigration*. Montreal, Canada: Encyclopedia on Early Childhood Development. www.child-encyclopedia.com/immigration/synthesis

Bornstein, M., & Bohr, Y. (2011). Immigration, acculturation and parenting. In Bornstein, M. (ed.), *Immigration*. Montreal, Canada: Encyclopedia on Early Childhood Development, pp. 15–20. www.child-encyclopedia.com/sites/default/files/textes-experts/en/664/immigration-acculturation-and-parenting.pdf

Brasfield, C. R. (2001). Residential school syndrome. *British Columbia Medical Journal* 43(2): 78–81.

Brave Heart, M. Y. H. (1999). Oyate Ptayela: rebuilding the Lakota nation through addressing historical trauma among Lakota parents. *Journal of Human Behavior in the Social Environment* 2(1/2): 109–26.

Brinkmeyer, M., & Eyberg, S. M. (2003). Parent–Child Interaction Therapy for oppositional children. In Kazdin, A. E., & Weisz, J. R. (eds.), *Evidence-Based Psychotherapies for Children and Adolescents*. New York: Guilford Press, pp. 204–23.

Campbell, F., Conti, G., Heckman, J. J., Moon, S. H., Pinto, R., Pungello, E., & Pan, Y. (2014). Early childhood investments substantially boost adult health. *Science* 343(6178): 1478–85.

Carter, A. S., Briggs-Gowan, M. J. & Davis, N. O. (2004). Assessment of young children's social-emotional development and psychopathology: recent advances and recommendations for practice. *Journal of Child Psychology and Psychiatry* 45(1): 109–34.

Cicchetti, D., Rogosh, F. A., & Toth, S. L. (2006). Fostering secure attachment in infants in maltreating families through preventive interventions. *Development and Psychopathology* 18(3): 623–49.

Cowen, P. S. (2001). Effectiveness of a parent education intervention for at-risk families. *Journal of the Society for Pediatric Nursing* 6(2): 73–82.

Crisante, L., & Ng, S. (2003). Implementation and process issued in using Group Triple P with Chinese parents: preliminary findings. *Australian e-Journal for the Advancement of Mental Health* 2(3): 226–35.

Dallaire, D. H., & Weinraub, M. (2005). The stability of parenting behaviors over the first six years of life. *Early Childhood Research Quarterly* 20: 201–19.

de Graaf, I., Speetjens, P., Smit, F., De Wolff, M., & Tavecchio, L. (2008). Effectiveness of the Triple P Positive Parenting Program on behavioural problems in children: a meta-analysis. *Behavior Modification* 32(5): 714–35.

Deater-Deckard, K., Ivy, L., & Smith, J. (2005). Resilience in gene-environment transactions. In Goldstein, S., & Brooks, R. (eds.), *Handbook of Resilience in Children*. New York: Springer US, pp. 49–63.

Dettlaff, A., & Earner, I. (2012). Children of immigrants in the child welfare system: characteristics, risk and maltreatment. *Families in Society* 93(4): 295–303.

Dionne, R., Davis, B., Sheeber, L., & Madrigal, L. (2009). Initial evaluation of a cultural approach to implementation of evidence-based parenting interventions in American Indian communities. *Journal of Community Psychology* 37(7): 911–21.

Dionne, R., & Dishion, T. (1998). *Indian Family Wellness Assessment Manual: A Culturally Sensitive, Family-Based Assessment for Native American Families*. Eugene, OR: Oregon Social Learning Center.

Duran, E., & Duran, B. (1995). *Native American Postcolonial Psychology*. Albany: State University of New York Press.

Evans-Campbell, T. (2008). Historical trauma in American Indian/Native Alaska communities: a multilevel framework for exploring impacts on individuals, families, and communities. *Journal of Interpersonal Violence* 23(3): 316–38.

Eurostat (2014). *Migration and Migrant Population Statistics*. ec.europa.eu/eurostat/statistics-explained/index.php/Migration_and_migrant_population_statistics

Falicov, C. J. (2007). Working with transnational immigrants: expanding meanings of family, community, and culture. *Family Process* 46(2): 157–71.

Farver, J. M., & Shinn, Y. L. (1997). Social pretend play in Korean- and Anglo-American pre-schoolers. *Child Development* 68(3): 544–56.

Gardner, F., Burton, J., & Klimes, I. (2006). Randomised controlled trial of a parenting intervention in the voluntary sector for reducing child conduct problems: outcomes and mechanisms of change. *Journal of Child Psychology and Psychiatry* 47(1): 1123–32.

Gardner, F., Montgomery, P., & Knerr, W. (2015). Transporting evidence-based parenting programs for child problem behavior (age 3-10) between countries: systematic review and meta-analysis. *Journal of Clinical Child & Adolescent Psychology* 0(0): 1–14.

Hartup, W. W. (1989). Social relationships and their developmental significance. *American Psychologist* 44(2): 120–6.

Heckman, J. J. (2011). The economics of inequality: the value of early childhood education. *American Educator* 35(1): 31–47.

Holigrocki, R. I., Kaminski, P. L., & Frieswyk, S. H. (2002). PCIA-II: Parent-Child Interaction Assessment Version II. Unpublished manuscript, University of Indianapolis, Indianapolis, IN.

IOM (International Organization of Migration) (2015). www.iom.int/countries

Jalali, M., Shaeeri, M. R., Tahmasian, K., & Pourahmadi, E. (2009). The effects of Triple P Positive Parenting Program on 7–10 year old children with oppositional defiant disorder (ODD). *Daneshvar Raftar* 1: 29–38.

Jent, J. F., Niec, L. N., & Baker, S. E. (2011). Play and interpersonal processes. In Russ, S. W., & Niec, L. N. (eds.), *Play in Clinical Practice: Evidence-Based Approaches*. New York: Guilford Press, pp. 23–47.

Johnston, J. R., & Wong, M. Y. A. (2002). Cultural differences in beliefs and practices concerning talk to children. *Journal of Speech, Language, and Hearing Research* 45(5): 916–26.

Juffer, F., Bakermans-Kranenburg, M. J., & Van IJzendoorn M. H. (2013). Attachment-based interventions: sensitive parenting is the key to positive parent-child relationships. In Holmes, P., & Farnfield, S. (eds.), *The Routledge Handbook of Attachment: Implications and Interventions*. New York: Routledge, pp. 83–103.

Kalinauskiene, L., Cekuoliene, D., Van IJzendoorn, M. H., Bakermans-Kranenburg, M. J., Juffer, F., & Kusakovskaja, I. (2009). Supporting insensitive mothers: the Vilnius randomized control trial of video feedback intervention to promote maternal sensitivity and infant attachment. *Child: Care, Health & Development* 35(5): 613–23.

Kim, E., Cain, K. C., & Webster-Stratton, C. (2008). The preliminary effect of a parenting program for Korean American mothers: a randomized controlled experimental study. *International Journal of Nursing Studies* 45(9): 1261–73.

Klein Velderman, M., Bakermans-Kranenburg, M. J., Juffer, F., Van IJzendoorn, M. H., Mangelsdorf, S. C., & Zevalkink, J. (2006). Preventing preschool externalizing behavior problems through video-feedback intervention in infancy. *Infant Mental Health Journal* 27(5): 466–93.

Kugler, E. G. (2009). *Partnering with Parents and Families to Support Immigrant and Refugee Children at School*. Washington, DC: George Washington University. www.healthinschools.org/Immigrant-and-Refugee-Children/~/media/48FDB9013C3C454AB6EC9E491D752AA0.ashx

La Fromboise, T. D. (1998). American Indian mental health policy. In Atkinson, D., Morten, G., & Sue, D. W. (eds.), *Counseling American Minorities: A Cross-cultural Perspective*, 5th ed.. Madison, WI: Brown & Benchmark, pp. 137–58.

Larsson, B., Fossum, S., Clifford, G., Drugli, M. B., Handegård, B. H., & Mørch, W.-T. (2009). Treatment of oppositional defiant and conduct problems in Norwegian children: results of a randomized controlled trial. *European Child & Adolescent Psychiatry* 18(1): 42–52.

Lau, A. S. (2006). Making the case for selective and directed cultural adaptations of evidence-based treatments: examples from parent training. *Clinical Psychology: Science and Practice* 13(4): 295–310.

Leung, C., Sanders, M. R., Leung, S., Mak, R., & Lau, J. (2003). An outcome evaluation of the implementation of the Triple P-Positive Parenting Program in Hong Kong. *Family Process*, 42(4), 531–544.

Leung, C., Sanders, M. R., Ip, F. & Lau, J. (2006). Implementation of Triple P-Positive Parenting Program in Hong Kong: predictors of program completion and clinical outcomes. *Journal of Children's Services* 1(2): 4–17.

Leung, C., Tsang, S., Heung, K., & Yiu, I. (2008). Effectiveness of Parent–Child Interaction Therapy (PCIT) among Chinese families. *Research on Social Work Practice* 19(3): 304–13.

LeVine, R. A., Miller, P. M., & West, M. M. (1988). *Parental Behavior in Diverse Societies*. San Francisco, CA: Jossey-Bass.

Lieberman A. F. (2008). *Psychotherapy with Infants and Young Children: Repairing the Effects of Stress and Trauma on Early Attachment*. New York: Guilford Press.

Lieberman, A. F., Ippen, C. G., & Van Horn, P. J. (2006). Child–parent psychotherapy: six month follow-up of a randomized control trial. *Journal of the American Academy of Child and Adolescent Psychiatry* 45(8): 913–18.

Lieberman, A. F., & Van Horn, P. J. (2004). *Don't Hit My Mommy: A Manual for Child–Parent Psychotherapy with Young Witnesses of Family Violence*. Washington, DC: Zero to Three.

Lieberman, A. F., & Van Horn, P. J. (2009). Child–parent psychotherapy: a developmental approach to mental health treatment in infancy and early childhood. In Zeanah, C. H. (ed.), *Handbook of Infant Mental Health* 3rd ed. New York: Guilford Press, pp. 439–49.

Lieberman, A. F., Van Horn, P. J., Ippen, C. G. (2005). Toward evidence-based treatment: child–parent psychotherapy with preschoolers exposed to marital violence. *Journal of the American Academy of Child and Adolescent Psychiatry* 44(12): 1241–8.

Lieberman A. F., Weston D. R., & Pawl J. H. (1991). Preventive intervention and outcome with anxiously attached dyads. *Child Development* 62(1): 199–209.

Lin, C.-Y. C., & Fu, V. R. (1990). A comparison of child-rearing practices among Chinese, immigrant Chinese, and Caucasian-American parents. *Child Development* 61(2): 429–33.

Little, M., Berry, V., Morpeth, L., Blower, S., Axford, N., Taylor, R., ... Tobin, K. (2012). The impact of three evidence-based programmes delivered in public systems in Birmingham, UK. *International Journal of Conflict & Violence* 6(2): 260–72.

Maher, E. J., Marcynyszyn, L. A., Corwin, T. W., & Hodnett, R. (2011). Dosage matters: the relationship between participation in the Nurturing Parenting Program for infants, toddlers, and preschoolers and subsequent child maltreatment. *Children and Youth Services Review* 33(8): 1426–34.

Masten, A. S., Gewirtz, A. H., & Sapienza J. K. (2013). *Resilience in Development: The Importance of Early Childhood*. Montreal, Canada: Encyclopedia on Early Childhood Development. www.child-encyclopedia.com/Pages/PDF/Masten-Gewirtz-SapienzaANGxp2.pdf

Matos, M., Bauermeister, J. J., & Bernal, G. (2009). Parent–Child Interaction Therapy for Puerto Rican preschool children with ADHD and behavior problems: a pilot efficacy study. *Family Process* 48(2): 232–52.

Matos, M., Torres, R., Santiago, R., Jurado, M., & Rodríguez, I. X. A. (2006). Adaptation of Parent–Child Interaction Therapy for Puerto Rican families: a preliminary study. *Family Process* 45(2): 205–22.

Matsumoto, Y., Sofronoff, K., & Sanders, M. R. (2007). The efficacy and acceptability of the Triple P-Positive Parenting Program with Japanese parents. *Behaviour Change* 24(4): 205–18.

Matsumoto, Y., Sofronoff, K., & Sanders, M. R. (2010) Investigation of the effectiveness and social validity of the Triple P Positive Parenting Program in Japanese society. *Journal of Family Psychology* 24(1): 87–91.

McCabe, K. M., & Yeh, M. (2009). Parent–Child Interaction Therapy for Mexican Americans: a randomized clinical trial. *Journal of Clinical Child & Adolescent Psychology* 38(5): 753–9.

McCabe, K. M., Yeh, M., Garland, A. F., Lau, A. S., & Chavez, G. (2005). The GANA Program: a tailoring approach to adapting Parent–Child Interaction Therapy for Mexican Americans. *Education & Treatment of Children* 28(2): 111–29.

McDonough, S. C. (1995). Promoting positive early parent–infant relationships through interaction guidance. *Child and Adolescent Psychiatric Clinics of North America* 4(3): 661–72.

McDonough, S. C. (2000). Interaction guidance: an approach for difficult-to-engage families. In Zeanah, C. H. (ed.), *Handbook of Infant Mental Health*, 2nd ed. New York: Guilford Press, pp. 485–93.

McDonough, S. C. (2004). Interaction guidance: promoting and nurturing the caregiving relationship. In Sameroff, A. J., McDonough, S. C., & Rosenblum, K. L. (eds.), *Treating Parent–Infant Relationship Problems: Strategies for Intervention*. New York: Guilford Press, pp. 79–96.

McNeil, C. B., & Hembree-Kigin, T. L. (2010). *Parent–Child Interaction Therapy* 2nd ed. New York: Springer US.

McQueen, A., Getz, J. G., & Bray, J. H. (2003). Acculturation, substance use, and deviant behavior: examining separation and family conflict as mediators. *Child Development* 74(6): 1737–50.

Merrell, K. W., Whitcomb, S. A., & Parisi, D. M. (2009). *Strong Start-PreK: A Social & Emotional Learning Curriculum*. Baltimore, MD: Paul H. Brookes.

Montañez, M., Devall, E., & Van Leeuwen, D. (2010). Social capital: strengthening Mexican-American families through parenting education. *Journal of Family and Consumer Sciences* 102(3): 27–33.

National Center for Mental Health Promotion and Youth Violence Prevention (2011). *Strategies in Engaging Immigrant and Refugee Families*. Waltham, MA:Education Development Center. www.promoteprevent.org/sites/www.promoteprevent.org/files/resources/strategies_for_engaging_immigrant_and_refugee_families_2.pdf

Navsaria, N. & Luby, J. L. (2015). Assessing the pre-school age child. In Dulcan, M. (ed.), *Dulcan's Textbook of Child and Adolescent Psychiatry*, 2nd ed. Arlington, VA: American Psychiatric Publishing.

Nowak, C., & Heinrichs, N. (2008). A comprehensive meta-analysis of Triple P-Positive Parenting Program using hierarchical linear modeling: effectiveness and moderating variables. *Clinical Child and Family Psychology Review* 11(3): 114–44.

Palusci, V. J., Crum, P., Bliss, R. & Bavolek, S. J. (2008). Changes in parenting attitudes and knowledge among inmates and other at-risk populations after a Family Nurturing Program. *Children and Youth Services Review* 30(1): 79–89.

Perry, B. D. (2002). Childhood experience and the expression of genetic potential: what childhood neglect tells us about nature and nurture. *Brain and Mind* 3 (1): 79–100.

Piquero, A. R., Farrington, D. P., Welsh, B., Tremblay, R., & Jennings, W. (2008). *Effects of Early Family/Parent Training Programs on Antisocial Behavior & Delinquency: A Systematic Review*. Stockholm: Swedish National Council for Crime Prevention.

Posthumus, J. A., Raaijmakers, M. A. J., Maassen, G. H., van Engeland, H., & Matthys, W. (2012). Sustained effects of Incredible Years as a preventive intervention in preschool children with conduct problems. *Journal of Abnormal Child Psychology* 40(4): 487–500.

Reid, M. J., Webster-Stratton, C., & Beauchaine, T. P. (2001). Parent training in Head Start: a comparison of program response among African American, Asian American, Caucasian, and Hispanic mothers. *Prevention Science* 2(4): 209–27.

Reid, M. J., Webster-Stratton, C., & Hammond, M. (2007) Enhancing a classroom social competence and problem-solving curriculum by offering parent training to families of moderate- to high-risk elementary school children. *Journal of Clinical Child and Adolescent Psychology* 36(4): 605–20.

Rusconi-Serpa, S., Sancho Rossignol, A., & McDonough, S. C. (2009). Video feedback in parent-infant treatments. *Child and Adolescent Psychiatric Clinics of North America* 18(3): 735–51.

Sanders, M. R. (2012). Development, evaluation, and multinational dissemination of the Triple P-Positive Parenting Program. *Annual Review of Clinical Psychology* 8: 345–79.

Sclafani, J. D. (2004). *The Educated Parent: Recent Trends in Raising Children*. West Port, CT: Praeger.

Scott, S., O'Connor, T. G., Futh, A., Matias, C., Price, J., & Doolan, M. (2010). Impact of a parenting program in a high-risk, multi-ethnic community: the PALS trial. *Journal of Child Psychology and Psychiatry* 51(12): 1331–41.

Scott, S., Spender, Q., Doolan, M., Jacobs, B., Aspland, H., & Webster-Stratton, C. (2001). Multicentre controlled trial of parenting groups for childhood antisocial behavior in clinical practice. *British Medical Journal* 323(7306): 194–8.

Shields, M. K., & Behrman, R. (2004). Children of immigrant families: analysis and recommendations. *Children of Immigrant Families* 14(2): 4–15.

Shonkoff, J. P., & Phillips, D. A. (2000). *From Neurons to Neighborhoods: The Science of Early Childhood Development*. Washington, DC: National Academy Press.

Sroufe, L. A., Egeland, B., & Kreutzer, T. (1990). The fate of early experience following developmental change: longitudinal approaches to individual adaptation in childhood. *Child Development* 61(5): 1363–73.

Steele, M., Steele, H., Bate, J., Knafo, H., Kinsey, M., Bonuck, K., & Murphy, A. (2014). Looking from the outside in: the use of video in attachment-based interventions. *Attachment & Human Development* 16(4): 402–15.

Stein, A., Woolley, H., Senior, R., Hertzmann, L., Lovel, M., & Lee, J. (2006). Treating disturbances in the relationship between mothers with bulimic eating disorders and their infants: a randomized, controlled trial of video feedback. *American Journal of Psychiatry* 163(5): 899–906.

Suárez-Orozco, C., & Suárez-Orozco, M. (2001). *Children of Immigration*. Cambridge, MA: Harvard University Press.

Sumargi, A., Sofronoff, K., & Morawska, A. (2014a). Evaluation of a brief format of the Triple P-Positive Parenting Program: a pilot study with Indonesian parents residing in Australia. *Behaviour Change* 31(2): 144–58.

Sumargi, A., Sofronoff, K., & Morawska, A. (2014b). A randomized-controlled trial of the Triple P-Positive Parenting Program seminar series with Indonesian parents. *Child Psychiatry and Human Development* (October): 749–61.

Thomas, R., & Zimmer-Gembeck, M. J. (2007). Behavioral outcomes of Parent-Child Interaction Therapy and Triple P-Positive Parenting Program: a review and meta-analysis. *Journal of Abnormal Child Psychology* 35(3): 475–95.

Toth, S. L., Maughan, A., Manly, J. T., Spagnola, M., & Cicchetti, D. (2002). The relative efficacy of two interventions in altering maltreated preschool children's representational models: Implications for attachment theory. *Developmental Psychopathology* 14(4): 877–908.

Veso, J. E., Cooper, D., & Behforooz, B. (2006). Effects of the Nurturing Curriculum on social, emotional, and academic behaviors in kindergarten classrooms. *Journal of Research in Childhood Education* 20(4): 275–85.

Vygotsky, L. S. (1978). *Mind in Society*. Cambridge, MA: Harvard University Press.

Webster-Stratton, C. (1984). A randomized trial of two parent-training programs for families with conduct-disordered children. *Journal of Consulting and Clinical Psychology* 52(4): 666–78.

Webster-Stratton, C. (1990). Enhancing the effectiveness of self-administered videotape parent training for families with conduct-problem children. *Journal of Abnormal Child Psychology* 18(5): 479–92.

Webster-Stratton, C. (1994). Advancing videotape parent training: a comparison study. *Journal of Consulting and Clinical Psychology* 62(3): 583–93.

Webster-Stratton, C. (1998). Preventing conduct problems in Head Start children: strengthening parenting competencies. *Journal of Consulting and Clinical Psychology* 66(5): 715–30.

Webster-Stratton, C., & Hammond, M. (1997). Treating children with early-onset conduct problems: a comparison of child and parent training interventions. *Journal of Consulting and Clinical Psychology* 65(1): 93–109.

Webster-Stratton. C., Hollinsworth, T., & Kolpacoff. M. (1989). The long-term effectiveness and clinical significance of three cost-effective training programs for families with conduct-problem children. *Journal of Consulting and Clinical Psychology* 57(4): 550–3.

Webster-Stratton, C., Reid, M. J., & Hammond, M. (2004). Treating children with early-onset conduct problems: intervention outcomes for parent, child, and teacher training. *Journal of Clinical Child & Adolescent Psychology* 33(1): 105–24.

Williams, C. L., & Berry, J. W. (1991). Primary prevention of acculturative stress among refugees: application of psychological theory and practice. *American Psychologist* 46(6): 632–41.

Yagmur, S., Mesman, J., Malda, M., Bakermans-Kranenburg, M. J., & Ekmekci, H. (2014). Video-feedback intervention increases sensitive parenting in ethnic minority mothers: a randomized control trial. *Attachment & Human Development* 16(4): 371–86.

Ying, Y.-W. (1999). Strengthening intergenerational/intercultural ties in immigrant families: a new intervention for parents. *Journal of Community Psychology* 27(1): 89–96.

Zeigler, K., & Camarota, S. A. (2014). *U.S. Immigrant Population Record 41.3 Million in 2013. Asian, Caribbean, and Middle Eastern Immigrant Populations Grew Most since 2010*. Washington, DC: Center for Immigration Studies. cis.org/immigrant-population-record-2013

Zigler, E., & Berman, W. (1983). Discerning the future of early childhood intervention. *American Psychologist* 38(8): 894–906.

17 Prevention of Academic, Cultural, and Behavioral Problems among International Student Populations

Hanako Suzuki, Nadia T. Hasan, & Kyle Rundles

Introduction

As the numbers of international students in higher education continuously grow throughout the world, it is becoming more important to deliver culturally sensitive, culturally appropriate services to meet the needs of the particular population. International students face many challenges during their study in a foreign country, including culture shock (e.g., McLachlan & Justice, 2009), language and accent difficulties (e.g., Chen, 1999; Lin, 2006), loss and/or reconstruction of identity (e.g., Kim, 2012; Ward & Searle, 1991), discrimination (e.g., Duru & Poyrazil, 2011; Lee & Rice, 2007), and separation from social support and feeling of isolation (e.g., Lin, 2006). These stressors are additional to developmental issues that domestic students also encounter. However, it has been widely reported that international students underutilize mental health services on campus (e.g., Hori et al., 2012; Hyun, Quinn, Madon, & Lustig, 2007; Nilsson, Berkel, Flores, & Lucus, 2004).

Providing services to reach international students and promote positive sojourn experiences is essential. Much of the literature on mental health services for international students suggests that service providers be open-minded about stepping out of counseling centers, proactive in reaching out, and flexible to offer nontraditional interventions (e.g., Chen, 1999; Komiya & Elles, 2001; Popadiuk & Arthur, 2004). One way to reach out to international students is delivering preventive interventions aimed at facilitating their well-being and preventing academic, cultural, and behavioral problems before the issues arise. Prevention strategies can not only reduce the incidence of emotional disturbances and minimize the long-term effects of psychological issues on educational, sociocultural, and vocational aspects of life, but also promote healthy adjustment in a new culture.

This chapter will present the descriptions of international student populations and the challenges that international students often face. It also explains the application of prevention efforts to international students as well as specific recommendations for prevention strategies and promotion of wellness. Furthermore, the chapter will touch upon preventive intervention on systemic levels. There are some limitations due to lack of literature on international students around the globe, because the previous research has been largely conducted in English-speaking countries; however, observations of international student services in the France, Japan, Malaysia, and the United States (U.S.) and some literature from non-English-speaking countries lead authors to conclude that international students around the world tend to face similar issues. Therefore, with some modification and adjustment to the cultural context where the prevention intervention is delivered, the prevention strategies introduced in this chapter can be effective with the international student population at large. The chapter is aimed at embracing the existing knowledge on prevention services for international students in higher education and at informing those who provide services to international students on university/college campus with comprehensive perspectives.

Description of International Students

The number of international students is steadily increasing, and in 2012 there were approximately 4.5 million international students worldwide (OECD, 2014). Approximately 75 percent of international students are studying in the United States, the United Kingdom, France, Germany, Australia, and Japan (World Education Services, 2010). International students originate from many countries, but the largest number of international students originate from China, India, Korea, Germany, Turkey, France, Russia, and Japan. China and India are predicted to continue as the top home country of international students worldwide (World Education Services, 2010). The United States had the largest number of international students with approximately 886,052 students studying there in 2014 (IIE, 2014).

There are several contributions that international students make to the educational institutes and host countries as well as to their home countries. Contributions to the host country and educational institute include enhanced cultural understanding, reduction of prejudice and biases by exposing people to cultural differences, promotion of the internationalization of education, and financial benefits (Hasan, Fouad, & Williams-Nickelson, 2008; Lin, 2000). Sometimes international students select majors that host countries have trouble filling with domestic students. This is another benefit for the host country. International students serve as cultural carriers and resources and links between cultures that increase international understanding and cooperation (Lin, 2000; Sam, 2001). When students return to their country of origin, they share their knowledge across cultures, increase cultural awareness at home, and challenge thoughts and personal biases of people. Many times, their degrees are assets to finding employment back home (Hasan et al., 2008).

International students begin their journey to study abroad in their home country by researching the country to which they plan to move, the educational degree they want to pursue, and the type of educational institution they would like to attend (Hasan et al., 2008). Then these individuals complete the required entrance exams for their programs and language proficiency tests, such as the Test of English as a Foreign Language (TOEFL). Once they are accepted to an institution of higher education, students need to request the appropriate visa and legal documents from their home country and the host country (Hasan et al., 2008).

Once students enter the country where they plan to study, they need to settle in, which often consists of acquiring basic living accommodations and figuring out tasks such as banking needs, currency issues, and degree and course requirements (Arthur, 2004; Hasan et al., 2008). Often, the host educational institution will have an office or department to assist international students in adjusting to their new country. This may include picking up students at the airport; aiding in housing accommodations; organizing welcoming socials and mixers; and planning academic orientations that include banking information, travel options, and health care plans. International students often continue to receive support from this office, which may also be responsible for their compliance with legal and academic criteria. For example, in the United States, this includes ensuring that the student is not employed and is making good progress toward his or her degree plan (Hasan et al., 2008).

Challenges That International Students Experience

International students are being recruited more and more throughout the world, thus the support for international students must also increase. It is the role of home and host universities and their staff to ensure that students are prepared and supported through this transition in order to tap into the positive side of stress. Because of the difficulties international students may encounter, it is important to take a closer look at this population and the ways in which they face challenges. Understanding specifics such as the differences between international graduate and international undergraduate students is important. Better understanding of difficulties and barriers that international students may face can help prevent these difficulties.

Academic Challenges

There are several academic challenges that many international students experience, and a language barrier is often named as one of the most isolating and difficult aspects of the experience of studying abroad (referred henceforth as the "study abroad experience"), especially for those whose first language is different from the host language (Hwang, Bennett, & Beauchemin, 2014; Mori, 2000; Smith & Khawaja, 2014; Tidwell & Hanassab, 2007). Struggling with a language barrier and lack of linguistic proficiency has been found to impact significantly the amount of culture shock an international student may experience and may lead to negative experiences with other students and professors from the host county (Lin, 2006). The language adjustment challenges impact both undergraduate and graduate students and include feeling comfortable reading in a different language, writing and speaking in a new language, and understanding the lectures in the host country language (Hasan et al., 2008; Lin, 2000; Sam, 2001). International students often report fear of talking in class in front of domestic classmates and faculty (Hasan et al., 2008), and speaking with an accent and performing at lower levels in school because of language difficulties can decrease a person's self-esteem. In this type of cross-cultural environment, students' methods of communication are drastically changed, which can contribute to a decrease in confidence and difficulty adjusting to life and study in a new country (Brown & Aktas, 2011; Hwang et al., 2014; Lin, 2006). Many international graduate students support themselves by working as teaching assistants, which can be challenging due to their lack of confidence in the host language speaking skills and the domestic students' reactions to their speaking skills and accents (Hasan et al., 2008). In a study by Mamiseishvili (2012), international students who required remedial English during their first year studying in the United States were less likely to persist in studying abroad than those who did not require remedial courses. With immersion in a different linguistic region, language proficiency can significantly improve very quickly, but the process can be quite stressful for less prepared students.

Differences in learning style, including understanding a new grading system, selecting courses, learning relevant study skills, adjusting to the different expectations of the instructors, and for some students getting used to the competitiveness of their classmates, are other academic challenges (Hasan et al., 2008; Lin, 2000; Sam, 2001). These differences may impact undergraduate and graduate students differently as graduate students usually have better study skills than undergraduates. Many international students need to adjust to a new style of learning; for instance, not only does the academic system in the United States require the memorization of key course materials, but also students must synthesize and draw conclusions from course materials (Hasan et al., 2008; Lin, 2000). Course participation differences, such as the expectation to either sit still and quiet or actively participate, can be a challenge to which international students need to adjust. Plagiarism is another challenge that impacts international students (Lin, 2000). In some countries, this is an accepted practice, and it may be seen as normal conduct in the student's home country. At times, international students feel pressured to perform well in a course in which they are unprepared and may make a deliberate decision to plagiarize.

Relationships with faculty members, staff, and authority figures on and off campus often require social skills that may vary from those required in their home country (Arthur, 2004; Hasan et al., 2008; Lin, 2000). The social code of behaviors is not clearly defined, and theses norms may vary from person to person and from culture to culture. One example includes how to address faculty members during class. Sometimes professors allow students to address them with their first name, though this practice may be considered too informal or even disrespectful in other countries (Lin, 2000). Although this may be true of domestic students as well, individuals from different cultural and social norms may struggle with this issue more than the individuals from the host culture. Other examples include interacting with faculty members during their office hours and meetings with faculty members that occur outside of the classroom (i.e., professional conferences, department social events, coffee shops, etc.). These situations are often unstructured, and social roles may be unclear to individuals from different countries, especially the ones that have very distinct cultural norms (Hasan et al., 2008).

A myth about international students is that they are wealthy and have unlimited finances to pay for courses, books, housing, and living expenses (Arthur, 2004). In reality, managing finances and paying for college is difficult, especially for international students who often experience employment restrictions in their host country. Added expenses due to their status in the host country, including high tuition fees, ineligibility for financial aid, or required health insurance costs (Hasan et al., 2008), may cast burdens on students and impede their academic success. Visa regulations and requirements are complex, and even the renewal process for the visa can be expensive, sometimes requiring a student to return home to complete the process (Hasan et al., 2008). International students often have an approved major of study and a strict timeline to complete their degree and need to find an employer to sponsor them for a work visa if they decide to remain in the host country for employment (Hasan et al., 2008). There are many challenges that students experience that may impact their ability to remain on track, and this can cause stress and unrealistic expectations for international students to complete their degrees.

Major and career decisions can be complicated for international students who come from cultures and mores that are different from those of the host country. Sometimes the educational degree program that they wanted to study originally is not what they decide to continue pursuing once they arrive in the new country. Other times, students do not make sufficient progress toward their original major and need to find a different career to remain in the country to continue their education. Making career decisions can be complicated for international students who are away from home and do not have their usual support network.

Cultural and Behavioral Challenges

Challenges with a new culture. When facing the challenges involved in cross-cultural exchanges, international students can experience acculturative stress, homesickness, and/or culture shock, which can be positive or negative (Thurber & Walton, 2012; Yakunina, Weigold, Hercegovac, & Elsayed, 2013; Yu et al., 2014). Brown and Aktas (2011) describe culture shock as "anxiety that results from losing the familiar signs and symbols of social intercourse, and their substitution by other cues that are strange," and "a period of mourning for the home world, characterized by feelings of grief and separation anxiety" (p. 340). These experiences can lead to depression, anxiety, withdrawal, physical health problems, and decreased ability to focus on other concerns, such as school work (Brown & Aktas, 2011; Smith & Khawaja, 2014; Thurber & Walton, 2012; Yakunina et al., 2013; Yan, Finn, Cardinal, & Bent, 2014). This reaction can impact a student's ability to fulfill the tasks of academic achievement and cultural exchange intended by the study abroad experience, but at certain levels is simply part of that experience. Homesickness, regardless of the student's reasons to study abroad, is a natural experience and can actually contribute to positive coping skills and healthy attachment at less distressing levels. "Those who feel efficacious, feel supported by their families, make host-country friends at school, and feel welcomed, connected, and 'at home' in their new school culture and climate are less likely to experience intense homesickness" (Thurber & Walton, 2012, p. 416), while those who feel inadequate during this process may suffer psychologically and physically (Smith & Khawaja, 2014).

There are many different aspects of the international sojourn that likely influence how well or poorly a student might adjust psychologically to a new culture while maintaining mental health. Lack of preparedness for the changes during the initial phase is a leading contributor to acculturative stress. Particular groups of students and those less prepared for the study abroad experience may be at increased risk for negative effects of acculturative stress (Brown & Aktas, 2011; Yu et al., 2014). In addition, students from countries with many differences from the host country may experience a greater challenge in adjusting to the new culture (Brown & Aktas, 2011; Brown & Brown, 2009). For instance, those from collectivistic cultures may be more sensitive to anxiety and dissatisfaction when studying in a country with an individualistic culture, and those from specific religious backgrounds may struggle to find a comparable community (Sümer, Poyrazli, & Grahame, 2008; Yu et al., 2014).

Research has shown that there is a pattern to the psychological adjustment of international students in the literature: adaptation problems are at their height in the early stages of the transition, the situation improves greatly during the first year, and then there are various outcomes in later stages depending on experiences and actions while dealing with the stress of the transition (Brown & Aktas, 2011; Brown & Holloway, 2008; Mathiesen & Lager, 2007). Of course, there are variations of this patterning, including sometimes experiencing a "honeymoon phase" when first arriving in the country and feeling excited about the new surroundings but not yet exposed to the challenges of living and studying abroad. Lin (2006) describes such a pattern as experiencing culture shock, reaching out to others to ameliorate this shock, and then developing a level of intercultural competence. Brown and Holloway's (2008) qualitative study of international postgraduates showed that the language used to describe the sojourner experience in the initial weeks was highly negative and included terms such as "... scared, frightened, unsure, nervous, anxious, stressed, and uncertain" (Brown & Holloway, 2008, p. 239), while later interviews elicited terms such as "open, open-minded, understand, and tolerant" (p. 242). Several different factors were associated with the intense initial period of stress, such as loneliness, personality factors, preparation, and interaction strategies (Brown & Holloway, 2008). An initial period of stress is not always detrimental to the study abroad experience overall, and a positive experience may result from being able to overcome difficulties.

Students are also faced with the loss of important social supports and familiar culture. The feeling of homesickness, or longing to be close to familiar people and environment and feeling distressed at the thought of or actual separation from home, can overwhelm students during their experience abroad if they do not feel connected to their surroundings (Brown & Holloway, 2008; Hwang et al., 2014; Thurber & Walton, 2012). When international students leave home, their access to established support systems is greatly limited in many cases, allowing for more vulnerability to negative adjustment factors (Charles-Toussaint & Crowson, 2010; Lin, 2006; Smith & Khawaja, 2014). In many cultures, individuals relate to family and friends for their sense of identity and well-being, and these sources may not be immediately present in a new country. The need to belong to a community is an essential part of the human experience, and access to and stability of such a community can be lost in the shuffle of moving abroad.

Challenges with minority status. Discrimination and prejudice are experiences that pose barriers to mental health and contribute to acculturative stress. The transition into a setting in which one is suddenly the minority can be jarring. Being marginalized by prejudice or microaggressions during the adjustment process or throughout the sojourn can lead to negative psychological and physiological reactions and often hinders students from healthy adaptation (Brown & Aktas, 2011; Lin, 2006; Smith & Khawaja, 2014; Yu et al., 2014). The level of difference in culture, especially being seen as more obviously distinct from individuals in the host community by way of skin color, financial status, religion, and dress, can significantly impact the level of culture shock and difficulty an international student may experience (Brown & Aktas, 2011; Lin, 2006). Prejudice and microaggressions can take the form of hostile communication, avoidance, making jokes about culture and norms, and even choosing different group members in class, all of which can contribute to alienation and poor adjustment (Lin, 2006).

The students subjected to prejudice and microaggressions express fear and anger about these situations (Lin, 2006). In addition, political stress between countries can negatively impact an entire group of people or students from particular countries. This variable is so influential that even the threat of being part of a stereotyped group can have negative effects on psychological well-being and academic success (Brown & Aktas, 2011; Charles-Toussaint & Crowson, 2010; Lin, 2006). Continued exposure to stereotype threat and, certainly, to acts of discrimination and prejudice has been closely associated with psychological stress and can exacerbate stressful situations, such as a transition to a new country (Charles-Toussaint & Crowson, 2010; Lin, 2006).

International students have reported less satisfaction and lower levels of acculturation when they perceive discrimination and experience rejection and opportunity deprivation due to prejudice and microaggressions (Lin, 2006; Yu et al., 2014).

Often, international status is not the only minority identity students studying abroad may possess. Differences in economic, political, academic ability and sexuality statuses may also contribute to barriers to trust, respect, and adjustment in a new country (Mathiesen & Lager, 2007). Students with multiple minority statuses are at risk for increased experiences of microaggressions, discrimination, and stress during the transition and throughout the study abroad experience. Needs and experiences also differ based on a student's minority statuses or cultural background (Tidwell & Hanassab, 2007). It is clear that microaggressions and discrimination are a detriment to the study abroad experience and deserve to be addressed in order to prevent the deleterious effects they could have on international students.

Religion and spirituality can be comforting cultural coping mechanisms that may not be as readily available or accepted in a new country. Students sometimes list involvement and connection with spiritual practices as helpful in their ability to persist throughout the experience abroad (Mamiseishvili, 2012). However, differences in religious or spiritual beliefs can contribute to culture shock and stress, which may lead students, despite their beliefs, to desire being perceived as a person from a culture or religion more associated with the host country (Brown & Aktas, 2011). The fact that international students sometimes feel the need to hide their religious beliefs or nationality indicates a systemic issue of the lack of acceptance of those who are actively recruited to other countries. The political environment related to religious issues can also deeply impact students from such backgrounds. For example, global tensions between the "West and Islam" have led to prejudicial action toward Muslim international students or even those presumed to be Muslim (Brown & Aktas, 2011). Religion and spirituality resources on campus could potentially serve as a source of comfort and resiliency among this population, but fear of prejudice may prevent international students from seeking out this valuable resource. It is the responsibility of host universities and staff to understand these global tensions and work to create an environment in which all students are able to engage actively in religious support networks, should they choose.

Basic Principle of Prevention and Its Application to International Students

Caplan (1964) categorized prevention of mental health issues into primary, secondary, and tertiary prevention, and Gordon (1983) categorized it into universal, selective, and indicated prevention. More recently, Romano and Hage (2000) conceptualized prevention with broader perspectives as intervention that "stops a problem behavior from ever occurring"; "delays the onset of a problem behavior"; "reduces the impact of an existing problem behavior"; "strengthens knowledge, attitudes, and behaviors that promote emotional and physical well-being"; and "supports institutional, community, and government policies that promote physical and emotional well-being" (pp. 740–1). Considering that international students in higher education face many more challenges than local students, prevention, in terms of risk reduction and strength promotion in particular, is a relevant and important concept to minimize the distress related to international relocation and to maximize their potential and the experiences of studying abroad. For example, providing knowledge about the educational system in a new culture and extending social support networks could prevent international students from experiencing maladjustment and feeling isolation and could promote academic achievement in the new environment. In sum, the aim of prevention is not only to decrease the incidence, prevalence, and impact of psychological disorders but also to reduce risks and facilitate well-being by promoting individual strengths and improving environments.

International students are known to be a hard-to-reach population on campus. The estimated mental health service utilization rate among international student populations around the world is between 2 and 17 percent (Hori et al., 2012; Hyun et al., 2007; Nilsson et al., 2004; Snider, 2001). A convenient sample study conducted in the United States showed that, among 33 percent of international graduate students who considered utilizing counseling services, only 17 percent actually sought counseling, which is significantly lower than that of domestic students (36 percent; Hyun et al., 2007). Another study conducted in the United States reported that only 2 percent of the institution's international student body sought counseling at the counseling center, which indicates underutilization of the services, and the percentage is lower compared to that of host country ethnic/racial minority students (Nilsson et al., 2004). A study conducted in an Australian university showed that only 17 percent of ethnic Chinese international students sought counseling (Snider, 2001). Finally, a study conducted in a Japanese university reported that the utilization rate of the psychiatric department in the student health center was around 2 percent, which is again significantly lower than that of domestic students (Hori et al., 2012).

Several reasons have been identified for this lower rate of mental health services utilization among international students. First, many of the mental health services available on campus lack considerations for the cultural and language differences of international students (Forbes-Mewett & Nyland, 2008; Mori, 2000). Second, some international students are unaware of the available services due to systemic differences or limited information when they need professional help (Mori, 2000; Sandhu, 1995). For instance, the types, locations, or even concepts of mental health services available on campus in a new country may be different from those in their home country. Third, stigmas are attached to mental health problems in some cultures, and seeking mental health services and disclosing their private issues to those outside of family may conflict with their cultural beliefs (Mori, 2000; Sandhu, 1995). Thus, students may feel afraid of being stigmatized and uncomfortable disclosing about personal issues in a counseling setting. Instead, some students may seek physical health care, as some cultures attribute emotional distress in the form of physical health issues, and physical health care is socially more acceptable. For these reasons, it is hard to expect international students to utilize professional mental health services even when they are faced with academic and/or cultural challenges in addition to developmental challenges unique to young adults.

Emotional distress can cause various psychological and behavioral problems and disorders, and without appropriate interventions, the behavioral problems may worsen. It has been reported that because of underutilization of mental health services, symptoms tend to be severe by the time an international student comes into the health center, and crisis intervention including hospitalization was required in some cases (Hori et al., 2012). The long-term consequences of mental health disorders can be burden to the students, in terms of academic attainment, social life, and vocational options.

Promotion of Wellness for International Students

In many cases, international students are only seen at times when the deleterious effects of the aforementioned various challenges have already begun to have a negative impact. Providing services to these students should not be confined to managing crises as they come up, but effort should be put into prevention strategies to set up international students for success in every way possible. Because of the overrepresentation of severe depression, incidence of microaggressions, underrepresentation among university staff, and limited awareness of appropriate services, international students are an important population to reach before problems develop into crisis (Boone et al., 2011).

Some programs have been developed to promote prevention for this population through preparation, orientation, and connection to appropriate resources. Excellence in Experiential Learning and Leadership (EXCELL), initially developed at University of Canberra and Griffith University in Australia, is a behavioral group approach focused on sociocultural adaptation that has been shown to increase social skills and social self-efficacy on college campuses (Mak, Westwood, Barker, & Ishiyama, 1998). Based on this program, Smith and Khawaja (2014) developed the STAR program at another Australian university. STAR is an acronym for Strengths, Transitions, Adjustment, and Resilience, which consists of cognitive-behaviorally based group meetings focused on developing healthy coping skills and enhancing the adjustment process. In this model, international students modify negative thoughts and learn about positive coping behavior, such as healthy interaction with local people, and develop problem-solving skills (Smith & Khawaja, 2014). The results of this particular trial indicated increased psychological adaptation and coping self-efficacy after participating in the STAR groups (Smith &

Khawaja, 2014). These results indicate that creative, thorough, and thought-out programs can be developed and implemented before crisis to meet the needs of international students.

Smith and Khawaja (2014) offer suggestions for these types of programs, such as including domestic students and experienced international students for modeling and "insider" information. In addition, they stress normalizing challenges, encouraging early help seeking, and addressing barriers to success in the adjustment process. Overall, programs for prevention and early intervention could focus on education about potential stressors during the study abroad experience, region-specific information, and culturally sensitive encouragement to seek support and knowledge about resources.

Before Going Overseas

As discussed earlier, a lack of preparation and anticipated separation from home can significantly impact an international student's mental health before traveling abroad. Thurber and Walton (2012) reported that 70 percent of self-reported homesickness of their sample of international students could be recognized and attended to prior to leaving their home country. Further, Lin's (2006) study of Chinese students coming to the United States found that the stress of the sojourn began for students before their move and continued to increase in the following weeks. In a qualitative study of Turkish students preparing to study abroad, Brown and Aktas (2011) report that students experienced heightened anxiety and fear about their upcoming trip, including worry about loneliness, accommodations, and language difficulty. Stress in the period before traveling can be related to logistical concerns, such as who will pick the student up from the airport, where they might live, and what expenses they should expect, as well as social and academic concerns, such as how to communicate and choose advisors (Brown & Aktas, 2011; Lin, 2006). These results indicate the necessity for prevention to take place predeparture in order to support students, alleviate stress, and help manage uncertainty that arises during this time

Before traveling to the host country and university, prevention efforts can focus on providing culture-specific information, building coping skills, and providing positive perspectives about the upcoming experience in a way that builds confidence before the stress of matriculation (Brown & Aktas, 2011; Thurber & Walton, 2012). Predeparture prevention strategies need not be expensive or complicated, as the advancement of technology has allowed for information and connection to be readily available cross-nationally. For instance, several studies recommend a detailed website and email/phone outreach from host universities to students before coming abroad (Brown & Aktas, 2011; Thurber & Walton, 2012). These websites could contain valuable information about the host country, the university and specific region, and where to find resources upon arrival, as well as forums for discussion and questions. An introduction to the culture, history, geography, and weather of the region in which students will be living should be as thorough as possible (Mathiesen & Lager, 2007). In addition, home universities, in the case of exchange programs, and recruiters could provide information on healthy coping skills and normalizing the difficulties of the experience beforehand (Thurber & Walton, 2012). Brown and Aktas (2011) reported that the students they interviewed found predeparture outreach helpful in easing the stress of the upcoming changes.

Connecting socially before traveling abroad can also boost a student's comfort before moving, knowing that a potential support system is in place (Lin, 2006; Thurber & Walton, 2012). One way to help establish this system is to connect incoming students to those who have already gone through the process. Lin (2006) gives a detailed description of a university's Chinese student organization with a thorough website that allowed incoming Chinese students to feel understood and more comfortable with the study abroad process before and during their travel. This organization, as Lin (2006) states, created a "cultural sanctuary" for students even before leaving their home country and provided helpful information about communication, housing, and the community available to students upon arrival. In return, the host university and potential support systems should inform themselves as much as possible about the political, social, and educational environment of the visiting students (Mathiesen & Lager, 2007). This proactive information-seeking by host universities can help inform culturally sensitive outreach and better prepare those interacting with international students.

After Arriving

As the chapter has discussed thus far, many difficulties and increased stress can await a student in his or her new country, and there are likely to be challenges in adjustment along the way. Upon arrival, students may struggle with how to get to the university from the airport, where to buy groceries, and even where to stay their first night (Lin, 2006; Mathiesen & Lager, 2007). Postarrival, international students are faced with managing their budgets, seeking out transportation, and dealing with language difficulties, along with adjusting to a new academic and cultural environment (Lin, 2006; Smith & Khawaja, 2014). Many times, the onus is put onto international students to "get themselves out" of culture shock, when the responsibility should also be placed on organizations. Most research on international students agrees that providing exemplary support depends on collaboration among different people and agencies (Lin, 2006; Mamiseishvili, 2012; Thurber & Walton, 2012). This includes the students themselves, as well as their family, home university, recruiters, advisors, chaplaincy, and student resources.

Because of patterns in difficulty during the initial adjustment process, it is important to focus on the first year abroad, although various support systems should be in place throughout the time a student is studying abroad (Brown & Aktas, 2011; Mamiseishvili, 2012; Smith & Khawaja, 2014). Orientation programs must be comprehensive, informative, and warm and provide opportunities to connect to the new country, culture, university, and peers. Further, connecting incoming students to campus and community resources, informing students about healthy coping skills, and providing opportunities to celebrate and engage in activities or traditions from their home culture can ease the transition. Promoting active coping strategies, such as language development, getting involved with organizations of interest, and knowing how and when to seek help can equip students with tools they may need during their experience abroad and in the future (Mamiseishvili, 2012; Smith & Khawaja, 2014; Yakunina et al., 2013).

For many challenges that international students might face, Lin (2006) recommends creating a connection with current students from the same country. These students can serve as mentors for new arrivals and help answer questions from the perspective of someone more experienced and familiar with the specific difficulties of students from that country. Students who have been through the matriculation and cross-cultural process can offer specific insight into culture shock and difficulties in the process, as well as healthy coping skills and tips. Domestic students who have traveled abroad may also be able to offer support from a different perspective, as well as connection to people from the host country. In addition, students who are connected with and meet regularly with advisors and study groups show better persistence in studying abroad (Mamiseishvili, 2012). Ideally, these connections could be promoted and set up from the first day a student arrives at his or her host university, so that a support system is there to assist students from the beginning.

Even if excellent orientation programs are in place, students are faced with an overwhelming amount of information, while not yet familiar with what challenges might lie ahead. Because of this, ongoing communication among international students and potential support systems is needed for feedback throughout the study abroad experience to catch issues before they begin or as early as possible (Mathiesen & Lager, 2007; Smith & Khawaja, 2014). With the knowledge of patterns in adjustment issues, as well as individual differences that arise, support networks at universities are responsible for not only orienting students to the new environment, but taking initiative to check in with students throughout the process and remind them of services available to them.

Academic Success Promotion

Building supportive relationships with academic advisors, international student office staff, faculty members, and mentors is important in providing international students with a circle of support to aid them as they pursue their education (Hasan et al., 2008). Having good relationships with these offices and individuals will help international students resolve their academic concerns that occur during their study. Establishing positive relationships with peers and students in their major is also important. Building relationships and friendships includes being proactive in meeting new people and using positive social skills to reach out to other people.

Another strategy is to enhance study skills by enrolling in a formal course or attending workshops offered by counseling centers or other university offices to provide strategies on how to study successfully. Skills that students learn are time management, test anxiety management, note taking, textbook reading and comprehension techniques, and critical thinking. Taking advantage of the university's library resources and writing center can also be useful for writing assignments and research papers. Participating in an informal conversation group can improve language use and confidence in speaking skills. These groups are often facilitated by the international student office or university counseling center or informally arranged by international and domestic peers. Students who are struggling to adapt to the host country language can enroll in language courses, such as English as a Second Language (ESL) courses.

International students often have time restrictions on completing their degree programs and finding employment. It is important to stay on track and in good standing with one's academic degree plan. The best way to be on track is to consult with academic advisors, program mentors, international student office staff, and relevant faculty members on progress each semester. If there are any problems or questions about courses, course assignments, or career opportunities, staff should encourage international students to contact them for support in resolving the issues. Some international students may realize that they want a different major or are uncertain about their degree of study. If these issues occur, students may reach out to university career centers or counseling centers where staff can help students resolve these concerns. Faculty members are also good resources for career specific development advice. University staff can encourage international students to be proactive in contacting faculty members and asking for help about these concerns.

Finally, career counseling can aid students in making career decisions such as changing majors and negotiating career decisions between them and their advisors as well as family members (Arthur, 2004; Bikos & Furry, 1999; Hasan et al., 2008; Yang, Wong, Hwang, & Heppner, 2002). Bikos and Furry (1999) found that job search clubs can influence international student's career self-efficacy, career decision making, and help to consolidate vocational identity. Job clubs can also increase practical skills, such as creating a resume and curriculum vita, writing cover letters for internships and externships, acquiring knowledge of specific job-related skills, and demonstrating professional behavior in the workplace.

Cultural Understanding and Adjustment Promotion

A major goal of prevention is to promote wellness and decrease instances of negative effects of certain experiences. For instance, experiences of perceived prejudice in a host country interfere with healthy adjustment (Duru & Poyrazil, 2011). Moreover, lower levels of acculturation and greater levels of perfectionism are related to increased level of stress (Nilsson, Butler, Shouse, & Joshi, 2008). These studies imply that environmental factors can influence one's adjustment, which in turn affects one's health among international students; therefore, facilitating cultural understandings of home and host country and promoting healthy cultural adjustment are integral to international students' academic, cultural, and social life in a host country.

Equipping international students with relevant information may be beneficial in promoting cross-cultural understandings. Making use of newly arrived student orientation is one way of promoting such information (Olivas & Li, 2006). Cultural values and expectations around educational and sociocultural scenes of a host country can be explained in an arrival orientation. Also, outreach programs by advanced students on common reactions to new language and culture and expected challenges may equip new students with information on the possible difficulties they may encounter in the near future (Nilsson et al., 2004). Mentoring or peer support programs have been shown to facilitate international students' adjustment (Matsumura & Abe, 2011). For example, a mentor program in which Japanese college students were coupled with newly arrived international students and provided informational support in addition to companion support helped international students adjust to the new social life and culture and provided them emotional security (Matsumura & Abe, 2011).

Another way of promoting cultural adjustment may be training international students on certain skills and competence. Chen (1999) suggested enhancing cultural skills and competence of international students using a social learning approach. Though Chen (1999) has originally developed the idea of helping clients understand certain cultural behaviors and practicing cultural skills in a therapy context, it can be adapted to a group or educational context where international students and domestic students discuss cultural implications of values and enhance reciprocal cultural understandings and multicultural competence. Differences in communications and behavioral expectations across cultures can potentially affect development and maintenance of relationships with classmates, faculty, and other individuals (Hwang et al., 2014). Multicultural Mental Wellness Workshop, a series of psychoeducational workshops on acculturation, cross-cultural communication, and other academic-related issues targeted at international students and domestic students implemented at University of Tsukuba in Japan, was shown to facilitate awareness of their cultural adjustment and competence among international student participants and cross-cultural awareness among domestic student participants (Shimada & Suzuki, 2014).

Behavioral Health Promotion

One major factor that has been consistently shown to contribute to psychological well-being is social support, as people thrive in environments where they are surrounded by a system that works well with and supports them. Social support appears to be essential in such potentially stressful situations as studying internationally. The sense of not belonging or being fundamentally different from the majority culture has been identified by some international populations as the most stressful part of transitioning to life in a new country (Charles-Toussaint & Crowson, 2010; Yu et al., 2014). The absence of support can increase the stress an international students is already experiencing (Kashima & Loh, 2006; Smith & Khawaja, 2014; Sümer, Poyrazli, & Grahame, 2008). The creation of social groups in the new country can help reestablish the sense of belonging that may have been lost in the transition and aid in the students' personal growth. A study by Brown and Holloway (2008) showed that the feeling of homesickness is likely mediated by creating friendship networks. The importance of interconnectedness among many international populations indicates that both intergroup and within-group socialization may make international students more at ease and better able to adapt to life in a new country (Brown & Aktas, 2011; Lin, 2006; Smith & Khawaja, 2014; Thurber & Walton, 2012). Brown and Aktas (2011) and Smith and Khawaja (2014) emphasize the variety of benefits from different social interactions: emotional support and shared history from students from the same region, cultural and language engagement from interacting with people from the host country, and the shared cross-cultural experience from other international populations. The Lin (2006) study on the aid of a Chinese student organization showed that this aid ultimately had a positive impact on the adjustment of incoming students, helping them feel understood and comfortable.

Support may come from various avenues, such as family, peer groups, mentors, and even larger social institutions. While students likely have a support system built up in their home country, this is suddenly missing, and international students may not have close support in place at a new university. People studying internationally tend to create a more familiar and personal co-ethnic group in the new country to provide a sense of belongingness and certainty (Brown & Holloway, 2008; Lin, 2006). Creating this type of community could supply a more acceptable replacement for close family social support while living away from their home country. In addition, the Internet and technology have created new opportunities for international students to keep in contact with their original (e.g., home country) support system, which may be extremely important in the early stages (Mathiesen & Lager, 2007). Not only does participating in a co-national community facilitate international students' adjustment to their life in a new country, but it also eases the transition of reentering their country of origin. However, research has also shown that exclusive co-national groups and too much contact with friends and family back home via the Internet may delay adjustment because of isolation and limiting time spent practicing interaction with host country nationals (Brown & Holloway, 2008; Lee, Lee, & Jang, 2011). One potential difficulty involved with exclusively interacting with those from the same background is limited familiarity with a new language, which as discussed previously can have a negative impact on adjustment.

Interaction with students from the host country has been shown to be another important contribution to healthy psychological adjustment of international students (Smith & Khawaja, 2014; Yan et al., 2014). Fostering positive interactions between two cultures can result in decreased prejudice and increased understanding and empathy on the part of the "in-group" and reduced anxiety and depression among members of the "out-group" (Charles-Toussaint & Crowson, 2010; Mori, 2000). In this way, both cultures have the opportunity to get the most out of international exchanges. Cross-cultural peer education has been shown to be valuable for language practice, cultural competence, and health promotion for international students (Yan et al., 2014). It seems that both inter- and intracultural friendship networks can offer a buffer for negative experiences and aid in healthy psychological adjustment for the sojourner. Staying with local families, or "homestays," can also be helpful in providing connections to and education about the host country. In well-regulated and successful homestays, international students are able to learn and practice the language, learn about host country culture, and benefit from the support of a family (Campbell, 2004; Richardson, 2003). However, students may experience stress, disappointment, and helplessness in families that are less warm and willing to really work with the student toward communication and cultural learning (Campbell, 2004). Often, this can occur when there are not clear guidelines or regulations for host families and/or lack of preparation for international students (Campbell, 2004; Richardson, 2003). More preparation, clarity, and regulations may allow homestay experiences to be more in line with the goals of such programs.

Another asset for prevention of problems for international students is having elements in place to help international students recognize their personal and cultural strengths as they relate to cross-cultural adjustment. For instance, academic, career, and mental health counselors could ask international students to reflect on the personal and multicultural strengths that they bring to the cross-cultural journey. Counselors could then help international students identify ways to use these strengths to reduce their acculturative stress and achieve optimal adjustment by promoting cultural heritage (Lin, 2006; Olivas & Li, 2006; Yakunina et al., 2013). While emphasizing multicultural strengths is important, understanding the finite nature of the study abroad experience can at times be helpful in accepting certain challenges and retaining a sense of one's own culture throughout the experience.

There is a clear need for comprehensive and empathetic research, counseling, and services, as well as outreach and awareness programs, available to international students before and during their stay, as well as through the reentry process. Research has shown time and again that utilization of counseling services is low for international students, and these students typically come in crisis (Boone et al., 2011; Hwang et al., 2014; Mori, 2000). This can be a vulnerable population; therefore, accessible, clear, and culturally competent counseling is necessary, as well as creative models for reaching students who are not coming in for help.

One possibility to decrease stigma and reach international students is for counseling centers to partner with resources and locations that this population might be more likely to access when distressed, such as advising offices, the international student office, and the health center (Boone et al., 2011; Hwang et al., 2014; Olivas & Li, 2006). This practice can decrease fear of being seen engaging in counseling and provides an accessible first interaction to demystify psychological services. In addition, culturally sensitive and flexible treatment should be offered to work with students who may not understand or work well with the traditional, regularly attended talk therapy model. Boone et al. (2011) offer suggestions based on the success of their Let's Talk program, initially implemented at Cornell University in New York (U.S.) and now at other universities throughout the United States, which provides walk-in support on an as-needed basis in alternate locations for college students. Boone et al (2011) emphasize the need for flexibility in terms of time, location, and length of sessions, as well as focusing on problem solving, connecting to resources, and advocacy in order to reach international students and meet the needs of this population. As globalization and recruitment of international students inevitably continues, universities can focus on prevention, flexibility, and early intervention in order to decrease crises and increase the academic and cultural goal of cross-cultural exchanges.

Reentry into the Country of Origin

Returning to the international student's home country after studying abroad and readjusting to their home culture can be challenging. The process of reentry and reverse culture shock is often addressed as more difficult than the original culture shock because international students may expect the relocation back home to be easier than initially moving abroad, assume that things have not changed since they left, and be taken by surprise (Young, 2014). When international students return home, they may experience grief for loss of their friends and experiences abroad, feel isolated and lonely, and face negative reactions from members of their home culture (Butcher, 2002; Young, 2014). They may have to reconstruct their worldview and lifestyles acquired while living abroad and may not be able to share their international and cross-cultural experiences in meaningful ways (Butcher, 2002). Moreover, the returning students may have changes in their cultural identity and communication styles, and people surrounding them may not be ready to accept these changes and their difficulties with reentry processes (Arthur, 2003). Although much of the previous literature focuses on the challenges of reentry, a study conducted by Kartoshkina (2015) found that reentry experiences for many were "bitter-sweet," in that students who studied abroad had both negative feelings, such as loss and frustration, as well as positive feelings, such as excitement and comfort.

The process of reentry begins when international students start preparing to leave the host country and continues after they return to their home country (Arthur, 2003). The severity of reentry shock depends on the length of stay in the host country and the degree of acculturation to the host culture, as well as the student's ability to keep home country traditions, language, and community intact, thus helping international students be better able to readjust upon return to their home country (Brown & Brown, 2009). Although educational institutions provide orientations upon arrival about what to expect in the new country, they rarely provide reentry orientations prior to returning to their home country. If offered, reentry sessions can prepare students for the demands of reentry shock and reverse culture shock. Young (2014) recommends that universities "help students understand and expect that returning home will involve an adjustment process similar to the one they experienced when first arriving abroad" (p. 62). One way to assist international students to prepare is to offer perspectives in which reentry shock should be taken as a positive challenge and an opportunity for personal growth and to remind them that they have overcome difficulties adjusting to the host culture and already have skill sets to manage culture shock (Young, 2014). In the case of students returning to their own university from an exchange program, Young (2014) provides some ideas for home universities, such as "Welcome Back Letter," "Faculty/Staff Dinners," and "Reentry Courses" (pp. 64–5), among others.

Prevention on Systemic Levels

In addition to providing preventive interventions to individuals studying overseas, promoting preventive intervention on systemic levels is equally critical. Conyne (1983) talks about "positive modification of those environmental conditions that have been shown to contribute negatively to the disorder in question" (p. 332) and "indirectly ensuring a greater degree of safety for the population at risk by removing or eliminating noxious environmental conditions" (p. 332) as some of the aims of primary prevention. Furthermore, Romano and Hage (2000) and the Guidelines for Prevention in Psychology (APA, 2014) underline the importance of prevention at the environmental level to promote systemic and institutional change and to foster well-being. Some of the challenges international students often face are rooted in universities, educational systems, and societies; thus, it is crucial to reduce the environmental factors that fuel international student challenges. Low tolerance and prejudice toward the differences in skin color, accent, visa status, religion, and other cultural aspects of an individual on campus need to be reversed. The professionals serving international students need to be not only aware of the systemic issues but also proactive about advocating for the students.

Creating a multicultural, accepting campus environment and intercultural communication and understanding is another key aspect that educational institutes that host international students need to consider (Lin, 2006; Mori, 2000; Yakunina et al., 2013). Intercultural understanding is often cited as helpful for all parties in the study abroad experience. Counselors, advisors, and other support systems in the host country need to be flexible with cultural differences and coping needs, and international students need to be open to diversity and be prepared properly for the specific culture in which they will be immersed (Boone et al., 2011; Brown & Aktas, 2011; Mathiesen & Lager, 2007). International students and host universities should be informed about global and political situations that might impact cultural exchange on campus. Striving for a place of mutual understanding and putting forth effort to consider different cultural approaches to coping can only benefit those involved.

It has been reported that conducting case conferences and creating conduct guidelines are effective for developing awareness of staff and faculty members to provide emotional and instrumental support proactively for international students and to relate continuously with international students (Moriya et al., 2012). Also, education about mental health issues among international student populations should be directed toward the whole campus and students leaders, in addition to faculty and staff members directly working with international students (Hyun et al., 2007). Because staff and faculty members as well as other students cast influences on international students' well-being, implementing preventive interventions on the systemic level, in addition to the international student populations, is an important way to prevent various issues that international students encounter at higher educational institutions.

Conclusions

International students are confronted with particular challenges in adjusting to life in a new country. Along with the difficulties of living abroad, international students are also required to manage academic pressures, new school systems, relationships with authority figures, financial difficulty, and studying material in a foreign language. Moreover, they may face culture shock, acculturation, loss and reconstruction of support systems, and discrimination and prejudice. It is particularly important to deliver services in forms that international students feel comfortable utilizing, especially for those whose cultural norms discourage them from using mental health services. Providing ample opportunities that target a population, rather than an individual, and making those opportunities nonthreatening would be beneficial.

Much of the currently available literature on international students' challenges and preventive efforts for this particular population is based on the international student populations in English-speaking countries (e.g., the United States, Australia, and Canada) where individualistic values are prevalent. It is important to keep in mind that the international students' experiences in collectivistic countries or non-English speaking countries may be somewhat different. In a study that compared factors relating to acculturation between individualistic students studying in collectivistic countries and collectivistic students studying in individualistic countries, it was revealed that learning social norms and values were related to acculturation among those in collectivistic countries while personality was associated with acculturation among those in individualistic countries (Jang & Kim, 2010). This implies that not only the cultural backgrounds of international students and the cultural climate of host countries but also the interaction of the two must be taken into consideration when international students' adjustment and wellness are discussed.

Nonetheless, it is evident that preventive interventions for international students in higher educational institutes are crucial to preclude unnecessary challenges, promote wellness, and facilitate positive study abroad experiences as the number of international students remains large in educational systems around the globe. Since the journey of international students starts before going abroad, preparation to ease the burden of initial adjustment in a new country should begin while they are still in their home country. Thereafter, prevention effort should be delivered continuously to meet the needs of international students throughout their stay, though more rigorous effort may be preferable during the early stages of the transition to studying abroad and reentry, which tend to be more intense periods of stress. Moreover, working with domestic students, staffs, and faculty members on campus is pivotal to reduce the negative environmental influences on international students that may otherwise hinder their adjustment to a new country as well as to facilitate multicultural competence of the educational institutes and communities. While some stress is useful and can ultimately be beneficial in this process, prevention of undue and harmful stress is important for retention and the creation of a meaningful experience and supportive community. International students are cultural carriers and can potentially bridge different cultures and values around the world. Thus, serving this particular hard-to-reach population with preventive perspectives and advocating the often marginalized population on campus will not only aid the international students' academic achievement and psychological well-being but also assist the advancement of globalization around the world.

References

APA (American Psychological Association) (2014). Guidelines for prevention in psychology. *American Psychologist* 69(3): 285–96.

Arthur, N. (2003). Preparing international students for the re-entry transition. *Canadian Journal of Counselling* 37(3): 173–85.

Arthur, N. (2004). *Counseling International Students: Clients from around the World.* New York: Kluwer Academic/Plenum.

Bikos, L. H., & Furry, T. S. (1999). The job search club for international students: an evaluation. *Career Development Quarterly* 48: 31–48.

Boone, M.S., Edwards, G.R., Haltom, M., Hill, J.S., Liang, Y., Mier, S., & Yau, T.Y. (2011). Let's talk: getting out of the counseling center to serve hard-to-reach students. *Journal of Multicultural Counseling and Development* 39: 194–205.

Brown, L., & Aktas, G. (2011). Fear of the unknown: a pre-departure qualitative study of Turkish international students. *British Journal of Guidance & Counseling* 39 (4): 339–55. doi: 10.1080/03069885.2011.576314

Brown, L., & Brown, J. (2009). Out of chaos, into a new identity: the transformative power of the international sojourn. *Existential Analysis* 20(2): 341–61.

Brown, L., & Holloway, I. (2008). The adjustment journey of international postgraduate students at an English university: an ethnographic study. *Journal of Research in International Education* 7(2): 232–49. doi: 10.1177/1475240908091306

Butcher, A. (2002). A grief observed: grief experiences of East Asian international students returning to their countries of origin. *Journal of Studies in International Education* 6(4): 354–68.

Campbell, N. (2004). Home(stay) is where the heart(ache) is: a study of Chinese international students living with local families in New Zealand. Paper presented at the Australian & New Zealand Communication Association Annual Conference, Sydney, Australia.

Caplan, G. (1964). *Principle of Preventative Psychiatry*. New York: Basic Books.

Charles-Toussaint, G.C., & Crowson, H.M. (2010). Prejudice against international students: the role of threat perceptions and authoritarian dispositions in U.S. students. *Journal of Psychology* 144(5): 413–28. doi: 10.1080/00223980.2010.496643

Chen, C. P. (1999). Common stressors among international college students: research and counseling implications. *Journal of College Counseling* 2: 49–65.

Conyne, R. K. (1983). Two critical issues in primary prevention: what it is and how to do it. *Personnel and Guidance Journal* 61(6): 331–4.

Duru, E., & Poyrazli, S. (2011). Perceived discrimination, social connectedness, and other predictors of adjustment difficulties among Turkish international students. *International Journal of Psychology* 46(6): 446–54.

Forbes-Mewett, H., & Nyland, C. (2008). Cultural diversity, relocation, and the scurity of international students at an internationalised university. *Journal of Studies in International Education* 12(2): 181–203.

Gordon, R. (1983). An operational classification of disease prevention. *Public Health Reports* 8: 107–9.

Hasan, N. T., Fouad, N. A., & Williams-Nickelson, C. (2008). *Studying Psychology in the United States: Expert Guidance for International Students*. Washington, DC: American Psychological Association.

Hori, T., Tachikawa, H., Ishii, T., Shimada, N., Takemori, T., Lebowitz, A., & Asada, T. (2012). An analysis of mental disorders of international students visiting the mental health services at Tsukuba University Health Center. *Psychiatria et Neurologia Japonica* 114(1): 3–12.

Hwang, B.J., Bennett, R., & Beauchemin, J. (2014). International students' utilization of counseling services. *College Student Journal* 48(3): 347–54.

Hyun, J., Quinn, B., Madon, T., & Lustig, S. (2007). Mental health need, awareness, and use of counseling services among international graduate students. *Journal of American College Health* 56(2): 109–18.

IIE (Institute of International Education) (2014). Open doors data: international students. www.iie.org/Research-and-Publications/Open-Doors/Data/International-Students

Jang, D., & Kim, D. -Y. (2010). The influence of host cultures on the role of personality in the acculturation of exchange students. *International Journal of Intercultural Relations* 34: 363–7.

Kartoshkina, Y. (2015). Bitter-sweet reentry after studying abroad. *International Journal of Intercultural Relations* 44: 35–45.

Kashima, E. S., & Loh, E. (2006). International students' acculturation: effects of international, conational, and local ties and need for closure. *International Journal of Intercultural Relations* 30: 471–85.

Kim, E. (2012). An alternative theoretical model: examining psychological identity development of international students in the United States. *College Student Journal* 46(1): 99–113.

Komiya, N., & Eells, G. T. (2001). Predictors of attitudes toward seeking counseling among international students. *Journal of College Counseling* 4: 153–60.

Lee, E. J., Lee, L., & Jang, J. (2011). Internet for the internationals: effects of Internet use motivations on international students' college adjustment. *Cyberpsychology, Behavior, and Social Networking* 14(7–8): 433–7. doi: 10.1089/cyber.2010.0406

Lee, J. Y., & Rice, C. (2007). Welcome to America? International student perceptions of discrimination. *Higher Education* 53: 381–409.

Lin, C. (2006). Culture shock and social support: an investigation of a Chinese student organization on a US campus. *Journal of Intercultural Communication Research* 35(2): 117–36. doi: 10.1080/17475750600909279

Lin, J-C. G. (2000). College counseling and international students. In Davis, D. C., & Humphrey, K. M. (eds.), *College Counseling: Issues and Strategies for a New Millennium*. Alexandria, VA: American Counseling Association, pp. 169–83.

Mak, A. S., Westwood, M. J., Barker, M. C., & Ishiyama, F. I. (1998). The Excel Program for developing international students' sociocultural competencies. *Journal of International Education* 9(1): 33–8.

Mamiseishvili, K. (2012). International student persistence in U.S. postsecondary institutions. *Higher Education* 64, 1–17. doi: 10.1007/s10734-011–9477-0

Mathiesen, S. G., & Lager, P. (2007). A model for developing international student exchanges. *Social Work Education* 26(3): 280–91. doi: 10.1080/02615470601049867

Matsumura, A., & Abe, Y. (2011). Supporting international students with the mentor program. *Student Counseling Journal [Gakusei Soudan kenkyu]* 31: 195–206.

McLachlan, D. A., & Justice, J. (2009). A grounded theory of international student well-being. *Journal of Theory Construction and Testing* 13(1): 27–32.

Mori, S. (2000). Addressing the mental health concerns of international students. *Journal of Counseling and Development* 78(2): 137–44.

Moriya, T., Ozeki, F., Sakata, R., Tanaka, A., Fukuike, A., & Kodaka, Y. (2012). The conduct guidelines and staff development in the support system for international students. *Waseda Nihongo Kyouiku Jissen Kenkyu[Waseda Practical Studies in Japanese Language Education]* 00(1): 39–54.

Nilsson, J. E., Berkel, L. V. A., Flores, L. Y., & Lucus, M. S. (2004). Utilization rate and presenting concerns of international students at a university counseling center: implications for outreach programming. *Journal of College Student Psychotherapy* 19(2): 49–59.

Nilsson, J. E., Butler, J., Shouse, S., & Joshi, C. (2008). The relationship among perfectionism, acculturation, and stress in Asian international students. *Journal of College Counseling* 11: 147–58.

OECD (Organization for Economic and Co-operation and Development) (2014). Education at a glance 2014: OECD indicators. dx.doi.org/10.1787/eag-2014-en

Olivas, M., & Li, C.S. (2006). Understanding stressors of international students in higher education: what college counselors and personnel need to know. *Journal of Instructional Psychology* 33(3): 217–22.

Romano, J. J., & Hage, S. M. (2000). Prevention and counseling psychology: revitalizing commitments for the 21st century. *Counseling Psychologist* 28(6): 733–63.

Popadiuk, N., & Arthur, N. (2004). Counseling international students in Canadian countries. *International Journal for the Advancement of Counselling* 26(2): 125–45.

Richardson, K. (2003). International education: the quality of homestay services. Paper presented at the 17th IDP Australian International Education Conference, Melbourne, Australia.

Sam, D. (2001). Satisfaction with life among international students: an exploratory study. *Social Indicators Research* 53: 315–37.

Sandhu, D. S. (1995). An examination of the psychological needs of the international students: implications for counseling and psychotherapy. *International Journal for the Advancement of Counselling* 17: 229–39.

Shimada, N., & Suzuki, H. (2014). Development and Implementation of a Multicultural Mental Wellness Psychoeducational Program: to promote the globalization of college environment. *Journal of Japanese Language Teaching [Nihongo Kyoiku Ronshu]* 29: 221–31.

Smith, R. A., & Khawaja, N. G. (2014). A group psychological intervention to enhance the coping and acculturation of international students. *Advances in Mental Health* 12(2): 110–24.

Snider, P. D. (2001). Counselling for international students in Western universities: a cross-cultural examination of counselling expectations and services. *International Education Journal* 2(5): 61–85.

Sümer, S., Poyrazli, S., & Grahame, K. (2008). Predictors of depression and anxiety among international students. *Journal of Counseling and Development* 86: 429–37.

Thurber, C. A., & Walton, E. A. (2012). Homesickness and adjustment in university students. *Journal of American College Health* 60(5): 415–19.

Tidwell, R., & Hanassab, S. (2007). New challenges for professional counselors: the higher education international student population. *Counseling Psychology Quarterly* 20(4): 313–24.

Ward, C., & Searle, W. (1991). The impact of value discrepancies and cultural identity on psychological and sociocultural adjustment of sojourners. *International Journal of Intercultural Relation* 15: 209–25.

World Education Services (2010). International student migration fact sheet. www.wes.org/ca/events/factsheet.pdf

Yakunina, E. S., Weigold, I. K., Weigold, A., Hercegovac, S., & Elsayed, N. (2013). International students' personal and multicultural strengths: reducing acculturative stress and promoting adjustment. *Journal of Counseling & Development* 91: 216–23. doi: 10.1002/j.1556-6676.2013.00088.x

Yan, Z., Finn, K., Cardinal, B. J., & Bent, L. (2014). Promoting health behaviors using peer education: a demonstration project between international and American college students. *American Journal of Health Education* 45: 288–96. doi: 10.1080/19325037.2014.932727

Yang, E., Wong, S. C., Hwang, M-H., & Heppner, M. J. (2002). Widening our global view: the development of career counseling services for international students. *Journal of Career Development* 28(3): 203–13.

Young, G. E. (2014). Reentry: supporting students in the final stage of study abroad. *New Directions for Student Services* 146: 59–67.

Yu, B., Chen, X., Li, S., Liu, Y., Jacques-Tiura, A. J., & Yan, H. (2014). Acculturative stress and influential factors among international students in China: a structural dynamic perspective. *PLOS ONE* 9(4): e96322. doi: 10.1382/journal.pone.0096322

18 Prevention of Adolescent Risk Behavior and Promotion of Positive Youth Development

A Beneficial Action Approach

John W. Toumbourou

Introduction

The chapter that follows defines adolescent risk behavior and the major health and social problems that arise as a consequence. The modifiable causes of adolescent risk behavior are described and prevention science approaches are outlined that are being increasingly applied to effectively prevent adolescent risk-behavior problems and encourage positive youth development. The chapter focuses on work completed by my research team in Australia, but also examines the relevance of this work within the broader international context.

In this chapter, I outline *beneficial action theory* to describe how positive youth development approaches can maximize their potential to prevent adolescent risk behavior. Beneficial action theory (Toumbourou, in press) is premised on evidence that healthy adolescent development leads to social trust and altruism (O'Connor et al., 2011a, 2014). Beneficial action theory argues that global adolescent health issues such as international inequality and the development of adolescent risk-behavior can be reduced in the coming years by increasing investment in effective positive youth development programs that also increase active youth involvement in the dissemination of effective prevention science programs. Through these means, beneficial action theory argues that it will be possible in the coming decades to encourage a greater number of adolescents to experience altruistic motivation to engage in effective actions to achieve prevention science outcomes that will result in a generational leap forward in healthy adolescent development across the world.

The Development of Adolescent Risk Behavior

Adolescence is a period of life that the World Health Organization (WHO) identifies as extending from puberty (at around age ten) to the end of the secondary school age period (around age nineteen) (Sawyer et al., 2012). With advances in science and technology, expectations have increased for young people to complete longer periods of education before they enter employment. These changes mean that increasing numbers of young people in Western societies do not achieve economic independence until the mid- to late twenties, extending the period youth spend in the adolescent context. Adolescence has in modern economies come to represent a unique culture and market that is aligned with risk behaviors such as hedonistic alcohol and drug use, unsafe sex, and health-compromising behaviors (Toumbourou, Olsson, Rowland, Renati, & Hallam, 2014).

Risk taking is defined as behavior that increases the probability of death, injury, and adverse health and social consequences (Tollit, Hemphill, & Toumbourou, 2016). In adolescence, examples of risk behavior include violence; antisocial behavior; dangerous recreational and occupational pursuits; self-harm; unsafe sex; health-compromising behavior; gambling; and substance abuse. Engaging in risk-taking behavior poses direct and indirect threats to the health, well-being, and safety of individuals and to the wider society.

Adolescence is a time when risk behavior emerges more prominently. During adolescence, physical maturity can lead to new potentiality to exert power, and, in the developed nations, young people enter a new sphere of social freedoms that require effective decision making. Due partly to both inexperience in decision making and neurological immaturity, adolescents can have unrealistic appraisal of risks and consequences during these years (Tollit et al., 2016). While risk behavior can result in harm, taking risks during adolescence and experiencing consequences is also important in learning to develop a more realistic understanding of acceptable limits of behavior and responsible decision making (Toumbourou et al., 2014).

Risk behaviors are interrelated during adolescence such that some individuals are known to engage in multiple forms of these behaviors (Tollit et al., 2016). The term "Problem Behavior Syndrome" was coined to describe the phenomena of different types of risk-behavior problems clustering in some individuals and groups (Donovan, Jessor, & Costa, 1988).

Risk-behavior problems in adolescents can lead to public health problems within populations as adolescents grow older. Because of population growth in the developing nations, adolescents (ten to nineteen) and young adults (twenty to twenty-four) now represent 24 percent of the world population and will continue to represent a disproportionate component in future decades (Sawyer et al., 2012). In the international context, adolescent health intervention is recognized as critical due to the potential to prevent the current trend for large international adolescent populations to take up lifestyle risk behaviors, such as tobacco and alcohol use and physical inactivity, that will have challenging future population health consequences across the world (Patton et al., 2012). Moreover, health intervention among adolescents is also argued to be critically important due to the potential for sexual behavior intervention and early family assistance to reduce the transfer of health and social problems to future generations (Catalano et al., 2012).

While a range of adolescent risk behaviors exist, some will have greater consequences for the future than others. The Youth Risk-Behavior Surveillance System (YRBSS[1]) monitors six types of health risk behaviors that contribute to the

1 www.cdc.gov/healthyyouth/yrbs.

leading causes of death and disability among youth and adults (Lowry, Eaton, Brener & Kann, 2011). These include behaviors that contribute to unintentional injuries and violence; sexual behaviors that contribute to unintended pregnancy and sexually transmitted diseases, including HIV infection; alcohol and other drug use; tobacco use; unhealthy dietary behaviors; and inadequate physical activity. The present chapter focuses on the potential to prevent these six YRBSS-monitored health risk behavior problems through interventions in adolescence.

The Prevention Science Approach

The field of prevention science synthesizes life course development research, community epidemiology, the evaluation of preventive intervention trials and service systems to develop recommendations to reduce health and social problems and encourage positive human development (Catalano et al., 2012). Prevention science approaches aim to direct evidence-based investment to modify the early developmental pathways and influences that lead to adolescent health and behavior problems (Catalano et al., 2012).

Defining Prevention

Prevention refers to strategies or programs that avert or delay the onset or severity of health, mental health, or social problems. Prevention responses can be classified as universal, where they apply to an entire population; selective, where they target groups with elevated risk; and indicative, where they target individuals already showing signs or symptoms of problems. This conceptualization of prevention addresses the etiological progression from risk factor to health problems within populations (National Research Council and Institute of Medicine, 2009).

As applied to the current context, prevention encompasses goals not just for reducing risk behavior but also for reducing underlying determinants or influences. For example, tobacco, alcohol, and drug policies typically include a broad set of goals. Their objective is not just to reduce demand for hazardous alcohol and drug use but also to reduce the supply of alcohol and drugs and to reshape the contexts where use results in harm (Toumbourou et al., 2014). Prevention approaches are attractive from an economic perspective, offering the potential to reduce problems that can otherwise overburden health and social systems.

A Systems Approach to Prevention

Prevention approaches targeting children and youth are often integrated within broader health and social system efforts to improve the health of the population (National Research Council and Institute of Medicine, 2009). A systems approach to prevention acknowledges the range of political and economic mechanisms operating at global, national, state, and community levels that can interact to influence adolescent health (Toumbourou et al., 2014).

Recognition of the importance of an integrated strategy for improving adolescent health has led to an increasing awareness of the need for developmentally focused intervention policies and programs within health and social systems (National Research Council and Institute of Medicine, 2009). Prevention can be used to deliver services and programs to reduce the incidence of health and social problems later in life, but to enable this possibility systems for monitoring healthy child and adolescent development are required. Examples of adolescent health monitoring systems include the YRBSS (Lowry et al., 2011) and the Communities That Care youth survey (Jonkman, Steketee, Toumbourou, Cini, & Williams, 2014). The Communities That Care youth survey measures the six adolescent risk behaviors in the YRBSS but additionally also measures a range of the modifiable factors that influence the development of risk behaviors, such as availability of tobacco, alcohol, and drugs; family conflict; low school commitment; and interactions with antisocial peers (Baheiraei et al., 2014).

Positive Youth Development

With growing prevention science understanding of adolescent development, options for encouraging positive health and social outcomes are increasingly being explored. Positive youth development refers in broad scope to childhood and adolescent development experiences that provide optimal life preparation for the attainment of human potential and well-being (Catalano, Toumbourou & Hawkins, 2014). Positive youth development identifies the characteristics of optimal development in areas such as connection, character, competence, confidence, and caring (Lerner, Almerigi, Thoeoksa & Lerner, 2005).

One of the first empirically tested models of positive youth development has emerged from the analysis of social and psychological adjustment within a large Australian longitudinal study (Hawkins et al., 2012). Data modeling yielded a measure of positive youth development that identified individual strengths that contribute to collective social capital, including civic action and altruistic engagement, such as volunteering, and trust and tolerance of others and organizations. These characteristics were found to associate with social competence and life satisfaction. Based on this measure Australian youth with high positive development at age nineteen were found at age twenty-three to have higher levels of emotional health, physical well-being, and friendship quality; reduced antisocial behavior; and higher positive development (Hawkins et al., 2012).

The identification of a measure of positive youth development has enabled investigations of the associations between positive development and risk behavior in the Australian context. Although there was not a complete division, most of those scoring high on positive youth development tended to have low levels of harmful risk behavior and mental health problems (O'Connor et al., 2011b). In examining the stability of positive development from age nineteen to twenty-three years, Hawkins et al. (2011) found that 35 percent of Australian young adults experience stable and high levels of positive development, while 12 percent were at consistent low levels and experienced considerable risk behavior and mental health problems. An important finding was that the majority (53 percent) of Australian young adults do not have harmful risk behavior but do not experience optimal levels of positive youth development over time (Hawkins et al., 2011). These findings suggest that there are two important goals in future youth development efforts: reducing harmful risk behavior and increasing positive youth development (including volunteering and social trust). Beneficial action theory outlined in later sections of the present chapter is a developmental theory that argues for the integration of these two goals within intervention responses.

The studies in positive youth development outlined in the preceding suggest a higher state of youth development can emerge where there is increased civic engagement volunteering and social trust (Hawkins et al., 2011). These findings suggest that positive youth development may lead to stronger altruistic motivation (Lerner, Almerigi, Thoeoksa, & Lerner, 2005).

The suggestion that when children and adolescents experience healthy social development they emerge into young adulthood with high levels of altruistic motivation (O'Connor et al., 2011a) is congruent with research identifying a strong social motivational and biological basis for altruism in human nature. Altruism is commonly defined as the motivation to engage in behavior that benefits others without regard to self-interest. In more formal terms, altruism is conceptualized as voluntary behavior enacted to benefit another and motivated by intrinsic values related to concerns for others, as opposed to hedonistic efforts to maximize personal rewards and minimize discomfort (Eisenberg & Mussen, 1989).

Although the egoistic traditions in philosophy and the social sciences have long refuted the existence of altruism, social psychological and cognitive neuroscience studies have provided more convincing evidence suggesting altruistic motivation exists and is quite widespread. Studies within the social psychology laboratory paradigm have shown that in experimental conditions that encourage feelings of empathy, participants provide assistance regardless of whether their actions are anonymous and increase their own discomfort (Batson, 2011). Neuroscience findings suggest that altruism is hard-wired within brain pathways associated with healthy social information processing and attachment. Thus, functional magnetic resonance imaging (fMRI) reveals that decisions to provide charitable donations trigger brain circuit activity typically associated with social attachment and bonding (Moll et al., 2006). Twin studies also suggest that altruism has a small to moderate genetically inherited component of between 20 percent (Cesarini, Dawes, Johannesson, Lichtenstein & Wallace, 2009) and 50 percent (Rushton, Fulker, Neale, Nias, & Eysenck, 1986) and has been recently observed in behavioral studies to associate with genetic allele variation (Avinun et al., 2011).

The evidence summarized in the previous paragraphs that altruism is evident in healthy human development suggests the potential to increase these characteristics within positive youth development programs. Beneficial action theory (outlined in more detail later in this chapter) argues that global adolescent health issues, such as international inequality and the development of adolescent risk behavior, can be maximally reduced in the coming years by increasing investment in positive youth development programs that are designed to increase youth altruistic involvement in the worldwide dissemination of effective prevention science programs. The next section considers modifiable factors that influence both the development of adolescent risk behavior and also positive youth development.

Modifiable Causal Factors for Adolescent Risk Behavior

Borrowing similar techniques to those used in the study of risk and protective factors for heart disease, researchers over the past four decades have identified risk and protective factors that influence the development of child and adolescent health and social problems. In the analysis of longitudinal studies, developmental risk factors are defined as independent predictors of particular health and/or social problems. Although protective factors are sometimes defined as the reverse of risk factors, they are more clearly differentiated as characteristics that buffer, mediate, or moderate the influence of risk factors, thereby reducing the likelihood of later problems. Researchers have identified several protective factors by studying children who have avoided problems after being exposed to difficult childhood experiences such as parental mental illness or extreme poverty (Catalano & Hawkins, 1996). In the sections that follow, biological and social development theories of behavioral development are outlined.

Behavioral Development Theories of Adolescent Risk Behavior

Behavior development theories refer to the tendency for the early introduction of behaviors to shape the later sequences in the development of adolescent risk behavior. For example, unhealthy eating and sedentary behavior in childhood and adolescence also increase the probability of developing adolescent and adult risk behaviors and lifestyles involving unhealthy food and inadequate physical activity (Mathews, Moodie, Simmons & Swinburn, 2010). Early behaviors shape later behavior due partly to skills that form into habits, which are then established in social identity and lifestyles (Toumbourou et al., 2014).

Biological Developmental Theories of Risk Behavior

Biological development theories can provide a complementary explanation for behavioral theories by describing the development of skills and preferences for risk behavior with reference to underlying neurological and biological changes. Biological theories can also partly explain the development of adolescent risk behaviors based on a range of factors, including genetic vulnerability, physical development problems, and early exposure to substances. These are briefly explained in the next sections.

Genetic risk factors can increase the probability of developing risk behaviors, such as tobacco, alcohol, and drug use, and antisocial behavior (Jones & Comer, 2015; Salvatore et al., 2015). Genetic factors can change the rewards experienced through substance use (Jones & Comer, 2015) and also indirectly increase risk behavior by influencing factors such as impulsivity that underlie self-control (Salvatore et al., 2015). Efforts to mediate biological risk factors include the use of medication in childhood and adolescence to address attention and impulsivity disorders (Salvatore et al., 2015).

Physical development problems refer to children and adolescents experiencing trauma such as physical injury and stressful negative experiences that can disrupt the course of healthy physical and neurological development (Middlebrooks & Audage, 2008). Physical injury, such as brain trauma, can increase some risk behavior by reducing effective decision making and self-control. The extended arousal of the nervous system and the release of stress hormones, such as cortisol, can result in damage to the development of the brain, and neurological systems that control stress reactions and immunity (Middlebrooks & Audage, 2008). There is evidence that stress-related risk processes have severe effects in the early years, when the brain and biological systems are rapidly developing and hence are more vulnerable to being permanently damaged (National Scientific Council on the Developing Child, 2005/2014). Because the development of biological stress response systems is influenced by early experience, early exposure to severe stress can result in physical, emotional, and cognitive problems that can increase adolescent risk behaviors (Shonkoff, Boyce, & McEwen, 2009).

Early exposure to alcohol, tobacco, and other substances is a further physical development problem that commonly leads to risk behaviors. Exposure to substances in the early years, such as fetal tobacco and alcohol exposure, can result in early neurological and physical damage that results in more severe risk-behavior problems in later life (Toumbourou et al., 2014).

Social Development Theories of Risk Behavior

Social development theories explain the development of risk behavior in terms of socialization and role modeling. Early socialization occurs in the family, then progresses later in childhood at school and with peers. In later stages, adolescent socialization is increasingly influenced by experiences in the wider community. As two examples, the risk of illicit drug problems is increased for children that grow up in families that use illicit drugs and for adolescents who form friendships with illicit drug using peers (Toumbourou & Catalano, 2005).

Social development theories of risk behavior are typically organized around social ecological theories (Bronfenbrenner, 2005). These theories recognize that child and adolescent socialization occurs most directly within the community social environment (in neighborhoods, schools, families, and peer groups) that are shaped by broader structural and societal determinants (e.g., state and national economic and political events) (Toumbourou et al., 2014).

The social development model (Catalano & Hawkins, 1996) is a theory of child and adolescent socialization that has grown out of behavioral and attachment research. The model provides a theoretical description of how social bonds within the social ecology of the family, school, peer, and neighborhood interact to influence the development of both adolescent risk behavior and positive youth development.

The review by Hawkins, Catalano, and Miller (1992) was influential in organizing what was known to that point of social developmental risk and protective factors for youth alcohol and drug abuse and concurs with subsequent reviews (e.g., Hong, Huang, Sabri, & Kim, 2011). The sections that follow summarize these risk and protective factors, beginning with those operating at the community level.

Community risk factors include neighborhood disadvantage (Toumbourou et al., 2007); community violence (Krug, Dahlberg, Mercy, Zwi, & Lozano, 2002); community prevalence and acceptance of substance use (e.g., Catalano & Hawkins, 1996; Hawkins et al., 1992), unhealthy role models for takeout food, and sedentary behavior (Mathews et al., 2010); and availability of substances and unhealthy food and lack of opportunities for physical activity (Toumbourou et al., 2014).

School risk factors include school behavior problems, school disorganization, academic failure, school disengagement, and exclusion (Hemphill et al., 2013; Tollit et al., 2016). In the developing nations, there are international efforts to reduce adolescent risk behaviors by ensuring access to educational opportunities (Catalano et al., 2012). In the developed nations with high levels of inequality, school risk factors are at higher levels for students in disadvantaged communities (e.g., Hemphill et al., 2010). In both the developing and developed nations, educational failure can associate with early pregnancy and adolescent risk behavior (Hemphill et al., 2010). Many teacher training programs do not include adequate student behavior management strategies, hence schools in recent decades have been noted increasingly to use suspension to address student discipline, resulting in this risk factor being prevalent cross-nationally in Australia and the United States (Hemphill et al., 2009).

Family risk factors include family conflict, parent engagement in and favorable attitudes toward risk behavior, harsh and inconsistent parenting behaviors, and poor family management (Hemphill et al., 2011). Family conflict is a highly prevalent and harmful influence on adolescent risk behavior internationally (Krug et al., 2002). In Australia, 33 percent of Australian adolescents are exposed to harmful levels of family conflict (Habib et al., 2014).

Peer and individual risk factors become increasingly important sources of developmental risk through the school-age period (Leung, Toumbourou & Hemphill, 2014; Vassallo et al., 2002). Peer risk factors include peer-influenced antisocial behaviors and attitudes; and peer rejection and bullying (Leung et al., 2014; Vassallo et al., 2002).

Protective Factors

While greater attention is often given to identifying risk factors, it is also useful to consider protective factors. Hawkins et al., (1992) organized protective factors into areas that included individual characteristics (e.g., a positive social orientation, high intelligence, and a resilient temperament), social bonding (e.g., warm relationships, social skills), adaptive stress coping (e.g., emotional control), healthy beliefs, and clear standards for behavior. More recent reviews note similar protective factors (O'Connor et al., 2014).

Cumulative Effects of Risk and Protective Factors

A consistent observation in prevention science is that risk factors have a cumulative impact (Newcomb & Felix-Ortiz, 1992; Toumbourou & Catalano, 2005). The more risk factors and the fewer protective factors that are present and the longer these conditions persist over time, the greater the subsequent developmental impact (e.g., Newcomb & Felix-Ortiz, 1992).

One heuristic proposed to describe the cumulative effect of adolescent risk factors is to use the analogy of a snowball (Toumbourou & Catalano, 2005). According to this view, risk processes that emerge early in life can lead to subsequent risk factors that tend to "adhere" and accumulate as a consequence of the experience of earlier problems (like a snow ball getting larger as it rolls down a mountain). For example, children with early behavior problems are more likely to develop school and peer risk factors through the school-age period (Leung et al., 2014). The snowballing accumulation of early risk factors is explained by the underlying behavioral, biological, and social developmental theories that were outlined previously.

Social and economic mobility patterns have increased socioeconomic differentials internationally and have led to a situation whereby children experiencing snowball risk trajectories tend to be disproportionately clustered within disadvantaged nations, geographic communities, and schools (Toumbourou et al., 2007; 2014). Using this analogy, the solution is to invest within these targeted areas to prevent the potential for an avalanching snowball by building protective factors and reducing early life risk factors in areas of disadvantage. For example, by increasing support to vulnerable mothers (Kemp et al., 2011), it may be possible to prevent the sequence of events that can result in the cumulative escalation of risk that leads to child-onset risk behaviors (Catalano et al., 2012).

In many cases, the cumulative effect of risk is more temporal and can be better described with the analogy of a snowstorm (Toumbourou & Catalano, 2005). According to this view, a healthy child can be put at risk by temporal events such as exposure to extreme weather. If such exposure continues for long enough and the child has few protective factors, adverse health outcomes can result (analogous to being in a blizzard without protective clothing). Where the adolescent has low protective factors (such as parents being unavailable to supervise activities or poor relationships with teachers) in communities with easily accessed hazards (e.g., access to alcohol, tobacco, and drugs), the likelihood of an adolescent succumbing to unhealthy outcomes such as substance use increases. The snowstorm risk process occurs in communities that have high levels of child and adolescent development hazards, such as injury risk factors (Hagel, Romanow, Enns, Williamson, & Rowe, 2015); community disorganization (Shapiro, Oesterle, & Hawkins, 2015); marketing by vested interests for substances (Rowland et al., 2014); and unhealthy foods (Carroll-Scott et al., 2013).

The protective advantages of positive relationships with adults suggest there is potential to protect health within risky social environments by increasing healthy adult relationships or other social developmental protective factors. From this perspective, solutions lie in improving social environments (by reducing peer risk factors, increasing protective social relationships, and reducing alcohol availability) through the course of development (Catalano & Hawkins, 1996; Leung et al., 2014).

Predictors of Positive Youth Development

Research examining factors that increase positive youth development is not as extensive as the research examining the development of risk behavior. Influences that have been shown in Australian longitudinal analyses to predict positive young adult development emerge in childhood and include parents' higher socioeconomic levels, easy childhood temperament, self-control, school adjustment, and positive social relationships with parents and peers. These factors influence positive adolescent adjustment and are also reinforced by community opportunities in adolescence (O'Connor et al., 2011a; 2014). In their absence, these life-course predictors act as the mirror opposite in influencing the development of adolescent antisocial risk behavior (Tollit et al., 2016).

The research summarized in the preceding sections reveals that risk and protective factors operating at the individual, family, school, peer, and neighborhood levels influence the development of both adolescent risk behaviors and positive youth development. In the sections that follow, evaluation research is summarized to describe interventions that can prevent adolescent risk behaviors and increase positive youth development.

Prevention Science Intervention Approaches to Reduce Adolescent Risk Behavior and Increase Positive Youth Development

Although it can be challenging to design and implement interventions and to complete evaluation trials, there is a mounting body of evidence indicating that intervening during the child and adolescent years can reduce risk behavior and enhance healthy youth development. Most of this evidence is of the highest quality, in the form of systematic reviews, meta-analyses, and economic syntheses of controlled trials (Aos et al., 2011; Catalano et al.,

2012; Toumbourou et al., 2014; Vos et al., 2010). In the sections that follow, policies, programs, and activities are briefly outlined that have evidence for efficacy (beneficial impacts in evaluations with high internal validity) or effectiveness (evaluation trials with high external validity) in reducing priority adolescent health and social problems. Interventions that have feasibility for implementation in the developing world are described together with those that have relevance in the developed nations.

In their review, Catalano et al. (2012) identified the potential to promote the implementation of prevention science programs in both the developed and developing nations with the goal of controlling fertility, reducing sexually transmissible disease, preventing alcohol and tobacco use, and preventing obesity. Their review identified the requirement to address structural policies at the national/state levels and to implement effective interventions at the community, school, family, and individual/peer levels. Relevant structural policies supported by at least quasi-experimental evidence in their review included adolescent access to contraception, taxation to reduce the economic availability of alcohol and tobacco, raising of the legal age for alcohol use and purchase to twenty-one, and graduated licensing to reduce road trauma. Effective interventions included mentorship at the community level, school reorganization and health curricula, parent education and family therapy, and web-based and interactive skill development interventions for individuals and peer groups (Catalano et al., 2012).

Although space limitations preclude a comprehensive overview, examples of these interventions and their evaluation evidence are summarized in the sections that follow. While many interventions aim to address only one outcome, it should be noted that adolescent interventions that address multiple risk factors often demonstrate preventive effects on more than one outcome (Toumbourou et al., 2014).

Structural and Macro Policy Interventions

Structural inequality and socioeconomic differentials are increasing internationally (OECD, 2012) and adversely impact children and adolescents and typically require national and state action to be effectively addressed (Toumbourou et al., 2007). The United Nations Millennium Development project achieved considerable success in recent years encouraging strategic support from the developed nations to reduce extreme poverty in the developing nations by encouraging universal access to basic education, health care, human rights, and income (United Nations, 2008).

Although community inequality has increased in many developed nations, prevention science intervention trials show evidence that they can reduce the intergenerational transfer of poverty and disadvantage by reducing behavioral, biological, and social development risk processes (Toumbourou et al., 2007). Strategies that have evidence from randomized trials include supportive home visiting to vulnerable mothers to reduce early risk factors (e.g., negative parent behavior [resulting in child neglect and abuse], substance use, mental health problems, and family conflict) and increase protective factors (e.g., breast feeding, reading to the child) (Kemp et al., 2011). Ensuring access to education is a central strategy for reducing poverty in the developing nations (United Nations, 2008). Intervention trials in the developed nations reveal that interventions to improve teacher effectiveness in primary school can improve school completion and reduce the intergenerational transfer of poverty (e.g., Hawkins, Kosterman, Catalano, Hill, & Abbot, 2005).

The major structural interventions that have been proposed to prevent adolescent risk behaviors are reforms to increase the price of alcohol and tobacco as well as industry regulation to control the marketing and availability of alcohol and tobacco (Toumbourou et al., 2014; Vos et al.. 2010).

Neighborhood Interventions

Neighborhood-level interventions are coordinated by government and nongovernment organizations. As will be summarized later in this chapter, there is evidence that adolescent alcohol and tobacco use can be prevented through community approaches that reduce supply (e.g., Rowland et al., 2014) and reduce demand by improving conditions for healthy child and youth development (Hawkins et al., 2009).

Reductions in adolescent alcohol use have been demonstrated using community interventions in the United States and Australia to reduce the sale and supply of alcohol to youth (Rowland et al., 2013). Strategies to monitor and enforce the legal minimum purchase age restrictions are important interventions for reducing adolescent tobacco and alcohol use (Toumbourou et al., 2014).

Sports clubs are an important social environment for adolescents, yet often have high rates of risk behavior among adults (Rowland, Allan, & Toumbourou, 2012). In Australia, the Good Sports program has been designed and widely disseminated to introduce effective alcohol harm reduction policies into sports clubs. Research examining the implementation of the Good Sports program has associated the program with lower levels of club member risky alcohol use and stronger adherence to responsible practices such as not supplying alcohol to under-age youth (Rowland et al., 2012).

Community interventions have been demonstrated to reduce adolescent risk factors for obesity in the areas of physical activity and healthy nutrition (Mathews et al., 2010). Local neighborhood redesign to increase opportunities for physical activity and healthy food has been proposed as a neighborhood strategy for encouraging healthy lifestyles (Carroll-Scott et al., 2013).

School Interventions

A Cochrane review (Waters et al., 2011) has identified that a number of strategies are effective in the school setting to tackle obesity, particularly for children between the ages of six and twelve. These strategies have been trialed in the developed nations and largely focus on increasing the capacity of schools and teachers to implement health promotion strategies and polices that reinforce healthier food and activity choices. Strategies used in these programs include school curriculum that includes content about healthy eating, physical activity and body image, increased sessions for physical activity and movement, environments and cultural practices that support children eating healthier foods and being active throughout the day, and support for teachers and staff to implement health promotion strategies and activities. Australian evaluations have demonstrated these programs are associated with reductions in adolescent overweight and obesity (Millar et al., 2013).

Although school health curricula can offer benefits in encouraging adolescent health behavior (Toumbourou et al., 2014), school reorganization whereby curricula are supported with teacher training and policy reform may offer greater advantages. The Gatehouse Project was delivered in Australian secondary schools and included staff support and training to develop healthy school policies, and teacher training to deliver student social and emotional competence curricula. A randomized trial revealed that exposure to the intervention was associated with reductions in a range of adolescent risk behaviors, including alcohol and tobacco use, antisocial behavior, and risky sexual behavior (Bond et al., 2004).

Family Interventions

Family interventions focus both on assisting the parents of adolescents and also assisting adolescents as they become parents. Increasing opportunities for parent education has been shown in Australian evaluation trials to be effective in reducing adolescent risk behaviors, including antisocial behavior and adolescent alcohol and drug use (Toumbourou & Greg, 2002). Intervening to increase parent education in the adolescent school context aims to enhance family management practices and reduce snowstorm risk factors such as parents supplying adolescents with alcohol (evident in 29 percent of Australian parents in 2004: Shortt, Hutchinson, Chapman, & Toumbourou, 2007). An Australian randomized school trial showed that an intervention strategy incorporating both student social competence training and parent education opportunities encouraged parents to set rules not to supply alcohol to adolescents and through this mechanism reduced schoolwide rates of adolescent alcohol misuse by 25 percent (Toumbourou, Douglas Gregg, Shortt, Hutchinson, & Slaviero, 2013).

The family environment has also been identified as an important domain in obesity prevention and physical health promotion. These interventions support parents to adopt family management practices that ensure that their children spend less time on screen-based activities, eat more nutritious food, and become more active. An Australian trial randomized parents to receive education in family management practices to encourage child health and demonstrated the intervention was effective in improving healthy weight in children aged from four to eleven (West, Sanders, Cleghorn & Davies, 2010).

Strategies shown to be effective in reducing snowball risk processes in vulnerable parents, including adolescent parents, include family home visiting aimed at supporting, good parenting practices, healthy child development, and secure child attachment with the parent (Kemp et al., 2011).

Individual and Peer-Based Interventions

As children enter adolescence, there is an increasing expectation that they will take responsibility for healthy choices relating to risk behavior. There is evidence that brief interventions including interactive online interventions can be effective in reducing risk behaviors. Effective brief interventions are based on behavior change theories and initiated following screening to assess levels of risk behavior. Behavior change strategies include motivational interviewing, cognitive behavior therapy, and feedback to encourage behavior change toward healthy peer norms (Toumbourou et al., 2014).

Evaluations reveal that alcohol education programs have been successfully implemented in secondary schools and universities in the United States using interactive online health interventions reinforced with policy strategies. Trials show that students randomized to complete these interventions show reduced alcohol use and harms (e.g., Croom et al., 2009).

Integrating and Disseminating Interventions at a System Level

A major problem recognized in efforts to disseminate effective prevention science programs is that health and social service delivery systems in the developed nations have not been based on evidence-based strategies and are frequently dominated by approaches that have low evidence for reducing adolescent risk behavior (Spoth et al., 2013). Popular but ineffective approaches to reducing adolescent risk behavior include the following (Toumbourou et al., 2014):

- The use of school suspension and exclusion to deter risk behavior that has the unintended consequence of increasing risk behavior by decreasing social developmental protective factors
- Peer group programs for adolescents exhibiting risk behavior that have the unintended consequence of increasing risk behavior by increasing bonding to deviant peers
- Encouragement of involvement in sports clubs that when poorly managed may increase alcohol use and violent behavior by increasing bonds to adults involved in these behaviors
- Poorly designed health curricula advertising the effects of and means of administering different types of drugs

Within the field of positive youth development, there is also evidence that the popularly supported strategy of character education in the United States has not resulted in improved motivational or behavioral outcomes (Catalano et al., 2014). Evidence-based strategies for improving positive youth development outcomes are available (Catalano et al., 2014) but have at this stage not been widely implemented.

Thus a major challenge for prevention science is to establish strategies to encourage wider investment both in the developed and developing nations in evidence-based approaches to preventing adolescent risk behavior and encouraging positive youth development (Catalano et al., 2012; Spoth et al., 2013). One strategy that is being increasingly used involves governments requiring service system investments to be based on evidence from systematic reviews.

Blueprints for Prevention[2] is a United States initiative initiated at the University of Colorado that reviewed over four hundred programs to identify prevention and intervention programs with evaluation evidence that met a high scientific standard and were also supported with implementation training and advice. A number of United States national and state justice agencies now require that their funds be exclusively used to support the Blueprints model programs or programs meeting equivalent evidence criteria (Toumbourou et al., 2015).

Economic analysis is a further method that is being increasingly used to synthesize the range of evaluation evidence to reach conclusions as to which investments would be most efficient in reducing risk behavior within a population (Aos et al., 2011; Vos et al., 2010). An example where economic analysis has been used in an effective system change effort occurred in Washington State in the United States. The Washington State Institute[3] has developed a unique model to synthesize scientific information required for evidence-based policy and for measuring implementation. The model rests on estimating economic "return on investment" to compare various policy options. Using this model, a complex range of scientific information has been synthesized in a form that is comprehensible to non-expert audiences within the Washington State legislature. The Institute has been successful in encouraging the Washington State legislature to increase investment in evidence-based prevention science programs. A notable achievement has been that the Washington State crime rate has steadily reduced over recent decades, while the use of incarceration has also fallen. In the 1980s, prior to the Institute, the crime and incarceration rates in Washington State were similar to those in the rest of the United States, and in recent decades the state crime rate has steadily fallen below the national rate (Toumbourou et al., 2015).

The Communities That Care framework provides a further example of a successful strategy for reorienting community investment toward effective prevention approaches. Communities That Care was developed in the United States to provide communities with training and support to increase community capacity to plan and deliver effective programs for reducing adolescent risk behavior and for increasing positive youth development (Greenberg, Feinberg, Brendan, Gomez & Osgood, 2005; Hawkins et al., 2009). The process

2 www.blueprintsprograms.com. 3 www.wsipp.wa.gov.

emphasizes both community development and the building of understanding and skills relevant to effective prevention strategies. Through the process, local community organizations use the Communities That Care youth survey to assess risk behaviors and factors that influence these behaviors within their community. This information is used to set priorities for selecting and implementing prevention strategies to reduce locally elevated risk factors and to increase locally depressed protective factors. Finally, monitoring and evaluation are implemented to ensure the effectiveness of the local community prevention plan. A randomized community trial across the United States (Hawkins et al., 2009) and a dissemination trial in the State of Pennsylvania (Greenberg at al., 2005) reveal the Communities That Care process is effective at increasing local community delivery of effective prevention strategies and in this way at reducing population rates of adolescent risk behavior (Hawkins et al., 2009). The framework has been adapted effectively for use in other countries internationally, including in Croatia, Germany, and Australia (e.g., Toumbourou et al., 2015).

Beneficial Action Theory and the Reduction of Adolescent Risk Behavior

The previous section summarized examples of effective strategies that are being used at the state and community levels within the developed nations to increase prevention science investments to reduce adolescent risk behavior and encourage positive youth development. An important current challenge that confronts prevention science is that of encouraging the international dissemination of prevention science to assist the majority of adolescents who live in the developing world (Sawyer et al., 2012). In the section that follows, I outline beneficial action theory (Toumbourou, in press) as an approach that integrates positive youth development and prevention science frameworks to develop a strategy to reduce international rates of adolescent risk behavior while also maximizing positive youth development.

As has been noted previously, higher levels of positive youth development have been shown in large Australian longitudinal studies to emerge from childhood and adolescent experiences characterized by healthy attachments, bonding to education, family and peer experiences reinforcing safety and security, and community opportunities (O'Connor et al., 2011a). Beneficial action theory proposes that where children and adolescents experience consistent conditions for healthy development, they emerge into adulthood with high levels of positive development characteristics that are required for building social capital, including altruistic behavior (indicated by civic engagement and volunteering), social trust, and competence (Hawkins et al., 2011; O'Connor et al., 2014). Beneficial action theory argues that worldwide adolescent health issues, such as international inequality, can be maximally reduced in the coming years by encouraging investment in programs that increase altruistic youth involvement in the international dissemination of effective prevention science programs.

There is evidence that encouraging youth volunteering and civic action can increase adult positive youth development characteristics associated with altruism. Adolescent volunteering has been found in longitudinal studies to predict higher levels of school completion and adult civic engagement (Zaff, Moore, Romano Papillo & Williams, 2003). Adolescent volunteering also appears to benefit physical health. An experimental trial randomly assigning adolescents to a weekly volunteering condition found that biological risk factors for heart disease, including cholesterol and body mass index, were reduced in the intervention group (Schreier, Schonert-Reichl, & Chen, 2013).

Although adolescents may individually experience enhanced development through participation in volunteering, current volunteering opportunities do not necessarily have beneficial outcomes for service recipients. The preceding summarized findings demonstrate that many currently popular health and social service programs (including peer group programs, sports clubs, and popular character education programs) do not have evidence that they contribute to reductions in adolescent risk behaviors or increased positive youth development (Catalano et al., 2014; Spoth et al., 2013). Beneficial action theory argues that altruistic action such as volunteering must be guided by knowledge from the evaluation sciences to maximize its contribution to positive human development outcomes.

A further limitation of many current health and social service programs, including youth civic engagement, volunteering, and positive youth development opportunities, is that they do not have an explicit objective of increasing social trust between different communities and countries internationally (O'Connor et al., 2014). By volunteering in local community programs youth, benefit by developing social bonds within the community they serve but may not necessarily increase understanding of community differences in factors such as international disadvantage and cultural diversity (O'Connor et al., 2014). Many altruistically inspired programs are designed to have benefits limited to specified populations (O'Connor et al., 2014) and "in-groups" (Tajfel & Turner, 1986). Beneficial action theory recognizes that a current human development challenge is to reduce international economic disparities, distrust, and conflict, hence adolescent development programs should deliberately seek to broaden adolescent social identity boundaries to increase trust for unfamiliar populations and identification with global citizenship (O'Connor et al., 2014).

Conceptions of thriving in positive youth development (Lerner et al., 2005; Magen, 1998) suggest the possibility that the developmental interests of adolescents may be best served where they are encouraged and supported to provide service to others and to deliberately broaden their boundaries of social competence and trust (Domitrovich, Cortes, & Greenberg, 2007). International plans to eliminate extreme poverty (United Nations, 2008) have led some youth-serving organizations to encourage a movement wherein young people within the developing nations have been supported to volunteer as "global citizens" and provide service in areas that can be measured against these ambitious plans[4] (Obeng-Odoom, 2010). Programs of this type offer an important means for adolescents of the future to be guided to engage and volunteer in constructive and well-designed programs that at the same time offer solutions to reducing global problems such as international inequality (United Nations, 2008).

Conclusion

This chapter has overviewed the development of adolescent risk behavior. The modifiable causes of adolescent risk behavior were described and an encouraging range of effective prevention science approaches was outlined that are being applied to prevent adolescent risk behavior problems and encourage positive youth development. The chapter outlined a beneficial action approach to the prevention of adolescent risk-behavior problems. Beneficial action theory forecasts that if investment is increased in effective adolescent development programs, a greater proportion of adolescents will emerge in future years with altruistic motivation and social trust. Beneficial action theory argues that by teaching prevention science to adolescents and by encouraging altruistic adolescents to achieve effective international and volunteering impacts, a generational leap forward in healthy adolescent development can be achieved across the world.

References

Aos, S., Lee, S., Drake, E., Pennucci, A., Klima, T., Miller, M., Anderson, L., Mayfield, J., & Burley, M. (2011). *Return on Investment: Evidence-Based Options to Improve Statewide Outcomes* (Document No. 11-07-1201). Olympia: Washington State Institute for Public Policy.

Avinun, R., Israel, S., Shalev, I., Gritsenko, I., Bornstein, G., Ebstein, R. P., & Knafo, A. (2011). AVPR1A variant associated with preschoolers' lower altruistic behavior. *PLoS One* 6: e25274. doi: 10.1371/journal.pone.0025274

Baheiraei, A., Soltani, F., Ebadi, A., Cheraghi, M. A., Foroushani, A. R., & Catalano, R. F. (2014). Psychometric properties of the Iranian version of "Communities That Care Youth Survey." *Health Promotion International*. dau062. doi: 10.1093/heapro/dau062

Batson, C. D. (2011). *Altruism in Humans*. New York: Oxford University Press.

Bond, L., Patton, G., Glover, S., Carlin, J. B., Butler, H., Thomas, L. & Bowes, G. (2004). The Gatehouse Project: can a multi-level school intervention affect emotional wellbeing and health risk-behaviours? *Journal Epidemiology and Community Health* 58: 997–1000. doi: 10.1136/jech.2003.009449

Bronfenbrenner, U. (2005). *Making Human Beings Human: Bioecological Perspectives on Human Development*. Thousand Oaks, CA: Sage.

4 www.globalcitizen.org/en/.

Carroll-Scott, A., Gilstad-Hayden, K., Rosenthal, L., Peters, S. M., McCaslin, C., Joyce, R., & Ickovics, J. R. (2013). Disentangling neighborhood contextual associations with child body mass index, diet, and physical activity: the role of built, socioeconomic, and social environments. *Social Science and Medicine* 95: 106–14. doi: 10.1016/j.socscimed.2013.04.003

Catalano, R. F., Fagan, A. A., Gavin, L. E., Greenberg, M. T., Irwin, C. E. Jr., Ross, D. A., & Shek, D. T. (2012). Worldwide application of prevention science in adolescent health. *Lancet* 379: 1653–64. doi: 10.1016/S0140-6736(12)60238-4

Catalano, R. F., & Hawkins, J. D. (1996). The social development model: a theory of antisocial behavior. In Hawkins, J. D. (ed.), *Delinquency and Crime: Current Theories*. New York: Cambridge University Press, pp. 149–97.

Catalano, R. F., Toumbourou, J. W., & Hawkins, J. D. (2014). Positive youth development in the United States: history, efficacy, and links to moral and character education. In Nucci, L., Krettenauer, T., & Narvaez, D. (eds.), *Handbook of Moral and Character Education*. Routledge: New York, pp. 423–40.

Cesarini, D., Dawes, C., Johannesson, M., Lichtenstein, P., & Wallace, B. (2009). Genetic variation in preferences for giving and risk taking. *Quarterly Journal of Economics* 124: 809–42. doi: 10.1162/qjec.2009.124.2.809

Croom, K., Lewis, D., Marchell, T., Lesser, M. L., Reyna, V. F., Kubicki-Bedford, L. M., Feffer, M., & Staiano-Coico, L. (2009). Impact of an online alcohol education course on behavior and harm for incoming first-year college students: short term evaluation of a randomized trial. *Journal of American College Health* 57: 445–54. doi: 10.3200/JACH.57.4.445–454

Domitrovich, C., Cortes, R., & Greenberg, M. (2007). Improving young children's social and emotional competence: a randomized trial of the preschool "PATHS" curriculum. *Journal of Primary Prevention* 28(2): 67–91.

Donovan, J. E., Jessor, R., & Costa, F. M. (1988). Syndrome of problem behavior in adolescence: a replication. *Journal of Consulting and Clinical Psychology* 56(5): 762–5. doi: 10.1037/0022–006x.56.5.762

Eisenberg, N., & Mussen, P. H. (1989). *The Roots of Prosocial Behavior in Children*. Cambridge, MA: Cambridge University Press.

Greenberg, M. T., Feinberg, M. E., Brendan J., Gomez, B. J., & Osgood, D. W. (2005). Testing a community prevention focused model of coalition functioning and sustainability: a comprehensive study of communities that care in Pennsylvania. In Stockwell, T., Gruenewald, P., Toumbourou, J. W., & Loxley, W. (eds.), *Preventing Harmful Substance Use: The Evidence Base for Policy and Practice*. London: Wiley, pp. 129–42.

Habib, C., Toumbourou, J. W., McRitchie, M., Williams, J., Kremer, P., McKenzie, D., & Catalano, R. F. (2014). Prevalence and community variation in harmful levels of family conflict witnessed by children: implications for prevention. *Prevention Science* 15: 757–66. doi: 10.1007/s11121-013–0416-4 PMID: 23812887

Hagel, B. E., Romanow, N. T., Enns, N., Williamson, J., & Rowe, B. H. (2015). Severe bicycling injury risk factors in children and adolescents: a case-control study. *Accident Analysis and Prevention* 78: 165–72. doi: 10.1016/j.aap.2015.03.002

Hawkins, J. D., Catalano, R. F., & Miller, J. Y. (1992). Risk- and protective factors for alcohol and other drug problems in adolescence and early adulthood:

implications for substance abuse prevention. *Psychological Bulletin* 112: 64–105.

Hawkins, J. D., Kosterman, R., Catalano, R. F., Hill, K., & Abbot, R. D. (2005). Promoting positive adult functioning through social development intervention in childhood: long-term effects from the Seattle Social Development Project. *Archives of Pediatric and Adolescent Medicine* 159: 25–31. doi: 10.1001/archpedi.162.12.1133

Hawkins, J. D., Oesterle, S., Brown, E. C., Arthur, M. W., Abbott, R. D., Fagan, A. A., & Catalano, R. F. (2009). Results of a Type 2 translational research trial to prevent adolescent drug use and delinquency: a test of Communities That Care. *Archives of Pediatric and Adolescent Medicine* 163: 789–98. doi: 10.1001/archpediatrics.2009.141

Hawkins, M. T., Letcher, P., Sanson, A., O'Connor, M., Toumbourou, J., & Olsson, C. (2011). Stability and change in positive development during the transition from adolescence to adulthood. *Journal of Youth and Adolescence* 40: 1436–52.

Hawkins, M. T., Villagonzalo, K., Sanson, A. V., Toumbourou, J. W., Letcher, P., & Olsson, C. (2012). Associations between positive development in late adolescence and social, health, and behavioral outcomes in young adulthood. *Journal of Adult Development* 19: 88–99. doi: 10.1007/s10804-011–9137-8

Hemphill, S. A., Heerde, J. A., Herrenkohl, T. I., Patton, G. C. Toumbourou, J. W., & Catalano, R. F. (2011). Risk and protective factors for adolescent substance use in Washington State, the United States and Victoria, Australia: a longitudinal study. *Journal of Adolescent Health* 49: 312–20.

Hemphill, S. A., Kotevski, A., Herrenkohl, T. I., Smith, R., Toumbourou, J. W., & Catalano, R. F. (2013). Does school suspension affect subsequent youth non-violent antisocial behaviour? A longitudinal study of students in Victoria, Australia and Washington State, United States. *Australian Journal of Psychology* 65: 236–49. doi: 10.1111/ajpy.12026

Hemphill, S. A., Smith, R., Toumbourou, J. W., Herrenkohl, T. I., Catalano, R. F., McMorris, B. J., & Romaniuk, H. (2009). Modifiable determinants of youth violence in Australia and the United States: a longitudinal study. *Australia and New Zealand Journal of Criminology* 42: 289–309.

Hemphill, S. A., Toumbourou, J. W., Smith, R., Kendall, G. E., Rowland, B., Freiberg, K., Williams, J. W. (2010). Are rates of school suspension higher in socially disadvantaged neighbourhoods? An Australian study. *Health Promotion Journal of Australia* 21: 12–18.

Hong, J. S., Huang, H., Sabri, B., & Kim, J. S. (2011). Substance abuse among Asian American youth: an ecological review of the literature. *Children and Youth Services Review* 33: 669–77. dx.doi.org/10.1016/j.childyouth.2010.11.015

Jones, J. D., & Comer, S. D. (2015). A review of pharmacogenetic studies of substance-related disorders. *Drug and Alcohol Dependence* 152: 1–14. doi: 10.1016/j.drugalcdep.2015.03.003

Jonkman, H., Steketee, M., Toumbourou, J. W., Cini, K., & Williams. J. (2014). Community variation in adolescent alcohol use in Australia and the Netherlands. *Health Promotion International. Health Promotion International* 29: 109–17. doi: 10.1093/heapro/das039

Kemp, L., Harris, E., McMahon, C., Matthey, S., Vimpani, G., Anderson, T., et al. (2011). Child and family outcomes of a long-term nurse home visitation programme: a randomised controlled trial. *Archives of Disease in Childhood* 96: 533–40. doi: 10.1136/adc.2010.196279

Krug, E. G., Dahlberg, L L., Mercy, J. A., Zwi, A. B., & Lozano, R. (eds.) (2002). *World Report on Violence and Health: Summary Report*. Geneva, Switzerland: World Health Organization. www.who.int/violence_injury_prevention/violence/youth/en/index.html.

Lerner, R. M., Almerigi, J. B., Thoeoksa, C., & Lerner, J. V. (2005). Positive youth development. *Journal of Early Adolescence* 25: 10–16.

Leung, R., Toumbourou, J. W., & Hemphill, S. (2014). The effect of peer influence and selection processes on adolescent alcohol use: a systematic review of longitudinal studies. *Health Psychology Review* 8: 426–57. doi: 10.1080/17437199.2011.587961

Lowry, R., Eaton, D. K., Brener, N. D., & Kann, L. (2011). Prevalence of health-risk-behaviors among Asian American and Pacific Islander high school students in the US, 2001–2007. *Public Health Reports* 126: 39–49.

Magen, Z. (1998). *Exploring Adolescent Happiness: Commitment, Purpose and Fulfillment*. Thousand Oaks, CA: Sage.

Mathews, L. B., Moodie, M. M., Simmons, A. N., & Swinburn, B. A. (2010). The process evaluation of It's Your Move! An Australian adolescent community-based obesity prevention project. *BMC Public Health* 10: 448 doi: 10.1186/1471–2458-10–448

Middlebrooks, J. S., & Audage, N. C. (2008). *The Effects of Childhood Stress on Health across the Lifespan*. Atlanta, GA: Centers for Disease Control and Prevention, National Center for Injury Prevention and Control.

Millar, L., Robertson, N., Allender, S., Nichols, M., Bennett, C., & Swinburn, B. (2013). Increasing community capacity and decreasing prevalence of overweight and obesity in a community based intervention among Australian adolescents. *Preventive Medicine* 56: 379–84. doi: 2-s2.0–84877588910

Moll, J., Krueger, F., Zahn, R., Pardini, M., de Oliveira-Souza, R., & Grafman, J. (2006). Human fronto-mesolimbic networks guide decisions about charitable donation. *Proceedings of the National Academy of Science* 103: 15623–8. doi: 10.1073/pnas.0604475103

National Research Council and Institute of Medicine (2009). *Preventing Mental, Emotional, and Behavioural Disorders among Young People: Progress and Possibilities*. Committee on the Prevention of Mental Disorders and Substance Abuse among Children, Youth, and Young Adults: Research Advances and Promising Interventions. Board on Children, Youth, and Families, Division of Behavioral and Social Sciences and Education. Washington, DC: National Academies Press.

National Scientific Council on the Developing Child (2005/2014). Excessive stress disrupts the architecture of the developing brain: Working Paper 3. developingchild.harvard.edu/resources/wp3/

Newcomb, M. D., & Felix-Ortiz, M. (1992). Multiple protective and risk-factors for drug use and abuse: cross-sectional and prospective findings. *Journal of Personality and Social Psychology* 63: 280–96.

Obeng-Odoom, F. (2010). Promoting human development through the Global Poverty Project. *Development* 53: 120–6.

O'Connor, M., Sanson, A., Hawkins, M. T., Letcher, P., Toumbourou, J. W., Smart, D., Vassallo, S., & Olsson, C. A. (2011a). Predictors of positive development in emerging adulthood. *Journal of Youth and Adolescence* 40: 860–74. doi 10.1007/s10964-010–9593-7

O'Connor, M., Sanson, A., Hawkins, M., Letcher, P., Toumbourou, J. W., Smart, D., Vassallo, S., & Olsson, C. (2011b). The relationship between positive development and psychopathology during the transition to adulthood: a person-centred approach. *Journal of Adolescence* 35: 701–12.

O'Connor, M., Sanson, A. V., Toumbourou, J. W., Hawkins, M. T., Letcher, P., Williams, P., & Olsson, C. (2014). Positive development and resilience in emerging adulthood. in Arnett, J. J. (ed.), *Oxford Handbook of Emerging Adulthood*. New York: Oxford University Press. doi: 10.1093/oxfordhb/9780199795574.013.19

OECD (Office of Economic Cooperation and Development) (2012). *Income Inequality and Growth: The role of Taxes and Transfers*. Economics Department Policy Notes, No. 9. Geneva, Switzerland: Office of Economic Cooperation and Development. oecd.org/tax/public-finance/49417295.pdf

Patton, G. C., Coffey, C., Cappa, C., Currie, D., Riley, L., Gore, F., Degenhardt, L., Richardson, D., Astone, N., Sangowawa, A. O., Mokdad, A., & Ferguson, J. (2012). Health of the world's adolescents: a synthesis of internationally comparable data. *Lancet* 379: 1665–75. doi: 10.1016/S0140-6736(12)60203–7

Rowland, B., Allan, F., & Toumbourou, J. W. (2012). Association of risky alcohol consumption and accreditation in the "Good Sports" alcohol management programme. *Journal of Epidemiology and Community Health* 66: 684–90. doi: 10.1136/jech- 2011-200334

Rowland, B., Toumbourou, J. W., Osborn, A., Smith, R., Hall, J., Kremer, P., Kelly, A., Williams, J., & Leslie, E. (2013). A clustered randomised trial examining the effect of social marketing and community mobilisation on the age of uptake and levels of alcohol consumption by Australian adolescents: study protocol. *BMJ Open* 3(1). doi: 10.1136/bmjopen-2012-002423

Rowland, B., Toumbourou J.W. Satyen, L., Tooley, G., Hall, J., Livingston, M., & Williams, J. (2014). Associations between alcohol outlet densities and adolescent alcohol consumption: a study in Australian Students. *Addictive Behaviors* 39: 282–8. dx.doi.org/10.1016/j.addbeh.2013.10.001

Rushton, J. P., Fulker, D. W. Neale, M. C., Nias, D. K. B., & Eysenck, H. J. (1986). Altruism and aggression: the heritability of individual differences. *Journal of Personality and Social Psychology* 50: 1192–8. doi: 10.1037/0022–3514.50.6.1192

Salvatore, J. E., Aliev, F., Bucholz, K., Agrawal, A., Hesselbrock, V., Hesselbrock, M., Bauer, L., Kuperman, S., Schuckit, M. A., Kramer, J., Edenberg, H. J., Foroud, T. M., & Dick, D. M. (2015). Polygenic risk for externalizing disorders: gene-by-development and gene-by-environment effects in adolescents and young adults. *Clinical Psychological Science* 3: 189–201.

Sawyer, S. M., Afifi, R. A., Bearinger, L. H., Blakemore, S. J., Dick, B., Ezeh, A. C., Patton, G. C. (2012). Adolescence: a foundation for future health. *Lancet* 379: 1630–40. doi: 10.1016/S0140-6736(12)60072-5

Schreier, H. M. C., Schonert-Reichl, K. A., & Chen, E. (2013). Effect of volunteering on risk-factors for cardiovascular disease in adolescents: a randomized controlled trial. *JAMA Pediatrics* 167: 327–32. doi: 10.1001/jamapediatrics.2013.1100

Shapiro, V. B., Oesterle, S., & Hawkins, J. D. (2015). Relating coalition capacity to the adoption of science-based prevention in communities: evidence from a randomized trial of Communities That Care. *American Journal of Community Psychology* 55: 1–12. doi: 10.1007/s10464-014–9684-9

Shonkoff, J. P., Boyce, W. T., & McEwen, B. S. (2009). Neuroscience, molecular biology, and the childhood roots of health disparities: building a new framework for health promotion and disease prevention. *JAMA* 301: 2252–9.

Shortt, A. L., Hutchinson, D. M., Chapman, R., & Toumbourou, J. W. (2007). Family, school, peer and individual influences on early adolescent alcohol use: first year impact of the Resilient Families program. *Drug and Alcohol Review* 26: 625–34.

Spoth, R., Rohrbach, L. A., Greenberg, G., Leaf, P., Brown, C. H., Fagan, A., Catalano, R. F., Pentz, M. A., Sloboda, Z., Hawkins, J. D., & Society for Prevention Research Type 2 Translational Task Force Members and Contributing Authors (2013). Addressing core challenges for the next generation of type 2 translation research and systems: the translation science to population impact (TSci Impact) framework. *Prevention Science* 14: 319–51. doi: 10.1007/s11121-012–0362-6

Tajfel, H., & Turner, J. C. (1986). The social identity theory of intergroup behaviour. In Worchel, S., & Austin, W. G. (eds.), *Psychology of Intergroup Relations*. Chicago, IL: Nelson-Hall, pp. 7–24.

Tollit, M. A., Hemphill, S., & Toumbourou, J. W. (2016). Understanding and responding to adolescent risk-taking behaviors and addictions. In Thielking, M., & Terjesen, M. (eds.), *The Australian Handbook of School Psychology: Bridging the Gaps in International Research, Practice, and Policy*. New York: Springer, ch. 22.

Toumbourou, J. W. (in press) Beneficial action within altruistic and prosocial behavior. *Review of General Psychology*. http://dx.doi.org/10.1037/gpr0000081.

Toumbourou, J. W., & Catalano, R. F. (2005). Predicting developmentally harmful substance use. In Stockwell, T., Gruenewald, P., Toumbourou, J. W., & Loxley, W. (eds), *Preventing Harmful Substance Use: The Evidence Base for Policy and Practice*. London: Wiley, pp. 53–66.

Toumbourou, J. W., Douglas Gregg, E., Shortt, A. L., Hutchinson, D. M., & Slaviero, T. M. (2013). Reduction of adolescent alcohol use through family-school intervention: a randomized trial. *Journal of Adolescent Health* 53: 778–84. doi: 10.1016/j.jadohealth.2013.07.005

Toumbourou, J. W., & Gregg, M. E. (2002). Impact of an empowerment-based parent education program on the reduction of youth suicide risk factors. *Journal of Adolescent Health* 31: 279–87.

Toumbourou, J. W., Hemphill, S. A., Tresidder, J., Humphreys, C., Edwards, J., & Murray, D. (2007). Mental health promotion and socio-economic disadvantage: lessons from substance abuse, violence and crime prevention and child health. *Australian Journal of Health Promotion* 18: 184–90.

Toumbourou, J. W., Leung, R. K., Homel, R., Freiberg, K., Satyen, L., & Hemphill, S. A. (2015). Violence prevention and early intervention: what works? In Day, A., & Fernandez, E. (eds.), *Preventing Violence in Australia: Policy, Practice and Solutions*. Australia: Federation Press, pp 45–62.

Toumbourou, J.W., Olsson, C., Rowland, B., Renati, S., & Hallam, B. (2014). Health psychology intervention in key social environments to promote adolescent health. *Australian Psychologist* 49: 66–74. doi: 10.1111/ap.12043

United Nations (2008). *Millennium Development Goals*. New York: United Nations.

Vassallo, S., Smart, D., Sanson, A., Dussuyer, I., McKendry, B., Toumbourou, J., Prior, M., & Oberklaid, F. (2002). *Patterns and Precursors of Adolescent Antisocial Behavior: The First Report*. Melbourne: Crime Prevention Victoria and Australian Institute of Family Studies.

Vos, T., Carter, R., Barendregt, J., Mihalopoulos, C., Veerman, J. L., Magnus, A., Cobiac, L., Bertram, M. Y., Wallace, A. L., & ACE–Prevention Team (2010). *Assessing Cost-Effectiveness in Prevention (ACE–Prevention): Final Report*. Melbourne: University of Queensland, Brisbane and Deakin University. public-health.uq.edu.au/assessing-cost-effectiveness-ace-prevention-study

Waters, E., de Silva-Sanigorski, A., Hall, B.J., Brown, T., Campbell, K. J., Gao, Y., Armstrong, R., Prosser, L., & Summerbell, C. D. (2011). *Cochrane Database of Systematic Reviews* 12. doi: 10.1002/14651858.CD001871.pub3

West, F., Sanders, M. R., Cleghorn, G. J., & Davies, P. S. W (2010). Randomised clinical trial of a family-based lifestyle intervention for childhood obesity involving parents as the exclusive agents of change. *Behaviour Research and Therapy* 48: 1170–9.

Zaff, J. F., Moore, K. A., Romano Papillo, A., & Williams, S. (2003). Implications of extracurricular activity participation during adolescence on positive outcomes. *Journal of Adolescent Research* 18: 599–630.

Expansion

19 Targeting Anxiety Sensitivity to Prevent the Development of Psychopathology

Ellen I. Koch, Barry D. Eye, Grant Ellison,
& Bethany Gourley

This chapter focuses on anxiety sensitivity (AS) as a risk factor for psychopathology and a potential target for universal, selective, and indicated prevention interventions. Specifically, this chapter reviews (a) the most prevalent psychological disorders and the burden that these conditions cause for individuals and society; (b) the conceptualizations, etiology, and dimensional properties of AS; (c) the relationship between AS and psychopathology; and (d) treatments affecting or targeting AS. In addition, the chapter provides suggestions for future prevention research. The goal of this chapter is to review the literature related to AS and the ability of this construct to help identify those who are at highest risk for mental health problems and would benefit from prevention and early intervention efforts.

Mental Health

Mental health difficulties, as defined by current diagnostic classification systems (e.g., DSM-5), are present in a significant proportion of the world's population. Based on the Global Burden of Disease Study (2010), it is estimated that mental and substance use disorders (including depressive, anxiety, substance abuse, eating, childhood behavioral, and pervasive developmental disorders) account for 7.4 percent of all mortality and morbidity worldwide (Whiteford et al., 2013). Disorders were classified based on diagnostic criteria and included only twenty major disorders, thereby providing an underestimate of the true global prevalence had other disorders (e.g., personality disorders) been included. Mental and substance use disorders ranked fifth behind cardiovascular/circulatory diseases, infectious diseases, neonatal disorders, and cancer in terms of combined morbidity and mortality, but ranked first in morbidity (22.9 percent) over all other physical health conditions (Whiteford et al., 2013).

The overall burden of the high prevalence of mental health disorders is estimated to be enormous. Of the twenty mental health disorders captured by the estimates in the Global Burden of Disease Study (2010), the highest prevalence rates were for depressive (42.5 percent), anxiety (15.3 percent), drug use (9.4 percent), and alcohol use (7.9 percent) disorders, when considering nonfatal disease burden (Whiteford et al., 2013). This estimate, however, is likely a significant underestimate of the total burden of mental health due to artificially low mortality (zero for almost all mental health disorders) because the cause of death is attributed to the specific (final) physical cause instead of any underlying mental health causes, including suicide.

In addition to the intangible estimates of burden due to disability and life lost, the annual estimated cost of mental health globally is around $2.5 trillion (3.5 percent of the world's gross domestic product), with roughly one-third of that cost consisting of direct treatment and the other two-thirds indirect costs such as lost income and productivity (Bloom et al., 2011). As such, improved treatments are needed for a host of mental health conditions, in formats that are both effective and efficient on a public health scale.

Mental Health Prevention

The Institute of Medicine (IOM: Mrazek & Haggerty, 1994) provided specific definitions for classifying prevention efforts that move beyond the previous labels of primary, secondary, and tertiary prevention. The proposed terms, based on Gordon (1983, 1987), include *universal* (targeting the general public or whole population without utilizing risk factors, similar to primary prevention), *selective* (interventions for individuals with an above-average risk to develop psychopathology), and *indicated* (treating individuals who are assessed as high-risk or who are displaying some symptoms without meeting diagnostic criteria for a disorder; generally, this involves early intervention). In addition to these three types of prevention, the IOM system has two levels of treatment that involve *case identification* and *standard treatment for known disorders* (similar to tertiary prevention) and two levels of maintenance covering *compliance with long-term treatment* and *after-care* (including rehabilitation; Mrazek & Haggerty, 1994).

Anxiety Sensitivity

AS is a construct that was originally identified by Reiss and McNally (1985) to represent the *fear of fear* and includes arousal-related thoughts and sensations (not the triggering stimuli) that arise from beliefs that these symptoms have adverse consequences such as death, insanity, or negative evaluation (Taylor & Fedoroff, 1999). As anxiety elevations become clinically significant, they can degrade performance and interfere with functioning. Sensitivity to anxiety can compound fear responding, increasing total anxiety experienced to severe levels.

The fear of fear is an idea that has been considered from multiple viewpoints within psychology, among them a behavioral model based on interoceptive conditioning (Goldstein & Chambless, 1978), a cognitive model focused on catastrophic misinterpretation of internal stimuli (Clark, 1986), and a trait characteristic conceptualization (the original coining of the term *anxiety sensitivity*; Reiss & McNally, 1985).

Conceptualizations

The earliest conceptualization of the fear of fear was formulated by Goldstein and Chambless (1978). They proposed that agoraphobia is a fear of fear, rather than a fear of public places, and posited that it may develop via a respondent conditioning process. They argued that experiencing a panic attack could sensitize people to related internal sensations (i.e., interoceptive experiences) via respondent conditioning. This associative learning then causes people to begin to interpret the internal sensations as cues for upcoming panic attacks, which then generates significant anxiety and, like a self-fulfilling prophecy, ends up triggering another attack. Critics of this model state that the theory conflates stimuli and responses and overpredicts panic attacks (McNally, 1999).

Clark (1986) proposed a cognitive model that focused on a person's *perception* of their reactions to stimuli, rather than their reactions or the original stimuli themselves. In this model, catastrophic misinterpretation of bodily sensations causes an overreaction that escalates in a positive feedback loop and culminates in a panic attack. Specifically, stimuli trigger catastrophic thoughts, which provoke anxiety, which produces anxious sensations, which are perceived as evidence of catastrophe, which escalates anxiety further, . . . and so on until panic ensues. Critics of this model, however, have shown that panic attacks can occur without precursor misinterpretations (Rachman, Lopatka, & Levitt, 1988).

A third model of the fear of fear proposed a construct, AS, which was conceptualized as an individual difference variable that is related to, but distinct from, trait anxiety (McNally, 1999). Whereas trait anxiety is the tendency toward fearful responding to stimuli, AS represents a person's fear of anxiety symptoms. The potential origins of this enduring tendency to react negatively to a severe extent toward such experiences included inherited disposition (Stein & Rapee, 1999) and cognitive behavioral learning mechanisms, such as conditioning, modeling, or even through verbal discussion (McNally, 1999).

Etiology

Three types of conditioning – respondent, operant, and vicarious (i.e., learning by observing a model) – have all been investigated as causes of AS via learning. Respondent conditioning, typically in a negative reinforcement paradigm (i.e., avoidance behavior leading to the reduction of unwanted symptoms, which then increases the likelihood of future avoidance behavior), was the first to be proposed (e.g., McNally, 2002). In part, this was due to AS's close links to panic phenomenon (and their shared element of misinterpretation of physical symptoms), as well as the significant literature supporting respondent learning of panic responses. However, one early study showed that a majority of participants with high AS were without any historical experience of panic, suggesting that other sources of AS likely exist (Donnell & McNally, 1990). Subsequent studies have found potential links between operant learning and AS. For instance, one investigation found a significant correlation between parental reinforcement of sick-role behavior related to somatic symptoms and higher levels of AS (Watt, Stewart, & Cox, 1998). Similar results have been shown for vicarious learning, with studies showing relationships between high levels of AS and social learning of arousal reactions, such as parent-modeled hypochondriasis (Watt & Stewart, 2000). Other studies, using sophisticated statistical analyses, have found that learning history (both operant and vicarious) appears to relate directly to high levels of AS, and high AS influences panic attack frequency above and beyond learning history in young adulthood (Stewart et al., 2001).

Attachment has also been investigated as a way AS can be learned. One form of attachment, insecure attachment (generally associated with psychopathology), has been found to correlate with higher levels of AS. For example, in one study a sample of high school and undergraduate students showed significantly higher levels of AS in those characterized by insecure attachment compared to secure, and even dismissing attachment styles (Weems, Berman, Silverman, & Rodriguez, 2002).

Parallel lines of research have investigated the heritability of AS and found that it does appear to have genetic contributions, though the exact mechanisms are yet unknown. For example, the initial study into the heritability of AS found higher correspondence in levels of AS in identical twins compared to fraternal twins (Stein, Jang, & Livesley, 1999). Their data suggested that roughly half of the variation in AS could be explained by genetic factors, but that this was only true in women. Subsequent studies have replicated and extended these findings, again showing gender differences with significant heritability in women and a complex relationship between genetics and AS severity, in which more severe AS may be genetically different from mild AS (Taylor, Jang, Stewart, & Stein, 2008). Multiple studies have also shown interaction effects between specific genotypes linked to mood and anxiety psychopathology and childhood maltreatment or trauma exposure that are related to high levels of AS in both males and females (Stein, Schork, & Gelernter, 2008).

Dimensional Properties of Anxiety Sensitivity

Originally, AS was viewed as a unitary construct (Reiss, Peterson, Gursky, & McNally, 1986) associated with behaviors that are experienced and carried out to escape and avoid anxious arousal. Accordingly, Reiss (1980, 1991) outlined the expectancy model, which included sensitivity to anxiety, negative evaluation, and injury/illness as the three fundamental fears contributing to anxiety. Of the three sensitivities in the expectancy model, AS has been studied extensively. Reiss et al. (1986) developed the Anxiety Sensitivity Index (ASI), a self-report questionnaire, to measure this construct. A similar measure, the Childhood Anxiety Sensitivity Index (CASI; Silverman, Fleisig, Rabian, & Peterson, 1991), was created to assess AS in children.

However, early studies into the factor structure of the ASI found varying results, including evidence of one to as many as four factors (see Zinbarg, Mohlman, & Hong, 1999, for a thorough review of the early factor analytic studies) without any clear indication of which was the most stable. As a result, Zinbarg et al. (1999) concluded that the ASI is best thought of as a hierarchical model, with three lower-order factors (physical, cognitive, and social) loading on a general higher-order AS construct.

Based on the accumulating evidence, Taylor and Cox (1998a, b) developed multidimensional scales of AS. Two longer measures of AS, the Anxiety Sensitivity Index-Revised 36 (ASI-R-36; Taylor & Cox, 1998a) and the Anxiety Sensitivity Profile (ASP; Taylor & Cox, 1998b), were developed to measure secondary factors potentially missed by the ASI. Similarly, the CASI was also revised, based on the ASI-R changes (Muris, 2002). Additionally, Laurent and Stark (1993) created another AS measure for children, Anxiety Sensitivity Index for Children (ASIC), covering physical and cognitive concerns.

The ASI-R-36 and ASP feature one higher-order factor with four lower-order factors, including, for both measures, fears of respiratory symptoms, cardiovascular symptoms, and cognitive dyscontrol, along with fears of publicly observable anxiety reactions (ASI-R only) and gastrointestinal symptoms (ASP only; Taylor & Cox, 1998a, b). Zvolensky et al. (2003) conducted a factor analysis on the ASI-R across six countries, and found the four- (Taylor & Cox, 1998a) and three-factor (Zinbarg et al., 1999) solutions fit the pooled data, but a two-factor solution (somatic and social-cognitive) fit across the data for each country.

Currently, the most prevalent model of AS includes three factors (Taylor et al., 2007): (1) *physical concerns* (physical AS), for example, fear that heart palpitations will lead to cardiac arrest; (2) *cognitive concerns* (cognitive AS), such as, worry that difficulties concentrating are precursors of insanity; and (3) *social concerns* (social AS), for example, concern that publicly observable anxiety will elicit social ridicule and rejection (see Figure 19.1). This current

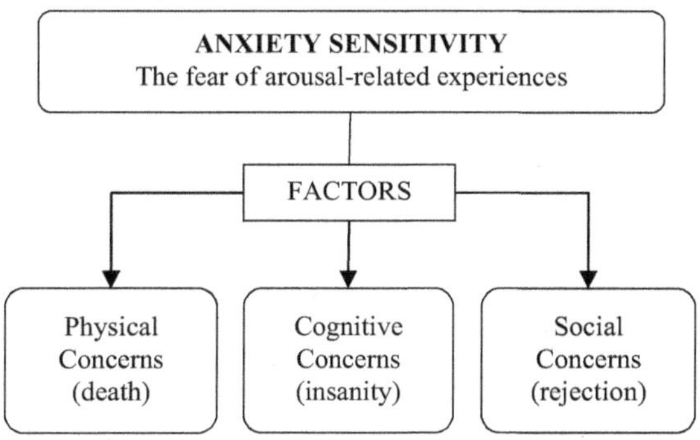

Figure 19.1. *A multidimensional model of anxiety sensitivity (Taylor et al., 2007.)*

factor model is reflected by the most recent measure for AS, the eighteen-item Anxiety Sensitivity Index-3 (ASI-3; Taylor et al., 2007).

Yet, recently taxometric and factor mixed modeling methods have been applied to evaluate the underlying properties of AS. Schmidt, Kotov, Lerew, Joiner, and Ialongo (2006) determined that a very large nonclinical sample demonstrated a taxonic (i.e., categorical) latent cognitive vulnerability for panic based on ASI scores. Bernstein, Zvolensky, Feldner, Lewis, & Leen-Feldner (2005a) identified the taxon of AS based on eight ASI items. The AS taxon demonstrates significant incremental validity over the dimensional full-scale ASI total, suggesting a cognitive vulnerability for adults (e.g., Bernstein et al., 2005a) and children (e.g., Bernstein, Zvolensky, Weems, Stickle, & Leen-Feldner, 2005b). However, other researchers found a dimensional structure for the ASI (Asmundson, Weeks, Carleton, Thibodeau, & Fetzner, 2011) and for the ASP and ASI-R (Broman-Fulks et al., 2008, 2010).

More recently, studies utilizing the ASI-3 suggest a taxon-dimensional structure in that dimensions within the AS taxon are associated with psychopathology (e.g., Bernstein et al., 2010). Factor analytic studies with nonclinically diagnosable or nontreatment-seeking individuals utilizing the ASI-3 have suggested one general overall AS factor and three independent group factors for the three subscales as a better fit than the three-factor model suggested by the developers of the ASI-3 (e.g., Ebesutani, McLeish, Luberto, Young, & Maack, 2013).

Taken together, research findings are inconclusive, although support is emerging for a taxometric-dimensional underlying structure, indicating that the dimensional structure among those with pathological AS (i.e., those possessing the AS taxon) may differ from those without pathological AS (i.e., complement class members). Future research utilizing factor mixture modeling is needed in order to better understand differences in AS in general and effectively target treatments to taxon members.

Despite the significant number of factor analytic studies of AS, further investigation to determine whether the ASI-3 maintains an overall and three independent subfactor structure in clinical populations, as recently demonstrated in nonclinical groups, would help indicate whether the ASI-3 results in a different factor structure compared to previous measures of AS. Additionally, the child measure of AS most widely used is based on the original ASI, and given the differences found across measures of adult AS, a version of the CASI consistent with the ASI-3 (as long as it contains similar strong psychometric properties) will allow for comparison between child/adolescent and adult AS experiences.

Anxiety Sensitivity and Psychopathology

Several psychological diagnoses and physical conditions have been associated with high AS across the various measures for children and adults. Numerous studies have also demonstrated the relationship between psychopathology and symptom clusters of psychological and physical conditions based on the three AS subfactors (see Figure 19.1).

Total Anxiety Sensitivity and Psychopathology

Three meta-analyses, two focused on adult populations and the other on children and adolescents, demonstrate the association between AS total score and anxiety disorders and depression. Olatunji and Wolitzky-Taylor (2009) conducted a meta-analysis of thirty-eight studies utilizing various measures for AS from several prominent databases, where at least one group of participants met diagnostic criteria for a mood or anxiety disorder. They found significantly greater levels of AS among clinically identified people who suffered from anxiety and mood disorders in general and specific anxiety disorders (i.e., panic disorder [PD]; social phobia; posttraumatic stress disorder [PTSD]; and generalized anxiety disorder [GAD]), compared to nonclinical controls. People suffering from anxiety disorders also demonstrated higher AS scores than those suffering from mood disorders, who also had higher scores than nonclinical control groups. However, levels of AS were moderated by gender, age, and assessment measure used in several comparisons (Olatunji & Wolitzky-Taylor, 2009). Another study conducted a meta-analysis of 117 studies, comparing differences on the ASI only for individuals with diagnosed depressive and anxiety disorders. The researcher found the strongest relationships between AS total and PTSD, GAD, and PD; only moderate relationships with depression, social phobia, and obsessive-compulsive disorder (OCD); and weak relationship with specific phobia (Naragon-Gainey, 2010). Finally, Noël and Francis (2011) conducted a meta-analysis for children and adolescents utilizing various measures for AS from fifteen studies and found higher levels of AS for youth with anxiety disorders, compared to nonclinical controls. Youth diagnosed with PD had higher levels of AS over those diagnosed with other anxiety disorders. Additionally, adolescents had a significantly higher correlation between AS and anxiety than children.

In addition to anxiety and mood disorders, elevated levels of AS have also been found for substance use disorders, physical conditions, and eating disorder symptoms. AS has been connected to various addictive behaviors, including use of nicotine, heroin, and alcohol. Recently Leventhal and Zvolensky (2015) presented a model for cigarette smoking that indicates anhedonia (an inability to feel pleasure), AS, and distress tolerance involved in multiple emotional pathologies interacting with smoking behaviors. Specifically, the anxiolytic effects of smoking may be highly negatively reinforcing for individuals with high AS (see Leventhal & Zvolensky, 2015, for a review). Schmidt, Buckner, and Keough (2007a) conducted a two-year prospective study and found both high AS and male gender uniquely associated with the later development of alcohol use disorders. Lejuez, Paulson, Daughters, and Bornovalova (2006) found significantly higher levels of AS, as well as the physical and social subscales, for individuals who utilize heroin over other substances. The authors suggest that for those with elevated AS, perhaps heroin serves an emotion regulation function, the bodily related withdraw symptoms make quitting more difficult, or psychological difficulties may be overrepresented in heroin users (Lejuez et al., 2006).

In terms of physical conditions, Asmundson, Wright, and Hadjistavropoulos (2000) thoroughly reviewed the relationship between elevated levels of AS and chronic health conditions (i.e., gastrointestinal dysfunction, asthma, vestibular dysfunction, and pain). They found that some chronic health conditions (functional dyspepsia, asthma in children, vertigo, etc.) are related to elevated levels of AS above the mean for the normal population (Asmundson et al., 2000). A meta-analysis of the connection between AS and chronic pain, utilizing forty-one studies of both clinical and nonclinical pain, indicated that elevated levels of AS are strongly associated with a greater fear of pain (Ocañez, McHugh, & Otto, 2010). High levels of AS are also associated with hypochondriasis and health anxiety, even after controlling for depression and negative affect, in a nonclinical sample (Olatunji et al., 2009).

In addition AS's association with physical conditions, Anestis, Holm-Denoma, Gordon, Schmidt, and Joiner (2008) found that AS is significantly related to eating disorder symptoms (i.e., bulimia and drive for thinness). Specifically, bulimia symptoms were mediated by interoceptive awareness in a clinical sample of college students after controlling for depression, anxiety, and impulsivity.

Finally, based on expectancy theory (Reiss, 1991), a recent study (Capron, Norr, & Schmidt, 2013) found that when controlling for gender and anxiety symptom severity, AS is significantly associated with the number of anxiety disorder diagnoses but not the number of nonanxiety disorder diagnoses (mood, substance use, eating, and somatoform). Capron et al. (2013) suggest that this study supports expectancy theory, in that higher levels of AS are associated with more anxiety comorbidity among individuals with anxiety disorder diagnoses; namely, that AS serves as a transdiagnostic factor, given the elevated levels across anxiety diagnoses.

Altogether, the accumulating findings regarding the association between AS total score and both psychopathology and physical health conditions have led researchers to explore the contribution of each of the AS subfactors (physical, social, and cognitive) to the emergence of these disorders.

Anxiety Sensitivity Subfactors and Psychopathology

Recently the subfactors of ASI-3 have also been connected to psychological disorders or symptoms within clinical samples. Specifically, for adults, a high physical subfactor is uniquely associated with PD, specific phobia diagnoses, and OCD symptoms while a low physical subfactor is related to a social phobia diagnosis (Allan, Capron, Raines, & Schmidt, 2014a). A high cognitive subfactor has consistently been related to GAD/worry and depression symptoms and diagnoses, PTSD diagnosis, OCD symptoms, and suicide ideation (Allan et al., 2014a). The social subfactor is associated with social phobia symptoms and diagnosis as well as symptoms of worry/GAD, OCD, and depression (Allan, 2014a). Capron, Cougle, Ribeiro, Joiner, and Schmidt (2012) found the interaction of high cognitive and low physical subscale scores significantly increased the likelihood for prior suicide attempts in outpatients with PTSD symptoms and suicide ideation prospectively in military cadets completing basic training.

In terms of the CASI for children and adolescents, high scores on the physical subfactor were significantly associated with the other six diagnoses measured (GAD, social phobia, physical fears, PD/agoraphobia, separation anxiety, and OCD) even when controlling for trait anxiety (McLaughlin, Stewart, & Taylor, 2007). The cognitive factor accounted for variance in PD/agoraphobia, separation anxiety, and OCD while the social factor was associated with GAD, social phobia, and physical injury fears (McLaughlin et al., 2007). This study found that the CASI total score was associated with all six diagnoses as well.

Interaction with Other Constructs

While elevated levels of AS total and subscale scores are related to various psychological disorders and physical conditions, several studies indicate that it is not the AS level by itself but rather that other related constructs are also involved, such as difficulties with emotion regulation and distress tolerance. Specifically, emotion regulation accounted for panic attack severity (not frequency) more than the ASI-R subfactors (Tull, 2006); PTSD, in a substance-dependent population, more than ASI-R social factor (McDermott, Tull, Gratz, Daughters, & Lejuez, 2009); and GAD (along with gender and panic disorder status) more than ASI physical and cognitive subscales (Tull, Stipelman, Salters-Pedneault, & Gratz, 2009). Two recent studies have looked at interaction effects of AS and emotion regulation with worry, panic, and social anxiety symptoms (Allan, Norr, Macatee, Gajewska, & Schmidt, 2015) and comorbid PTSD and alcohol dependence (Sippel et al., 2015). These explorations indicated that and found AS and emotion regulation interact most strongly at low levels, but not when either the AS or the emotion regulation is high. Given the overlap between emotion regulation and AS, further investigation of how these constructs interact in different populations could help identify the most appropriate prevention treatment to pursue.

Along with emotion regulation, distress tolerance has also been linked to AS (Leyro, Zvolensky, & Bernstein, 2010). Similar to the interaction with emotion regulation, low levels of distress tolerance or high levels of AS weakened the effect of the other risk factor for worry, GAD, and major depressive disorder (Allan, Macatee, Norr, & Schmidt, 2014b). It should be noted that the findings regarding the singular role of AS, in comparison to other aforementioned variables, are inconsistent. For example, Bernstein, Zvolensky, Vujanovic, and Moos (2009) completed an exploratory factor analysis and determined that AS and distress tolerance are related lower-order factors to an overall distress and sensitivity factor. However, Mitchell, Riccardi, Keough, Timpano, and Schmidt (2013) conducted a confirmatory factor analysis and found AS to be a component of distress tolerance for both clinical and nonclinical samples. Thus, further conceptual and empirical discriminant analyses of AS and distress tolerance are needed. This is particularly important in light of the prevalence and burden of these conditions and potential impact of transdiagnostic interventions.

Intervention for Anxiety Sensitivity

Treatment research involving AS followed a similar path to theoretical research; namely, initially AS was indirectly investigated alongside psychopathology and eventually became a direct focus of interventions that address indicated prevention.

Indirect Intervention Research

The earliest treatment research showing improvements in AS levels did not target AS directly; instead, the improvements were coincident to changes in symptoms of disorders that were the actual targets of interventions. For instance, multiple studies targeting PD have shown parallel recovery alongside reductions in AS levels compared to controls (see Otto & Reilly-Harrington, 1999, for a review). Ollendick (1995), utilizing a multiple baseline across participants design, found similar results with adolescents. Next, AS was examined in relation to changes in target symptoms of disorders. For instance, one study showed reductions in key panic symptoms as a result of reducing overall fear of fear (Smits, Powers, Cho, & Telch, 2004).

Direct Interventions to Reduce Anxiety Sensitivity

Gradually, AS has been established as a clinical variable of interest, demonstrating some role related to clinical disorders. Following that, researchers began interventions targeting AS directly. Given the relationship between AS and PD, initial interventions utilized cognitive-behavior therapy (CBT) to treat AS (e.g., Barry, Tart, & Powers, Smits, 2008b). The most common components include (a) psychoeducation regarding the development and maintenance of AS and the impact on anxiety and related symptoms and (b) some form of interoceptive exposure involving direct confrontation of physiological/anxiety sensations leading to habituation.

Advanced AS interventions include active treatment components such as interoceptive exposure (e.g., Vujanovic, Bernstein, Berenz, & Zvolensky, 2012), relaxation training (e.g., Kenardy, McCafferty, & Rosa, 2003), psychoeducation (Schmidt et al., 2007b), cognitive restructuring (e.g., Watt, Stewart, Lefaivre, & Uman, 2006), motivational enhancement (e.g., Korte & Schmidt,

2013b), and relapse prevention (e.g., Kenardy et al., 2003) to sustain intervention gains. Some dismantling studies have compared psychoeducation, interoceptive exposure, and/or cognitive restructuring components to control conditions to determine the most efficacious treatment components. For example, one study found that even a single fifty-minute session including psychoeducation and interoceptive exposure techniques showed significant reductions in AS compared to a physical health education control group, with results maintained at a six-month follow-up (Keough & Schmidt, 2012). In another study, a computerized intervention, involving psychoeducation and interoceptive exposure, targeted AS cognitive concerns specifically in a sample of veterans and civilians with various conditions including anxiety, PTSD, and depression (Mitchell, Capron, Raines, & Schmidt, 2014). Cognitive AS and PTSD symptom severity were successfully reduced in both groups compared to the health-information control condition at one-month follow-up, with no differences between veteran and civilian participants.

Overall, AS appears to be amenable to direct treatment, with large effect sizes for treatment-seeking samples (g = 1.40) and moderate to large effect sizes for at-risk samples (g = 0.74; Smits, Berry, Tart, & Powers, 2008b). Studies have shown improvements in AS whether the control group involved waitlist (e.g., Gardenswartz & Craske, 2001), minimal contact (e.g., Broman-Fulks & Storey, 2008), or psychological placebo (e.g., Schmidt et al., 2007a, b). Furthermore, improvements in AS levels due to treatment have been maintained through follow-up periods, with long-term outcomes maintained as far as two years post-intervention (Schmidt et al., 2007b).

More recently, modern transdiagnostic approaches such as the Unified Protocol (e.g., Boswell et al., 2013) and motivational enhancement techniques such as Motivational Interviewing (e.g., Korte, Brown, & Schmidt, 2013) have successfully reduced AS across anxiety disorders and depression. Specifically, the Unified Protocol involves the following modules: motivational enhancement, psychoeducation and tracking of emotions, emotional awareness, cognitive reappraisal, reduction of emotional and behavioral avoidance, awareness and tolerance of physical sensations, interoceptive and situational exposure, and relapse prevention (Barlow et al., 2011). Although CBT transdiagnostic treatment approaches demonstrate preliminary evidence for anxiety disorders and depression, more research with larger sample sizes is still needed (Rector, Man, & Lerman, 2014), as well as efficacy studies utilizing these approaches targeting AS specifically.

Intervention Design Variation

Intervention studies targeting AS have had significant variation in their design and structure, including targeting both individuals (e.g., Capron, Norr, Zvolensky, & Schmidt, 2014) and groups (e.g., Watt et al., 2006). They have been delivered in person as traditional psychotherapy (e.g., Boswell et al., 2013), guided exercise (e.g., Broman-Fulks, Berman, Rabian, & Webster, 2004), workshop interventions (e.g., Gardenswartz & Craske, 2001), video or PowerPoint presentations (Schmidt et al., 2007a, b; Keough & Schmidt, 2012), and computer-delivered interventions (e.g., Mitchell et al., 2014). They have also been delivered remotely in the form of telephone-delivered psychotherapy (Olthuis, Watt, Mackinnon, & Stewart, 2014), computer-delivered interventions over the Internet (e.g., Kenardy et al., 2003), and via a self-help manual (Watt & Stewart, 2008). Interventions have been as long as eighteen weekly, sixty-minute sessions (e.g., Boswell et al., 2013) and as brief as a single, fifty-minute intervention (e.g., Keough & Schmidt, 2012). AS has been significantly reduced within a number of treatment modalities and levels of intervention intensity and typically involves psychoeducation, interoceptive exposure, and relapse prevention components.

Diversity of Target Populations

AS interventions have also been used on a range of populations including nonclinically diagnosed college students (e.g., Kenardy et al., 2003) and those with identified psychopathology. Investigations of groups with identified psychological disorders have included community members seeking treatment for anxiety or mood disorders (e.g., Boswell et al., 2013) as well as veterans with PTSD (e.g., Mitchell et al., 2014). Notably absent from the AS intervention literature is a study targeting AS directly in children or adolescents. To date, AS has only been measured in a multiple baseline treatment study targeting PD in four adolescents (Ollendick, 1995). This lack of AS-related studies among children and adolescents especially needs to be addressed in light of the already existing theory and scales dealing with AS among children and youth and significant support for CBT approaches with children that parallel adult populations.

Prevention-Focused Treatment

In light of the growing attention that AS gets, as a significant psychological construct by itself, one would expect researchers and practitioners, in the field of prevention related to mental health disorders, to draw more attention to AS, both as a potential moderator variable as well as a goal for direct prevention efforts. Recent AS intervention studies have started to target individuals at high risk to develop psychopathology with indicated prevention. At-risk groups have included general samples with elevated AS levels recruited from college students (e.g., Keough & Schmidt, 2012) and the community (e.g., Smits et al. 2008a) alongside specific groups that research shows are at risk for psychopathology, such as smokers (e.g., Capron, Norr, Zvolensky, & Schmidt, 2014) and victims of multiple traumatic events (e.g., Vujanovic et al., 2012). The two main components of indicated prevention programs targeting AS are psychoeducation and interoceptive exposure, but other interventions (e.g., transdiagnostic and motivational approaches) may also prove useful. Although these indicated prevention studies have shown efficacy even with only one session, utilization of universal prevention approaches is lacking.

Huberty (2012) identified nine principles for effective prevention programs, including (1) comprehensiveness, (2) varied teaching methods, (3) sufficient dosage, (4) theory-driven programs, (5) positive relationships, (6) appropriate timing, (7) sociocultural relevance, (8) outcome evaluation, and (9) well-trained staff. The use of prevention interventions should incorporate these nine principles. Additionally, intervention should occur at the universal, selective, and indicated levels given the prevalence of elevated AS in the general population and the relationship between AS and common psychological disorders that are burdensome and problematic for individuals. Investigating the most effective timing for indicated, selective, and universal prevention interventions could outline when individuals are most likely to benefit from prevention, either prior to developing any symptoms or when more motivated to address an emerging difficulty. Finally, prevention interventions should track diagnostic status at follow-up to determine whether treatment produced the intended prevention of psychopathology. A large-scale, longitudinal study, comparing a group receiving one of the brief, convenient treatments with empirical support (e.g., the one-hour computer protocol by Keough & Schmidt, 2012) with a control group would demonstrate directly the importance of AS for prevention.

Universal prevention interventions. Considering universal prevention interventions could be beneficial in potentially reducing stigma involved with psychopathology or singling out individuals for selective or indicated interventions since these would be applied broadly at the population level. One particular challenge with universal prevention interventions could be having individuals motivated to participate particularly when they are not experiencing problematic symptoms. Motivational enhancement therapy (Miller, Zweben, DiClemente, & Rychtarik, 1999) is effective as an adjunct to AS-targeted treatment for increasing motivation for treatment (Korte & Schmidt, 2015) as well as a stand-alone intervention for reducing AS (Korte & Schmidt, 2013b). Adding motivation enhancement procedures before the universal intervention may increase motivation, compliance, and possibly treatment outcome. Accordingly, Korte and Schmidt (2013a) found that providing feedback on high-risk status for psychopathology, based on AS scores, produces significant increases in confidence and importance of changing their anxiety. Although feedback was provided to participants with elevated levels of AS, the ability for generic high-risk feedback to improve motivation for change within individuals who have yet to develop high AS could be valuable for effective universal interventions.

Indicated prevention interventions. In terms of future research focused on improving treatment of AS, an increased focus on indicated early interventions for those with elevated AS can provide a particularly efficient intervention to prevent, or at least delay, the development of psychopathology or problematic responses to chronic health conditions. Given that brief treatments are available targeting AS directly, determining how best to administer these treatments in the most cost-efficient and effective manner for individuals across diverse cultures will inform indicated intervention programs. Additionally, despite a significant amount of research focused on adults with elevated AS, very little research has been conducted to address elevated AS in children and adolescents. Selective or indicated prevention efforts could involve the development of interventions directly created for children and adolescents informed from the effective treatment components in adult AS indicated prevention programs.

Another focus of intervention could involve targeting elevated AS subfactors with treatment matching (i.e., interoceptive exposure for those with high physical AS and cognitive restructuring for high cognitive AS) may produce an efficient way to reduce AS. Additionally, comparing interoceptive exposure to acceptance-based approaches may help determine which prevention efforts could be most beneficial to particular individuals and under which conditions.

Summary

A significant amount of research has been conducted related to AS in terms of assessment, prediction, and treatment. As a result of the extensive amount of this research, AS is a significant risk factor for the development of psychopathology, particularly those disorders that are emotion-based, in addition to having a negative impact on chronic health conditions.

Despite the significant amount of research available regarding AS, additional focus on assessment of AS could improve prevention of psychopathology. Given the concerns with relying solely on self-report measures, other multimodal options with strong psychometric properties would contribute significantly to the assessment of AS.

Finally, assessing the impact of AS within multicultural and international samples will significantly improve our understanding of potentially common and culturally unique mental health experiences. Despite measure validation studies being conducted in various countries, little is known about similarities and differences in AS total and subscale scores across cultures.

Efficacy research has found several brief interventions that reduce AS and subsequently delays or prevents the development of psychopathology. Future research should continue to focus on improving prevention efforts and determining whether universal, selective, or indicated prevention provides the most effective and efficient means of addressing elevated AS.

References

Allan, N. P., Capron, D. W., Raines, A. M., & Schmidt, N. B. (2014a). Unique relations among anxiety sensitivity factors and anxiety, depression, and suicidal ideation. *Journal of Anxiety Disorders* 28: 266–75. doi: 10.1016/j.janxdis.2013.12.004

Allan, N. P., Macatee, R. J., Norr, A. M., & Schmidt, N. B. (2014b). Direct and interactive effects of distress tolerance and anxiety sensitivity on generalized anxiety and depression. *Cognitive Therapy and Research* 38: 530–40. doi: 10.1007/s10608-014–9623-y

Allan, N. P., Norr, A. M., Macatee, R. J., Gajewska, A., & Schmidt, N. B. (2015). Interactive effects of anxiety sensitivity and emotion regulation on anxiety symptoms. *Journal of Psychopathology and Behavioral Assessment*. Advance online publication. dx.doi.org/10.1007/s10862-015–9484-z

Anestis, M. D., Holm-Denoma, J. M., Gordon, K. H., Schmidt, N. B., & Joiner, T. E. (2008). The role of anxiety sensitivity in eating pathology. *Cognitive Therapy and Research* 32: 370–85. doi:1 0.1007/s10608-006–9085-y

Asmundson, G. J. G., Weeks, J. W., Carleton, R. N., Thibodeau, M. A, & Fetzner, M. G. (2011). Revisiting the latent structure of the anxiety sensitivity construct: more evidence of dimensionality. *Journal of Anxiety Disorders* 25: 138–47. doi: 10.1016/j.janxdis.2010.08.013

Asmundson, G. J. G., Wright, K. D., & Hadjistavropoulos, H. D. (2000). Anxiety sensitivity and disabling chronic health conditions state of the art and future directions. *Scandinavian Journal of Behaviour Therapy* 29: 100–17. doi: 10.1080/028457100300049719

Barlow, D. H., Farchione, T. J., Fairholme, C. P., Ellard, K. K., Boisseau, C. L., Allen, L. B., & Ehrenreich-May, J. T. (2011). *Unified Protocol for Transdiagnostic Treatment of Emotional Disorders: Therapist Guide*. New York: Oxford University Press.

Bernstein, A., Stickle, T. R., Zvolensky, M. J., Taylor, S., Abramowitz, J., & Stewart, S. (2010). Dimensional, categorical, or dimensional-categories: testing the latent structure of anxiety sensitivity among adults using factor-mixture modeling. *Behavior Therapy* 41: 515–29. doi: 10.1016/j.beth.2010.02.003

Bernstein, A., Zvolensky, M. J., Feldner, M. T., Lewis, S. F., & Leen-Feldner, E. W. (2005a). Anxiety sensitivity taxonicity: a concurrent test of cognitive vulnerability for post-traumatic stess symptomatology among young adults. *Cognitive Behaviour Therapy* 34: 229–41. doi: 10.1080/16506070510041176

Bernstein, A., Zvolensky, M. J., Vujanovic, A. A., & Moos, R. (2009). Integrating anxiety sensitivity, distress tolerance, and discomfort intolerance: a hierarchical model of affect sensitivity and tolerance. *Behavior Therapy* 40: 291–301. doi: 10.1016/j.beth.2008.08.001

Bernstein, A., Zvolensky, M. J., Weems, C., Stickle, T., & Leen-Feldner, E. W. (2005b). Taxonicity of anxiety sensitivity: an empirical test among youth. *Behaviour Research and Therapy* 43: 1131–55. doi: 10.1016/j.brat.2004.07.008

Bloom, D. E., Cafiero, E. T., Jané-Llopis, E., Abrahams-Gessel, S., Bloom, L. R., … Weinstein, C. (2011). *The Global Economic Burden of Non-communicable Diseases*. Geneva, Switzerland: World Economic Forum. www.weforum.org/reports/global-economic-burden-non-communicable-diseases

Boswell, J. F., Farchione, T. J., Sauer-Zavala, S., Murray, H. W., Fortune, M. R., & Barlow, D. H. (2013). Anxiety sensitivity and interoceptive exposure: a transdiagnostic construct and change strategy. *Behavior Therapy* 44(3): 417–31. doi: 10.1016/j.beth.2013.03.006

Broman-Fulks, J. J., Berman, M. E., Rabian, B. A., & Webster, M. J. (2004). Effects of aerobic exercise on anxiety sensitivity. *Behaviour Research and Therapy* 42: 125–36. doi: 10.1016/S0005-7967(03)00103–7

Broman-Fulks, J. J., Deacon, B. J., Olatunji, B. O., Bondy, C. L., Abramowitz, J. S., & Tolin, D. F. (2010). Categorical or dimensional: a reanalysis of the anxiety sensitivity construct. *Behavior Therapy* 41: 154–71. doi: 10.1016/j.beth.2009.02.005

Broman-Fulks, J. J., Green, B. A., Olatunji, B. O., Berman, M. E., Arnau, R. C., Deacon, B. J., & Sawchuk, C. N. (2008). The latent structure of anxiety sensitivity – revisited. *Assessment* 15: 188–203. doi: 10.1177/1073191107311284

Broman-Fulks, J. J., & Storey, K. M. (2008). Evaluation of a brief aerobic exercise intervention for high anxiety sensitivity. *Anxiety, Stress, and Coping* 21: 117–28. doi: 10.1080/10615800701762675

Capron, D. W., Cougle, J. R., Ribeiro, J. D., Joiner, T. E., & Schmidt, N. B. (2012). An interactive model of anxiety sensitivity relevant to suicide attempt history and future suicidal ideation. *Journal of Psychiatric Research* 46: 174–80. doi: 10.1016.j.psychires.2011.10.009

Capron, D. W., Norr, A. M., & Schmidt, N. B. (2013). Risk of co-occurring psychopathology: testing a prediction of expectancy theory. *Journal of Anxiety Disorders* 27: 79–83. doi: 10.1016/j.janxdis.2012.10.011

Capron, D. W., Norr, A. M., Zvolensky, M. J., & Schmidt, N. B. (2014). Prospective evaluation of the effect of an anxiety sensitivity intervention on suicidality among smokers. *Cognitive Behaviour Therapy* 43: 72–82. doi: 10.1080/16506073.2013.777466

Clark, D. M. (1986). A cognitive approach to panic. *Behaviour Research and Therapy* 24: 461–70. doi: 10.1016/0005–7967(86)90011-2

Donnell, C. D., & McNally, R. J. (1990). Anxiety sensitivity and panic attacks in a nonclinical population. *Behavior Research and Therapy* 28: 83–5. doi: 10.1016/0005–7967(90)90058-Q

Ebesutani, C., McLeish, A. C., Luberto, C. M., Young, J., & Maack, D. J. (2013). A bifactor model of anxiety sensitivity: analysis of the Anxiety Sensitivity Index-3. *Journal of Psychopathology and Behavioral Assessment* 36: 452–64. doi: 10.1007/s10862-013–9400-3

Gardenswartz, C. A., & Craske, M. G. (2001). Prevention of panic disorder. *Behavior Therapy* 32: 725–37. doi: 10.1016/S0005-7894(01)80017-4

Goldstein, A. J., & Chambless, D. L. (1978). A reanalysis of agoraphobia. *Behavior Therapy* 9: 47–59. doi: 10.1016/S0005-7894(78)80053-7

Gordon, R. (1983). An operational classification of disease prevention. *Public Health Reports* 98: 107–9.

Gordon, R. (1987). An operational classification of disease prevention. In Steinberg, J. A., & Silverman, M. M. (eds.), *Preventing Mental Disorders*. Rockville, MD: Department of Health and Human Services, pp. 20–6.

Huberty, T. J. (2012). Building resilience through prevention. In *Anxiety and Depression in Children and Adolescents: Assessment, Intervention, and Prevention*. New York: Springer, pp. 345–68.

Kenardy, J., McCafferty, K., & Rosa, V. (2003). Internet-delivered indicated prevention for anxiety disorders: a randomized controlled trial. *Behavioural and Cognitive Psychotherapy* 31: 279–89. doi: 10.1017/S1352465803003047

Keough, M. E., & Schmidt, N. B. (2012). Refinement of a brief anxiety sensitivity reduction intervention. *Journal of Consulting and Clinical Psychology* 80: 766–72. doi: 10.1037/a0027961

Korte, K. J., Brown, M.-A. S., & Schmidt, N. B. (2013). Anxiety sensitivity and impairment: evidence for a direct association and partial mediation by subclinical anxiety symptoms. *Journal of Affective Disorders* 151: 875–81. doi: 10.1016/j.jad.2013.07.026

Korte, K. J., & Schmidt, N. B. (2013a). High-risk feedback: a brief intervention to increase motivation to change anxiety. *Cognitive Therapy and Research* 37: 332–39. doi: 10.1007/s10608-012–9464-5

Korte, K. J., & Schmidt, N. B. (2013b). Motivational enhancement therapy reduces anxiety sensitivity. *Cognitive Therapy and Research* 37(6): 1140–50. doi: 10.1007/s10608-013–9550-3

Korte, K. J., & Schmidt, N. B. (2015). The use of motivation enhancement therapy to increase utilization of a preventative intervention for anxiety sensitivity. *Cognitive Therapy and Research* 39: 520–30. doi: 10.1007/s10608-014–9668-y

Laurent, J., & Stark, K. D. (1993). Testing the cognitive content-specificity hypothesis with anxious and depressed youngsters. *Journal of Abnormal Psychology* 102: 226–37. doi: 10.1037/0021–843x.102.2.226

Lejuez, C. W., Paulson, A., Daughters, S. B., & Bornovalova, M. A. (2006). The association between heroin use and anxiety sensitivity among inner-city individuals in residential drug use treatment. *Behavior Research & Therapy* 44: 667–77. doi: 10.1016/j.brat.2005.04.006

Leventhal, A. M., & Zvolensky, M. J. (2015). Anxiety, depression, and cigarette smoking: a transdiagnostic vulnerability framework to understanding emotion – smoking comorbidity. *Psychological Bulletin* 141: 176–212. doi: 10.1037/bul0000003

Leyro, T. M., Zvolensky, M. J., & Bernstein, A. (2010). Distress tolerance and psychopathological symptoms and disorders: a review of the empirical literature among adults. *Psychological Bulletin* 136: 576–600. doi: 10.1037/a0019712

McDermott, M. J., Tull, M. T., Gratz, K. L., Daughters, S. B., & Lejuez, C. W. (2009). The role of anxiety sensitivity and difficulties in emotion regulation in posttraumatic stress disorder among crack/cocaine dependent patients in residential substance abuse treatment. *Journal of Anxiety Disorders* 23: 591–9. doi: 10.1016/j.janxdis.2009.01.006

McLaughlin, E. N., Stewart, S. H., & Taylor, S. (2007). Childhood Anxiety Sensitivity Index factors predict unique variance in DSM-IV anxiety disorder symptoms. *Cognitive Behaviour Therapy* 36: 210–19. doi: 10.1080/16506070701499988

McNally, R. J. (1999). Theoretical approaches to the fear of anxiety. In Taylor, S. (ed.), *Anxiety Sensitivity: Theory, Research, and Treatment of the Fear of Anxiety*. Mahwah, NJ: Lawrence Erlbaum, pp. 3–16.

McNally, R. J. (2002). Anxiety sensitivity and panic disorder. *Biological Psychiatry* 52: 938–46. doi: 10.1016/S0006-3223(02)01475-0

Miller, W. R., Zweben, A., DiClemente, C. C., & Rychtarik, R. G. (1999). *Motivational Enhancement Therapy Manual: A Clinical Research Guide for Therapists Treating Individuals with Alcohol Abuse and Dependence (NIH Publication No. 94-3723)*. Rockville, MD: U.S. Department of Health and Human Services.

Mitchell, M. A., Capron, D. W., Raines, A. M., & Schmidt, N. B. (2014). Reduction of cognitive concerns of anxiety sensitivity is uniquely associated with reduction of PTSD and depressive symptoms: a comparison of civilians and veterans. *Journal of Psychiatric Research* 48: 25–31. doi: 10.1016/j.jpsychires.2013.10.013

Mitchell, M. A., Riccardi, C. J., Keough, M. E., Timpano, K. R., & Schmidt, N. B. (2013). Understanding the associations among anxiety sensitivity, distress tolerance, and discomfort intolerance: a comparison of three models. *Journal of Anxiety Disorders* 27: 147–54. doi: 10.1016/j.janxdis.2012.12.003

Mrazek, P. J., & Haggerty, R. J. (1994). *Reducing Risks for Mental Disorders: Frontiers for Preventive Intervention Research*. Washington, DC: National Academy Press.

Muris, P. (2002). An expanded Childhood Anxiety Sensitivity Index: its factor structure, reliability, and validity in a non-clinical adolescent sample. *Behaviour Research and Therapy* 40: 299–311. doi: 10.1016/S0005-7967(00)00112–1

Naragon-Gainey, K. (2010). Meta-analysis of the relations of anxiety sensitivity to the depressive and anxiety disorders. *Psychological Bulletin* 136: 128–50. doi: 10.1037/a0018055

Noël, V. A., & Francis, S. E. (2011). A meta-analytic review of the role of child anxiety sensitivity in child anxiety. *Journal of Abnormal Child Psychology* 39: 721–33. doi: 10.1007/s10802-011–9489-3

Ocañez, K. L. S., McHugh, R. K., & Otto, M. W. (2010). A meta-analytic review of the association between anxiety sensitivity and pain. *Depression and Anxiety* 27: 760–7. www.ncbi.nlm.nih.gov/pubmed/20336798

Olatunji, B. O., & Wolitzky-Taylor, K. B. (2009). Anxiety sensitivity and the anxiety disorders: a meta-analytic review and synthesis. *Psychological Bulletin* 135: 974–99. doi: 10.1037/a0017428

Olatunji, B. O., Wolitzky-Taylor, K. B., Elwood, L., Connolly, K., Gonzales, B., & Armstrong, T. (2009). Anxiety sensitivity and health anxiety in a nonclinical sample: specificity and prospective relations with clinical stress. *Cognitive Therapy and Research* 33: 416–24. doi: 10.1007/s10608-008–9188-8

Ollendick, T. H. (1995). Cognitive behavioral treatment of panic disorder with agoraphobia in adolescents: a multiple baseline design analysis. *Behavior Therapy* 26: 517–31. doi: 10.1016/S0005-7894(05)80098-X

Olthuis, J. V, Watt, M. C., Mackinnon, S. P., & Stewart, S. H. (2014). Telephone-delivered cognitive behavioral therapy for high anxiety sensitivity: a randomized controlled trial. *Journal of Consulting and Clinical Psychology* 82: 1005–22. doi: 10.1037/a0037027

Otto, M. W., & Reilly-Harrington, N. A. (1999). The impact of treatment on anxiety sensitivity. In Taylor, S. (ed.), *Anxiety Sensitivity: Theory, Research, and Treatment of the Fear of Anxiety*. Mahwah, NJ: Lawrence Erlbaum, pp. 321–36.

Rachman, S., Lopatka, C., & Levitt, K. (1988). Experimental analysis of panic – II. Panic patients. *Behaviour Research and Therapy* 26: 33–40.

Rector, N. A., Man, V., & Lerman, B. (2014). The expanding cognitive-behavioural therapy umbrella for the anxiety disorders: disorder-specific and transdiagnostic approaches. *Canadian Journal of Psychiatry* 59: 301–9.

Reiss, S. (1980). Pavlovian conditioning and human fear: an expectancy model. *Behavior Therapy* 11: 380–96. doi: 10.1016/S0005-7894(80)80054-2

Reiss, S. (1991). Expectancy model of fear, anxiety, and panic. *Clinical Psychology Review* 11: 141–53. doi: 10.1016/0272–7358(91)90092-9

Reiss, S., & McNally, R. J. (1985). Expectancy model of fear. In Reiss, S., & Bootzin, R. R. (eds.), *Theoretical Issues in Behavior Therapy*. New York: Academic Press, pp. 107–21.

Reiss, S., Peterson, R. A., Gursky, D. M., & McNally, R. J. (1986). Anxiety sensitivity, anxiety frequency and the prediction of fearfulness. *Behaviour Research and Therapy* 24: 1–8. doi: 10.1016/0005–7967(86)90143-9

Schmidt, N. B., Buckner, J. D., & Keough, M. E. (2007a). Anxiety sensitivity as a prospective predictor of alcohol use disorders. *Behavior Modification* 31: 202–19. doi: 10.1177/0145445506297019

Schmidt, N. B., Eggleston, A. M., Woolaway-Bickel, K., Fitzpatrick, K. K., Vasey, M. W., & Richey, J. A. (2007b). Anxiety Sensitivity Amelioration Training (ASAT): a longitudinal primary prevention program targeting cognitive vulnerability. *Journal of Anxiety Disorders* 21: 302–19. doi: 10.1016/j.janxdis.2006.06.002

Schmidt, N. B., Kotov, R., Lerew, D. R., Joiner, T. E., & Ialongo, N. S. (2006). Evaluating latent discontinuity in cognitive vulnerability to panic: a taxometric investigation. *Cognitive Therapy and Research* 29: 673–90. doi: 10.1007/s10608-005–9632-y

Silverman, W. K., Fleisig, W., Rabian, B., & Peterson, R. A. (1991). Child Anxiety Sensitivity Index. *Journal of Clinical Child Psychology* 20: 162–8.

Sippel, L. M., Jones, R. E., Bordieri, M. J., Dixon, L. J., May, A. C., Malkin, M. L., . . . Coffey, S. F. (2015). Interactive effects of anxiety sensitivity and difficulties in emotion regulation: an examination among individuals in residential substance use treatment with comorbid posttraumatic stress disorder. *Cognitive Therapy and Research* 39: 245–52. doi: 10.1007/s10608-014–9648-2

Smits, J. A. J., Berry, A. C., Rosenfield, D., Powers, M. B., Behar, E., & Otto, M. W. (2008a). Reducing anxiety sensitivity with exercise. *Depression and Anxiety* 25: 689–99. doi: 10.1002/da.20411

Smits, J. A. J., Berry, A. C., Tart, C. D., & Powers, M. B. (2008b). The efficacy of cognitive-behavioral interventions for reducing anxiety sensitivity: a meta-analytic review. *Behaviour Research and Therapy* 46: 1047–54. doi: 10.1016/j.brat.2008.06.010

Smits, J. A. J., Powers, M. B., Cho, Y., & Telch, M. J. (2004). Mechanism of change in cognitive-behavioral treatment of panic disorder: evidence for the fear of fear mediational hypothesis. *Journal of Consulting and Clinical Psychology* 72: 646–52. doi: 10.1037/0022–006X.72.4.646

Stein, M. B., Jang, K. L., & Livesley, W. J. (1999). Heritability of anxiety sensitivity: a twin study. *American Journal of Psychiatry* 156: 246–51.

Stein, M. B., & Rapee, R. M. (1999). Biological aspects of anxiety sensitivity: is it all in the head? In Taylor, S. (ed.), *Anxiety Sensitivity: Theory, Research, and Treat ment of the Fear of Anxiety*. Mahwah, NJ: Lawrence Erlbaum, pp. 199–215.

Stein, M. B., Schork, N. J., & Gelernter, J. (2008). Gene-by-environment (serotonin transporter and childhood maltreatment) interaction for anxiety sensitivity, an intermediate phenotype for anxiety disorders. *Neuropsychopharmacology* 33: 312–19. doi: 10.1038/sj.npp.1301422

Stewart, S. H., Taylor, S., Jang, K. L., Cox, B. J., Watt, M. C., Fedoroff, I. C., & Borger, S. C. (2001). Causal modeling of relations among learning history, anxiety sensitivity, and panic attacks. *Behaviour Research and Therapy* 39: 443–56. doi: 10.1016/S0005-7967(00)00023–1

Taylor, S., & Cox, B. J. (1998a). An expanded Anxiety Sensitivity Index: evidence for a hierarchic structure in a clinical sample. *Journal of Anxiety Disorders* 12: 463–83. doi: 10.1016/S0887-6185(98)00028-0

Taylor, S., & Cox, B. J. (1998b). Anxiety sensitivity: multiple dimensions and hierarchic structure. *Behaviour Research and Therapy* 36: 37–51. doi: 10.1016/S0005-7967(97)00071–5

Taylor, S., & Fedoroff, I. C. (1999). The expectancy theory of fear, anxiety, and panic: a conceptual and empirical analysis. In Taylor, S. (ed.), *Anxiety Sensitivity: Theory, Research, and Treatment of the Fear of Anxiety*. Mahwah, NJ: Lawrence Erlbaum, pp. 17–33.

Taylor, S., Jang, K. L., Stewart, S. H., & Stein, M. B. (2008). Etiology of the dimensions of anxiety sensitivity: a behavioral-genetic analysis. *Journal of Anxiety Disorders* 22: 899–914. doi: 10.1016/j.janxdis.2007.09.005.

Taylor, S., Zvolensky, M. J., Cox, B. J., Deacon, B., Heimberg, R. G., Ledley, D. R., ... Cardenas, S. J. (2007). Robust dimensions of anxiety sensitivity: development and initial validation of the Anxiety Sensitivity Index-3. *Psychological Assessment* 19: 176–88. doi: 10.1037/1040–3590.19.2.176

Tull, M. T. (2006). Extending an anxiety sensitivity model of uncued panic attack frequency and symptom severity: the role of emotion dysregulation. *Cognitive Therapy and Research* 30: 177–84. doi: 10.1007/s10608-006–9036-7

Tull, M. T., Stipelman, B. A., Salters-Pedneault, K., & Gratz, K. L. (2009). An examination of recent non-clinical panic attacks, panic disorder, anxiety sensitivity, and emotion regulation difficulties in the prediction of generalized anxiety disorder in an analogue sample. *Journal of Anxiety Disorders* 23: 275–82. doi: 10.1016/j.janxdis.2008.08.002

Vujanovic, A. A., Bernstein, A., Berenz, E. C., & Zvolensky, M. J. (2012). Single-session anxiety sensitivity reduction program for trauma-exposed adults: a case series documenting feasibility and initial efficacy. *Behavior Therapy* 43: 482–91. doi: 10.1016/j.beth.2012.03.005

Watt, M. C., & Stewart, S. H. (2000). Anxiety sensitivity mediates the relationships between childhood learning experiences and elevated hypochondriacal concerns in young adulthood. *Journal of Psychosomatic Research* 49: 107–18. doi: 10.1016/S0022-3999(00)00097-0

Watt, M. C., & Stewart, S. H. (2008). *Overcoming the Fear of Fear: How to Reduce Anxiety Sensitivity*. Oakland, CA: New Harbinger.

Watt, M. C., Stewart, S. H., & Cox, B. J. (1998). A retrospective study of the learning history origins of anxiety sensitivity. *Behaviour Research and Therapy* 36: 505–25. doi: 10.1016/S0005-7967(97)10029–8

Watt, M. C., Stewart, S. H., Lefaivre, M.-J., & Uman, L. S. (2006). A brief cognitive-behavioral approach to reducing anxiety sensitivity decreases pain-related anxiety. *Cognitive Behaviour Therapy* 35: 248–56. doi: 10.1080/16506070600898553.

Weems, C. F., Berman, S. L., Silverman, W. K., & Rodriguez, E. T. (2002). The relation between anxiety senstivity and attachment style in adolescence and early adulthood. *Journal of Psychopathology and Behavioral Assessment* 24: 159–68.

Whiteford, H. A., Degenhardt, L., Rehm, J., Baxter, A. J., Ferrari, A. J., Erskine, H. E., ... Vos, T. (2013). Global burden of disease attributable to mental and substance use disorders: findings from the Global Burden of Disease Study 2010. *Lancet* 382: 1575–86. doi: 10.1016/S0140-6736(13)61611-6

Zinbarg, R. E., Mohlman, J., & Hong, N. N. (1999). Dimensions of anxiety sensitivity. In Taylor, S. (ed.), *Anxiety Sensitivity: Theory, Research, and Treatment of the Fear of Anxiety*. Mahwah, NJ: Lawrence Erlbaum, pp. 83–114.

Zvolensky, M. J., Arrindell, W. A., Taylor, S., Bouvard, M., Cox, B. J., Stewart, S. H., … Eifert, G. H. (2003). Anxiety sensitivity in six countries. *Behaviour Research and Therapy* 41: 841–59. doi: 10.1016/S0005-7967(02)00187-0

20 Prevention in the Context of Cross-Cultural Neuroscience

Addressing Insomnia with EEG Biofeedback

Genomary Krigbaum & Nancy L. Wigton

Insomnia is a pervasive symptom in many health disorders, and it could merit a chapter in its relation to each disorder. Consequently, the focus of this chapter is solely on insomnia as a primary concern, and electroencephalography biofeedback (EBF) will be presented as a generalized modality for insomnia treatment, with evidence of clinically significant results (Koyanagi et al., 2014). The goals are to address the following: overview of the incidence and prevalence of insomnia; negative impact of insomnia and considerations of underlying physiological mechanisms; EBF background; EBF as a preventive intervention for insomnia; and benefits of addressing insomnia with EBF as a feasible cross-cultural intervention.

Overview of the Incidence and Prevalence of Insomnia

Insomnia is often referred to as a significant public health concern that merits close attention due to its high incidence, prevalence, and morbidity (Ferrie, Kumari, Salo, Singh-Manoux, & Kivimaki, 2011; Gagnon, Belanger, Ivers, & Morin, 2013; Morin, Belleville, Bélanger, & Ivers, 2011). Insomnia does not discriminate among the population. It is perceived as psychosocially and financially burdensome, since it negatively affects overall quality of life, disrupting daily routines as well as overall functionality. Thus it merits increased knowledge regarding risk/protective factors, epidemiology, course, prognosis, and treatment (Calem et al., 2012; Morin & Jarrin, 2013; Stranges, Tigbe, Gómez-Olivé, Thorogood, & Kandala, 2012).

Insomnia is frequently categorized as a potential epidemic in Canada and the United States (U.S.), affecting as many as 25 to 30 percent of the population, at a mild or moderate level, chronic/severe insomnia affecting over 10 percent of the global population, as well as 4 to 40 percent of incidence reported in youths; and it is considered to be on the rise (APA, 2013; Calhoun, Fernandez-Mendoza, Vgontzas, Liao, & Bixler, 2013; CDC, 2011; Cunnington, Junge, & Fernando, 2013; Hammer, Colbert, Brown, & Ilioi, 2011; Kim et al., 2012; Pallesen, Sivertsen, Nordhus, & Bjorvatn, 2014; Voinescu & Orasan, 2014). In the DSM-5 (APA, 2013), insomnia is a symptom of clinical concern that is accounted for in at least ten sleep-wake disorder groups; it is comorbid with other mental health, medical, and substance use disorders.

Current trends show there is great variation in the makeup of the symptom profile and negative effects of insomnia among sufferers, entailing non-restorative sleep and not being able to initiate or maintain sleep, plus subsequent symptoms of sleepiness, fatigue, cognitive difficulties, and mood disturbances, negatively affecting the functionality of individuals. More so, as a clinically significant symptom, it is a useful indicator of potential mental health, neurological, as well as other medical concerns/disorders (APA, 2013). Insomnia is pervasive across demographics, including life span, socioeconomic status, culture, and sex/gender, yet the prevalence increases with age, to the extent that insomnia is considered to have an emerging high cross-cultural incidence and prevalence rate (Green, Espie, & Benzeval, 2014; Green, Espie, Hunt, & Benzeval, 2012; Hysing, Pallesen, Stormark, Lundervold, & Vertsen, 2013; Kim et al., 2012; Koyanagi, et al., 2014; Matthews et al., 2014; Mindell et al., 2013; Salo et al., 2012; Sanchez-Ortuno, Edinger, & Wyatt, 2011; Suh et al., 2014). Thus, preventive measures and cost-effective interventions are needed in order to counteract and/or offset the negative impact of insomnia as a growing concern (Baglioni, et al., 2013; Pallesen et al., 2014).

Negative Impact of Insomnia and Considerations of Underlying Physiological Mechanisms

The impact of insomnia is as pervasive as its prevalence. In cutting across national, cultural, and socioeconomic borders, it negatively impacts quality of life regardless of geographic setting. This impact leads to increased risk for accidents, absenteeism, cognitive-affective dysregulation, and greater need for physical as well as mental health care, with an overall negative effect on quality of life (Buckelew, DeGood, Roberts, Butkovic, & MacKewn, 2009; Gagnon et al., 2013; Hammer et al., 2011; Morin et al., 2011). For example, insomnia has been reported as the third most common reason for seeking psychological services; it can double the risk for depression; increase medical concerns (including issues of hypertension as well as reduced metabolism); and lead to hypothalamus-pituitary-adrenal, thyroid, and gonadal axes depletion as well as hormone dysregulation (e.g. cortisol, adrenaline, and adrenocorticotropic hormone) (Cunnington et al., 2013; Kassi & Chrousos, 2013; Riemann et al., 2011; Vgontzas et al., 2012; Vgontzas, Fernandez-Mendoza, Liao, & Bixler, 2013; Xia, Chen, Li, Jiang, & Shen, 2013).

Researchers concur that the negative impact of insomnia is counterproductive to effective functionality and performance as reflective on decreased learning capacity/memory consolidation retrieval, potential judgment limitation, mood disturbances and disorders, endocrine dysregulation (so hormones that modulate stress, such as growth releasing hormone, are inhibited/limited), reduced motor coordination, decreased alertness, increased propensity for medical concerns and chronic diseases (e.g., diabetes, obesity, cardiovascular problems), less productivity, and suppressed immune function, thus reducing life expectancy (Cunnington et al., 2013; Ferrie et al., 2011; Kassi & Chrousos, 2013; Matthews et al., 2014; Suh et al., 2014; Vgontzas et al., 2012; Vgontzas et al., 2013; Xia et al., 2013). Due to the biopsychosocial negative effect of insomnia on individuals, it is important to consider the physiological mechanisms underlying it.

Insomnia encompasses biopsychosocial factors, exacerbated by underlying physiological mechanisms that are centered at a neurophysiological level of dysregulation, signaling hyperarousal, which in turn can enable stress and emotional reactivity that contributes to perpetuating insomnia (Baglioni, Spiegelhalder, Nissen, & Riemann, 2011). This process is summed up in the understanding of the predisposition, precipitation, and perpetuation that contribute to and maintain the symptom of insomnia (Bonnet & Arand, 2010; Harvey, Gehrman, & Espiea, 2013; Riemann et al., 2010). Even though predisposition can be understood as a genetic factor, little is known about the genetic underpinnings of insomnia aside from epigenetic dynamics that have been noted to be at play in the gene and environment interaction, which, to an extent, are considered to enable or disable predisposing and perpetuating factors (Palaginia, Biberb, & Riemann, 2014; Pigeon & Cribbet, 2012; Riemann, Kloepfer, & Berger, 2009; Vandekerckhove & Cluydts, 2010). The dearth of information on predisposing factors and the limited understanding on its etiology present the need for an intervention that can address insomnia and its underlying factors, at a neurophysiological level, without medication associated side effects, such as EBF.

EBF Background

EBF is considered an operant conditioning of brain frequency oscillations. It is also termed neurofeedback or brainwave biofeedback. The procedure consists of recording EEG, through sensors placed on the scalp, processing that data via computer software, and then providing feedback information to the trainee about his or her own brain functioning. When specified brain frequencies (e.g., delta, theta, alpha, beta) change in the targeted manner, an auditory reward tone is presented together with movement in a visual animation display. Therefore, through the use of conscious feedback signals, volitional control is achieved over unconscious physiological processes (Ros, Baars, Lanius, & Vuilleumier, 2014). In other words, when more rewards are presented (e.g., tones, visual animations), training happens through implicit learning such that a change toward more efficient brain (wave frequency) functioning occurs.

In 1929, Hans Berger's findings that brainwaves could be detected and measured paved the way for researchers to explore brainwave regulation through operant conditioning in the 1960s and 1970s. During this period, Kamiya's (1968) work was focused on humans' ability to sustain (over time) an increase in alpha (8–12Hz) waves to induce feelings of well-being. Instead, Sterman, Howe, and Macdonald's (1970) initial experiments involved investigations of cats' ability to increase a distinctive 12 to 15Hz brainwave frequency originating in the sensorimotor cortex, termed sensory motor rhythm (SMR), and its relation to sleep spindles. They did not expand this research into human sleep improvement, as their focus developed toward the investigation of seizure remediation in humans, through the enhancement of the SMR frequency (Sterman & Egner, 2006). Later, Lubar and Shouse (1976) furthered Sterman's work in applying EBF beginning technology to attention concerns. This led to clinical applications of EBF for the condition of attention deficit/hyperactivity disorders (ADHD) (Robbins, 2000) and a framework of EBF protocols (e.g., targeting theta/beta ratio frequencies), which are still in use, consequently opening the field to research applications in other areas of health concern, such as insomnia. In the 1990s, there was an advent of quantitative EEG (qEEG) technology, wherein an individual's EEG is compared to a normative database, resulting in scientifically objective normalization metrics (expressed as z-scores) such that the development of individualized approaches to EBF was possible (Hammond, 2010).

Currently, EBF technology has expanded to include various modalities addressing an array of concerns and neurophysiological dysregulation; these can generally be classified as traditional, qEEG-guided, and z-score (Krigbaum & Wigton, 2014). The vast majority of EBF research is centered on traditional approaches. Traditional EBF encompasses models that either apply a standardized (e.g., one-size-fits-all) protocol or take into account symptom reports to determine which EEG frequencies to target. These frequencies include theta/beta ratio (inhibit theta and enhance beta), SMR enhancement, and slow cortical potential models/frameworks. In qEEG-guided EBF, the protocol is informed by the qEEG data to identify individually which brain frequencies to target, increasing or decreasing the frequency of brain oscillations. Z-score EBF incorporates real-time qEEG data to enable operant conditioning of qEEG z-scores in the normalization of brain frequencies. These modalities include four-channel and nineteen-channel z-score EBF, as well as low resolution electromagnetic tomography (LORETA) z-score EBF. For a complete discussion of the various EBF modalities and their clinical relevance, see Krigbaum and Wigton (2014).

EBF as a Preventive Intervention for Insomnia

In the context of prevention, some have begun to discuss EBF as a relevant and feasible intervention. For example, Stokes and Lappin (2010) evaluated the efficacy of EBF in migraines, with thirty-seven participants who had on average forty sessions of EBF and thermal biofeedback. The results were that twenty-six (70 percent) of participants achieved 50 percent reduction in headache frequency; and this benefit was maintained 14.5 months after the discontinuation of treatment. Of note, during this study, participants reported that EBF helped them to gain control over their symptoms and prevent the onset of headaches. The authors stated EBF could be viewed as an intervention used to prevent episodic migraines from progressing to chronic migraines, and thus avert the progression of other comorbid symptoms, for example, insomnia. Similarly, Trudeau, Sokhadze, & Cannon (2009) suggest that EBF for ADHD in childhood could be a valuable preventive intervention for those at risk of developing substance use disorders. They also believe that qEEG data could be used to predict those at risk for relapse, wherein EBF could be used to train and improve dysregulated brain frequencies.

Dysregulation of brain frequencies was also noted in the 1970s, when researchers indicated that the (neurophysiological) regulation of brain waves in the awake state can be related to brainwave activity while asleep (Sterman et al., 1970). For instance, when awake, most individuals exhibit EEG patterns that can be classified into beta and alpha brainwaves. However, in the stages of sleep, individuals transition into theta/delta brainwaves and REM (associated with an idiosyncratic brain wave frequency pattern). More so, Sterman and colleagues (Sterman, et al., 1970; Sterman & Egner, 2006) were among the first to identify the relationship between the functions of the SMR frequency with quality of sleep. As such, using EBF to enhance SMR, and thereby increase sleep spindles, led to a framework of insomnia being related to brain function dysregulation. Hauri, Percy, Hellekson, Hartmann, and Russ (1982) sought to expand on this work and found evidence supporting the identified relationship between insomnia and sleep spindle deficit. However, Hauri (2008) suggested that the 1980s technology was too cumbersome to facilitate the empirical exploration of the relationship. Now, with the advent of newer technology, in terms of higher-quality EEG amplifiers as well as faster and more powerful computers, researchers have recently revived a focus on a connection between neurophysiological dysregulation and insomnia. Thus, being that EBF targets brainwave frequency dysregulation, it is important when considering relevant preventive interventions for insomnia.

Research Supporting EBF as an Intervention

As the evidence of EBF efficacy increases and correlated symptomatology (including insomnia) is identified, EBF becomes a viable choice of intervention and prevention to address insomnia-related concerns. EBF research has been actively pursued for decades, addressing conditions such as ADHD, epilepsy, and other mental health/medical concerns. Interestingly, many ADHD EBF studies report improvements in sleep and/or insomnia being the most frequently reported supplemental benefit. This improvement is frequently framed as a positive and preventive side effect of EBF (Arns & Kenemans, 2014).

In the last ten years, there has been an emergence in EBF research with a focus on insomnia, such as the work of Hoedlmoser et al. (2008). In a randomized, placebo-controlled study, twenty-seven participants were evaluated after ten sessions of EBF targeting an increase in SMR. The experimental group size was $n = 16$, with the control group being $n = 11$. This study yielded results demonstrating that EBF increased SMR amplitude ($p = 0.014$, Cohen's $d = 0.7$) and number of sleep spindles ($p = 0.004$, Cohen's $d = 0.6$), as well as decreasing sleep onset latency ($p = 0.006$, Cohen"s $d = 0.7$); thus, insomnia was addressed and sleep quality was improved. In another study, Cortoos, DeValck, Arns, Breteler, and Cluydts (2010) hypothesized cortical hyperarousal to impair normal sleep. As such, they propose interventions, such as EBF, targeting hyperarousal dysregulation, to positively address insomnia. To test this hypothesis, they conducted a randomized control study comparing EBF ($n = 9$) and electromyography (EMG) biofeedback ($n = 8$) to healthy controls ($n = 12$). In this study, they used traditional EBF targeting an inhibition of theta and high beta with an increase of the SMR frequency, and the primary outcome measure was *Total Sleep Time*, as measured by polysomnography (e.g. diagnostic testing to detect sleep disorders) and home sleep logs. The main results indicated only the EBF group achieved pre-post *Total Sleep Time* improvement ($p<0.05$) on both the polysomnography and sleep logs, corroborating the positive effect of EBF as a beneficial intervention for insomnia.

Likewise, Hammer et al. (2011) conducted a randomized, parallel group, single-blind study, using z-score EBF to evaluate the efficacy of two different EBF protocols (two-electrode sites to normalize SMR z-scores versus four-electrode sites to normalize highest z-scores) for insomnia. The primary findings suggest z-score EBF as a beneficial intervention for insomnia, measured by assessments such as the *Insomnia Severity Index* (ISI) and *Pittsburgh Sleep Quality Inventory* (PSQI). While the sample size for each group was small ($n = 5$ and $n = 3$), for the combined group, all insomnia-related pre-post outcome measure comparisons yielded symptom improvement (ISI; $p<0.005$; PSQI $p<0.0001$), and all participants improved their quality of (or achieved normal) sleep. Additionally, intervention response (relapse prevention) was sustained at six to nine months' follow-up for $n = 5$ of the participants (over 50percent), since one of the participants reported perimenopause complications and two participants were unreachable. On the other hand, Schabus et al. (2014) studied EBF with twenty-four participants, who reported symptoms of primary insomnia, in a counterbalanced within-subject design. The participants received ten EBF sessions targeting an increase in SMR amplitude at a single electrode location (C3; per the International 10-20 System). The EBF was counterbalanced against a sham EBF condition, where the participants received the sham condition either before or after the true EBF condition. Analysis of pre-to post-EBF data yielded an increased SMR amplitude ($p = 0.02$) and number of sleep spindles ($p = 0.033$), while decreasing number of awakenings ($p = 0.025$), as well as a reduction in self-reported sleep complaints ($p<0.001$). Thus, the study yielded results supporting to EBF as being beneficial for addressing symptoms of insomnia and improving overall quality of sleep. However, due to the newness in the development of research methodologies to suit EBF technology, the results from these studies need cautionary interpretation.

Ros et al. (2014) reviewed the underlying mechanisms of EBF and posited that healthy brain function requires a delicate balance between low and high oscillatory synchronization, such that psychobiological dysfunction can be viewed as homeostatic plasticity disorders. They go on to support EBF as an upcoming intervention having therapeutic advantages over interventions, such as medication with associated side effects, in its ability to safely promote long-lasting stability of brain frequency oscillations; the authors also support EBF as a natural approach that can lead to neurophysiological improvement and neuroplasticity. As such, EBF represents a promising evidence-based intervention to address the underlying dysregulation and factors of insomnia.

EBF Addressing Underlying Factors of Insomnia

In the review of ADHD literature as related to insomnia, Arns and Kenemans (2014) affirm the connection between increased sleep spindles and sleep quality to include increased sleep time duration and decreased sleep latency. They further propose EBF as an intervention that operates on the cortical and subcortical level to regulate sleep onset through sleep spindle production. In other words, EBF addresses the neurophysiological dysregulation underlying sleep spindle deficits and, in turn, insomnia. Advancing their work of investigating the role of sleep problems in the manifestation of ADHD, Arns, Feddema, and Kenemans (2014) found a positive relationship between sleep problems and inattention, as well as SMR EBF reducing sleep onset latency and self-reported sleep problems sooner than theta/beta ratio EBF in the intervention process.

Buckelew et al. (2009) proposed an EEG dysregulation model of insomnia, which they later redefined as an impaired neuroflexibility model (Buckelew et al., 2013). On the premise of the neuroflexibility model, it is believed there is cortical inflexibility such that individuals' brains are unable to match activity to the situational demands of the immediate environment. An example applicable to insomnia would be a cortical inability to shift to slower EEG frequencies necessary for sleep induction. To test this framework further, Buckelew et al. (2013) studied ten *good* and ten *poor* sleepers with an alpha EBF protocol. They propose that self-regulation of the alpha frequency represents neuroflexibility and hypothesize that *good* sleepers would demonstrate better self-regulation of the alpha frequency than *poor* sleepers. Across two trial sessions, results indicated significant differences between good and poor sleepers for alpha activation ($p = 0.006$, $p = 0.015$) as well as for alpha suppression ($p = 0.04$, $p = 0.027$). Moreover, good sleepers demonstrated better alpha control (defined as ability to both reduce and increase alpha) in the first trial session ($p = 0.02$), with a pattern of better alpha control among good sleepers in the second trial. Therefore, they believe their results support a model of impaired neuroflexibility as an underlying cause of insomnia.

Thus, it can be concluded that EBF is an intervention that has yielded initial evidence of addressing underlying neurophysiological dysregulation in insomnia. The research and work of Buckelew et al. (2009; 2013), Cortoos et al. (2010), Hammer et al. (2011), Hauri et al. (1982), Hoedlmoser et al. (2008), Ros et al. (2014), Schabus et al. (2014), and Sterman et al. (1970) collectively yield promising results positioning EBF as a preventative intervention suitable to address insomnia, in part due to its neurocortical etiology. As EBF continues to be developed and strengthened as a preventive intervention, further research is needed to validate its efficacy in comparison trials with other interventions, including medications and psychotherapy.

Benefits of Addressing Insomnia with EBF as a Feasible Cross-Cultural Intervention

In recent years, there has been a surge of EBF studies, with more researchers collaborating at a global scale, resulting in a cross-cultural focus (Van Boxtel & Gruzelier, 2014). This collaboration has been facilitated in part by memberships to professional guilds with an international focus, including the Association for Applied Psychophysiology and Biofeedback[1]; the International Society for Neurofeedback and Research,[2] with members from more than thirty countries worldwide as well as individuals from more than thirty countries certified through the Biofeedback Certification International Alliance.[3] Through the years, and as EBF cross-cultural empirical evidence mounts, researchers such as Myers and Young (2012) discuss the evidence of EBF efficacy as being a "cultural currency within the mental health field" and call for the field to "include brain-based measures/metrics in research and practice. . ."(p. 26).

In their scientific review of replicated qEEG metrics/databases, Hughes and John (1999) report these metrics have been found to be independent of ethnic and cultural factors in "studies from Barbados, China, Cuba, Germany, Holland, Japan, Korea, Mexico, Netherlands, Sweden, the United States, and Venezuela. . ."(p. 192). Thus, they contend qEEG metrics are applicable to persons of any origin or ethnic background. As a result, Hammond (2010) has discussed qEEG assessments as being a culture-free method of brain function evaluation. Thus, EBF is posed as a suitable cross-cultural intervention, since it operates at an individual neurophysiological level, separate from language or cultural influences. This is evident in EBF research conducted yielding similar results in various regions of the world, such as in North America and Europe (Arns, de Ridder, Strehl, Breteler, & Coenen, 2009; Buckelew et al., 2013; Cortoos et al., 2010; Hammer et al., 2011; Hoedlmoser et al., 2008; Schabus et al., 2014); China (Zhonggui, Shuhua, & Haiqing, 2005); Latin America (Fernández et al., 2007); the Middle East (Moghanloo, Vafaie, Rostami, & Farahani, 2014); and Russia (Bazanova & Aftanas, 2010).

1 www.aapb.org. 2 www.isnr.org. 3 www.bcia.org.

Additionally, in a meta-analysis by Arns et al. (2009), EBF efficacy was evaluated at a global scale, including the following countries, as well as number of studies and sum of participants: the United States (five studies; n = 771), Germany (six studies; n = 295), Canada (one study; n = 20), Switzerland (one study; n = 30), Russia (one study; n = 18), and China (one study; n = 60). The findings indicated that EBF is both efficacious and specific as an intervention for ADHD, with large to medium effect sizes for inattention and impulsivity, respectively. Subsequently, Arns and Kenemans (2014) and Arns, Feddema, and Kenemans (2014) documented a significant linkage between ADHD and sleep disorders. Furthermore, in contemporary research cross-sectional correlates between symptoms of attention, inattention, impulsivity, mood disorders (e.g., anxiety, depression), migraines, and insomnia are highlighted, where prevention and/or decrease in symptoms of insomnia offset any of the other symptoms noted (Calhoun et al., 2013; Goldman-Mellor et al.,2014; Green et al., 2014; Koyanagi et al., 2014; Pallesen, Sivertsen, Nordus, & Bjorvatn, 2014; Riemann et al., 2010). In all studies, there is a consensus that the benefits of addressing insomnia are many, including the improvement of overall quality of life and longevity (Ellis, Perlis, Neale, Espie, & Bastien, 2012).

Conclusion

Insomnia is a significant problem worldwide; to a degree, it is considered a growing concern of epidemic proportions in the United States and abroad. The cumulative negative impact on overall quality of life is significant in terms of safety/fiscal risks and increased need for mental as well as physical health care. The benefits of adequate sleep outweigh the lack thereof. Thus, EBF shows potential as an efficacious cross-cultural preventive intervention for addressing the underlying physiological factors involved, symptom relief, and management as well as prevention of further complications (to include comorbid symptoms) aggravated and perpetuated by insomnia. The gains and benefits of addressing and preventing further perpetuation of insomnia would have a net positive global impact in secondary health gains.

References

APA (American Psychiatric Association) (2013). *Diagnostic and Statistical Manual of Mental Disorders*, 5th ed. Arlington, VA: American Psychiatric Publishing.

Arns, M., de Ridder, S., Strehl, U., Breteler, M., & Coenen, A. (2009). Efficacy of neurofeedback treatment in ADHD: the effects on inattention, impulsivity and hyperactivity: a meta-analysis. *Clinical EEG & Neuroscience* 40: 180–9.

Arns, M., Feddema, I., & Kenemans, J. (2014). Differential effects of Theta/Beta and SMR neurofeedback in ADHD on sleep onset latency. *Frontiers in Human Neuroscience* 8: 1019. doi: 10.3389/fnhum.2014.01019

Arns, M., & Kenemans, J. L. (2014). Neurofeedback in ADHD and insomnia: vigilance stabilization through sleep spindles and circadian networks. *Neuroscience & Biobehavioral Reviews* 44: 183–94. doi: 10.1016/j.neubiorev.2012.10.006

Baglioni, C., Regen, W., Teghen, A., Spiegelhalder, K., Feige, B., Nissen, C... Riemann, D. (2013). Sleep changes in the disorder of insomnia: a meta-analysis of polysomnographic studies. *Sleep Medicine Reviews* 18: 195–213.

Baglioni, C., Spiegelhalder, K., Nissen, C., & Riemann, D. (2011). Clinical implications of the causal relationship between insomnia and depression: how individually tailored treatment of sleeping difficulties could prevent the onset of depression. *EPMA Journal* 2: 287–93. doi: 10.1007/s13167-011-0079-9

Bazanova, O. M., & Aftanas, L. I. (2010). Individual EEG alpha activity analysis for enhancement neurofeedback efficiency: two case studies. *Journal of Neurotherapy* 14(3): 244–53. doi: 10.1080/10874208.2010.501517

Berger, H. (1929). Über das elektroenkephalogramm des menschen [About the elektroenkephalogram of humans]. *Archiv für Psychiatrie und NerveMrankheilen* 87: 527–70.

Bonnet, M., & Arand, D. (2010). Hyperarousal and insomnia: state of the science. *Sleep Medicine Reviews* 14(1): 9–15. doi: 10.1016/j.smrv.2009.05.002

Buckelew, S. P., DeGood, D. E., Roberts, K. D., Butkovic, J. D., & MacKewn, A. S. (2009). Awake EEG disregulation in good compared to poor sleepers. *Applied Psychophysiology and Biofeedback* 34: 99–103. doi: 10.1007/s10484-009-9080-7

Buckelew, S. P., DeGood, D. E., Taylor, J., Cunningham, N. B., Thornton, J., & MacKewn, A. (2013). Neuroflexibility and sleep onset insomnia among college students: Implications for neurotherapy. *Journal of Neurotherapy* 17(2): 106–15. doi: 10.1080/10874208.2013.784681

Calem, M., Bisla, J., Begum, A., Dewey, M., Bebbington, P., Brugha, T., ... Stewart, R. (2012). Increased prevalence of insomnia and changes in hypnotics use in England over 15 years: analysis of the 1993, 2000, and 2007 national psychiatric morbidity surveys. *Sleep* 35(3): 377–84.

Calhoun, S., Fernandez-Mendoza, J., Vgontzas, A., Liao, D., & Bixler, E. (2013). Prevalence of insomnia symptoms in a general population sample of young children and preadolescents: gender effects. *Sleep Medicine* 15: 91–5.

CDC (Centers for Disease Control and Prevention) (2011). Effect of short sleep duration on daily activities –United States, 2005–2008. *Morbidity and Mortality Weekly Report* 60: 239–42.

Cortoos, A., DeValck, E., Arns, M., Breteler, M. H. M., & Cluydts, R. (2010). An exploratory study on the effects of tele-neurofeedback and tele-biofeedback on objective and subjective sleep in patients with primary insomnia. *Applied Psychophysiology and Biofeedback* 35: 125–34. doi: 10.1007/s10484-009-9116-z

Cunnington, D., Junge, M. F., & Fernando, A. T. (2013). Insomnia: prevalence, consequences and effective treatment. *Medical Journal Australia* 199: S36–S40. doi: 10.5694/mja13.10718

Ellis, J., Perlis, M., Neale, L., Espie, C., & Bastien, C. (2012). The natural history of insomnia: focus on prevalence and incidence of acute insomnia. *Journal of Psychiatric Research* 46: 1278–85.

Fernández, F., Harmony, T., Fernández-Bouzas, A., Díaz-Comas, L., Prado-Alcalá, R., Valdés-Sosa, P., ... García-Martínez, F. (2007). Changes in EEG current sources induced by neurofeedback in learning disabled children: an exploratory study. *Applied Psychophysiology and Biofeedback* 32(3–4): 169–83. doi: 10.1007/s10484-007-9044-8

Ferrie, J., Kumari, M., Salo, P., Singh-Manoux, A., & Kivimaki, M. (2011). Sleep epidemiology – a rapidly growing field. *International Journal of Epidemiology* 40: 1431–7. doi: 10.1093/ije/dyr203

Gagnon, C., Belanger, L., Ivers, H., & Morin, C. (2013). Validation of the insomnia severity index in primary care. *Journal of the American Board of Family Medicine* 26: 701–10.

Goldman-Mellor, S., Caspi, A., Gregory, A., Harrington, H., Poulton, R., & Moffitt, T. (2014a). Is insomnia associated with deficits in neuropsychological functioning? Evidence from a population-based study. *Sleep* ISSN: 0161–8105

Green, M., Espie, C., & Benzeval, M. (2014). Social class and gender patterning of insomnia symptoms and psychiatric distress: a 20-year prospective cohort study. *BMC Psychiatry* 14: 152.

Green, M., Espie, C., Hunt, K., & Benzeval, M., (2012). The longitudinal course of insomnia symptoms: inequalities by sex and occupational class among two different age cohorts followed for 20 years in the west of Scotland. *Sleep* 35(6): 815–23.

Hammer, B. U., Colbert, A. P., Brown, K. A., & Llioi, E. C. (2011). Neurofeedback for insomnia: a pilot study of Z-score SMR and individualized protocols. *Applied Psychophysiology and Biofeedback* 36(4): 251–64.

Hammond, D. C. (2010). The need for individualization in neurofeedback: heterogeneity in QEEG patterns associated with diagnoses and symptoms. *Applied Psychophysiology and Biofeedback* 35: 31–6. doi: 10.1007/s10484-009-9106-1

Harvey, C., Gehrman, P., & Espiea, C. (2013). Who is predisposed to insomnia: a review of familial aggregation, stress-reactivity, personality and coping style. *Sleep Medicine Reviews* 18(3): 237–47. doi: 10.1016/j.smrv.2013.11.004

Hauri, P. J. (2008). EEG biofeedback in the treatment of insomnia: a historical perspective. *Applied Psychophysiology and Biofeedback* 33(4): 246.

Hauri, P. J., Percy, L., Hellekson, C., Hartmann, E., & Russ, D. (1982). The treatment of psychophysiologic insomnia disorder with biofeedback: a replication study. *Biofeedback and Self-Regulation* 7(2): 223–35.

Hoedlmoser, K., Pecherstorfer, T., Gruber, E., Anderer, P., Doppelmayr, M., Klimesch, W., . . . Schabus, M. (2008). Instrumental conditioning of human sensorimotor rhythm (12–15 Hz) and its impact on sleep as well as declarative learning. *Sleep* 31(10): 1401–8.

Hughes, J. R., & John, E. R. (1999). Conventional and quantitative electroencephalography in psychiatry. *Journal of Neuropsychiatry and Clinical Neurosciences* 11(2): 190–208.

Hysing, M., Pallesen, S., Stormark, K., Lundervold, A., & Vertsen, B. (2013). Sleep patterns and insomnia among adolescents: a population-based study. *Journal of Sleep Research* 22: 549–56.

Kamiya, J. (1968). Conscious control of brainwaves. *Psychology Today* 1: 56–60.

Kassi, E. N., &Chrousos, G. P. (2013). The central CLOCK system and the stress axis in health and disease. *Hormones* 12(2): 172–91.

Kim, B., Jeon, H. J., Hong, J. P., Bae, J. N., Lee, J., Chang, S. M., . . . Cho, M. J. (2012). DSM-IV psychiatric comorbidity according to symptoms of insomnia: a nationwide sample of Korean adults. *Social Psychiatry and Psychiatric Epidemiology* 47: 2019–33. doi: 10.1007/s00127-012-0502-0

Koyanagi, A., Garin, N., Olaya, B., Ayuso-Mateos, J. L., Chatterji, S., Leonardi, M., ... Haro, J. M. (2014). Chronic conditions and sleep problems among adults aged 50 years or over in nine countries: a multi-country study. *PLoS One* 9(12): e114742. doi: 10.1371/journal.pone.0114742

Krigbaum, G., & Wigton, N. L. (2014). When discussing neurofeedback, does modality matter?*NeuroRegulation* 1(1): 48–60. doi: 10.15540/nr.1.1.48

Lubar, J. F., & Shouse, M. N. (1976). EEG and behavioral changes in a hyperkinetic child concurrent with training of the sensorimotor rhythm (SMR): a preliminary report. *Biofeedback & Self-Regulation* 1: 293–306.

Matthews, K., Changd, Y., Kravitze, H., Brombergera, J., Owensa, J., Buyssea, D., ... Halla, M. (2014). Sleep and risk for high blood pressure and hypertension in midlife women: the SWAN (Study of Women's Health across the Nation) Sleep Study. *Sleep Medicine* 15(2): 203–8. doi: 10.1016/j.sleep.2013.11.002

Mindell, J. A., Bartle, A., Ahn, Y., Ramamurthy, M. B., Huong, H. T. D., Kohyama, J., ... Goh, D. Y. T. (2013). Sleep education in pediatric residency programs: a cross-cultural look. *BioMed Central Research Notes* 6(130): 1–5. doi: 10.1186/1756-0500-6-130

Moghanloo, M., Vafaie, M. E. A., Rostami, R., & Farahani, H. (2014). Determination of the effects of neurofeedback training in the neuropsychological rehabilitation in inattentive and combined subtypes of attention deficit/hyperactivity disorder. *NeuroRegulation* 1(2): 131–50. doi: 10.15540/nr.1.2.131

Morin, C., Belleville, G., Bélanger, L., & Ivers, H. (2011). The insomnia severity index: psychometric indicators to detect insomnia cases and evaluate treatment response. *Sleep* 34(5): 601–8.

Morin, C., & Jarrin, D. (2013). Epidemiology of insomnia – prevalence, course, risk factors, and public health burden. *Sleep Medicine Clinic* 8: 281–97. dx.doi.org/10.1016/j.jsmc.2013.05.002

Myers, J. E., & Young, J. S. (2012). Brain wave biofeedback: benefits of integrating neurofeedback in counseling. *Journal of Counseling and Development* 90: 20–8.

Palaginia, L., Biberb, K., & Riemann, D. (2014). The genetics of insomnia –evidence for epigenetic mechanisms? *Sleep Medicine Reviews* 18(3): 225–35. doi: 10.1016/j.smrv.2013.05.002

Pallesen, S., Sivertsen, B., Nordhus, I., & Bjorvatn, B. (2014). A 10-year trend of insomnia prevalence in the adult Norwegian population. *Journal of Sleep Medicine* 15: 173–9.

Pigeon, W., & Cribbet, M. (2012). The pathophysiology of insomnia from models to molecules (and back). *Current Opinion in Pulmonary Medicine* 18(6): 546–53. doi: 10.1097/MCP.0b013e328358be41

Riemann, D., Kloepfer, C., & Berger, M. (2009). Functional and structural brain alterations in insomnia: Implications for pathophysiology. *European Journal of Neuroscience* 29(9): 1754–60. doi: 10.1111/j.1460-9568.2009.06721.x

Riemann, D., Spiegelhalder, K., Espie, C., Pollmächer, T., Léger, D., Bassetti, C., ... van Someren, E. (2011). Chronic insomnia: clinical and research challenges – an agenda. *Journal of Pharmacopsychiatry* 44: 1–14.

Riemann, D., Spiegelhaldera, K., Feigea, B., Voderholzera, U., Bergera, M., Perlisb, M., ... Nissena, C. (2010). The hyperarousal model of insomnia: a review of the concept and its evidence. *Sleep Medicine Reviews* 14(1): 19–31.

Robbins, J. (2000). *A Symphony in the Brain*. New York: Grove Press.

Ros, T., Baars, B. J., Lanius, R. A., & Vuilleumier, P. (2014). Tuning pathological brain oscillations with neurofeedback: a systems neuroscience framework. *Frontiers in Human Neuroscience* 8(1008): 1–37. doi: 10.3389/fnhum.2014.01008

Salo, P., Vahtera, J., Ferrie, J., Akbaraly, T., Goldberg, M., Zins, M., . . . Kivimaki, M. (2012). Trajectories of sleep complaints from early midlife to old age: longitudinal modeling study. *Sleep* 35(11): 1559–68.

Sanchez-Ortuno, M. M., Edinger, J. D., & Wyatt, J. K. (2011). Daytime symptom patterns in insomnia sufferers: is there evidence for subtyping insomnia? *Journal of Sleep Research* 20: 425–33. doi: 10.1111/j.1365-2869.2010.00905.x

Schabus, M., Heib, D. P. J., Lechinger, J., Griessenberger, H., Klimesch, W., Pawlizki, A., . . . Hoedlmoser, K. (2014). Enhancing sleep quality and memory in insomnia using instrumental sensorimotor rhythm conditioning. *Biological Psychology* 95: 126–34. doi: 10.1016/j.biopsycho.2013.02.020

Sterman, M. B., & Egner, T. (2006). Foundation and practice of neurofeedback for the treatment of epilepsy. *Applied Psychophysiology and Biofeedback* 31(1): 21–35.

Sterman, M. B., Howe, R. C., & Macdonald, L. R. (1970). Facilitation of spindle-burst sleep by conditioning of electroencephalographic activity while awake. *Science* 167(921): 1146–8.

Stokes, D. A. & Lappin, M. S. (2010). Neurofeedback and biofeedback with 37 migraineurs: a clinical outcome study. *Behavioral and Brain Functions* 6: 9–19. doi: 10.1186/1744-9081-6-9

Stranges, S., Tigbe, W., Gómez-Olivé, F., Thorogood, M., & Kandala, N. (2012). Sleep problems: an emerging global epidemic? Findings from the indepth WHO-SAGE study among more than 40,000 older adults from 8 countries across Africa and Asia. *Sleep* 35(8): 1173–81.

Suh, S., Yang, H., Fairholme, C., Kim, H., Manber, R., & Shin, C. (2014). Who is at risk for having persistent insomnia symptoms? A longitudinal study in the general population in Korea. *Sleep Medicine* 15(2): 180–6. doi: 10.1016/j.sleep.2013.09.024

Trudeau, D. L., Sokhadze, T. M., & Cannon, R. L. (2009). Neurofeedback in alcohol and drug dependency. In Budzynski, T. H., Budzynski, H. K., Evans, J. R., & Abarbanel, A. (eds.), *Introduction to Quantitative EEG and Neurofeedback: Advanced Theory and Applications,* 2nd ed. Burlington, MA: Elsevier, pp. 241–67.

Van Boxtel, G. J. M., & Gruzelier, J. H. (2014). Neurofeedback: introduction to the special issue. *Biological Psychology* 95: 1–3.

Vandekerckhove, M., & Cluydts, R. (2010). Physiological review –the emotional brain and sleep: an intimate relationship. *Sleep Medicine Review* 14(4): 219–26.

Vgontzas, A. N., Fernandez-Mendoza, J., Bixler, E. O., Singareddy, R., Shaffer, M. L., Calhoun, S. L., . . . Chrousos, G. P. (2012). Persistent insomnia: the role of objective short sleep duration and mental health. *Sleep* 35(1): 61–8. doi: 10.5665/sleep.1586

Vgontzas, A. N., Fernandez-Mendoza, J., Liao, D., & Bixler, E. O. (2013). Insomnia with objective short sleep duration: the most biologically severe phenotype of the disorder. *Sleep Medicine Reviews* 17: 241–54. doi: 10.1016/j.smrv.2012.09.005

Voinescu, B. I., & Orasan, R. (2014). Sleep disturbance in relation to alcohol misuse. *Journal of Evidence-Based Psychotherapies* 14(1): 95–104.

Xia, L., Chen, G-H., Li, Z-H., Jiang, S., & Shen, J. (2013). Alterations in hypothalamus-pituitary-adrenal/thyroid axes and gonadotropin-releasing hormone in the patients with primary insomnia: a clinical research. *PLoS One* 8(8): e71065. doi: 10.1371/journal.pone.0071065

Zhonggui, X., Shuhua, S., & Haiqing, X. (2005). A controlled study of the effectiveness of EEG biofeedback training on children with attention deficit hyperactivity disorder. *Journal of Huazhong University of Science and Technology* 25(3): 368–70.

21 Prevention of Disaster Impact and Outcome Cascades

James M. Shultz, Maria Espinola, Andreas Rechkemmer, Madeline A. Cohen, & Zelde Espinel

Overview: The Intersection of Prevention Science and Disaster Health

When disasters strike, human populations are exposed to a variety of hazards during impact and to a multiplicity of hazards, losses, and life changes in the aftermath (Reissman, Schrieber, Shultz, & Ursano, 2009; Shultz, Espinel, Flynn, Hoffman, & Cohen, 2007a; Shultz, Espinel, Galea, & Reissman, 2007b; Shultz, Neria, Allen, & Espinel, 2013c). Once set in motion, disasters frequently trigger a succession of compounding consequences (Buldyrev, Parshani, Paul, Stanley, & Havlin, 2010; Lorenz, Battiston, & Schweitzer, 2009). Disasters are complex, nonlinear phenomena, and for the disaster-affected community, the situation tends to go from bad to worse and often very fast (Cavallo, 2010, 2013, 2014; Cavallo & Ireland, 2014; Ramalingam, Jones, Toussainte, & Young, 2008).

This chapter considers the "prevention potential" for disasters through the lens of prevention science. The application of prevention science offers the prospect of diminishing the severity of extreme events' impacts and perhaps reducing the frequency of disaster occurrence. While extreme events are not usually preventable, it may be possible to reduce the preimpact "risk landscape" and thereby minimize the disastrous impacts of an event. To limit the degree of human exposure and the extent of disaster consequences, it is possible to intervene preventively at various points along the disaster risk and impact cascades when

Authors' Note: Figures 21.1–5 adapted from Shultz, Espinel, Cohen, Smith, & Flynn, 2006a. Figure 21.6 prepared for this chapter.

James M. Shultz. Director, Center for Disaster & Extreme Event Preparedness (DEEP Center), University of Miami Miller School of Medicine, Miami FL 33136, USA, 305-219-9011. jamesmichaelshultz@gmail.com.
Maria Espinola. Assistant Professor of Clinical Psychiatry, Department of Psychiatry and Behavioral Neuroscience, University of Cincinnati College of Medicine, Cincinnati OH, USA. 513-558-7607. maria.espinola@uc.edu.
Andreas Rechkemmer. Professor and American Humane Endowed Chair, Graduate School of Social Work (GSSW), University of Denver, Denver, CO 80208, USA. 303-871-2493. andreas.rechkemmer@du.edu.
Madeline A. Cohen. The Mailman School of Public Health, Columbia University, New York, NY, USA. 561-346-3212. madelineacohen@gmail.com.
Zelde Espinel. Department of Psychiatry and Behavioral Health, University of Miami Miller School of Medicine and Jackson Memorial Hospital, Miami FL 33136, USA. 786-202-7450. z.espinel@med.miami.edu.

natural hazards occur and along the disaster outcome cascade in the aftermath. This approach integrates complexity sciences into disaster risk reduction (DRR) and disaster risk management (DRM) (Cavallo, 2010, 2014; Cavallo & Ireland, 2014; Helbing, 2013; Helbing et al., 2015; Johnson, 2007; Shi et al., 2011).

Aligned with the goals of the *Cambridge Handbook of International Prevention Science*, this chapter focuses on disaster prevention and interweaves discussion of the psychological dimensions of disasters and extreme events (Reissman et al., 2009; Shultz, 2007a, b; 2013a, b, c).

Prevention of disasters is a continuum concept. Some disasters may truly be prevented. Strategies can be applied to prevent some human-generated (anthropogenic) disasters, such as climate change impacts – assuming that what is "human-generated" has the potential to be "human-prevented." In other instances, harm to human populations may be prevented even though the "forces of harm" cannot be deterred, as examples, by evacuating persons away from barrier islands prior to landfall of an approaching hurricane or through "preventive resettlement" of entire populations at extreme risk for disaster. More commonly, it is possible to blunt the impact of extreme events when human populations cannot be separated from the hazards.

This chapter consists of narrative interspersed with illustrative case examples. Beginning with the central theme of this *Handbook*, we ask whether disasters can be prevented and respond by providing a case study where prevention was achieved (Shultz et al., 2013b). We next present a primer of disaster basics and follow this with the description of an internationally significant "hybrid" disaster involving both natural and human-generated technological components (Shultz et al. 2011, 2013a). Details are then presented describing how disasters produce psychological consequences. Expanding on this point, the final case study describes an armed conflict disaster that has evolved into a long-duration humanitarian crisis (Shultz et al., 2014a, b, c). With each case example, the prevention perspective is discussed following the synopsis of the event.

Part 1: Can Disasters Really Be Prevented?

Responding to the question, "Can disasters be prevented?" Muralee Thummarukudy, Chief of Disaster Risk Reduction at the United Nations Environment Programme, apparently thinks so. His popular TEDx talk is unequivocally titled "All Disasters Are Preventable."[1] The title is phrased to attract viewers to give a listen and consider Thummarukudy's thesis. In his presentation, Thummarukudy does not actually suggest that all disasters can be prevented outright (most cannot), but he demonstrates that the magnitude of harmful consequences to human populations and the natural environment can be substantially reduced in many cases.

1 www.youtube.com/watch?v=GTm7564Vyg.

Part 1 Case Example

Successful prevention of flooding along the Red River of the North at Fargo, North Dakota, USA, 2009.

Disaster Classification: Natural hydrological river valley and overland flood disaster related to seasonal thawing of winter snowpack.

Considering whether disasters can be prevented, we present a case illustration describing community-involved mitigation of river flooding (Shultz et al., 2013b).

To achieve "universal" prevention, sparing an entire community from disaster impact and consequences despite an imminent threat, requires two uncommon ingredients: (1) the ability to precisely predict the future occurrence of a hazard in terms of time, place, and impact and (2) the availability and timely application of effective risk reduction interventions to neutralize the threat. The coincidence of these two necessary conditions is extraordinarily rare, but instances of successful universal disaster prevention have occurred. We present a case in point, involving the coincidence of disaster predictability and successful mitigation leading to impact prevention.

Natural hazards usually cannot be eliminated, but sometimes their impacts on humans can be deflected. In the case study to be presented, the hazard was present and threatening, but human populations were successfully shielded.

In 2009, during an episode of historic flooding, a river community of one hundred thousand residents was able to safeguard its citizens and infrastructure by erecting a system of levees that held back floodwaters that ringed the city on all sides. Fargo, North Dakota, USA, is an exemplar of the practical application of prevention science and a showcase for community resilience.

The Red River of the North originates in northerly latitudes and then flows much farther north, one of very few rivers worldwide with this distinction. The Red River meanders in a loopy ribbon along the eastern flanks of the cities of Fargo and Grand Forks, North Dakota, before entering the province of Manitoba, Canada, bypassing the capital of Winnipeg via the Red River Floodway diversion, spilling into Lake Winnipeg, and eventually emptying into Hudson Bay.

Flood specialist, Dr. Donald Schwert, lucidly describes the geographic features that shape the springtime Red River flood threats at Fargo:

> Fargo lies at the center of the Red River Valley, which is the lakebed of ancient Glacial Lake Agassiz and one of the flattest land surfaces on Earth. When the Red River of the North floods, waters spill out of its shallow floodplain onto the old lake plain, creating vast floods that are slow-flowing and shallow. But spring flooding is predictable, based on the depth of the developing snowpack over the winter; hence, major flooding can be predicted weeks in advance of the actual event (Shultz et al., 2013b, p. 40).

Since the memorable and devastating Red River Valley Flood of 1997, when Grand Forks was almost completely submerged and Fargo sustained significant inundation, Fargo has successfully activated its citizens every March and April to engage in sandbagging and construction of dikes and levees to prevent flooding of the city. In local parlance, citizens transform themselves into "Flood Fighters" for several weeks each spring. Fargo citizens faced their greatest challenge in 2009 when the Red River waters rose to unprecedented heights, twenty-four feet above flood stage. The 2009 "flood fight" relied upon the strong backs and energized efforts of eighty-five thousand individuals. Working nonstop shifts inside the Fargo Dome (dubbed "Sandbag Central"), students, community citizens, and volunteers collectively filled 8.5 million sandbags. Concurrently, with precision coordination, brigades of citizens were deployed to vulnerable sections of riverbanks, where they were met by flatbed trucks laden with palletized sandbags. Since subfreezing temperatures are the norm, sandbags had to be stored inside the heated Fargo Dome and then transported just in time to rendezvous with the waiting teams. Parka-clad citizens had just minutes to stack the bags, while the sand remained sufficiently malleable to sculpt into tight-packed levees. For weeks, Fargo's Flood Fighters braved blizzard conditions to construct sandbag fortifications.

Stress was palpable and rising steadily along with the river level. The levees required continuous monitoring; Fargoans knew that a single breech in the barricades would result in widespread flooding. Fortunately, the levees did not fail and the icy waters of the engorged Red River of the North were held back.

The prevention perspective. As illustrated, when the opportunity presents, invoking effective "universal" prevention measures can effectively short-circuit a major disaster threat. Hence, the cascade of harmful impacts was averted. So too were the series of consequences that an impacting flood disaster would trigger. Citizens were spared from exposures to glacially cold waters filling their homes and to the attendant damage, destruction, infrastructure disruption, resource loss, displacement, physical harm, and psychological distress.

Savvy to both stress and psychological distress inherent in the flood operation and the uncertainty of success during a year when the river reached record heights, Fargo developed contingency plans that incorporated universal, selective, and indicated components of prevention. Plans were in place to shelter children, frail elderly, and other subpopulations of persons with special needs, as well as to maintain services and safeguard psychiatric medications for the subpopulation of persons with severe and persistent mental illness. The North Dakota director of medical services, a psychiatrist, was at the table with the mayor of Fargo, civic leaders, and emergency managers. He was frequently broadcasting messages on themes of resilience and coping – and identifying available resources and support services – to Fargo and Red River Valley communities via a range of media channels.

Having experienced widespread flooding in 1997, the citizens of Fargo responded with grit and determination to prevent a recurrence. Beginning in 1998, Fargo had fourteen consecutive years when the Red River rose above flood stage, and every year the flood fighters emerged victorious. The city has not flooded again. This year-over-year success of Fargo's citizens supports the notion that DRR prevention coupled with mitigation, preparedness, and risk governance) deserves increasing prioritization relative to the traditional emergency management emphasis on the crisis management phases (response and recovery).

The natural phenomenon of river flooding was not prevented in 2009. Indeed, at Fargo, the Red River rose to a historical record of forty-two feet and overflowed its banks, with water extending for miles across the shallow floodplain. Fortunately, the flat landscape made it possible to erect a levee fortress around the city of Fargo, even as the flood submerged large expanses of farmland on all sides. Aerial views showed Fargo appearing like a dry island encircled by a vast liquid landscape of floodwaters. What was prevented was the disastrous impact of floodwaters inundating the neighborhoods of Fargo. Over years of coming together for a common purpose, the annual Fargo citizen flood response has melded into the community's identity and solidified with the creation of a not-for-profit organization entitled Red River Resilience.

Part 2: Disaster Basics and Conceptual Building Blocks

This section provides a primer of disaster terms and concepts (Shultz, et al. 2007a, b).

Disaster. What is a disaster? Among many definitions for the term "disaster," here are two:

1. "A disaster is characterized as an encounter between forces of harm and a human population in harm's way, influenced by the ecological context, in which demands exceed the coping capacity of the disaster-affected community" (Center for Disaster and Extreme Event Preparedness [DEEP Center], quoted in Shultz et al., 2007a, p. 18).
2. "A disaster is an occurrence that causes damage, ecological disruption, loss of human life, deterioration of health and health services on a scale sufficient to warrant an extraordinary response from outside the affected community area."[2]

Across a spectrum of definitions, including these two examples, five commonalities emerge (see Table 21.1). First, disasters are social-ecological phenomena, typically affecting human populations, often entire communities, and the ecosystems they rely on, often spanning large regions (Walker & Westley, 2011). Second, disasters are frequently notable for the extraordinary magnitude of harm inflicted. Third, disasters produce differential and often disproportionate effects on subpopulations of vulnerable groups and persons. Fourth, in a disaster, the demands exceed the community's capacity to respond. Fifth,

2 www.who.int/gender/gwhgendernd2.pdf.

Table 21.1 *Disaster Definitions: Five Common Elements*

1.	Disasters are socio-ecological phenomena
2.	Magnitude of harm
3.	Disproportionate effects on vulnerable populations
4.	Demands exceed affected community's capacity to respond
5.	Disaster-affected communities typically require outside help

affected communities require outside help. The two upcoming case illustrations possess all five of these defining characteristics.

Disaster Ecology Model. The DEEP Center definition for disaster was developed in tandem with the creation of the Disaster Ecology Model (DEM) (Shultz et al., 2007a, b). The model diagram embodies the definition, concurrently displaying the three pillars of the DEM: forces of harm, affected populations in harm's way, and the ecological context.

Forces of harm refer to exposures to disastrous hazards, losses, and changes. The *affected population in harm's way* is comprised of multiple tiers of persons and communities that, directly or indirectly, are threatened or impacted by the forces of harm, or sustain losses and changes associated with the disaster event. Finally, the *ecological context* is made up of an array of risk and resiliency factors, operating at many levels (Shultz et al., 2007a, b). These factors interact collectively, and in a complex manner, to influence the degree of physical and psychological harm sustained during a disaster and in the aftermath. The DEM provides a framework for simultaneously considering the interrelationships among these three components (Figure 21.1). As a socioecological model, the DEM attempts to better understand how disasters affect human communities and provides a guiding structure for how to enhance resiliency for communities that are threatened or impacted by disasters (Shultz, et al., 2007a, b).

Disaster frequency. Disasters are locally rare but globally common. Natural disasters occur with an average frequency of more than one per day. For the period 2003 to 2012, an average of 388 natural disasters was registered annually (Guha-Sapir, Hoyos, & Below, 2014). Nonintentional anthropogenic/technological disasters also occur, on average, more often than daily.

Disaster continuum. Extreme events affect communities differentially, depending in part on the seesaw balance between the demands imposed by the event and the response capacity of the community. Three terms – emergency, disaster, and catastrophe – describe a continuum that interrelates demand and capacity (Shultz et al., 2007a). An *emergency* is an event where community assets are able, and sufficient, to respond to the demands. In a *disaster*, demands exceed the coping capacity of the disaster-affected community. The term *catastrophe* is reserved for the uncommon disaster of such magnitude that not only do demands exceed capacity, but also the impact actually destroys response capacity. Examples of catastrophes include the

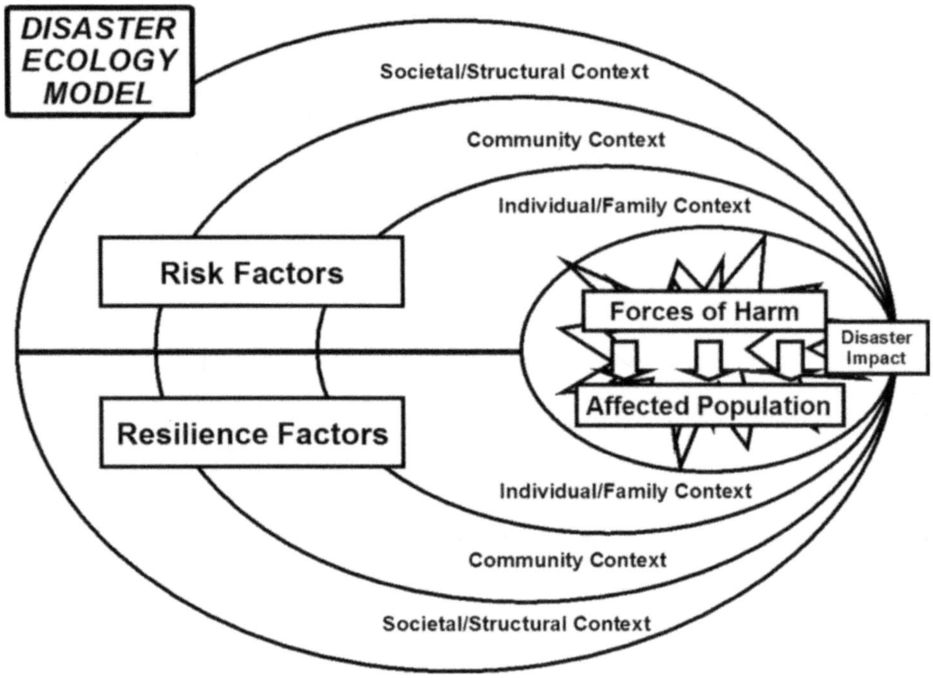

Figure 21.1. *Disaster Ecology Model.*

2010 Haiti Earthquake, the 2011 Great East Japan Disaster, and the 2013 Super Typhoon Haiyan in the Philippines.

Disaster classification. Disasters are characteristically subdivided into natural disasters (acts of nature) and human-generated or "anthropogenic" disasters. Some disasters have prominent natural and anthropogenic elements combined, leading to their description as "hybrid" disasters. The Centre for Research on the Epidemiology of Disasters (CRED), based in Brussels, Belgium, maintains the official international tallies of natural disasters (Guha-Sapir et al., 2014) and what CRED describes as "technological" human-generated disasters. CRED has recently introduced a database to tabulate "complex emergencies."

Natural disasters. CRED's disaster taxonomy distinguishes five subcategories of natural disasters: (1) *meteorological,* "events caused by short-to-medium term atmospheric events," including winter storms, tornadoes, cyclones, and hurricanes; (2) *hydrological,* "events caused by deviations in the normal water cycle," including river and flash floods, storm surges, and mudslides; (3) *geophysical,* "events originating from solid earth," including earthquakes, landslides, and volcanoes; (4) *climatological,* "events caused by medium-to-long-term climate change processes," including extremes of heat and cold, wildfires, and droughts; and (5) *biological:* "disasters caused by exposure of living organisms to pathogens and toxins," including epidemics/pandemics, insect infestations, animal diseases, and plant blights (Guha-Sapir et al., 2014).

Anthropogenic disasters. Within anthropogenic disasters, the DEEP Center specifically differentiates nonintentional/technological disasters, including transportation crashes and hazardous materials spills, from intentional events, including armed conflicts and acts of mass violence (Shultz et al., 2007a, b). Moreover, many potentially disastrous phenomena of global environmental change, including climate change, are considered anthropogenic (IPCC, 2012).

Disaster consequences. Disasters produce excess mortality, morbidity (injury and disease), and economic costs (Shultz et al., 2007a, b). During the decade 2003 to 2012, an annual average of 107,000 deaths were attributed to disasters, 215 million persons were affected each year, and annual economic costs associated with these natural events were estimated at U.S. $156.7 billion (Guha-Sapir et al., 2014).

An expanded array of disaster consequences includes (1) morbidity and mortality (injury, disease, death); (2) material losses (damage, destruction, economic losses); (3) social disruption (damage to infrastructure, lack of survival necessities, population displacement); (4) psychosocial impact (distress, detrimental behavior change, psychopathology, loss, bereavement and grief); and (5) socioecological impact, including cultural impact (Shultz et al., 2007a, b).

Disaster prevention. The fields of disaster management, disaster public health, disaster medicine, and disaster nursing routinely address prevention using the classical approach to the topic: primary, secondary, and tertiary prevention. In contrast, throughout this volume, a more contemporary conceptualization of prevention is used. Based on the seminal work of Gordon (1983), prevention is conceived at three levels: universal, selective, and indicated. The National Research Council (U.S.) and Institute of Medicine (2009) provide the following concise descriptions that distinguish universal, selective, and indicated prevention:

> *Universal prevention* includes strategies that can be offered to the full population, based on the evidence that it is likely to provide some benefit to all (reduce the probability of disorder), which clearly outweighs the costs and risks of negative consequences. *Selective prevention* refers to strategies that are targeted to subpopulations identified as being at elevated risk for a disorder. *Indicated prevention* includes strategies that are targeted to individuals who are identified (or individually screened) as having an increased vulnerability for a disorder based on some individual assessment but who are currently asymptomatic. Selective and indicated prevention strategies might involve more intensive interventions and thus involve greater cost to the participants, since their risk and thus potential benefit from participation would be greater (National Research Council and Institute of Medicine, 2009, p. 61).

Cascading disaster risks, impacts, and consequences. Disasters expose human populations to harm and produce consequences. For many disaster events, the timeline can be simplified into three phases: preimpact, impact, and postimpact. This before-during-after sequence has great utility for organizing disaster risk management strategies. Furthermore, the DRR approaches of prevention, mitigation, and preparedness are best applied preimpact, while the crisis management strategies, response and recovery, are initiated during impact and extend far into the postimpact periods.

We can also describe cascades in a tripartite fashion. Preimpact, the "risk landscape" may be comprised of a complex set of risks that mutually interdepend and build upon each other. When disaster strikes, the impact cascades are foremost. In the aftermath, consequence cascades come to prominence.

While some disasters involve a one-time single impact, many disasters involve multiple simultaneous, sequential, or cascading impacts. Disaster consequences typically occur in multiples. Furthermore, in relation to the exposures experienced, disaster consequences interact, synergize, compound, amplify, exacerbate, and cascade.

Major disasters are frequently distinguished by their multidimensionality and their interrelated and interacting components (hallmarks of complexity). The next case example, the Great East Japan Disaster, is notable for its composite of cascading events. The storyline consists of three parts: an underwater earthquake set off a tsunami that caused a radiation release at a nuclear power plant. Natural phenomena (earthquake, tsunami) and human-generated/technological elements (radiation disaster) combined to create a hybrid disaster of daunting scope and complexity that required remarkable ingenuity to counteract.

Part 2 Case Example

A multiple impact "hybrid disaster": The Great East Japan Disaster, 2011.

Disaster Classification: Natural geophysical earthquake/tsunami disaster triggering anthropogenic (nonintentional human-generated) radiation release leading to a complex humanitarian crisis.

On the afternoon of March 11, 2011, an extreme seismic phenomenon – a 9.0 moment magnitude (Mw) earthquake – precipitated multiple cascading events leading to what would collectively be called the Great East Japan Disaster (Shultz et al. 2011, 2013a). The undersea megathrust earthquake involved the subduction of the Pacific plate beneath the tectonic plate that supports Japan's largest island, Honshu. Originating at profound ocean depths about one hundred kilometers from Japan's eastern coastline, the earthquake was the strongest ever to hit Japan – and the fourth most powerful in recorded earthquake history. Earthquake shock waves were experienced on the Japanese mainland within seconds. The earthquake set off a massive tsunami at the ocean's surface, directly above the epicenter, sending waves toward the coastline, traveling at the flight speed of a commercial jet aircraft. The "run-up" of the tsunami waves inundated hundreds of kilometers of coastal territory, toppling structures and bulldozing piles of debris far inland. Towering tsunami waves came ashore in the Fukushima Prefecture and overtopped the protective seawalls buttressing the Fukushima Dai-ichi nuclear power plant. Surging seawater scuttled the plant's safety systems, ultimately triggering meltdowns in three reactors. Radiation releases resulted in limited direct exposure of human populations in the area and contaminated the water supplies, agricultural products, and ocean fish and shellfish populations (Shultz et al., 2013a).

Populations in the area of the power plant experienced a triple threat situation during the impact phase: powerful earthquake ground shaking within seconds of the underwater event, tsunami waves rushing ashore with deadly effect within the first hour, and radiation exposure over days and weeks (Shultz et al., 2011).

In the aftermath, many survivors were dealing with psychological trauma while grieving their lost loved ones, some of whom were swept away by the waves. Many of these survivors were concurrently recovering from physical injuries sustained during harrowing escapes from the onrushing tsunami. Near the power plant, populations in closest proximity were evacuated and displaced with almost no chance of return to their radiation-contaminated properties. To this day, disaster survivors in the hardest hit areas, as well as their products and services, have been victims of stigma, ostracism, and discrimination.

A detailed "trauma signature analysis" of the Great East Japan Disaster has been published, detailing the multiplicity of psychological risk factors operating in relation to each and all of the three hazards comprising this catastrophic event (Shultz et al., 2013a). The Japanese population was subjected to multiple impacting hazards, with each one ranked at extreme magnitude on the respective rating scales (Shultz et al., 2013a).

The prevention perspective – enriched by complexity sciences. This brief synopsis presents a streamlined account of the events. Even so, this description highlights the cascading, amplifying, aggravating sequence of impacts and outcomes that distinguished the Great East Japan Disaster.

Disasters are complex and nonlinear events. There is increasing recognition that disasters need to be viewed as such to better respond to the intricate web of challenges posed once an event, such as the Great East Japan Disaster, is rolling onshore – in the most literal sense. Complexity scientists are grappling with how best to deal with the richly populated disaster "risk landscape" and how to infuse preparation for the "unknown unknowns" into emergency management planning and response (Cavallo, 2010, 2014; Cavallo & Ireland, 2014). Traditional, regimented, hierarchical, compartmentalized approaches to disaster management are rigid and antiquated. Paradigmatic change is necessary at this critical juncture.

The application of complexity sciences, defined as "the study of the phenomena which emerge from a collection of interacting objects" (Johnson, 2007, p. 3), is highly relevant. More than most complex phenomena, disasters routinely break the mold of predictability, logical sequences, and linear causality. Major disasters tend to be dynamic, complex, unpredictable, nonlinear, cascading events. In order to integrate prevention science into DRR and DRM planning and operations, and to forge a path toward community disaster resilience, it is necessary to grapple with the complexities of disaster events.

In the case of the Great East Japan Disaster, the fact that an undersea earthquake could give rise to a surface-riding tsunami was anticipated. A similar scenario played out seven years earlier when the deadly 2004 Southeast Asia tsunami originated from a 9.2–9.3 moment magnitude (Mw) earthquake with its submarine epicenter close to Aceh, Indonesia. Tsunamis are generated by sudden displacements in the seafloor, landslides, or volcanic activity. In the language of complexity science, the highly predictable occurrence of a tsunami that was produced by the powerful earthquake of March 11, 2011, was not "emergent." To be emergent, a phenomenon needs to be unpredictable, trigger a downward causal sequence, and create organization or order on an unexpected scale.

Instead, what was "emergent" was the tsunami-induced radiation disaster at the Fukushima Dai-ichi nuclear power plant. Once the tsunami waves surmounted the protective seawalls, the generators for the cooling systems were submerged in salt water and shut down. This led to system failures and ultimately to the meltdown of three nuclear reactors. The Fukushima Dai-ichi nuclear power plant disaster was an unpredictable encounter with "unknown unknowns" (e.g., unanticipated tsunami wave heights) leading to a downward causal sequence that was unstoppable but orderly (the meltdown and local area contamination unfolded in stages, progressively and inevitably).

What was also "emergent" was the stranding of pockets of coastal residents who became geographically isolated by the tsunami waters that pooled onshore. Unreachable for days by rescue personnel, these populations were exposed to harsh March winter conditions without access to shelter or survival supplies.

What was also "emergent" were the psychological effects for persons exposed to three compounding impacts from earthquake, tsunami, and radiation. We have previously described these phenomena as a "triple threat trauma" (Shultz et al., 2011).

Nevertheless, despite the extraordinary demands and the level of complexity, Japan mounted a model disaster mental health response that we have previously documented (Kim, 2011; Kim & Akiyama, 2011; Shultz et al., 2013a; Suzuki & Kim, 2012; Takeda, 2011). This response incorporated elements of universal, selective, and indicated prevention (Gordon, 1983; National Research Council and Institute of Medicine, 2009).

Part 3: Psychological Dimensions of Disasters

We are now at a pivot point to move the conversation into a domain where prevention science and complexity science have not met previously – examining the psychological dimensions of disasters. Prevention science has been applied effectively to the promotion of psychological health and the prevention of psychological consequences of a variety of exposures throughout the lifespan. This *Handbook* is a testament to the state of the science. Complexity science has not been fully infused into the social sciences generally or into the psychological dimensions of disasters. This is an unexplored frontier. Moreover, within the domain of the psychological aspects of disasters, prevention science and complexity science have yet to shake hands. Part 3 of this chapter is intended to make this introduction, presenting two interrelated sections – on the psychological consequences of disasters and on disaster behavioral health concepts – before providing a third case example that exemplifies a very high degree of complexity.

Psychological Consequences of Disasters

When applying prevention science to the area of disaster health, it is useful to understand the four primary attributes of the psychological consequences of disaster (Shultz, 2013a, b). This section summarizes key teachings from disaster behavioral health trainings conducted for more than twenty thousand public health, mental health, health care, hospital, and emergency management professionals throughout the United States and Canada, and in a series of international venues, by DEEP Center professionals (Shultz et al., 2006b, 2007a, Shultz, Allen, Bustamant, & Espinel, 2009). This information has been previously published, upon invitation, by the Substance Abuse and Mental Health Services Administration's (SAMHSA) Disaster Technical Assistance Center (U.S.), and the following discussion closely parallels our previous writing (Shultz, 2013a, b).

In a disaster, the psychological consequences (1) are widespread, (2) extend across a spectrum of severity, (3) persist for a prolonged duration, and (4) reflect the unique and defining features of the specific disaster event. These distinguishing psychological features relate directly to exposure of a population to the physical forces of harm in a natural or anthropogenic disaster and to perpetrated actions during situations of armed conflict.

Psychological consequences of disaster are widespread and pervasive. The most basic premise is that in a disaster, more people are affected psychologically than are harmed physically (see Figure 21.2). This can be illustrated by showing that the "psychological footprint" of a disaster is larger than the "medical footprint" (Shultz, 2013a, b).

The application of multiple levels of prevention – universal, selective, and indicated – provides an excellent starting point. When preparing for disasters, it is very important to identify a range of special populations that are more vulnerable when disasters strike. What is unappreciated is the fact that disasters produce "new" special populations. Persons who, prior to impact, were healthy, functional, and "needs-free" may suddenly become candidates for a disaster-created "special population" of persons who have sustained, as examples, traumatizing exposures to the forces of harm, loss of home leading to displacement, loss of a loved one and subsequent bereavement, personal life-changing injury, or disruption of ecosystem services. Each of these instances creates needs that did not previously exist and cause psychological distress. Psychological repercussions may occur for persons far from the scene who are socially

In a disaster, the size of the psychological "footprint" greatly exceeds the size of the medical "footprint."

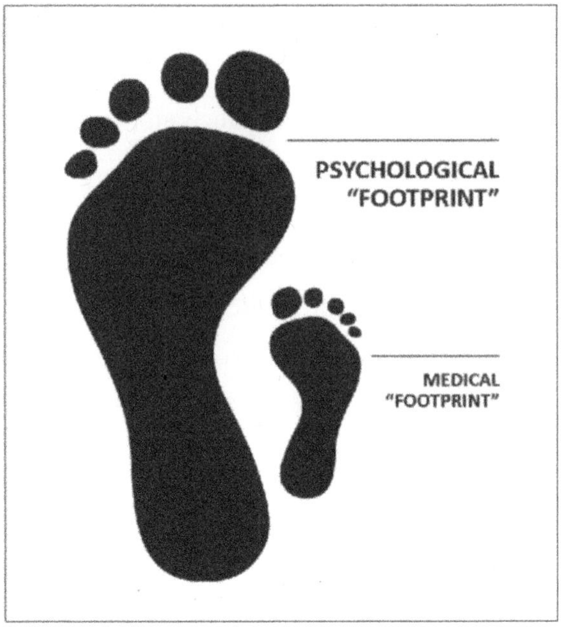

Figure 21.2. *Psychological consequences of disasters: widespread and pervasive.*

connected to direct victims of the disaster. So, following a disaster, persons who may need psychological support tend to be larger in number and geographically more dispersed than persons sustaining harm at the epicenter of destruction.

Psychological consequences of disaster are arrayed across a spectrum of severity. Almost everyone exposed to a disaster experiences fear and distress. This is a common, expectable, and nearly universal reaction. Many who are initially affected will rebound rapidly and regain full functioning without need for intervention. However, some disaster-exposed persons will exhibit detrimental behavior changes such as when unharmed-but-fearful citizens converge on area hospitals. A smaller proportion of persons, especially those with the most intense exposures, will experience more pronounced psychological consequences, leading to diagnosis of common mental disorders (CMDs) such as posttraumatic stress disorder (PTSD), major depression, generalized anxiety disorder, panic reactions, somatic complaints, and/or increased use of substances. Persons who have lost a loved one are likely to experience traumatic bereavement or complicated grief. There are individual differences, but a general rule of thumb is that the intensity of exposure to the disaster event predicts where disaster survivors fall along this continuum from transient distress to psychopathology (Shultz, 2013a, b). There are higher rates of severe psychological consequences and diagnosable psychiatric disorders among those who have a "ground zero" exposure to the disaster compared to survivors who are more peripherally exposed.

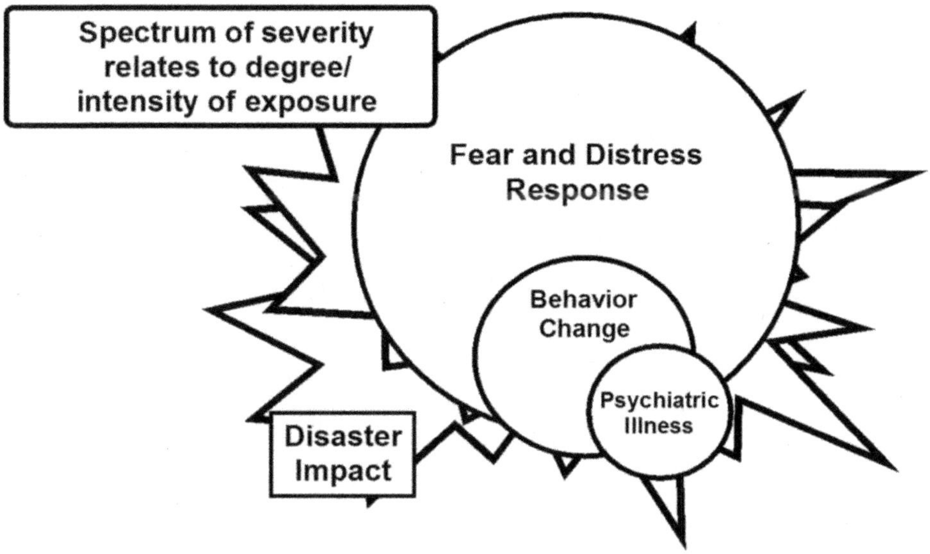

Figure 21.3. *Psychological consequences of disasters: spectrum of severity.*

From a prevention science vantage point, it is possible, based on historic disaster experiences, to plan and prepare for the magnitude and extent of psychological needs for persons exposed to common disasters across a spectrum of intensity (see Figure 21.3). Based on experience, disaster mental health professionals can estimate the proportions of survivors exposed to varying levels of injurious or potentially traumatizing events and to provide active outreach to persons in geographic areas or shelter environments who are most likely to need mental health and psychosocial support.

Psychological consequences of disaster extend across a range of duration. While the exposure to disaster hazards during impact may be relatively brief, hardships in the aftermath, associated with losses, lifestyle changes, and socio-ecological disruptions, often persist for extended periods of time (Shultz, 2013a, b). Accordingly, psychological stressors maintain even after the physical forces have ceased to do harm (see Figure 21.4). Disaster survivors who have lost loved ones must cope with the tasks of disaster recovery and reconstruction while grappling with traumatic bereavement and, often, with prolonged grief disorder.

Psychological consequences of disaster relate to the defining features of the event. The type of disaster matters. Each disaster creates a unique composite of psychological risk factors unlike any other event (see Figure 21.5). What survivors experience and witness in a particular disaster event shapes what becomes consolidated into traumatic memories of the event. The novelty of each disaster episode, leading to a specific pattern of potentially traumatizing exposures, has been operationalized into an evidence-based method called trauma signature (TSIG) analysis (Shultz & Neria, 2013).

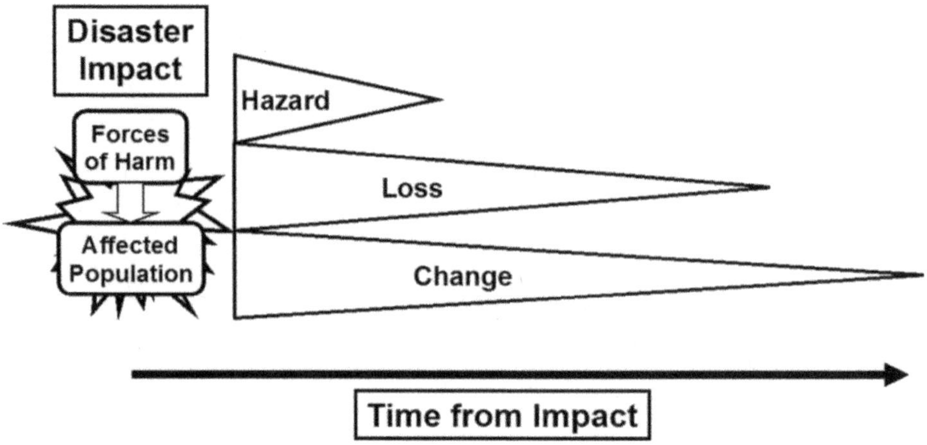

Figure 21.4. *Psychological consequences of disasters: range of duration.*

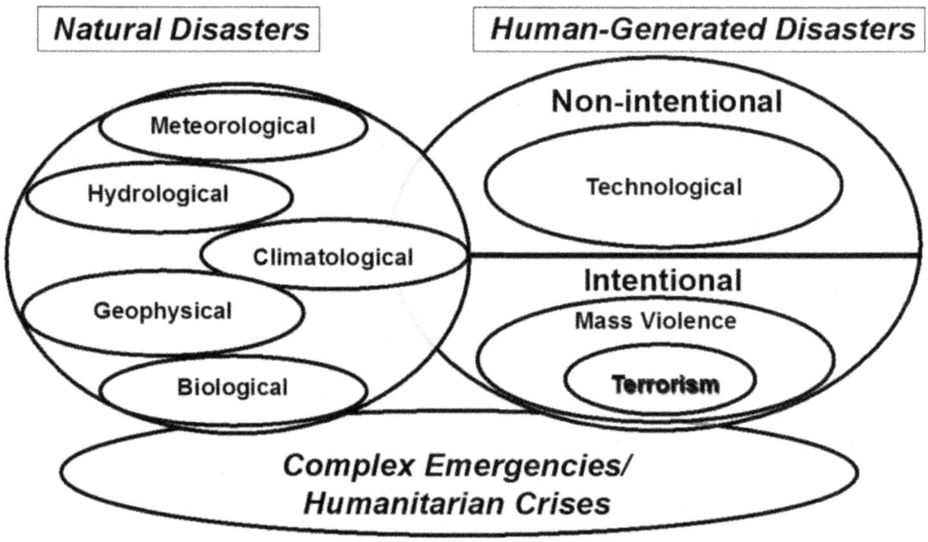

Figure 21.5. *Psychological consequences of disasters: type of disaster.*

Disaster Behavioral Health Concepts: A Review of the Scientific Evidence

Disasters can be traumatic via three interacting pathways: (1) disasters can be perceived as threats of bodily injury and potential death (Neria, Nandi, & Galea, 2008); (2) disasters can lead to temporary or permanent loss of assets, resources, and services (McFarlane, Van Hooff, & Goodhew, 2009; Norris, Friedman, Watson, Byrne, & Kaniasty, 2002); and (3) disasters can lead those affected to experience physical and/or psychological disorders (Neria & Galea, 2008).

Studies have suggested that anthropogenic disasters can lead to more, and more complex, psychological problems than natural disasters (Galea, Nandi, &

Vlahov, 2005; Norris et al., 2002; Shultz, 2013a, b). However, since natural disasters impact wide geographic areas, researchers often based their findings on the report of individuals with very different levels of exposure. Galea et al. (2005) proposed that communities affected by natural disasters have lower rates of PTSD than communities impacted by anthropogenic disasters due to lower average levels of exposure.

Most individuals who experience traumatic incidents do not develop mental health disorders as a result of trauma exposure (Breslau et al.,1998; Norris, Tracy, & Galea, 2008), and most are able to maintain or regain their pre-exposure level of functioning (Bonanno, 2005; Bonanno & Gupta, 2009). The adaptive capacity to cope with trauma is a prerequisite to achieving "resilience" (Bonanno & Gupta, 2009; Norris et al., 2008). Although resilient people may experience psychological symptoms during and after a disaster, they typically recover within a brief period of time (Norris et al., 2002).

PTSD is a psychological disorder caused by exposure to a traumatic incident. Symptoms of PTSD include reexperiencing the traumatic event (e.g., nightmares, flashbacks); alterations in arousal (e.g., hypervigilance, exaggerated startle response); avoidance of reminders of the trauma; and negative alterations in cognition and mood (e.g., negative beliefs and expectations about oneself and the world) (American Psychiatric Association, 2013).

PTSD is the only disorder whose diagnostic criteria include exposure to a traumatic incident. Thus, it is one of the most common psychological disorders experienced by people who have been exposed to a disaster. It is also one of the most widely researched postdisaster psychopathologies (Galea et al., 2005; Neria, Nandi, & Galea, 2008). During the first year after a disaster, the prevalence of PTSD ranges between 30 percent and 40 percent among individuals who were directly exposed to the disaster; between 10 percent and 20 percent among first responders; and between 5 percent and 10 percent among the general population (Neria et al., 2008). However, certain factors can place people at a higher risk of developing psychopathology if exposed to a disaster, including (1) extent of exposure (measured by severity of physical injuries, possibility of death, magnitude of property destruction, and rate of casualties) (Neria et al., 2008); (2) female gender (Green et al., 1991; Hagstrom, 1995; Pulcino et al., 2003); (3) younger age (Kar, 2009); (4) history of previous traumatic experiences and life stressors (Galea et al., 2003; Maes, Mylle, Delmeire, & Janca, 2001); (5) history of previous psychiatric conditions (Smith, North, & Spitznagel, 1993; Udwin, Boyle, Yule, Bolton, & O'Ryan., 2000); (6) low social support (Dalgleish, Joseph, Thrasher, Tranah, & Yule, 1996; Weiss, Marmar, Metzler, & Ronfeldt, 1995); (7) low socioeconomic status (Bonanno & Gupta, 2009; Norris et al., 2002); (8) ethnic minority status (Galea et al., 2005; Norris et al., 2002); and (9) exposure to the disaster through media outlets (Ahern et al., 2002; Pfefferbaum et al., 2000; Schlenger et al., 2002). Longitudinal studies have shown changes – typically declines – in PTSD rates over time (Carr et al., 1997; Sloan, 1988).

Following PTSD, depression is the second most commonly researched post-disaster mental health disorder. Symptoms of major depressive disorder (MDD) include depressed mood, loss of interest or pleasure, changes in eating and sleeping patterns, decreased energy, and difficulty concentrating. After the September 11 attacks in New York City, 10 percent of the city residents reported experiencing symptoms of MDD (Galea et al., 2002), while 5 percent of Texans impacted by Hurricane Ike met diagnostic criteria for MDD thirty days after the disaster (Tracy, Norris, & Galea, 2011).

Several studies have indicated that the substance use increases in communities that have been impacted by disasters. For example, after the September 11 attacks, 10 percent of New Yorkers reported increased use of cigarettes, 3 percent reported increased use of marijuana, and close to 25 percent reported increased consumption of alcohol (Vlahov et al,. 2002). After the Oklahoma City bombing, 32.4 percent of survivors with comorbid PTSD reported using alcohol, and 73 percent reported using prescription medications as a coping mechanism (North et al., 1999).

Other mental health disorders that have been studied in the disaster research field have included generalized anxiety disorder (McFarlane, Van Hooff, & Goodhew, 2009) and panic disorder (Norris et al., 2002).

After examining two longitudinal data sets from populations impacted by 1999 floods in Mexico and the September 11 attacks, Norris (2009) proposed that postdisaster symptomatology can follow four trajectories: (1) resistance (absence of symptoms or stable and mild symptoms); (2) resilience (moderate or severe symptoms immediately after the disaster that decrease significantly within a circumscribed period of time); (3) recovery (moderate or severe symptoms immediately after the disaster that gradually decrease over an extended period of time); and (4) chronic dysfunction (moderate or severe symptoms that remain stable over time).

Mental health interventions. In 1980, critical incident stress debriefing (CISD) was developed as an early intervention for populations exposed to traumatic incidents. Used within forty-eight hours of the traumatic exposure, survivors are encouraged to give detailed accounts of their experiences and to share their emotional reactions associated with the trauma. CISD also includes providing survivors with psychoeducation and steps to manage their reactions (Bryant & Litz, 2009). Research on CISD has shown that this intervention may cause survivors to solidify their memories of their trauma and experience more severe symptoms than those who do not participate in CISD (McNally, Bryant, & Ehlers, 2003). Consequently, many experts no longer recommend the use of CISD (Bryant & Litz, 2009; Norris et al., 2002).

Currently, the most popular intervention for survivors of disaster-related traumas is psychological first aid (PFA). The World Health Organization (WHO) defines PFA as "a humane, supportive response to a fellow human being who is suffering and who may need support" (WHO, WTF, WVI, 2011, p. 3). Some authors argue that PFA is a universal intervention because it could be used with the entire population affected by a disaster (Goldenberg, Benedeck, & Ursano, 2012). However, other experts in the field believe that PFA is an intervention for selective and indicative prevention to be used only with high-risk subpopulations or with people who exhibit distress or impairment after a disaster (Nash & Watson, 2012).

PFA seeks to offer the following protections for survivors: (1) improves survivors' safety and access to basic needs (e.g., shelter, food, medical aid); (2) decreases stress; and (3) provides survivors with appropriate resources. Survivors are not asked to speak about their trauma; instead, PFA seeks to increase survivor's ability to cope with issues that have emerged in their lives as a result of the disaster. Since the goal of PFA is not to treat severe mental health symptoms, laypeople can be trained to conduct PFA. Through the use of PFA, survivors who need psychiatric services can be identified and referred to trained mental health professionals. Although PFA has been endorsed by organizations worldwide, research that supports PFA's effectiveness is lacking (Dieltjens, Moonens, Van Praet, Buck, & Vanderkerckhove, 2014; Shultz & Forbes, 2013).

As previously mentioned, most people who survive disasters are expected to return to their previous level of functioning without receiving mental health services. However, survivors who develop severe mental health symptoms can benefit from professional treatments such as cognitive behavioral therapy, exposure therapy, narrative exposure therapy, and/or psychopharmacology. However, access to appropriate treatments in the aftermath of a disaster can be challenging. It has been reported that only 6 percent of survivors of Hurricane Katrina were able to access mental health services within six months of the disaster (Elhai & Ford, 2009). Some barriers to accessing services include (1) difficulty identifying survivors, (2) insufficient referral sources, (3) damaged infrastructure (Reifels et al., 2013), (4) gender issues, (5) oppressive patterns and/or racism, (6) stigma, and (7) socioeconomic status (Dückers, 2013).

Experts in the field of disaster mental health endorse a "multidimensional approach to psychosocial care ranging from the provision of broad-based, low intensity support to specialized high-intensity interventions" (Reifels et al., 2013, p. 6). Some examples of this approach include the responses after the 2011 Great East Japan earthquake, tsunami, and nuclear disaster and after the Sandy Hook, Connecticut (U.S.), school shooting. In Japan, the response included the provision of social support, PFA, psychoeducation, assessments, and high-intensity interventions for people with severe mental illness who were disaster-displaced. In the aftermath of the Sandy Hook shooting, the response included universal prevention services (e.g., psychoeducation), selective prevention services (e.g., practical assistance), and indicated prevention services (e.g., crisis and grief counseling services, referrals for people who were identified as in need of intensive services) (Reifels et al., 2013).

Part 3 Case Example: Armed Conflict in Colombia, South America, Leading to Forced Migration, 1960–2015.

Disaster Classification: Intentional anthropogenic (human-generated) armed conflict disaster with multiple armed actors and massive internal displacement, leading to a prolonged humanitarian crisis.

Colombia has experienced the world's longest continuous, ongoing armed conflict.[3] Multiple armed actors, including left-wing guerrilla and right-wing paramilitary, have been battling with Colombian military and National Police since 1948. Complexity science studies indicate that one of the keys to the longevity of the conflict has been the ability of the armed insurgents to "right-size" their units for optimal invisibility, mobility, and strategic advantage. A complicating factor is the ability of armed actors to support themselves with proceeds from the lucrative illicit drug trade, supplemented by other activities such as kidnapping for ransom.

The Colombian nation has paid a heavy toll, estimated at 250,000 deaths and millions forced to abandon homes and property (Shultz et al., 2014a). Guerrilla forces move into a region and establish property rights, and when a critical mass of comrades arrive, they rearrange the community power structure, setting strict codes of conduct and displacing homeowners and landholders as it suits them.

As an outcome of decades of conflict and forced migration, Colombia currently has the second highest tally of internally displaced persons (IDPs) in the world, estimated at 6.04 million in 2014 (Bilak et al., 2015; Shultz et al., 2014a, b). This number does not count the millions of children who have been born into displacement. In fact, Colombia has ranked either first or second in numbers of IDPs every year since 2004; no other nation holds this distinction. Seventy percent of IDPs in Colombia are women or children. One-quarter are of Indian or Afro-Colombian descent. Internal displacement is predominantly rural to urban and unidirectional; once displaced, IDPs cannot return to their homes of origin (Shultz et al., 2014a, b).

IDPs are frequently forced to leave after witnessing or directly experiencing extreme violence – warfare, massacres, assassinations, kidnappings, physical and sexual assaults, disappearances, and forced recruitment of youth into the armed groups (Bilak et al., 2015; Shultz et al., 2014a, b, c). Trauma and violence exposure are almost universal in this population. Permanent displacement comes with staggering losses, including but not limited to loss of home, land, animals, possessions, schools, social bonds to family and friends, livelihood, status and stature in the community, personal identity, and reputation as a landholding citizen. All these are left behind on the day of "the departure" (*la salida*). Researchers describe such experiences as "loss cascades," and scientific evidence strongly ties resource loss to high risk for progression to psychopathology (Hobfoll, Tracy, & Galea, 2006).

The magnitude of loss coupled with fear of the unknown explains why so many families have delayed their departures until they have experienced direct, often deadly, victimization.

After a period of migration, IDPs arrive in the large cities devoid of urban survival or job skills. They arrive anonymous and without resources, driven by the survival imperative of staying alive in harsh, impoverished urban settings.

3 www.theguardian.com/world/2015/mar/15/colombia-end-in-sight-longest-running-conflict.

Fully 95 percent are unable to find stable employment and work instead in the "informal sector" (Shultz et al., 2014b).

Phases of displacement. Psychologically, internal displacement involves an ever-changing but always challenging trajectory. We have distinguished six phases of internal displacement in Colombia: (1) months or years of pre-departure vulnerability in the home community, including witnessing atrocities and receiving threats of harm; (2) the day of departure or expulsion; (3) migration away from danger, often without a specific destination; (4) initial relocation and adaptation to life as an IDP; and (5) longer-term resettlement and, for some, achievement of durable solutions for the family. The final phase, (6) return to the community of origin, is extremely rare in Colombia (Shultz et al., 2014a).

Psychological consequences of internal displacement. "Abrupt and coerced displacement is one of the harshest multiple-loss experiences imaginable" (Shultz et al., 2014a). At each stage along the pathway of displacement, IDPs are exposed to hazards, losses, and changes (see Figure 21.6). The specific stressors change by phase, but there is never a period when IDPs are able to

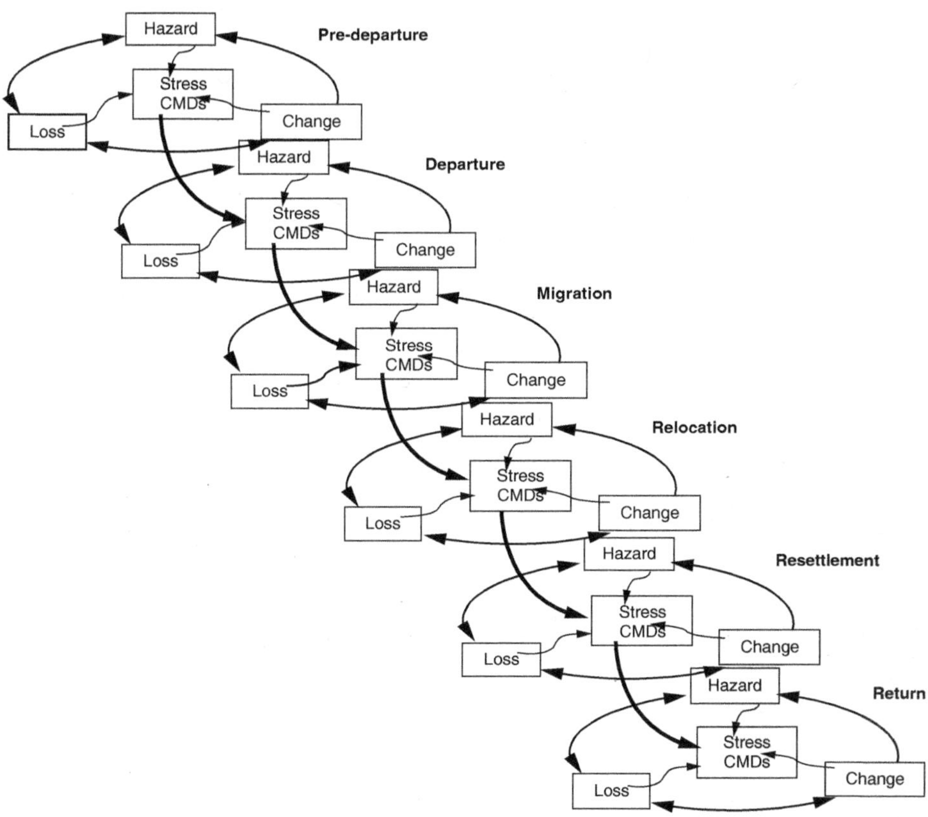

Figure 21.6. *Phases of armed-conflict-induced internal displacement in Colombia.*

escape from danger. There are varying degrees of safety, but exposure to violence is a lifelong constant for most IDPs.

The experiences of forced migration combine the stressors of multiple traumas with irrecoverable losses, thereby elevating risks for progression to CMDs. This includes increased risks for major depression, PTSD, and generalized anxiety disorder, as well as somatic complaints and increased consumption of alcohol and illicit drugs (Doctors without Borders, 2006, 2010; Londoño, Romero, & Casas, 2012; Richards et al., 2011; Shultz et al., 2014a, b, c).

The prevention perspective. In relation to the psychological repercussions of the extended armed conflict in Colombia, the situation is both complicated and complex. Three generations have been born during the period of armed insurgency; two generations of children have been born into internal displacement. Exposure to violence is a common occurrence in Colombia, and most citizens have witnessed or been directly victimized by multiple traumas.

In Colombia, violence comes in many forms and at multiple levels: intrafamilial violence, gender-based violence, and community violence (at the hands of gangs and criminal bands – BACRIM) occur daily with apparent impunity. Domestic and community violence are overlaid upon the substrate of conflict-associated terrorism and violence, intermixed with drug and human trafficking. Frequently, the daily news cycle is punctuated with stories of assaults, homicides, kidnappings, landmine injuries, and massacres.

How is prevention science relevant here? Not in the conventional sense certainly. Prevention needs to be as multifaceted, complex and textured as the challenges presented by Colombia's prevalent, pervasive, protracted, and prolonged violence exposure. The "peace" is being formally negotiated. If successful, a signed agreement will officially shift Colombia to "postconflict" nation status for the first time in sixty years. Recent legislation, including Law 1448, the Law of the Victims, accords protected status and opens up a range of programs, including psychosocial programs, to more than seven million victims. The human rights violations and the psychological impact of the armed conflict are acknowledged and slated for redress. Support and restitution are legally guaranteed, although the programming is slow to take shape and far more political than scientific in its inaugural form. Still, there is now a legal and programmatic framework for providing psychological support within a broader structure that includes jobs training and support for achieving economic self-sufficiency through, for example, microenterprises. Gainful employment and economic stability is one component of the new programs that also confers a degree of psychological well-being. From the vantage of prevention, these services serve as protections. Ultimately, prevention will need to be multigenerational, healing the current generation that has been exposed lifelong to conflict while preparing proactively to raise the next generation, the first to grow up in an era of declared peace, in a manner that is psychologically healthy and that diminishes traumatic exposures. To achieve this will require invoking prevention science in highly creative ways. This will require incorporation of multiple facets of preventive governance that target, as examples, the macro-societal and political realities and ecosystems.

Concluding Comments

What we have attempted to establish is the fact that disasters typically set in motion a concatenation of consequences. We describe this phenomenon in terms of disaster cascades. By making this case, we then ask ourselves, given that disasters can only rarely be prevented outright, can impacts and consequences be mitigated? Can we intervene at various points along the cascade to halt or dampen the consequences? Can we remove a "domino" or short-circuit a destructive sequence? Can we "disaster-cascade-proof" a community or population? How do we enhance personal and community resilience? How do we prevent postdisaster violence? How do we implement "force protection" for first responders?

Prevention science is very applicable to the outright prevention of some anthropogenic disasters and to the development of approaches to intervene on disaster impact and outcome cascades to diminish the magnitude of consequences. In the process of developing our theses, we have introduced three case examples, progressively increasing in complexity. Concurrently, we have incorporated the psychological dimensions of disaster exposure and response.

First, the community response to the 2009 Red River flood in Fargo, North Dakota, provided evidence that some disasters can be prevented. Here, prevention depends upon having (1) the ability to predict the time and place when the hazard would occur and (2) the means to protect the community, in this case, by building levees to keep the floodwaters out. What has been emergent here is the development of a community identity based on the successful "flood fights" – Fargo residents promote and exude resilience. This community knows how to create protections.

Second, the Great East Japan Disaster illustrated the disaster impact cascade – earthquake, tsunami, and nuclear radiation event – and the need to match the comprehensiveness of the response to the complexities posed by the disaster. This multi-impact event, combining three extreme-intensity hazards, demonstrated how prevention sciences must incorporate some elements of complexity sciences to handle the "unknown unknowns" and the emergent properties of hybrid disasters. The exceptional mental health and psychosocial support response was nimble, evidence-based, and adept at addressing the psychosocial needs of the Japanese population (Shultz et al., 2013a).

Third, the prolonged armed conflict, compounded by pervasive societal violence throughout Colombia, South America, provided an example of how trauma exposure accumulates over time and throughout multiple phases for such experiences as forced internal displacement. The peace process that is progressing, coupled with recent initiatives for "victims of the armed conflict" (including "psychosocial" interventions), together holds promise for addressing the conflict-induced, populationwide symptom elevations for PTSD, depression, and generalized anxiety disorders. This optimism assumes that evidence-based interventions will be adapted to Colombia. Meanwhile, for future "peacetime" generations, prevention science can help guide the development of programs for violence- or trauma-proofing the youth of Colombia.

Recognizing that disasters are complex and consequences are plentiful, prevention science, in tandem with complexity sciences, has a major future role to play in increasing the sophistication and effectiveness of DRR and DRM.

References

Ahern, J., Galea, S., Resnick, H., Kilpatrick, D., Bucuvalas, M., Gold, J., & Vlahov, D. (2002). Television images and psychological symptoms after the September 11 terrorist attacks. *Psychiatry* 65(4): 289–300.

APA (American Psychiatric Association) (2013). *Diagnostic and Statistical Manual of Mental Disorders: DSM-5™*, 5th ed. Arlington, VA: American Psychiatric Publishing.

Bilak, A., Caterina, M., Charron, G., Crozet, S., Díaz-Leal, L. R., Foster, F., et al. (2015). *Global Overview 2015: People Internally Displaced by Conflict and Violence*. Geneva, Switzerland: Internal Displacement Monitoring Centre.

Bonanno, G. A. (2005). Resilience in the face of potential trauma. *Current Directions in Psychological Science* 14: 135–8.

Bonanno, G. A., & Gupta, S. (2009). Resilience after disaster. In Neria, Y., Galea, S., & Norris, F. H. (eds.), *Mental Health and Disasters*. New York: Cambridge University Press, pp. 145–60.

Breslau, N., Kessler, R. C., Chilcoat, H. D., Schultz, L. R., Davis, G. C., & Andreski, P. (1998). Trauma and posttraumatic stress disorder in the community: the 1996 Detroit Area Survey of Trauma. *Archives of General Psychiatry* 55: 626–32.

Bryant, R. A., & Litz, B. (2009). Mental health treatments in the wake of disaster. In Neria, Y., Galea, S., & Norris, F. H. (eds.), *Mental Health and Disasters*. New York: Cambridge University Press, pp. 321–35.

Buldyrev, S. V., Parshani, R., Paul, G., Stanley, H. E., & Havlin, S. (2010). Catastrophic cascade of failures in interdependent networks. *Nature* 464: 1025–8. doi: 10.1038/nature08932

Carr, V. J., Lewin, T. J., Webster, R. A., Kenardy, J. A., Hazell, P. L., & Carter, G. L. (1997). Psychosocial sequelae of the 1989 Newcastle earthquake: II. Exposure and morbidity profiles during the first 2 years post-disaster. *Psychological Medicine* 27: 167–78.

Cavallo, A. (2010). *Risk Management in Complex Projects: An Exploratory Study to Managing Unknown Unknowns in Uncertain Environments*. Saarbruecken, Germany: Lambert Academic.

Cavallo, A. (2014). Integrating disaster preparedness and resilience: a complex approach using system of systems. *Australian Journal of Emergency Management* 29: 46–51.

Cavallo, A., & Ireland, V. (2014). Preparing for complex interdependent risks: a system of systems approach to building disaster resilience. *International Journal of Disaster Risk Reduction* 9: 181–93. dx.doi.org/10.1016/j.ijdrr.2014.05.001

Dalgleish, T., Joseph, S., Thrasher, S., Tranah, T., & Yule, W. (1996). Crisis support following the Herald of Free Enterprise disaster: a longitudinal perspective. *Journal of Traumatic Stress* 9: 833–45.

Dieltjens, T., Moonens, I., Van Praet, K., De Buck, E., & Vandekerckhove, P. (2014). A systematic literature search on psychological first aid: lack of evidence to develop guidelines. *PLoS ONE* 9(12): e114714. doi: 10.1371/journal. pone. 0114714

Doctors without Borders/Médecins Sans Frontières. (2010). *Three Times Victims: Victims of Violence, Silence and Neglect: Armed Conflict and Mental Health in the Department of Caquetá, Colombia.* www.lekari-bez-hranic.cz/cz/downloads/Three_time_victims.pdf

Doctors without Borders/Médecins Sans Frontières–Holland. (2006). Living in fear: Colombia's cycle of violence. www.msf.org.au/resources/reports/report/article/living-in-fearcolombias-cycle-of-violence.html

Dückers, M. L. A. (2013). Five essential principles of post-disaster psychosocial care: looking back and forward with Stevan Hobfoll. *European Journal of Psychotraumatology* 4: doi: 10.3402/ejpt.v4i0.21914

Elhai, J. D., & Ford, J. D. (2009). Utilization of mental health services after disasters. In Neria, Y., Galea, S., & Norris, F. H. (eds.), *Mental Health and Disasters.* New York: Cambridge University Press, pp. 366–86.

Galea, S., Ahern, J., Resnick, H., Kilpatrick, D., Bucuvalas, M., Gold, J., & Vlahov, D. (2002). Psychological sequelae of the September 11 terrorist attacks in New York City. *New England Journal of Medicine* 346: 982–7. doi: 10.1056/NEJMsa013404

Galea, S., Nandi, A., & Vlahov, D. (2005). The epidemiology of post-traumatic stress disorder after disasters. *Epidemiologic Reviews* 27: 78–91.

Galea, S., Vlahov, D., Resnick, H., Ahem, J., Susser, E., Gold, J., ... Kilpatrick, D. (2003). Trends of probable post-traumatic stress disorder in New York City after the September 11 terrorist attacks. *American Journal of Epidemiology* 158: 514–24.

Goldenberg, M. N., Benedeck, D., & Ursano, R. (2012). Disaster victims and the response to trauma. In McQuistion, H. L., Sowers, W. E., Ranz, J. M., & Feldman, J. M. (eds.), *Handbook of Community Psychiatry.* New York: Springer, pp. 435–46.

Gordon, R. (1983). An operational classification of disease prevention. *Public Health Reports* 98: 107–9.

Green, B. L., Korol, M., Grace, M. C., Vary, M. G., Leonard, A. C., Gleser, G. C., & Smitson-Cohen, S. (1991). Children and disaster: age, gender, and parental effects on PTSD symptoms. *Journal of the American Academy of Child and Adolescent Psychiatry* 30(6): 945–51.

Guha-Sapir, D., Hoyois, P., & Below, R. (2014). *Annual Disaster Statistical Review 2013: The Numbers and Trends.* Brussels, Belgium: Centre for Research on the Epidemiology of Disasters (CRED).

Hagstrom, R. (1995). The acute psychological impact on survivors following a train accident. *Journal of Traumatic Stress* 8: 391–402.

Helbing, D. (2013). Globally networked risks and how to respond. *Nature* 497: 51–9. doi: 10.1038/nature12047

Helbing, D., Brockmann, D., Chadefaux, T., Donnay, K., Blanke, U., Woolley-Meza, O., & Perc, M. (2015). Saving human lives: what complexity science and information systems can contribute. *Journal of Statistical Physics* 158: 735–81

Hobfoll, S. E., Tracy, M., & Galea, S. (2006). The impact of resource loss and traumatic growth on probable PTSD and depression following terrorist attacks. *Journal of Traumatic Stress* 19: 867–78.

IPCC (Intergovernmental Panel on Climate Change) (2012). *Managing the Risks of Extreme Events and Disasters to Advance Climate Change Adaptation. A Special Report of Working Groups I and II of the Intergovernmental Panel on Climate Change*. Field, C. B., Barros, V., Stocker, T. F., Qin, D., Dokken, D. J., Ebi, K. L., Mastrandrea, M. D., Mach, K. J., Plattner, G.-K., Allen, S. K., Tignor, M., & Midgley, P.M. (eds.). Cambridge, UK, and New York: Cambridge University Press.

Johnson, N. (2007). *Simply Complexity: A Clear Guide to Complexity Theory*. London: Oneworld.

Kar, N. (2009). Psychological impact of disasters on children: review of assessment and interventions. *World Journal of Pediatrics* 5: 5–11.

Kim, Y. (2011). Great East Japan earthquake and early mental-health response. *Psychiatry and Clinical Neurosciences* 65: 539–48.

Kim, Y,. & Akiyama, T. (2011). Post-disaster mental health care in Japan. *Lancet* 378 (9788): 317–18. doi: 10.1016/S0140-6736(11)61169-0

Kim, Y., Abe, Y., Araki, H., Fujita, M., Iwai, K., Kato, H., ... Yamamoto, K. (2004). *Guideline for Local Mental Health Care Activities after a Disaster*. Kodaira, Japan: National Institute of Mental Health, National Center of Psychiatry and Neurology. www.ncnp.go.jp/nimh/seijin/EnglishDisasterMentalHealth.pdf

Londoño, A., Romero, P., & Casas, G. (2012). The association between armed conflict, violence and mental health: a cross sectional study comparing two populations in Cundinamarca department, Colombia. *Conflict and Health* 6: 12.

Lorenz, J., Battiston, S., & Schweitzer, F. (2009). Systemic risk in a unifying framework for cascading processes on networks. *European Physical Journal B* 71, 441–60.

Maes, M., Mylle, J., Delmeire, L., & Janca, A. (2001). Pre- and post-disaster negative life events in relation to the incidence and severity of post-traumatic stress disorder. *Journal of Psychiatry Research* 105: 1–12.

McFarlane, A. C., Van Hooff, M., & Goodhew, F. (2009). Anxiety disorders and PTSD. In Neria, Y., Galea, S., & Norris, F. H. (eds.), *Mental Health and Disasters*. New York: Cambridge University Press, pp. 47–66.

McNally, R. J., Bryant, R. A., & Ehlers, A. (2003). Psychological debriefing and its alternatives: a critique of early intervention for trauma survivors. *Psychological Science in the Public Interest* 4: 45–79.

Nash, W. P., & Watson, P. J. (2012). Review of VA/DOD clinical practice guideline on management of acute stress and interventions to prevent posttraumatic stress disorder. *Journal of Rehabilitation Research & Development* 49(5): 637–48.

National Research Council and Institute of Medicine (2009). *Preventing Mental, Emotional, and Behavioral Disorders among Young People: Progress and Possibilities*. Committee on the Prevention of Mental Disorders and Substance Abuse among Children, Youth, and Young Adults: Research Advances and

Promising Interventions. O'Connell, M. E., Boat, T. & Warner, K. E. (eds.), Board on Children, Youth, and Families, Division of Behavioral and Social Sciences and Education. Washington, DC: National Academies Press.

Neria, Y, Nandi, A, & Galea, S. (2008). Post-traumatic stress disorder following disasters: a systematic review. *Psychological Medicine* 38: 467–80.

Norris, F. H. (2009). The impact of disasters and political violence on mental health in Latin America. *PTSD Research Quarterly* 20(4): 1–7. www.ptsd.va.gov/professional/newsletters/research-quarterly/V20N4.

Norris, F., Friedman, M. J., Watson, P. J., Byrne, C., & Kaniasty, K. (2002). 60,000 disaster victims speak: Part I. An empirical review of the empirical literature: 1981–2001. *Psychiatry* 65: 207–39.

Norris, F. H., Tracy, M., & Galea, S. (2008). Looking for resilience: understanding the longitudinal trajectories of responses to stress. *Social Science & Medicine* 68: 2190–8.

North, C. S., Nixon, S. J., Shariat, S., Mallonee, S., McMillen, J. C., Spitznagel, E. L., & Smith, E. M. (1999). Psychiatric disorders among survivors of the Oklahoma City bombing. *Journal of the American Medical Association* 282(8): 755–62.

Pfefferbaum, B., Seale, T. W., McDonald, N. B., Brandt, E. N., Rainwater, S. M., Maynard, B. T., . . . Miller P. D. (2000). Posttraumatic stress two years after the Oklahoma City bombing in youths geographically distant from the explosion. *Psychiatry* 63: 358–70.

Pulcino, T., Galea, S., Ahern, J., Resnick, H., Foley, M., & Vlahov, D. (2003). Post-traumatic stress in women after the September 11 terrorist attacks in New York City. *Journal of Women's Health* 12: 809–20.

Ramalingam, B., Jones, H., Toussainte, R., & Young, J. (2008). *The Science of Complexity. Ideas and Implications for Development and Humanitarian Efforts* 2nd ed. London: Overseas Development Institute.

Reifels, L., Pietrantoni, L., Prati, G., Yoshirahu, K., Kilpatrick, D. G., Dyb G.,. . . O'Donnell, M. (2013). Lessons learned about psychosocial responses to disaster and mass trauma: an international perspective. *European Journal of Psychotraumatology* 4. doi: 10.3402/ejpt.v4i0.22897

Reissman, D. E., Schreiber, M. D., Shultz, J. M., & Ursano, R. J. (2009). Disaster mental and behavioral health. In Koenig, K. L., & Schultz, C. H. (eds.), *Disaster Medicine*. Cambridge, UK: Cambridge University Press, pp. 103–10.

Richards, A., Ospina-Duque, J., Barrera-Valencia, M., Escobar-Rincón. J., Ardila-Gutiérrez, M., Metzler, T., et al. (2011). Posttraumatic stress disorder, anxiety and depression symptoms, and psychosocial treatment needs in Colombians internally displaced by armed conflict: a mixed-method evaluation. *Psychological Trauma* 3: 384–93.

Schlenger, W. E., Caddell, J. M., Ebert, L., Jordan, B. K., Rourke, K. M., Wilson, D., . . . Kulka, R. A. (2002).Psychological reactions to terrorist attacks: findings from the national study of Americans' reactions to September 11. *Journal of the American Medical Association* 288(5): 581–8.

Shi, P., Zu, W., Ye, T., He, C., Jing'ai, W., Li, N. (2011). Developing disaster risk science: discussion on the disaster reduction implementation science. *Journal of Natural Disaster Science* 32: 79–88.

Shultz, J. M. (2013a). Perspectives on disaster public health and disaster behavioral health integration. *Disaster Health* 1(2): 1–4.

Shultz, J. M. (2013b). Perspectives on disaster public health and disaster behavioral health integration. *Dialogue* 9(2): 2–6.

Shultz, J. M., Allen, A., Bustamante, H., & Espinel, Z. (2009). *Safety Function Action for Disaster Responders: Training Module Guidebook*. Miami, FL: DEEP Center, University of Miami Miller School of Medicine.

Shultz, J. M., Espinel, Z., Cohen, R. E., Smith, R. G., & Flynn, B. W. (2006a). *Disaster Behavioral Health: All-Hazards Training*. Miami, FL: DEEP Center, University of Miami Miller School of Medicine.

Shultz, J. M., Espinel, Z., Flynn, B. W., Hoffman, Y., & Cohen, R. E. (2007a). *DEEP PREP: All-Hazards Disaster Behavioral Health Training*. Tampa, FL: Disaster Life Support.

Shultz, J. M., Espinel, Z., Galea, S., Hicks, J., Shaw, J. A., & Miller, G. T. (2006b). *SURGE, SORT, SUPPORT: Disaster Behavioral Health for Health Care Professionals*. Tampa, FL: Disaster Life Support.

Shultz, J. M., Espinel, Z., Galea, S., & Reissman, D. E. (2007b). Disaster ecology: implications for disaster psychiatry. In Ursano, R. J., Fullerton, C. S., Weisaeth, L., & Raphael, B. (eds.), *Textbook of Disaster Psychiatry*. Cambridge, UK: Cambridge University Press, pp. 69–96.

Shultz, J. M., & Forbes, D. (2013). Psychological first aid: rapid proliferation and the search for evidence. *Disaster Health* 1(2): 1–10. doi: dx.doi.org/10.4161/dish.26006

Shultz, J. M., Forbes, D., Wald, D., Kelly, F., Solo-Gabriele, H. M., Rosen, A., Espinel, Z., McLean, A., Bernal, O., & Neria, Y. (2013a). Trauma signature of the Great East Japan Disaster provides guidance for the psychological consequences of the affected population. *Disaster Medicine and Public Health Preparedness* 7(2): 201–14.

Shultz, J. M., Garfin, D. R., Espinel, Z., Araya, R., Oquendo, M. A., Wainberg, M. L., Chaskel, R., Gaviria, S. L., Ordoñez, A. E., Espinola, M., Wilson, F. E., Muñoz Garcia, N., Gomez Ceballos, A. M., Garcia-Barcena, Y., Verdeli, H., & Neria, Y. (2014a). Internally displaced "victims of armed conflict" in Colombia: the trajectory and trauma signature of forced migration. *Current Psychiatry Reports* 16(10): 475. doi: 10.1007/s11920-014-0475-7

Shultz, J. M., Gomez Ceballos, Á. M., Espinel, Z., Oliveros, S. R., Fonseca, M. F., & Hernandez Florez, L. J. (2014b). Internal displacement in Colombia. *Disaster Health* 2(1): 13–24. doi: 10.4161/dish.27885

Shultz, J. M., Kelly, F., Forbes, D., Leon, G. R., Verdeli, H., Rosen, A., & Neria, Y. (2011). Triple threat trauma: evidence-based mental health response for the 2011 Japan disaster. *Prehospital and Disaster Medicine* 26(3): 141–5.

Shultz, J. M., McLean, A., Herberman Mash, H. B., Rosen, A., Kelly, F., Solo-Gabriele, H. M., Youngs, G. A. Jr., Jensen, J., Bernal, O., & Neria, Y. (2013b). Mitigating flood exposure: reducing disaster risk and trauma signature. *Disaster Health* 1(1): 30–44.

Shultz, J. M., Muñoz García, N., Gomez Ceballos, Á. M., Hernandez Florez, L. J., Araya, R., Verdeli, H., Espinel, Z., Cipaguata Bolivar, S. P., & Neria, Y. (2014c). Outreach to internally displaced persons in Bogotá, Colombia: challenges and potential solutions. *Disaster Health* 2(2): 75–81. doi: 10.4161/21665044.2014.954500

Shultz, J. M., & Neria, Y. (2013) Trauma signature analysis: state of the art and evolving future directions. *Disaster Health* 1(1): 4–8. doi: dx.doi.org/10.4161/dish.24011

Shultz, J. M., Neria, Y., Allen, A., & Espinel, Z. (2013c). *Psychological Impacts of Natural Disasters*. In Bobrowsky, P. (ed.), *Encyclopedia of Natural Hazards*. Dordrecht, Heidelberg, London, New York: Springer, pp. 779–91.

Sloan, P. (1988). Post-traumatic stress in survivors of an airplane crash-landing: a clinical and explanatory research intervention. *Journal of Traumatic Stress* 1: 211–29.

Smith, E. M., North, C. S., & Spitznagel, E. L. (1993). Post-traumatic stress in survivors of three disasters. *Journal of Social Behavior and Personality* 8: 353–68.

Suzuki, Y., & Kim, Y. (2012). The Great East Japan earthquake in 2011: toward a sustainable mental health care system. *Epidemiology and Psychiatric Sciences* 21: 7–11.

Takeda, M. (2011). Mental health care and East Japan great earthquake. *Psychiatry and Clinical Neurosciences* 65: 207–12.

Tracy, M., Norris, F. H., & Galea, S. (2011). Differences in the determinants of posttraumatic stress disorder and depression after a mass traumatic event. *Depression and Anxiety* 28: 666–75.

Udwin, O., Boyle, S., Yule, W., Bolton, D., & O'Ryan, D. (2000). Risk factors for long-term psychological effects of a disaster experience in adolescence: predictors of posttraumatic stress disorder. *Journal of Child Psychology and Psychiatry* 41(8): 969–79.

Vlahov, D., Galea, S., Resnick, H., Ahern, J., Boscarino, J. A., Bucuvalas, M., ... Kilpatrick, D. (2002). Increased use of cigarettes, alcohol, and marijuana among Manhattan, New York, residents after the September 11th terrorist attacks. *American Journal of Epidemiology* 155(11): 988–96.

Walker, B., & Westley, F. (2011). Perspectives on resilience to disasters across sectors and cultures. *Ecology and Society* 16(2): 4. www.ecologyandsociety.org/vol16/iss2/art4/

Weiss, D. S., Marmar, C. R., Metzler, T. J., & Ronfeldt, H. M. (1995). Predicting symptomatic distress in emergency services personnel. *Journal of Consulting and Clinical Psychology* 63: 361–8.

WHO, WTF, WVI (World Health Organization, War Trauma Foundation, and World Vision International) (2011). *Psychological First Aid: Guide for Field Workers*. Geneva, Switzerland: World Health Organization.

22 Forgiveness Interventions and the Prevention of Poor Health, Hostile Relationships, and Societal Hatred and Violence

Everett L. Worthington, Jr., Brandon J. Griffin, Caroline R. Lavelock, Nathaniel G. Wade, & Katherine Kulick

The thesis of this chapter is that promoting forgiveness by individuals and within society may prevent problems both at individual and societal levels. Thus, we (a) discuss forgiveness interventions as one way to alleviate unforgiveness and its associated problems and (b) demonstrate that preventive use of forgiveness interventions might benefit both individuals and society. Namely, we argue that prevention of poor health outcomes, hostile relationships, and societal hatred and violence occurs as forgiveness alleviates problems associated with unforgiveness through healing past harms, dealing with present injustices, and enriching relationships.

We believe that societal conflict is inevitable; however, this conflict becomes unproductive when not aimed at creating solutions that are acceptable to multiple stakeholders. One reason for this is that when people experience injustices that they perceive as not rectified, negative, unforgiving emotions can develop and become lasting grudges. Those grudges evoke vengeful and avoidant motives that threaten peace at individual, relational, and societal levels.

Forgiveness promotes resolution of conflict and forges lasting peace both in individuals and in society by (1) fostering healthier individuals, (2) healing past damage done by conflict, and (3) promoting reconciliation within and between groups. In the present chapter, forgiveness is discussed as not simply a single exchange between individuals (i.e., saying "I forgive you") or a governmental proclamation that some debt is forgiven. Rather, *forgiveness* is the intrapersonal experience of a victim who makes a decision to inhibit vengeful and avoidant motives toward an offender or experiences an emotional change that replaces negative emotions related to suffering wrongdoing with more positive (or less negative) emotions.

In society, Brounéus (2008) reported that during the years 1989 – 2006, the global number of armed intrastate conflicts recorded in the Uppsala Conflict Data Program ranged between twenty-five and fifty annually. However, the global number of armed interstate conflicts ranged between zero and two. Thus, recovery efforts after armed conflict frequently involve people *within* a country who have killed or harmed their fellow citizens – not people perpetrating harm on citizens of a different country. This is not surprising given that people more often hurt, and are hurt by, people they know (for a review and meta-analysis, see Fehr, Gelfand, & Nag, 2010). Romantic partners, family members, coworkers, friends, and members of our religious and social groups are the people with whom we interact most, and those relationships have the potential to harm us because they are meaningful to us. Others in our communities and societies – such as police, officials in the judicial system, and elected or appointed leaders – control our resources or behaviors, sometimes using methods that we oppose. Forgiveness may heal wounds and prevent escalation of conflict by interrupting cycles of reactionary violence by stimulating positive public health outcomes and promoting relational reconciliation. Indeed, though precarious peace may be compelled by governmental policies backed by strong leadership or militant power, enduring peace likely must involve change in societal structures and in internal personal processes of the people – from leaders to citizens.

Definitions

Decisional and Emotional Forgiveness

People respond to transgressions and offenses in many ways (Worthington, 2006). For example, people might seek to excuse (e.g., "You couldn't help it because you are a jerk") or justify (e.g., "You hurt me because I hurt you yesterday") wrongdoing. People might condone what was done ("What you did wasn't really wrong"), or people might seek legal justice or pursue vigilante justice. People might turn the issue over to a higher power, either hoping for divine justice or simply relinquishing the issue. People might forbear (seek to not express anger or resentment to preserve group harmony), or people might simply accept that injustice happens. None of these are forgiveness.

But people also might forgive. Forgiveness is viewed by virtually all social scientists as occurring within, not between, individuals (Worthington, 2005). While reconciliation is the restoration of trust between people (Worthington & Aten, 2010), forgiveness entails cognitive and affective changes that occur within one person in pursuit of either reconciliation or personal peace (or both). Still, while being localized within a person's body, expressions of forgiveness of two types – decisional or emotional forgiveness – occur within a social context (for a review, see Exline, Worthington, Hill, & McCullough, 2003; Worthington, 2006).

Decisional forgiveness. *Decisional forgiveness* is a behavioral intention to act prosocially toward the offender in the future (Davis et al., 2015). Victims who make a decision to forgive inhibit negative and vengeful acts directed toward offenders. Avoidance of an offender might or might not be discouraged, depending on whether interaction with the offender(s) is safe and prudent. Under conditions where it is safe for the victim to interact with the offender, decisional forgiveness creates opportunities for victims to experience empathy and perhaps act benevolently toward offenders.

Emotional forgiveness. Even though a victim may decide to forgive an offender, feelings of emotional unforgiveness may persist. The emotionally unforgiving victim harbors resentment, bitterness, hostility, hatred, anger, and fear, which are called unforgiving emotions (Worthington, 2006). The victim, thus, may experience a second type of forgiveness called emotional forgiveness. *Emotional forgiveness* is the emotional replacement of negative, unforgiving emotions with positive, other-oriented emotions, such as empathy, sympathy, compassion, or love for the offender. For example, a soldier involved in and wounded during a civil war, through perspective shifting, may begin to see the shared humanity of the soldier who wounded him, despite disagreeing with the offending soldier's political convictions.

Reconciliation

Reconciliation is the restoration a relationship where trust has been violated, often repeatedly (Worthington, 2006). Unlike forgiveness, reconciliation is not an individual phenomenon. It is a social or societal phenomenon. Reconciliation cannot be granted to someone else. Rather, all parties, through mutually trustworthy behaviors, contribute to reconciliation. Certainly, reconciliation may be initiated by one party, who may labor more for reconciliation than does the other. But, eventually, if reconciliation is to occur, it requires mutually trustworthy behaviors from both offenders and victims.

Talking about Transgressions

During reconciliation, people often talk about *transgressions* or offenses during a series of interchanges (Goffman, 1969). When a transgressor commits an offense against a victim, the victim will often make a reproach to the transgressor. A *reproach* is a request to explain the cause of the offense (Schönbach, 1990), which may encourage mitigating or aggravating accounts. For example, a forthright accusation of wrongdoing typically elicits defensiveness from the transgressor, but a gentle reproach might elicit apology

Transgressors respond to reproaches with an account. Schönbach (1990) identified four unique responses. *Refusals* or *denials* reject the idea of wrongdoing or deny that anything offensive happened. *Justifications* admit to responsibility for one's actions but claim that the actions were not wrong, possibly blaming the victim for previous offenses. *Excuses* admit to wrongdoing but claim that mitigating circumstances should be considered. That is; because the offender's actions were not motivated by harmful intent, the offender does not believe that their actions are worthy of blame. Finally, *concessions* or *confessions* admit to wrongdoing and may attempt to repair the relationship through apology or offer of restitution.

Justice

Justice is a social and societal construct (Pittman, 2008). Procedures are established and followed so that fairness is made more likely. *Distributive justice* describes how resources are equitably distributed. That is, it describes whether resources are equitably available, equitably distributed, and equitably allocated, and this considers both social costs for producing the goods, responsibility, power over the goods, level of need, and receipt of the goods. *Forensic justice* describes how civil disputes and putative criminal acts are adjudicated. *Procedural justice* stipulates the specific procedures by which people attempt to bring about distributive and forensic justice. Whereas justice is social and societal, individuals judge the degree that justice has occurred (Pittman, 2008). We will call this one's *perception of justice* to differentiate between justice as social construct and as individual construct.

When injustices are perceived, the perception of net injustice is represented mentally by the injustice gap. The *injustice gap* is the perception of the difference between the way that a person might wish a perceived injustice to be resolved relative to the way the person perceives the situation at present (Exline et al., 2003). The injustice gap is thus an ongoing, frequently changing subjective evaluation of the degree of residual injustice. It is affected by actions taken by transgressor, victim, and observers and events (such as, e.g., changes in leadership after a workplace inequity) after the original transgression. Thus, this concept is particularly relevant for ongoing conflicts between individuals and people groups because it is, in a way, a summary that is affected by the other changes that occur as well as changes in the attitudes of participants toward each other. Sometimes, new transgressions can be factored into an original injustice gap, increasing the sense of injustice. At other times, a subsequent additional injustice might be considered separate and require its own resolution for a perception of justice to reign. Overall, the injustice gap may be reduced through ways that move a person's evaluation of the current situation closer to the person's idealized situation (e.g., seeing civil or criminal justice realized) or by changing one's idea about how the situation might be resolved (e.g., accepting and moving on, deciding to turn the matter over to God, etc.; Worthington, 2006).

Unforgiveness Is Associated with Negative Effects

In Individuals

Unforgiveness and physical health. A variety of reviews have summarized physical health costs of not forgiving (but have established a bit less strongly the benefits of physical health of forgiving). For example, Toussaint, Worthington, and Williams (2015) edited a recent volume in which fourteen teams of investigators reviewed research evidence in different areas of forgiveness and health.

Other reviews have included Worthington, Witvliet, Pietrini, and Miller (2007), who looked at different effects on health of emotional forgiveness and decisional forgiveness.

In summarizing the research in Toussaint et al. (2015) and Worthington et al. (2007), we find that some of the major health-related effects of unforgiveness include cardiovascular strain, which shows up as vascular diseases, risky spikes in blood pressure, inflammation of bifurcations in arteries, hypertension, and increased risk of stroke and myocardial infarction. Other effects of not forgiving include dysregulation of the immune system. Additionally, persistent unforgiveness has been found to be related to elevated cortisol (Berry & Worthington, 2001; Tabak & McCullough, 2011; Worthington et al., 2015), and Sapolsky (2004) has shown ways that chronically high levels of cortisol seriously affect virtually every physical system in the body, including shrinking the brain, affecting digestion and elimination, dysregulating the immune system, and undermining sexual functioning. Witvliet, DeYoung, Hofelich, and DeYoung (2011) have shown that forgiving improves parasympathetic functioning (as shown by increased heart rate variability, a measure of ability to respond effectively to stress), increases vagal tone (which is the physical self-soothing function of the parasympathetic nervous system), and produces better psychophysiological well-being. Also, Tabak, McCullough, Szeto, Mendez, and McCabe (2011) found that, when women experienced a transgression, their oxytocin levels decreased, suggesting that they were less attached to the transgressor.

Unforgiveness and mental health. Likewise, multiple reviews have summarized substantial research showing that unforgiveness is related to mental health problems and that forgiveness is related to better mental health. For example, Toussaint and Webb (2005) initially reviewed the nascent research on forgiveness and mental health. About ten years later, Griffin, Worthington, Wade, Hoyt, and Davis (2015c) and Lavelock, Griffin, and Worthington (2013) reviewed further research on forgiveness and mental health. They found that the salutary effects of forgiveness among victims of offense could be represented by four propositions: (1) unforgiveness is a stress reaction related to poor mental health; (2) forgiveness is a coping strategy related to improved mental health; (3) individual differences (e.g., the Big Five, especially neuroticism and agreeableness, trait rumination, age, sex, and willingness to forgive) moderate the impact of forgiveness on health; and (4) psychological states mediate the impact of forgiveness on health; these psychological states include anger, fear, and depression, which generate rumination, hopelessness, negative affect, and self-esteem. In addition, they considered perpetrators of offense who (a) seek and receive forgiveness, (b) forgive themselves, (c) retain self-condemnation, or (d) reduce self-condemnation without accepting responsibility for their wrongdoing. They concluded that empirical evidence supports the application of forgiveness of others and oneself as mechanisms to promote better mental health among victims and perpetrators of interpersonal harm, respectively (for a review and meta-analysis, see Davis et al., 2015).

Much of the cost of not forgiving is due to rumination. Rumination (i.e., angry, anxious, or depressed worry) has been associated with increased depression, anxiety, anger, obsessive-compulsive disorders, posttraumatic stress disorders, and psychosomatic disorders. Thus, it becomes one mechanism by which the effect of unforgiveness on mental health subsequently affects physical health. In addition, poor mental health is related to poorer physical health (for a review, see Worthington et al. 2007). It can affect physical health through many mechanisms, but one in particular is participation in high health-risk behaviors, including smoking, overeating, reduced exercise and sleeping, and self-medicating through drugs or alcohol (Vermeulen-Smit, Ten Have, Van Laar, & De Graaf, 2015).

Unforgiveness and relationships. Riek and Mania (2012) meta-analyzed 158 samples of participants within from 103 articles regarding forgiveness and relationships. This meta-analysis revealed that people in relationships characterized by low levels of security and satisfaction have been prone to be more unforgiving when wronged. Also, unforgiveness of an event has been found to further weaken poor relationships. Forgiveness of transgressions has usually been related to improved relationships; however, McNulty and Fincham (2012) have found that, in some cases, forgiving can be counterproductive if it reinforces harmful couple interactions and patterns. Riek and Mania (2012) conclude that there are direct positive benefits to most relationships when partners forgive frequently. Not only are there usually direct benefits to relationships when forgiveness occurs, but there are often indirect benefits as well. For instance, some higher-quality relationships have been related indirectly to better mental and physical health (Riek & Mania, 2012).

Riek and Mania identified distal and proximal predictors of forgiveness and also outcomes of forgiving using effect sizes (reported as r). In each case, the 95 percent confidence interval does not contain zero, suggesting a reliable relationship exists. Sometimes (usually involving personality constructs), the effect size is small (i.e., usually considered to be below $r = 0.15$). At the most distal level of relation, personality qualities – agreeableness ($r = 0.37$), neuroticism ($r = -0.27$), religiosity ($r = 0.25$), trait empathy ($r = 0.24$), narcissism ($r = -0.17$), self-esteem ($r = 0.16$), conscientiousness ($r = 0.14$), openness ($r = 0.08$), and extraversion ($r = 0.06$) – predicted forgiveness. At an intermediate level of relationship, relationship commitment predicted forgiveness ($r = 0.34$) and, at the offense level, apology ($r = 0.33$) and severity of offense ($r = -0.24$) predicted forgiveness. At the proximal, social-cognitive level, state empathy ($r = 0.50$) strongly predicted forgiving, and the empathy was not merely a matter of perspective taking ($r = 0.25$). How people attributed the offense (i.e., accidental, personal) ($r = 0.37$) and how they emotionally reacted to the offense – such as in anger ($r = -0.37$) and with angry, hurt, or depressed rumination ($r = -0.35$) predicted forgiveness. In turn, forgiveness predicted less negative affect ($r = -0.47$), depression ($r = -0.26$), stress ($r = -0.23$), and anxiety ($r = -0.18$), and also forgiveness predicted more positive affect ($r = 0.32$) and life satisfaction ($r = 0.25$).

Forgiveness and religious/spiritual experiences. Forgiveness has long been advocated by organized religions (see Rye et al., 2000), but empirical evidence has recently solidified this as an empirically supported relationship (Davis, Worthington, Hook, & Hill, 2013). Davis et al. meta-analyzed studies of religion/spirituality and trait forgivingness (k = 64; i.e., k indicated the number of samples analyzed), state forgiveness (k = 50), and self-forgiveness (k = 23). While forgiveness of others was related differently to religiousness than to spirituality, it was positively related to each. (Note that in the following results, all effect sizes, rs, have 95 percent confidence intervals that do not contain 0.) For example, trait forgivingness was related to religiousness (k = 39; r = 0.35), spirituality (k = 9; r = 0.23), intrinsic religious motivation (k = 8; r = 0.24), quest motivation (k = 3; r = 0.38), religious well-being (k = 7; r = 0.28), and existential well-being (k = 7; r = 0.29). State measures of forgiveness were related (less strongly than were trait measures) to religiousness (k = 35; r = 0.14), spirituality (k = 5; r = 0.12), intrinsic religious motivation (k = 8; r = 0.12), religious well-being (k = 5; r = 0.14), and existential well-being (k = 5; r = 0.23). Although Davis et al. did not compare people from different religions as to their levels of endorsement of forgiveness, these have frequently been compared in the past. The findings have been reliable (for reviews, see Maamri, Nevin, & Worthington, 2010). Because forgiveness is one of two central concepts in Christianity, forgiveness has tended to be most often highly endorsed by Christians, and people describe themselves as highly forgiving (Rye et al., 2000). However, for Islam and Judaism, forgiveness is valued, yet other competing values tend to reduce the high endorsement of forgiveness. For Islam, that tends to be justice; for Judaism, that tends to be repentance (i.e., *teshuvah*), which contextualizes forgiveness within apologies, amends making, and assurance of nonoffense. For Buddhism, forgiveness is not frequently endorsed, but compassion often is. For Hinduism, whether forgiveness is endorsed often depends on one's specific religious beliefs.

In the meta-analysis by Davis et al., self-forgiveness was neither related to religiousness (k = 9; r = 0.04, 95 percent confidence interval contains 0) nor spirituality (k = 6; r = 0.05, 95 percent confidence interval contains 0). Secular interventions to promote self-forgiveness have also been found efficacious for both religious and nonreligious people (Griffin et al., 2015a).

Furthermore, the connection between religiousness/spirituality and forgiveness provides a useful avenue for prevention science that may target religious groups across the globe to help create the optimal conditions under which explicit forgiveness interventions may have the strongest effect. For instance, people tend to take more offense when offended by a member of their in group than when offended in the same way by an out-group member; however, people tend to forgive in group members much more readily for the same type of offense than they do out-group members (Van Tongeren, Burnette, O'Boyle, Worthington, & Forsyth, 2014). Group interventions aimed at people across cultures (Lin et al., 2014) and at people within their religious in-group have been found to be efficacious (Greer, Worthington, Lin, Lavelock, & Griffin, 2014).

Public Health Costs of Unforgiveness

Health costs for individuals related to the ill effects of unforgiveness accumulate to yield public health costs. Worthington, Kulick, and Griffin (2014) presented data on potential public health benefits of forgiving. Their analyses were based on the conceptualization of unforgiveness as an emotional stress reaction, which many people experience as chronic stress. That leads to stress reactions, which are well documented to be related to physical health and mental health outcomes (for a review, see Sapolsky, 2004). Two indirect effects also occur that link forgiveness and better health. Forgiveness affects relationships – like good romantic relationships (Worthington et al., 2015), good family relationships (Kramer, Kavanaugh, Trentham-Dietz, Walsh, & Yonker, 2010), and good workplace relationships (Fehr & Gelfand, 2012). In each case, forgiveness promotes stronger emotional bonds between partners, family members, or workers, leading to stronger relationships overall. Sometimes, when people mistakenly believe that forgiveness most necessarily entails reconciliation, harm can occur to individuals or relationships; however, in that case, it is not forgiveness that leads to poor relational outcomes but a misunderstanding of what forgiveness is. Genuine forgiveness has consistently been found to be related to more positive physical health (for reviews, see Toussaint, Worthington, & Williams, 2015) and mental health (for a review, see Griffin et al., 2015b). Finally, forgiveness affects spirituality (Davis et al., 2013). There is a strong relationship between spiritual dwelling (i.e., stable and satisfying spiritual relationships), forgiveness, and positive health indices for most people (McCullough, Hoyt, Larson, Koenig, & Thoresen, 2000). Similarly, negative physical and mental health is often correlated with unforgiveness and with spiritual struggle, anger with God, or disappointment with God (Wood et al., 2010). Thus, stress-related disorders due to unforgiveness can affect people's religion and spirituality, their relationships, their mental health, and their physical health. These relationships can be causal, but they are often, at a minimum, correlational. The accumulation of effects among individuals presents a public health concern, and stresses can spread through networks and communities.

Beyond the mere accumulation of individual problems, though, other public health issues might be experienced to the degree that society is characterized by more conflict, intractable disagreement, uncivil discourse, and conflict. When people within a society are likely to have frequent conflicts, social systems become crucibles of conflict, unforgiveness, interpersonal aggression, and intrapersonal stress-related disorders. Worthington et al. (2014) identified social and societal systems likely to be negatively affected by a general atmosphere of unforgiveness (see also Worthington & Berry, 2004). These include the following: police enforcement; the civil justice system; the criminal justice system; the prison system; health care systems and iatrogenic illness; workplace conflicts; domestic violence; alcoholism and substance-related problems; divorce; civility in domestic politics (i.e., Democrats vs. Republicans); and civility in socially divisive issues such as abortion, immigration, and health care. Perhaps these conflicts can be mitigated, and perhaps even prevented, with the practice and promotion of forgiveness.

Solutions

People Can Be Helped to Forgive

In seeking to provide contributions of prevention science to healing individual and societal unforgiveness (and thus preventing many of the problems we outlined in the preceding), we begin with the individual. Numerous clinical scientists have put forth interventions to promote forgiveness in individuals, and many have tested them empirically. These will be crucial to our argument because we suggest that these interventions can be used for psychotherapeutic and psychoeducational goals in communities and groups to deal with long-standing or acute problems within the communities, groups, or larger society in which communities are ensconced.

Wade, Hoyt, Kidwell, and Worthington (2014) conducted a meta-analysis of interventions, with individuals, couples, families, and groups. Most of the interventions were based on either the Enright and Fitzgibbons (2015) process model or the REACH Forgiveness (Worthington, 2006; see www.EvWorthington-forgiveness.com) model, which are conducted either in groups or individually. Wade et al. (2014) found that, on the average, most interventions produced increased forgiveness. When different kinds of interventions were compared (if severity of offense and duration of intervention were controlled), interventions did not differ in their efficacy. Instead, efficacy was generally dependent on (a) modality (individual treatment was better than group treatment ($p = 0.021$) but not couple treatment ($p = 0.251$) and (b) dosage. The average effect size was about 0.1 standard deviations of forgiveness experienced per hour of intervention. Worthington's (2006) REACH Forgiveness ($n = 22$ comparisons) and Enright's (Enright & Fitzgibbons, 2015) Forgiveness Process ($n = 23$ comparisons) had been tested as often as all others combined ($n = 22$ comparisons). Both of the frequently tested models sought to define forgiveness as an intrapersonal experience and contrast forgiveness and other easily confused processes (such as reconciliation or saying, "I forgive you"). They then promoted a decision to forgive or to work toward forgiving a specific transgression. They walked people through forgiveness exercises that emphasized empathizing with the offender to get a better understanding of the offender's situation, pressures, and thought processes. Then forgiveness experiences were discussed.

Forgiveness interventions produced other outcomes besides forgiveness. For example, when studies treated forgiveness but measured both forgiveness and depression ($k = 10$), forgiveness had a larger effect size (expressed as Δ_{+}, roughly the number of standard deviations the measure changed) than did depression, but there were, nevertheless, strong improvements in depression, $\Delta_{+} = 0.34$

(95 percent confidence interval, CI: 0.17, 0.52), compared to forgiveness in those same ten studies $\Delta_+ = 0.60$, (95 percent CI: 0.26, 0.94). Similarly, when treating anxious people for forgiveness ($k = 7$), the aggregate effect size for anxiety was $\Delta_+ = 0.63$ (95 percent CI: 0.0003, 1.26), compared to forgiveness $\Delta_+ = 1.34$ (95 percent CI: 0.55, 2.12) in those same seven studies. In both cases, without addressing depression or anxiety, the gains were half as many standard deviations as the gains in forgiveness. Looking at the gains in emotion-centered measures in relationship to the gains that typically occur with cognitive-behavior therapy (CBT) for depression and anxiety, they were about one-quarter to one-third as much as are produced in twelve to twenty weeks of CBT full psychotherapy targeted at depression or anxiety. For hope as an outcome ($k = 6$), the aggregate effect size for hope was $\Delta_+ = 1.00$ (95 percent CI: 0.38, 1.62) compared to forgiveness in those same 6 studies, $\Delta_+ = 0.94$ (95 percent CI: 0.16, 1.73). In summary, from the meta-analysis, we can conclude that forgiveness intervention studies will produce substantial forgiveness and a fairly high accompanying change in emotional functioning.

Wade et al. (2014) concluded three things from their review and analyses. First, forgiveness interventions efficaciously promote forgiveness. Second, time spent trying to forgive is more important than is specific program or even modality (individual, couple, or group). Third, when people participate in forgiveness interventions, their depression and anxiety get better but at a reduced rate relative to the forgiveness experienced (about half the effect size). Conversely, hope improved at about the same rate (equal effect size) as forgiveness, even though the intervention did not address hope per se.

Recent Developments in Forgiveness Treatment

New developments have recently occurred. First, the range of problems that forgiveness is targeted to help has consistently expanded. Forgiveness interventions have been sculpted to apply to medical settings (Green, Decourville, & Sadava, 2012), educational settings (Enright, Rhody, Litts, & Klatt, 2014), Christian churches (Greer et al., 2014), divorce recovery (Rye et al., 2012), and many others. Second, the efficacy of nontargeted psychoeducational interventions – those that seek to help people wanting help forgiving a variety of unspecified transgressions – have been well established. Those interventions can be used in a variety of settings, with populations that are diverse and those that are narrowly focused on a particular transgression. Third, the treatment of individuals (Freedman & Enright, 1996), couples (Ripley et al., 2014), and psychoeducational groups (for a review and meta-analysis, see Wade et al., 2014) is effective, though individual treatment tends to be slightly preferred. Fourth, targeted (at a specific problem) and nontargeted interventions are both efficacious. Fifth, people can forgive without involving a mental health provider. Recently, Harper et al. (2014) and Greer et al. (2014) used self-administered workbooks that take from six to seven hours (on the average) to complete. Much like the psychoeducational groups, the workbooks take participants through a series of individual exercises that people complete in writing (rather than through interactions with group members, partners, or a psychotherapist). Sixth, for psychoeducational groups, peer-led groups are almost as effective as professional-led groups (Lin et al., 2014).

Two Frequently Used Methods for Forgiving

The REACH Forgiveness approach (Worthington, 2006) is one of two methods that have most consistently been associated with successful administration. Both methods – the REACH Forgiveness and Enright's process method – are typically implemented in a group psychoeducational format. However, the content of the treatment is well specified, so both have been implemented in individual counseling or with couples conjointly present. The REACH Forgiveness model has also recently been implemented using do-it-yourself workbooks. The five steps to REACH Emotional Forgiveness are as follows: R = *Recall* the Hurt (without blaming the offender or ruminating about negative consequences of the offense); E=*Empathize* (Sympathize, Feel Compassion for, Love) with the Transgressor (sometimes also referred to as E = *Emotionally Replace* Negative Unforgiving Emotions with Positive Other-Oriented Emotions); A = Give an *Altruistic* Gift of Forgiveness (rather than a solely embracing a self-enhancing motive of forgiving because it has positive physical health, mental health, relational, and spiritual consequences); C = *Commit* to the Emotional Forgiveness One Has Experienced; and H = *Hold on* to Forgiveness When Doubts Arise.

Enright's (Enright & Fitzgibbons, 2015) approach has four phases comprised of twenty discrete steps. In the Uncovering Phase, people experience both the pain and reality of the injury and how it has affected them. In the Decision Phase, the person commits to forgive. In the Work Phase, the person experiences emotional replacement through empathic reframing, empathy, compassion, and acceptance. In the Deepening Phase, people seek meaning in suffering and forgiveness, realize that they have needed others' forgiveness, achieve insight that they are not alone, embrace purpose, and become attuned to more positive affect.

Forgiveness Interventions in Non-USA Contexts and Their Effects

Studies of the efficacy of group interventions have mostly been done in the United States. In the meta-analysis of Wade et al. (2014), which restricted their analyses to randomized clinical trials, only seven of fifty-four studies were conducted outside the United States. In the present chapter, we are concerned with preventing problems in communities and societies and across societies. By crossing "forgiveness intervention" and twenty-five countries in PsychINFO, we located a total of eight additional forgiveness intervention studies for a total of fifteen. Most trials of explicit forgiveness interventions occurred in some of the higher income nations, such as England (n = 4; e.g., Egleston et al., 2004),

Northern Ireland (n = 1; Magnusson, 2010), Canada (n = 3; e.g., Greenberg, Warwar, & Malcolm, 2010), Hong Kong (n = 2; e.g., Hui & Chau, 2009), Taiwan (n = 1; Lin, Enright, & Klatt, 2013), South Korea (n = 1; Park, Enright, Essex, Zahn-Waxler, & Klatt., 2013), and Israel (n = 1; Shnabel, Halabi, & Moore, 2013). Others were done in the Philippines (Worthington et al., 2010) and Brazil (van der Meer Sanchez, & Nappo, 2008), (n = 1 each). Searches such as this are imprecise and undoubtedly miss many studies, but they give a picture of the distribution of studies available. Some of the adaptations needed were, first and foremost, proper (i.e., spoken-language) translation. Typically, the secular version of a U.S.-developed intervention was used, but some attention was paid to local pressures and situational events (e.g., adaptation both to religion and culture in Worthington et al., 2010) specific to the country. In addition, quotes from leaders in the country spice up the manuscripts, and in some cases, the authors used indigenous concepts of terms related to forgiveness. Mostly, the changes were cosmetic rather than content-oriented, but importantly, the changes invited participants into a culture-congruent intervention involving language, situations, and people with which the participants were often familiar.

In the present chapter, we are concerned with preventing problems in communities and societies and across societies. However, it is important to know more about how well the intervention programs that have been developed within the United States can work in other countries across the globe, given the influence of culture on expressions of forgiveness (Hook, Worthington, & Utsey, 2009).

The Effects of Forgiveness Intervention within Close Relationships

Forgiveness interventions with couples. Several forgiveness interventions have been developed for use with couples. Greenberg et al. (2010) concluded that emotionally focused couple therapy as a means of promoting forgiveness are successful and may support other therapeutic gains. DiBlasio and Benda (2008) compared couples in treatment that received a three-hour pretherapy intervention focused on hard-to-forgive offenses. The brief intervention proved effective, but it appeared more effective for Christian couples than for those who did not espouse a religious position. Worthington has sought to treat marriages in both enrichment and couple therapy to promote forgiveness (Ripley et al., 2014; Worthington et al., 2015) using a method called FREE (Forgiveness and Reconciliation through Experiencing Empathy), which included within it the REACH Forgiveness model. The FREE model has also been used effectively with parents forgiving each other or their children due to offenses they experienced in the family (Kiefer et al., 2010).

Efficacy of couple interventions. Wade et al. (2014), within their meta-analysis of forgiveness interventions, found six randomized clinical trials testing the efficacy of interventions with couples. Cohen's d is a statistic that compares the amount of change for a treatment when compared with no-treatment control. Cohen's *d* is expressed as a standard score – the number of standard deviations that the treatment score is superior to the control condition. Wade et al. found that Cohen's *d* was 0.75 (k = 6, 95 percent CI: 0.44, 1.06). When compared with alternative treatments, *d* was 0.22, and the 95 percent CI included zero (k = 3, CI: –0.27, 0.71). Neither of the *d*s for comparisons of individual interventions to alternative treatments (k = 2, d = 1.98, CI: 1.03, 2.92) and group interventions to alternative treatments (k = 17, d = 0.37, CI: 0.15, 0.60) contained zero. To provide a context to interpret the magnitude of these changes, meta-analyses for psychotherapy are often around $d \sim 1$. For example, in one recent meta-analysis, which compared Acceptance and Commitment Therapy (ACT) to various alternatives, the standardized effect size was 0.82 of ACT compared to waitlist, 0.51 compared to a placebo, and 0.64 compared to treatment as usual. In the comparisons in Wade et al. (2014), the alternatives in the three studies on couples were against strong, bona fide communication-training treatments; thus, finding that forgiveness training did not differ from the alternatives is hardly surprising.

The Effects of Forgiveness Interventions within Communities

Often, we think of forgiveness as an individual experience. But societal and social wrongdoing can create an atmosphere in which many members of a community or entire society adopt similar attitudes toward a transgressor. Virtually any war or armed conflict will involve each side's attempts to focus the perceptions of their own in-group members and of the world as a whole on the wrongdoing of the out-group and the virtuous beliefs and behavior of their in-group (Van Tongeren et al., 2014).

Warfare or active ideological conflict is a strong case of community unforgiveness, but often after conflicts or wars cease, the community may value or even sanctify forgiveness (Bell et al., 2014). However, communities strongly affect each of the members even if the leaders are not trying actively to organize opposition to common enemies. For example, any community develops norms (Lenzi, Vieno, Santinello, & Perkins, 2013). Those norms are standards that prescribe (informally and not often explicitly) what the group's stance is toward others who are different. Religious groups might, for example, strongly preach inclusion, acceptance, and toleration of differences. Just as easily, though, the religious group could see itself as being in opposition to another religious group that embraces terrorism and encourages hatred or unforgiveness toward members of the out-group. Or, less dramatically, through advocating the value of forgiveness, a religious group could set people's attention on forgiveness and its importance, which could influence the members' willingness to consider forgiveness for personal transgressions they experience, domestic transgressions, workplace transgressions, or even racial and ethnic microaggressions (Owen, Tao, Imel, Wampold, & Rodolfa, 2014).

Awareness-raising campaigns in communities. In the research on forgiveness, until recently most research has been focused on forgiveness in individuals and in various types of dyadic relationships (i.e., couples, parent–child, workplace, etc.). Few interventions have been aimed at changing communities. Recently, Griffin et al. (2015a) examined an awareness-raising campaign for forgiveness as a community intervention at a private Midwestern, religiously affiliated university (see Table 22.1). Numerous students (N = 877) of a student body of about 2,500 completed measures immediately before and after the two-week administration of the multimodal campaign. The campaign employed activities such as articles in the campus newspaper, speakers, essay contests, banners, signs on dining hall tables, groups offered within dormitories, and others (see Table 22.1). Students reported on the activities in which they participated using a checklist of activities that were available the two weeks. The mean dose encountered by students was about 2.5 hours of exposure per individual over the two-week period. Griffin et al. (2015a) found an effect size of 0.02 standard deviations of change in forgiveness per hour of exposure on the average. Thus, the total change was about 0.05 per person over the two weeks. Recall that the mean change in a psychotherapy study involving unlimited psychotherapy is usually about 1.00 (twenty times as great). However, the community awareness campaign clearly did not engage some people, and yet, averaged over all students completing the measures (i.e., about one-third of the student body), the change was about one-twentieth as much. There were some participants who were very engaged. Others might not even have realized the campaign was ongoing, but in a community, the high number of participants suggests substantial change campus- or communitywide.

We can estimate the amount of generalizable change likely from wider, more secular awareness-raising community campaigns. First, the Griffin et al. (2015a) research occurred at a Christian college. Because Christians have been found to embrace forgiveness more than the general population, including other religions (Davis et al., 2013), we assume that a forgiveness awareness-raising intervention in a secular society would likely engender less forgiveness on average than was found in the religiously affiliated university sample. Intervention research on forgiveness involving secular samples produces only slightly less change than in Christian samples. Therefore, we conservatively estimate about half the effect size for general societies. (Obviously, there might be small pockets of people who abhor forgiveness, and an awareness-raising campaign might produce negative change. But the numbers available suggest that, on the average, the changes in secular society will be slightly less than in Christian communities.) Second, most intervention research involves people who have explicitly sought forgiveness intervention. But, in a societal forgiveness-awareness-raising campaign, not everyone exposed to general awareness raising will desire to use or increase forgiveness. We estimate that the intervention affects only one-fifth the number of people in a secular setting, similar to the proportion of the population reported by Griffin et al. (2015a). Our conclusion is this: $d \sim 0.05 \times \frac{1}{2} \times 1/5 = 0.005$ for a two-week public health intervention in a secular society. This is an average. It obscures the range of responses, which are likely to vary from zero effect to large positive effects. Now, imagine that this campaign had

Table 22.1 *A Few Activities for a Campus Forgiveness Blitz plus Those (Marked with *) That Could Be Used in a Citywide Public-Relations Blitz*

Universitywide Interventions Requiring Substantial Coordination

- Symposium talks on forgiveness, relationships, and related topics at libraries.*
- Guest speakers giving lectures.*
- Debates or dialogues involving clergy of different religions, people from different professional or business employment sites.*
- Research Team makes a video record of all activities to document the Blitz; edited into one or a set of YouTube four-minute summaries.*

Things Students Can Do Alone

- Books reviewed in the school (or city*) newspaper.
- Email blasts from administration to students or to special interest groups' lists.*
- Website postings.*
- Talks, such as TED Talks, that are available to download.*
- A website established in which people can post forgiveness stories* (the site would have to be monitored and moderated).
- Professors encouraged to assign their classes projects related to forgiveness (e.g., journaling and have them watch forgiveness-related films, read forgiveness-related books or journal articles, and participate in forgiveness discussion groups).

Group Activities

- Movie nights to watch and discuss forgiveness-themed movies (e.g., *Les Miserables, The Unforgiven, You've Got Mail*), tragedies that raise issues about the limits of forgiveness (e.g., *Schindler's List, Hotel Rwanda*), or documentary movies (*The Big Question*, Paulist Productions; *The Power of Forgiving,* Journey Films) – on campus or at public libraries.*
- An area designated the Forgiveness Rock Garden, with the letters "F-O-R-G-I-V-E" outlined in paint. Students or citizens* are challenged to view a grudge they are holding as a heavy weight, like a rock. When they forgive, during the forgiveness blitz, they should take some rock to the Forgiveness Rock Garden as a symbolic act of forgiveness, or they might place the rock in one of the letters. By the end of the blitz, the letters might be full of rocks.*
- Psychoeducational groups offered to students in libraries,* dormitories, in fraternities, in academic departments, in religiously oriented groups,* or other free-standing groups.*
- Blogs from the site coordinator.*
- Op-ed articles* including targeted articles on topics like forgiveness and parents, forgiveness and your roommate, forgiveness and your coursework, health and forgiveness,* mental health and forgiveness,* spiritual issues in forgiving.*
- Reading and discussion of Simon Wiesenthal's *The Sunflower* in a class, as a university summer reading project, as a civic public interest project.*
- Invitation to local professors or thought leaders (like television personalities, columnists, magazine writers) to respond to *The Sunflower* as did essayists in the book.*
- Discussion groups in the dormitories and fraternities/sororities or other existing groups on campus.

Table 22.1 (*cont.*)

- Groups challenged to come up with a creative project for the group to accomplish related to forgiveness.
- Agreements among professors to discuss forgiveness in class.

Student or Civic Competitions
- Poster competition. Posters can be chosen to decorate a public space for two weeks.*
- Essay contests, song-writing contests, art contests, video contests. Winners might receive some prize and might perform or demonstrate their project publicly.*
- One-act play writing contest in the English Department or at a local cultural arts center* to solicit entries and the Drama Department or drama group* could perform.*
- Banner competition among groups on campus; banners displayed in public space.*
- *The Sunflower* (Simon Wiesenthal) essay competition (college or city).*
- Competitions dorm versus dorm for the best forgiveness project.
- Air-band competition for performing a song with a forgiveness theme.

occurred in a major city with a population over one million people! The total amount of forgiveness experienced and the sheer number of people affected may be extremely large with a relatively low cost of providing awareness-raising interventions. We freely admit that this is the rawest speculation. However, we do base it on research available all over the world that suggests that most people respond positively to the concept of forgiveness, so – admitting to local reversals – we suspect that, *on the average*, there will be a relative strong effect in most communities within society.

Recall also that forgiveness interventions tend to produce changes in depression, anxiety, and hope (Wade et al., 2014). So, we might legitimately estimate effect sizes of $d \sim 0.0025$ for depression and anxiety and $d \sim 0.005$ for hope. Thus, we might expect changes in mental health within a large community. In addition, we have already shown that changes in individuals' forgiveness and their mental health are related to changes in physical health, relationships, and even religion and spirituality; each of these may also improve as a result of a large-scale community intervention to promote forgiveness.

Costs to promote the change in communities. The costs of conducting a large public relations campaign within a large city are quite modest. For example, such a campaign would require a public relations effort; advertising for special events; distribution of free resources; costs of professional time to run groups, write talks, and educate the public; resources devoted to raising money (or allocating it) for sponsorship; time and money to organize special events and to engage organizations that can use volunteers to run forgiveness groups or provide forgiveness workbooks; time to evaluate the outcomes; printing costs for hardcopy information; website preparation; and costs of electronic dissemination. Such costs are likely minimal compared to the current public health costs being incurred as a result of stress and aggression related to unforgiveness. (For examples of activities, see Table 22.1.)

Political Forgiveness

In a recent meta-analysis of intergroup forgiveness, Van Tongeren et al., (2014) meta-analyzed 43 studies with 13,371 total participants from 20 different nationalities. Van Tongeren et al. meta-analyzed studies from more countries than did Wade et al. (2014), who meta-analyzed intervention studies. Van Tongeren et al. (2014) examined both intracountry (65 percent) and intercountry (35 percent) conflicts. They examined correlates of intergroup forgiveness regardless of whether the conflict was a political conflict within a country (i.e., Rwanda) or between countries. They examined nine potential predictors of forgiveness between conflicting groups, and they investigated study characteristics as moderators of these effects (i.e., sex of victim and conflict type). *Collective guilt* ($r = 0.49$, $k = 3$, 95 percent CI: 0.21, 0.69), *trust* ($r = 0.42$, $k = 11$, 95 percent CI: 0.33, 0.51), the *outgroup attempts to make amends* ($r = 0.39$, $k = 11$, 95 percent CI: 0.28, 0.49), *empathy for the outgroup* ($r = 0.37$, $k = 13$, 95 percent CI: 0.30, 0.44), *contact* ($r = 0.31$, $k = 5$, 95 percent CI: 0.26, 0.35), and *sharing a common identity* ($r = 0.29$, $k = 14$, 95 percent CI: 0.25, 0.32) were the strongest facilitators of forgiveness across groups. *Negative emotions* ($r = -0.33$, $k = 9$, 95 percent CI: –0.19, –0.45), *strong in-group identity* ($r = -0.32$, $k = 20$, 95 percent CI: –0.24, –0.40), and *perceived victimhood* ($r = -0.28$, $k = 16$, 95 percent CI: –0.21, –0.35) most strongly inhibited forgiveness across groups.

Van Tongeren et al. (2014) arrived at several additional conclusions based on their analyses. First, forgiveness has effects on intracountry and intercountry conflict. Second, offenses by an out-group member relative to an in-group member were perceived as less severe and as inflicting less hurt. Third, however, people were less willing to forgive an out-group member than they were to forgive an in-group member. The implications are that in the beginning, when wounds are raw, peacemakers are better served by emphasizing group differences – perhaps by promoting empathy for differences. But, as the interactions continue and parties are willing to work toward repair of the relationships, peacemakers are better served to emphasize group similarities and similar group identities. Fourth, the contact hypothesis – that more peaceful contact with an out-group member whose group had offended would lead to better relationship with (i.e., more forgiveness of) the out-group was not well supported. In fact, when people were highly sensitized to political differences, more contact with an out-group member reduced the forgiveness relative to less contact. The likelihood is that politicized people selectively looked for behavior that confirmed their suspicions that the out-group member was neither penitent nor trustworthy. They would thus be less likely to forgive. Thus, policy makers should not think that merely bringing former enemies together peacefully will initiate forgiveness. Rather, fifth, close relations with a group (i.e., trust, shared identity, empathy), one's own collective guilt, and whether the out-group had made efforts to repair the damage done predicted forgiveness, but forgiveness was hard to come by from the people who were most injured and upset.

Forgiveness in Conflicted Society – within and between Countries – through Peacemaking

Forgiveness can affect whole societies by healing wounds from conflict. Conflicts bring out concerns with justice and therefore with *forgiveness.* Recall that forgiveness is a specific individual's response to injustice, but expressions of forgiveness, societal forgiveness, granting forgiveness, saying "I forgive you," and so forth are all part of reconciliation.

Track-one diplomacy. To bring about healing after conflict, we suggest a three-tier use of forgiveness (Worthington & Aten, 2010). When hostilities are under way, they must be brought to an end (Botcharova, 2001; Montville, 1990). *Track-one diplomacy* is negotiation at the level of a state's leaders and the leaders of peacekeeping bodies (such as nongovernmental organizations or intervening nations) that work together to craft agreements that will end violence and promote peace. Strategies for bringing about peace as an end to hostile (or even armed) conflict are often imposed by peacekeeping bodies – and they need to be imposed. Track-one diplomacy usually is aimed at established leaders, who have decision-making power. Governmental leaders are usually entrenched – as are conflicting individuals in any relationship. But with governmental leaders, political structures, not just individual interests, often provide a level of inertia opposing change that means that to change their stance is highly unlikely unless external pressure is applied. Track-one diplomacy can sometimes stop conflict, but it can rarely, by itself, promote forgiveness, reconciliation, and peaceful stability.

Track-two diplomacy. To forgive and reconcile, *track-two diplomacy* is needed. Track-two diplomacy attempts to promote understanding, cooperation, empathy, and goodwill among opinion leaders of the formerly divided communities. The hopes are twofold. First, opinion leaders – such as community leaders, clergy, university professors, or local politicians – who meet with and develop empathy for members of the other side and understand and gain respect for them can apply pressure on national, party, or tribal leaders to work out agreements. Second, and perhaps more importantly, opinion leaders can carry their empathy back to the communities that they represent. Opinion leaders gain a different experiential view about the other group members and bring that experience-based knowledge back into their local communities. There, they might set in motion groups and experiences that would promote healing within their community.

Track-three diplomacy. To forgive and reconcile, track-three diplomacy should be utilized to provide either direct or indirect avenues for healing within communities. Once opinion leaders are on board for promoting societal rehabilitation, then programs and persuasion can be employed in the community. These community meetings are open to the public and invite the participation of members in the community. Track-three diplomacy programs may be aimed directly at some sort of justice, truth-telling, or forgiveness and reconciliation.

Justice-based track-three diplomacy. There are several examples of justice-based track-three diplomacy. First, there are truth commissions. A single accepted narrative will not usually arise from a truth commission; the truth commission can at best summarize major perspectives and yield a more balanced view of the perspectives than any individual is likely to hold. The South African Truth and Reconciliation Commission (SA TRC) was perhaps one of the most innovative peacemaking strategies (Chapman & Spong, 2003). It consisted of three types of hearings: (1) human rights hearings sought victims' stories; (2) hearings considered amnesty for people who agreed to tell the whole truth (they were promised amnesty for politically motivated crimes); and (3) hearings that considered reparation about fair ways to compensate people who had been damaged through apartheid. Another example is the Rwandan *gacaca* hearings. In Rwanda, the solution to their problem was different from in South Africa. About eight hundred thousand people were massacred in one hundred days, and many people participated in those massacres, thus making hearings modeled on the SA TRC practically impossible. Thus, amnesty hearings were moved into the local communities. The hearings were called *gacaca* hearings, which were public hearings for amnesty within the communities in which the violence took place. Brounéus (2008) has described some of the problems that have arisen with the *gacaca* hearings.

Forgiveness-based track-three diplomacy. Some efforts at track-three diplomacy use forgiveness education to promote intrastate healing after conflict. For example, Staub, Pearlman, Gubin, and Hagengimana (2005) have conducted a number of groups in Rwanda to bring Rwandians from different tribal background together. Narváez Gómez (2005) conducted forgiveness education in at least ten South American countries to promote intrastate forgiveness and reconciliation. Narváez Gómez typically has people on both sides of a conflict go through an educative process of fifty or more hours to learn forgiveness and reconciliation skills. He has used this with warring parties, criminals who have confessed to political crimes, and other people who have done violence. The approach is tailored to the country in which the problem exists. His methods drew liberally from Worthington's REACH Forgiveness and Enright's process model.

Forgiveness in Society through Promoting Research Infrastructure

An additional way to promote more attention to forgiveness and perhaps more world peace is to foster research and its dissemination in countries throughout the world. In 1997, the John Templeton Foundation (JTF) funded three million U.S. dollars in grants to promote forgiveness throughout the world. Because of the strong response to the grant, *A Campaign for Forgiveness Research*, a 501c

(3) nonprofit corporation was formed.[1] It raised, through fourteen funding partners, an additional $6.4 million to fund research projects and disseminate results through two international conferences for basic and applied scientific investigations. Virtually all of the projects funded in these initiatives were from research teams in the United States, with some in western Europe and one successful project from South Africa.

The amount of change in the United States, Canada, Australia, New Zealand, England, and other United Kingdom societies from the aforementioned funding initiative is astounding. For example, scientific publications on forgiveness increased from 58 in 1998 to more than 2,500 in 2015.[2] Public awareness was increased through thousands of media exposures. Television and documentary movies have increased substantially. Suppose that something similar to this could be enacted in Africa, South America, the Middle East, western Asia, the Indian subcontinent and surroundings (i.e., India and Pakistan), and Southeast Asia. A need exists to adapt th successful domestic initiatives to promote forgiveness in some well-developed countries to garner international interest.

Barriers to a Vibrant Prevention Science of Forgiveness

There are at least six barriers to furthering prevention science of forgiveness and the societal implementation of the evidence-based practices of forgiveness toward preventing problems. These include (1) misunderstandings about what forgiveness is, (2) limited access to forgiveness interventions, (3) limited use of forgiveness interventions (even when access is available), (4) limited expertise to provide interventions or scientific study of interventions in local areas, (5) limited resources available to promote widespread application, and (6) lack of leadership.

Misunderstandings about What Forgiveness Is

The first barrier to a thriving prevention science of forgiveness is that many people hold misconceptions about what forgiveness is, and those misconceptions interfere with people's choices to use, provide, or recommend forgiveness interventions. For example, some people think that to forgive, one must follow up by seeking reconciliation. This is not a correct understanding of forgiveness and reconciliation. Forgiveness is intrapersonal and occurs within a person's own skin. It can affect people's attitudes toward the offender, and it can promote conciliatory motives. However, reconciliation is interpersonal and need not follow forgiveness, especially if continued contact between parties places the victim at greater than normal risk for continued injustice and abuse. In fact, some forgiveness might even follow reconciliation. In some cases, of

1 www.forgiving.org. 2 www.forgivenessresearch.org.

course, what is leading what is difficult to decipher. For example, when a nation or community's interest is piqued, the entire community can seem to be forgiving. But this is best thought of an aggregation of individuals of similar mindedness who are forgiving; it is not really a "group" that is forgiving. Another misunderstanding is to think that forgiveness is opposed to justice. Some people mistakenly believe that if one forgives an offender, it is inappropriate to seek justice or fairness. Yet, justice is a societal and social construct, and forgiveness is an intrapersonal construct. Both may occur simultaneously.

Sometimes people misunderstand forgiveness to be a weak response to injustice. This might be thought to have two potential consequences. It might be thought that to advocate forgiveness, one is perceived (often by the offender) to condone injustice, and thus the offender might take advantage of the perceived weakness and perpetrate further injustices. Behind this misbelief is the belief that forgiveness is the only response to injustice in which one could engage. That is, one might believe that if one is forgiving, one cannot also be courageous in standing against injustice. The other misunderstanding is that forgiveness is perceived to be a moral escape valve and thus does not hold an offender morally responsible for offenses. Some people perceive that forgiveness inherently condones injustice, conveying that nothing was done wrong. To the contrary, forgiveness implies that a moral wrong was done. To say, "I forgive you," inherently conveys that *you have done some wrong* that I choose to forgive.

One might also believe that one should not forgive in the midst of a conflict, assuming that forgiveness is appropriate only after all hostilities cease. But how would one know that hostilities had, for all time, ceased? Instead, forgiveness can occur at any time after an offense – even if one is likely to be offended again. Any human relationship can be the locus of numerous offenses over time; humans almost inevitably will at some time offend the other, and thus, to forgive, one does not have to wait until all offenses have ceased. Because forgiveness is often understood somewhat differently across cultures, "misunderstanding forgiveness" is especially crucial once cross-cultural applications are made or once forgiveness interventions are adapted to a new culture. It is tempting, of course, to want to impose a Western scientific understanding of forgiveness. But, in the spirit of multiculturalism, sometimes we must simply let local norms and understandings rule and trust that different cultures will adapt interventions and understandings to best represent each one.

Limited Access to Forgiveness Interventions

A second barrier to the expansion of the prevention science of forgiveness is limited access to forgiveness interventions. Forgiveness interventions are widely available, and they are available in many forms. But one must know where and how to gain access to them. For example, forgiveness interventions through books, the Internet, workbooks, and other written materials are inaccessible if they have not been translated into the vernacular of the people. Others might live in rural nondeveloped locales and do not have access to mental health practitioners who are familiar with the prevention science of forgiveness interventions.

Limited Use of the Science of Forgiveness Interventions

A third barrier to the expansion of a prevention science of forgiveness is that some people might not value the information of mental health providers or prevention scientists. For example, some very restrictive religious communities, some military and police forces, many traditional societies, and some civic organizations do not seek forgiveness interventions. Custom or stigma can prevent societies from forgiving. While some societies prefer one or more of the many alternative ways to handle offenses (e.g., in China people tend to think more about forbearance, which is responding to an offender by not emotionally reacting and not showing emotional upset so that social harmony is maintained), the empirical study of forgiveness may be used to help create the optimal conditions under which religious and cultural forgiveness rituals affect people.

Limited Local Expertise to Provide or Study Interventions

The fourth barrier to expanding a prevention science of forgiveness is the limited expertise to provide interventions to promote forgiveness and, as related, limited expertise in the scientific study of interventions within local areas. The United States and Europe are well supplied with numerous research-oriented and applied mental health professionals. However, in many areas throughout the world, such resources are simply not available. This is true throughout lower-income nations (i.e., throughout Africa, South America, Southeast Asia) and in many rural areas in large countries that are, on the whole, industrial and informational powerhouses (i.e., China, India, Brazil, Russia). Deficits often include (a) few practitioners who might have knowledge of and access to evidence-based practices or, more likely, (b) few basic and clinical scientists who have done research on forgiveness. Often there is a general paucity of both clinical and scientific resources.

Limited Resources Available to Promote Wider Application

The fifth barrier to a flourishing prevention science of forgiveness is limited resources to promote a wide application of the knowledge we have about forgiveness. Although forgiveness interventions typically do not require much in tangible resources to run groups – other than personnel costs – there can be other expenses to advertise, market, track participants, and provide materials and access to tangible resources, and those can make widespread dissemination throughout a community or society quite expensive. Thus, sometimes, resource limitations are important. For example, in lower-income nations, there are often insufficient funds to purchase training materials and professorial or researcher time to do research, or funds to permit professionals to get degrees that build skills to deliver high-quality forgiveness interventions.

Lack of Effective Leadership in Promoting Forgiveness

The sixth barrier to expanding the prevention science of forgiveness is lack of effective leadership in promoting forgiveness. In today's socially interconnected environment, networks of people are needed to transmit information about forgiveness. Some people serve as nodes of information transmission, and network analyses can reveal how some people serve as funnels that seem to affect many others (Christakas & Fowler, 2009). These nodes can be either formal leaders or informal leaders. Informal leaders seem to know a lot of people, often communicate in ways that followers can retain and use practical wisdom, continue to influence others, and provide entrees into networks of other opinion leaders. Formal leaders have position authority, and by virtue of their platform as an appointed leader with credentials, they are able to convey information, shape policy, influence decisions, and shape evaluations and opinions. Currently, there is a lack of effective formal and informal leadership to form the coalitions needed to promote forgiveness widely.

Leaders are needed across many areas. For example, leaders are needed among the basic and applied forgiveness researchers and in the treatment community to organize treatments and direct large programmatic efforts to promote forgiveness. Leaders are needed in public advocacy by politicians, celebrities, news anchors, website operators, communications media, and so on. Leaders also are needed among philanthropy and funding agencies. Philanthropists and governmental agencies can have huge effects on the direction of science, businesses, nonprofits, and even charitable organizations and churches. They can set a general agenda and, with funds, direct people's efforts toward achieving the vision of the philanthropist or agency.

Conclusions Relevant to Prevention Science

In this chapter, we have been aiming at several important points. First, unforgiveness is a problem for individuals, resulting in negative physical health, mental health, relationship, and spiritual effects, and socially costly outcomes in larger units of society. Prevention science is concerned with all of these. The effects in individual lives are reflected in other negative effects in relationships, communities, and societies – and once we get beyond effects on individuals, the effects are hard to quantify. We have addressed forgiveness as a preventive intervention on a broad societal front, so we relied in most part on existing meta-analyses and making logical extensions from the findings within those meta-analytic reviews. Our analysis of the impact of forgiveness on preventing problems is thus imprecise.

Second, positive, clinical, community, political, and peace psychologies have developed interventions that can help people forgive. A variety of interventions are available to people who wish to forgive offenses and hurts. Their use can have many positive benefits to promote health and social benefits and to prevent poor health or maladjusted social outcomes. These interventions have the potential to benefit individuals, families, groups, communities, and societies.

Third, barriers to widespread application of these interventions are numerous, including lack of awareness, misunderstanding about what forgiveness is, literacy of many people who might benefit by forgiveness intervention, resources available to promote wider application, use of resources that are available, and lack of effective leadership to form the coalitions needed to promote forgiveness widely.

We believe that world prosperity and peace demand that we take forgiveness seriously as a prevention goal. Thus, we recommend that prevention scientists to take seriously the public health risks of unforgiveness, seek new and innovative intervention strategies, and seek to eliminate barriers to international applications. If we can do those things, perhaps the world will become a better place.

Acknowledgments

This publication was made possible through the support of a grant from Templeton World Charity Foundation (e.g., Forgiveness in Africa) with other support from a grant from the John Templeton Foundation (e.g., Relational Humility). The opinions expressed in this publication are those of the authors and do not necessarily reflect the views of Templeton World Charity Foundation or the John Templeton Foundation.

References

Bell, I. C., Woodruff, E., Davis, D. E., Van Tongeren, D. R., Hook, J. N., & Worthington, E. L., Jr. (2014). Community sanctification of forgiveness. *Journal of Psychology and Theology* 42(3): 243–51.

Berry, J. W., & Worthington, E. L., Jr. (2001). Forgivingness, relationship quality, stress while imagining relationships events, and physical and mental health. *Journal of Counseling Psychology* 48: 447–55.

Botcharova, O. (2001). Implementation of track two diplomacy: developing a model of forgiveness. In Helmick, R. G., & Petersen, R. L. (eds.), *Forgiveness and Reconciliation: Religion, Public Policy, and Conflict Transformation*. Philadelphia, PA: Templeton Foundation Press, pp. 269–94.

Brounéus, K. (2008). Reconciliation in the Great Lakes region: some thoughts on key topics, agendas, and challenges. Paper presented at the meeting of the John Templeton Foundation ad hoc Task Force on the Possibility of Research in Rwanda, Nassau, Bahamas, June 3.

Chapman, A. R., & Spong, B. (eds.). (2003). *Religion and Reconciliation in South Africa*. Philadelphia, PA: Templeton Foundation Press.

Christakas, N. A., & Fowler, J. H. (2009). *Connected: The Surprising Power of Our Social Networks and How They Shape Our Lives*. New York: Little, Brown.

Davis, D. E., Ho, M. Y., Griffin, B. J., Bell, C., Hook, J. N., Van Tongeren, D. R., Worthington, E. L., Jr.. DeBlaere, C., & Westbrook, C. (2015). Forgiving the self and physical and mental health correlates: a meta-analytic review. *Journal of Counseling Psychology* 62(2): 329–35.

Davis, D. E., Hook, J. N., Van Tongeren, D. R., DeBlaere, C., Rice, K. G., & Worthington, E. L., Jr. (2015). Making a decision to forgive. *Journal of Counseling Psychology* 62(2): 280–8.

Davis, D. E., Worthington, E. L., Jr., Hook, J. N., & Hill, P. C. (2013). Research on religion/spirituality and forgiveness: a meta-analytic review. *Psychology of Religion and Spirituality* 5: 233–41.

DiBlasio, F. A., & Benda, B. B. (2008). Forgiveness intervention with married couples: two empirical analyses. *Journal of Psychology and Christianity* 27: 150–8.

Egleston, P. N., Lee, K. H., Brown, W. H., Green, R. D. J., Farrow, T. F. D., Hunter, M. D., Parks, R. W., Spence, S. A., & Woodruff, P. W. R. (2004). Treatment induced brain changes during forgiveness tasks in patients with schizophrenia. *Schizophrenia Research* 67: 193.

Enright, R. D., & Fitzgibbons, R. P. (2015). *Forgiveness Therapy: An Empirical Guide for Resolving Anger and Restoring Hope*, 2nd ed. Washington, DC: American Psychological Association.

Enright, R. D., Rhody, M., Litts, B., & Klatt, J. S. (2014). Piloting forgiveness education in a divided community: comparing electronic pen-pal and journaling activities across two groups of youth. *Journal of Moral Education* 43: 1–17.

Exline, J. J., Worthington, E. L., Jr., Hill, P. C., & McCullough, M. E. (2003). Forgiveness and justice: a research agenda for social and personality psychology. *Personality and Social Psychology Review* 7: 337–48.

Fehr, R., & Gelfand, M. J. (2012). The forgiving organization: a multilevel model of forgiveness at work. *Academy of Management Review* 37: 664–88.

Fehr, R., Gelfand, M. J., & Nag, M. (2010). The road to forgiveness: a meta-analytic synthesis of its situational and dispositional correlates. *Psychological Bulletin* 136: 894–914.

Freedman, S. R., & Enright, R. D. (1996). Forgiveness as an intervention with incest survivors. *Journal of Consulting and Clinical Psychology* 64: 983–92.

Goffman, E. (1969). *Social Interaction*. Oxford, UK: University of Pennsylvania Press.

Green, M., Decourville, N., & Sadava, S. (2012). Positive affect, negative affect, stress, and social support as mediators of the forgiveness-health relationship. *Journal of Social Psychology* 152: 288–307.

Greenberg, L. S., Warwar, S., & Malcolm, W. (2010). Emotion-focused couples therapy and the facilitation of forgiveness. *Journal of Marital and Family Therapy* 36: 28–42.

Greer, C. L., Worthington, E. L., Jr., Lin, Y., Lavelock, C. R., & Griffin, B. J. (2014). Efficacy of a self-directed forgiveness workbook for Christian victims of within-congregation offenders. *Spirituality in Clinical Practice* 1: 218–30.

Griffin, B. J., Toussaint, L. L., Worthington, E. L., Jr., Coleman, J. A., Lavelock, C. R., Hook, J. N., Wade, N. G., Sandage, S. J., & Rye, M. S. (2015a). *Forgiveness Blitz: A community-based forgiveness initiative*. (Unpublished manuscript under editorial review). Virginia Commonwealth University.

Griffin, B. J., Worthington, E. L., Jr., Lavelock, C. R., Greer, C. L., Lin, Y., Davis, D. E., & Hook, J. N. (2015b). Efficacy of a self-forgiveness workbook: a randomized controlled trial with interpersonal offenders. *Journal of Counseling Psychology* 62(2): 124–36.

Griffin, B. J., Worthington, E. L., Jr., Wade, N. G., Hoyt, W. T., & Davis, D. E. (2015c). Forgiveness and mental health. In Toussaint, L., Worthington, E. L., Jr., & Williams, D. (eds.), *Forgiveness and Health: Scientific Evidence and Theories Relating Forgiveness to Better Health*. New York: Springer, pp. 77–90.

Harper, Q., Worthington, E. L., Jr., Griffin, B. J., Lavelock, C. R., Hook, J. N., Vrana, S. R., & Greer, C. L. (2014). Efficacy of a workbook to promote forgiveness: a randomized controlled trial with university students. *Journal of Clinical Psychology* 70: 1158–69.

Hook, J. N., Worthington, E. L., Jr., & Utsey, S. O. (2009). Collectivism, forgiveness, and social harmony. *Counseling Psychologist* 37: 821–47.

Hui, E. K. P., & Chau, T. S. (2009). The impact of a forgiveness intervention with Hong Kong Chinese children hurt in interpersonal relationships. *British Journal of Guidance & Counselling* 37(2): 141–56.

Kiefer, R. P., Worthington, E. L., Jr., Myers, B. J., Kliewer, W. L., Berry, J. W., Davis, D. E., Kilgour, J. M., Jr., Miller, A. J., Van Tongeren, D. R., & Hunter, J. L. (2010). Training parents in forgiving and reconciling. *American Journal of Family Therapy* 38: 32–49.

Kramer, B. J., Kavanaugh, M., Trentham-Dietz, A., Walsh, M., & Yonker, J. A. (2010). Predictors of family conflict at the end of life: the experiences of spouses and adult children of persons with lung cancer. *Gerontologist* 50: 215–25.

Lavelock, C. R., Griffin, B. J., & Worthington, E. L., Jr. (2013). Forgiveness, religion, spirituality, and mental health in people with physical challenges: a review and a model. *Research in the Social Scientific Study of Religion* 24: 53–92.

Lenzi, M., Vieno, A., Santinello, M., & Perkins, D. D. (2013). How neighborhood structural and institutional features can shape neighborhood social connectedness: a multilevel study of adolescent perceptions. *American Journal of Community Psychology* 51(3–4): 451–67.

Lin, W. N., Enright, R. D., & Klatt, J. S. (2013). A forgiveness intervention for Taiwanese young adults with insecure attachment. *Contemporary Family Therapy: An International Journal* 35(1): 105–20.

Lin, Y., Worthington, E. L., Jr., Griffin, B. J., Greer, C. L., Opare-Henaku, A., Lavelock, C. R., Hook, J. N., Ho, M. Y., & Muller, H. (2014). Efficacy of REACH forgiveness across cultures. *Journal of Clinical Psychology* 70: 781–93.

Maamri, M. M., Nevin, N., & Worthington, E. L., Jr. (eds.). (2010). *A Journey through Forgiveness*. Oxford, UK: Inter-Disciplinary Press. www.inter-disciplinary.net/publishing/id-press/ebooks/a-journey-through-forgiveness/

Magnuson, C. M. (2010). The forgiving family: effects of a parent-led forgiveness program on mental and relational health. *Dissertation Abstracts International, Section A: Humanities and Social Sciences* 70(11-A): 4178.

McCullough, M. E., Hoyt, W. T., Larson, D. B., Koenig, H. G., & Thoresen, C. (2000). Religious involvement and mortality: a meta-analytic review. *Health Psychology* 19: 211–22.

McNulty, J. K., & Fincham, F. D. (2012). Beyond positive psychology: toward a contextual view of psychological processes and well-being. *American Psychologist* 67(2): 101–10.

Montville, J. V. (1990). *The Arrow and the Olive Branch: A Case for Track-Two Diplomacy*. Lexington, MA: Lexington.

Narváez Gómez, L. (2005). Elementos básicos del perdón y la reconciliación. In Villamizar, D., Cuesta, J., Sánchez, C., & Morales, R. (eds.), *Desmovilización, un camino hacia la paz*. Bogotá, D.C., Colombia: Librería y Editorial Filigrana, pp. 73–86.

Owen, J., Tao, K. W., Imel, Z. E., Wampold, B. E., & Rodolfa, E. (2014). Addressing racial and ethnic microaggressions in therapy. *Professional Psychology: Research and Practice* 45: 283–90.

Park, J.-H., Enright, R. D., Essex, M. J., Zahn-Waxler, C., & Klatt, J. S. (2013). Forgiveness intervention for female South Korean adolescent aggressive victims. *Journal of Applied Developmental Psychology* 34: 268–76.

Pittman, C. T. (2008). The relationship between social influence and social justice behaviors. *Current Research in Social Psychology* 13: 243–54.

Riek, B. M., & Mania, E. W. (2012). The antecedents and consequences of interpersonal forgiveness: a meta-analytic review. *Personal Relationships* 19: 304–25.

Ripley, J. S., Leon, C., Worthington, E. L., Jr., Berry, J. W., Davis, E. B., Smith, A., Atkinson, A., & Sierra, T. (2014). Efficacy of religion accommodative strategic hope-focused theory applied to couples therapy. *Couple and Family Therapy: Research and Practice* 3(2): 83–98.

Rye, M. S., Fleri, A. M., Moore, C. D., Worthington, E. L., Jr., Wade, N. G., Sandage, S. J., & Cook, K. M. (2012). Evaluation of an intervention designed to help divorced parents forgive their ex-spouse. *Journal of Marriage, Divorce, and Remarriage* 53: 231–45.

Rye, M. S., Pargament, K. I., Ali, M. A., Beck, G. L., Dorff, E. N., Hallisey, C., Narayanan, V., & Williams, J. G. (2000).Religious perspectives on forgiveness. In McCullough, M. E., Pargament, K. I., & Thoresen C. E. (eds.), *Forgiveness: Theory, Research, and Practice*. New York: Guilford Press, pp.17–40.

Sapolsky, R. M. (2004). *Why Zebras Don't Get Ulcers*, 3rd ed. New York: Henry Holt.

Schönbach, P. (1990). *Account Episodes: The Management or Escalation of Conflict*. New York: Cambridge University Press.

Shnabel, N., Halabi, S., & Noor, M. (2013). Overcoming competitive victimhood and facilitating forgiveness through re-categorization into a common victim or perpetrator identity. *Journal of Experimental Social Psychology* 49(5): 867–77.

Staub, E., Pearlman, L. A., Gubin, A., & Hagengimana, A. (2005). Healing, reconciliation, forgiving, and the prevention of violence after genocide or mass killing: an intervention and its experimental evaluation in Rwanda. *Journal of Social and Clinical Psychology* 24(3): 297–334.

Tabak, B. A., & McCullough, M. E. (2011). Perceived transgressor agreeableness decreases cortisol response and increases forgiveness following recent interpersonal transgressions. *Biological Psychology* 87: 386–92.

Tabak, B. A., McCullough, M. E., Szeto, A., Mendez, A., & McCabe, P. M. (2011). Oxytocin indexes relational distress following interpersonal harms in women. *Psychoneuroendocrinology* 36: 115–22.

Toussaint, L., & Webb, J. R. (2005). Theoretical and empirical connections between forgiveness, mental health, and well-being. In Worthington, E. L. (ed.), *Handbook of Forgiveness*. New York: Brunner-Routledge, pp. 349–62.

Toussaint, L. L., Worthington, E. L., Jr., & Williams, D. R. (eds.). (2015) *Forgiveness and Health: Scientific Evidence and Theories Relating Forgiveness to Better Health*. New York: Springer.

van der Meer Sanchez, Z., & Nappo, S. A. (2008). Religious treatments for drug addiction: an exploratory study in Brazil. *Social Science & Medicine* 67 (4): 638–46.

Van Tongeren, D. R., Burnette, J. L., O'Boyle, E., Worthington, E. L., Jr., & Forsythe, D. (2014). A meta-analysis of inter-group forgiveness. *Journal of Positive Psychology* 9: 81–95.

Vermeulen-Smit, E., Ten Have, M., Van Laar, M., & De Graaf, R. (2015). Clustering of health risk behaviours and the relationship with mental disorders. *Journal of Affective Disorders* 171: 111–19.

Wade, N. G., Hoyt, W. T., Kidwell, J. E. M., & Worthington, E. L., Jr. (2014). Efficacy of psychotherapeutic interventions to promote forgiveness: a meta-analysis. *Journal of Consulting and Clinical Psychology* 82: 154–70.

Witvliet, C. V. O., DeYoung, N. J., Hofelich, A. J., & DeYoung, P. W. (2011). Compassionate reappraisal and emotion suppression as alternatives to offense-focused rumination: implications for forgiveness and psychophysiological well-being. *Journal of Positive Psychology* 6(4): 286–99.

Wood, B. T., Worthington, E. L., Jr., Exline, J. J., Yali, A. M., Aten, J. D., & McMinn, M. R. (2010). Development, refinement, and psychometric properties of the Attitudes toward God Scale (ATGS-9). *Psychology of Religion and Spirituality, 2*, 148–167.

Worthington, E. L., Jr. (ed.). (2005). *Handbook of Forgiveness*. New York: Brunner-Routledge.

Worthington, E. L., Jr. (2006). *Forgiveness and Reconciliation: Theory and Application*. New York: Brunner-Routledge.

Worthington, E. L., Jr., & Aten, J. D. (2010). Forgiveness and reconciliation in social reconstruction after trauma. In Mantz, E. (ed.), *Trauma Rehabilitation after War and Conflict*. New York: Springer, pp. 55–71.

Worthington, E. L., Jr., & Berry, J. W. (2004). Can society afford not to promote forgiveness and reconciliation? In Hampton, R. L., & Gullotta, T. P. (eds.), *Promoting Racial, Ethnic, and Religious Understanding and Reconciliation*. Washington, DC: Child Welfare League of America, pp. 159–92.

Worthington, E. L., Jr., Berry, J. W., Hook, J. N., Davis, D. E., Scherer, M., Griffin, B. J., Wade, N. G., Yarhouse, M., Ripley, J. S., Miller, A. J., Sharp, C. B., Canter, D. E., & Campana, K. L. (2015). Forgiveness-reconciliation and communication-conflict-resolution interventions versus rested controls in early married couples. *Journal of Counseling Psychology* 62(1): 14–27.

Worthington, E. L., Jr., Hunter, J. L., Sharp, C. B., Hook, J. N., Van Tongeren, D. R., Davis, D. E., Miller, A. J., Gingrich, F. C., Sandage, S. J., Lao, E., Bubod, L., & Monforte-Milton, M. M. (2010). A psychoeducational intervention to promote forgiveness in Christians in the Philippines. *Journal of Mental Health Counseling* 32(1): 82–103.

Worthington, E. L., Jr., Kulick, K., & Griffin, B. J. (2014). Public health and promoting forgiveness of self and other. Invited talk presented at Harvard School of Public Health, Cambridge, MA, April 16.

Worthington, E. L., Jr., Witvliet, C. V. O., Pietrini, P., & Miller, A. J. (2007). Forgiveness, health, and well-being: a review of evidence for emotional versus decisional forgiveness, dispositional forgivingness, and reduced unforgiveness. *Journal of Behavioral Medicine* 30: 291–302.

PART II

The Globalization of Prevention Science

Asia & Australia

23 South Korea's Efforts to Prevent Internet Addiction

Cheung-Moon Cho

South Korea is located in the northeast of Asia continent, with a population of 50.22 million people. South Korea's per capita gross national income (GNI) in 2013 was $25,920 (U.S.) (World Bank, 2015). Most of the people (91 percent) live in urban areas, and life expectancy is 81.9 years (males = 78.5, females = 85.1) (Statistics Korea, 2014). Many South Korean people are religious, as 50 percent belong to a religion; the most popular religion is Buddhism (44 percent), followed by Protestantism (41 percent), and Roman Catholicism (14 percent) (Korea Gallup, 2015). South Korea's education achievement is very high, as 70.9 percent of high school graduates entered college/university in 2014 (Korea Education Development Institute, 2014). South Korea is a very industrialized nation, with leading exports being petroleum products, semiconductors, cars, ships and liquid crystal devices. However, South Korea's strong economic development has more recently occurred during last decades after the Korea War (1950–1953); in 1970, the per capita GNI per capita was only $225 (U.S.), and the urbanization rate was also low, as 39.2 percent of the population lived in urban areas in 1960 (World Bank, 2015).

Current Status of Internet and Smart Phone Addiction in South Korea

Penetration of the Internet and smart phones is very high across the population of South Korea, as 83.6 percent were Internet users and 78.6 percent owned smart devices (including smart phones and smart pads) in 2014, according to a nationwide survey on 25,000 households and their 63,583 members (Ministry of Science, Information Communication Technology [ICT] and Future Planning, Korea Internet & Security Agency, 2014). In recent

Dr. Cho is currently working for the Korea Information Society Agency as an Executive Principal Researcher in charge of developing safe and healthy environments using information communication technology (ICT), such as prevention of Internet addiction and awareness of cyber humanity. He received his Ph.D. from University of Maryland (U.S.), majoring in sociology. He has also worked as a consultant with the Economic and Social Commission for Asia and the Pacific and the World Bank in the field of ICT for development. In addition to the preceding experiences, he has held the Vice Chairmanship of Telecommunication Development Advisory Group of International Telecommunication Union from 2002 to 2010.

Table 23.1 *Rates of Internet Use and Smart Device Ownership by Age in 2014*

Age (yrs)	6–19	20–29	30–39	40–49	50–59	60–69	Over 70
Internet use	99.7* (10–19)	99.9	99.8	97.5	86.1	50.6	14.1
Smart device ownership	81.6	99.8	99.0	96.1	82.7	26.4** (over 60)	

*This figure was based on age group of ten to nineteen years old.
**This figure was based on age group of over sixty years old.
Source: Ministry of Science, ICT and Future Planning, Korea Internet & Security Agency (2014).

years, smart media addiction has been getting more attention due to changing life and communication styles, resulting from a rapidly rising use of smart media, especially the smart phone (National Information Society Agency, 2011). Further, Internet use and smart device ownership rates among youths are almost 100 percent (see Table 23.1).

Internet addiction has appeared as one of the adverse effects in South Korea due to the country's advance into the information society with a wide diffusion of Internet use. Although a common definition of Internet addiction has not been agreed upon by scholars in the psychological and medical fields, Internet addiction is generally referred to as an infliction of hard-to-recover damages to people's physical, mental, and social functions that occur as a result of excessive use of an electronic network service. A more formal definition of Internet addiction is as follows: "due to a severe overuse of telecommunication services delivered over telecommunication network, users' physical and social function are damaged to the unrecoverable condition" (National Informatization Basic Act, article 3). Most people with Internet addictions tend to have withdrawal and tolerance symptoms such as extreme anxiety or depression, resulting in serious impediment in their daily life. So deeply hooked up with the cyber world, excessive Internet users show diverse forms of Internet addiction, such as game playing, chatting, and accessing pornography. For the purposes of this chapter, Internet use includes all kinds of online activities delivered by various types of electronic media, including personal computers and pads, smart phones, and other electronic devices.

About 7.0 percent of Internet users aged five to fifty-four years were the risk group for Internet addiction,[1] according to the 2013 National Survey on Internet addiction (released in March 2014 by Ministry of Science, ICT and Future Planning, and National Information Society Agency). While Internet addiction among the total number of Internet users has been reduced from 7.7 percent in 2011 to 7.2 percent in 2012 to 7.0 percent in 2013, teenage

1 The term "risk group of Internet addiction" rather than "Internet addict" is preferred, since there is no academically agreed-upon standardized tool to distinguish addicts from nonaddicts. Thus it is believed that the Korean tool for measuring Internet addiction is just to discern the "risk group of Internet addiction," not "Internet addicts."

Table 23.2 *Status of Internet Addiction in 2013*

Category	High Risk for Addiction (%)	Potential Risk for Addiction (%)	General Users (%)
Total sample (n = 17,500)	1.7	5.3	93.0
Children (5–9 yrs; n = 1,036)	0.8	5.6	93.6
Adolescents (10–19 yrs; n = 3,301)	2.8	8.9	88.3
Adults (20–54 yrs; n = 13,163)	1.5	4.4	94.1
20–29 yrs; n = 3,631	2.7	6.8	90.5
30–39 yrs; n = 4,244	1.4	4.2	94.4
40–49 yrs; n = 4,028	0.5	2.9	96.6
50–54 yrs; n = 1,260	0.8	3.0	96.2
Males (n = 9,225)	2.1	5.7	92.2
Females(n = 8,275)	1.1	5.0	93.9

*Definition of high-risk and potential risk-groups of Internet addiction will be provided in the section "Surveys and Research on the Prevention of Internet Addiction" in this chapter.
Source: Ministry of Science, ICT and Future Planning, National Information Society Agency (2014).

Internet addiction has increased from 10.4 percent in 2011 to 10.7 percent in 2012 to 11.7 percent in 2013, according to National Surveys on Internet Addiction (Ministry of Science, ICT and Future Planning, and National Information Society Agency, 2012, 2013, 2014). Internet addiction is highest in teens, and followed by adults in their twenties and thirties (see Table 23.2).

Meanwhile, smart phone addiction increases were found to be steeper than those of Internet addiction. About 11.8 percent of smart phone users aged ten to fifty-four years were a risk group of smart phone addiction, up 3.4 percent from 8.4 percent in 2011, when the smart phone addiction survey started. Teenage users were the highest risk group, as about 25.5 percent of South Korean adolescents (age ten to nineteen) were a risk group of smart phone addiction, compared to 8.9 percent of South Korean adults (see Table 23.3).

Gender differences were found for Internet addiction, showing that the percentage of females in the risk group (6.1 percent) is lower than that of the male group (7.8 percent). However, in the smart phone addiction group, the female high-risk group is slightly higher than the male high-risk group (1.4 percent versus 1.2 percent) (see Table 23.3). Comparison of smart phone addiction by gender and age also shows that female students in the elementary and high schools are more likely to be addicted than their male counterparts (see Table 23.4). Personal computer–based (PC) Internet addiction has been mainly caused by online games; however, much smart phone addiction is caused by chatting. Thus, female smart phone users may be more likely to be addicted than male users.

Table 23.3 *Status of Smart Phone Addiction in 2013*

Category	High Risk for Addiction (%)	Potential Risk for Addiction (%)	General Users (%)
Total (n=15,978)	1.3	10.5	88.2
Adolescents (10–19 yrs; n = 2,749)	2.4	23.1	74.5
Adults (20–54 yrs; n = 13,229)	1.0	7.9	91.1
20–29 yrs; n = 3,858)	2.0	13.0	85.0
30–39 yrs; n = 4,349)	1.0	7.2	91.8
40–49 yrs; n = 3,786)	0.3	4.7	95.0
50–54 yrs; n = 1,236)	0.3	4.7	95.0
Males (n = 8,495)	1.2	11.3	87.5
Females (n = 7,483)	1.4	9.8	88.8

Source: Ministry of Science, ICT and Future Planning, National Information Society Agency (2014).

Table 23.4 *Status of Smart Phone Addiction by Gender and Age in 2013*

Category		High Risk of Addiction (%)	Risk Group of Addiction (%)	General User (%)
Elementary (1–6 grade, n = 1,849)	Male	1.8	20.3	77.9
	Female	2.2	21.0	76.8
Middle (7–9 grade, n = 1,368)	Male	2.2	28.2	69.6
	Female	3.0	25.1	71.9
High (10–12 grade; n = 1,041)	Male	2.4	20.3	77.3
	Female	2.6	22.1	75.3
College(n = 1,034)	Male	2.3	18.0	79.7
	Female	1.6	13.2	85.2

Source: Ministry of Science, ICT and Future Planning, National Information Society Agency (2014).

South Korea is not the only Asian nation that is experiencing Internet addiction. For example, recently Taiwan banned children under the age of two from using electronic devices such as smart phones, Tablet PCs, and televisions. Parents who allow their young children to play with their devices face fines up to $1,500 (U.S.). The new law also states that parents must ensure that those under eighteen years old use electronic devices only for a "reasonable" length of time (*Daily Mail*, 2015). In addition, the International Society of Internet Addiction (ISIA) was established in 2012 for Asian regional cooperation in preventing Internet addiction. The countries of Hong Kong, Taiwan, Japan, Singapore, the Philippines, Malaysia, and South Korea participate in ISIA and in ISIA's annual conference.

South Korea's Efforts to Prevent and Reduce Internet and Smart Phone Addiction

South Korea's first government initiative to prevent Internet addiction was the establishment of the first Internet Addiction Prevention Center (IAPC) in 2002. Since then, the number of IAPCs has expanded to fifteen in order to provide nationwide services and provide one IAPC per each of seventeen metropolitan cities/provinces. In the early years, Internet addiction was handled only by the Ministry of Science, ICT and Future Planning (MSIP, formerly the Ministry of Information and Communication). However, social concerns about Internet addiction has increased due to several bad incidents, as described in the following examples: (a) middle school student in Gwangju killed his younger brother to mimic the online game that he had been playing; (b) Mr. Lee in Gyungnam Province died while he was playing Internet games for ninety hours; (c) frustrated, Mr. Joe jumped to his death after he was expelled from a certain online game community; (d) Mr. Kim, in his twenties, an online gamer, had his neck twisted to one side at a 70 degree angle; (e) a baby was choked to death while his parents were playing a game at a PC-bang café; and (f) Mr. Kim died suddenly while he was playing an online game for ten days. Due to these and other incidents, South Korean ministries such as the Ministry of Education, Ministry of Health and Welfare, and Ministry of Gender Equality and Family have joined the efforts to prevent Internet addiction. A Master Plan to Prevent and Treat Internet Addiction was first developed in 2010 jointly by all related ministries.

In June, 2013, eight ministries[2] and seventeen metropolitan cities/provinces jointly announced a Second Master Plan to Prevent and Treat Internet Addiction. The Plan identifies a full range of preventive, counseling, psychiatric, and aftercare assistances available to all age groups of children, adolescents, and adults. The Second Master Plan also paid special attention to new social media, where smart phones rather than PCs are becoming the main social media. Therefore, special features of the Second Master Plan included extension of preventive education and counseling service for children through adults. In addition, the plan promotes closer cooperation among ministers, local governments, and private sectors in policy development and service delivery.

Table 23.5 shows the South Korean policy shifts responding to the change of the electronic environment. In the early days, the main addiction causing agents were PC-based online games and adult material. Therefore, early policies targeted mainly youth, and addiction prevention services were delivered by the Internet Addiction Prevention Center. However, as the addiction expanded, the causing agents have widened to include online communities and chat rooms; the media has also moved from PCs to smart phones. Policies

2 The Ministry of Science, ICT and Future Planning; Ministry of Education; Ministry of Justice; Ministry of National Defense; Ministry of Culture Sports and Tourism; Ministry of Health and Welfare; Ministry of Gender Equality and Family; and the Korea Communications Commission.

Table 23.5 *Change of Policy Structure for the Prevention of Internet Addiction*

Years	2002–9	2010–12	2013–15
Policy framework	No governmentwide Master Plan	1st Master Plan (2010)	2nd Master Plan (2013)
Main addiction-causing agents	PC-based online games, adult material	PC-based online contents (e.g., chatting, communities)	Diversity of content and media including smart phones
Main services	Prevention education, public awareness campaign, and counseling	Prevention education, public awareness campaign, counseling, and medical treatment	Prevention education, public awareness campaign, counseling, medical treatment, and aftercare services
Main target groups	Adolescents	Adolescents, children	All age groups
Service delivering organization	IAPC	IAPC and Youth and Welfare Centers	Inclusion of community service organizations
Leading ministry	Ministry of Information and Communication (Currently Ministry of Science, ICT and Future Planning)	Participation of 7 related ministries	Close cooperation among all related ministries
Training of counselors	Retraining of existing counselors	Advancement of counselor training	Certification of Internet addiction counselors

Sources: Ministry of Public Administration and Security, etc. (2010); Ministry of Science, ICT and Future Planning, etc. (2013).

now cover all age groups, and Internet addiction is not handled only by one Internet Addiction Prevention Center and one ministry. Internet addiction has become a social issue requiring close cooperation among various ministries and community organizations.

Second Master Plan to Prevent and Treat Internet Addiction

The Second Master Plan identified six policy domains: Compulsory Prevention Training, Healing, Aid, Evaluation, Governance, and Environment.

- Compulsory Prevention Training means to oblige all social groups, including children, adolescents, and adults, to participate in Internet Addiction Prevention Training. This training is described later in this chapter.
- Healing is to provide customized professional counseling services fitted to the different populations of the risk group of Internet addiction.

- Aid means to strengthen the systematic harmonization of psychological and medical treatment of various institutes for the risk group of Internet addiction.
- Evaluation indicates a need for efforts to prevent reoccurrence of Internet addiction through careful follow-up services for those who have recovered from Internet addiction.
- Governance is intensive cooperation between central and local governments and private and international societies.
- Environment means to build a policy environment for supporting financial, social, and human assistance to prevent Internet addiction.

South Korea's Second Master Plan covers not only prevention of Internet addiction but also medical treatment of the high-risk group of Internet addiction; however, the purpose of this chapter is to show South Korea's policy on the prevention of Internet addiction. Therefore, the following sections will describe prevention-related activities such as preventive education, counseling services, training of internet addiction counselors, social campaign to prevent addiction, legal control of minor's access to online games, and surveys and research on the prevention of internet addiction.

Preventive Education

Considering the importance of education in preventing Internet addiction, preventive education has become compulsory by law. Article 30, item 8 of National Information Basic Act (revised May 2013) states that all kindergartens, elementary through high schools, universities, and public institutions must provide Internet addiction prevention training, and central and local governments shall support preventive training financially and administratively.

The goal of preventive education is to enhance public consciousness about the potential or actual risk of addiction and help Internet users be better able to cope with excessive desires to use the Internet and smart phones. In order to increase the effectiveness of preventive education, the curriculum is modified to the need of each age group.

Specialized counselors are sent to schools as lecturers giving a special (one-hour) class. An intensive (two-hour) education program has also been available for primary, middle, and high school students since 2013. Both one-hour and intensive classes are designed for different age groups, emphasizing student participation and discussion through class activities. In the course, each student uses his or her own workbook as a self-diagnosis tool and keeps a self-monitored record of Internet and smart phone use. Students may make a resolution to reduce Internet use, if they are found to be excessive users. Table 23.6 shows the number of students and adults who participated in preventive education since 2002.

Since 2014, the Addiction Prevention Play for preschool children and lower-grade primary school students has been performed in order to deliver the

Table 23.6 *Number of Participants in Preventive Education**

Category	2002–9	2010	2011	2012	2013	2014
Preschool		-	31,279	18,200	47,890	85,703
Teenager	1,795,752	645,981	954,425	621,621	970,696	941,018
Adult	136,540	33,753	90,363	93,001	105,363	76,288
Total	**1,932,292**	**679,734**	**1,076,067**	**732,822**	**1,123,949**	**1,103,009**

*Numbers include only participants in the programs offered by National Information Society Agency.
Source: National Information Society Agency (2015).

prevention message easily and effectively in a way that engages these children. In the program, child and students watch a play (for lower-grade primary students) or a puppet show (for preschool children) that tells stories about animal engagement in Internet addiction or Internet addiction in familiar daily life. After watching the play, the teacher talks about the danger of Internet addiction and how to prevent Internet addiction. Since 2014, the play has been performed forty-five times and more than ten thousand children have watched the play. This program is effective in making children easily understand the risk of Internet addiction without feeling uncomfortable.

Since 2014, twenty-three middle and high schools have been designated as a Smart Media Clean School. These schools have received financial and technical assistance to enact school activities/campaigns for promoting sound habits using the Internet and smart media and for preventing Internet addiction by cooperating with parents, teachers, and experts.

In order to facilitate compulsory preventive Internet addiction education, school curricula have been modified to include components of Internet addiction prevention education. The components have included five e-learning courses (primary, middle, high school, and university students and adults) to help schools, universities, and public/community institutions provide prevention training to students and adults.

Another tool that was developed for preventive education is a smart media addiction guidebook, which was distributed to all schools from kindergarten through high school. The guidebook consists of four weekly sections of strategy/guides to prevent smart media addiction. The first week guide is designed to motivate readers to control their use of smart media and to make a plan. The second week guide is to help students put their plan into action and make a self-assessment and to give them feedback. The third week guide is designed to help students make a habit of controlling their smart media use. The fourth week guide consists of how to keep sound habits for smart media use. If readers use this guidebook well, they will be able to prevent smart media addiction and acquire a healthy habit of using smart media. Parental guidance is necessary for kindergarteners and first- and second-grade students in the primary schools to use the guidebook. Other students can use it by themselves.

Examples of guidebook pages can found at www.iapc.or.kr/english/preventivediscipline/smartmediauserguidebook.do And a diversity of educational materials, such as preventive guide books, flash animation, videos, standard teaching books, and counseling tools, has been developed and posted to be available at the website (www.iapc.or.kr).

Counseling Services

Counseling services to prevent and treat Internet addiction have been provided since 2002. Currently, in order to provide nationwide services, the South Korean government operates fifteen Internet Addiction Prevention Centers (IAPCs) at fourteen metropolitan cities/provinces nationwide. The centers are equipped with individual and group counseling rooms and office space. Each center employs three fulltime counselors

The IAPC provides counseling services that are delivered through a diversity of channels, including home visits, online counseling services at www.iapc.or.kr, and a nationwide call-in service center. Table 23.7 summarizes the numbers who have used IAPC counseling services since 2002.

To provide nationwide services, the IAPC also offers counseling services in collaboration with forty-eight related centers, such as the Healthy Family Support Centers and Youth Support Centers. In addition, other institutes such as the Youth Counseling and Welfare Centers (Ministry of Gender Equality and Equity), We Centers for students not performing well in school (Office of Education), and Mental Health Promotion Centers (Ministry of Health and Welfare) provide Internet addiction counseling services throughout South Korea. The yearly counseling services provided by these centers reaches more than 800 persons by Youth Counseling and Welfare Centers, approximately 350,000 persons by We Centers, and 3,000 persons by Mental Health Promotion Centers.

Home visit counseling services merit special mention as they provide free counseling services to families who are not able to visit the centers. The program is particularly effective for the risk group of Internet addiction from marginal social groups such as low-income or interracial families and for children living with a single parent or grandparents. After receiving a request for a home visit, the counselor visits the applicant's home at a mutually agreeable time and date. The service consists of six sessions of home visits

Table 23.7 *Number of IAPC Counseling Services by Service Type*

Category	2002–9	2010	2011	2012	2013	2014
Face-to-face (home visit)	79,205	15,037	10,522 (6,089)	20,701 (10,595)	24,623 (19,519)	22,041 (15,891)
Online	8,226	1,916	569	866	489	257
Telephone	24,280	9,569	7,915	16,138	11,512	11,853
Total	**111,711**	**26,522**	**19,006**	**37,705**	**36,624**	**34,151**

Source: National Information Society Agency (2015).

and two sessions of phone counseling. Each home visit service lasts ninety minutes or less. All the sessions are free of charge. After completing the home visit counseling sessions, applicants can continue to receive counseling by visiting the IAPC if needed.

Training of Internet Addiction Counselors

A training program to produce specialized counselors for Internet addiction has started in 2002. The training program has been customized for the diversity of specialized counselors, such as teachers and home visiting counselors. The training teaches not only technical skills for counseling practice but counseling theory so that they can practice as a specialized counselor for Internet addiction clients.

Training for current counselors is also provided. This training is designed to offer specialized skills for Internet addiction counseling for counselors new to Internet addiction counseling. Most current counselors have not received any training related to Internet addiction during their programs of study to become a counselor. Therefore, this training is necessary to those who want to provide Internet addiction counseling services. Eligible participants of the training program for current counselors are those who have studied at least three semesters in a graduate program of counseling, hold a counseling license, and have more than five years of counseling experience. The training covers theory and practice related to Internet addiction over five days for forty hours.

A follow-up continuing education program for certified counselors for Internet addiction is also provided. The program helps counselors to update their knowledge and skills with new trends and to improve their counseling techniques during the course. Eligible participants of this program are those who have completed the forty hours of intensive training for Internet addiction counseling. The training length is thirteen hours over two days.

A specialized training course is also provided for current counselors who want to provide home visit counseling. Target recipients for this course are current counselors with at least three years of counseling experience and who have completed the Internet addiction certified counselor training course. The training length is eight hours over one day.

Training for school teachers who want to become Internet addiction counselors is also provided. The training program is available for current school teachers so that they can also practice as school counselors for preventing and reducing Internet addiction of their students. This training is provided in both of offline and online modalities. The offline course training length is thirty hours (over five days) and the online course is composed of thirty lectures. Both courses give teachers two credits, which count as continuing education credits required for teachers.

Table 23.8 summarizes the number of participants who have participated in training for Internet addiction counselor since 2002.

Table 23.8 *Participants of Training for Internet Addiction Counselor*

Category		2002–9	2010	2011	2012	2013	2014
Counselor	General counselor	1,179	273	831	1,195	688	923
	Home visit counselor	-	-	129	73	99	-
Teacher	Offline	659	120	457	227	175	311
	Online	-	-	-	1,363	1,494	2,561
Continuing education		-	52	263	235	890	377
Total		**1,838**	**445**	**1,680**	**3,093**	**3,346**	**4,172**

Source: National Information Society Agency (2015).

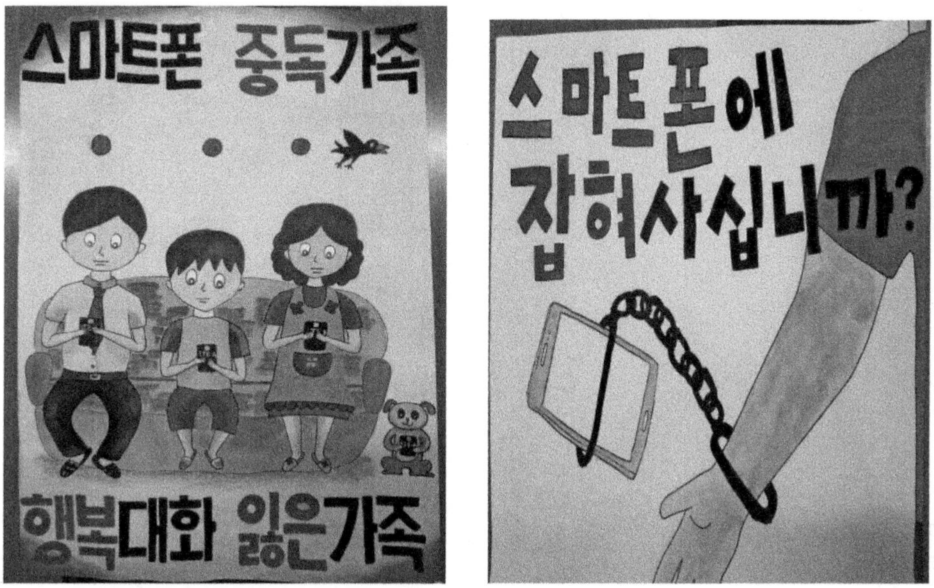
스마트폰 중독가족
행복대화 잃은가족
스마트폰에
잡혀사십니까?

Figure 23.1. *Best poster in the Internet Addiction Prevention Poster Competition.*

Social Campaign to Prevent Internet Addiction

The Smart Break Campaign for preventing Internet addiction has been initiated jointly by all related entities such as the South Korean central and local governments, the Office of Education, mass media, telecom operators, and subway operators. In subways, poster or video clips that deliver a message to ask citizens to use the Internet or smart phone in an appropriate manner are posted or shown. To promote awareness of the risk of Internet addiction among students, a competition for writing the best essay or poster was initiated. Figure 23.1 shows award-winning posters (*Money Today*, 2015). The left figure suggests that all family members are using smart phones all the time, and therefore they do not talk and lose happiness as a result of less face-to-face communication. The right figure suggests that persons have become captive and a slave to the smart phone.

Another special luminous poster was developed to encourage people not to use smart phones in bed before sleeping. This poster shows the shape of a brain; the right side of the brain is not shown in daylight under the sunshine, but it grows in the dark. It could be hung from the ceiling or on a wall. Therefore, when turning off the light before sleeping, the right side of the poster grows with the wording, "it is the time to use the right side of brain." The meaning of this message is to end the use of smart phones in bed before sleeping (*Joongang Daily*, 2015).

Another poster shows a smart phone–shaped transparent plastic poster with the phrase "WiFi-Free," which could be hung in a cafe. Instead of typical sign of "Free-WiFi," a cafe or restaurant can hang a "WiFi-Free" poster. This poster was designed to encourage cafe and restaurant clients to talk with each other or read a book instead of using smart phones (*Joongang Daily*, 2015).

Technical tools for the prevention of Internet addiction are also available to the public. Mobile apps to monitor and control the hours and contents using the Internet were developed by telecom operators and distributed to users. Most applications are installed in smart phones and used for self-control purposes; some applications can be installed in both parents' and children's smart phones, then parents can monitor children's use of the smart phone upon the consent of the child. Parents' monitoring children's smart phone use is not legally binding, therefore it is possible only when children accept parents' request to monitor. Some apps are free to use, but some are pay-based service. In order to promote the use of these apps, several outreach programs exist to make citizens aware of the benefits of these apps.

In South Korea, schools can prohibit the use of smart phones in the classroom by school regulation. One survey showed that 65 percent of schools in South Korea prohibit the use of smart phones in the classroom. To enforce this regulation, teachers collect students' smart phones before class and return them after class. Prohibition rate is the highest in middle schools, as 91 percent of middle schools prohibit the use of smart phones in the classroom; the rate in elementary schools is only 46 percent (see Table 23.9).

In order for Internet service providers to participate in efforts to prevent Internet addiction, the South Korean government has initiated an incentive program giving a certificate to Internet service providers who are active in preventing Internet addiction. The criteria to issue the certificate are abiding

Table 23.9 *Prohibition of Smart Phone in the Classroom by School Grade*

	Prohibited	Not Prohibited
Elementary School	532 (46%)	633 (54%)
Middle School	801 (91%)	81 (9%)
High School	728 (66%)	372 (34%)
Total	**2,061 (65%)**	**1,086 (35%)**

Source: Korean Federation of Teachers' Association (2013).

by laws for the prevention of Internet addiction, providing appropriate service contents, encouraging clients to assess their habit to use Internet through tools to assess Internet addiction, and advertising IAPCs and counseling services to consumers.

Legal Control of Minors' Access to Online Gaming

Strong legal enforcement has been enacted in South Korea so that that minors under sixteen years old are not allowed to access online games from midnight to 6 A.M., and parents can monitor and block their children's access (if the child is under eighteen years old) to online games by making a request to service providers. Game service providers have to fulfill various measures to prevent the excessive use of Internet games, such as confirmation of real name; age of user; consent of parents to access games when children are under eighteen years old; placement of warning notices, such as showing dangers of overuse of online games; indication of the passage of time spent gaming; and so on. These regulations are detailed in South Korea's Juvenile Protection Act and Game Industry Promotion Act.

Blocking of minors' online games at midnight has led to a hot debate about the validity and effectiveness of this measure and the legal rights of minors who use the Internet. Dissidents of this measure assert that minors can avoid this enforcement by using another person's ID, and the law infringes on minors' rights to decide about their usage of online games, and also infringes on parental rights to guide their children's usage of online games. Therefore, the Ministry of Gender Equality and Family, which initiated the legal measure, is considering a revision of the Juvenile Protection Act to allow parents to permit their children to access online games after midnight if they desire.

Surveys and Research on the Prevention of Internet Addiction

Since 2004, an annual survey has been conducted to measure the status of Internet addiction in South Korea. In the early days, sample size was small at 2,000 persons and it surveyed people from nine to thirty-nine years old. However, in 2013 the sample size was enlarged to 17,500 persons and it surveyed people from five to fifty-four years old. The measurement tool for Internet addiction was developed by the Ministry of Science, ICT and Future Planning and the National Information Society Agency with the following stages. The first stage is to identify symptoms associated with Internet addiction. The four symptoms of Internet addiction, identified by experts, are withdrawal symptoms, tolerance to addiction, orientation to the cyber world, and disturbances in daily life. The second stage is to develop a survey to measure the four symptoms; fifteen questions were developed to measure the symptoms. The third stage is to set criteria to distinguish the risk group of addiction from the nonrisk group. Expert opinion and statistical distributions were used to identify people as the risk group for addiction. The measure also distinguishes between the high-risk and potential-risk groups among the addiction group.

Three different sets of questionnaires to measure Internet addiction were developed for children, adolescents, and adults. Preschool children cannot fill out questionnaires by themselves, thus a third-party observation tool was developed to be used by parents or counselors to measure the children's level of Internet addiction. Recently, smart phones have becoming a dominant source for addiction, thus two sets of questionnaires to measure smart phone addiction for adolescents and adults also have been developed. See Appendices 1 and 2 for examples of the Self-Rating Internet and Smart Phone Addiction Scales for Adolescents.

Characteristics of the High-Risk Group of Addiction

Those in this group show a serious disorder suffering withdrawal symptoms and disturbance in their daily life due to the overuse of the Internet. Most of their personal relations are based on cyberspace and they are more comfortable with meetings online than offline. Most of them know they are addicted to the Internet and have difficulties in studying and other activities that require concentration. In addition, it is common that they are anxious or depressed. They also tend to act impulsively and be aggressive. Socially, many of them have problems in personal relations and feel lonely. These observations were gathered from the self-rating scales.

Characteristics of the Potential-Risk Group for Addiction

Although having lower levels of addiction than those in the high-risk group, the potential-risk group tends to have disorders in their daily life. Their hours on the Internet have increased, and they tend to have an obsession about the Internet. Some of them might have difficulties studying and show mental instability, yet they feel that they have no problems. However, most of them are not good at planning things, have self-control problems, and tend to have low confidence. These observations were also gathered from the self-rating scales.

Other Research

It has been widely acknowledged that Internet addiction is related to various factors such as the individual's intrinsic psychological dysfunction or social maladaptation, excessive exposure to addiction-leading content, and lack of proper guidance from parents and the larger community on youth Internet use habits. However, research has not shown causalities between sociopsychological problems and Internet addiction, since most of studies show coexistence between Internet addiction and various factors without conducting causality investigations through longitudinal surveys or experimental studies.

Lee (2013) reviewed 145 Internet addiction articles published from 2005 to 2013 in South Korea in order to identify factors that are associated with Internet addiction. The study grouped the factors into five categories: psychological, family and school, social interaction, demographic, and habit or mode of Internet use. Among psychological factors, self-esteem, self-competency, depression, anxiety, social stress, lack of social control, compulsivity, aggressiveness, attachment anxiety, narcissism, Attention Deficit and Hyperactivity Disorder (ADHD), and lack of achievement motivation were related to Internet addiction. Thus, people are more likely than others to be addicted if they suffer from lower self-esteem and self-competency; higher depression, anxiety, and social stress; loss of social control; higher compulsivity and aggression; higher attachment anxiety and narcissism; higher ADHD; and lack of achievement motivation. These results imply that the risk group of Internet addiction may also suffer psychological problems caused by social maladaptation.

Lee (2013) also found that in terms of family factors, Internet addiction was related to lack of supportive parental discipline or excessive use of physical discipline or control, amount/quality or openness of interaction with parents, level of family cohesion or affectionate environment in family, conflict between parents, and lack of emotional attachment with parents. School factors related to being less likely to be addicted to the Internet included a satisfied school life, a supportive relationship with teachers, and good school achievement. Interpersonal relationship factors related to Internet addiction included lack of proper interpersonal communication skills, lack of supportive peer relationships, and being excessively oriented to the cyber world. Sociodemographic factors such as gender and deviant behaviours such as smoking or drug usage were also found to be related to Internet addiction. Delinquent youths and males and adolescents who smoke or abuse drugs are more likely to be addicted. However, smart phone addiction is more salient among female than male youth. In terms of the habit or mode of Internet use, hours and frequency, purpose, and place (e.g., a cyber café) when not monitored by parents were found to be related to addiction. Persons who use the Internet longer and more frequently, with the purpose of fun or gaming and in a place not controlled by parents, are more likely to be addicted than others.

An issue that has been addressed through survey research is the question of responsibility for the prevention of Internet addiction. Responsibility may vary depending upon the characteristics or nature of each addict. Survey results show that the most important factor for the prevention of Internet addiction is the addict (66.2 percent), followed by the family (13.0 percent), school (8.6 percent), corporation (5.6 percent), and government (2.3 percent). South Korean society is a strong family- and collectivistic-oriented culture compared to Western individually oriented nations, thus family is the second most important factor for the prevention of Internet addiction. Table 23.10 summarizes this survey conducted in 2014.

In a qualitative study, Cho (2014) interviewed Internet addiction counselors in order to reveal how the counselors perceived the causes and prevention of

Table 23.10 *Importance of Each Factor for the Prevention of Internet Addiction*

Category	Addict Oneself	Family	School	Corporation (Service Provider)	Government	Medical Entity	Other Public, Religious, Civic Organization
%	66.2	13.0	8.6	5.6	2.3	1.6	2.6

Source: Ministry of Science, ICT and Future Planning, and National Information Society Agency (2014).

Table 23.11 *Perceived Causes of Internet Addiction by Gender and Age*

Gender & Age \ Perceived Cause*	Intrinsic Psychological Traits	Negative Emotional Sentiment	Social Maladaptation	Addiction-Causing Content
Female adolescents	15.75	32.5	35.75	15.5
Male adolescents	21.25	22.75	35	20.5
Female adults	16.75	34	35	14.25
Male adults	19.75	26.5	33.25	20

*Counselors (n = 20) were asked to judge the relative importance of each perceived cause by assigning points to each cause, based on a point total of 100.

Internet addiction. A total of twenty Internet counselors were interviewed, and their average counseling experience was 2.5 years. Counselors were asked the question, "Reflecting on your counseling experiences, what are the most important causes of Internet addiction?" The responses were grouped into four categories: the addict's intrinsic psychological traits (e.g., sensation seeking, excessive reward dependence, impulsivity), negative emotional sentiment (e.g., depression, anxiety, low self-esteem), social maladaptation, and excessive exposure to addiction-causing contents (e.g., online games, adult material, chatting). Counselors were also asked to respond to the question across four types of risk groups of Internet addiction: female and male adolescents and female and male adults. Adolescents (not graduated from high school) were distinguished from adults (graduated from high school).

Table 23.11 shows that the counselors believe that Internet addiction is more likely to be caused by sociopsychological dysfunction led by social maladaptation rather than intrinsic biological or psychological traits or by addiction-causing Internet content. Gender differences were also perceived by the counselors, as males are more likely addicted by addiction-causing content, and females are more likely to be addicted by negative psychological sentiments such as depression, anxiety, and low self-esteem.

Table 23.12 *Perceived Prevention of Internet Addiction by Gender and Age*

Gender & Age \ Perceived Prevention*	Efforts of the Individual with Addiction	Support of Family	Support of School/ Organization	Control by Legal Authority
Female adolescents	33	36.75	18.25	11.25
Male adolescents	34.75	35.5	18	12.75
Female adult	44.5	29.75	15	11.25
Male adult	45	28	15.25	12.25

*Counselors (n=20) were asked to judge the relative importance of each perceived cause by assigning points to each cause, based on a point total of 100.

During the same interviews with addiction counselors, counselors were asked: "Reflecting on your counseling experiences, which is the most important for the prevention of Internet addiction?" Counselor responses were grouped into four categories: efforts of the individual with addiction, support of the family, support of the school/organization, and control by legal authorities. Table 23.12 shows that Internet addiction counselors believe that efforts of the addict himself or herself and support of the family are more important than the efforts of the school/organization and legal authorities in preventing Internet addiction. Some difference was found between adolescent and adult groups of Internet addiction regarding the roles of the individual with addiction and family for the prevention of Internet addiction. The role of the individual with addiction was perceived to be more important in the case of adults; however, the individual and family are equally important among adolescents.

Summary and Conclusions

Characteristics and Challenges of South Korea's Policy

The Internet and smart phones are widely used in South Korea across all age groups. While electronic devices provide many benefits, the dark side of Internet use, Internet addiction, has becoming a major social issue in South Korea. Annual surveys show that the overall Internet addiction rate in 2013 was 7.0 percent for all ages, and 11.7 percent for adolescents (Ministry of Science, ICT and Future Planning, and National Information Society Agency, 2014). The smart phone addiction rate is higher across all ages at 11.8 percent, and much higher for adolescents at 25.5 percent (Ministry of Science, ICT and Future Planning, and National Information Society Agency, 2014). Therefore, South Korea has implemented a Master Plan to Prevent Internet Addiction. The plan includes many components, such as IAPCs, prevention education, and counseling services, training for Internet addiction counselors, Internet addiction public prevention campaigns, legal controls on minors' access to online games, and surveys and research on the prevention of Internet addictions.

In South Korea, most of the activities are initiated by the government. The South Korean government is supporting public and private organizations financially and technically in order for them to engage in the prevention of Internet addiction. The government's strong involvement with preventing Internet addiction is also exemplified by banning minors' use of online games during the night. In addition, Parliament has also tried to pass the law called "Act to Prevent, Manage and Treat Addiction." The main feature of this proposed Act is to manage various addictions such as alcohol, drug, gambling, and online game addictions with one organization, called the National Addiction Management Committee. The Act would establish a nationwide Addiction Management Center to treat all addictions in one place. This proposed Act triggered a major debate concerning the necessity and effectiveness of treating different types of addictions in one place, as the effectiveness of this approach may depend on the similarity or differences of types of addictions. Table 23.13 shows that most people with Internet addiction are under thirty years old; however, most of the others with addictions are over thirty years old. Furthermore, Internet activity is not a prohibited or illegal activity as are drugs and gambling. Therefore, it seems appropriate to treat Internet addiction separately rather than to treat all those with different addictions in one place. The Act is still being debated in Parliament at the writing of this chapter.

Challenges faced by the South Korean government is to keep a balance between promotion of the ICT industry, especially the online game industry, and the protection of game users to prevent Internet addiction. The Ministry of Culture, Sports, and Tourism, which is in charge of the development of the

Table 23.13 *Percentage of Addictions by Age in South Korea*

Age (yrs)	5–9	10–19	20–29	30–39	40–49	50–59	60–69	Over 70	Unknown
Internet addiction	5.4	31.7	28.3	19.5	11.2	3.9			
Heavy drinkers			17.5	22.1	22.7	16.5	13.2	8.0	
Illegal drug criminals		0.6	10.3	25.6	36.2	18.8	6.6 (over 60)		1.8
Gambling addictions		0.4	22.0	38.1	19.4	13.9	6.2 (over 60)		

Sources: Alcohol Project Supporting Committee. (2011); Ministry of Science, ICT and Future Planning, National Information Society Agency (2014); National Gambling Control Commission (2013); Prosecution Service (2013).

online game industry, does not want to hurt the game industry while preventing game addiction; however, the Ministry of Gender Equality and Family, in charge of the protection of adolescents, wants to keep strong policy measures to protect adolescents from addiction. One measure against addiction is a proposal by members of Parliament for an Addiction Prevention Fund (1 percent of revenue of game providers) to be used for the operation of Internet Addiction Treatment Centers and to help fund the various projects for the prevention and treatment of Internet addiction. However, this proposal has not been passed at the time of writing this chapter due to objections of the game industry.

Another challenge in South Korea is to motivate all related stakeholders to participate in efforts to prevent Internet addiction. Due to the government-driven initiatives, the participation of private sectors such as civil society and service providers is relatively rare. In order to stimulate service providers' participation, an Internet Addiction Prevention Certificate was introduced to be awarded to good service providers who are active in the prevention of Internet addiction. However, awareness and recognition of this certificate are still low, thus service providers are not eager to obtain it. Therefore, South Korea is still encountering challenges to promote the civic sector's participation in Internet addiction prevention activities. Internet addiction cannot be overcome by the efforts of government alone, since the prevention of Internet addiction requires the close cooperation among family, school, community, workplace, and online content providers. Thus, through the success of all prevention efforts initiated by the government such as preventive training, counseling, and operating the IAPCs, the government can play more of a coordination role by supporting the relevant stakeholders rather than actually carrying out the Internet addiction prevention activities by itself.

Appendix 1

Self-Rating Internet Addiction Scale for Adolescents

No.	Items	Strongly Disagree	Disagree	Agree	Strongly Agree
1	I feel my health get worse than before because of the use of the Internet.				
2	I get recognized more while online than offline.				
3	My life is boring and not fun without the Internet.				
4	After I'm done using the Internet, I want to be with the Internet again.				
5	I have a headache because I use the Internet too much.				
6	I understand those I meet on the Internet better than those I meet in real life.				
7	If I cannot use the Internet, I get nervous and anxious.				
8	I tried to reduce the time I spend on the Internet but failed.				
9	I failed to fulfill things I planned to do because of the Internet.				
10	I'm not nervous even though I cannot use the Internet.				
11	I always think that I should cut back the time I spend on the Internet.				
12	I tried to lie about the hours I spend on the Internet.				
13	When I'm not using the Internet, I don't think about the Internet.				
14	People around me point out that I use the Internet too much.				
15	I spend more money because of the Internet.				

The scale consists of four factors: Disturbance of daily life (1, 5, 9, 12, 15), cyberspace-oriented (2, 6), withdrawal symptom (3, 7, 10, 13), tolerance (4, 8, 11, 14).

Appendix 2

Self-Rating Smart Phone Addiction Scale for Adolescents

No.	Items	Strongly Disagree	Disagree	Agree	Strongly Agree
1	My school grades dropped due to excessive smart phone use.				
2	Using a smart phone is more enjoyable than spending time with family or friends.				
3	I cannot imagine my life without a smart phone.				
4	I tried to reduce the time I spend on a smart phone but failed.				
5	I have a hard time doing what I have planned (study, do homework, or go to after-school classes) due to using smart phone				
6	When I cannot use a smart phone, I feel like I have lost the entire world.				
7	I get anxious and nervous without a smart phone.				
8	I can control my smart phone usage time.				
9	People frequently comment on my excessive smart phone use.				
10	I am not anxious without a smart phone.				
11	Even when I know I should stop, I continue to use my smart phone.				
12	Family or friends complain that I use my smart phone too much.				
13	My smart phone does not distract me from studying.				
14	I panic when I cannot use my smart phone.				
15	Spending a lot of time on a smart phone has become my habit.				

The scale consists of four factors: disturbance of daily life (1, 5, 9, 12, 13), cyberspace-oriented (2, 6), withdrawal symptom (3, 7, 10, 14), tolerance (4, 8, 11, 1).

References

Alcohol Project Supporting Committee (2011). *Whitepaper on Alcohol Statistics.* Goyang: Alcohol Project Supporting Committee.

Cho, Cheung Moon (2014). Interview of Internet addiction counselor on cause and prevention of Internet addiction. (Unpublished article).

Daily Mail (2015). Does YOUR toddler play on an iPad? Taiwan makes it ILLEGAL for parents to let children under two use electronic gadgets ... and under-18s must limit use to "reasonable" lengths. January 1. www.dailymail.co.uk/news/article-2929530/Does-toddler-play-iPad-Taiwan-makes-ILLEGAL-parents-let-children-two-use-electronic-gadgets-18s-limit-use-reasonable-lengths.html

Joongang Sunday (2015). Game OFF, Right Brain ON, Illuminating poster: more effective than coercive banning of online game. January 11. http://sunday.joins.com/archives/8278.

Korea Education Development Institute (2014). *Analysis of Education Statistics.* Seoul: Korea Education Development Institute.

Korea Gallup (2015). *Religion and Religious Rituals of Koreans.* Seoul: Korea Gallup.

Korean Federation of Teachers' Association (2013). *Survey on Management of Smart-phone Use in Classroom.* Seoul: Korean Federation of Teachers' Association.

Lee, Soo Sang (2013). *Review of Internet Addiction-Related Articles.* Seoul: National Information Society Agency.

Ministry of Public Administration and Security, etc. (2010). *1st Master Plan to Prevent and Treat Internet Addiction.* Seoul: Ministry of Public Administration and Security, etc.

Ministry of Science, ICT and Future Planning, etc. (2013). *2nd Master Plan to Prevent and Treat Internet Addiction.* Seoul: Ministry of Science, ICT and Future Planning, etc.

Ministry of Science, ICT and Future Planning, Korea Internet & Security Agency (2014). *2014 National Survey on Internet Use.* Seoul: Korea Internet & Security Agency.

Ministry of Science, ICT and Future Planning, National Information Society Agency (2012). *2011 Annual Survey on Internet Addiction.* Seoul: National Information Society Agency.

Ministry of Science, ICT and Future Planning, National Information Society Agency (2013). *2012 Annual Survey on Internet Addiction.* Seoul: National Information Society Agency.

Ministry of Science, ICT and Future Planning, National Information Society Agency (2014). *2013 Annual Survey on Internet Addiction.* Seoul: National Information Society Agency.

Money Today. (2015). U Clean campaign. uclean.mt.co.kr/together/ucWorksView.html?cnt=10&part1=post&part2=ele&part3=4;uclean.mt.co.kr/together/ucWorksView.html?cnt=10&part1=post&part2=mid&part3=2

National Gambling Control Commission (2013). *Statistics on Gambling Industry.* Seoul: National Gambling Control Commission.

National Information Society Agency (2011). *Development of Smartphone Addiction Measuring Tool.* Seoul: National Information Society Agency.

National Information Society Agency (2014). *Smart Off Campaign Plan.* Seoul: National Information Society Agency.

National Information Society Agency (2014). *2014 Action Plan to Prevent and Treat Internet Addiction*. Seoul: National Information Society Agency.

National Information Society Agency (2015). *Report of 2014 Activities to Prevent and Treat Internet Addiction*. Seoul: National Information Society Agency.

National Information Society Agency (2015). *2014 Activity Report of Internet Addiction Prevention Center*. Seoul: National Information Society Agency.

Prosecution Service (2013). *Whitepaper on the Illegal Drug Crime*. Seoul: Prosecution Service.

Statistics Korea (2014). *2013 Life Table*. Seoul: Statistical Korea.

World Bank. (2015). *World Development Indictors*. Washington, DC: World Bank. data.worldbank.org/country/korea-republic

24 Implementation of an Early Childhood Prevention Program from a Health Care to Community-Based Setting in Singapore

Lessons from "Mission: I'm Possible"

Wan Har Chong[1], Hui Nee Tang[2], Patricia A. L. Koh,[3] & Sylvia H. T. Choo[4]

In countries throughout the developed world, increasing proportions of children and young people have been shown to display various patterns of health and developmental problems. These include a range of learning and behavior problems such as attention deficit disorder, hyperactivity and dyslexia, aggression and antisocial behavior (Gettinger, Ball, Mulford, & Hoffman, 2010). Additionally, these problems associated with development appear to be occurring at younger ages and with more severity and complexity (Moore, 2006). Some may begin subtly. Poor developmental trajectories of very young children have been commonly associated with health and social problems in later life (Shonkoff & Bales, 2011). In Singapore, the Child Development Program under the Ministry of Health has observed about a twofold increase of new referrals from 2004 to 2011 (SingHealth, 2011). Although this may not be indicative of the prevalence rate, the increased number could be suggestive of the interplay of a number of factors such as better community and parental awareness and community resource availability.

From a health care perspective, primary prevention is crucial to address these problems early. With changing patterns of health and illness, however, health care interventions in Singapore can no longer center on major causes of child and adolescent morbidity and mortality of diseases and need to move beyond a predominantly medical perspective (Ho, 2009; Lantos & Ward, 2013). There is a need to focus on interventions related to potentially preventable behaviors that are socially situated (such as within the family). One way of providing a more encompassing service delivery model is to increase service accessibility to

1 National Institute of Education, Nanyang Technological University, Singapore.
2 Department of Child Development, KK Women's and Children's Hospital, Singapore.
3 Department of Child Development, KK Women's and Children's Hospital, Singapore.
4 Department of Child Development, KK Women's and Children's Hospital, Singapore.

more specialized populations that are in need of specific preventive services. This can be achieved by engaging the community at sites where such problems are most likely to be presented, thus making these easier to detect. In this chapter, we present an example of an innovative service delivery model in Singapore to meet the learning needs of young children who are potentially at risk in their growth and development.

The chapter begins with introducing the "Mission: I'm Possible" (MIP) project, which strives to facilitate young children's poor attendance of therapeutic services from a major health care center. We provide an overview of the Singapore context to place the problem in perspective, outline the development of the project, and delineate factors that relate to its implementation. We also highlight critical components of the program that differ from other early intervention programs and the challenges posed during its implementation. We reason that this discussion of implementation factors provides important learning points in prevention science, particularly in the field of early childhood intervention.

Understanding the Development of MIP in the Singapore Context

Singapore is an island city-state situated at the southern tip of the Malay Peninsula. About 700 square kilometer in size, it has a population of just over 5 million people of which about 18 percent are below the age of fourteen years. Its diverse multiracial make-up consists of three major ethnic groups: ethnic Chinese, who comprise about 77 percent; Malays 14 percent; Indians 7.6 percent; and other ethnic groups 1.4 percent. A highly urbanized country, its major economic activities are diversified to include international banking and finance, as well as capital-intensive, high-wage, and high-technology activities that provide the infrastructures for manufacturing, financial, and communications facilities for multinational firms. Singapore has very limited natural resources except for its people. The economy is, therefore, highly sensitive and dependent on the world economic environment. Education is seen as a critical pathway through which the nation may maximize its advantage in the global economy.

Educators in Singapore, a small nation with a colonial past, tend to look west for successful tested models and ideas from which to adapt many of its educational initiatives and child psychological services. Singapore's education system provides a strong academic-focused curriculum. Nevertheless, as is the case with many developed nations in the West and East, it has increasingly recognize that an education based on a traditional rationalist, subject-based curriculum with expected academic standards to be achieved is no longer adequate to give school children the added advantage in today's technological age (Chong & Lee, 2014). To prepare children and young people for successful learning and living in the twenty-first century, the Singapore education system has therefore developed a diversified and flexible program for students with different interests and ways of learning. However, even with this diversification in educational structure, there will remain children who continue to experience difficulties in school, some as early as in the preschool years. Early interventions aimed at addressing these difficulties would be pertinent if these young ones are to have a good head start.

In Singapore, preschool education is not compulsory and preschool centers are largely operated by private and voluntary sectors. The government maintains both an administrative and regulatory role. A government estimate that about 99 percent of children in grade one at six years of age attended "at least one year of pre-school" (Ministry of Education, 2012). For young children under the age of six years and diagnosed with a broad range of disabilities, most are referred by doctors during medical follow-up to the Early Intervention Programs for Infants and Young Children (EIPIC) run by voluntary welfare organizations (VWOs). These children have developmental challenges, and current regular preschools may not be able to cater to their needs adequately. Many eventually enroll in special needs schools run by VWOs with partial funding from the government. Inclusive education whereby children with special needs attend preschool alongside typical peers (i.e., mainstreaming) is relatively new and slowly expanding in Singapore. Young children with mild and/or emerging learning difficulties are often identified when they start attending preschool and/or about to enter into mainstream schools at seven years of age. Their struggles are often overlooked and deemed transitory by parents and early childhood teachers. These difficulties can predispose many to learning challenges when they begin elementary school without the skills necessary in school. The current range of early intervention programs is therefore not designed to address kindergarten children with special needs. This gap is also exacerbated by a lack of trained early child educators and allied health professionals to screen, diagnose, and provide additional support, instruction, or therapy in the community.

Importance and Rationale for Early Childhood Intervention

Aptly termed "the formative years," the first years of life have been regarded as a critical period of development in a child's life. This is a period of rapid growth and development within the cognitive, socioemotional, and physical domains of functioning in which the quality of brain architecture constructed through this early and ongoing process of development will either establish a firm or fragile foundation for all of the individual's capabilities and behaviors that follow. This contention is backed by a wealth of research in contemporary science (e.g., Fox, Levitt, & Nelson, 2010; Shonkoff & Bales, 2011). In particular, advances in neuroscience have provided substantial evidence that rapid maturation of the brain structure and functionality occurs during the first few years of life (Shonkoff & Bales, 2011). Of significance is that this window of opportunity for optimal development is crucial to a child's long-term adaptation and adjustment as brain plasticity and the ability to change behaviors have been shown to decrease over time. Consequently, problems arising from a poor early foundation would be more difficult to circumvent and costly to fix in later years.

Genetic factors, of course, exert an important influence on the developmental trajectories of young children, but environmental factors have the potential to alter this biological influence. However, research has indicated that the interaction between adverse environment and genetic factors can increase a child's risk for long-term negative developmental trajectories (Shonkoff & Bales, 2011). In particular, children from economically disadvantaged homes can face significant challenges in learning because of a lack of supportive resources, and those with developmental and learning concerns and/or interfering behaviors have been shown to be significantly compromised developmentally when they enter preschools (Arnold & Doctoroff, 2003; Gettinger et al., 2010). Additive risk factors resulting from an accumulation of multiple factors can further increase the susceptibility of children to poor developmental outcomes. Extant research has already indicated the effects of such risks on language and literacy development, self-regulatory behaviors, social competence, and positive learning behaviors. These factors undermine the child's readiness for school and may continue to work in concert to produce poor academic and social outcomes (Cadima, McWilliam, & Leal, 2010; Reynolds, Ou, & Topitzes, 2004; Rouse & Fantuzzo, 2009). In the same way, protective and growth-enhancing mechanisms in the child's environment have the potential to modify the developmental outcomes of young children in positive directions. The preschool provides such a protective context if early detection and intervention are implemented.

Early identification of children who are at risk is therefore critical in early prevention and remediation. Early childhood interventions refer to the array of services that incorporate these goals in education, health care, and therapy services for young children between birth and school age, with developmental disabilities or delays. The primary aim of these interventions is to remediate existing developmental problems or to minimize later developmental problems from occurring (Ramey & Ramey, 2006). Despite methodological limitations, evaluation of large-scale early childhood programs shows that intensive and high-quality early intervention consistently brings about impressive short-term effects in cognitive, emotional, and social development. Two-generation programs in the United States such as the Abecedarian Project (Ramey & Ramey, 1999) and Perry Preschool project (Barnett, 1992) have shown long-term effects for disadvantaged preschoolers in a range of cognitive, language, and social-emotional functioning (Arnold & Doctoroff, 2003; Odom et al., 2010), with continuing positive outcomes sustained to age thirty (Campbell, Ramey, Pungello, Sparling, & Miller-Johnson, 2002; Ramey & Ramey, 1998, 1999). Furthermore, these U.S.-based early childhood interventions seem to show them to contribute toward two of the most important long-term outcomes: higher educational attainment and lower rate of delinquency (Reynolds et al., 2004).

International research has shown that successful programs require that the program considers an ecological perspective that integrates child, family, school, and community factors into the intervention package (e.g., Guralnick, 1999; Guralnick, Neville, Hammond, & Connor, 2008). That is, they should best occur in the child's natural learning environment and involve significant people in the child's daily life to enable learning to continue with these people. Such community-based programs work to exploit the interventions' potentiality by ensuring that gains are sustained over time (Lloyd, Steinberg, & Wilhelm-Chapin, 1999; Willson & Hughes, 2009). For sustainability, effective early childhood programs also seek to address the "whole child" in preparing children for transition to schools (Shonkoff & Bales, 2011). After all, school success necessarily involves more than academic skills, and a combination of social-emotional, health, language, motivational, and other cognitive factors are equally important in contributing to school engagement (Moore, 2006).

Early intervention programs are, however, not a "one-size-fits-all" approach. Ramey and Ramey (2006) highlighted that some children show greater benefits from participation in early educational interventions than do others. These individual differences appear to relate to various aspects of the children's risk condition. It could also be related to the extent to which the early intervention program meets the child's needs, as well as the nature of services the child receives in order to prevent the negative consequences of those risk conditions over time (Barnett, 1992). The approach proposed by Guralnick et al. (2008) calls for maximized inclusion of children and families as the core principle in any community-based early intervention program or system.

In summary, a wealth of empirical evidence attests to the effectiveness of early childhood interventions in major programs undertaken in the West and suggests that they can make a difference to the long-term developmental trajectories of children at risk. Considerable evidence indicates too that effective implementation of prevention programs must pay attention to the contextual conditions under which the program is introduced (e.g., Berkel, Mauricio, Schoenfelder, & Sandler, 2011). Cultural assumptions and beliefs underpinning these perspectives may differ from those that operate in non-Western settings. As such, in designing MIP, the developers were mindful that their conceptualization of a workable program should be guided by sound theoretical underpinnings but remain flexible in critical aspects of the program to allow for responsiveness to the context of implementation.

The MIP Model: An Ecological Perspective

MIP is aimed at addressing the initial concern with parents' persistent failure to bring their young children, who have seemingly mild problems associated with developmental delays, to the needed psychoeducational sessions at the Department of Child Development, KK Women's and Children's Hospital, in Singapore (Chong et al., 2014). Allied health professionals have identified many of these emerging concerns to be keystone competencies necessary to prepare young children for learning in school (Gettinger et al., 2010). They are, however, often disregarded or may not be recognized by parents to warrant early attention. Also, a significant number of these children come from low socioeconomic families that may not be aware of the need and/or have the financial resources to obtain services. Making a commitment to attend psychoeducational sessions can be cumbersome for many of these parents who need to work, are unable to find alternate care arrangements for other children, and/or live far away from the hospital. In attempting to address these issues, MIP reasoned that the hospital can address these children's learning needs by moving its hospital-based therapeutic services to the contexts where the child and family live. By bringing the psychoeducational services to the community, the program seeks to extend children's learning beyond the traditional therapeutic model and situate such support within the children's contexts of development.

Conceptually, this project rests on an extensive body of family and early childhood research that has demonstrated the importance of early development of family processes, early childhood quality, and the adequacy of social and economic resources to meet children's basic physical and social needs and their psychological need for responsive care and nurturance (Barbarin et al., 2006). Additionally, MIP recognizes that children live in complex environments involving multiple caregiving systems, and MIP therefore works at developing a program that is responsive to changing demands of the environment. To respond appropriately and in a timely manner, MIP adopts an ecological perspective that is probably best characterized by the work of Bronfenbrenner (1977; Landry, Zucker, Solari, Crawford, & Williams, 2012). Bronfenbrenner argued that to understand how the environment affects children's social and cognitive outcomes, it is crucial to look beyond single predictors into the more comprehensive interrelationships between factors that might affect the child's development over time (Hirsh-Pasek & Burchinal, 2006). Specifically, child development is seen within the context of five structures of relationship, namely the *microsystem*, *mesosystem*, *exosystem*, *macrosystem,* and *chronosystem*. The family, school, teachers, peers, workplace, community, and influence of time on development are examples of these respective systems. Each system present factors, experiences, and challenges that come to influence and be shaped by other levels of the system to affect the developmental trajectories of the child.

This perspective recognizes individual differences and proposes that an effective program needs to stay responsive by remaining flexible and adaptable and not adopting a "one-size-fits-all" approach to resolving the developmental problems experienced by young children. Its multidisciplinary approach with built-in support to facilitate transitions across various contexts is a response to meet these demands and the needs of the growing child. The ecological model encapsulates many of the central ideas in successful early intervention programs described in Western early intervention models. However, it needs to be adapted to the cultural demands of the Singapore context so that families can be appropriately supported in their efforts to engage their children.

An Overview of the Development of the MIP Project

The MIP project is the brainchild of the Department of Child Development at the KK Women's and Children's Hospital, a major children's hospital in Singapore. The project's intent is to bring hospital-based psychoeducational services to young preschool children attending ordinary kindergartens. The department offers consult and therapeutic services to children below ten years of age with a wide range of developmental and learning issues (such as emergent literacy, language delays, and gross and fine motor skills) through a multidisciplinary team consisting of various allied health professionals (psychologists, speech language therapists, and occupational therapists, and learning support facilitators). Initiated in 2010, the project began as a pilot community-based project that represented a collaborative attempt with PAP Community Foundation (PCF), a major public preschool operator in Singapore, and the Lien Foundation, a philanthropic organization. The stakeholders agreed that early detection and intervention are crucial for such children's development in pursuit of minimizing their future referrals for support and healing services.

Preschool children with learning issues are first identified and screened by their class teachers. A learning support educator (LSEd) from MIP makes classroom observations to verify the teacher's assessment of the problem. The team then meets to discuss whether the emergent problem relates to development in language, speech, or gross or fine motor skills – the three different psychoeducational interventions offered by MIP. These intervention packages are undertaken by the learning support facilitator for literacy, a speech language therapist for those with speech problems, and an occupational therapist for those with fine and gross motor problems. A LSEd is also assigned to work alongside the specialist and oversee the work with each child. In 2011, LSEds themselves offered four support packages – literacy support, language development, social skill support, and motor skills (handwriting) – for those children whose identified learning problems were assessed to be readily amendable without specialized support.

Intervention by therapists primarily consists of ten individual forty-five-minute sessions at the preschool. Instruction is carried out in English, the medium of instruction in the Singapore education system. The LSEd sits in at the sessions to observe the interactions and follows up on the learning issues during five in-class support sessions that take place immediately after one-on-one sessions end. During in-class support, the LSEd works in the class of the target child for between half an hour and an hour per week for five consecutive weeks. The intent is to work with both the child and class teacher to facilitate opportunities for the child to use and extend what were learned in the individual sessions to typical classroom interactions. Parents are invited to observe their children in the weekly sessions and encouraged to carry out homework activities with them.

From a systemic perspective, the MIP service model recognizes and pays attention to the importance of creating pathways to enable the learning gained in the sessions to be extended and supported in the contexts where the children live. A pivotal and integral component of the MIP model is the strategic deployment of the LSEd to support the child and teacher to ensure sustainability of learning gains outside of the intervention context. In addition, they form the critical link to parents to enable and support their efforts with the child in learning-related matters at home. This is a new component created from a conceptual framework that departs from the traditional special education models in Western countries that incorporate teacher aides or support the teacher in an inclusive classroom. This also differs from hospital-based models whereby therapeutic interventions are predominantly carried out by allied health professionals with the child and/or parents in the medical facility, and collaboration and consultation with the preschool to integrate the child's learning in real-life contexts are often limited and can pose challenges.

The Role of Learning Support Educators

The LSEd is a new breed of senior early childhood educators with recognized qualifications in early childhood education and who have been principals or senior teachers in PCF preschools or other preschools. They have been specifically recruited to serve as LSEds for the duration of the MIP project. These educators have extensive experience working with children having special needs and have an in-depth understanding and appreciation of the idea of inclusive education. They therefore have the capability to work in preschools and to use collaborative problem-solving processes to facilitate change for children and families and in preschool with teachers. Although LSEds share many similar functions with itinerant special education teachers in the United States in enabling atypical children to benefit from community early childhood programs (Sadler, 2003), their role is multifaceted and they are expected to come with more skills that allow them to work collaboratively and consultatively with various stakeholders to support the child's learning in the classroom.

Indeed, their role is similar to that of resource teachers in learning and behavior (RTLB) in New Zealand elementary schools (Thomson et al., 2003). LSEds are seen as enablers of change for the children they support. Essentially, they provide the critical scaffolds for generalization of learning by the targeted children from one-on-one sessions to the classroom setting. They are resource teachers with the capacity to facilitate structural changes in the classroom. Their role is further extended to working with parents to support home efforts. LSEds' training and experience in working with preschools make them cognizant of the myriad influences on the teaching-learning process: the sociocultural background of the children; policies, regulations, and management systems; and the preschool teachers themselves (Thomson et al., 2003). This strengthens their ability to negotiate, facilitate, and coordinate changes in school and in routine. Indeed, the MIP project presents a different perspective on the nature of community service delivery, and this requires the LSEd, as key support worker, to remain highly flexible and versatile to the changing demands of classroom situations, the teacher, and the individual child. This role versatility has made it difficult to set down a list of prescriptive tasks undertaken by them and consequently for the program to isolate and evaluate their specific contributions to the learning outcomes of the children.

Teacher support and professional development. MIP recognizes that effective program implementation must provide preschool teachers intensive training and establish in them the competencies that are needed for supporting the children. Strengthening teacher competencies would also give them the confidence to work with new or unfamiliar learning problems in the future, thus reducing the need for external intervention. Indeed, Gettinger et al. (2010), in a review of the extant international literature, have identified professional development and support as keys to prevention program success.

Two important aspects of professional development were specifically highlighted. First, the training should align preschool teachers' learning with their classroom experiences. Additionally, the development program should be ongoing with opportunities offered for collaborative learning, mentoring, and feedback (Gregoire, 2003; Hochberg & Desimone, 2010). In this regard, MIP schedules regular workshops focusing on children development in physical, literacy, and language development. Furthermore, LSEds provide ongoing support and consultation to teachers to foster these theory-practice linkages. For instance, they work with teachers in rearranging classroom contingencies to ensure learning opportunities are embedded in the curricular activities to benefit not just the child but other children in the class as well.

A three-tiered pyramid intervention model. In 2011, the role of LSEds was reviewed with the view to optimize their competencies in meeting the increasing number of referrals for MIP support. To improve service efficiency, MIP broadly adopted principles underpinning the Response to Intervention (R*t*I) framework. Such a framework has been widely embraced in Western schools and child and family support models as a basis for delivery of evidence-based interventions (Ball & Trammell, 2011). The R*t*I framework represents a comprehensive model for the prevention of delays in learning and behavior, in promoting young children's academic and social competence, and in ameliorating behavior problems. Working within this framework, the MIP team pitches instructional intensity and therapeutic support to match the level of children's needs. The approach optimally exploits the capabilities of the LSEds by leveraging their work scope in the following ways:

- At the universal prevention level, LSEds continue to provide expert resources and consultation to preschool teachers. They work with the aim of ensuring an inclusive and more effective classroom environment and to minimize barriers to learning.
- At the selective prevention level, where problems emerge, LSEds work to support children with minimal intervention at the class level. These interventions are largely group-based and delivered within classrooms. With their

experience with preschool teachers and parents, much of their work involves seeking collaboration from these people to facilitate and sustain the child's learning in the classroom environment and provide appropriate support from the home.
- At the indicated level of prevention, LSEds continue to identify, screen, and monitor the class for children who experience difficulty in keeping pace in class. Where screening suggests a need for specialist help or when the problem persists despite selective and indicated levels of intervention, the child is referred for more specialized intervention by the therapist(s).

The LSEds increased their involvement at the selective preventive level of the R*t*I pyramid model of care to intervene in the classrooms and to support teachers with children who have emerging learning and behavior problems. They received supervisory support from the therapists. In addition, they continue to work with parents on home activities that they can later carry out to support their children. This revised model worked to reduce delays arising from the referral process by one to two months and enables LSEds to intervene early, during class time and/or in partnership with the preschool teachers. As such, they start to work with identified children earlier than the therapy packages.

Relatively few models have highlighted the contribution of how this personnel resource can make a difference to service outcomes. Western models emphasize the provision of itinerant support within an inclusive learning environment that is natural and least restrictive and preclude pull-out interventions (Dinnebeil, McInerney, Roth, & Ramaswamy, 2001; Sadler, 2003). However, we reason that a key difference between MIP and many of these established models may be with the former's attempt to move the focus of intervention from a hospital-based and therapist-centered approach to one that is ecological and inclusive in outlook by targeting primary caregivers with the capacity to influence the developmental trajectories of disadvantaged children in their everyday life. As pull-out sessions are perceived to be disruptive to classroom routines for the target child, the decision to do so is carefully evaluated by the team and in consultation with the preschool personnel and parents. The sessions are deemed necessary to remediate the learning needs of targeted children only when teachers do not have the capacity and ability to support them in their large classes where the teacher–student ratio is about 1:20. The LSEd therefore functions as the "bridging liaison" to provide the scaffolds of change for the child and teacher.

Engaging parents and families. The literature has highlighted the importance of enriching home experiences in influencing the development of school readiness competencies in children (Chazan-Cohen et al., 2009; Van Steensel, McElvany, Kurvers, & Herppich, 2010). In particular, parents' sensitive interactions with their children are an important developmental "input" to the growth of preacademic as well as social behavioral competencies (Duncan & Magnusson, 2005; Hindman, Skibbe, Miller, & Zimmerman, 2010; Hirsh-Pasek & Burchinal, 2006). Of note is that where young children are found to be better supported at home by their parents, there are associated increased levels of cooperation, conformity, peer sociability, and confidence, with the strongest effect demonstrated on cognitive development. Parents who afford their children varied opportunities and enriching experiences in the early years are likely to prepare them well for school. Those with fewer economic or educational resources are often less likely to provide a home environment that supports their children's development. Indeed, such differential exposures to learning experiences from home have been shown to be associated with large individual differences in a range of important cognitive, language, and social development of the growing child by the age of three (Morrison & Connor, 2010).

Children from low SES backgrounds do not begin preschool and kindergarten with differing levels in their self-confidence and school attitudes compared with their peers from better-resourced backgrounds (Arnold & Doctoroff, 2003). Multiple factors work to decrease their competence beliefs and school interest over the course of their early school years. One important contributing factor is their increasing recognition and understanding that they are deficient in skills to handle preschool learning effectively (Arnold & Doctoroff, 2003). As demands of the tasks increase, the challenges resulting from these early skill deficits can be more difficult to remediate, suggesting the importance for prevention and early intervention. As such, for early intervention programs to be impactful and sustained over time, parent engagement to enhance the positive early experiences of children at home must be built in to strengthen positive child outcomes. This should require parent and family involvement to take place in all phases of the program.

MIP Parent Literacy Program

MIP similarly aims to capitalize on these early years of development to equalize the learning opportunities of the children who may either have some specific challenges with emergent literacy or come from disadvantaged families. Although MIP intervention is available to children with other learning issues, it targeted emergent literacy for a parent education program as part of MIP because reading difficulties were more prevalent among children identified by their teachers. Many of the children come from low socioeconomic backgrounds where parents are not strong readers. Furthermore, the other specialized programs (that is, speech language and occupational therapy programs) require expert knowledge and skills that do not lend themselves well to parent training. This focus on the parent education component of the program sits well with the large body of research on early literacy and its relationship to school readiness, particularly in the United States (e.g., National Early Literacy Panel Report, 2010). In particular, longitudinal studies showed that typical children who remain poor readers by the end of the first grade will almost never acquire average-level reading skills by the end of elementary school (Lonigan & Shanahan, 2010). Early intervention for children from low-income families, on the other hand, had helped them to attain better school progress up to middle school years. In these families, household composition (e.g., single-parent families) and low income, and low maternal education and occupation, have been shown to assert a poor influence on preschool skills and subsequent first-grade literacy skills (Cadima et al., 2010). MIP reasoned that for children at risk for reading failure and whose parents do not have supportive resources, reading engagement will very much reside with the preschool. However, this will remain insufficient if the home environment does not provide the reinforcing support.

In designing the parenting program, the approach has two foci. The first is on teaching specific activities that parents can do with their children at home to support and reinforce their learning in the classroom. Parents are provided with the knowledge base to further their children's learning around these "school readiness" skills that form the basis of the parenting education curriculum goals. The second focus looks to support parents in their learning participation that would lead to specific and increased competencies in oral language, vocabulary and background knowledge, emerging literacy skills, comprehension, fluency and interest in literacy, and motivation to read. Teachers of the children's respective classes are expected to support these parents with teaching them both *how* to best contribute to their children's literacy development and *what* developing competencies they can intentionally reinforce in their interactions with their children.

In developing the literacy package, key team members and a reading expert first discuss and map out the core competencies and learning strategies considered to be most helpful to parents. The team then worked on materials for each session as well as the teaching resources and take-home kits designed to cover print and phonological awareness and reading and writing activities. A preliminary run was carried out to ensure that the materials were appropriate for use by parents. Professional development training was undertaken to prepare the teachers for participation in the literacy component of the MIP project. About thirty teachers attended the half-day session. However, when the workshops were rolled out with parents, the response was exceptionally poor, with five parents who signed up. The plan had to be aborted. Instead of using the group-based workshop approach involving parents in developing their children's reading competencies, the materials were redesigned and adapted for more one-on-one coaching with parents and children. Parents were encouraged during their meetings with the MIP team to meet with the teacher and LSEd to work out a feasible take-home plan. This approach was also slow to take off with the parents. The LSEds then began to approach and work with parents on an individual and just-in-time basis. These parents were found to be more comfortable and receptive to this way of engagement.

To summarize, the MIP adopts an R*t*I framework in which instructional intensity and therapeutic support are pitched at a level to match the target children's learning needs. Intervention packages are undertaken by allied health professionals or the LSEd, depending on the nature and severity of the learning issue. A pivotal component of MIP in the deployment of the LSEd is to facilitate transition from the individual sessions by engaging the teacher in the classroom so that learning gains made by the child are sustained in class. Additionally, the LSEd works to ensure that parents are supported in their efforts to carry out activities to reinforce the child's learning in the home.

Evaluation of MIP Program

MIP was implemented between 2010 and 2012, involving thirty-three preschool centers and about two hundred preschool children. The team consisted of three allied professionals for each of the specialist packages and four LSEds. A feasibility study was undertaken in 2008 and 2009 to map out the implementation plan. An evaluation of the program was also planned at the time of the program implementation. The intent of the evaluation was to generate information on the profiles of the children and families involved, review the program effectiveness, and identify barriers and challenges encountered in the process. Although two hundred children participated in MIP, complete information on both the profiles of parents and their children were obtained from only 149 of them and 281 other children who were attending the same classes as those identified for the program. This latter group of children serves as a comparison group, and those children are typical in their development.

Children and family profiles. The preliminary profiles of the children and their families suggested that they were in many ways different from the comparison group, indicating that there were developmental issues and concerns that place them at risk for successful school outcome(s). Children with the MIP Project (n = 149) and their peers (n = 281) in the respective classrooms were evaluated on various measures: *Peabody Picture Vocabulary Test, Fourth Edition* (PPVT-4; Dunn & Dunn, 2007); *Woodcock-Johnson III Tests of Achievement, Third Edition* (WJ-III: Woodcock, McGrew, Mather, & Schrank, 2001); *The Strengths and Difficulties Questionnaire* (SDQ, Goodman, 2001); and *The Behavior Assessment System for Children* (BASC-2; Reynolds & Kamphaus, 2004). Children in the MIP program obtained 'borderline' scores in various aspects of social, interpersonal, and behavioral competence on teacher-rated scales. Specifically, these children were comparably less prosocial and adaptable, and displayed less adequate social skills than their peers in the comparison group. Furthermore, they were reported to display significantly more behavioral and attention problems. They did not differ significantly from their peers with respect to any display of emotional symptoms.

Parents of children attending MIP and those of their peers also completed a take-home parent questionnaire at the beginning of the program implementation with the following composite scales: *Family Environment Scale* (FES; Moos & Moos, 2002); *Parenting Sense of Competence Scale* (PSOC; Johnston & Mash,1989); *Parental Warmth and Hostility Scale* (PWHS; Melby et al., 1991); and *Parent-Teacher Involvement Questionnaire* (PTIQ; Corrigan, 2002).

The following profile was obtained of these families at the time of the children's enrollment in the program:

- MIP families were comparably lower in social-economic and educational statuses according to various indicators. These parents attained lower educational qualifications and family income as compared to the other group of parents.
- The home environment appeared to have fewer resources to promote the child's learning and educational development. A lower proportion of their parents spoke English at home. Fewer books were available in these homes and the children tended to spend less time being engaged in reading or literacy-related activities.
- The parents have comparably lower educational expectations of their children compared to the other group of parents. However, they did not differ significantly in the family orientation toward achievement or competitiveness, the level of interest in intellectual and cultural activities, and the amount of participation in social and recreational activities.
- Both groups of parents perceived themselves to be adequate as parents, although more parents whose children are in the comparison group felt they were doing better than average. However, it was noted that parents whose children were attending MIP reported less consistency in the management of their children's behavior and tended to display more hostile behaviors when provoked by the latter. They did not differ significantly in the reported frequency of displayed affectionate behavior toward their children.
- Both groups of parents did not differ significantly in the extent of their involvement in preschool. They had high confidence in the adequacy of the preschool to prepare their children for the future. They were also reasonably positive about their relationship with teachers, perceiving the latter to have an interest in them and their children. Both groups, however, reported low levels of interest in initiating contact with the school and in involving themselves with various school activities.

MIP outcomes and effectiveness. The MIP program has brought about improvement in the specific areas of developmental deficits identified by preschool teachers and LSEds. As occupational and speech language therapies addressed problems that were highly individualized and required specialist input, it was not feasible to obtain objective measures to evaluate child outcomes. Neither was it possible to obtain comparable control group measures since presenting problems vary with each child. Similarly, the LSEd support packages were not amendable to objective evaluation considering the variability of each package with each child.

In overcoming this challenge, common benchmarks were used to evaluate the extent to which the children's identified learning issues were adequately addressed. Individual Educational Plans (IEP) and the Goal Attainment Score (GAS) (Turner-Stokes, 2009) were used to evaluate the extent to which the children achieved their developmental goals in these interventions. Interviews with parents, together with survey and focus group feedback from teachers and the principals, provided additional social validity to the program effectiveness.

The findings from the IEPs and GAS suggested that specialized therapists, in general, set modest goals that can be realistically achieved within a fifteen-week intervention time frame and that children in the program made good progress in attaining them. The baseline scores obtained across the preschools for the individual sessions and LSEd support packages suggested that children identified for MIP were performing below expectations in the respective skill areas evaluated at the time of goal development for IEP. After all the respective interventions were completed, the children obtained scores indicating that they were able to achieve the goals as expected in the respective packages.

The psychoeducational packages were designed to resolve targeted learning issues, and the IEP goals were developed with this purpose in mind. Once the identified issue was resolved, there was no necessity to develop further goals in the specific areas. Also, the fifteen-week time frame may have made it difficult to identify and work on new goals pitched at the next developmental level (as in speech development) that can be achieved within this period of time. For those children on the literacy package, there were more accomplished goals that exceeded the expectations of the therapists, suggesting that the children may have preexisting or foundational skills to support their learning of more advanced reading skills. The LSEds identified and helped the children attain comparably more goals compared to the specialized therapy packages. Compared to the two specialized therapy packages, they were somewhat conservative in identifying challenging goals for the children's accomplishment.

Although the LSEd packages were intended to maximize the expert resources of the MIP team, the specialized programs offered by allied health professionals remained critical in serving those children whose delays cannot be ameliorated through LSEd support packages. The findings arising from IEP goal development in the LSEd support packages suggested that LSEds may not have sufficient specialized skills to enable more pertinent assessment of children's physical, speech, and language competencies and skill levels. Further coaching and supervision from the therapists were found necessary to support their emerging competencies in these areas.

Effectiveness of the MIP literacy therapy program for children. We evaluated the literacy program to establish whether there were positive shifts in aspects of literacy among children who underwent the program as compared to a comparison group comprised of their peers in the same class (Chong et al., 2014). A nonequivalent group design was used to evaluate the impact of the program on those children identified with early reading difficulties. Pre- and posttests measures on the PPVT-4 and WJ-III showed that significant gains in aspects of literacy were indeed made with the intervention group (n = 35). At pretest, children in the program obtained significantly lower scores for age norms in comparison with their peers (n = 39). At posttest, within- and between-group analyses indicated the most significant gains were made by the MIP group in the following areas: vocabulary based on PPPVT-4 (11 months gain), passage comprehension (12.7 months gain), understanding directions (8.8 months gain), and letter-word Identification (6.9 months gain). Their performances on letter-word identification, spelling, and passage comprehension approximated the age norms at posttest. On the average, the children in the MIP program made a mean gain of about 6.5 months within 10 weeks of intervention followed by five sessions of graduated in-class support, compared to 2.9 month for their peers who did not receive extra support. Effect sizes obtained on the various tests ranged from 0.65 to 0.85 for the MIP group, compared to between 0.31 and 0.63 for the comparison group.

Preexisting differences in the pretest scores of the SDQ and BASC-2 were noted between the two groups, with children in the comparison group obtaining significantly lower scores on the scales measuring emotional, attentional, and behavioral problems. Paired-sample tests showed a significant positive shift from pre- to posttest in the MIP group on the SDQ score for prosocial behavior, with an effect size of 0.35. Social validity measures were also obtained from parents on their perceptions of the children's social, interpersonal, and behavioral functioning after MIP intervention. Anecdotal feedback from both parents and teachers suggested positive shifts in the children's prosocial behaviors during and after the intervention. We hypothesize that while there is a strong possibility that the children normally develop and mature over time, the specificity in the positive shift in prosocial behavior is related to the intervention. As the children acquired more skills, it is possible that they grew more confident in making friends, interacting with peers, and participating in social exchanges.

Program Challenges

As a pioneering effort, MIP faces challenges that are not unlike those faced in other interventions as they work to translate a conceptual model into practice. In identifying effective pathways underpinning program implementation, Berkel et al. (2011) have singled out participant responsiveness as a key moderator or mediator in determining the quality of program outcomes. With MIP, parent and teacher engagement have been identified as key components that are crucial in contributing to the sustenance of the intervention after it has ended. Finding collaborative platforms to work with these stakeholders has been a challenging undertaking but must be resolved so as not to temper program effectiveness.

Working with parents. Soliciting parental support and involvement poses considerable challenges. Parental engagement began with procuring their consent for the child's participation in MIP. The failure of parents to recognize the child's developmental concerns, their difficulty with appreciating the magnitude of the problem, parent work commitments, and/or fear of stigmatization were commonly encountered by the team. Additionally, it was difficult getting parents to cooperate and work with their child at home in the assigned activities. Feedback from the preschools involved and various team members suggested that some parents may not have the competencies to support their children, particularly for those in the literacy and speech language programs. Although we do not have empirical evidence, anecdotal accounts suggest that this lack of parental response may also have to do with the Asian mindset in the view toward education. In Asian societies where education is highly valued, it is largely perceived as the school's domain of responsibility, and parents often deem the expert knowledge and skills of these "educational" tasks to reside in the teachers and educators. Many Asian parents do not have a sense of shared responsibility for education with the school. This perception has similarly been noted by Willson and Hughes (2009) when they evaluated the role of home environment of preschool children in first grade retention in the United States.

Although MIP planned to capitalize on the family as a primary context of intervention to promote literacy skills in the long run, the various encounters in engaging parents draw important learning points for MIP to reconsider other ways to foster parent involvement. In retrospection, MIP recognizes the need for greater sensitivity to the social and cultural conditions of child development, which are important when the family and MIP and preschool cultures differ. MIP may have presupposed skills and knowledge that are not necessarily present in the parents and that cannot be developed simply by their participation in training. Also, MIP may not have paid sufficient attention to parent characteristics that can hinder the transfer of the training content. First of all, many parents may have left school early or not have significant positive schooling experiences. Second, busy work schedules of the families often make it difficult for them to carry out activities at home. As such, MIP recognizes the importance of ensuring cultural congruence, particularly to those features that emanate from a different socioeconomic perspective.

In redesigning this component of parent intervention, MIP repositioned the LSEd as an advocate for the child in a different way. Instead of approaching parent involvement from an instructional perspective and as a group for training, LSEds now focus on strengthening their interactions and relationships with parents on an individual basis to build trust first. This way of intervening appeared to have given some parents greater confidence in that they were more forthcoming in seeking help with challenges faced at home. A just-in-time model rather than an anticipatory approach to parent collaboration and problem solving seems to suggest this approach to be a more amenable platform to engage parents productively. We need to explore this avenue further to obtain a better understanding of how parent training can be translated in practical and acceptable ways (Van Steensel et al., 2010).

Engaging preschool teachers. Preschool teachers often lack core skills and knowledge necessary to enable their incorporation of developmentally appropriate practices in working with children with somewhat atypical development. One of the ways to circumvent this problem in MIP was to create opportunities for just-in-time sessions to dialogue with teachers. Therapists came in for the pullout sessions with the children once a week and were on the lookout for opportunities between sessions with the children to monitor the children's progress and to assess teacher support for practice of the new learned skills in class. However, teachers, preoccupied with the demands of ongoing classroom activities, were often not able to avail themselves for discussion or consultation. Anecdotal accounts suggest that many teachers and some preschools continued to assume that it is the responsibility of MIP to "see" the child through and failed to appreciate the school's contributions to the success of the child. This suggests that a set of organizational supports has to be in place for teachers and preschools to implement new ideas adequately from the project and ensure effective partnerships (Landry et al., 2012; Odom, 2009).

Another key area identified by MIP as critical for program effectiveness is the ability of the teachers to identify learning issues as accurately and as early as possible. This calls for better training in the way initial screening is to be carried out by them. Additionally, the team recognizes that professional development activities must also attend to "core" or essential elements of teacher practice to facilitate the teachers' productive engagement of the children after intervention has ended (Odom, 2009). Professional development workshops were organized in response to these needs and were well received, indicating that MIP was able to identify and meet a real training need. As identified in the literature (Gregoire, 2003; Hochberg & Desimone, 2010), short bursts of training may not be sufficient to ensure new teaching practices are in place. Mentoring and/or coaching have been identified as necessary ongoing activities for teachers to bridge the theory–practice gap. Access to the specialist support, though needed, had proven to be difficult as the therapists are hospital-based and not as readily available for consultations. Thus, the LSEds, as community-based workers, have proven to be crucial in bridging this gap to initiate teachers into the processes critical to the program's effectiveness.

Program Limitations and Implications

From a research perspective, methodological problems pose significant challenges to establish unequivocal evidence regarding the effectiveness of interventions (Gettinger et al., 2010). Evaluation of MIP has, however, provided evidence to suggest that it has been successful in reducing the disparity in preschool children's developmental needs by promoting skills they will need for school. Specifically, it demonstrated the malleability of young children's learning capacities despite mild delays and indicated the efficacy of a short-term pullout program when efforts to promote skill development were intentional and strategic and must necessarily solicit the collaboration of teachers and peers in the classroom. These improvements were not specific to the problems identified by teachers, therapists, and/or LSEds. Positive effects on other aspects of their development and functioning have also been documented as summarized previously. The MIP findings reiterated those established in Western countries by demonstrating the effectiveness of early childhood interventions in mitigating the risk factors that some children face in their learning and development.

Despite the impressive gains made in the course of literacy intervention, children in the MIP program continued to lag marginally behind their peers in literacy-related skills. This suggests that MIP may need to reexamine whether specific intervention intensity parameters such as program frequency, duration and dosage, and level of parent engagement have been adequately addressed (Justice & McGinty, 2012). This notwithstanding, Arnold and Doctoroff (2003) and Gettinger et al. (2010) have cautioned that even though children do benefit from such programs, it may be unrealistic to expect the positive effects to continue over time without restructuring their contextual experiences following the early intervention program. Empirical evidence suggests that positive effects arising from early intervention will diminish over time, as the result of experiences following the program (Gettinger et al., 2010). In particular, classroom, school, and home factors have been identified to play increasingly significant roles in predicting the developmental trajectories of children after intervention has ended (Burchinal, Peisner-Feinberg, Pianta, & Howes, 2002). It appears that if learning gains are to continue over time, more strategic involvement from the preschool and home must be incorporated. Additionally, although the MIP evaluation indicates a need to strengthen the channels through which to engage parents and the existing preschool structure to support these children, it may not be realistic to expect a preschool intervention to have a long-lasting impact on children's academic, behavioral, and social functioning without extending intervention through the elementary school years. The literature identifies this to be an inherent problem with many early childhood interventions when their impact may become apparent only in the later school years (Gettinger et al., 2010).

To our understanding, no local study in Singapore has been undertaken to examine the impact of an intervention program for preschool children with mild developmental delays. The MIP project represents an important milestone in the development of early childhood intervention programs in Singapore, considering that most of the others focus interventions on special needs populations (Goh, Chong, Chan, & Tang, 2010). MIP shows how best to make use of empirical evidence to develop a service model that is culturally relevant to children and families in an Asian context. In particular, it has articulated a cogent conceptual framework by shifting intervention from a clinical hospital-based to a community-based model where young children gain access to support in their natural learning environment. In adapting an ecological perspective in this service model, MIP has worked to address this problem by introducing well-trained early childhood personnel – the LSEd – to engineer the child's environment to ensure sustainable gains. Specifically, MIP highlighted a key ingredient that is crucial to provide supportive and consultative services to the children, their teachers and families. This "facilitator behavior" (Berkel et al., 2011, p. 25) has been seen as a critical component when attempting to establish quality outcome(s) in program implementation.

As with any pioneering program, continuing fine-tuning is essential to ensure quality program implementation and delivery (Landry et al., 2012). We have learned from critical feedback of the need to determine the pathways in strengthening parent engagement and teacher capacity to sustain implementation. For the field of prevention science in early intervention programs in Singapore to move forward, these are critical to address. This notwithstanding, the success of MIP has attracted the attention of the government ministry, and in the year 2013, it secured state funding support for a nationwide scale-up. The program has since been renamed the Developmental Support Program. As it undertakes this new venture, the diverse preschool landscape in the country will potentially challenge the program's fidelity and integrity. To ensure that program outcomes are not compromised, yet meet the demands of educational realities, MIP will need to strike a balance with adaptation and reinvention so as to remain responsive to the needs of those children it first set out to address (Berkel et al., 2011). This would essentially require MIP to focus its efforts in strengthening the capability and capacity of the program's linchpin – the LSEd – as the liaison bridge between the child, family, and the preschool.

Reference

Arnold, D. H., & Doctoroff, G. L. (2003). The early education of socioeconomically disadvantaged children. *Annual Review of Psychology* 54: 517–45.

Ball, C. R., & Trammell, B. A. (2011). Response-to-intervention in high-risk preschools: critical issues for implementation. *Psychology in the Schools* 48: 502–12.

Barbarin, O., Bryant, D., McCandies, T., Burchinal, M., Early, D., Clifford, R., & Pianta, R. (2006). Children enrolled in public pre-K: the relation of family life, neighborhood quality, and socioeconomic resources to early competence. *American Journal of Orthopsychiatry* 76: 265–76.

Barnett, S. W. (1992). Benefits of compensatory preschool education. *Journal of Human Resources* 27: 279–312.

Berkel, C., Mauricio, A. M., Schoenfelder, E., & Sandler, I. N. (2011). Putting the pieces together: an integrated model of program implementation. *Prevention Science* 12: 23–33.

Bronfenbrenner, U. (1977). Toward an experimental ecology of human development. *American Psychologist* 32: 513–31.

Burchinal, M. R., Peisner-Feinberg, E., Pianta, R., & Howes, C. (2002). Development of academic skills from preschool through second grade: family and classroom predictors of developmental trajectories. *Journal of School Psychology* 40: 415–36.

Cadima, J., McWilliam, R. A., & Leal, T. (2010). Environmental risk factors and children's literacy skills during the transition to elementary school. *International Journal of Behavioral Development* 34: 24–33.

Campbell, F. A., Ramey, C. T., Pungello, E. P., Sparling, J. J., & Miller-Johnson, S. (2002). Early childhood education: young adult outcomes from the Abecedarian Project. *Applied Developmental Science* 6: 42–57.

Chazan-Cohen, R., Raikes, H., Brooks-Gunn, J., Ayoub, C., Alexander Pan, B., Kisker, E. E., Roggman, R., & Fuligni, A. S. (2009). Low-income children's school readiness: parent contributions over the first five years. *Early Education and Development* 20: 958–77 doi: 10.1080/10409280903362402

Chong, W. H., & Lee, B. O. (2014). Social-emotional learning: promotion of youth wellbeing in Singapore schools. In Wright, K., & McLeod, J. (eds.). *Rethinking Youth Wellbeing: Critical Perspectives.* Melbourne: Springer, pp. 161–77.

Chong, W. H., Moore, D., Nonis, K. P., Tang, H. N., Koh, P., & Wee, S. (2014). Mission I'm Possible (MIP): effects of a community-based project on the basic literacy skills of at-risk kindergarteners. *Infants and Young Children* 27: 60–73.

Corrigan, A. (2002). *Fast Track Project Technical Report.* September 26. www.fasttrackproject.org

Dinnebeil, L. A., McInerney, W. F., Roth, J., & Ramaswamy, V. (2001). Itinerant early childhood special education services: service delivery in one state. *Journal of Early Intervention* 24: 35–44.

Duncan, G. J., & Magnusson, K. (2005). Can family socioeconomic resources account for racial and ethnic test score gaps? *Future of Children* 15(1): 35–54.

Dunn, L. M., & Dunn, D. M. (2007). *The Peabody Picture Vocabulary Test*, 4th ed. Bloomington, MN: NCS Pearson.

Fox, S. E., Levitt, P., & Nelson III, C. A. (2010). How the timing and quality of early experiences influence the development of brain architecture. *Child Development* 81: 28–40.

Gettinger, M., Ball, C., Mulford, L., & Hoffman, A. (2010). Prevention and early intervention for preschool children at risk for learning and behavior problems. In Doll, B., Pfohl, W., & Yoon, J. (eds.). *Handbook of Youth Prevention Science.* New York: Routledge.

Goh, W., Chong, W. H., Chan, W. P., & Tang, H. N. (2010). *Baseline Study of the Early Intervention Programme for Infants and Young Children (EIPIC).* Singapore: National Council of Social Service and KKH.

Goodman, R. (2001). Psychometric properties of the Strengths and Difficulties Questionnaire (SDQ). *Journal of the American Academy of Child and Adolescent Psychiatry* 40: 1337–45.

Gregoire, M. (2003). Is it a challenge or a threat? A dual-process model of teachers' cognition and appraisal processes during conceptual change. *Educational Psychology Review* 15: 147–79.

Guralnick, M. J. (1999). The nature and meaning of social integration for young children with mild developmental delays in inclusive settings. *Journal of Early Intervention* 22: 70–86.

Guralnick, M. J., Neville, B., Hammond, M. A., & Connor, R. T. (2008). Continuity and change from full-inclusion early childhood programs through the early elementary period. *Journal of Early Intervention* 30: 237–50.

Hindman, A. H., Skibbeb, L. E., Miller, A., & Zimmerman, M. (2010). Ecological contexts and early learning: contributions of child, family, and classroom factors during Head Start, to literacy and mathematics growth through first grade. *Early Childhood Research Quarterly* 25: 235–50.

Hirsh-Pasek, K., & Burchinal, M. (2006). Mother and caregiver sensitivity over time: predicting language and academic outcomes with variable- and person-centered approaches. *Merrill-Palmer Quarterly* 52: 449–85.

Ho, L. Y. (2009). Raising children in Singapore: a paediatrician's perspective. *Annals Academy of Medicine* 2: 158–62.

Hochberg, E. D., & Desimone, L. M. (2010). Professional development in the accountability context: building capacity to achieve standards. *Educational Psychologist* 45: 89–106.

Johnston, C., & Mash, E. J. (1989). A measure of parenting satisfaction and efficacy. *Journal of Clinical Child Psychology* 18: 167–75.

Justice, L. M., & McGinty, A. S. (2012). Early literacy intervention intensity and its relation to child outcomes. In Howes, C., Hamre, B. K., & Pianta, R. C. (eds.). *Effective Early Childhood Professional Development: Improving Teacher Practice and Child Outcomes*. Baltimore, MD: P. H. Brookes.

Landry, S. H., Zucker, T. A., Solori, E., Crawford, A. D., & Williams, J. M. (2012). In Howes, C., Hamre, B. K., & Pianta, R. C. (eds.). *Effective Early Childhood Professional Development: Improving Teacher Practice and Child Outcomes*. Baltimore, MD: P. H. Brookes.

Lantos, J. D., & Ward, N. A. (2013). A new pediatrics for a new century. *Pediatrics* 131 (Suppl. 2): S121–S126.

Lloyd, J. W., Steinberg, D. R., & Wilhelm-Chapin, M. K. (1999). Research on the transition to kindergarten. In Pianta, R. C., & Cox, M. J. (eds.). *The Transition to Kindergarten*. National Center for Early Development & Learning. Baltimore, MD: Paul H. Brookes.

Lonigan, C. J., & Shanahan, T. (2010). Developing early literacy skills: things we know we know and things we know we don't know. *Educational Researcher* 39: 340–6.

Melby, J., Conger, R. D., Book, R., Rueter, M., Lucy, L., Repinski, D., Rogers, S., Rogers, B., & Scaramella, L. (1991). *The Iowa Family Interaction Rating Scales*. Ames: Iowa State University.

Ministry of Education (2012). List of MOE-Registered Kindergartens. www.moe.gov.sg/education/preschool/find-a-kindergarten

Moore, T. (2006). *Early Childhood and Long Term Development*. Perth: Australian Research Alliance for Children and Youth.

Morrison, F. J., & Connor, C. M. (2010). Literacy development in the transition to school. In Meece, J. L., & Eccles, J. S. (eds.). *Handbook of Research on Schools, Schooling, and Human Development*. New York: Routledge.

Moos, R., & Moos, B. (2002). *The Family Environment Scale*, 3rd ed. Menlo Park, CA: Mind Garden.

National Early Literacy Panel Report (2010). Summary, commentary, and reflections on policies and practices to improve children's early literacy. *Educational Researcher* 39 (Special Issue).

Odom, S. L. (2009). The tie that binds: evidence-based practice, implementation science, and outcomes for children. *Topics in Early Childhood Special Education* 29: 53–61.

Odom, S. L., Hanson, M., Lieber, J., Diamond, K., Palmer, S., Butera, G., & Horn, E. (2010). Prevention, early childhood intervention, and implementation science. In Doll, B., Pfohl, W., & Yoon, J. (eds.). *Handbook of Youth Prevention Science*. New York: Routledge.

Ramey, C. T., & Ramey, S. L. (1998). Early intervention and early experience. *American Psychologist* 53: 109–20.

Ramey, C. T., & Ramey, S. L. (1999). Beginning school for children at risk. In Pianta, R. C., & Cox, M. J. (eds.). *The Transition to Kindergarten; National Center for Early Development & Learning*. Baltimore, MD: Paul H. Brookes.

Ramey, S. L., & Ramey, C. T. (2006). Early educational interventions: principles of effective and sustained benefits from targeted early education programs. In Dickinson, D. K., & Neuman, S. B. (eds.). *Handbook of Early Literacy Research*, vol. 2. New York: Guilford Press, pp. 445–59.

Reynolds, A. J., Ou, S., & Topitzes, J. W. (2004). Path effects of early childhood intervention on educational attainment and delinquency: a confirmatory analysis of the Chicago child–parent centers. *Child Development* 75: 1299–328.

Reynolds, C. R., & Kamphaus, R. W. (2004). *BASC-2: Behavior Assessment System for Children*, 2nd ed. Circle Pines, MN: American Guidance Service.

Rouse, H. L., & Fantuzzo, J. W. (2009). Multiple risks and educational well being: a population-based investigation of threats to early school success. *Early Childhood Research Quarterly* 24: 1–14.

Sadler, F. H. (2003). The itinerant special education teacher in the early childhood classroom. *Teaching Exceptional Children* 3: 8–15.

Shonkoff, J. P., & Bales, S. N. (2011). Science does not speak for itself: translating child development research for the public and its policymakers. *Child Development* 82: 17–32.

SingHealth (2011). More children diagnosed with special needs. www.healthxchange.com.sg/News/Pages/More-Children-Diagnosed-With-Special-Needs.aspx

Thomson, C., Brown, D., Jones, L., Walker, J., Moore, D. W. …, & Glynn, T. L. (2003). Resource teachers learning and behavior: collaborative problem solving to support inclusion. *Journal of Positive Behavior Interventions* 5: 101–11.

Turner-Stokes, L. (2009). Goal attainment scaling (GAS) in rehabilitation: a practical guide. *Clinical Rehabilitation* 23: 362–70.

Van Steensel, R., McElvany, N., Kurvers, J., & Herppich, S. (2010). How effective are family literacy programs? Results of a meta-analysis. *Review of Educational Research* 81: 69–96.

Willson, V. L., & Hughes, J. N. (2009). Who is retained in first grade? A psychosocial perspective. *Elementary School Journal* 109: 251–66.

Woodcock, R. W., McGrew, K. S., Mather, N., & Schrank, F. A. (2001). *Woodcock-Johnson III*. Itasca, IL: Riverside.

25 Prevention of Illegal Substance Use and Abuse in Bhutan

Tshering Dolkar

Introduction

Bhutan is in the Eastern Himalayas, between India and Tibet, sharing border with China in the north and India on the other three sides. It is a landlocked country with a total land area of 38,394 square kilometers and measures approximately 150 kilometers north to south and 300 kilometers east to west. It is roughly the size of Switzerland but far more sparsely populated and geographically remote. Bhutan's geographical position, mountainous landscape, and restricted numbers of tourists until the late 1980s have protected the country's values and cultural heritage.

The influence of Buddhism is highly visible in everyday life and is a major reason for Bhutan's spiritual and cultural legacy. The Buddhist philosophical foundations based on the four noble truths, eightfold noble path, and Karma – the law of cause and effect that is generally known as the karmic cycle of life and death – basically form the social structure, value system, and lifestyle of the Bhutanese people. Buddhism has since long played an important role in the political, economic, and social lives of Bhutanese.

Even in the twenty-first century, Bhutan remains a mystical country to many who are not even remotely associated with the country and the people. Bhutan still remains hidden in the vastness of the great Himalayas. However, Bhutan's development philosophy of Gross National Happiness (GNH) over gross domestic product is gaining international recognition. Gross National Happiness (GNH) is the central development philosophy of Bhutan.[1] This unique philosophy aims at maximizing well-being and minimizing suffering by balancing economic needs with spiritual and emotional needs. Bhutan's fourth king, His Majesty Jigme Singye Wangchuck, propounded the term "Gross National Happiness" in the 1970s. His Majesty's vision was to create a society in which happiness and well-being are the ultimate purpose of governance.

Strongly influenced by the Buddhist concepts and cultural consciousness, the GNH framework is supported by four principal pillars:

1. Good governance. This is considered a pillar for happiness because it determines the conditions in which Bhutanese thrive. While policies and programs

1 www.grossnationalhappiness.com/.

that are developed in Bhutan are generally in line with the values of GNH, there are also a number of tools and processes employed to ensure the values are indeed embedded in social policy.

2. Sustainable socioeconomic development. This means a thriving GNH economy must value social and economic contributions of households and families, free time, and leisure given the roles of these factors in happiness.
3. Preservation and promotion of culture. Happiness is believed to be contributed to by preserving the Bhutanese culture. Developing cultural resilience can be understood as the culture's capacity to maintain and develop cultural identity, knowledge, and practices and ability to overcome challenges and difficulties from other norms and ideals
4. Environmental conservation. This pillar is considered a key contribution to GNH because in addition to providing critical services such as water and energy, the environment is believed to contribute to aesthetic and other stimuli that can be directly healing to people who enjoy vivid colors and light, untainted breeze, and silence in nature's sound.

These four pillars are further elaborated into nine domains that articulate the different elements of GNH in detail and form the basis of GNH measurement, indices, and screening tools: (1) living standards; (2) education; (3) health; (4) environment; (5) community vitality; (6) time use; (7) psychological well-being; (8) good governance; and (9) cultural resilience and promotion.

According to the Center for Bhutan Studies (2009), the level of happiness among Bhutan citizens is evident once the level of entropy (i.e., the level of state's dysfunction; Evans, 2010) is compared to that of other nations – with only 4 percent of entropy feelings in Bhutan, in comparison to 60 percent in Argentina, 53 percent in the United States, 32 percent in Canada, and 21 percent in Denmark. Accordingly, results of Bhutan's national survey of happiness (Gross National Happiness, 2011) indicated that on a scale ranging from 0 (not at all) to 10 (extremely happy), only 9 percent of the population reported low levels (0–4) of happiness, 25 percent reported an average level(5) of happiness, and 66 percent of the population reported being happy (6–10). Thus, unsurprisingly the happiness philosophy that governs Bhutan's definition of well-being attracts much attention from scholars from various disciplines (e.g., Burns, 2011), who were astonished by its equilibrium and achievements (e.g., Metz, 2014). Evans (2010) attributes the achievement of such a high level of happiness to the values and tradition that the Bhutanese society holds, especially the one of friendship and communality.

Bhutan is a small, low-income country with 80 percent of the people dependent on agriculture and livestock rearing for their livelihood. Poverty is still high in remote rural areas of Bhutan (Santos, 2013). However, within the last few decades, modernization has set in and is making its way, generating urban settlements and introducing computers, mobile phones, televisions, and other Western amenities. Indeed, Bhutan is going through a transition from a primarily agrarian country to a more technology-based one, reflected in the changing lifestyle of the population and related public health issues, one of which is psychotropic substance use.

The population of Bhutan is approximately 760,643 people, with about 60 percent of the population below the age of twenty-five years. Bhutan's policy of Gross National Happiness aims at the overall well-being and happiness of each one of its people rather than the state's economic growth. Ironically, today Bhutan is faced with a challenging situation of increasing drug and alcohol abuse among its youth.

History of Substance Use in Bhutan

Culturally Doma Pani and Ara are two commonly used substances by the Bhutanese. They are the traditional forms of offerings and greetings during any occasion, whether religious, ceremonial celebrations or funerals. A piece of areca nut (locally known as *doma*) is folded in betel leaf (locally termed *pani*), to which lime (locally called *tsuni*) is applied and then chewed. The *doma-pani* is also called *doma* in abbreviated form, the juice of which is either swallowed after chewing or spat out. Chewing doma gives a sensation of heat and sometimes it can give a high too. Ara, an alcohol distilled from locally produced rice, barley, and maize, is the traditional form of alcohol used in Bhutan. It is usually more popular in the eastern part of Bhutan. Ara is brewed locally in the home and is easily available. Alcohol use is common and deeply rooted in Bhutan's custom and culture. Drinking alcohol is widely accepted in the Bhutanese society. It is used during all social occasions, including childbirth, religious ceremonies, festivals, social gatherings, and funerals. It is also a cultural practice to offer ara as a gesture of hospitality in the homes. Alcohol is believed to reduce body ache and pain and is used for initiation of breast feeding during the postpartum recovery period. Accordingly, in a study of prevalence, patterns, and predictors of alcohol consumption in a mountainous district of Bhutan, Subady, Assanangkornchai, and Chongsuvivatwong (2013) found that 38.5 percent of the participants in their study reported at least one standard daily drink in the past year (52 percent in men and 30 percent in women). Belief in the medicinal use of alcohol was reported by 34.8 percent of the men and 58 percent of the women as the reason to start drinking and was the strongest independent predictor for current drinking, even after adjustments for age and sex. Yet, it should be mentioned that according to findings presented to the Members of Parliament of Bhutan by RENEW (Respect, Educate, Nurture, Empower Women, July 12, 2015), a Bhutanese nongovernmental organization (NGO) that addresses domestic violence and gender-based violence (discussed later in this chapter), 80 percent of domestic violence cases in Bhutan are due to alcohol abuse.

Marijuana grows wildly in Bhutan throughout the subtropical to subtemperate to temperate climatic zones of the country. It was traditionally fed to the pigs to fatten them. However, the concern is that many of our school children may be experimenting with it and moving into the habit of using harder drugs. The problem seems to be more concentrated in urban areas. Data on other types of psychotropic substance use in the country are sparse.

The first psychotropic narcotic drug abuse case in Bhutan was recorded in 1989 by the police, after the police caught a man abusing marijuana. Bhutan has seen an increase in the number of cases of substance use reaching the police ever since. The National Baseline Assessment of Drugs and Controlled Substance Use in Bhutan–2009 (NBA-2009) indicated that the majority of those engaging in harmful drug use were students, with a mean age of onset at sixteen years of age. Increasing drug use in recent years, especially by youths who comprise more than half of the population of Bhutan (56 percent below the age of twenty-four years), has been a major concern among policy makers, agencies, and civil societies in Bhutan. Alcohol and cannabis have been the most common drugs of use among youths in Bhutan. According to the NBA-2009, cannabis use and glue sniffing were reported from all the fourteen dzongkhags (districts) out of the twenty dzongkhags studied under the assessment (BNCA & UNODC, 2009). Pharmaceutical use was reported from all except one (Zhemgang in Central Bhutan). Brown sugar (crude heroin) smoking within the last one month was reported from six dzongkhags (Bumthang, Paro, SamdrupJongkhar, Samtse, Trashigang, and Thimphu). The types of pharmaceuticals use reported codeine-containing cough syrups, benzodiazepine or nitrazepam tablets, dextropropoxyphene, and antihistaminic tablets. Sixty percent of the respondents for the NBA-2009 reported ever using alcohol. Both male (84 percent) and females (88 percent) had reported ever using alcohol (BNCA & UNODC, 2009).

Drug and controlled substance use by school students was also examined under the same study. Daily tobacco use was found to be 5 percent among students in classes VII and VIII and 8t percent among male students (classes IX and X), while in case of female students from these same classes, it was found to be less than 1 percent. However, higher prevalence of use was reported from classes XI and XII (13 percent and 1 percent in males and females respectively). Daily volatile solvent use (sniffing) was reported only by 1 percent of male students from classes IX and X, and the proportion of daily use was less than 1 percent for the rest across the classes (BNCA & UNODC, 2009).

As per the police report, in 2010, the Narcotic Drugs Law Enforcement Unit of Bhutan arrested seventy-two people for illegal transaction of psychoactive substances. Although the drug use epidemic is still considered in its early phase, the potential for a widespread epidemic remains a real threat. In 2014 alone, police arrested 950 people in connection with drugs, out of which 58 percent were youth. There was a 30 percent increase in cases involving possession of controlled substances, such as pharmaceuticals and prescription drugs, and a 10 percent increase in its illegal transaction of drugs, such as pharmaceuticals, prescription drugs, and narcotics. There are 284 drug traffickers serving their sentences in Bhutan today as abusers as per the national newspaper (Kuensel, 2015).

Policy on Illegal Substance Use Regulation and Prevention

Bhutan regulates drugs – from pharmaceuticals to narcotics – through the Narcotic Drugs and Psychotropic Substances and Substance Abuse Act 2005 ("Narcotics Act"). Its stated legislative purpose is "to ensure that drugs are available exclusively for medical, veterinary and scientific purposes." To this end, the Narcotics Act emphasizes education and treatment as means of combating illegal drug use. The Act sets forth a fivefold schedule for substances under which Schedule I includes the most restricted substances and plants having no medical use, and Schedule V includes substances "liable for abuse but [not falling] under International control" (National Assembly of Bhutan, 2005; 2015).

To address drug-related issues, the Bhutan Narcotics Control Board and the Narcotics Control Agency were created by the Narcotics Act. The Narcotics Control Board, made up entirely of government appointees and chaired by "a relevant Cabinet Minister," is responsible for formulating drug policy while its ancillary Narcotics Control Agency is chiefly responsible for implementing the Board's policy and advising the Board. The Narcotics Act provides enforcement and investigation powers to drug enforcement agencies, including the Royal Bhutan Police and Narcotics Control Agency. Under the Narcotics Act, every person and entity is subject to inspection by competent authorities.

The Narcotics Act mandates drug treatment under the auspices of the Narcotics Control Board and punishes repeat offenders and those who otherwise fail to abide by the terms of treatment. The Board is bound to ensure treatment, rehabilitation, and social reintegration of drug-dependent persons, through interventions, counseling, and detoxification; it is thus required by law to maintain adequate personnel and institutions to provide such services. Records of treatment must be kept confidential. Persons dependent on drugs are subject to compulsory treatment and rehabilitation; those who refuse to submit voluntarily must be confined in criminal custody. The Act authorizes courts to impose treatment as part of sentencing in cases related to drugs and provides for probation-like "periodic attendance before a panel for review and evaluation of treatment and progress." Successful compliance with such a regimen allows courts to discharge other penalties related to narcotics, such as prison terms and fines. The Narcotics Act further sets forth about a dozen offenses and penalties regarding compliance with the Act, further supplementing the Penal Code.

The Tobacco Control Act, 2009, bans the sale of tobacco, taxes imports, and places restrictions on quantities individuals may possess for personal consumption only. Smoking in public places is banned. The Act also authorizes the Tobacco Control Board, through the Tobacco Control Office, to provide cessation programs in health facilities and to work with rehabilitation centers in diagnosing and counseling tobacco dependence. The Ministry of Health, Ministry of Economic Affairs, Ministry of Finance, Ministry of Education, and Ministry of Home and Cultural Affairs are all responsible for implementing the laws in the Act and the policies of the Board in specified arenas (RGoB, 2009).

However, since the tobacco control act, there has been a significant increase of tobacco-related activity on the black market, and survey evidence demonstrates that tobacco use is still a major health concern for the adults and especially the youth of Bhutan (Givel, 2011).

Bhutan Narcotics Control Agency (BNCA), established in November 2006, is the agency of the government responsible for all matters related to narcotic drugs, psychotropic substances, and tobacco. BNCA is mandated to coordinate, monitor, regulate, and provide support to all those government and nongovernmental organizations that address substance use and abuse problems, (OAG, 2005).

Future of Substance Abuse Prevention in Bhutan

In recent years, Bhutan has come a long way in addressing the illegal substance use and abuse in the country, especially among our youth. In spite of all the mechanisms and strategies in place, the drug abuse problem is increasing and will continue to increase. Alongside drug and alcohol abuse, tobacco use also continues to present a major health concern for the youth of Bhutan (Givel, 2011). The problem of addiction is becoming increasingly complex in Bhutan. This complexity is evidenced by the shift from psychotropic drugs to narcotic drugs; the associated social problems, such as suicide, depression, and other mental health disorders; the repeated admissions for substance use disorders; and the costs of detoxification.

There is an increasing percentage of youth using multiple drugs, including intravenous drug use (IDU). There is a gross underreporting of drug use and abuse because of the stigma attached to publicly acknowledged addiction. The full nature of the situation is not known.

Geographical proximity to high IDU prevalence areas, such as Nepal and the Indian states such as West Bengal and Assam, render Bhutan potentially vulnerable to IDU and its consequences. Several factors – free and unregulated trade with India; open, porous borders; and the presence of Bhutanese, Indian, and Nepalese refugees in each other's countries – make Bhutan vulnerable to drug trafficking, particularly amphetamines and benzodiazepines smuggled from India.

Concerns regarding youth resorting to drug use due to unemployment, poor academic performance, peer pressure, urbanization, migration from rural areas to urban cities for employment, and education have been constantly raised by representatives from the highest legislative body of Bhutan, Gyalyong Tshogdu (the National Assembly). Currently there are no updated data available on drug and alcohol abuse in Bhutan, but the government and policy makers recognize the seriousness of the potential problem.

Bhutan Education Blueprint 2014–2024 is a 172-pages document in which the Ministry of Education presents its plans in pursuit of providing Bhutan children with "the necessary knowledge and skills to meet the new challenges" (*Bhutan*

Education Blueprint, 2014, p. 12) of encountering the complementary needs of national identity alongside current globalization. The document outlines several "Shifts" that should be made in order to meet these goals. "Shift Seven" focuses on the "enhancement of values education and wellbeing." Under this title the Ministry of Education states that there is a need "to scale up schools in integrating values in curricular and extracurricular contexts in the development of student responsibility, social skills, resilience and wellbeing" (p. 85). Outlining such a goal is justified by the notion that Bhutanese youth are increasingly exposed to "hundreds-even-thousands-of images and ideas," leading them to rising trends in various problem areas, such as substance abuse, suicide, crime, and violence. Recognizing the increasing problems of youth in Bhutan, and referring to the emerging system of counseling and guidance in Bhutan (Lorelle & Guth, 2013), several initiatives have been suggested in order to meet the increasing challenges of Bhutan youth issues. Among them are parenting education; school-based counseling programs; encouragement of massive participation of children in sports and physical activities; and strengthening of life skills education in schools (Lorelle & Guth, 2013, p. 86). These initiatives are already being implemented and carried out for children both in school and out of school.

Due to these declarations, the Bhutan education system is facing major challenges (e.g., VanBalkom & Sherman, 2010) that have to be resolved (e.g., keeping up with the GNH framework/philosophy and educating to it, while opposing substance abuse). Yet, appropriately and successfully encountering these educational challenges – such as those initiated under the *Bhutan Education Blueprint 2014–2024* – would have major implications on Bhutan's future, including the control over substance abuse among its youth.

Personal Conclusion

As a certified counseling professional who worked both in the school system as well as with various communities,[2] with experiences working with youth, substance abuse, education, domestic violence, and gender-based violence in Bhutan, I feel confident to say that, unfortunately, the trends of substance abuse in Bhutanese youth will continue to rise despite the increasing investment in prevention programs, interventions, and policies. It is therefore, my recommendation that while evidence-based prevention is important, we may need to give equal importance to treatment and interventions too. In pursuit of these two goals (i.e., prevention and treatment of substance abuse), Bhutan needs to give more importance to developing professionalism among service providers by developing our own certification process and establishing standards and qualifications of our own professionals. Currently, the training of

2 www.nbcc.org/assets/newsletter/issues/fall08.pdf.

counselors in Bhutan is limited and not well established. However, the Bhutan Board for Certified Counselors (BBCC), which was established in 2015 under the auspices of Her Majesty the Queen Mother of Bhutan Gyalyum Sangay Choden Wangchuck, is working to provide this platform to professionalize counseling services and provide support across all the helping professions.[3] Thus, it is evident that in spite of the increasing challenges in the field of substance abuse prevention and treatment, the people of Bhutan are committed to working together as a country to create a healthy and sustainable future for our youth.

References

Bhutan Ministry of Education (2014). Bhutan education blueprint. sites.google.com/a/gov.bt/blueprint/home

Bhutan Majestic Travel (BMT) (2007). Marijuana grows in abundance. www.bhutanmajestictravel.com/news/2007/marijuana-grows-in-abundance.html

BNCA (Bhutan Narcotics Control Agency and UNODC (United Nations Office on Drugs and Crime (2009).*National Baseline Assessment of Drugs and Controlled Substance Use in Bhutan –2009*. www.unodc.org/documents/southasia/reports/National_Baseline_Assessment_of_Drugs_and_Controlled_Substance_use_in_Bhutan_2009.pdf

BNCA (Bhutan Narcotics Control Agency) (2015). Narcotic Drugs, Psychotropic Substances and Substance Abuse Act. http://www.bnca.gov.bt/wp-content/uploads/2015/05/NDPSSA-2015.pdf

Burns, G. W. (2011). Gross National Happiness (GNH) is more important than gross domestic product: a gift from Bhutan to the world. In Biswas-Diener, R. (ed.), *Positive Psychology as Social Change*. New York: Springer Science, pp. 73–87.

Center for Bhutan Studies (CBS) (2009). Gross National Happiness: coronation address of his majesty King Khesar, The 5th Druk Gyalpo of Bhutan. www.thersa.org/discover/publications-and-articles/rsa-logs/2013/02/understanding-your-values–a-group-exercise–new-uk-values-report

Evans, S. (2010). The impact of cultural folklore on national values: a preliminary study with a focus on Bhutan. *Storytelling, Self, Society: An Interdisciplinary Journal of Storytelling Studies* 6: 8–18.

Givel, M. S. (2011). History of Bhutan's prohibition of cigarettes: implications for the neo-prohibitions and their critics. *International Journal of Drug Policy* 22: 306–10.

Gross National Happiness (2011). *Bhutan – Results of the Second Nationwide 2010 Survey on Gross National Happiness*. www.grossnationalhappiness.com/survey-results/index/

National Assembly of Bhutan (2005). Narcotic Drugs, Psychotropic Substances and Substance Abuse Act. www.nab.gov.bt/assets/uploads/docs/acts/2014/Narcotic_Drugs_act_of_Bhutan,_2005Eng.pdf

3 //counselinginbhutan.blogspot.com/.

National Assembly of Bhutan (2015). Narcotic Drugs, Psychotropic Substances and Substance Abuse Act. www.nab.gov.bt/assets/uploads/docs/acts/2015/Substance_Abuse_Act_2015.pdf

Kuensel (2015). Not too late for Bhutan to address drug abuse problem. www.kuenselonline.com/not-too-late-for-bhutan-to-address-drug-abuse-problem/

Lorelle, S., & Guth, L. J. (2013). Establishing the school counseling profession in Bhutan: reflections from the field. *Journal for the International Counselor Education* 5: 1–13

Metz, T. (2014). Gross national happiness: a philosophical appraisal. *Ethics and Social Welfare* 8: 218–32. dx.doi.org/10.1080/17496535.2014.932420

OAG (Office of the Attorney General) (2005).Narcotic Drugs and Psychotropic Substance Abuse Act of Bhutan. http://oag.gov.bt/wp-content/uploads/2010/05/Narcotic-DrugsPsychotropic-Substance-Substance-Abuse-Act-of-BhutanDE.pdf

Royal Government of Bhutan (RGoB) (2009). Tobacco Control Act of the Kingdom of Bhutan, 2009.

Santos, M. E. (2013). Tracking poverty reduction in Bhutan: income deprivation alongside deprivation in other sources of happiness. *Social Indicators Research* 112: 259–90. dx.doi.org/10.1007/s11205-013–0248-4

Subady, B. N., Assanangkornchai, S., & Chongsuvivatwong, V. (2013). Prevalence, patterns and predictors of alcohol consumption in a mountainous district of Bhutan. *Drug and Alcohol Review* 32(4): 435–42. dx.doi.org/10.1111/dar.12015

UNODC (United Nations Office on Drugs and Crime) (2009). Drug use situation and responses in schools and communities: a rapid assessment in Phuentsholing, Bhutan. Publication of Project RAS/H13 (prevention of transmission of HIV among drug users in SAARC countries) in collaboration with the Bhutan Narcotics Control Agency (BNCA), Bhutan. Project RAS/H13, a joint initiative of UNODC, the United Nations Programme on HIV/AIDS (UNAIDS), and the World Health Organization (WHO). www.unodc.org/documents/southasia/reports/Drug_use_situation_and_responses_in_schools_and_communities.pdf

VanBalkom, W. D., & Sherman, A. (2010).Teacher education in Bhutan: highlights and challenges for reform. *Asia Pacific Journal of Education* 30: 43–55. dx.doi.org/10.1080/02188790903503585

26 Promoting Coping Skills in Children, Adolescents, and Parents

What We Have Learned in the Australian Context

Erica Frydenberg

Coping has been a useful heuristic device once operationalized in that it is possible to identify the elements of helpful and unhelpful coping. The language that represents the constructs can be used to teach people what to do and what not to so as to achieve best outcomes.

In this chapter, coping is operationalized as a resource that is underpinned by the transactional theory of Richard Lazarus and his colleagues (Lazarus & Folkman, 1984) and the resource theory promulgated by Stevan Hobfoll (Hobfoll, 1989). The theory of coping is introduced, followed by the measurement of coping in children, adolescents, and adults. Intervention programs with both short-term and long-term benefits for children and adolescents are presented, and finally a parenting program that incorporates coping skills for parents of young children is reported.

Introduction

The Context

Australia is a Western democratic industrialized country of 23 million people. The population is made up of the indigenous inhabitants, dating back at least fifty thousand years, followed by British colonists who arrived after 1788 when Sydney was established as a penal settlement. In 2013, about 27.7 percent of Australians were born overseas (6.4 million people). The predominant proportion of people are from European backgrounds and estimated to be 85 percent; Asian Australians make up 12 percent of the population and Aboriginal and Torres Strait Islander population about 3 percent. Even though English is Australia's national language, due to cultural diversity over three hundred languages are spoken in the community. Approximately 81 percent of people speak English in the home. While the dominant culture is Anglo-Celtic, and Christianity is the most widely reported religion (61 percent), the country cannot be described as a religious one. A keen interest and pursuit of sports is evident in the leisure activities of the community and in the sporting representations in international meetings such as the Olympics. There is a strong awareness of mental illness, including anxiety-related disorders, with regular reporting that one in five Australians will experience mental illness (ABS, 2014a, b).

School education in Australia is compulsory between the ages of six and fifteen years (sixteen years in Tasmania and recently South Australia, which equates to year ten of schooling), and can then be followed by two senior years of schooling (years eleven and twelve), which are necessary for those students wishing to proceed to higher education (ACARA, 2013). In 2013, there were 3,645,519 students attending school in Australia. Despite the continuing growth in the nongovernment sector, government schools remain the major provider of school education in Australia in 2013, with nearly twice as many students attending government schools (2,375,024) as were attending nongovernment schools (1,270,495) (ACARA, 2013).

The research reported in this chapter has been in the main conducted in Australia, with adolescents, adults, and young people in various school settings and in early childhood settings. There is generalizability of findings beyond the Australian context, particularly to like communities, such as United States of America, United Kingdom, Canada, and New Zealand, but the reader is always encouraged to adapt both instruments and programs to their own settings. Coping research is considered to be useful tool in the prevention armory.

Coping

In the Australian context, there has been a substantial focus on stress and coping research and publications output since the 1980s mirroring the output in the international literature. Coping has emerged as one of the most highly researched areas of psychology, and it is reflected through countless publications appearing across the globe since the 1960s (Frydenberg, 2014). The abundant output in the field may be due to the fact that coping is firmly embedded in theory, there are accessible measurement tools, and there are ready applications to professional practice, particularly in the promotion of healthy development and prevention of mental illness. Additionally, coping fits comfortably into the contemporary psychological landscape, where there has been a shift from an emphasis on a deficit model of human endeavor, that is, what people can't do, to one that is positive in focus and considers what people can do and how they can do it better. It is about adaption and closely related to self-regulation, health, and well-being. Thus it fits well with prevention science that focuses on skilling people with resources.

Theoretical Frameworks

Although coping as a construct has had its origins in psychodynamic theory, with an emphasis on conscious and unconscious processes in human behavior, the two major complementary theoretical frameworks that underpin contemporary coping research are the transactional theory of Richard Lazarus and resource theory as articulated by Stevan Hobfoll. Richard Lazarus launched the transactional theory of coping with his seminal book, *Psychological Stress and the Coping Process* (Lazarus, 1966) where he focused on maximizing immune functioning and removing harmful effects on the cardiovascular system. However, the impact of his interest in coping went well beyond health and adult populations to almost every facet of human endeavor, and now coping has become part of everyday vernacular.

The most frequently cited definition of coping is that of Lazarus and his colleague Susan Folkman, who define coping "as constantly changing cognitive and behavioral efforts to manage specific external and/or internal demands that are appraised as taxing or exceeding the resources of the person" (Lazarus & Folkman, 1984, p. 141). This definition addresses the cognitive and behavioral aspects of the coping process and also focuses on the effort associated with an individual‘s response. Lazarus and Folkman (1984) also point out that managing stress includes accepting, tolerating, avoiding, or minimizing the stressors as well as the more traditional view of coping as mastery over the environment. Moreover, coping is not limited to successful efforts but includes all purposeful attempts to manage stress regardless of their effectiveness. That is, the coping response is initiated as a response to a stressful event that is personally significant and taxes or exceeds an individual's resources.

An important complementary theory, the Conservation of Resources (COR; Hobfoll, 1989, 2010) is based on a single motivational tenet that individuals strive to obtain, retain, and protect that which they value. Like Lazarus, Hobfoll explains that stress occurs when resources are threatened, but then goes on to emphasize what happens when resources are actually lost or when the individual invests resources without getting adequate return for effort. When there is adequate return for investment, the resource pool is built up and self-esteem and confidence are boosted, and the converse also holds true.

Resources are defined as objects such as possessions that are valued for their physical nature, but they can often be associated with socioeconomic status or status in general; personal characteristics such as seeing things as predictable and happening in one's best interest and being optimistic; mastery; conditions such as marriage, employment, or tenure; and promotion or energies, examples of which are networks, power, money, time, knowledge, and such that allow you to obtain other resources. COR theory posits that people do not wait for disaster to strike: they invest in resources, that is, they take out insurance and purchase future protection, for example, by investing time and energy in relationships. In that sense, this aspect of the framework is proactive rather than reactive.

According to Hobfoll (1989), the emphasis of COR theory is on objective elements of threat and loss and "common appraisals" by people who share a biology and culture. He challenges the neglect of the environment in the appraisal approach and emphasizes the importance of the social context in which coping occurs. The emphasis is on the circumstances that occur rather than the appraisals. There is an importance placed on loss and gain cycles. While COR theory was born out of trauma and disaster research, today Hobfoll

(2010) sees it as being aligned with positive psychology with a focus on how it contributes to resilience and capacity to thrive beyond surviving.

While Hobfoll and Lazarus developed their theorizing based on adult populations, the reach of their work has gone well beyond adults into the world of children and adolescents (e.g., Roubeni, De Haene, Keatley, Shah, & Rasmussen, 2015). Our work in Australia largely rests upon these two theoretical underpinnings. According to the transactional model, coping is a function of situational determinants and the individual's characteristics, perception of the situation, and coping intentions. Following an appraisal of the situation, the individual assesses whether the consequences are likely to lead to "loss," "harm," "threat," or "challenge," and also assesses the resources available to deal with the stressor. Following a response, the outcome is reviewed or reappraised (tertiary appraisal or reappraisal), and another response may follow. Individuals with greater resources will be safer from threats to resources and in a stronger position to make further gains.

Substantial research in child and adolescent coping has revealed that coping in children and adolescents shares similarities with adult adaptation in that temperament, developmental, and environmental factors all play a part (Frydenberg, 2008; Frydenberg & Lewis, 1993a). This means there is no right or wrong coping, but the situation determines what is likely to achieve the desired outcomes. Nevertheless, there are broad dimensions that can be construed as helpful or unhelpful coping (Frydenberg & Lewis, 2011).

The Measurement of Coping

Measurement provides the first step in operationalizing a construct so as to enable research and applications to follow. Early measurement of coping focused on adult populations. Interest in the assessment of how younger people cope emerged in the late 1980s, when the coping literature turned its attention to coping in childhood (Compas, 1987). In her comprehensive review of coping scales, Carolyn Aldwin (2007) identified two hundred references to different coping scales, with fifty-one of these being in the child and adolescent arena. Generally, coping instruments have been developed through self-reports, semi-structured interviews, daily diary recordings, observation of behavior, and the reports of significant others, such as parents, teachers, and peers.

The many ways to assess coping generally have in common a set of descriptions or single actions that are grouped into coping strategies where there is a similarity of concept or ideation. These in turn can be further grouped more broadly into commonality of practice. The most common categorization or grouping of approaches to coping is the dichotomous grouping of strategies by Lazarus and Folkman (1984) and Lazarus (1993), which identifies problem- and emotion-focused coping. Alternative categorizations range from groupings of eight to ten strategies or scales (e.g. Stark, Spirito, Williams, & Guevremont, 1989). For example, in the work of Frydenberg and Lewis we have identified eighteen strategies in the Adolescent Coping Scale (ACS; Frydenberg & Lewis,

1993a) and nineteen strategies in the Coping Scale for Adults (CSA; Frydenberg & Lewis, 1997) and sixty strategies in both the ACS-2 (Frydenberg & Lewis, 2011) and CSA-2 (Frydenberg & Lewis, 2014). The second level of grouping characterizes coping styles that represent functional and dysfunctional aspects of coping (Cox, Gotts, Boot, & Kerr, 1985; Frydenberg & Lewis, 1997, 2011; Seiffge-Krenke & Shulman, 1990). The functional styles represent direct attempts to deal with the problem, with or without reference to others, whereas the dysfunctional styles relate to the use of nonproductive strategies. Coping is influenced by person and situation characteristics (Skinner, Edge, Altman, & Sherwood, 2003). Thus, like others, we have found that there is both consistency and variation in coping (Frydenberg & Lewis, 1994) with an "inherently variable" concept like coping. This is reflected in when asking individuals how they cope in general and how they cope with a specific situation under consideration.

In the work of Frydenberg and Lewis, we have conceptualized the rubric of coping as thoughts, behaviors, and actions that arise in response to demands placed upon an individual. Some strategies attempt to remove or to remedy the source of the demand (e.g., problem solving), others help individuals to accommodate to it (e.g., wishful thinking), and there are strategies that demonstrate an inability to deal with the demand (e.g., despair and illness) (Frydenberg, 2008). The tools that Frydenberg & Lewis[1] have developed provide measures of all three types of responses and have been used to both identify correlates and determine outcomes.

Thus far, Frydenberg and Lewis's research has identified conceptual areas of coping for three age groups. Firstly, we identified coping dimensions used by the adolescent population with the ACS (Frydenberg & Lewis, 1993a) and the ACS-2 (Frydenberg & Lewis, 2011). Secondly, we considered coping in adult populations (CSA; Frydenberg & Lewis, 1997) and the CSA-2 (Frydenberg & Lewis, 2014) and more recently in young children (Yeo, Frydenberg, Northam & Deans, 2014).

The ACS was developed to assist with understanding adolescent coping behavior, both generally and in response to particular stressors, and as a means for determining how adolescents cope with a range of life concerns and circumstances. Based on two studies of Australian youth undertaken in the early 1990s (Frydenberg & Lewis, 1991, 1993b), two forms of the ACS were produced: a long form that could be used in both a general and specific manner, and a short form that consisted of one item from each group of strategies that could be used as an indicator of coping strategies used by adolescents. The seventy-nine items were grouped into eighteen strategies, and three styles of coping were common among Australian adolescents. The first of these three styles is comprised of coping based on problem solving while attempting to remain physically active and socially connected; the second grouping relies on reference to others in an effort

1 acer.edu.au.

to deal with concerns; and the last, which indicated the use of avoidance strategies, is generally associated with an inability to cope with stresses.

Since context is all-important in coping, it seemed relevant to be able to examine how adults in the young person's world cope, so we developed the Coping Scale for Adults.

Similar to the ACS, there are two forms of the CSA: a long form, which could be used with either a general or specific focus; and a short form, which consisted of one item from each group of strategies that could be used as an indicator of the coping strategies used by adults. It was found that in addition to nineteen coping strategies, four styles of coping were common among adults: the first emphasized productive coping based on attempting to solve the problem while remaining physically active and socially connected; the second operated on reference to others in an effort to deal with concerns; the third related to optimism, where individuals focus on the positives and seek spiritual support or relaxing diversions; and the last highlighted the use of avoidance strategies generally associated with an inability to cope with stressors. A range of other variables were also found to impact on adult coping, from perceptions of the self, perception of the ability by others, supportive workplace climates, and the experience of stress in the family. The original CSA was distinct from other similar instruments in that it identified a wider array of conceptual areas of coping, allowing administrators essentially to profile an individual or group's coping styles and strategies, providing a basis upon which adults could be assisted to reflect upon their coping actions in a meaningful way, thus providing the opportunity for functional behavioral change.

The number of items in each of the strategies of the ACS-2 and CSA-2 has been reduced from the earlier iterations of the ACS and CSA from as many as five to three, making a total of sixty items. Thus the sixty items of both the ACS-2 and the CSA-2 are organized into twenty reliable scales or coping strategies of three items each and contain a total of sixty items that can be grouped into three subscales based on second-order factors, namely productive coping, nonproductive coping, and problem-solving coping.

The conceptualizations of the adolescent and the adult constructs are presented in Figure 26.1 along with the definitions of the coping strategies and the groupings that have been reported and are helpful for interpreting the findings. The figure presents the ACS and CSA categorizations or groupings in their original form, as much of the research discussed in this chapter is based on those categorizations.

Children's Coping

Children's coping in the early years has been tackled in multiple ways. For many years, the ACS has been adapted and used for children ten to twelve years old. However, we thought it would be helpful to develop a parent report instrument for children in the early years. To develop the Children's Coping Scale (CCS), we generated items that were drawn from the literature and

Figure 26.1 *Coping strategies on ACS-2 (Frydenberg & Lewis, 2011) and CSA-2 (Frydenberg & Lewis, 2014).*

ACS-2

Productive [Problem Solving] Style: 11 coping strategies

SOCIAL SUPPORT (*SocSup*) is represented by items that indicate an inclination to share the problem with others and enlist support in its management, e.g., *Look for support and encouragement from others.*

FOCUS ON SOLVING THE PROBLEM (*SolvProb*) is a strategy that tackles the problem systematically by learning about it and taking into account different points of view or options, e.g., *Work out a way of dealing with the problem.*

PHYSICAL RECREATION (*PhysRec*) is characterized by items that relate to playing sports and keeping fit, e.g., *Keep fit and healthy, e.g. play sport.*

SEEK RELAXING DIVERSIONS (*Relax*) is about relaxation in general rather than about sport. It is characterized by items that describe leisure activities such as reading and painting, e.g., *Relax,* e.g., *watch TV, play computer games, go for a walk.*

INVEST IN CLOSE FRIENDS (*Friends*) is about engaging in a particular intimate relationship, e.g., *Spend more time with a good friend.*

WORK HARD & ACHIEVE (*Work*) is a factor describing commitment, ambition (achieve well) and industry, e.g., *Work hard.*

FOCUS ON THE POSITIVE (*FocPos*) is represented by items that indicate a positive and cheerful outlook on the current situation. This includes seeing the "bright side" of circumstances and seeing oneself as fortunate, e.g., *Look on the bright side of things and think of all that is good.*

ACCEPT ONE'S BEST EFFORTS (*Accept*) is characterized by items that indicate an acceptance of having done one's best and therefore there is nothing further to be done,

CSA-2

Productive Coping Style: 8 coping strategies

WISHFUL THINKING (*WishThink*) is characterized by items that are based on hope and anticipation of a positive outcome, e.g., *Imagine that things will work out well.*

IMPROVE RELATIONSHIPS (*ImpRel*) is about improving close relationships, e.g.,*Get into or improve on existing special relationships; for example, partner, spouse, boy-/girlfriend.*

IGNORE THE PROBLEM (*Ignore*) is characterized by items that reflect a conscious blocking out of the problem, e.g. *Put the problem out of my mind.*

HUMOR (*Humor*) consists of items involving entertaining others, e.g.,, *Try to be funny.*

SEEK SPIRITUAL SUPPORT (*Spirit*) is comprised of items that reflect prayer and belief in the assistance of a spiritual leader or higher power, e.g. *Pray for help and guidance so that everything will be all right.*

PROTECT SELF (*ProtSelf*) involves improving one's self image by looking after oneself, particularly through one's appearance, e.g., *Improve my appearance.*

FOCUS ON THE POSITIVE (*FocPos*) is represented by items that indicate a positive and cheerful outlook on the current situation. This includes seeing the "bright side" of circumstances and seeing oneself as fortunate, e.g., *Look on the bright side of things and think of all that is good.*

SEEK RELAXING DIVERSIONS (*Relax*) is about relaxation in general rather than about sport. It is characterized by items that describe leisure time with friends and family, such as reading, watching a movie, or listening to music, e.g. *Make time for friends or family.*

Figure 26.1 (*cont.*)

ACS-2	*CSA-2*
e.g., *Accept things as they are, because I've done my best.*	
SOCIAL ACTION (*SocAct*) is about letting others know your concerns and enlisting support by writing petitions or organizing an activity such as a meeting or a rally, e.g., *Join with others to deal with the problem,* e.g., *organize a petition, attend a meeting.*	
SEEK PROFESSIONAL HELP (*ProfHelp*) denotes the use of a professional adviser, such as a teacher or counselor, e.g.,, *Ask a teacher or other professional person for help.*	
HUMOR (*Humor*) is characterized by items that involve entertaining others, e.g., *Try to be funny.*	
Nonproductive [Passive Avoidant] style: 9 strategies	**Nonproductive coping style: 5 strategies**
WORRY (*Worry*) is characterized by items that indicate concern about the future in general terms or more specifically concern with happiness in the future, e.g., *Worry about what will happen to me.*	DWELL ON THE NEGATIVE (*DwellNeg*) is a strategy whereby a person focuses on the negative, e.g., *I keep thinking about my failures.*
WISHFUL THINKING (*WishThink*) is characterized by items that are based on hope and anticipation of a positive outcome, e.g., *Wish a miracle would happen to make things turn out well.*	SELF-BLAME (*SelfBlame*) is characterized by items that indicate that an individual sees himself or herself as responsible for the concern or worry, e.g., *Blame myself.*
NOT COPING (*NotCope*) consists of items that reflect the individual's inability to deal with the problem and the development of psychosomatic symptoms, e.g., *I get sick.*	WORRY (*Worry*) is described by items that indicate concern about what is happening and what may happen in the future, e.g., *Worry about what is happening.*
IGNORE THE PROBLEM (*Ignore*) is a style that reflects a conscious blocking out of the problem and resignation coupled with an acceptance that there is no way of dealing with it, e.g., *Shut myself off from the problem so I can try and ignore it.*	NOT COPING (*NotCope*) consists of items that reflect the individual's inability to deal with the problem and the development of psychosomatic symptoms, e.g., *I get sick.*
KEEP TO SELF (*KeepSelf*) is characterized by items that reflect the individual's withdrawal from others and wish to keep others from	TENSION REDUCTION (*TensRed*) is a strategy that focuses on making oneself feel better by releasing tension, e.g., *Find a way*

Figure 26.1 (*cont.*)

ACS-2	*CSA-2*
knowing about concerns, e.g., *Don't let others know about my problem.*	*to let off steam; for example, cry, scream, drink, take drugs.*
SELF-BLAME (*SelfBlame*) is characterized by items that indicate that an individual sees himself or herself as responsible for the concern or worry, e.g., *Blame myself.*	
ACT UP (*ActUp*) is characterized by items which reflect an attempt to make oneself feel better by releasing tension, e.g., *Act up and make life difficult for those around me.*	**Problem-Solving Style: 4 strategies**
SEEK SPIRITUAL SUPPORT (*Spirit*) is comprised of items that reflect prayer and belief in the assistance of a spiritual leader or Lord, e.g., *Pray for God to look after me.*	FOCUS ON SOLVING THE PROBLEM (*SolvProb*) is a strategy that analyzes and tackles the problem, e.g., *Develop a plan of action.*
TENSION REDUCTION (*TensRed*) is an attempt to make oneself better by, e.g., *Letting off steam; crying; screaming; using alcohol, cigarettes, or drugs.*	SEEK PROFESSIONAL HELP (*ProfHelp*) denotes consultation with a professional adviser, such as a counselor, e.g., *Discuss the problem with qualified people.*
	SOCIAL ACTION (*SocAct*) is about letting others know what is of concern and enlisting support by attending or organizing activities such as meetings or rallies, e.g., *Go to meetings that look at the problem.*
	SOCIAL SUPPORT (*SocSup*) is represented by items indicating an inclination to share the problem with others and enlist support in its management, e.g., *Talk to other people about my concern to help me sort it out.*
	OTHER
	WORK HARD & ACHIEVE (*Work*) is a factor describing increasing one's focus on his or her work, commitment, ambition (achieve well), and industry, e.g., *Focus on my work.*
	PHYSICAL RECREATION (*PhysRec*) is characterized by items that relate to playing sports and keeping fit, e.g., *Play sport.*
	KEEP TO SELF (*KeepSelf*) is characterized by items that reflect the individual's wish to keep concerns to himself or herself, e.g., *Don't let others know how I am feeling.*

experience with children in early childhood settings. We found that children four to five years old were able to articulate up to thirty-six different coping responses. These responses were categorized conceptually into three groupings: active (what children do), passive (how they withdraw or avoid difficult situations), and relational (how they deal with situations involving others) (Deans, Frydenberg, & Tsurutani, 2010).

In a recent study using the CCS with a population of four- to five-year-olds at an Early Learning Centre in Metropolitan Melbourne (N = 94) and whose parents completed the questionnaire, Yeo et al. (2014) reported one positive coping style and two negative coping styles: emotional expression and emotional inhibition. The positive coping style included emotion-focused strategies such as "be happy with the way things are" and included a number of coping-by-distraction strategies such as "go out and play and forget about their problem," "chat with friends," and "have fun, play sport, draw, play games." These distraction strategies would typically be considered secondary-control coping in adult research whereas the current results suggest that for preschoolers, both primary- and secondary-control strategies can be categorized under a single positive coping style. This lack of distinction between problem-focused and emotion-focused or primary control and secondary control is consistent with coping research in both preschoolers and school-age children (Ayers, Sandier, West, & Roosa, 1996; Tsurutani, 2009). This suggests that the dichotomies between problem- versus emotion-focused coping and primary- versus secondary-control coping replicated in many adult studies (Skinner et al., 2003) are not universally applicable for preschoolers. This may represent an important developmental difference in coping. Children learn the distinction between coping efforts directed at solving the problem and those that manage their reactions to the problem as they mature cognitively. Such a conclusion is supported by studies that demonstrate that emotion-focused coping emerges in later childhood and early adolescence (Band & Weisz, 1988; Compas, Malcarne, & Fondacaro, 1988).

Coping Research

Measurement is a first step to understanding the variables that operate in relationship to helpful coping and unhelpful coping and as a precursor to prevention research. Thus, from our research in Australia and using the ACS and CSA, we have learned how coping is associated with a range of factors such as age, gender, culture, family, problem solving, well-being, school connectedness, and different types of aggression. Some of these findings are reported here, and for a full summary of findings, see Frydenberg and Lewis (2011, 2014).

Age and Gender

Age and gender differences in coping have been consistently identified in the Australian context both in cross-sectional (Frydenberg & Lewis, 1999) and longitudinal studies (Frydenberg & Lewis, 2000). In the main, it is females who turn to each other and utilize more social support than boys, and at the same time girls are more inclined to declare their inability to cope and are more likely to utilize strategies such as tension reduction, self-blame, and worry. In contrast, boys, at least in the Australian context, are more likely to utilize physical recreation and relaxation strategies than are girls. Older adolescents, particularly girls, are more inclined to report their use of nonproductive coping strategies (Frydenberg & Lewis, 2000). When the same young people are followed through from age twelve to fifteen, and from fifteen to seventeen years, it was found that girls particularly report a greater inability to cope during the fourteen- to sixteen-year period than they did two years previously (Frydenberg & Lewis, 2000). That is one of the reasons why we recommend teaching coping skills in the early adolescent years and then providing booster sessions in the later adolescent years with a particular focus on what is of greatest importance to young people at that time.

Coping Resources

Coping resources are determined by what is valued in a culture. In order to explore the relationship between the resources identified by young people and their coping styles, a sample of 172 secondary students in Metropolitan Melbourne, Australia, completed the modified version of Hobfoll's (1989) Conservation of Resources Evaluation (M-CORE) (McKenzie & Frydenberg, 2004) and the long version of the ACS, focused on a specific self-nominated concern. The modified instrument was validated in the study, and a relationship was found between the degree to which students had the resources under consideration and the coping styles they used. Resources for that particular age group included having friends, parental support, adequate home, and adequate food and being able to speak up for oneself. Young people high in resources tended to use productive ACS strategies, while those young people with fewer resources report using fewer and more nonproductive ACS strategies. The implications are that both a focus on facilitating the augmenting of young people's resources and the building up of coping skills is important in that the two are closely interrelated. Both development of productive coping skills, such as working hard to achieve and the reduction in use of nonproductive coping strategies such as self-blame, along with resources, such as a supportive family or healthy interpersonal relationships, are important for prevention work.

Positive and Negative Coping Strategies

The coexistence of positive and negative coping strategies was explored with 1,219 students from 11 government and nongovernment schools who completed the ACS (Lewis & Frydenberg, 2002). Predictably, a positive relationship was found between the use of problem-focused coping and ability to cope, and an inability to cope was related to greater use of a nonproductive coping style. Young people who were coping less successfully were those utilizing more emotion-focused strategies. Further, students' usage of emotion and problem-focused coping strategies was intercorrelated. This suggests that failure to cope triggers increased coping activities of all kinds and that overuse of nonproductive strategies interferes with the capacity to use productive coping. The findings also showed that adolescents who use more productive strategies also used more nonproductive strategies rather than the expected logic of those who used greater productive coping strategies would use decreased levels of nonproductive strategies. Tackling both sets simultaneously is recommended so as to build up young people's coping resources in order to develop their resilience. What we need to do is to raise awareness of the fact that attention to only one of these (that is, productive or nonproductive) to the exclusion of the other is likely to be of limited benefit.

Self-efficacy

Self-efficacy is intrinsically related to coping, although the two bodies of theory have not been frequently linked in the literature. A belief in one's capacity to change behavior has implications for how coping skills are acquired and subsequently employed. Self-efficacy is a regulatory process through which an individual shapes his or her responses to the environment (Bandura, 2012).

Given the probable links of coping with self-efficacy and importance of problem solving in the educational context, Frydenberg and Lewis (2009) examined the relationship between adolescents' sense of problem solving and their use of productive and nonproductive coping strategies. Using data from two studies, namely Study 1 sample comprising of 1,047 (460 males and 587 females) and Study 2 sample of 870 (392 males and 478 females) where coping was measured using the ACS, it was found that there was a significant positive relationship between self-perceived efficacy of problem solving and a productive coping style. These findings suggest that focusing on the positive and accepting one's best effort can assist in problem-solving efficiency in adolescents. It is not only problem-solving skills per se that are important but the belief in one's efficacy and the capacity to judge one's coping as efficacious that are also of benefit.

Well-being and Coping

Well-being and coping were examined with a sample of 870 students (age twelve through sixteen) from eight Metropolitan Government schools (55 percent female) completed the short form of the ACS and the twelve-item State of Being questionnaire (Reynolds, 2001). The effectiveness of coping and the frequency of coping strategy use were also considered (Frydenberg & Lewis, 2009). Inherent in the State of Being scale was one construct that referred to well-being and used positive coping styles such as "I had fun with my friends" and a second construct related to items that were associated with a more negative terminology and strategies (e.g., "I felt depressed, I was very lonely"). There was a significant relationship between the use of negative avoidant coping styles with both well-being and distress. It was not just about the frequency of the coping strategy but once again the perceived effectiveness of the coping strategy that was also deemed to be important (Frydenberg & Lewis, 2009).

A second study explored the interrelationships between coping styles, emotional well-being, and school connectedness using path analysis (Frydenberg, Care, Freeman, & Chan, 2009). A total of 536 (241 boys and 295 girls) were included in this study. A productive coping style was positively related both to student-reported sense of well-being and to a lesser extent to school connectedness. A nonproductive coping style was inversely related to students' sense of well-being and connection to school. Students' sense of emotional well-being was positively related to school connectedness.

The negative relationship between nonproductive coping with emotional well-being, and to a lesser extent with school connectedness, highlights the importance of taking into account the influence of risk factors that may be interpersonal or environmental, as well as positive factors when focusing on well-being. Furthermore, it is likely that enhancing coping skills will both increase well-being and to a lesser extent increase young people's sense of connectedness in the school setting. Overall, it is posited that young people could be expected to cope better following a coping skills program.

Bullying

Bullying has always been a concern in school settings, but our alertness to it has grown in recent years (Coggan, Bennett, Hooper, & Dickinson, 2003). With the advent of the Internet and mobile technology, bullying has been transformed into new forms. Cyber-bullying can occur over the Internet though the means of Instant Messenger, chat rooms, personalized web pages, blogs and social networks such as MySpace and Facebook, and mobile phones (Beran & Li, 2004).

Lodge and Frydenberg (2007) conducted a study to examine the prevalence of cyber-bullying and real world (general) bullying for adolescents between the ages of eleven to seventeen years. The sample consisted of 652 students (204 male and 378 female) from two independent schools and three government and nongovernment schools. In addition to investigating gender differences in cyber and general bullying, the study sought to determine the coping strategies used by students who had generally experienced bullying as compared to the coping profiles of their cyber-victimized peers. Peer victimization was measured with a nine-item, self-administered questionnaire (alpha = 0.82) in the students' classroom setting. The items tapped cyber-bullying (e.g., receiving nasty messages from peers via email or Short Message Service [SMS]) and general bullying experiences, which included physical bullying (e.g., attacks, property damage), social bullying (e.g., exclusion), and verbal bullying (e.g., teasing). Using a five-point Likert type scale (1 = never; 2 = less than once a term; 3 = several times a term; 4, = about once a week; and 5 = every day), participants indicated how often they had experienced each of the bullying behaviors from peers. Higher scores indicated higher levels of peer victimization. It was found that, 91 percent (n = 596) of students reported real-world bullying of some description and 22 percent (n = 134) reported that they have been victims of cyber-bullying.

Gender differences in coping with bullying were identified. Girls reported greater use of relating to others, social support, social action, tension reduction, and self-blame; boys reported using more coping actions such as working hard to solve the problem and engaging in relaxing diversions and physical activity. Girls who expressed cyber-bullying concerns reported using coping actions such as excessive worry, tension reduction, and self-blame. Boys were more inclined to ignore the problem and keep the problem to themselves and less likely to seek professional help.

The implication of these findings is that a large number of young people do experience bullying, particularly cyber-bullying, which is increasingly becoming of concern. Therefore, there is a need to develop resilience and the capacity for both the community and the individual to deal with the problem. It is recommended that coping skills programs incorporate some instruction on the management of the cyber-world and ways to deal with cyber-bullying when it occurs such as focusing on deleting cyber-harassment by skill development (see Frydenberg, 2010). The study once again highlights the different ways that boys and girls cope and how they might change their coping practices to address the situation. This can then become part of the coping skills instruction since the application of theory has to be relevant to the world of the contemporary adolescent.

Proactive Coping

Proactive coping and proactive aggression were explored because it was postulated that the profile of the proactive aggressor is very similar to the proactive coper in that he or she also uses aggression to obtain goals and makes a deliberate choice of how to act (Larkins & Frydenberg, 2004). While proactive coping is seen as positive and proactive aggression is seen as negative, we thought that there may be some underlying characteristics that are the same but are manifested differently in the proactive copers and proactive aggressors. Two hundred and six participants from fifteen nongovernment regional schools in Victoria, Australia (nine to thirteen years of age), most of whom were from Anglo-European and middle to low socioeconomic backgrounds, took part in the study. The participants completed an adapted version of the ACS. Responses from teachers' checklists were used to identify children as reactive aggressors (troubled by others), proactive aggressors (troubling to others), or nonaggressors.

The group of children identified by their teachers as reactive aggressive obtained a higher score on nonproductive coping. Of the factors underlying the nonproductive scale, not coping and tension reduction were significant. All groups reported using a similar number of productive coping strategies, but the reactive group had a higher mean score for nonproductive coping strategies than the other groups. This suggests that they do know and use productive coping strategies but may also use nonproductive strategies. This supports recommendations for interventions and prevention to focus on reducing nonproductive coping strategies rather than just increasing productive coping strategies, which is what has been the approach in education (Frydenberg & Lewis, 2002a).

Adult Coping

Adult coping research has reinforced much of what we have learned in our research with adolescents. There has been a range of studies that have focused both on individual and group responses of adults in a variety of contexts. They include studies relating to workplace, domestic violence, eating disorders, teachers, and populations like the hearing impaired. See Frydenberg and Lewis (2014) for a summary.

Using the CSA, we examined the coping behavior of a group of 137 Australian middle managers and 236 community based adults, none of whom were managers. In general, the managers, irrespective of gender and age, were more likely to respond to their general concerns by applying themselves and engaging in problem solving. They are less likely to engage in nonproductive strategies such as worrying, letting off steam, and wishful thinking. The findings suggest that managers rely less on nonproductive forms of coping, and consequently perhaps they are coping more effectively than others. Whether they are self-selected as a group or the choice of workplace influences which coping strategies to use is interesting to consider. When it comes to age, there were clear-cut differences. Adults in the younger group (under forty-five years) used more protections of self, worry, social support, relaxing diversions, tension reduction, humor, and physical recreation (Frydenberg & Lewis, 2002b). These were not an entirely surprising range of findings.

Early Years Coping

Yeo and colleagues reported the coping skills that preschoolers used as reported by their parents (Yeo et al. (2014). Using a sample of ninety-four parent reports, two forms of negative coping that were predominantly emotion-focused reflected whether emotions were expressed or inhibited. Negative coping–emotional expression consisted of strategies such as "lose it," "cry or scream," and "get mad with themselves," where emotional expression can usually be observed by caregivers. In contrast, negative coping–emotional inhibition consisted of strategies such as "keep feelings to self," "don't let others know how they are feeling," and "do nothing," where emotional inhibition is inferred by caregivers based on their understanding of their child's behavior. Both forms of negative coping are primarily emotion-focused as opposed to some of the problem-solving-type strategies in positive coping.

Prevention Coping Programs

Having determined the merit of coping theory, identified the constructs, and developed an understanding of how different populations cope, we were ready to incorporate coping skills into a prevention framework. A three-tier public health model of prevention and intervention approaches has fit well with our framework for prevention and intervention (Gordon, 1983, 1987; Simeonsson, 1991). The first tier provides a universal intervention focus with professionals such as teachers and counselors delivering programs to all students. Tier 2 is the implementation of such a program to young people at risk (selective prevention), such as those with learning difficulties or health-related difficulties such as diabetes. Finally, Tier 3 allows the intervention to focus on a particular individual or group that has an identified need (indicated prevention). Programs that promote coping with normative stress, delivered to the whole population (universal prevention), represent a promising direction for the prevention of social-emotional difficulties. The American Psychological Association has recently developed a resource with guidelines for prevention practices (APA, 2014), such as the need for theory-driven, evidence-based interventions that are culturally relevant and that focus on strengths. The programs described in the following subsections incorporate many of these guidelines.

Adolescent Coping Programs

Three universal coping skills programs that draw on the aforementioned earlier coping research – namely *The Best of Coping* (BOC; Frydenberg & Brandon, 2007), a CD-ROM *Coping for Success* (CFS, Frydenberg, 2007), and *Think Positively* (Frydenberg, 2010) – each targeted the adolescent population. The elements of the three programs are described in Figure 26.2. The BOC program is a pencil and paper program with an instructor's manual and a student workbook; *Coping for Success* is a CD-ROM that can be completed in a self-paced format; and *Think Positively* is a stand-alone book where instructors can move through the activities and provide the students with worksheets. The core content of the three formats is similar, and the programs are generally delivered over ten to twelve weeks in a one-classroom session (generally forty to fifty minutes long). They have been adapted and trialed with different populations. For example, groups such as young people with diabetes and with learning difficulties and children who have relationship difficulties have completed the adapted BOC program, which has been subsequently evaluated.

The principle that underscores the programs is that we can all do what we do better. If we do not like how we cope in certain contexts, we can learn new strategies. It is possible to enhance and develop one's coping if we have a framework within which to do that. Thus, the programs are universal in that they are suitable for all students and young people rather than those with

Figure 26.2. *Teaching coping: the twelve modules (Frydenberg, 2010).*

1: The language of coping
Aim: To introduce the concept of coping, explore individual styles, and facilitate an understanding of the various coping strategies.
2: Positive thinking
Aim: To facilitate an awareness of the connection between thoughts and feelings and to introduce basic skills in thought evaluation and change thinking.
3: Strategies that don't help
Aim: To raise awareness of the ineffective coping strategies that people use and to explore some productive alternatives.
4: Getting along with others
Aim: To explore and practice aspects of communicating and listening.
5: Asking for help
Aim: To raise awareness of the importance of reaching out to others and to available networks and supports.
6: Dealing with conflict
Aim: To explore conflict in your life and how to resolve conflicts.
7: Problem solving
Aim: To learn and practice the six-step problem-solving model.
8: Social problem solving
Aim: To deal with situations in relationships. handling and avoiding teasing, rejection, etc.
9: Decision making
Aim: To teach students how to make considered decisions through evaluating options.
10: Coping in the cyber-world
Aim: To create awareness of the risks and benefits of the cyber-world and how to manage it.
11: Goal setting
Aim: To build awareness about the relationship between goals and achievement and to explore and set individual achievable goals.
12: Time management
Aim: To evaluate how we spend our time and learn to manage it in effective way.

specific needs. Instructors bring their own experience and adaptations to the sessions using drawing, modeling, direct teaching, and roleplay as appropriate. Generally, all students receive the program with an emphasis on analysis of outcomes for students in relationship to coping.

In a series of studies, Frydenberg, Bugalski, Firth, Kamsner, and Poole (2006) set out to assess the usefulness of BOC for young people in the context of providing a generic program to all students. There was a focus on understanding those who were "at risk." Risk included depression, learning problems, and anxiety, which are the most common mental health problems for adolescents in Western communities such as Australia (DoHA, 2010). Additionally, students who show low academic achievement are associated with an increased likelihood of encountering a number of problems and stressors (e.g., hyperactivity, social-behavioral, low self-esteem, and depression (Gresham, Macmillan, & Bocian, 1996; Valas, 1999).

Three separate studies using BOC were conducted. The first study by Buglaski (Frydenberg et al., 2006) was completed with a sample of 115 students (57 males and 56 females) aged fifteen to seventeen years. Students were divided into three groups: at risk for depression (n = 22), not that vulnerable to depression (n = 68), and resistant to depression (n = 220. Students deemed to be at risk for depression were identified using the criteria determined by the Children's Attribution Styles Questionnaire (CASQ; Seligman, 1995) and the Perceived Control of Internal States Questionnaire (PCIS; Pallant, 1998). Using a pre-posttest design, students completed the ACS. All three groups completed the BOC program. To determine whether program participants made the hypothesized changes in coping styles over time, a repeated measures multivariate analysis of variance (MANOVA) was conducted. Significant differences were found over time for all groups – Wilks' Lambda = 0.78, $F(4,107) = 7.39$, $p < 0.001$ – and over time between groups – Wilks' Lambda 0.86, $F(8,214) = 2.08$, $p < 0.05$. There were significant differences, across all groups, in reference to others coping over the time the program had been conducted. There were also significant differences between the groups in non-productive coping over time. No significant differences were found in productive coping styles across time or between the groups. The most significant insight regarding prevention is that when a universal program is implemented, those who need it most – in this case, those being at risk for depression – benefit the most from the program.

In a second study by Firth (Frydenberg et al., 2006) comprised of a sample of ninety-eight participants (age range twelve to sixteen years) who had some form of a specific learning disability. Participants were divided into four groups, according to the nature of the intervention. Group 1 received an adapted coping program; Group 2 received the teacher feedback program (that is, each student received individual feedback) as well as the adapted BOC program; Group 3 received teacher feedback only; and Group 4 was the control group. Additionally, there was a two-month follow-up of the program.

Analysis of pre- and postprogram and two- month follow-up data were undertaken for all measures using one-way between-group analyses of covariance where the means were adjusted for preprogram levels for each group. The analyses investigated the difference in the means between the intervention and the control groups.

The coping group reported increased productive coping at postprogram, and this was maintained at follow-up reporting. Adjusted postprogram mean scores were 16.77 for the control group and 17.41 for the coping group. Follow-up adjusted means were slightly lower at 16.07 for the control group but remained at a level similar to postprogram for the coping group at 17.71.

Further analysis of these differences for the coping and combined coping and teacher feedback groups was undertaken to compare means of the productive coping strategies. Increases were found for these groups in the strategies of working hard and focusing on solving the problem. The adjusted control group mean for use of working hard on the problem at postprogram testing was 3.31, the coping group mean was 3.67 ($p < 0.05$), and the combined teacher feedback and coping group mean was 3.71 ($p < 0.05$). This difference was maintained to follow-up testing for the coping group only. The control group adjusted mean at follow-up was 3.30, and the coping group mean was 3.72 ($p < 0.02$). Follow-up responses also indicated that the coping group reported higher use of working at solving the problem compared to the control group. The control group adjusted mean was 2.70 for this strategy, and the coping group mean was 3.39 ($p < 0.001$).

Study three by Kamsner (Frydenberg et al., 2006) participants comprised of 112 students (thirteen to seventeen years of age) who were deemed to be performing poorly academically and were enrolled in a special literacy program. These students subsequently participated in the BOC program. Males reported a significant increased use of investing in close friends, $F (1,112) = 12.55$, $p < 0.01$, and a significant decreased use of wishful thinking, $F (1,112) = 7.66$, $p < 0.01$. Females reported a significant increased use of tension reduction, $F (1,112) = 9.04$, $p <0.01$.

Overall, the implications of these findings are that it is possible to facilitate the development of coping skills in young people, particularly those at risk of depression or those who have learning disabilities. However, the findings are not always consistent and may be related to the particular needs and characteristics of a population of young people. We can help young people to appraise their circumstances differently and help to build up their coping resources. Nevertheless, there are resources over and above coping skills, such as teacher and parent support, that remain important, particularly for certain populations. Thus, for prevention and intervention, it is the building up of both personal and interpersonal resources that is important.

Following development of the pencil and paper version of the BOC program, it was possible to incorporate similar learning objectives into a self-administered CD-ROM version of the program called *Coping for Success* (Frydenberg, 2007).

Two studies evaluated the efficacy of the coping skills programs (BOC and the CD-ROM) in different populations (Frydenberg, Eacott, & Clark, 2008). In the first study by Clark, we were interested in examining the impact of coping skills training on a population of senior secondary school students, ranging in age from fifteen to eighteen years, with a mean age of 16.8 years, who were deemed to have few resources. It had been established in previous studies that adolescents who have access to few resources are more likely to use nonproductive coping strategies and are particularly vulnerable to stress (McKenzie & Frydenberg, 2004; Wojcik, McKenzie, Frydenberg, & Poole, 2004). This is all the more so for senior school students who face many stressors in their final years of high school, such as high expectations of academic success by parents, teachers, and society (Metilkovic, 2007), while trying to complete their studies and are also impacted by other factors, such as financial or family pressure, trauma, or illness (physical or mental). Out of 206 students (75 male and 131 female) from a senior secondary government school in metropolitan Melbourne, Australia, students who scored in the lowest quartile on the modified version of the Conservation of Resources Evaluation (M-CORE; McKenzie & Frydenberg, 2004) were classified to be in the lowest resourced group (n = 52). This select population (n = 38) was placed into either the Experimental (n = 16) or the Wait List (control) group (n = 16). The M-CORE is a forty-eight-item questionnaire that assesses identification of resources and evaluates the impact of loss or gain of resources. Examples of items include having a stable family, achieving at school, having adequate food, having friends, and so on. For each item, respondents were required to rate four questions according to the following:

Are these resources important in your life? (1 = always, 2 = sometimes, 3 = never)
How much of this item do you have? (1 = none to 5 = a lot)
How stressful would it be to lose this item? (1 = no stress, to 5 = great stress)
If you gained on this item, what effect would it have? (1 = none, to 5 = great impact).

Students in the lowest quartile based on scores from the "Have Resources" scale were identified as low in resources.

The Experimental group completed the *Coping for Success* CD-ROM. Both groups completed the ACS two weeks prior to the program being implemented and postprogram. In addition, the experimental group completed the CFS evaluation form.

To assess the effects of the intervention program, gains and losses in coping style scores for the experimental and control groups from preintervention to postintervention were calculated. The changes in the reported use of coping styles from preintervention to postintervention were significant for the following nonproductive strategies: ignoring the problem, reducing tension, not coping, self-blaming, and keeping to self, where frequency of use decreased. Encouragingly, use of the productive coping strategies were also increasing in the expected direction. In the qualitative responses, the experimental group indicated an increase in their knowledge and understanding of coping strategies. Students also reported that they would recommend the *Coping for Success* program to other senior high school students.

The second of these studies by Eacott (Frydenberg et al., 2008) was conducted in a rural setting with two cohorts of students aged fifteen to sixteen years, fifty in 2006, and sixty in 2007. The sample comprised 53 males and 64 females and 97.5 percent were Anglo-Australian. Students identified as low in resources, based on scores from the M-CORE, were of particular interest in terms of their response to the program. A total of thirty students were identified as low in resources. Again, pre- and posttesting with the ACS (Frydenberg & Lewis, 1993a) was used to evaluate the program. All students participated in the BOC program.

The eighty-item Adolescent Coping Scale (ACS) – Specific Form (Frydenberg & Lewis 1993a) has each item rated on a five-point Likert scale according to use; higher scores indicate higher frequency of use. The M-CORE (McKenzie & Frydenberg, 2004) was used to assess students' possession of relevant resources and the ACS (Frydenberg & Lewis, 1993a) to measure pre- and postchanges in coping. A selection of students from Study 1 and all participants from Study 2 responded to qualitative questions after completing the program.

To investigate how participants responded to the program according to their level of resources, the students were categorized according to reported ownership of resources. Groups were formed on the basis of quartiles, where four groups were identified: Group 1 (low resources) represented the lowest quartile (N = 30), and Group 4 (high resources) the highest (N = 29). Group 2 (low average resources) and Group 3 (high average resources) represented the middle band (N = 30 and N = 29 respectively). A series of analyses were run to examine the relationship between level of identified resources and responses to the program using coping gain scores. Significant group differences between Groups 1 and 4, the low and high resource groups, were found for gains on reference to others coping, where the low resource group reported significant increases in use of professional help.

Again, of particular interest in that study were those students who were low in resources. The low resource group made particular gains in being able to turn to others for professional help when required. Six months following the students' participation in the ten-session CD-ROM version of the coping program, the at-risk group members maintained their reduction in nonproductive coping but felt they would benefit from further intervention. Over 80 percent of the students indicated that it is helpful to be reminded of the coping skills that they had learned twelve months earlier, highlighting that in addition to one-off interventions there is benefit from providing booster sessions.

The BOC program was adapted for a group of adolescents with Type 1 diabetes to include information and motivational sessions targeting that particular population. The BOC program was evaluated in a randomized control trial with seventy-nine young people (age thirteen to sixteen years) being offered the program and seventy-seven being offered standard care in a randomized controlled trial. The primary outcome measure was glycemic control at three and twelve months posttreatment, and secondary measures were stress, self-efficacy, and quality of life at three and twelve months. While participation in the intervention arm was poor, with only thirty participants (38 percent) attending all five BOC sessions (which were equivalent to the ten-session regular BOC program) and there being little evidence of differences in glycemic control between the intervention and control group at either time point, the intervention group had greater self-efficacy than the control group at three- and twelve-month follow-up as well as higher quality of life at three months. Although the program did not improve glycemic control in youth with type 1 diabetes, it showed promise for improving psychosocial well-being when all BOC sessions offered (five sessions with two-hours of contact time) were attended (Serlachius et al., 2014).

Families Coping Program

Initially in the Early Years Coping project, we identified preschool children's coping responses and matched these with parent understandings of their children's coping responses. We then developed visual images of challenging situations and the age-appropriate coping strategies. The visual representations of young people's concerns and coping were trialed with children, parents, and teachers. The Early Years Coping Cards comprise a set of Situation Cards that depict the following situations: "losing something or someone special," "saying goodbye to someone you love," "being in trouble with an adult," "scared of the dark," "afraid of trying something new," "being teased or bullied," "being left out by your friends," "broken toy," and "getting hurt." The set of cards also includes Coping Cards that depict both productive and nonproductive coping strategies. The productive coping strategies include "think happy thoughts," "hug a toy," "play," "help others," "talk to an adult," and "work hard." The nonproductive coping strategies include "worry," "run away," "hide," "scream," "complain of pain," "keep feelings to self," and "blame yourself."

Having developed the tools to teach coping skills to children and parents, it was then possible to incorporate these skills into a universal parenting program. The content of the parenting program, *Families Coping* (Frydenberg, 2015), incorporates positive psychology, communication, and coping skills as well as an introduction to mindfulness.

We have evaluated the program on numerous occasions including in 2013 (Gulliford, Frydenberg, Deans, & Liang, 2015) with fourteen parents and again in 2014 with an additional nine parents added to the sample. The data were analyzed to consider whether when both parents participated there were different outcomes (Thomson, 2014). Parents rated their children's coping on the CCS and their own coping on the CSA pre- and postprogram. Additionally, parents responded to five open questions postprogram to provide a qualitative response of their experience of the program. The participant group was comprised of fourteen parents of preschoolers in an early learning setting located in the inner-metropolitan Melbourne area. Parents were provided with effective communication skills, developed an understanding of their own coping and that of their children, and learned how to engage their child actively in shared conversations about coping. To assess change, a mixed methods design was employed, where parents completed pre- and postprogram paper and pencil surveys and open-ended responses. Parents reported greater use of productive coping and a concurrent reduction in nonproductive coping skills. Despite there being no statistically significant change in child coping or parent and child well-being, written responses indicated that most parents perceived a trend toward the development of more positive parenting practices and use of productive coping by their child, as well as some aspect of improvement in both parent and

Figure 26.3. *Overview of the five sessions comprising the Families Coping Parenting Program.*

Session 1 *Positive Psychology of Parenting*	• History and core principles of positive psychology and positive parenting. • Family health and well-being. • Parents review subjective well-being and personal strengths.
Coping with Stress in the Family	• Everyday stresses associated with family life. • Social learning theory and the transactional model of stress and coping. • Parenting styles and the building blocks of healthy and happy families.
Session 2 *Parents Dealing with Difficult Situations*	• How adult coping can be operationalized. • Productive and nonproductive coping. • Social learning and what it means to cope as a parent. • Parents examine their own styles of coping by reflecting on their CSA profiles specific to the parenting role.
Everyday Worries and Anxieties of Children	• Ages and stages of social emotional development. • Children's worries and how they cope. • How to help children identify stressors and the physical symptoms of stress in the body.
Session 3 *Listening to Children: The Neuroscience of Communication*	• Neuroscience of communication • Reflective listening and barriers to communication. • How to respond to children's concerns and worries in a helpful way.
Purposeful Behavior of Children: When Assertiveness Helps	• Self-reflection of own parenting style as parents explore the skill of assertiveness. • Understanding children's behavior, needs, and wants.
Session 4 *How Children Deal with their Worries and Talking about Challenging Situations with Children*	• Open questioning and reflective listening as helpful communication tools. • The Early Years Coping cards

Figure 26.3. (*cont.*)

Collaborative Problem Solving	• Problem solving; a core skill that can be drawn on in diverse contexts. • Applying the skill to their own problems and children's problems. • How problem solving can be used with children as a collaborative process.
Session 5 *Mindfulness as a Way of Achieving Well-being*	• Origins of mindfulness and contemporary evidence-based applications in relation to well-being. • Mindfulness activities and resources to benefit both the child and their parent.
Putting It Together	• Core messages from the five sessions are drawn together. • Parents reflect on their personal experiences from during program in relation to parenting, coping, and well-being for both themselves and their child. • Parents share highlights and areas they will continue to focus on to improve family life.

child well-being. Thomson also employed a mixed methods design in which parents completed pre- and postprogram questionnaires (including the CSA) and an open-ended question on their perception of coping and well-being change upon program completion. Results were considered with respect to gender and partner attendance. A one-way repeated-measures multiple analysis of variance (RM-MANOVA) showed a significance increase in one productive parenting style (dealing with the problem), a significant decrease in nonproductive parent coping, and a significant increase in parent well-being. Comparison of results between gender and partner attendance groups showed minimal differences in program effectiveness. Qualitative data mostly confirmed the key findings.

What We Have Learned

We know from our work in Australia, and that of others, that coping can be meaningfully measured across the lifespan. We have firmly established that both in the adult and adolescent populations there are age, gender, and cultural differences in coping. Those who are high in resources are most likely to cope productively. There are some family patterns of coping, with some similarities but many differences. For example, mothers and fathers are more likely to use problem solving than their children, and daughters are more likely to use tension reduction than their parents. While both problem- and emotion-focused coping are used simultaneously, the more emotion-focused coping that is used, the less successful the coping. Ultimately, it is the belief in one's capacity, such as problem-solving efficacy, that is important rather than the capacity itself. Well-being is associated with a use of productive coping and a reduced use of nonproductive coping, as is school connectedness. When it comes to aggression, reactive aggressive young people are more inclined to use nonproductive coping strategies than proactively aggressive young people. Cyberbullying is responded to differently by boys and girls, with boys more likely to ignore the problem and girls more likely to worry, blame themselves, and resort to tension-reduction strategies.

While there is no right or wrong coping, there are ways to review one's coping and change it to achieve the best outcomes. Generally, it is about reducing the use of nonproductive coping strategies and increasing the use of productive ones. Whether this is done in a self-help format or through a universal or targeted program for a group or for an individual, there are benefits to be gained. The benefits can be achieved through the building up of a pool of coping resources for occasions when the individual is challenged and needs to draw upon coping strategies that they have in store, that is, resilience. Universal and targeted programs provide the opportunity to be proactive. Parenting programs that incorporate coping skills have been demonstrated to be a helpful way of enhancing parents' confidence, well-being, and relationship with their children. It is an ideal way to strengthen parent–child relationships and to be a tool for prevention and scaffolding against difficulties in the later years.

Conclusions

From more than twenty years of research, we have learned that coping is a highly useful construct. Having a theory and model to work with and being able to measure the elements enables communication and reflection to occur so as to enhance healthy development across the lifespan. Coping skills can be learned. A coping skills program such as the BOC can be adapted for particular groups. And at least in the school setting, when a universal program is implemented, at-risk students benefit most. Professional psychologists or an instructor who is supported by a psychologist get the best results. Booster or refresher sessions are important for changes to be maintained.

Our understanding of coping in recent years has grown, and there is growing evidence of what works and what does not, so it has become timely to incorporate coping skills into parent programs. It is possible to provide parents with tools so that they can achieve helpful coping and maintain their level of well-being and at the same time increase the well-being of their children. To date, we have done this most successfully in the early years, where it is likely to have the greatest impact for prevention and early intervention.

References

ABS (Australian Bureau of Statistics) (2014a). *Schools, Australia, 2013* (cat. no. 4221.0). Retrieved from www.abs.gov.au

ABS (Australian Bureau of Statistics) (2014b). *Mental Health of Young People* (cat. no. 4840.0.55.001). Retrieved from www.abs.gov.au

ACARA (Australian Curriculum, Assessment and Reporting Authority) (2013). *National Report on Schooling in Australia 2011*. Sydney: ACARA.

Aldwin, C. M. (2007). *Stress, Coping, and Development: An Integrative Perspective*. Foreword by Werner, E. E. New York: Guilford Press,

APA (American Psychological Association) (2014). Guidelines for prevention in psychology. *American Psychologist* 69(3): 285–96. doi: 10.1037/a0034569

Ayers, T. S., Sandier, I. N., West, S. G., & Roosa, M. W. (1996). A dispositional and situational assessment of children's coping: testing alternative models of coping. *Journal of Personality* 64: 923–58.

Band, E. B., & Weisz, J. R. (1988). How to feel better when it feels bad: children's perspectives on coping with everyday stress. *Developmental Psychology* 24: 247–53.

Bandura, A. (2012). On the functional properties of self-perceived efficacy revisited. *Journal of Management* 38: 9–44. doi: 10.1177/0149206311410606

Beran, T., & Li, Q. (2004). *Is Cyber-Harassment a Significant Problem? A Report on Children's Experiences*. Calgary: University of Calgary.

Coggan, C., Bennett, S., Hooper, R., & Dickinson, P. (2003). Association between bullying and mental health status in New Zealand adolescents. *International Journal of Mental Health Promotion* 5: 16–22.

Compas, B. E. (1987). Coping with stress during childhood and adolescence. *Psychological Bulletin* 101: 393–403.

Compas, B. E., Malcarne, V. L., & Fondacaro, K. M. (1988). Coping with stressful events on older children and young adolescents. *Journal of Consulting and Clinical Psychology* 56: 405–11.

Cox, T., Gotts., G., Boot. N., & Kerr, J. (1985). Physical exercise, employee fitness and the management of health at work. *Work and Stress* 2: 71–7.

Deans, J., Frydenberg, E., & Tsurutani, H. (2010). Operationalising social and emotional coping competencies in kindergarten children. *New Zealand Research in ECE Journal* 13: 113–24.

DoHA (Department of Health and Ageing) (2010). *National Mental Health Report 2010: Summary of 15 Years of Reform in Australia's Mental Health Services under the National Mental Health Strategy 1993–2008*. Canberra: Department of Health and Ageing.

Frydenberg, E. (2007). *Coping for Success*. Melbourne: Australian Council for Educational Research.

Frydenberg, E. (2008). *Adolescent Coping: Advances in Theory, Research and Practice*. London: Routledge.

Frydenberg, E. (2010). *Think Positively: A Course for Developing Coping Skills in Adolescents*. London: Continuum.

Frydenberg, E. (2014). Coping research: historical background, links with emotion, and new research directions on adaptive processes. *Australian Journal of Psychology* 66: 82–92. doi: 10.1111/ajpy.12051

Frydenberg, E. (2015). *Families Coping*. Melbourne: Australian Council for Educational Research.

Frydenberg, E., & Brandon, C. (2007). *The Best of Coping: Instructors Manual*. Melbourne: Oz Child.

Frydenberg, E., Bugalski, K., Firth, N., Kamsner, S., & Poole, C. (2006). Teaching young people to cope: benefits and gains for at risk students. *Australian and Developmental Psychologist* 23: 91–110.

Frydenberg, E., Care, E., Freeman, E., & Chan, E. (2009). Interrelationships between coping, school connectedness and wellbeing. *Australian Journal of Education* 17: 338–45.

Frydenberg, E., & Deans, J. (2011). *The Early Years Coping Cards*. Melbourne: Australian Council for Educational Research.

Frydenberg, E., Eacott, C., & Clark, N. (2008). Teaching coping skills: from distress to success. *Prevention Researcher* 15(4): 8–12.

Frydenberg, E., & Lewis, R. (1991). Adolescent coping styles and strategies: is there functional and dysfunctional coping? *Australian Journal of Guidance and Counselling* 1: 1–8.

Frydenberg, E., & Lewis, R. (1993a). *Manual: The Adolescent Coping Scale*. Melbourne: Australian Council for Educational Research.

Frydenberg, E., & Lewis, R. (1993b). Boys play sport and girls turn to others: age, gender and ethnicity as determinants of coping. *Journal of Adolescence*, 16: 253–66.

Frydenberg, E., & Lewis, R. (1994). Coping with different concerns: consistency and variation in coping strategies used by adolescents. *Australian Psychologist* 29: 45–8.

Frydenberg, E., & Lewis, R. (1997). *Coping Scale for Adults*. Melbourne: Australian Council for Educational Research.

Frydenberg, E., & Lewis, R. (1999). Things don't get better just because you're older: a case for facilitating reflection. *British Journal of Educational Psychology* 69: 81–94.

Frydenberg, E., & Lewis, R. (2000). Teaching coping to adolescents: when and to whom. *American Educational Research Journal* 37: 727–45.

Frydenberg, E., & Lewis, R. (2002a). Adolescent wellbeing: building young people's resources. In Frydenberg, E. (ed.), *Beyond Coping: Meeting Goals, Visions and Challenges*. New York: Oxford University Press, pp.175–94.

Frydenberg, E., & Lewis, R. (2002b). Do managers cope productively? A comparison between Australian middle level managers and adults in the general community. *Journal of Managerial Psychology* 17 (8).: 640–54.

Frydenberg, E., & Lewis, R. (2009). The relationship between wellbeing, negative avoidant coping, and active coping in a large sample of Australians adolescents. *Psychological Reports*: 745–58.

Frydenberg, E., & Lewis, R. (2011). *Adolescent Coping Scale-2*. Melbourne: Australian Council for Educational Research.

Frydenberg. E., & Lewis, R. (2014). *Coping Scale for Adults CSA-2)*. Melbourne: Australian Council for Educational Research.

Gordon, R. (1983). An operational classification of disease prevention. *Public Health Reports* 98: 107–9.

Gordon, R. (1987). An operational classification of disease prevention. In Steinberg, J. A., & Silverman, M. M. (eds.), *Preventing Mental Disorders*. Rockville, MD: Department of Health and Human Services, pp. 20–6.

Gresham, F. M., Macmillan, D. L., & Bocian, K. M. (1996). Learning disabilities, low achievement and mild retardation: more alike than different? *Journal of Learning Disabilities* 29: 570–81.

Gulliford, H., Frydenberg, E., Deans, J., & Liang (2015). Teaching coping skills in the context of positive parenting. *Australian Psychologist*. doi: 10.1111/ap.12121

Hobfoll, S. E. (1989). Conservation of resources, a new attempt at conceptualising stress. *American Psychologist* 44: 513–24.

Hobfoll, S. E. (2010). Conservation of resources theory: its implication for stress, health, and resilience. In Folkman, S. (ed.), *The Oxford Handbook of Stress, Health, and Coping*. Oxford, UK: Oxford University Press, pp. 127–47. doi: 10.1093/oxfordhb/9780195375343.013.0007

Larkins, G., & Frydenberg, E. (2004). Two types of aggression and the relationship with coping: implications for educational practice. In Frydenberg, E. (ed.), *Thriving, Surviving or Going Under: Coping with Everyday Lives*. In series, Research on stress and coping in education. Greenwich, CT: Information Age, pp. 135–66.

Lazarus, R. S. (1966). *Psychological Stress and the Coping Process*. New York: McGraw-Hill.

Lazarus, R. S. (1993). Coping theory and research: past, present and future. *Psychosomatic Medicine* 55: 234–47.

Lazarus, R. S., & Folkman, S. (1984). *Stress, Appraisal and Coping*. New York: Springer.

Lewis, R., & Frydenberg, E. (2002). Concomitants of failure to cope: what we should teach adolescents. *British Journal of Educational Psychology* 72: 419–31.

Lodge, J., & Frydenberg, E. (2007). Profiles of adolescent coping and cyber-bullying: insights for school practitioners. *Australian Educational and the Developmental Psychologist* 24: 45–58.

McKenzie, V., & Frydenberg, E. (2004). Young people and their resources. In Frydenberg, E. (ed.), *Thriving, Surviving, or Going Under: Coping with Everyday Lives*. Greenwich, CT: Information Age, pp. 79–108.

Metilkovic, J. (2007). Exam pressures rattle students. *Herald Sun*, October 19, p. 11.

Pallant, J. (1998). Perceived control of internal states. (Unpublished Ph.D thesis). University of Melbourne, Melbourne.

Reynolds, W. M. (2001). *Reynolds Adolescent Adjustment Screening Inventory*. Odessa, FL: Psychological Assessment Resources.

Roubeni, S., De Haene, L., Keatley, E., Shah, N., & Rasmussen, A. (2015). "If we can't do it, our children will do it one day": a qualitative study of West African immigrant parents' losses and educational aspirations for their children. *American Educational Research Journal* 52(2): 275–305. dx.doi.org/10.3102/0002831215574576

Seiffge-Krenke, I., & Shulman, S. (1990). Coping style in adolescence: a cross cultural study. *Journal of Cross-Cultural Psychology* 21: 351–77.

Seligman, M. E. (1995). *The Optimistic Child*. New South Wales, Australia: Random House Australia.

Serlachius, A., Scratch, S. E., Northam, E. A., Frydenberg, E., Lee, K. J., & Cameron, F. J. (2014). A randomized controlled trial of cognitive behaviour therapy to improve glycaemic control and psychosocial wellbeing in adolescents with type 1 diabetes. *Journal of Health Psychology*. doi: 10.1177/1359105314547940.

Simeonsson, R. J. (1991). Primary, secondary, and tertiary prevention in early intervention. *Journal of Early Intervention* 15: 124–34.

Skinner, E. A., Edge, K., Altman, J., & Sherwood, H. (2003). Searching for the structure of coping: a review and critique of category systems for classifying ways of coping. *Psychological Bulletin* 129: 216–69.

Stark, L. J., Spirito, A., Williams, C. A., & Guevremont, D. C. (1989). Common problems and coping strategies I: findings with normal adolescents. *Journal of Abnormal Child Psychology* 17: 203–12.

Thomson, S. (2014). Parents coping: developing coping skills and enhanced wellbeing in a parenting program. (Unpublished master's thesis). University of Melbourne, Melbourne Graduate School of Education.

Tsurutani, H. (2009). A multi-informant approach to understanding the coping behaviours of preschool children: a comparative study of teachers' and parents' observations. (Unpublished master's thesis). University of Melbourne, Melbourne Graduate School of Education.

Valas, H. (1999). Students with learning disabilities and low-achieving students: peer acceptance, loneliness, self-esteem, and depression. *Social Psychology of Education* 3: 173–92.

Wojcik, Z., McKenzie, V., Frydenberg, E., & Poole, C. (2004). Resources loss, gain, investment, and coping in adolescents. *Australian Educational and Developmental Psychologist* 19: 52–77.

Yeo, K., Frydenberg, E., Northam, E., & Deans, J. (2014). Coping with stress among preschool children and associations with anxiety level and controllability of situations. *Australian Journal of Psychology* 66: 93–101. doi: 10.1111/ajpy.12047

27 Prevention of Drug Abuse in Chinese Adolescents in Hong Kong

The Role of Positive Youth Development

Daniel T. L. Shek

Drug Abuse in Hong Kong

Although there are many definitions of the term "drug abuse," it is commonly conceived as the use of drugs not for medicinal purpose and where the related drugs are usually not prescribed by medical professionals. Besides, such drugs create physical and/or psychological dependence over time. According to the National Institute on Drug Abuse (2014) in the United States, drugs of abuse include drugs that are sold legally (such as tobacco, alcohol, and drugs sold over the counters) and illegally (such as heroin and cocaine). In the field of substance abuse, drugs of abuse commonly refer to the use of alcohol, tobacco, and other drugs (ATOD) that "harms or threatens to harm the physical, mental or social well-being of an individual, in doses above or for periods beyond those normally regarded as therapeutic" (Central Registry of Drug Abuse, 2013, p. 3). In this chapter, we review the prevalence of smoking, drinking, and abuse of illicit drugs in Hong Kong.

Hong Kong is an international financial center situated on the southern coast of China. In mid-2013, the population of Hong Kong was 7.1875 million. The majority of the population was ethnic Chinese. According to the 2011 Hong Kong Population Census, the population of adolescents (aged from fifteen to twenty-four) was approximately 861,400 (Census and Statistics Department, 2013). After reunification, the education system in Hong Kong was changed from the British system (i.e., five years of high school education, two years of matriculation study, and three years of university study) to the North American system (i.e., three years of junior secondary school education, three years of senior secondary school education, and four years of university education) starting from 2006. Historically, Hong Kong was ceded to Britain after the Opium War in the nineteenth century, and the sovereignty of Hong Kong was handed over to China in 1997. Under the Basic Law, Hong Kong is a Special Administrative Region that has a capitalistic economy and a common law legal system. Probably because of the Opium War, people in Hong Kong generally hold conservative attitudes toward substance abuse.

Regarding abuse of illicit drugs, several observations can be highlighted. First, compared to Western societies, data based on the Central Registry of Drug

Abuse in Hong Kong and school surveys on adolescent substance abuse in Hong Kong suggest that substance abuse is not as serious as in the West (Shek, 2006a; Shek & Leung, 2014). Based on the survey of substance abuse among Hong Kong students in 2011–12 school year, lifetime prevalence rates were 1.1 percent, 2.3 percent, and 3.3 percent for upper primary, secondary school, and other postsecondary school students, respectively (Narcotics Division, 2013). Second, ketamine abuse among Hong Kong adolescents is the highest in the global context. Ketamine is surgical anesthetic that can produce a dissociative state, and prolonged use can lead to damage in the neural and urinary systems. Third, the duration between the first time when an individual takes drugs and the first time the individual seeks help has increased. Finally, as Hong Kong is close to China, cross-border substance abuse is a source of concern.

Studies investigating the problem of alcohol use in Hong Kong adolescents are sparse (Lou & Shek, 2006). In most related studies, drinking was examined in the context of substance use or delinquent behavior (e.g., Cheung, 2014; Lee & Tsang, 2004; Lou & Shek, 2006; Shek & Ma, 2011), with a few studies focusing exclusively on youth drinking in Hong Kong (Griffiths et al., 2006; Kim et al., 2009; Lo & Globetti, 2000; Wang, Ho, & Lam, 2013).

For the prevalence of drinking among adolescents, Lo and Globetti (2000) conducted a study on 101 high school adolescents and found that about 36 percent of females and 43 percent of males had consumed alcohol in the preceding year. In another study involving 15,448 adolescents, Lee, Tsang, Lee, and To (2001) showed that 16.0 percent and 7.7 percent of prevocational school students reported having current alcohol use and episodic heavy drinking, respectively, while 11.3 percent and 4.0 percent of adolescents in mainstream schools reported having current alcohol use and episodic heavy drinking, respectively. Based on the responses of 26,111 students aged from ten to nineteen, Lee and Tsang (2004) reported that 45.2 percent reported having at least one drink of alcohol during their lifetime, 9.4 percent currently reported using alcohol, and 3.4 percent reported having episodic heavy drinking.

Some recent studies showed that there has been a growing concern about alcohol consumption in secondary school students (Ong, Wong, Lee, Holroyd, & Huang, 2013; Wang et al., 2013). Based on 3,328 Secondary 1 students (grade 7 students with an average age of twelve years old), Shek and Ma (2012) revealed that 28 percent of the respondents had consumed alcohol in the past year. Based on the longitudinal data, findings from Shek and Leung's (2014) study showed that drinking gradually increased in the adolescent years.

Alcohol consumption in university students has also been examined. In a study with 1,197 undergraduates, Abdullah, Fielding, and Hedley (2002) showed that 61 percent reported current and past use of alcohol. In another study based on 2,630 first-year university students, Griffiths et al. (2006) reported that 62 percent of respondents reported that they had "ever drank" alcohol, and 7 percent reported having engaged in binge drinking. Using longitudinal data collected from 2,630 university students, Kim and colleagues (2009) showed that the percentage of respondents who reported "ever drinking" increased from 71.8 percent to 86.6 percent among men and 53.0 percent to 80.6 percent among women from the first year to the second year. Moreover, 7.0 percent of males and 1.6 percent of females in the second year reported at least one symptom of alcohol abuse in the past year.

Regarding smoking, studies in Hong Kong generally showed that the smoking rates increased with age in adolescents. The proportion of adolescents who had ever tried smoking under fourteen years old was over 10 percent, and the proportion was over 15 percent in those who were above sixteen years old (Lai, Ho, & Lam, 2004; Lam, Chung, Betson, Wong, & Hedley, 1998; Lam, Stewart & Ho, 2001; Lam et al, 2005; Lee & Tsang, 2004). These findings suggest that the prevalence rates of smoking in young people in Hong Kong were relatively lower than those reported in the West.

Positive Youth Development and Adolescent Drug Abuse

While there are many approaches that have been used to conceptualize, explain, treat, and prevent adolescent drug abuse, a growing number of researchers have used the positive youth development (PYD) approach to explain how adolescent substance abuse can be prevented. PYD focuses on the talents, assets, and potentials in young people (Benson, Scales, Hamilton, & Sesma, 2006; Catalano, Berglund, Ryan, Lonczak, & Hawkins, 2004). PYD places emphasis on the intrinsic competencies (including both intra- and interpersonal competencies) that should be nurtured and developed through holistic and systematic training.

In an early review conducted by Hawkins, Lishner, Catalano, and Howard (1986), it was proposed that PYD attributes, particularly behavioral and interpersonal attributes, had influence on prevention of substance abuse in the Western context. In recent decades, there is growing evidence from Asia and North America that adolescents who possessed PYD attributes were less likely to engage in substance abuse risk behaviors (Flay et al., 2004; Lerner et al., 2005; Oman et al., 2004; Phelps et al., 2007; Shek & Ma, 2012; Shek & Yu, 2012a; Tebes et al., 2007; Zimmerman, Phelps, & Lerner, 2008). Catalano et al. (2012) reviewed effective adolescent prevention in the field and identified several effective programs in North America (Botvin, Griffin, & Nicholas, 2006; Griffin, Botvin, & Nichols, 2004) and Hong Kong (Shek & Ma, 2012; Shek & Yu, 2012) contexts.

Several PYD attributes have been found to prevent adolescent substance abuse. First, sound decision-making skills were negatively related to substance abuse in U.S. adolescents (e.g., Tebes et al., 2007). Second, good self-esteem might help adolescents stay away from drugs. For example, in a cross-national longitudinal study involving adolescents in the United States and New Zealand, higher self-esteem was negatively related to the risk of adolescent substance abuse (Donnellan, Trzesniewski, Robins, Moffitt, & Caspi, 2005). Third, positive hope and goals for the future were negatively related to substance abuse in

U.S. adolescents (Oman et al., 2004). Fourth, bonding (such as parental support and caring mentors) was found possibly to help U.S. adolescents overcome adversity and improve their self-efficacy while reducing their risk of engaging in substance abuse behavior (Nash, McQueen, & Bray, 2005; Scales et al., 2005).

There are research findings showing that PYD can help to reduce adolescent drinking behavior. In Caplan et al.'s (1992) study, they implemented a structured PYD program that provided social competence sessions and substances/health information for sixth and seventh graders in the United States. They found that social competence significantly reduced excessive drinking rather than experimental drinking. In the School Health and Alcohol Harm Reduction Project (SHAHRP), McBride, Farringdon, Midford, Meuleners, and Phillips (2004) showed that higher levels of emotional competence minimized adolescent drinking in Australian youths.

Studies also showed that psychosocial competencies were related to adolescent drinking in Hong Kong. There are studies showing that low self-control and impaired self-esteem significantly predicted strong permissiveness toward heavy use of alcohol and alcohol abuse among high school students (Bagley, 1992; Cheung, 2014). Drinking behavior (i.e., episodic heavy alcohol drinking) of secondary school students was positively related to their emotional and behavior problems, such as hopelessness, depression, and suicidal behavior (Bagley, 1992; Lam, 2010; Lee et al., 2001, 2009). Based on a study of 6,776 students, Yuen et al. (2006) showed that avoidance of excessive drinking was correlated with higher positive youth development indexed by self-realization, leadership and teamwork, emotional and social wellness, interests and life goals, and interpersonal relationships.

With specific reference to tobacco, findings showed that adolescent smoking was related to a number of positive youth development attributes. First, negative relationship between adolescent smoking and psychosocial competence in U.S. adolescents was reported (e.g., Scheier, Botvin, Diaz, & Griffin, 1999). It has been shown that behavioral and cognitive self-management skills were negatively related to adolescent smoking in the United States (Griffin, Scheier, Botvin, & Diaz, 2001), Hong Kong (Lam et al., 2001), and Hungary (Piko, Luszczynska, Gibbons, & Teközel, 2005). Although results from Pederson, Koval, and O'Connor's (1997) study did not show the relationship between the total score of coping strategy and smoking behavior in Canadian adolescents, nonsmokers showed better problem-solving skills than did the smokers. Research studies have also shown that decision-making skills and personal efficacy influenced refusal assertiveness, which further affected intention to smoke in future among U.S. adolescents (Epstein, Griffin, & Botvin, 2000).

Some studies showed that cigarette use was associated with emotional stress and management, where higher negative emotionality was associated with smoking more cigarettes while positive affect was associated with less smoking in adolescents in Iran (Anbari et al., 2014) and Slovakia (Veselska, Geckova, Reijneveld, & van Dijk, 2011). Some researchers argued that adolescents used smoking to cope with stress and negative emotions (Veselska et al., 2011).

Regarding the role of social competence, although the competence to resist substance and peer pressure was negatively related to smoking in U.S. adolescents (Epstein et al., 2000; Jackson, Henriksen, Dickinson, & Levine, 1997), social assertiveness and self-efficacy in social interactions were found to be positively related to smoking in United States (Lillehoj, Trudeau, Spoth, & Wickrama, 2004) and Slovakian adolescents (Veselska et al., 2011).

Adolescent smoking behavior was also negatively related to future life orientation, assertion, self-determination, self-esteem, positive self-image, resilience, spirituality, and general youth development qualities in different countries, including Iran (Anbari et al., 2014), Greenland (Edvardsson, Geisler, & Lendahls, 2014), the United States (Ladapo et al., 2014; Simons-Morton & Haynie, 2003), Hungary (Piko et al., 2005), and Slovakia (Veselska et al., 2009). Life satisfaction and subjective well-being were also negatively related to the smoking behavior in the United States (Griffin et al., 2001; Zullig, Valois, Huebner, Oeltmann, & Drane, 2001) and Hong Kong (Sun & Shek, 2010, 2013) contexts. Schwartz et al. (2010) examined the 4H program (Head, Heart, Hands, and Health) on substance abuse prevention with 5,305 U.S. middle-class children (grade 5 to grade 10) and found that the girls in the program had a significant reduction in tobacco use.

The Project P.A.T.H.S. in Hong Kong

Initial Phase of the Project (P.A.T.H. I)

Despite the growing adolescent developmental problems in Hong Kong (Shek & Leung, 2013; Shek, Sun, & Merrick, 2012a), particularly adolescent substance abuse, there are very few validated adolescent prevention and positive youth development programs in Hong Kong. Among the available prevention programs, they are rather scattered without strong theoretical foundations. Besides, most of them are deficit-oriented programs aiming at reduction of adolescent problems. Most important of all, evaluation utilizing multiple strategies, including long-term evaluation, is almost nonexistent in Hong Kong (Shek & Yu, 2011b).

Against this background, the Hong Kong Jockey Club Charities Trust earmarked H.K. $400 million (roughly equivalent to U.S. $51.2 million) to embark on a 2004 project entitled "P.A.T.H.S. to Adulthood : A Jockey Club Youth Enhancement Scheme" (Project P.A.T.H.S.) to promote holistic development of young people in Hong Kong. The acronym P.A.T.H.S. denotes "Positive Adolescent Training through Holistic Social Programs." With Daniel Shek as the Principal Investigator, a research team was formed with scholars from five universities in Hong Kong serving as co-principal investigators or co-investigators. There were several tasks for the Research Team. First, they developed Chinese and English versions of the program, with twenty hours of programs for each grade in Secondary 1 to Secondary 3 levels (grade 7 to grade 9 in the North American system with students aged from around twelve to fifteen). This is an indigenously developed program utilizing fifteen positive youth development constructs identified in the successful PYD programs (i.e., not translated from programs in the West). Second, the research team developed the training programs and trained the potential program implementers. Third, the team developed training programs for teachers and social workers during the program implementation process. Finally, the research team utilized multiple evaluation strategies to examine the impact of the program. Preceding the Full Implementation Phase (2006–7 to 2008–9 school years) in which more than 250 schools participated in the project, there was an Experimental Implementation Phase in which 52 schools joined to become familiar with the program details and operations. The background details of the study can be found in Shek and Sun (2013a, b).

There were two tiers of programs in the Project P.A.T.H.S. (Tier 1 and Tier 2 programs). For the Tier 1 Program, all Secondary 1 to Secondary 3 students in the participating schools joined the program developed by the research team, with ten to twenty hours of training at each grade (i.e., universal program). For the Tier 2 Program, roughly one-fifth of the students showing greater psychosocial needs at each grade joined the program developed by the school social workers because the problems of the students varied across schools (i.e., selective program). To adopt an evidence-based strategy to develop the program, fifteen adolescent developmental constructs based on successful PYD programs (Catalano et al., 2004) were adopted for the project. These PYD constructs included bonding, resilience, psychosocial competencies (i.e., social competence, emotional competence, cognitive competence, behavioral competence, moral competence, self-determination, spirituality, self-efficacy, clear and positive identity, beliefs in the future, recognition for positive behavior, opportunities for prosocial involvement, and prosocial norms). As the program was conducted in Hong Kong, which is a Chinese society, the application of the constructs was made with particular reference to the Chinese cultural context. It is our assumption that while the PYD constructs covered in the program are universally applicable, their manifestations may differ across cultures. The relationship between these constructs and the Chinese culture can be seen in Shek, Sun, and Merrick (2012b).

As P.A.T.H.S. is a pioneer PYD project in Hong Kong as well as mainland China that also upholds the importance of evidence-based practice, systematic evaluation is a hallmark of the project. Guided by the spirit of triangulation, multiple evaluation strategies were used to examine program effects of the Tier 1 Program, including objective outcome evaluation, subjective outcome evaluation, process evaluation, qualitative evaluation, and repertory grid evaluation. Taken as a whole, evaluation findings collected by different methods revealed that different stakeholders generally had positive views about the Tier 1 Program, program implementers, and benefits of the program (Shek, Ma, & Merrick, 2012). With specific reference to the longitudinal randomized group trial, results showed that compared with the control participants, students in the experimental schools showed better psychosocial competencies and slower development in drug abuse, delinquent behavior, and behavioral intention to engage in problem behavior (Shek & Sun, 2013a, b). The evaluation findings are further presented in the later sections of this chapter.

Extension Phase of the Project (P.A.T.H.S. II)

As there was an overwhelming success in the initial phase of the project and the program gained much recognition from international, regional, and local professionals as well as academic communities, the Hong Kong Jockey Club Charities Trust decided in 2009 to extend the project for another three years, with an additional earmarked grant of H.K. $350 million (approximately equivalent to U.S. $44.8 million). The Project P.A.T.H.S. was extended for another cycle from the 2009–10 to 2011–12 school years. Similar to the initial phase of the project, there were several tasks undertaken by the research team, including implementation of the Tier 1 and Tier 2 programs, arrangement of training programs for social workers and teachers, development of e-learning curriculum and training packages, and development of systematic evaluation. To understand the development of adolescents in Hong Kong, a six-year longitudinal study as part of the P.A.T.H.S. Project focusing on the influence of personal and family factors on adolescent development was conducted to establish a pioneer longitudinal database on Chinese adolescent development in Hong Kong (e.g., Shek, 2013).

Unique Features of Project P.A.T.H.S.

There are several unique features of the Project P.A.T.H.S. in Hong Kong. First, this project is pioneering and groundbreaking in Hong Kong and other Chinese societies. In terms of dosage, it provides sixty hours of universal prevention training on positive youth development in the junior secondary school years based on positive youth development attributes identified in the successful programs. Second, both universal programs (i.e., the Tier 1 Program) and selective programs (i.e., the Tier 2 Program) are included in the project. Third, it is a multiyear positive youth development program spanning from Secondary 1 to Secondary 3. Fourth, more than 280 schools have joined the project and more than 7,000 social workers and teachers were trained in the past decade. Fifth, intersectoral and interdisciplinary collaboration were intrinsic to the project, with the involvement of five universities, different government departments, nongovernmental organizations (NGOs) providing school social work service, and the education sector. The money injected in this project is also substantial. Sixth, a longitudinal evaluation over six years involving the collection of different data from different sources was conducted. Finally, the project has generated many curriculum manuals, training manuals, as well as academic publications recognized by international academic and professional communities that can be downloaded from the project website.[1]

1 www.paths.hk.

Positive Youth Development and Drug Abuse: Insight from P.A.T.H.S. I

As mentioned previously, multiple evaluation strategies were used in P.A.T.H.S I to evaluate the intervention. In particular, a longitudinal evaluation study was conducted, with eight waves of data collected from nineteen experimental schools and twenty-four control schools over five years to assess the long-term impact of the project. At each wave, students responded to measures assessing their use of alcohol, tobacco, ketamine, cannabis, cough mixture, organic solvent, ecstasy, and heroin during the previous six months. While the details of the related analyses can be seen in Shek and Yu (2011a) and Shek and Yu (2012b), a summary of the findings follows.

In an initial study involving six waves of data collected (i.e., Secondary 1 to Secondary 3), Shek and Yu (2011a) found that the participants from the experimental group generally showed slower development in drug abuse as compared to the control students. For example, while the experimental and control groups did not differ at initial status, the growth of ketamine use was faster in the control group than in the experimental group. To further understand the effect of the program, experimental subjects who perceived the program to be beneficial to them were compared with control subjects. Similar to the original findings, control subjects showed faster growth in drug abuse behaviors, including smoking, drinking, and use of illicit drugs (ecstasy, ketamine, cannabis, and heroin).

Based on all eight waves of data collected, Shek and Yu (2012b) reported similar findings. First, using overall substance abuse as an indicator, results showed that while there was no initial difference between the experimental group and the control group participants, control group participants showed a faster rate of increase and a slower rate of deceleration than did the experimental group in substance abuse. Second, the experimental group also performed better than the control group when different types of substance abuse (such as ketamine, cannabis, solvent, ecstasy, and heroin) were used. Finally, in conjunction with the findings based on the previous six waves of data (Shek & Yu, 2011a), results showed that the beneficial effect of the program in preventing drug abuse persisted after Secondary 3 (grade 7 in North American system with the mean age of the students around fifteen years), hence giving support to the long-term effect in preventing these adolescent problem behaviors.

To further understand the impact of the program on substance abuse behavior, the data were reanalyzed by comparing those experimental students who perceived the program to be effective with the control participants. Results showed that experimental participants who expressed positive subjective evaluation about the program showed significantly slower increase in substance abuse behaviors than did the control group participants (Shek & Yu, 2013). Similar to the original analyses, the findings also support the long-term effect of the program in reducing adolescent drug abuse.

Positive Youth Development and Substance Abuse: Insight from P.A.T.H.S. II

In the extension phase of Project P.A.T.H.S., a six-year longitudinal study was conducted to examine the prevalence of substance abuse in the adolescent years and the related psychosocial correlates. Among all secondary schools in Hong Kong (around 400+ schools), 28 randomly selected secondary schools in Hong Kong joined the study. With particular reference to the junior secondary school students, there were 3,325 (mean age = 12.6), 2,904 (mean age = 13.6), and 2,885 (mean age = 14.7) secondary school students who responded to the questionnaire at Waves 1, 2, and 3, respectively. As far as substance abuse was concerned, reported frequencies of using different types of substances over the previous year were assessed, including tobacco, alcohol, ketamine, cannabis, cough mixture, organic solvent, heroin, and pills (such as ecstasy and methaqualone). For the assessment of positive youth development, the Chinese Positive Youth Development Scale (CPYDS) was used to assess positive youth development in the respondents (Shek, Siu, & Lee, 2007). Modeled after the fifteen PYD constructs identified in the successful PYD programs (Catalano et al., 2004), this scale assessed the following attributes: bonding, resilience, cognitive competence, emotional competence, social competence, behavioral competence, moral competence, self-determination, self-efficacy, clear and positive identity, spirituality, beliefs in the future, prosocial norms, prosocial involvement, and recognition for positive behavior. Previous studies have consistently showed that the CPYDS possessed good psychometric properties (Shek & Ma, 2010; Shek et al., 2007).

Based on the three waves of data in the junior secondary school students, Shek and Leung (2014) showed that Wave 1 PYD negatively predicted overall substance abuse, smoking, and drinking at Wave 3. Multiple regression analyses also showed that Wave 1 PYD attributes predicted Wave 3 smoking, drinking, and overall substance abuse. Furthermore, utilizing four waves of data, while PYD at Time 1 (i.e., the baseline assessment) did not predict overall substance abuse, Wave 1 PYD predicted smoking at Wave 4 (Shek & Liang, 2015).

Issues Encountered and Lessons Learned

Since Project P.A.T.H.S. is a pioneering positive youth development program in Hong Kong and mainland China, it is important to consider the related issues and the lessons learned in the project.

Lesson 1: Understand the political context of PYD program development and implementation. At the time when Project P.A.T.H.S. was conceived in 2004, Hong Kong faced major changes in its education and welfare systems. For education, Hong Kong was planning to change the education system from a 5+2+3 format to a 3+3+4 format. That is, secondary and university education would be changed from five years of secondary school education plus two years advanced-level education plus three years of university education to three years of junior secondary school education plus three years of senior secondary school education plus four years of university education. Obviously, frontline teachers and school administrators had skepticism and resistance toward the Project P.A.T.H.S. initially. For the welfare sector, the Project P.A.T.H.S. was viewed as a replacement for the Understanding the Adolescent Project, which had been in the field for quite some time; it also met with resistance from the social workers because they would implement the Tier 1 and Tier 2 programs. Besides, social workers were also stressed by the change in the subvention model in the welfare field to a lump-sum grant system (i.e., salary-based on the midpoint of the salary scale). To reduce the burden of the workers in the education and welfare sectors, two initiatives were carried out. First, an Experimental Implementation Phase involving fifty-two schools was added in the 2005–6 school year so that schools and welfare agencies had more time to prepare for the program. Second, financial assistance given to the schools and welfare agencies was made in a more flexible manner where schools can use the subsidy to hire different professionals to run the program (Shek & Sun, 2012).

Lesson 2: Positive focus instead of negative focus. In the traditional Chinese culture, adolescent misbehavior was a serious matter. If a child misbehaved, it was usually assumed that parents were not doing their part well. As such, it is not easy for parents to "wash the dirty linen in public" ("jia chou bu ke wai yang"). Therefore, if an "antidrug" program is offered at a school, parents usually do not allow their children to join because they simply believe that their children do not have drug problems; they might also be afraid that young people will take drugs if they know more about drugs. Even if their children have drug abuse problem, they usually do not admit to it easily. The same problem applies to schools in Hong Kong. If we run "antidrug" programs, the school principal usually rejects them because he or she will simply say that no students in the school abuse drugs. They may also decline such programs because accepting a drug abuse program easily creates a poor image for the school and invites challenges from parents. Therefore, focusing on positive youth development attributes in the Project P.A.T.H.S. is not stigmatizing because it focuses on the strengths and developmental assets of the students. Some schools joined the project because they realized that the program is not specifically targeted at adolescent developmental problems. Besides, the refocus on strengths in young people is attractive (Shek & Wu, 2013). In short, packaging the program in terms of positive youth development can help to engage schools and parents.

Lesson 3: Inner strengths and developmental assets are appealing. Although Chinese medicine focuses on "treating disease when the problem is not serious" ("bing xiang jian zhong yi"), it is not the case for youth problems in Hong Kong. Typically, youth services in Hong Kong are rather remedial in nature, focusing on social rehabilitation and treatment. While remedial programs are necessary, they have two problems. First, such programs may be too late, as adolescent problems such as drug abuse may create problems that cannot be readily treated. Second, indicative prevention programs are very expensive. Hence, there is a growing call for universal prevention initiatives that can save money and lives in the long run. In the case of the Project P.A.T.H.S., we have spent much effort to publicize this philosophy and its attractiveness. Consistent with the philosophy of Chinese medicine of "strengthening the inner resources" ("gu ben pei yuan"), the Project P.A.T.H.S. is appealing to colleagues in the education and social work contexts. Our experience is that we have to promote this concept and induce a paradigm shift in principals, teachers, social welfare agency administrators, and social workers. One way to do this is to publish work on positive youth development (Shek, 2006b; Shek et al., 2012b).

Lesson 4: There are arguments for developing one's own PYD program. One question we faced at the beginning of the project was whether we should "import" Western PYD programs or develop our own programs (Shek, Ma, & Sun, 2011a). In the Western contexts, there is no shortage of related programs for prevention of substance abuse. Besides, it is more convenient to use Western programs that have been commonly validated. However, we considered several questions during the process. First, was copyright an issue to be addressed? Second, would we be charged and was the program expensive? Third, were the programs developed in the West (which were more individualistic) suitable for Chinese people, who were more collectivistic in their behavior? Finally, did we need to adapt the program, and would the adaptation be extensive? After much discussion within the research team, we eventually decided to develop our own program in Hong Kong. There were several advantages of doing this. First, there would not be any copyright issue. Second, there was no need to pay the publisher. Third, instead of working on adaptation, effort could be put into developing new curriculum materials. Fourth, the curriculum materials could be developed with specific reference to the social and cultural contexts of Hong Kong. Of course, the chief disadvantage of developing an indigenous program is that we were not sure about its effectiveness. To answer the questions on the program's validity, quantitative and qualitative evaluations were carried out.

Lesson 5: Teachers and school social workers within the school are ideal program implementers. Within the school context, a question emerges regarding who should teach the developed program. Primarily, it would be intuitive to argue that teachers should teach the developed program because they are familiar with the students and they can incorporate the PYD program within the formal curriculum. However, there are two difficulties for teachers to teach. First, teachers are usually not trained to conduct experiential learning activities in the Chinese context, such as conducting experiential learning activities for the students. In the traditional Chinese culture, teachers and students occupy very different positions in the relationship. Second, asking teachers to identify the strengths of young people is not easy because of an overemphasis on academic excellence in the Chinese culture. Similarly, there are pros and cons of inviting external social workers to teach. While social workers have flexibility in delivering the program, they usually do not have classroom management skills and knowledge. Besides, since social workers do not come to the school every day, their work is more "airborne" (i.e., engaging workers outside schools to run the program in the school premises) than "marine" (i.e., engaging workers within schools to run the program in the school premises) in nature. After roughly a decade of program implementation, our experience tells us that teachers and school social workers in the school are in a much better position to teach the program. In other words, the effect of "airborne" mode (i.e., external social workers) is relatively less desirable as compared to the "marine" mode (i.e., internal social workers).

Lesson 6: Training is of paramount importance. Our experience in the Project P.A.T.H.S. tells us that training is of paramount importance to program effectiveness. Our conclusion is that even if we have a perfect evidence-based program, it would be a failure if we cannot obtain the support and foster the skills of frontline teachers and school social workers. Before the program was implemented, we put strong emphasis on training professionals to carry out the program. For each grade, workers had to join a twenty-hour training program. According to Shek and Wai (2008), twelve principles were used to design the training programs: theory-based training programs, help for workers to acquire knowledge about adolescents, program philosophy, curriculum design, help for workers to cultivate appropriate implementation skills, development of self-reflection skills, appreciation of the importance of role models, promotion of efficacy and motivation of workers, hands-on practice and demonstration, provision of adequate training to empower the potential program implementers, sensitivity to the cultural context of the implementation, and focus on training evaluation. From the evaluation findings, we realized that the potential program implementers welcomed the training program and felt that the training program helped them align with the philosophy of the program and enabled them to teach in an efficient manner (Shek, Sun & Merrick, 2011).

Lesson 7: Paradigm shift in teaching is necessary. As experiential learning was emphasized in the Project P.A.T.H.S., it was important to rethink the teaching and learning process. In the traditional Chinese culture, several unique features of education could be identified, including rote memorization, teacher orientation, punishment orientation, deemphasis on play, and strong emphasis on teacher authority. In contrast, active learning, student-centered learning, reward orientation, emphasis on fun in the learning process, and strong emphasis on meeting the needs of the students are intrinsic to contemporary education. Therefore, one of the purposes of training programs was to create a paradigm shift in the mindset of the teachers, enabling them to teach in accordance with the spirit of experiential learning. We did this by devoting twenty hours of training for each grade, developing training manuals, providing adequate practice opportunities, inviting potential implementers to reflect on the needs of young people, and providing positive models. Systematic evaluation showed that the training programs were effective in helping teachers to reflect on their teaching style (Shek & Merrick, 2010).

Lesson 8: Giving continued support to the program implementers. In view of the initial opposition of teachers and social workers to the program, the research team was aware of the importance of providing adequate support to the program implementers and several measures were carried out. First, a Co-Walker system was developed. For each school, a colleague from the research team was assigned to be a Co-Walker to provide support to the school. Through regular Co-Walker visits to the schools, the link between program implementers and the schools was strengthened. To minimize skepticism, the information collected from the schools was not directly channeled to the Hong Kong Jockey Club Charities Trust. Evaluation data based on the Co-Walker scheme showed that the scheme was effective (Shek, Sun, & Kan, 2009). Second, we issued a biweekly newsletter to the workers so that they understood the latest development of the project and points of view of different stakeholders. Third, we organized regular workshops to promote sharing among colleagues who were participating in the program.

Lesson 9: Timely feedback to the frontline workers is important. For most intervention research, the evaluation findings are typically reported after the project is completed. This approach has two problems. First, the workers know nothing about the program impact during the process (i.e., black box experience). Second, there is no way we can improve the program and implementation once the project is completed. Hence, timely publication and feedback to workers were the hallmarks of this project. There were three strengths of doing this. First, workers were motivated by the positive findings, and this helped to sustain their passion and involvement. Second, the workers could feel a sense of ownership in a promising program. Third, the research team could identify the factors that promoted or impeded the program's success, and this served as a useful pointer for program refinement. For example, based on several case studies, we identified people, program, process, policy, and place factors that promoted or impeded program success (Shek & Sun, 2008).

Lesson 10: Developing positive attitude in evaluation. One major hurdle in the implementation of the Project P.A.T.H.S. was evaluation. In the project, we emphasized the importance of evidence-based practice and evaluation. In particular, we encouraged workers to conduct their own evaluation. In addition, as the Hong Kong Jockey Club Charities Trust financially supported the project, it also expected workers to conduct proper evaluation. As such, there was strong initial resentment and tension from workers. We did three things to deal with this problem. First, we conducted special workshops to help workers write proposals for the Tier 2 Program based on the unique needs of the students and reiterated the importance of evaluation. Second, we devoted time to discuss the value and plans for evaluation during the training programs. As far as the value of evaluation is concerned, we emphasized the importance of treating "evaluation as part of practice" and that practice evaluation should be treated as routine activities of practice. Regarding the plans for evaluation, step-by-step explanations on how evaluation data should be collected were covered in the training program. To reduce the workload of the workers, we also developed standardized subjective outcome evaluation forms, data entry forms, report templates, and sample reports for workers to use. Third, the research team provided support to teachers and school social workers when they encountered difficulties in completing evaluation tasks and writing reports (Shek, 2008).

Lesson 11: Multiple evaluation strategies should be used to evaluate PYD programs. As mentioned previously, to give a more comprehensive view of the program effects, multiple evaluation strategies were used. There are several reasons why multiple evaluation strategies were used. First, consistent with the spirit of triangulation, the utilization of different evaluation methods can help generate a more comprehensive picture about the program's effect. Second, as there are strengths and weaknesses of different evaluation strategies, the inclusion of different evaluation approaches can complement the limitations of each other. Third, the involvement of different stakeholders can help give a sense of fairness in the evaluation process. For example, to reduce the skepticism of teachers and social workers on the use of subjective outcome evaluation to understand the views of the students, subjective outcome evaluation was also carried out to understand the views of the program implementers. This approach can give different stakeholders an impression that evaluation would be fairly conducted taking into account the views of different stakeholders. In this project, besides randomized group trials (the "gold standard" in program evaluation) and subjective outcome evaluation (which is commonly used in human service evaluation), different forms of qualitative evaluation were used to give alternative perspectives on the program's effects.

The research findings of the different evaluation methods and processes are reported elsewhere (Shek et al., 2012; Shek & Sun, 2013a, b). They are briefly summarized as follows:

- *Objective Outcome Evaluation:* At the initial stage, twenty-four experimental schools and twenty-four control schools joined a randomized group trial. Eight waves of data were collected over five years to examine the impact of the program. Longitudinal findings showed that students in the experimental schools performed better than did students in the control schools on indices of positive youth development, drug use, delinquent behavior, and intention to engage in problem behavior.
- *Subjective Outcome Evaluation:* To assess the views and experiences of the students and program implementers, they completed subjective outcome evaluation forms at the end of the program. Students and implementers generally had positive perceptions of the program, workers, and benefits of the program.
- *Process Evaluation:* Schools were randomly selected to join process evaluation where trained observers observed the classes to determine the degree of adherence and implementation quality. Results showed that program adherence and implementation quality were good.
- *Interim Evaluation:* Roughly half of the schools were randomly selected to join the interim evaluation whose purpose was to understand the

implementation issues and quality. The findings showed that the implementation quality was good and positive feedback from students was observed.
- *Qualitative Evaluation Based on Program Participants:* We randomly selected students to join focus groups to discuss their experience and perceived impact of the program. Results showed that students had positive experiences with the program and its benefits.
- *Qualitative Evaluation Based on Program Implementers:* We randomly selected teachers and social workers to join focus groups to discuss their teaching experience, experience of the participants, and the perceived impact of the program. The workers generally had positive experiences with the program and its impacts.
- *Qualitative Evaluation (Case Study):* A case study examining the implementation experience of several schools that had incorporated the Tier 1 Program into school formal curriculum was conducted. Facilitating factors and barriers affecting the implementing process were identified (Shek & Sun, 2008).
- *Qualitative Evaluation (In-depth Interviews with Program Implementers):* Prolonged in-depth interviews with several teachers were conducted. The teachers generally had positive experiences with program implementation, and they saw the program to be beneficial to the students.
- *Qualitative Evaluation (Student Logs):* Randomly selected students were invited to share their experiences regarding how to apply the knowledge gained from the Project P.A.T.H.S. to real-life challenges. The students generally had positive experiences with the program.
- *Qualitative Evaluation (Student Products):* More than one thousand pieces of weekly diaries written by the students were collected after completion of the program. Students had positive views about the program, workers, and benefits of the program.
- *Management Information Collected from the Co-Walker Scheme:* In the Co-Walker Scheme, colleagues visited schools and conducted observations. The gathered information was analyzed to give an overall picture about the implementation quality of the program. The related findings showed that the implementation quality was good and the program was able to promote positive changes in the students.
- *Evaluation Based on the Repertory Grid Tests:* Repertory grid tests were administered to assess the change in the self-identity systems of the students before and after joining the program. Students were randomly selected to join this part of the evaluation study. Students generally showed positive changes in the self-identity system.

With specific reference to the evaluation based on the longitudinal randomized group trial, findings showed that compared with the control schools, students in the experimental schools developed better in terms of positive youth development indicators and they had slower growth trajectories in smoking, drinking, use of illicit drugs, delinquency, and intention to engage in problem behavior.

Lesson 12: Maximization of the impact of the developed program. To enhance the sustainability of the program, we encouraged the schools to incorporate the program in the formal curriculum. By the end of the second cycle of program implementation, roughly half of the schools had incorporated the program P.A.T.H.S. in the formal curriculum so that the program can have impact in the long run. We also promoted the program in the context of substance abuse. The program was regarded as a key youth enhancement program by the Social Welfare Department in Hong Kong. It was also regarded as a primary adolescent prevention program by the Panel on Child Fatality Review and the Task Force on Youth Drug Abuse in Hong Kong. The program was listed as an effective program in the Resource Kit for Teachers on Anti-Drug Education. Outside Hong Kong, the program had been piloted in Macau and mainland China. For example, with positive evaluation outcomes (Shek, Han, Lee & Yu, 2014a), the project will be promoted among Tin Ka Ping schools in China by the Tin Ka Ping Foundation (Shek et al., 2014). The project was also listed as an effective program in a recent review in *Lancet* (Catalano et al., 2012).

Summary and Conclusion

This chapter focuses on the prevention of drug abuse (alcohol, tobacco, and other drugs) in Chinese adolescents in Hong Kong. In the first section, the situation of drug abuse in Hong Kong is reviewed. In the second section, the relationship between positive youth development and adolescent drug abuse is examined. In the third section, the Project P.A.T.H.S. in Hong Kong is introduced. In the initial phase (P.A.T.H.S. I), a curricula-based PYD program (Tier 1 Program), was developed and implemented in more than 250 high schools. An evaluation based on multiple strategies showed that the program participants and implementers perceived the program, implementers, and benefits of the program in a favorable light. With specific reference to the five-year longitudinal evaluation study, results showed that the program participants had better holistic development and showed slower growth trajectories in drug use and delinquency behavior than did the control participants. In the extension phase (P.A.T.H.S. II), the findings from the longitudinal study showed that PYD attributes were negatively related to adolescent risk behavior, including drug abuse.

With specific reference to the initial phase (P.A.T.H.S. I), several lessons can be learned. These include the importance of understanding the political context in program development and implementation, positive program orientation, focus on inner strengths and developmental assets, need for indigenous program development, teachers and school social workers as ideal program implementers, emphasis on training, the need for paradigm shift, continued support given to program implementers, importance of timely feedback, promotion of positive attitude in evaluation, use of multiple evaluation strategies, and the importance of maximizing the impact of developed programs.

References

Abdullah, A. S., Fielding, R., & Hedley, A. J. (2002). Patterns of cigarette smoking, alcohol use and other substance use among Chinese university students in Hong Kong. *American Journal on Addictions* 11: 235–46.

Anbari, A., Mostafavi, M., Asadi, S., Mirzaee, A., Hashemzadeh, A., & Nahr, R. R. (2014). The role of risky and protective individual, psychological, familial, scholastic and social factors in health promotion and substance abuse prevention in adolescents. *MAGNT Research Report* 2: 1197–1208.

Bagley, C. (1992). Development of an adolescent stress scale for use by school counsellors: construct validity in terms of depression, self-esteem and suicidal ideation. *School Psychology International* 13: 31–49. doi: 10.1177/0143034392131003

Benson, P. L., Scales, P. C., Hamilton, S. F., & Sesma, A. (2006). Positive youth development: theory, research, and applications. In Damon, W., & Lerners, R. (eds.), *Handbook of Child Psychology*, vol. 1. Hoboken, NJ: John Wiley & Sons, pp. 894–941.

Botvin, G. J., Griffin, K. W., Nichols, T. D. (2006). Preventing youth violence and delinquency through a universal school-based prevention approach. *Prevention Science* 7: 403–8. doi: 10.1007/s11121-006-0057-y

Caplan, M., Weissberg, R. P., Grober, J. S., Sivo, P. J., Grady, K., & Jocoby, C. (1992). Social competence promotion with inner-city and suburban young adolescents: effects on social adjustment and alcohol use. *Journal of Consulting and Clinical Psychology* 60: 56–63.

Catalano, R. F., Berglund, M. L., Ryan, J. A., Lonczak, H. S., & Hawkins, J. D. (2004). Positive youth development in the United States: research findings on evaluations of positive youth development programs. *Annals of the American Academy of Political and Social Science* 591: 98–124. doi:10.1177/0002716203260102

Catalano, R. F., Fagan, A. A., Gavin, L. E., Greenberg, M. T., Irwin, C. E., Ross, D. A., & Shek, D. T. L. (2012). Worldwide application of prevention science in adolescent health. *Lancet* 379: 1653–64.

Census and Statistics Department. (2013). *Hong Kong 2011 Population Census Thematic Report: Youths*. Hong Kong: Government of the Special Administrative Region, P.R.C. www.censtatd.gov.hk/press_release/ press ReleaseDetail.jsp?charsetID=1&pressRID=3345

Central Registry of Drug Abuse. (2013). *Drug Abuse Situation in Hong Kong in 2012*. Hong Kong: Security Bureau.

Cheung, N. W. T. (2014). Low self-control and co-occurrence of gambling with substance use and delinquency among Chinese adolescents. *Journal of Gambling Studies* 30: 105–24. doi: 10.1007/s10899-012–9351-8

Donnellan, M. B., Trzesniewski, K. H., Robins, R. W., Moffitt, T. E., & Caspi, A. (2005). Low self-esteem is related to aggression, antisocial behavior, and delinquency. *Psychological Science* 16: 328–35.

Edvardsson, I., Geisler, D., & Lendahls, L. (2014). Experiences of being non-smoking among adolescents in a smoking context. *Health* 6: 1133–42. doi: 10.4236/health.2014.611140

Epstein, J. A., Griffin, K. W., & Botvin, G. J. (2000). Competence skills help deter smoking among inner city adolescents. *Tobacco Control* 9: 33–9. doi: 10.1136/tc.9.1.33

Flay, B. R., Graumlich, S., Segawa, E., Burns, J. L., Holiday, M. Y., & Aban Aya (investigators). (2004). Effects of 2 prevention programs on high-risk behaviors among African American youth. *Archives of Pediatrics & Adolescent Medicine* 158: 377–84.

Griffin, K. W., Botvin, G. J., & Nichols, T. R. (2004). Long-term follow-up effects of a school-based drug abuse prevention program on adolescent risky driving. *Prevention Science* 5: 207–12.

Griffin, K. W., Scheier, L. M., Botvin, G. J., & Diaz, T. (2001). Protective role of personal competence skills in adolescent substance use: psychological well-being as a mediating factor. *Psychology of Addictive Behaviors* 15: 194–203. doi: dx.doi.org/10.1037/0893–164X.15.3.194

Griffiths, S., Lau, J. T., Chow, J. K., Lee, S. S., Kan, P. Y., & Lee, S. (2006). Alcohol use among entrants to a Hong Kong university. *Alcohol Alcoholism* 41: 560–5. doi: dx.doi.org/10.1093/alcalc/agl047

Hawkins, J. D., Lishner, D. M., Catalano, R. F. Jr., & Howard, M. O. (1986). Childhood predictors of adolescent substance abuse: toward an empirically grounded theory. *Journal of Children in Contemporary Society* 18: 11–48.

Jackson, C., Henriksen, L., Dickinson, D., & Levine, D. W. (1997). The early use of alcohol and tobacco: Its relation to children's competence and parents' behavior. *American Journal of Public Health* 87: 359–64.

Kim, J. H., Chan, K. W. C., Chow, J. K. W., Fung, K. P., Fong, B. Y. F., Cheuk, K. K., & Griffiths, S. M. (2009). University binge drinking patterns and changes in patterns of alcohol consumption among Chinese undergraduates in a Hong Kong university. *Journal of American College Health* 58: 255–65. doi: 10.1080/07448480903295318

Lai, M. K., Ho, S. Y., & Lam, T. H. (2004). Perceived peer smoking prevalence and its association with smoking behaviours and intentions in Hong Kong Chinese adolescents. *Addiction* 99: 1195–1205.

Lam, P. K. (2010). Values and problem behaviors in Hong Kong adolescents (Unpublished doctoral dissertation). Wayne State University, Detroit, MI.

Lam, T. H., Chung, S. F., Betson, C. L., Wong, C. M., & Hedley, A. J. (1998). Tobacco advertisement: one of the strongest risk factors for smoking in Hong Kong students. *American Journal of Preventive Medicine* 14: 217–23.

Lam, T. H., Stewart, S. M., & Ho, L. M. (2001). Prevalence and correlates of smoking and sexual activity among Hong Kong adolescents. *Journal of Adolescent Health* 29: 352–8. doi: 10.1016/S1054-139X(01)00301–9

Lam, T. H., Stewart, S. M., Ho, S. Y., Lai, M. K., Mak, K. H., Chau, K. V., . . ., Salili, F. (2005). Depressive symptoms and smoking among Hong Kong Chinese adolescents. *Addiction* 100: 1003–11. doi: 10.1111/j.1360-0443.2005.01092.x

Ladapo, J. A., Elliott, M. N., Kanouse, D. E., Tortolero, S. R., Windle, M., Cuccaro, P. M. . . ., Schuster, M. A. (2014). Tobacco use and smoking intentions among U.S. fifth-grade students. *Journal of Adolescent Health* 55: 445–51. doi: 10.1016/j.jadohealth.2014.03.008

Lee, A., & Tsang, C. K. K. (2004). Youth risk behavior in a Chinese population: a territory-wide youth risk behavior surveillance in Hong Kong. *Public Health* 118: 88–95.

Lee, A., Tsang, C. K., Lee, S. H., & To, C. T. (2001). A YRBS survey of youth risk behaviors at alternative high schools and mainstream high schools in Hong Kong. *Journal of School Health* 71: 443–7.

Lee, A., Wong, S. Y. S., Tsang, K. K., Ho, G. S. M., Wong, C. W., & Cheng, F. (2009). Understanding suicidality and correlates among Chinese secondary school students in Hong Kong. *Health Promotion International* 24: 156–65. doi: 10.1093/heapro/dap011

Lerner, R. M., Lerner, J. V., Almerigi, J. B., Theokas, C., Phelps, E., Gestsdottir, S., . . . & von Eye, A. (2005). Positive youth development, participation in community youth development programs, and community contributions of fifth-grade adolescents: findings from the first wave of the 4-H study of positive youth development. *Journal of Early Adolescence* 25: 17–71. ase.tufts.edu/iaryd/documents/pubPositiveYouth.pdf

Lillehoj, C. J., Trudeau, L., Spoth, R., & Wickrama, K. A. (2004). Internalizing, social competence, and substance initiation: influence of gender moderation and a preventive intervention. *Substance Use & Misuse* 39: 963–91. doi: 10.1081/JA-120030895

Lo, C. C., & Globetti, G. G. (2000). Gender differences in drinking patterns among Hong Kong Chinese youth: a pilot study. *Substance Use & Misuse* 35: 1297–1306.

Lou, V. W. Q., & Shek, D. T. L. (2006). Alcohol use and abuse amongst adolescents in Hong Kong. *International Journal of Adolescent Medicine and Health* 18: 69–79.

McBride, N., Farringdon, F., Midford, R., Meuleners, L., & Phillips, M. (2004). Harm minimization in school drug education: final results of the School Health and Alcohol Harm Reduction Project (SHAHRP). *Addiction* 99: 278–91. doi: 10.1046/j.1360-0443.2003.00620.x

Narcotics Division (2013). *A Review of Estimation Methods on Prevalence of Drug Abuse Population in Hong Kong: Executive Summary*. Hong Kong: Narcotics Division, Security Bureau, Government of Hong Kong Special Administrative Region.

Nash, S. G., McQueen, A., & Bray, J. H. (2005). Pathways to adolescent alcohol use: family environment, peer influence, and parental expectations. *Journal of Adolescent Health* 37: 19–28.

National Institute on Drug Abuse. (2014). Drugs of abuse. www.drugabuse.gov/drugs-abuse

Oman, R. F., Vesely, S., Aspy, C. B., McLeroy, K. R., Rodine, S., & Marshall, L. (2004). The potential protective effect of youth assets on adolescent alcohol and drug use. *American Journal of Public Health* 94: 1425–30.

Ong, J., Wong, W., Lee, A., Holroyd, E., & Huang, S. Y. (2013). Sexual activity and adolescent health risk behaviors amongst high school students in three ethnic Chinese urban populations. *Journal of Clinical Nursing* 22: 3270–9. doi: 10.1111/jocn.12267

Pederson, L. L., Koval, J. J., & O'Connor, K. (1997). Are psychosocial factors related to smoking in grade-6 students? *Addictive Behaviors* 22: 169–81.

Phelps, E., Balsano, A. B., Fay, K., Peltz, J. S., Zimmerman, S. M., Lerner, R. M., & Lerner, J. V. (2007). Nuances in early adolescent developmental trajectories of positive and problematic/risk behaviors: findings from the 4-H study of positive youth development. *Child and Adolescent Psychiatric Clinics of North America* 16: 473–96.

Piko, B. F., Luszczynska, A., Gibbons, F. X., & Teközel, M. (2005). A culture-based study of personal and social influences of adolescent smoking. *European Journal of Public Health* 15: 393–8. doi: dx.doi.org/10.1093/eurpub/cki008

Scales, P. C., Foster, K. C., Mannes, M., Horst, M. A., Pinto, K. C., & Rutherford, A. (2005). School-business partnerships, developmental assets, and positive outcomes among urban high school students: a mixed-methods study. *Urban Education* 40: 144–89. uex.sagepub.com/content/40/2/144.full.pdf

Scheier, L. M., Botvin, G. J., Diaz, T., & Griffin, K. W. (1999). Social skills, competence, and drug refusal efficacy as predictors of adolescent alcohol use. *Journal of Drug Education* 29: 251–78.

Schwartz, S. J., Phelps, E., Lerner, J. V., Huang, S., Brown, C. H., Lewin-Bizan, S., . . . & Lerner, R. M. (2010). Promotion as prevention: positive youth development as protective against tobacco, alcohol, illicit drug, and sex initiation. *Applied Developmental Science* 14: 197–211. doi: 10.1080/10888691.2010.516186

Shek, D. T. L. (2006a). Adolescent developmental issues in Hong Kong: relevance to positive youth development programs in Hong Kong. *International Journal of Adolescent Medicine and Health* 18: 341–54.

Shek, D. T. L. (ed.). (2006b). Positive youth development program in Hong Kong. *International Journal of Adolescent Medicine and Health* 18(special issue): 299–558.

Shek, D. T. L. (2007). Tackling adolescent substance abuse in Hong Kong: where we should and should not go. *Scientific World Journal* 7: 2021–30. doi: 10.1100/tsw.2007.315

Shek, D. T. L. (2008). Enthusiasm-based or evidence-based charities: personal reflections based on the Project P.A.T.H.S. in Hong Kong. *Scientific World Journal* 8: 802–10. doi: 10.1100/tsw.2008.111.

Shek, D. T. L. (2013). Sexual behavior and intention to engage in sexual behavior in junior secondary school students in Hong Kong. *Journal of Pediatric and Adolescent Gynecology* 26: S33–S41. doi: 10.1016/j.jpag.2013.03.013

Shek, D. T. L., Han, X. Y., Lee, T. Y., & Yu, L. (2014a). Subjective outcome evaluation of a positive youth development program in China. *International Journal on Disability and Human Development* 13: 275–83.

Shek, D. T. L., & Leung, J. T. Y. (2013). Adolescent developmental issues in Hong Kong: phenomena and implications for youth service. In Shek, D. T. L., & Sun, R. C. F. (eds.), *Development and Evaluation of Positive Adolescent Training through Holistic Social Programs (P.A.T.H.S.)*. Heidelberg, Germany: Springer, pp. 1–14.

Shek, D. T. L., & Leung, J. T. Y. (2014). Substance abuse in junior secondary school students in Hong Kong. In Shek, D. T. L., Sun, R. C. F., & Ma, C. M. S. (eds.), *Chinese Adolescents in Hong Kong - Family Life, Psychological Well-being and Risk Behavior*. New York: Springer, pp.133–54.

Shek, D. T. L., & Liang, J. (2015). Risk factors and protective factors in substance abuse in Chinese Adolescents in Hong Kong. In Lee, T. Y., Shek, D. T. L., & Sun, R. C. F. (eds.), *Student Well-being in Chinese Adolescents in Hong Kong*. Singapore: Springer, pp. 237–53.

Shek, D. T. L., & Ma, C. M. S. (2010). Dimensionality of the Chinese Positive Youth Development Scale: confirmatory factor analyses. *Social Indicators Research* 98: 41–59.

Shek, D. T. L., & Ma, C. M. S. (2011). Impact of the Project P.A.T.H.S. in the junior secondary school years: individual growth curve analyses. *Scientific World Journal* 11: 253–66. doi: 10.1100/tsw.2011.6

Shek, D. T. L., & Ma, C. M. S. (2012). Substance abuse in junior secondary school students in Hong Kong: prevalence and psychosocial correlates. *International Journal of Child Health and Human Development* 4: 433–42.

Shek, D. T. L., Ma, H. K., & Merrick, J. (eds.) (2012). Evaluation of the Project P.A.T.H.S. in Hong Kong: findings based on multiple methods. *Scientific World Journal* (special issue): Article ID 427801.

Shek, D. T. L., Ma, H. K., & Sun, R. C. F. (2011a). Development of a new curriculum in a positive youth development program: the Project P.A.T.H.S. in Hong Kong. *Scientific World Journal* 11: 2207–18. doi: 10.1100/2011/289589

Shek, D. T. L., & Merrick, J. (eds.) (2010). Positive youth development and training. *International Journal of Adolescent Medicine and Health* 22 (special issue): 341–447.

Shek, D. T. L., Siu, A. M. H., & Lee, T. Y. (2007). The Chinese Positive Youth Development Scale: a validation study. *Research on Social Work Practice* 17: 380–91. doi: 10.1177/1049731506296196

Shek, D. T. L., & Sun, R. C. F. (2008). Implementation quality of a positive youth development program: cross-case analyses based on seven cases in Hong Kong. *Scientific World Journal: TSW Holistic Health & Medicine* 8: 1075–87. doi: 10.1100/tsw.2008.130

Shek, D. T. L., & Sun, R. C. F. (2012). Epilogue: the Project P.A.T.H.S. in Hong Kong: lessons learned and implications for positive youth development programs. *Scientific World Journal*: Article ID 687536. doi: 10.1100/2012/687536

Shek, D. T. L., & Sun, R. C. F. (2013a). The Project P.A.T.H.S. in Hong Kong: development, training, implementation, and evaluation. *Journal of Pediatric and Adolescent Gynecology* 26: S2–S9.

Shek, D. T. L., & Sun, R. C. F. (eds.) (2013b). *Development and Evaluation of Positive Adolescent Training through Holistic Social Programs (P.A.T.H.S.)*. Heidelberg, Germany: Springer.

Shek, D. T. L., Sun, R. C. F., & Kan, V. W. M. (2009). Full implementation of the Secondary 1 program of Project P.A.T.H.S.: observations based on the Co-Walker scheme. *Scientific World Journal: TSW Child Health & Human Development* 9: 982–91. doi: 10.1100/tsw.2009.116

Shek, D. T. L., Sun, R. C. F., & Merrick, J. (eds.) (2011). Training and program implementation in project P.A.T.H.S. in Hong Kong. *International Journal of Adolescent Medicine and Health* 23(special issue): 303–83.

Shek, D. T. L., Sun, R. C. F., & Merrick, J. (eds.) (2012a). *Developmental Issues in Chinese Adolescents*. New York: Nova Science.

Shek, D. T. L., Sun, R. C. F., & Merrick, J. (eds.). (2012b). Positive youth development constructs – conceptual review and application. *Scientific World Journal* (special issue).

Shek, D. T. L., & Wai, C. L. Y. (2008). Training workers implementing adolescent prevention and positive youth development programs: what have we learned from the literature? *Adolescence* 43: 823–45.

Shek, D. T. L., & Wu, F. K. Y. (2013). Conceptual framework underlying the development of a positive youth development program in Hong Kong. In Shek, D. T. L., & Sun, R. C. F. (eds.), *Development and Evaluation of Positive Adolescent Training through Holistic Social Programs (P.A.T.H.S.)*. Heidelberg, Germany: Springer, pp. 15–28.

Shek, D. T. L., & Yu, L. (2011a). Prevention of adolescent problem behavior: longitudinal impact of the Project P.A.T.H.S. in Hong Kong. *Scientific World Journal* 11: 546–67. doi: 10.1100/tsw.2011.33

Shek, D. T. L,. & Yu, L. (2011b). A review of validated youth prevention and positive youth development programs in Asia. *International Journal of Adolescent Medicine and Health* 23: 317–24. doi: 10.1515/IJAMH.2011.028

Shek, D. T. L., & Yu, L. (2012a). Longitudinal impact of the Project PATHS on adolescent risk behavior: what happened after five years? *Scientific World Journal* 2012: Article ID 316029. doi: 10.1100/2012/316029

Shek, D. T. L., & Yu, L. (2012b). A longitudinal study of substance abuse in Hong Kong adolescents. In Shek, D. T. L., Sun, R. C. F., & Merrick, J. (eds.), *Drug Abuse in Hong Kong: Development and Evaluation of a Prevention Program*. New York: Nova Science, pp. 171–98.

Shek, D. T. L., & Yu, L. (2013). Impact of the Project P.A.T.H.S. on adolescent risk behavior: a five-year longitudinal study. In Shek, D. T. L., & Sun, R. C. F. (eds.), *Development and Evaluation of Positive Adolescent Training through Holistic Social Programs (P.A.T.H.S.)*. Heidelberg, Germany: Springer, pp. 85–106.

Shek, D. T. L., Yu, L., Sun, R. C. F., Lee, T. Y., Han, X. Y., Li, X. X., & Zhao, X. (2014b). Objective outcome evaluation of a positive youth development program in China. *International Journal on Disability and Human Development* 13: 255–65. doi: 10.1515/ijdhd-2014-0311

Simons-Morton, B. G., & Haynie, D. L. (2003). Psychosocial predictors of increased smoking stage among sixth graders. *American Journal of Health Behavior* 27: 592–602. doi: dx.doi.org/10.5993/AJHB.27.6.2

Sun, R. C. F., & Shek, D. T. L. (2010). Life satisfaction, positive youth development, and problem behaviour among Chinese adolescents in Hong Kong. *Social Indicators Research* 95: 455–74. doi: 10.1007/s11205-009–9531-9

Sun, R. C. F., & Shek, D. T. L. (2013). Longitudinal influences of positive youth development and life satisfaction on problem behaviour among adolescents in Hong Kong. *Social Indicators Research* 114: 1171–97. doi: 10.1007/s11205-012–0196-4

Tebes, J. K., Feinn, R., Vanderploeg, J. J., Chinman, M. J., Shepard, J., Brabham, T., Genovese, M., & Connell, C. (2007). Impact of a positive youth development program in urban after-school settings on the prevention of adolescent substance use. *Journal of Adolescent Health* 41: 239–47. doi: 10.1016/jadohealth.2007.02.016

Veselska, Z., Geckova, A. M., Orosova, O., Gajdosova, B., van Dijk, J. P., & Reijneveld, S. A. (2009). Self-esteem and resilience: the connection with risky behavior among adolescents. *Addictive Behaviors* 34: 287–91. doi: 10.1016/j.addbeh.2008.11.005

Veselska, Z., Geckova, A. M., Reijneveld, S. A., & van Dijk, J. P. (2011). Self-efficacy, affectivity and smoking behavior in adolescence. *European Addiction Research* 17: 172–7. doi: 10.1159/000326071

Wang, M. P., Ho, S. Y., & Lam, T. H. (2013). Underage alcohol drinking and medical services use in Hong Kong: a cross-sectional study. *BMJ Open* 3. doi: 10.1136/bmjopen-2013-002740.

Yuen, M., Hui, E. K. P., Lau, P. S. Y., Gysbers, N. C., Leung, T. K. M., Chan, R. M. C., & Shea, P. M. K. (2006). Assessing the personal-social development of Hong Kong Chinese adolescents. *International Journal for the Advancement of Counseling* 28: 317–30. doi: 10.1007/s10447-006–9017-2

Zimmerman, S. M., Phelps, E., & Lerner, R. M. (2008). Positive and negative developmental trajectories in U.S. adolescents: where the positive youth development perspective meets the deficit model. *Research in Human Development* 5: 153–65. doi: 10.1080/15427600802274001

Zullig, K. J., Valois, R. F., Huebner, E. S., Oeltmann, J. E., & Drane, J. W. (2001). Relationship between perceived life satisfaction and adolescents' substance abuse. *Journal of Adolescent Health* 29: 279–88. doi: dx.doi.org/10.1016/S1054-139X(01)00269–5

28 Suicidal Behavior and Its Prevention in India

Solomon Renati & Shreeletha Solomon

Suicide is a complex problem with no single cause or reason. It results from a complex interaction of biological, genetic, psychological, social, cultural, and environmental factors. It is difficult to explain why some people decide to commit suicide while others, in a similar or even worse situation, do not. It is estimated that one in sixty persons in India are affected by suicide. This estimate includes both those who have attempted suicide and those who have been affected by the suicide of a close family or friend (Vijayakumar, 2007). However, most suicides can be prevented. The recent spate of farmers' suicides in India has raised societal and governmental concern to address this growing tragedy. In India, suicide rates have increased particularly among rural male farmers following changes to farming practices that made farming less economically viable (Beautrais, 2006) Factors contributing to the high rate of suicide in this vulnerable population include economic adversity, exclusive dependence on rainfall for agriculture, and possibly monetary compensation to the family following suicide (Behere & Behere, 2008).

There is a growing recognition that prevention strategies need to be tailored to the region-specific demographics of a country and to be implemented in a culturally sensitive manner (Radhakrishnan & Andrade, 2012). Preventive strategies implemented at a community level and identifying vulnerable individuals may be more effective than global strategies. This chapter presents the suicide prevalence in India and explores the historical and cultural roots of suicide in India. It also identifies the unique risk and protective factors for suicides in India and examines the effective strategies aimed at preventing suicide.

Prevalence of Suicide in India

Because suicide is mostly a private and personal act, a wide disparity exists in the rates of suicide across the nation. Further, India is a nation of people from divergent religious, ethnic, racial, linguistic, caste, and cultural backgrounds with each group representing unique beliefs and lifestyles. (Hence a greater understanding of region-specific factors related to suicide would enable prevention strategies to be more culturally sensitive.)

An estimated eight hundred thousand people die worldwide by suicide every year (WHO, 2014). India and China together represent 54 percent of the global total of suicides (Vijayakumar, 2004b), and India accounted for the highest estimated number of suicides in the world in 2012 (WHO, 2014). The increasing rates of suicide in India during recent decades are consistent with the global trend. Increases in suicide rates are a global phenomenon, and rates have increased over the past forty-five years (WHO, 2012a).

The annual data on suicides in India are available from National Crime Research Bureau (NCRB), the Ministry of Home Affairs, the Government of India. The number of suicides in the country during the last decade (2003–13) has recorded an increase of 21.6 percent (from 110,851 in 2003 to 134,799 in 2013). In 2013, five states including the states of Maharashtra, Tamil Nadu, Andhra Pradesh, West Bengal, and Karnataka together accounted for 53.5 percent of the total suicides reported in the country. The remaining 46.5 percent of suicides were reported in the rest of the twenty-three states and seven union territories. The rate of suicides for all of India was 11 per 100,000 of the population during the year 2013. The Union Territory of Puducherry reported the highest rate of suicide (35.6 per 100,000 of the population), while Bihar reported the lowest rate (1.1 per 100,000 of the population), indicating wide variations in suicide rates among states.

The NCRB data are based on police records. Sociocultural factors undermine the veracity of these records. Section 309 of the Indian Penal Code (IPC) clearly states as follows: "Whoever attempts to commit suicide and does any act towards the commission of such offence, shall be punished with simple imprisonment for a term which may extend to one year or with fine or both." This results in underreporting. The process of registering a death is particularly inefficient in rural areas (Gajalakshmi & Peto, 2007). Only about 25 percent of deaths are registered, and only about 10 percent are medically certified (WHO, 2001; Zonda, 2006). Death by suicide is frequently reported as due to illness or accident to avoid police investigation and due to family and social stigma. Statistics derived from police records hence underreport suicides (Radhakrishnan & Andrade, 2012). In India, studies using verbal autopsies and covering catchment areas of a comprehensive community health program have documented rates of 95 per 100,000, about 9 times the national average (Aaron et al., 2004; Abraham, Abraham, & Jacob, 2005; Gajalakshmi & Peto, 2006; Joseph et al., 2003; Prasad et al., 2006).

Suicide rates in the high-income countries are low compared to high rates reported from the low-income countries (Aaron et al., 2004; Abraham, et al., 2005; Gajalakshmi & Peto, 2007; Joseph et al., 2003; Prasad et al., 2006; Vijayakumar, Nagaraj, Pirkis, & Whiteford, 2005). The stigma of mental disease and psychiatric help-seeking further compounds the problem, leading to underreporting of suicides. There are no reliable figures relating to the true scale of the problem of deaths by suicide in India, although reporting of deaths in the media suggest a sharp increase in the past decade (Jones & Keenan, 2014).

Thus several factors, such as social stigma, local beliefs, and legal consequences, result in many suicides being declared natural or accidental deaths. Developing and implementing appropriate suicide prevention programs for India requires both an understanding of the limitations of the available data and a commitment to improving data quality to reflect more accurately the effectiveness of specific interventions.

Historical and Cultural Roots of Suicide in India

Exploration of the historical and epidemiological aspects of suicide in India will facilitate universal, indicated, and selective prevention planning. An understanding of suicide in the Indian context calls for an appreciation of the literary, religious, and cultural ethos of the subcontinent because tradition has always influenced the lives of people in India. Ancient Indian texts contain stories of valor in which suicide as a means to avoid shame and disgrace was glorified. Upanishads, the Holy Scriptures, on the other hand, condemn suicide. However, the Vedas, the most revered scriptures of Hindus, permit suicide for religious reasons and consider that the best sacrifice was that of one's own life (Bhugra, 2005; Braun, 2008; Vijayakumar, 2004a). Suicide by starvation was linked by Hindus to the attainment of liberation from the cycle of life and death and is still practiced to this day (Gururaj, Isaac, Subbakrishna, & Ranjani, 2004). According to Durkheim (1951), India is the classic example for both obligatory and optional altruistic suicides. Sati, a medieval Hindu practice involving concremation of the living wife along with the dead husband, was for a long time thought to be intimately connected with the religious beliefs of the Hindus. Even now, stray cases of Sati (i.e., widow burning) are being reported in the press, although the practice as such has disappeared (Manoranjitham et al., 2007). A notable example of altruistic suicide is Jauhar, a kind of mass suicide committed by the women of the community when their men folk faced defeat. To avoid intolerable shame and escape sexual dishonor, the women used to build a huge pyre and all the women and children jumped into it. When performed, a whole tribe became extinct within a few hours. Jauhar was in a sense a spontaneous outburst of violent reaction against the atrocities perpetrated by the conquerors (Vijayakumar, 2004a) While social facts influence patterns of suicidal behavior in societies, it is also clear that there are individual differences to their response to social circumstances.

The influence of social conditions is mediated by not only individual-level differences but also cultural differences. When looking for explanations for differences between countries or cultures in their suicide rates, there is much emphasis in the literature on the role of cultural influences in shaping attitudes to suicidal behavior (De Leo, 2003). A cultural point of view of suicides focuses on the interaction of the individual and his or her larger context. Culture shapes not only the nature and perception of stressful conditions but also the responses to stressors. Several studies show that the same risk factors across cultures are of varying relevance for individuals who engage in suicidal behaviors (Aubert, Daigle, & Daigle, 2004; Bhui & McKenzie, 2008; Pritchard & Hean, 2008). Increasing evidence shows that the context is imperative to understanding the risk of suicide (WHO, 2014).

Salient Features of Suicides in India

Jacob (2008) observed that the differences between Indian and Western suicide data are probably a reflection of the many differences in the government supports and populations, including the social security net and national health service systems in the West, and the rapidity of social and economic change, growth and development, cultures, and so on. These support systems are scarcely available in India. Severe mental illness seems to be related to suicide when the rates are low (i.e., 10 per 100,000 population) but does not seem to contribute significantly when the suicide rates are high, as in India, where social, economic, and cultural factors play a much greater part (Manoranjitham et al., 2010). Recent studies in several low- and middle-income countries such as China and India suggest the occurrence of suicidal behaviors may differ markedly from high-income countries (Phillips & Cheng, 2012; Vijayakumar, 2004b). The prominent among the salient features that distinguish suicides in India with those in high-income countries are discussed in the following sections.

Gender Difference in Suicide Attempts and Completion

Like many countries in the world (Bertolote et.al., 2005), suicide deaths in India have been increasing progressively (NCRB, 2013). However, certain observations are diametrically opposite to those of the West. According to the WHO (2000), it is generally accepted that more males commit suicide, while more females attempt suicide (Sadock & Sadock, 2008).

Studies from high-income countries typically show male-to-female suicide death ratios of about three to one (Dombrovski et al., 2008). According to the Million Death Study in India (Patel et al., 2012), the male-to-female suicide death ratio was about one and a half to one at all ages. These differences may be due to sociocultural and economic variations (Canetto, 2008).

In an attempt to trace the trend of sex differences in completed suicides in India during the last 100 years, Nandi, Banerjee, and Boral (1978) found that females outnumbered males in every part of India in 1872, but in 1972 the data were just the reverse.

Globally, attempted suicides are more among women, while completed suicide is more common among men (Phillips, Yang, Li, & Li, 2004). Studies in India have showed a male-predominant, male/female ratio for completed suicide ranging from 1.13:1 (Das et al., 2008) to 1.63:1 (Latha, Bhat, & D'Souza, 1996). These differences may be reconciled by an appreciation of social changes in India, with a shift toward nuclear families and the cultural emphasis on the male stereotype that the individual tries to fulfill in vain. The changing sociodemographic profile, such as increased participation of women in the workforce and the gradual change of health delivery systems in the region, call for a periodic reevaluation of gender paradox in suicide attempters and making cross-cultural comparisons (Menon, Kattimani, Sarkar, & Muthuramalingam, 2015).

Marital Status

Distinct from global demographic risk factors, in India, marital status is not necessarily a protective factor for suicide (Radhakrishnan & Andrade, 2012). This protective effect of marriage in India is seen more for men than for women, and rates of suicide decreased in order from widowers to divorced, single, and married men. Young widowers were at highest risk. The vast majority of regular marriages in India are still parent-made, arranged marriages. In such marriages, the social and familial pressure on a woman to stay married even in abusive relationships appears to be one of the factors that increases the risk of suicide in women (Gururaj et al., 2004; Patel et al., 2012). Dowry, which involve a continuing series of gifts before and after marriage, complicates the problem. When dowry expectations are not met, young brides can be harassed to the point where they are driven to suicide (Kumar, 2004). According to Government of India data, 69.4 percent of the suicide victims in India were married while 23.6 percent were never married. Divorcees and separated have accounted for about 3.2 percent, and widowed and widower were about 3.7 percent of the total suicide victims (NCRB, 2013).

Rural–Urban Difference in Suicide

A growing body of research indicates that suicide is a public health concern in rural areas. Rural areas often suffer from social fragmentation, which may contribute to their higher rates of suicide (Durkheim, 1952; Kurosu, 1991; Lingren, 1995; Middleton et al., 2004). The agricultural communities that comprise many rural areas often necessitate a challenging and strenuous lifestyle (e.g., caring for crops and animals, working long days and nights, and weather concerns) that can contribute to rural suicides (Dyer, 1997; Gunderson et al., 1993; Thu et al., 1989). Pesticide self-poisoning is a largely rural phenomenon and the most common method of rural suicide (WHO in collaboration with UNEP, 1990).

By definition, rural areas have decreased population density and encompass wide geographic areas, resulting in expanses of land that are sparsely populated and potentially isolating. Further, the gradual depopulation of rural areas results in a loss of primary relationships, culture, and sense of community, as well as loneliness, for many rural residents (Gerrard, 2003), which are, in turn, associated with suicide (Dorling & Gunnell, 2003; Renwick, Olsen, & Tyrrell, 1982; Shajahan & Cavanagh, 1998). Workforce migration, an aging population, and economic decline have eroded the infrastructure of rural communities, resulting in a loss of land and livelihood, political power and status, and personal control for many rural residents (Beeson, 2000; Center for Suicide Prevention, 2002; Klaber, 2006). Together with all these changes in rural life, there is a greater likelihood of increasing rates of suicide in rural areas as the nation is rapidly transforming with migration from rural to urban areas. This global rural scenario is also reflected in India.

Suicide rates are generally higher in urban than in rural areas in most countries (Qin, 2005; WHO, 1989). Studies from Western countries have demonstrated that urban dwellers are at increased risk of suicide because of a variety of stressors related to living and working in cities, including overcrowding and social isolation (Heikkinen, Aro, & Lonnqvist, 1994; Isometsa et al., 1997; Johansson, Sundquist, Johansson, & Bergman, 1997; Mortensen, Agerbo, Erikson, Qin, & Westergaard-Nielsen, 2000).

In India, however, the suicide rate in rural areas is found to be three times higher than the overall national rate (Gajalakshmi, Peto, Kanimozhi, Whitlock, & Verramani, 2007; Joseph et al., 2003; NCRB, 2000). There are numerous aspects of rural life, such as cultural ideals, geographic and interpersonal isolation, and economic and sociopolitical distress, that may contribute to increased rates of suicide in rural areas (Hirsch, 2006). Those who have studied the problem in rural areas suggest that this may relate to the difficulties associated with making a living in rural areas, particularly in the face of stressors such as drought, fire, and flood. They provide evidence from studies of particular occupational groups, noting particularly high rates of suicide among agricultural and fishery workers (Sundar, 1999). Problems facing rural workers may be exacerbated by a lack of health services in rural areas. As noted previously, the migration of youth from rural to urban areas may also mean that those left behind, especially older people, are particularly vulnerable because of poverty, loneliness, and lack of family support. The rural folks may also have greater access to more lethal means of suicide (e.g., pesticides), with the result that many impulsive, low-intent suicide "attempts" become fatal because of the lethality of the method and the lack of high-quality resuscitation services (Eddleston & Phillips, 2004).

Mental Health and Suicide

It is important to note that the association of mental disorders with suicides has been well established by many researchers in India (Srivastava, 2013) and other countries (Beautrais et al., 1996; Cheng 1995; Lesage et al., 1994; Phillips et al., 2002; Pirkis, Burgess, & Jolley, 2002). Therefore, the component of mental disorders should not be ignored in an effort for suicide prevention. Yet, suicides in India are suggested to be mainly linked with social and economic factors (Manoranjitham et al., 2010, Radhakrishnan & Andrade, 2012).

Globally, more than 90 percent of suicide attempts are linked to a psychiatric disorder and most often to a major depressive disorder (Cavanagh, J. T., Carson, A. J., Sharpe, M., & Lawrie, S. M. 2003, Demyttenaere et al., 2004; Miret, Ayuso-Mateos, Sanchez-Moreno, & Vieta, 2013). Data from high-income countries also argue for a high prevalence of mental illness in those who complete suicide. The Indian experience suggests that many suicides are impulsive and related to stress (Manoranjitham et al., 2010; Radhakrishnan & Andrade, 2012). Recent studies using verbal autopsy data have shown that suicide is often related to socioeconomic circumstances and to interpersonal, social, and cultural conflicts (Prasad et al., 2006). Other Indian studies using psychological autopsies have supported the conclusion that suicide is related to interpersonal conflicts, marital discord, alcoholism, financial problems, and unemployment (Gururaj et al., 2004) and with adverse economic circumstances among farmers (Sainath, 2007). Etzersdorfer, Vijayakumar, Schony, Grausgruber, and Sonneck (1998) in their study indicated that a range of social stressors were strongly associated with both suicidal thoughts and attempts. In fact, it was social stressors that appeared to be providing the added stimulus behind suicide attempts (Armstrong et al., 2014). Many suicides occur impulsively in moments of crisis and, in these circumstances, ready access to the means of suicide – such as pesticides – can determine whether a person lives or dies (WHO, 2014). Qualitative data suggest that many among Indian population view suicide as an option when faced with apparently insoluble personal difficulties and misfortune (Manoranjitham et al., 2007). These findings are relevant to the claim that impulsivity and social stressors play an equally or more important role in suicide deaths in India than psychopathology.

A case-control study on risk factors for suicide in India, although documenting the association between suicide and psychopathology, highlighted its association with adverse life events (Srivastava et al., 2004). Suicide ideation, attempts, and completions may occur in the absence of underlying overt psychiatric disorders. A state of hopelessness (which includes difficulty in believing that there are nonsuicidal alternatives to life problems) has been reported to be more predictive of suicide than depression in India (Greydanus, Bacopoulou, & Tsalamanios, 2009).

The majority of those who commit suicide in India have experienced a number of stressful life events in the three months prior to suicide (NCRB, 2013). Those stressful life events may be interpersonal problems, such as quarrels with spouses, family, friends, or lovers; a rejection, such as separation from family and friends; loss events, such as financial loss or bereavement; work or financial problems, such as job loss, retirement, or financial difficulties; changes in society, such as rapid political and economic changes; as well as various other stressors, such as shame or the threat of being found guilty of a crime.

Income and Educational Determinants

Increased individual or household income has been associated with significantly lower suicide rates in several countries (Phillips, Li, & Zhang, 2002; Registrar General of India, 2007). More suicide deaths occurred in richer states (many of which are in the south) and among individuals with higher levels of education than those who have less than primary education (NCRB, 2013; Patel et al., 2012). By contrast with these findings, in high-income countries, suicide death rates are greater in individuals with lower education (Manoranjitham et al., 2010; Phillips et al., 2002; Rehkopf & Buka, 2006).

Suicide among Youth

Globally, suicide rates among adolescents and young adults are worrying (Minino, 2010), and this is an important public health issue in India as well (Jena & Sidhartha, 2004; Vijayakumar, 2010). The India Million Death study using the RHIME (Representative, Re-sampled, Routine Household Interview of Mortality with Medical Evaluation) method revealed that suicide has become the second leading cause of death for youth aged fifteen to twenty-nine years, with an age-standardized rate per 100,000 population as 25.5 years among males and 24.9 years among females (Patel et al., 2012).

Among young people, suicidal behavior was found to be associated with female gender, not attending school or college, independent decision making, premarital sex, physical abuse at home, lifetime experience of sexual abuse, and probable common mental disorders. Factors associated with gender disadvantage increased vulnerability, particularly in rural women (Pillai, Andrews, & Patel, 2009). Adolescents as an age group are more vulnerable to pressures related to educational expectations from parents and teachers, relationship issues, and peer pressure, thus becoming primary targets of suicide (Bhola, Rekha, Sathyanarayanan, Daniel, & Thomas, 2014). The pressure to do well on exams and the shame associated with failure have been cited as the cause for suicide among young people in India (Vijayakumar, Pirkis, & Huong, 2008). Pressure to achieve in exams is cited as a precipitant in adolescent suicide deaths in Japan and India, where population pressures lead to intense competition for admission to prestigious schools (Beautrais, 2006).

Marital Status

A review of available data in India concluded that marital status alone was not predictive of suicide, suggesting instead that family and social integration were more significant (Rao, 1991). Family is the core of Indian social fabric and the key source of care and social inclusion (Mullatti, 1995). Narratives of distress are almost exclusively located within the domain of the family with particular emphasis on family problems, role strain, and difficulties associated with marriage (Karasz, 2005).

Marriage is usually understood to protect against suicide, particularly for men, based on findings from studies in Western settings (Kposowa, 2000). However, research undertaken in India yields mixed findings regarding the relationship between marital status and suicide for both men and women, suggesting that either marriage is not a protective factor for suicide attempts or indeed that the risk of suicide is higher among those who are married (Latha et al., 1996.; Srivastava et al., 2004).

Several factors associated with higher suicidal behavior in women in India include early age at marriage, lack of autonomy in choosing male partner (arranged marriage), pressure to have children early in marriage (in many cases for a male offspring), economic dependence on husband, and the joint family system. Domestic violence is also a serious problem leading to suicides in India (Gururaj et al., 2004; Vizcarra et al., 2004). Under these circumstances, the young married woman's position is severely compromised, making her vulnerable to psychiatric morbidity and suicidal behaviour (Mayer & Ziaian, 2002).

Suicide and the Elderly

There is a global trend toward increased suicide in late life, again mainly in men (Adamek & Kaplan, 1996; Crepet et al., 1991). Traditionally, the old are revered and well cared for in India, and the suicide rates among them are lower than those of younger age groups (Badrinarayan, 1977). Also, life expectancy in the elderly is lower in India than elsewhere, contributing to the comparatively lower suicide rate (Rao, 1991). However, with gradual neglect of the older population due to modernization and globalization factors, the rates tend to change to those found in Western countries. Thus, the rising mortality from suicide among the aged in some areas in India may reflect the rapid socioeconomic changes influencing the family ties in contemporary Indian society (Rao, 1971).

Risk and Protective Factors for Suicide in India

Risk Factors for Suicide

Although suicide is a deeply personal and an individual act, suicidal behavior is determined by a number of individual and social factors. Suicide is best understood as a multidimensional, multifactorial malaise (Vijayakumar, 2007). According to the 2013 India NCRB data, the reason for suicide is not known for about 16 percent of suicides while illness and family problems contribute to about 44 percent of suicides. The act of suicide depends most importantly on the presence of risk factors and the lack of protective factors. Empirical research has identified and confirmed hundreds of suicide-specific risk factors or characteristics that may increase the likelihood that individuals will desire, attempt, or die by suicide at some point in their lives (O'Connor & Nock, 2014).

Results of such studies consistently suggest that the presence of risk factors can highlight whether someone is more likely to engage in suicide-related behaviors at some point throughout his or her life (i.e., "chronic" risk). Understanding the interactive relationship between risk and protective factors in suicidal behavior and how this interaction can be modified are challenges to suicide prevention (Móscicki, 1997). Variations in suicide risk factors in different cultures and periods have been observed in India (Bhatia et al., 2006). The detection and management of risk factors is an important step in suicide prevention.

Alcohol as Risk Factor

Although social drinking is not a way of life in India, alcoholism plays a significant role in suicide in India. An ecological study in India showed a high correlation between levels of alcohol consumption and suicide rates, with areas such as the state of Pondicherry ranking among the highest on both (NCRB, 2000). Alcohol dependence and abuse were found in 35 percent of suicides in Puducherry. Around 30 to 50 percent of male suicides were under the influence of alcohol at the time of suicide, and many wives have been driven to suicide by their alcoholic husbands. Not only were there a large number of alcoholic suicides, but also many had come from alcoholic families, started consumption of alcohol early in life, and were heavily dependent on alcohol. The odds ratio (OR) for alcoholism was 8.25 (confidence interval: CI 2.9–3.2) in the city of Chennai (Vijayakumar & Rajkumar, 1999) and 4.49 (CI 2.0–6.8) in the city of Bangalore (Gururaj et al., 2004)

Clusters of Suicides

A small portion of suicides consists of vulnerable adolescents who are exposed to suicide through the media and who may be influenced to engage in suicidal behavior. The media sometimes give intense publicity to "suicide clusters" – a series of suicides that occur mainly among young people in a small area within a short period of time. These have a contagious effect, especially when they have been glamorized, provoking imitation or "copycat suicides." This phenomenon has been observed in India on many occasions, especially after the death of a celebrity, most often a movie star or a politician. The tragic death of Dr. Rajashekar Reddy, Chief Minister of State of Andhra Pradesh, is a classic example, in that it was followed by numerous suicides of both young and old people. The wide exposure given to these suicides by the media has led to suicides in a similar manner. Copying methods shown in movies is also not uncommon. This is a serious problem, especially in India, where film stars enjoy an iconic status and wield enormous influence, particularly over the young, who often look up to them as role models (Vijayakumar, 2007).

Protective Factors for Suicide

It is important in suicide prevention to identify broader sociocultural, environmental, and individual protective factors that may reduce a person's vulnerability to suicidal behaviors. Protective factors are quite varied and include an individual's attitudinal and behavioral characteristics, as well as attributes of the environment and culture (Plutchik & Van Praag, 1994). It is very important to consider and strengthen factors that have been shown to increase resilience and connectedness and that protect against suicidal behavior. Resilience has a buffering effect on suicide risk; for persons who are highly resilient, the association between the risk of suicide and suicidal behavior is diminished (Johnson, Wood, Gooding, Taylor, & Tarrier, 2011). Some protective factors counter specific risk factors while others protect individuals against a number of different suicide risk factors.

Social Integration

Social integration refers to the bonds and links that attach individuals to social groups outside of themselves. These bonds create a feeling of allegiance to the wider group (e.g., national identity or religious groups) and are manifested in devotion toward common goals and shared beliefs and sentiments. Social integration – such as through participation in sport, religious organizations, clubs and other activities, good relationships with schoolmates or work colleagues, good relationships with teachers or superiors, and support from relevant people – can also be found among protective factors. However, the social reality of India is determined by competing factors such as caste (an endogamous and hereditary social group limited to persons of the same rank, occupation, or economic position), religion, ethnic, and regional factors that restrict greater social interaction. If people are able to overcome these barriers and learn to build bridges with others, a feeling of unity and integrity can be achieved that leads to universal brotherhood.

Religious or Spiritual Beliefs

Religion may be protective against suicide, both at the individual and societal level, and this effect may be mediated by the degree to which a given religion sanctions suicide (Vijayakumar, 2002). This view coincides with individual-level studies that have found variables such as lack of religious conviction to be a risk factor for suicide in India (Gururaj et al., 2004). A study in Chennai found that the OR for lack of belief in God was 6.8 (CI 2.88–19.69) (Vijayakumar, 2002). It was found, in this study, that those who committed suicide had less belief in God, changed their religious affiliation, and rarely visited places of worship. Eleven percent had lost their faith in the three months prior to suicide. Gururaj et al. (2004) also found that lack of religious belief in India was a risk factor (OR 19.18, CI 4.17–10.37).

Obstacles to Suicide Prevention

Negative Attitudes toward Suicide Prevention

While major determinants for suicide are considered to be social and environmental factors such as unemployment over which an individual has relatively little control, a belief has emerged in India even among health professionals that suicide cannot be prevented. Such beliefs explain the apathy and negative attitude toward suicide prevention.

Legal Issues

Until 2014, attempted suicide was a punishable offense in India. Suicide is illegal, and a survivor could face a jail term of up to one year and a fine under Section 309 of the Indian Penal Code. However, the aim of the law to prevent suicide by legal methods has proved to be counterproductive. Emergency care to those who have attempted suicide is denied as many hospitals, and practitioners hesitate to provide the needed treatment fearful of legal hassles. The Government of India has decided to delete the Section 309 of Indian Penal Code to decriminalize suicide attempts (Jain, 2014).

Taboo on Suicide

The strong taboo on suicide that still exists and the distress it arouses and has aroused throughout history make it difficult to approach the problem of suicide in an open way or through prevention. To this day, suicidal behavior is associated with shame, uneasiness, and guilt. However, by openly discussing suicidal thoughts they turn from a problem to be hidden to a problem to be solved. Raising community awareness and breaking down taboos are important in making efforts to prevent suicide.

Stigma on Mental Illnesses

The reduction of the stigma that is still attached to people with mental disorders helps these people coming forward to receive treatment at early stages of the disease, when treatment is more efficient.

Gaps in Suicide Prevention in India

Insufficient Funds

Recently, the Government of India has acknowledged the growing concerns over the alarming rate of suicide and has allocated funds and resources for mental health services in the affected regions in South India. However, the government funding for mental health services are mostly restricted to the development of hospitals, payment of salaries, and the cost of medication, while funds for suicide prevention are not explicitly allocated, suggesting their low priority. The lack of funding for services and programs renders these important suicide prevention services inaccessible to the community. Therefore, the vast majority of the rural and urban population is deprived of specialty services in suicide intervention despite the dire need for them in the region.

Shortage of Trained Mental Health Professionals

One of the major gaps in suicide prevention is the lack of trained mental health professionals in the rural communities where most suicides occur. There are approximately 4,000 psychiatrists, 1,000 clinical psychologists, 3,000 psychiatric social workers, and 1,500 mental health nurses in India, which has a population of about 1.25 billion people (Sinha & Kaur, 2011). Thus, the ratio of mental health professional to population is extremely low. It is almost impossible for the existing mental health resources to provide psychiatric services and suicide intervention to all rural communities.

According to Rural Health Survey conducted in 2011, there are 148,124 subcenters, 23,887 primary health centers, and 4,809 community health centers functioning in India. This report revealed a significant shortage of trained human resources such as health care workers, auxiliary nurses, midwives, medical doctors, and specialists in primary and community health centers (Pandve & Pandve, 2013).

Since India is facing a severe shortage of primary care providers, it is almost impossible for the country to develop infrastructure and resources within a reasonable timeline to meet the need of people living in the rural areas. The acute shortage of psychiatrists in India, and of mental health services generally in that nation, suggests that others must become involved in service improvements.

Most medical school and residency programs do not provide adequate training in suicide prevention. Thus, primary care providers lack proper knowledge of risk factors and feel unprepared to manage suicidal patients (Taliaferro & Borowsky, 2011). A recent study has highlighted the existing gaps in core competencies in primary care professionals related to suicide risk identification, assessment, and management in India (Shah et al., 2015). There is an urgent need to provide training for primary care providers and equip them with knowledge of identification and management of suicidal patients to ensure that patients receive the early care they need. Therefore, initiatives from various sectors (the government, medical universities, the medical council and other regulatory bodies, nongovernmental organizations [NGO] and international nongovernmental organizations [INGO], and community-based programs) are required to achieve a satisfactory goal in suicide prevention in the region (Shah et al., 2015).

Health Inequalities

In the last few decades, Indian society has experienced rapid economic growth. However, large proportions of the population have not benefited from this progress. Key features of health inequities are that they are socially produced, systematic in their distribution across the population, and unfair (Withhead & Dahlgren, 2006). Balarajan, Selvaraj, and Subramanian (2011) describe how insufficient allocation of public spending on health between rural and urban areas and between preventative and curative services in India, access to quality care among the poor, and high out-of-the pocket expenditures act as key barriers to increased equitable access to health care in India. Health inequalities in India also pose serious ethical challenges. The lack of a moral framework for religious values and ethical reasoning prevents the general public from responding and the government from taking initiatives to achieve the goal of health justice for all.

The Challenge of Suicide Prevention in India

Prevention scientists in India are divided on how to focus on suicide prevention efforts. While some are agitating for greater attention to mental health services and treatment (Vijayakumar, 2005), others argue that the predominant focus should be on policies to ensure that the basic human needs and rights of the population are met and that we avoid medicalizing personal and social distress (Jacob, 2008). In India, a few mental disorders are significantly associated with suicide. Mood disorders, alcohol and other substance misuse, schizophrenia, and personality disorders are particularly relevant in this respect (Bhatia et al., 2006). Therefore, some people argue that the early identification and the appropriate treatment of those mental disorders are important strategies for the prevention of suicide.

A previous case-control study on risk factors for suicide in India, although documenting the association between suicide and psychopathology, highlighted its association with adverse life events (Vijayakumar & Rajkumar, 1999). Qualitative data suggest that many in the general population view suicide as an option when faced with apparently insoluble personal difficulties and misfortune (Manoranjitham et al., 2007).

Western data argue for a high prevalence of mental illness in those who complete suicide (Hawton & Heeringen, 2001). The Indian experience, however, suggests that many suicides are impulsive and related to stress (Manoranjitham et al., 2010; Radhakrishnan & Andrade, 2012).

In literature and in practice, evidence-based interventions for suicide prevention are usually organized in a theoretical framework that distinguishes among universal, selective, and indicated interventions on the basis of how their target groups are defined (Mrazek & Haggerty, 1994).

Universal Interventions

Universal interventions target whole populations with the aim of favorably shifting proximal or distal risk factors across the entire population. Thus, "universal" prevention strategies may aim to increase access to health care, promote mental health, reduce harmful use of alcohol, limit access to the means for suicide, promote responsible media reporting, strengthen protective processes such as social support, and alter the physical environment (WHO, 2014).

In India, high rates of suicide are due to economic difficulties (Sainath, 2007) and social, cultural, and interpersonal conflicts among people without known mental illness (Gururaj et al., 2004; Manoranjitham et al., 2007; Prasad et al., 2006). Poverty, unemployment, illiteracy, lack of civic facilities, poor access to health facilities, and the absence of health insurance or of welfare are factors that adversely impact the overall mental health status of the population. There is a need to focus on underlying causes of human suffering, including poverty, economic inequality, and lack of social justice (Jacob, 2008).

In India, where nearly 30 percent of people live below the poverty line (as of 2014), the Indian government should introduce such social policies that are fair, just, and equitable and that attempt to bring down the disparity. Sustained economic policies that include the concept of distributive justice will need to be pursued. It is further stated that the reductions in suicide rates reported in some countries have more to do with secular trends and improvements in living standards than specific prevention programs (Bellanger, Jourdain, & Batt-Moillo, 2007).

Selective Interventions

Selective interventions target subgroups whose members are not yet manifesting suicidal behavior but exhibit risk factors that predispose them to do so in the future. "Selective" prevention strategies target vulnerable groups such as persons who have suffered trauma or abuse, those affected by conflict or disaster, refugees and migrants, and persons bereaved by suicide, by training "gatekeepers" who assist the vulnerable and by offering helping services such as helplines.

Preventive strategies implemented at a community level and identifying vulnerable individuals may be more effective in India than global strategies. A greater understanding of region-specific factors related to suicide would enable prevention strategies to be more culturally sensitive (Radhakrishnan & Andrade, 2012). Similarly, Jacob (2008) argues for psychosocial interventions for vulnerable sections of society that provide social support and challenge a culture in India that accepts suicide as a way out of personal misery. These interventions at community level are basic and mandatory requirements in addition to population-based interventions in reducing the suicides.

Indicated Interventions

Indicated interventions are designed for people already beginning to exhibit early signs of suicide potential or who have made a suicide attempt., "Indicated" prevention strategies target specific vulnerable individuals with community support, follow-up for those leaving health care facilities, education and training for health workers, and improved identification and management of mental and substance use disorders (WHO, 2014).

Reducing risk will go only part of the way toward reducing suicide. Furtherance of protective factors will help build much needed resilience. This is achieved when community organizations provide support and appropriate referrals to those in need of assistance, families and social circles enhance resilience and intervene effectively to help loved ones, and there is a social climate where help-seeking is no longer a taboo and public dialogue is encouraged.

Prevention programs need to be eclectic, since no single theory or framework can explain or provide effective interventions for all potential suicides. The many components of comprehensive suicide programs are difficult to implement in practice, given the numerous competing demands on limited governmental resources in the developing world.

The following are some of the other population-based interventions that should form the core of suicide prevention programs in India (Jacob, 2008):

1. Prevention, apart from dealing with risk factors for suicide, can also be strengthened by encouraging protective factors such as strong personal relationships, a personal belief system, and positive coping strategies.
2. Capitalism, urbanization, and migration have led to a breakdown in traditional support mechanisms and social connectedness that need to be revived or replaced. Communities can organize themselves to provide social support to vulnerable individuals and engage in follow-up care, fight stigma, and support those bereaved by suicide.
3. There is an urgent need to devise and implement an essential pesticide list that excludes compounds that are extremely lethal, and to regulate the manufacture, packaging, and sale of pesticides that are lethal to humans. Preventing suicide by restricting access to suicide methods is one of the few evidence-based suicide prevention strategies (Mann et al., 2005).
4. The concerns of women, gender justice, and violence, as well as changing the culture that undervalues women and providing legal recourse for problems, are issues that need to be addressed on a national scale.
5. Increase in public awareness through the mass media is needed with controls for portrayal of suicide that currently borders on the voyeuristic. The media should be recruited to fight stigma and discrimination related to mental illness and suicide. The mass media should also be recruited to argue for social justice and for the need for governments to meet the basic needs of populations. There is a need for intensive explorations of the various aspects of suicidal behavior and possible ways of prevention, within the Indian society, as a necessary preliminary step toward an efficient prevention strategy.

Need for National Suicide Prevention Strategy

The creation of a national response provides a rallying point for bringing together a diversity of stakeholders in suicide prevention and for building on their expertise through a participatory approach. The result is a convergence of stakeholders from government, NGOs, and health and non-health sectors that can contribute to country-specific, national long-term strategies that follow a public health model (WHO, 2014).

Several NGOs have been formed in India by concerned citizens who have come together to design programs that create awareness and support individuals dealing with emotional stresses and help save lives. These NGOs essentially work to raise awareness about mental health and promote mental well-being. The services are provided over the phone; face-to-face, at the address; and over email. Some of these NGOs based in major Indian cities include 1life Hyderabad, Aasra Navi Mumbai, Befrienders India Chennai, National Association Chennai, Connecting India Pune, Lifeline Foundation Kolkata, Maitreyi Puducherry, Roshni Secunderabad, Saath Ahmedabad, Sneha Chennai, the Samaritans Sahara Mumbai, Sumaitri New Delhi, and Maithri Cochin.

A systematic way of developing a national response to suicide is to create a national suicide prevention strategy. A national strategy indicates a government's clear commitment to dealing with the issue of suicide. Typical national strategies should comprise a range of prevention strategies such as surveillance, means restriction, media guidelines, stigma reduction, and the raising of public awareness as well as training for health workers, educators, police, and other gatekeepers. The strategy should also include crisis intervention services and postvention. A comprehensive strategy allows for the transparent identification of stakeholders who are accountable for specific tasks and outlines ways to coordinate between them effectively (WHO, 2012b).

Key elements in developing a national suicide prevention strategy in India are to make prevention a multisectoral priority that involves not only the health sector but also education, employment, social welfare, the judiciary, and others. The strategy should be tailored to India's cultural and social context, establishing best practices and evidence-based interventions in a comprehensive approach. Resources should be allocated for achieving both short-to-medium and long-term objectives; there should be effective planning; and the strategy should be regularly evaluated, with evaluation findings feeding into future planning. The national suicide prevention strategy should be tailored for diversity, taking into consideration specific social and cultural contexts.

Conclusions

Suicide prevention programs in India should involve a whole series of activities, ranging from the environmental control of risk factors and means, through the early identification and effective treatment of people with mental and substance use disorders, to the responsible reporting of suicide in the media. Many diverse approaches, taking into consideration the cultural diversity of India, focusing on population interventions, and being tailored to the regional context, will need to be implemented simultaneously in order to produce any reduction in suicide rates for populations. The involvement of various sectors (e.g., health, education, labor, agriculture) needs to be sought as well as the engagement of various partners (e.g., governments, NGOs).

The different risk and protective factors and the scarcity of human and economic resources necessitate the development of integrated suicide prevention strategies in India. Specially designed programs for vulnerable populations, such as the women and the young, need to be initiated. More importantly, suicide prevention programs need to be locally relevant, culturally appropriate, and cost effective. Thus suicide prevention in India is more a social and public health objective than a traditional exercise in the mental health sector. A comprehensive suicide prevention program should employ a combination of prevention strategies at the general population level, for vulnerable subpopulations at risk, and for those specific vulnerable individuals who are already beginning to exhibit early signs of suicide potential.

References

Aaron, R., Joseph, A., Abraham, S., Muliyil, J., George, K., Prasad, J., ... Bose, A. (2004). Suicides in young people in rural southern India. *Lancet* 363: 1117–18.

Abraham, V. J., Abraham, S., & Jacob, K. S. (2005). Suicide in the elderly in Kaniyambadi block, Tamil Nadu, South India. *International Journal of Geriatric Psychiatry* 20: 953–5.

Adamek, M. E., & Kaplan, M. S. (1996). The growing use of firearms by suicidal older women, 1979–1992: a research note. *Suicide Life Threat Behavior*. 26: 71–8.

Armstrong, G., Jorm, A. F., Samson, L., Joubert, L., Singh, S., & Kermode, M., (2014). Suicidal ideation and attempts among men who inject drugs in Delhi, India: psychological and social risk factors. *Social Psychiatry and Psychiatric Epidemiology* 49: 1367–77.

Aubert, P., Daigle, M. S., & Daigle, J. G. (2004). Cultural traits and immigration: hostility and suicidality in Chinese Canadian students. *Transcultural Psychiatry* 41: 514–32.

Badrinarayan, A. (1977). Suicide attempts in Gulbarga. *Indian Journal of Psychiatry* 19: 69–70.

Balarajan, Y., Selvaraj, S., & Subramanian, S. V. (2011). Health care and equity in India. *Lancet* 377: 500–15.

Beautrais, A. L. (2006). Suicide in Asia. *Crisis* 27(2): 55–7. doi: dx.doi.org/10.1027/0227-5910.27.2.55

Beautrais, A. L., Joyce, P. R., Mulder, R. T., Fergusson, D. M., Deavoll, B. J., & Nightingale, S. K. (1996). Prevalence and comorbidity of mental disorders in persons making serious suicide attempts: a case-control study. *American Journal of Psychiatry* 153: 1009–14.

Beeson, P. G. (2000). Some notes and data on rural suicide. *Rural Mental Health* 25: 13–15.

Behere, P. B., & Behere, A. P. (2008). Farmers' suicide in Vidarbha region of Maharashtra state: a myth or reality? *Indian Journal of Psychiatry* 50: 124–7.

Bellanger, M. M., Jourdain, A., & Batt-Moillo, A. (2007). Might the decrease in the suicide rates in France be due to regional prevention programmes? *Social Sciences & Medicine* 65: 431–41.

Bertolote, J. M., Fleischmann, A., De Leo, D., Bolhari, J., Botega, N., De Silva, D., ... Wasserman, D. (2005). Suicide attempts, plans, and ideation in culturally diverse sites. *Psychological Medicine* 35: 1457–65.

Bhatia, T., Thomas, P., Semwal, P., Thelma, B. K., Nimgaonkar, V. L., & Deshpande, S. N. (2006). Differing correlates for suicide attempts among patients with schizophrenia or schizoaffective disorder in India and USA. *Schizophrenia Research* 86: 208–14.

Bhola, P., Rekha, D. P, Sathyanarayanan, V., Daniel, S., & Thomas, T. (2014). Self--reported suicidality and its predictors among adolescents from a pre-university college in Bangalore, India. *Asian Journal of Psychiatry* 7: 38–45.

Bhugra, D. (2005). Sati: A type of nonpsychiatric suicide. *Crisis* 26: 73–7.

Braun, W. (2008). Sallekhana: the ethicality and legality of religious suicide by starvation in the Jain religious community. *Med Law* 27: 913–24.

Canetto, S. S. (2008) Women and suicidal behavior: a cultural analysis. *American Journal of Orthopsychiatry* 78: 259–66.

Cavanagh, J. T., Carson, A. J., Sharpe, M., & Lawrie, S. M. (2003) Psychological autopsy studies of suicide: a systematic review. *Psycholgical Medicine* 33: 395–405.

Center for Suicide Prevention (2002). *Rural Stress: Suicide Information and Education Collection (Rep. No. 50)*. Calgary, Alberta, Canada: Center for Suicide Prevention, Canadian Mental Health Association.

Cheng, A. T. (1995). Mental illness and suicide. a case-control study in East Taiwan. *Archives of General Psychiatry* 52: 594–603.

Crepet, P., Caracciolo, S., Casoli, R., Fabbri, D., Florenzano, F., Grassi, G. M., et al. (1991). Suicidal behavior in Italy: data, trends and guidelines for a suicide intervention/prevention policy. *Suicide Life Threat Behavior* 21: 263–78.

Das, P. P., Grover, S., Avasthi, A., Chakrabarti, S., Malhotra, S., & Kumar, S. (2008). Intentional self-harm seen in psychiatric referrals in a tertiary care hospital. *Indian Journal of Psychiatry* 50: 187–91.

De Leo, D. (2003). The interface of schizophrenia, culture and suicide. In Vijayakumar, L., (eds.), *Suicide Prevention: Meeting the Challenge Together*. Hyderabad, India: Orient Longman, pp. 11–41.

Demyttenaere, K., Bruffaerts, R., Posada-Villa, J., Gasquet, I., Kovess, V., Lepine, J. P. ... & Chatterji, S. (2004). Prevalence, severity, and unmet need for treatment of mental disorders in the World Health Organization World Mental Health Surveys. *Journal of American Medical Association* 291: 2581–90.

Dombrovski, A. Y., Szanto, K., Duberstein, P., Conner, K. R., Houck, P. R., & Conwell, Y. (2008). Sex differences in correlates of suicide attempt lethality in late life. *American Journal of Geriatric Psychiatry* 16: 905–13.

Dorling, D., & Gunnell, D. (2003). Suicide: the spatial and social components of despair in Britain, 1980–2000. *Transactions of the Institute of British Geographers* 28: 442–60.

Durkheim, E. (1951 [1897]). *Suicide: A Study in Sociology*. Trans. Spaulding, J. A., & Simpson, G.. New York: Free Press

Durkheim, E. (1952). *Suicide*. London: Routledge and Kegan Paul.

Dyer, J. (1997). *Harvest of Rage*. Boulder, CO: Westview Press.

Eddleston, M., Phillips, M. R. (2004). Self poisoning with pesticides. *British Medical Journal* 328: 42–4.

Etzersdorfer, E., Vijayakumar, L., Schony, W., Grausgruber, A., & Sonneck, G. (1998). Attitudes towards suicide among medical students – comparison between Madras (India) and Vienna (Austria). *Social Psychiatry Psychiatric Epidemiolpgu* 33: 104–10.

Gajalakshmi, V., & Peto, R. (2006). Commentary: verbal autopsy procedure for adult deaths. *International Journal of Epidemiology* 35: 748–50. doi: 10.1093/ije/dyl112

Gajalakshmi, V., & Peto, R. (2007). Suicide rates in rural Tamil Nadu, South India: verbal autopsy of 39 000 deaths in 1997–98. *International Journal of Epidemiology* 36: 203–7.

Gajalakshmi, V, & Peto, R., Kanimozhi, C. V., Whitlock, G., & Veeramani, D. (2007). Cohort profile: the Chennai prospective study of mortality among 500 000 adults in Tamil Nadu, South India. *International Journal of Epidemiology* 36: 1190–5.

Gerrard, N. (2003). *Farm Stress: Resiliency in Rural People*. Regina, Saskatchewan, Canada: Saskatchewan Agriculture and Food.

Government of India (1976). *Suicides in India, 1964–1972*, New Delhi: Government of India.

Greydanus, D. E., Bacopoulou, F., & Tsalamanios, E. (2009). Suicide in adolescents: a worldwide preventable tragedy. *Keio Journal of Medicine* 58: 95–102.

Gunderson, P., Donner, D., Nashold, R., Salkowicz, L., Sperry, S., & Wittman, B. (1993). The epidemiology of suicide among farm residents or workers in five north-central states, 1980–1988. *American Journal of Preventive Medicine* 9: 26–32.

Gururaj, G., Isaac, M. K., Subbakrishna, D. K., & Ranjani, R. (2004). Risk factors for completed suicides: a case-control study from Bangalore, India. *Injury Control and Safety Promotion* 11: 183–91.

Hawton, K., & Heeringen, K. V. (2001). *The International Handbook of Suicide and Attempted Suicide*. New York: Wiley

Heikkinen, M., Aro, H., & Lönnqvist, J. (1994). Recent life events, social support and suicide. *Acta Psychiatrica Scandinavica* 377: 65–72.

Hirsch, J. K. (2006). A review of the literature on rural suicide: risk and protective factors, incidence, and prevention. *Crisis* 27: 189–99. dx.doi.org/10.1007/978-81-322-1674-2_11

Isometsa, E., Heikkinen, M., Henriksson, M., Marttunen, M., Aro, H., & Lonnqvist, J. (1997). Differences between urban and rural suicides. *Acta Psychiatrica Scandinavica* 95: 297–305.

Jacob, K. S. (2008). The prevention of suicide in India and the developing world: the need for population-based strategies. *Crisis* 29: 102–6.

Jain, B. (2014). Government decriminalizes attempt to commit suicide, removes section 309. *Times of India,* December 10. Retrieved from timesofindia.indiatimes.com/india/Government-decriminalizes-attempt-to-commit-suicide-removes-section-309/articleshow/45452253.cms

Jena, S., & Sidhartha, T. (2004). Non-fatal suicidal behaviors in adolescents. *Indian Journal of Psychiatry* 46: 310–18.

Johansson, L. M., Sundquist, J., Johansson, S., & Bergman, B. (1997). Ethnicity, social factors, illness and suicide: a follow-up study of a random sample of the Swedish population. *Acta Psychiatrica Scandinavica* 95:125–31.

Johnson, J., Wood, A. M., Gooding, P., Taylor, P. J., & Tarrier, N. (2011). Resilience to suicidality: the buffering hypothesis. *Clinical Psychology Review* 31: 563–91.

Jones, S., & Keenan, P. (2014) Comparisons of attempted suicide between India and UK. *Mental Health Nursing* 34: 14–17.

Joseph, A., Abraham, S., Muliyil, J. P., George, K., Prasad, J., Minz, S., . . . Jacob, K. S. (2003). Evaluation of suicide rates in rural India using verbal autopsies, 1994–9. *British Medical Journal* 326(7399): 1121–2.

Karasz, A. (2005). Cultural differences in conceptual models of depression. *Social Science & Medicine* 60: 1625–35.

Klaber, A. (2006). *Trends in Suicide Rates in Urban and Rural Areas across Trent Region, 1988–1998*. University of Sheffield, UK: Public Health GIS Unit.

Kposowa, A. J. (2000). Marital status and suicide in the National Longitudinal Mortality Study. *Journal of Epidemiology and Community Health* 54: 254–61.

Kumar, V. (2004). Poisoning deaths in married women. *Journal of Clinical Forensic Medicine* 11: 2–5.

Kurosu, S. (1991). Suicide in rural areas, the case of Japan 1960–1980. *Rural Sociology* 56: 603–18.

Latha, K. S., Bhat, S. M., & D'Souza, P. (1996). Suicide attempters in a general hospital unit in India: their socio-demographic and clinical profile – emphasis on cross-cultural aspects. *Acta Psychiatrica Scandinavica* 94: 26–30.

Lesage, A. D., Boyer, R., Grunberg, F., Vanier, C., Morissette, R., Menard-Buteau, C., et al. (1994). Suicide and mental disorders: a case-control study of young men. *American Journal of Psychiatry* 151: 1063–8.

Lingren, H. (1995). *Rural Families Facing Economic and Emotional Stress (Rep. No. NF93–155)*. Lincoln: Cooperative Extension, Institute of Agriculture and Natural Resources, University of Nebraska–Lincoln.

Mann, J. J., Apter, A., Bertolote, J., Beautrais, A., Currier, D., Haas, A., . . . Marusic, A., et al. (2005). Suicide prevention strategies, a systematic review. *JAMA – Journal of the American Medical Association* 294: 2064–74.

Manoranjitham, S. D., Charles, H., Saravanan, B., Jayakaran, R., Abraham, S., & Jacob, K. S. (2007). Perceptions about suicide, a qualitative study from southern India. *National Medical Journal of India* 20: 176–9.

Manoranjitham, S. D., Rajkumar, A. P., Thangadurai, P., Prasad, J., Jayakaran, R., & Jacob, K. S. (2010). Risk factors for suicide in rural South India. *British Journal of Psychiatry* 196: 26–30.

Mayer, P., & Ziaian, T. (2002). Suicide, gender, and age variations in India: are women in Indian society protected from suicide? *Crisis* 23: 98–103.

Menon, V., Kattimani, S., Sarkar, S., & Muthuramalingam, A. (2015). Gender differ ences among suicide attempters attending a crisis intervention clinic in South India. *Industrial Psychiatry Journal* 24: 64.

Middleton, N., Whitley, E., Frankel, S., Dorling, D., Sterne, J., & Gunnell, D. (2004). Suicide risk in small areas in England and Wales, 1991–1993. *Social Psychiatry & Psychiatric Epidemiology* 39: 45–52.

Minino, A. M., (2010). *Mortality among Teenagers Aged 12–19 Years: United States 1999–2006*. NCHS Data Brief, No. 37. Hyattsville, MD: National Center for Health Statistics.

Miret, M., Ayuso-Mateos, J. L., Sanchez-Moreno, J., & Vieta, E. (2013). Depressive disorders and suicide: epidemiology, risk factors, and burden. *Neuroscience and Biobehavioral Reviews* 37: 2372–4.

Mortensen, P. B., Agerbo, E., Erikson, T., Qin, P., & Westergaard-Nielsen, N. (2000). Psychiatric illness and risk factors for suicide in Denmark. *Lancet* 355: 9–12.

Moscicki, E. K. (1997). Identification of suicide risk factors using epidemiologic studies. *Psychiatric Clinics of North America* 20: 499–517.

Mrazek, P. J., & Haggerty, R. (1994). *Reducing Risks for Mental Disorders: Frontiers for Preventive Intervention Research*. Washington, DC: National Academy Press.

Mullatti, L. (1995). Families in India, beliefs and realities. *Journal of Comparative Family Studies* 26: 11–25.

Nandi, D. N., Banerjee, G., & Boral, G. C., (1978). Suicides in West Bengal: a century apart. *Indian Journal of Psychiatry* 20: 155.

NCRB (National Crime Records Bureau) (2000). *Accidental Deaths and Suicide in India*. New Delhi: Ministry of Home Affairs, Government of India.

NCRB (National Crime Records Bureau) (2013). *Accidental Deaths and Suicides in India 2012*, 46th ed. New Delhi: National Crime Records Bureau, Ministry of Home Affairs, Government of India.

O'Connor, R. C., & Nock, M. K. (2014). The psychology of suicidal behavior. *Lancet Psychiatry* 1: 73–85. doi: 10.1016/S2215-0366(14)70222-6

Pandve, H., & Pandve, T. (2013). Primary healthcare system in India: evolution and challenges. *International Journal of Health System and Disaster Management* 1: 125–8.

Patel, V., Ramasundarahettige, C., Vijayakumar, L., Thakur, J. S., Gajalakshmi, V., & Gururaj, G. et al. for the Million Death Study Collaborators (2012). Suicide mortality in India, a nationally representative survey. *Lancet* 379 (9834): 2343–51.

Phillips, M. R., & Cheng, H. C. (2012). The changing global face of suicide. *Lancet* 379: 2318–9.

Phillips, M. R., Li, X., Zhang, Y. (2002). Suicide rates in China, 1995–99. *Lancet* 359: 835–40.

Phillips, M. R., Yang, G., Li, S., & Li, Y. (2004). Suicide and the unique prevalence pattern of schizophrenia in mainland China: a retrospective observational study. *Lancet* 364: 1062–8.

Phillips, M. R., Yang, G., Zhang, Y., Wang, L., Ji, H., & Zhou, M. (2002). Risk factors for suicide in China: a national case-control psychological autopsy study. *Lancet* 360(9347): 1728–36.

Pillai, A., Andrews, T., & Patel, V. (2009). Violence, psychological distress and the risk of suicidal behaviour in young people in India. *International Journal of Epidemiology* 38: 459–69.

Pirkis, J., Burgess, P., & Jolley, D. (2002). Suicide among psychiatric patients: a case-control study. *Australian and New Zealand Journal of Psychiatry* 36: 86–91.

Plutchik, R., & Van Praag, H. M. (1994). Suicide risk: amplifiers and attenuators. In Hillbrand, M., & Pollone, N. J. (eds.), *The Psychobiology of Aggression*. Binghamton, NY: Haworth Press.

Prasad, J., Abraham, V. J., Minz, S., Abraham, S., Joseph, A., Muliyil, J. P., et al. (2006). Rates and factors associated with suicide in Kaniyambadi Block, Tamil Nadu, South India, 2000–02. *International Journal of Social Psychiatry* 52: 65–71.

Pritchard, C., & Hean, S. (2008). Suicide and undetermined deaths among youths and young adults in Latin America, comparison with the 10 major developed countries – a source of hidden suicides? *Crisis* 29: 145–53.

Qin, P. (2005). Suicide risk in relation to level of urbanicity – a population-based linkage study. *International Journal of Epidemiology* 34(4): 846–52.

Radhakrishnan, R., & Andrade, C. (2012). Suicide: an Indian perspective. *Indian Journal of Psychiatry* 54: 304–19.

Rao, A. V. (1971). Suicide attempters in Madurai. *Journal of Indian Medical Association* 57: 278–83.

Rao, A. V. (1991). Suicide in the elderly: a report from India. *Crisis* 12: 33–9.

Registrar General of India (2007). *Medically-Certified Causes of Death, Statistical Report: 2004*. New Delhi: Government of India.

Rehkopf, D. H., Buka, S. L. (2006). The association between suicide and the socio-economic characteristics of geographical areas, a systematic review. *Psychological Medicine* 36: 145–57.

Renwick, M. Y., Olsen, G. G., & Tyrrell, M. S. (1982). Suicide in rural New South Wales: comparison with metropolitan experience. *Medical Journal of Australia* 1: 377–80.

Sadock, B. J., & Sadock, V. A. (2008). *Kaplan & Sadock's Concise Textbook of Clinical Psychiatry*, 3rd ed. Philadelphia, PA: Wolters Kluwer/Lippincott Williams and Wilkins.

Sainath, P. (2007). Nearly 1.5 lakh farm suicides from 1997 to 2005. *Hindu*, November 12. www.hindu.com/2007/11/12/stories/2007111257790100.htm

Shah, R., Eynan, R., Srivastava, A., Reiss, L., Rao, T. S., Parkar, S., Dutt, L., Kadam, K., & Links, P. S. (2015). Indo–Canadian collaboration for suicide prevention: training needs assessment for healthcare professionals in India. *Community Mental Health Journal*. doi: 10.1007/s10597-015–9895-z [Epub ahead of print]

Shajahan, P. M., & Cavanagh, J. T. O. (1998). Admission for depression among men in Scotland, 1980–95, retrospective study. *British Medical Journal* 316: 1496–7.

Sinha, S. K., & Kaur, J. (2011). National mental health programme: manpower development scheme of eleventh five-year plan. *Indian Journal of Psychiatry* 53: 261–5.

Srivastava, A. (2013). Psychological attributes and socio-demographic profile of hundred completed suicide victims in the state of Goa, India. *Indian Journal of Psychiatry* 55: 268–72.

Srivastava, M. K., Sahoo, R. N., Ghotekar, L. H., Dutta, S., Danabalan, M., Dutta, T. K., & Das, A. K. (2004). Risk factors associated with attempted suicide: a case control study. *Indian Journal of Psychiatry* 46: 33–8.

Sundar, M. (1999). Suicide in farmers in India. *British Journal of Psychiatry* 175: 585–6.

Taliaferro, L. A., & Borowsky, I. W. (2011). Perspective, physician education: a promising strategy to prevent adolescent suicide. *Academic Medicine* 86: 342–7.

Thu, K., Lasley, P., Whitten, P., Lewis, M., Donham, K. J., Zwerling, C., et al. (1989). Stress as a potential risk factor for agricultural injuries: comparative data from the Iowa Farm Family Health and Hazard Survey (1994) and the Iowa Farm and Rural Life Poll (1989). *Journal of Agromedicine* 4: 181–92.

Vijayakumar, L. (2002). Religion: a protective factor in suicide. *Suicidologi* 2: 9–12.

Vijayakumar, L. (2004a). Altruistic suicide in India. *Archives of Suicide Research* 8: 73–80. doi: 10.1080/13811110490243804

Vijayakumar, L. (2004b). Suicide prevention, the urgent need in developing countries. *World Psychiatry* 3: 158–9.

Vijayakumar, L. (2005). Suicide and mental disorders in Asia. *International Review of Psychiatry* 17: 109–14.

Vijayakumar, L. (2007). Suicide and its prevention: the urgent need in India. *Indian Journal of Psychiatry* 49: 81–4. doi: 10.4103/0019–5545.33252

Vijayakumar, L. (2010). Indian research on suicide. *Indian Journal of Psychiatry* 52: S291–S296.

Vijayakumar, L., Nagaraj, K.., Pirkis, J., & Whiteford, H. (2005). Suicide in developing countries (1), frequency, distribution, and association with socioeconomic indicators. *Crisis* 263: 104–11. doi: 10.1027/0227–5910.26.3.104

Vijayakumar, L., Pirkis, J., & Huong, T. T. (2008). Socio-economic, cultural and religious factors affecting suicide prevention in Asia. In Hendin, H., Phillips, M. R., & Vijayakumar, L. (eds.), *Suicide and Suicide Prevention in Asia*. Geneva, Switzerland: World Health Organization, pp. 19–30.

Vijayakumar, L., & Rajkumar, S. (1999). Are risk factors for suicide universal? A case-control study in India. *Acta Psychiatria Scandinavia* 99: 407–11.

Vizcarra, B., Hassan, F., Hunter, W. M., Muñoz, S. R., Ramiro, L., & Paula, C. S. (2004). Partner violence as a risk factor for mental health among women from communities in the Philippines, Egypt, Chile, and India. *Injury Control and Safety Promotion* 11: 125–9.

WHO (World Health Organization) (1989). *World Health Statistics Annual*. Geneva, Switzerland: World Health Organization.

WHO (World Health Organization) (2000). *Preventing Suicide. A Resource for General Physicians*. Geneva, Switzerland: World Health Organization.

WHO (World Health Organization) (2001). *World Health Report 2001: Mental Health, New Understanding, New Hope*. Geneva, Switzerland: World Health Organization.

WHO (World Health Organization) (2012a). *Global Burden of Mental Disorders and the Need for a Comprehensive, Coordinated Response from Health and Social Sectors at the Country Level. A65/10*. Geneva, Switzerland: World Health Organization.

WHO (World Health Organization) (2012b). *Public Health Action for the Prevention of Suicide: A Framework.* Geneva, Switzerland: World Health Organization. apps.who.int/iris/bitstream/10665/75166/1/9789241503570_eng.pdf

WHO (World Health Organization). (2014). *Preventing suicide, A global imperative.* Geneva, Switzerland: World Health Organization.

WHO (World Health Organization) in collaboration with the United Nations Environment Programme (UNEP) (1990). *Public Health Impact of Pesticides Used in Agriculture.* Geneva, Switzerland: World Health Organization.

Withhead, M., & Dahlgren, G. (2006). *Levelling Up (Part 1): A Discussion on Concepts and Principles for Tackling Social Inequities in Health.* Studies on Social and Economic Determinants of Population Health No. 2. Report no. WHOLIS E89383. Copenhagen: WHO Regional Office for Europe, p. 44. Retrieved from who.int/social_determinants/resources/leveling_up_part1.pdf

Zonda, T. (2006). One-hundred cases of suicide in Budapest, a case-controlled psychological autopsy study. *Crisis* 27: 125–9.

29 Prevention Psychology and Counseling Services in Thailand

Happy and Healthy University Students

Arunya Tuicomepee & Skultip Sirikantraporn

Introduction

Thailand is a country in Southeast Asia, south of China, and bordering Myanmar, Laos, and Cambodia. Thailand's population is approximately 67 million, with nearly 10 million residing in Bangkok, its capital. Thailand's political system is a constitutional monarchy and its economic system is capitalist. Thailand has made substantial social and economic progress since 1970s, especially at its peak in 1980s and early 1990s, which brought Thailand up from a low-income country to middle-upper-income country before being interrupted by the Asia's financial crisis in late 1990s and later intermittent political instability and turmoil. According to World Bank (2015), Thailand is expected to regain its economic growth rate to 3.5 percent by the end of 2015 from 0.4 percent in 2014, as the low 2014 rate was due to political turmoil.

Almost 95 percent of Thais endorse Buddhism as their religious belief and practice (Newman, Shell, Li, & Innadda, 2006). With Buddhism being such a prevailing religion in Thailand, it is important to understand happiness and well-being within the Buddhist context. Buddhist concept of happiness (Buddhist term is *Sukha*) refers to state of mental balance and insight into the nature of reality. Consequently, individuals have experienced pleasure and satisfaction. Buddhists generally believe that individual happiness can be cultivated by refining attention, emotional balance, and mindfulness (Ekman et al., 2005). For example, a study of four hundred Thais found strong relationships among the observance of the five precepts of the Buddhist code of moral conduct, life satisfaction, and well-being, suggesting that happiness starts by not transgressing upon self and others, based on the Buddhist precepts of no hurting others and self (Ariyabuddhiphongs & Jaiwong, 2010). Buddhist philosophy is the foundation of Thai life, happiness, and mental health. Therefore, many psychological and counseling services in Thailand, including university counseling services, are largely informed and guided by both Buddhist and psychological perspectives on happiness enhancement and prevention of mental health problems.

Psychological and counseling services in Thailand have proliferated since the 1990s, partly due to issues such as HIV/AIDS prevention and control, the 1997 economic crisis, the 2004 Asian tsunami, and political unrest. These services, along with other forms of mental health relief, help people with their emotional and psychological concerns. Although Thai psychological and counseling services have improved significantly, many Thais still either decline to seek services or end treatment prematurely, perhaps because of the stigma associated with using the services. Another complication in Thailand is that clients receive insurance reimbursement for mental health services that are provided in the public sector, if they can present evidence that the mental health condition is related to a physical condition. Even then, clients may prefer to pay privately for mental health services instead of seeking a medical referral and insurance reimbursement, thus avoiding stigma associated with seeking mental health services, especially among university students, although students may not be able to afford private mental health services.

Positive emotion, like happiness, has been increasingly studied in the context of mental health prevention, mostly under the overarching topic of positive psychology. The synergy between positive psychology and public health is the study that generally aims to understand what is "right" about people and ways in which psychologists can strengthen these assets to prevent the development and/or severity of mental health illness (Kobau et al., 2011). The concept of happiness has been studied as a salient factor that is associated with positive outcomes in various settings, including educational institutions (King, Vidourek, Merianos, & Singh, 2014). This chapter reviews the current state of psychological and counseling services for college students in Thailand. It details the status of prevention psychology in Thailand, concerns and services related to psychological and counseling prevention, and examples of culturally relevant prevention initiative projects for college students, specifically the application of the concept of happiness in college-based prevention services.

Prevention Psychology Initiatives in a University Setting

Prevention has been conceptualized in terms of reducing individual risks and promoting individual strengths while attending to systemic and policy interventions that enhance the development and well-being of large segments of the population (Romano & Hage, 2000). Psychological and counseling services that emphasize personal well-being (e.g., health promotion) and social and political change initiatives to improve environments where people learn, live, and work are prevention interventions. The prevention initiatives that strengthen knowledge, attitudes, and behaviors to promote emotional and physical well-being are examples of health promotion interventions. Such programs and strategies inoculate against harmful and potentially destructive behaviors. There are also risk-reduction strategies (RRS) that can mitigate the characteristics, variables, or hazards that increase a person's vulnerability to a disorder or strengthen factors that are protective against the disorder (Romano & Hage, 2000; Romano & Netland, 2008).

While many universities and schools in Thailand have counseling centers and guidance offices for their students, these services are largely underutilized. Mental health stigma continues to be a barrier for individuals seeking mental health services. Having contacts with mental health staff is still considered a stigma (Romano, & Pokaeo, 2012, Tapanya, 2010;Tuicomepee). In addition, this stigma is also prevalent among primary health care doctors (WHO, 2006), who are typically the first professionals to see individuals with potential mental health needs, resulting in lack of appropriate mental health referrals for these individuals. If students become more familiar with the importance of mental health and counseling services as a student, they may become more likely to access those services after graduation. Thailand's universities have undergraduate and graduate programs in psychology and counseling psychology. At the graduate level, counselors have been trained in Thailand for over fifty years.

Thai researchers have paid substantial attention to the prevalence of psychological distress among Thai university students. University students are prone to problems with their mental health and well-being. According to a 2009 survey, Thai people aged fifteen to twenty-four years old scored lower on mental health assessment as measured by the Thai Mental Health questionnaire than any other age group (National Statistical Office of Thailand, 2009). Mental health problems could affect every aspect of their lives. People with difficulty managing and adjusting to life stressors may experience an overwhelming sense of despair, loss of interest, and lack of energy or motivation. Their relationships with friends and family suffer, as do students' academic work. Like university students in other countries, many Thai students suffer from distress. Ramasoot (2004) conducted a survey of 869 Thai undergraduates to investigate sources and perceived levels of stress. Findings revealed that approximately 52 percent of students agreed that they experienced stress, often due to exams and grades.

Although many college students in Thailand complain about being stressed, they rarely take advantage of professional counseling. Page, Taffel, Ruammake, and Reed (1994), for example, studied Thai college students' perceptions of counseling and reported that a majority of them expressed minimal confidence in the usefulness of psychotherapy and were therefore reluctant to use services. It has been noted that the majority of Thai people in general are reluctant to use mental health services even though Thai counselors are available for telephone and face-to-face counseling (Weisz, McCarty, Eastman, Chaiyasit, & Suanlert, 1997). This is also true for the college student population. Factors such as lack of awareness of counseling services, familial and cultural values, religious beliefs, and social restrictions may contribute to limited help-seeking behavior among Thai college students, especially for emotional and psychological problems (Christopher, Skillman, Kirkhart, & D'Souza, 2006; Pinyuchon, Gray, & House, 2003).

Despite help-seeking challenges, the mental health field is steadily growing as the general public is more aware of the importance of mental health and well-being. Counseling psychology and counseling services in Thailand, especially at universities, continue to expand. In 2001, the Thai Health Promotion Foundation[1] was established as a health promotion funding mechanism. It is funded by a 2 percent surcharge levied on alcohol and tobacco excise tax, approximately U.S. $50 to 60 millions a year. The Foundation is a catalytic funding agency for civil movements that improve the well-being of the Thai people. According to the Thai Health Promotion Foundation, universities are important sites to develop best practices in becoming healthy places, as encouraged by the World Health Organization (Thai Health Promotion Foundation, 2001). Most universities have a counseling office to assist students with academic, career, and personal issues, and some universities, such as Chulalongkorn University, are integrating student wellness and prevention programs into their student affairs services. Chulalongkorn University (CU) is Thailand's oldest institution of higher education, founded nearly a century ago. Chulalongkorn University Strategies 2012–2016 has six strategies to formulate guidelines for the university's development plan. The first strategy is "Advancement" to a world-class university whose graduates, research, and academic functions attain and maintain high standards of quality and service to Thai society. The second is "Admiration" to become a center of knowledge for Thailand's people, in order to produce highly qualified graduates for Thailand and global society. The third strategy is "Efficiency" to become a university whose management is efficient, effective, and transparent and that takes a participative approach in its administrative activities. The fourth strategy is "Sustainability" to sustainably manage both its financial and intellectual properties in the short and long terms. The fifth strategy is "Care" to promote equal access to education and to support all students, employees, and the community. The last strategy is "Happiness" to promote energy conservation, build a livable environment, and establish good relationships with and support career advancement of the university personnel (Stitmannaithum, 2014). Drawing from prevention and happiness studies, the "Happiness" strategy is at the center of a comprehensive student psychological and counseling service, with emphasis on student happiness. The service recently has been expanded to include wellness and preventive services for students and university personnel. Happiness Research and CU Happy and Healthy University Students

Happiness is often defined as the state of mind that involves satisfaction in one's ability to develop one's potential, work productively and creatively, build strong and positive relationships with others, and contribute to their community (Bar-On, 2005; Centreforum Commission, 2014). Studies on happiness in the United States and other countries received much attention through the positive psychology movement. Since then there has been rapid growth in the study of happiness and subjective well-being and its association with positive physical health and mental health outcomes, such as longevity (Levy, Slade,

1 en.thaihealth.or.th/.

Kunkel, & Kasl, 2002), and productivity (Binkley, 2014; McDonald & O'Callaghan, 2008). Happiness is often seen to benefit individuals in preventing psychopathology from developing. However, even in the population that has already been affected by mental health problems (e.g., anxiety, depression, substance abuse), research contends that happiness may still play a significant role in recovery and preventing the severity of the symptoms from increasing (Bergsma & Veenhoven, 2011), as higher happiness is associated with better self-esteem, higher energy levels, and more relaxed attitude (Bergsma, Ten, Veenhoven, & De Graaf, 2011).

Along with the growth of happiness research in the field of psychology, interest in interdisciplinary research on happiness has been growing, particularly in sociology and philosophy. While psychology studies tend to examine salient factors associated with the increase and decrease of happiness (e.g., altruism, optimism, personality, meaning in life) and outcomes, sociology studies attempt to contextualize the research and ground this concept within cultural specificity and contingency (Becker & Maracek, 2008; Christopher & Hickinbottom, 2008; Frawley, 2015). This intersection contributes substantially to the understanding of happiness in non-Western societies, such as Thailand, in that it positions local culture at the center when discussing happiness and well-being in societies outside of Western cultures.

Clinical and counseling psychology researchers have become interested in the science of happiness and prevention. The literature shows that happiness is correlated with positive health outcomes, productivity, and longevity (Oswald, Proto, & Sgroi, 2009). The literature has shown development in the Eastern and Western hemispheres. With cultural sharing between Eastern and Western researchers, the study of happiness has begun to incorporate Eastern perspectives, especially Buddha Dhamma (Ekman, Davidson, Ricard, & Wallace, 2005; Wallace, 2005). In addition, considering the academic interest in the role of happiness throughout the lifespan, studies of young adults (i.e., college students) in the Eastern context deserve further attention.

Regarding the concept of Buddhist happiness among college students, Phongvarin, Tuicomepee, Kotajaras, and Pokaew (2012) used qualitative research to study the conceptual frame of happiness among twenty-six Thai undergraduates. Findings revealed that Thai university students' happiness in Buddha Dhamma context consists of five themes: life satisfaction, interdependence, faith, peaceful mind, and wisdom and understanding. Life satisfaction is pleasure derived from doing what one loves, self-sufficiency, and doing one's best. Interdependence is the appreciation of values and meanings of relationships; understanding oneself and others; openness to new things; ability to live happily in a diverse society with the sense of intimacy and involvement; consideration and compassion toward others; and desire to see others happy, successful, and free from suffering. In addition, the students indicated that their happiness was derived from their response "virtuous happiness" by leading a benevolent life benefiting both themselves and others and having the peaceful mind, wisdom, and understanding of the true nature of life. This leads to life satisfaction and internal well-being. The conceptual framework of happiness is consistent with the Buddhist philosophy of the self as constantly in a state of flux and is interdependent with other people and the environment (Ekman, et al., 2005; PhraphomKhunaphon, Phraphom Khunaphon (P.A.Payitto), 2009).

Faith in living with integrity means having principles or models to stick to in living, being optimistic, and behaving with integrity. A peaceful mind is free from any disturbances, and one that is so still and empty that it perceives everything accurately and dispassionately. Individuals with a peaceful mind are ready to face reality and solve problems with an unwavering mind. These results, particularly the spiritual state, support the finding that happiness in Eastern cultures requires interdependence and social harmony (Uchida & Kitayama, 2009).

Application of Prevention Psychology Based on Buddhism at Chulalongkorn University

Drawing from the literature on Thai Buddhism, happiness and health, and prevention psychology concepts and research, two Chulalongkorn University (CU) projects have been developed: the CU Happiness Index Project and the CU Happiness Enhancement Project (Imsupasit, Suttiwan, Tuicomepee, & Loapoonpat, 2011).

Project One: The CU Student Happiness Index

There were two phases to Project One. Phase 1, a qualitative study conducted in the 2010–11 academic year, examined the conceptual framework of happiness among CU students (Imsupasit et al., 2011). In this phase, 246 students from 14 faculties were asked to define happiness. After receiving approval from the Ethics Review Committee for Research Involving Human Research Subjects, Health Science Group, Chulalongkorn University, the researcher contacted the gatekeepers to recruit participants. Then appointments were scheduled to offer participants information about the study and their rights. Those who were willing to participate in the study were asked to sign the consent form. After that, the students either joined the focus group or had a one-hour individual interview. The interview guideline included the students' definition of happiness, the characteristics of a happy person, and the factors supporting students' happiness. The "definition of student's happiness" was submitted to content analysis. After the interviews were transcribed, the scripts were analyzed by coding messages with similar meanings together. Then those with the same themes were grouped into categories and subcategories. Two experts in qualitative research evaluated the trustworthiness and validity of analysis on the findings, interpretation, and summary from supportive data.

Findings revealed four main themes of student happiness: Meanings and Experience of Happiness, Characteristics of a Happy Person, Happiness in an

Academic Institution, and Ranking the Importance of Happiness. These themes were later incorporated into the CU Happiness Scale.

Theme 1: Meanings and Experience of Happiness

1.1 *Happiness from self-discovery:* This kind of happiness occurs when a person can express himself or herself freely, do what he or she pleases, and handle difficulties. Acting freely, a person can take his or her dream paths to the desired goal, leading to satisfaction, elation, pride, and happiness. The intermediate effects include social approval, in which the person's actions are seen as good, right, and respectable. This is exemplified in the following statements:
- *Ability to do what one wants or likes without bothering others*
- *To express oneself, to do what is good and right*
- *Gaining approval, whether in education, work, or hobby*
- *Feeling sated, elated, impressed, and smiley after certain actions*
- *Willing and content to do whatever it is*
- *Heart beating with happiness when we are doing what makes us content*

1.2 *Happiness from creating a good future for oneself:* This type of happiness arises from seeing a bright future, owing to successful experience in coping with life crises. This contributes to the sense of confidence and determination, clarity of future goals, and ability to handle whatever happens. A person can see his or her future clearly and without worry.
- *Able to get through a critical period in life, leading to the feeling of determination and success*
- *Happiness after suffering with support from parents*
- *Seeing oneself ahead without worry about the future*

1.3 *Happiness from harmony with people*: This kind of happiness is the result of good rapport. It is a calm form of happiness. It follows from seeing other people smiling, whether the causes of those smiles are the students or others' actions. This happiness also arises from enjoyable activities with families, relatives, and friends.
- *Making others happy, which, in turn, makes us happy*
- *Making the family proud*
- *Making the people we love happy with our actions*
- *Peaceful happiness when seeing others happy*

Theme 2: Characteristics of a Happy Person

2.1 *Friendliness*: The students described a happy person as friendly, considerate, kind, vivacious, and lighthearted. The happy person can bring joy to other people. He or she is always laughing or smiling. He or she can enjoy simple pleasures.
- *A good-humored, congenial person without a serious countenance*
- *A considerate person who is a good company*
- *A vivacious person who can put smiles on the faces of other people*

2.2 *Realistic life management with optimism*: A happy person, according to the students, can manage his or her life realistically with feet firmly on the ground. He or she has unwavering resolution and is a self-made achiever with clear identity and is content with what he or she has. Such a person in self-sufficient, can create happiness for himself or herself, and has a right attitude toward happiness. He or she has a positive outlook and enjoys the simple things in life. A happy person lives by the Dharma principles (loving kindness, compassion, empathetic joy, and equanimity).

- *An optimistic person who views the world rationally*
- *While others see problems or crises, happy people cope*
- *A person who can accept whatever happens in life*
- *A self-sufficient person who craves nothing more than to be happy*

Theme 3: Happiness in an Academic Institution

3.1 *Pride in oneself and family:* Being enrolled in a higher academic institution is a source of pride to the student participants and their families. The students feel a sense of responsibility to do the best they can.
- *Study what I like and my family is proud of me*
- *Success on the entrance examination brought happiness to me, and especially to my family.*
- *Proud of the university's reputation, and developing inspiration to perform well academically, to behave well, and to make myself and my family proud. This achievement brought greater happiness to the family. My family and I are proud of myself.*

3.2 *Happiness at being a student of a reputable institution:* The students admitted that the reputation, the uniforms, and above all the school insignia make them proud. They were happy when someone complimented them for attending one of the best universities in the country.
- *Being part of a well-known academic institution, the uniform, its emblem*
- *My highest ambition was to be part of this university. Being here makes me happy.*
- *This institution is thought of as the most reputable in the country. This makes me confident that a bright future will await me after my graduation.*
- *As everyone thinks that this university is the best, everyone who can pass in must be good. This inspires me to achieve good performance.*

3.3 *Close-knit relationship of junior and senior students:* The university community, according to the students, has a seniority system called SOTUS (Seniority, Order, Tradition, Unity, Spirit), in which senior and junior students and friends show loving goodwill to one another. The result is a warm network.
- *As everyone accepts this university as the best, everyone who can pass in must be good. This inspires me to achieve good performance.*
- *I like the harmonious relationship between senior and junior students.*

3.4 *Academic atmosphere and environment:* The students reported that the university's academic environment, academic knowledge, and their access to comprehensive information contributed to happy feelings.
- *Central library is large and vast, full of books. During the exam period, the place will be arranged for studying, enabling me to concentrate. If not, I don't know where I would go to study.*

3.5 *Campus activities enabling social networking for students:* According to the students, freshman-welcoming activities or camping offer opportunities to be good citizens, show generosity, and help one another.

- *In the university, we know a wide, wide range of people, lots of them. Stepping into the faculty can evoke the warm feeling.*
- *A vast array of activities on the campus, so I can try my hand at many things.*
- *I also love participating in a camp, for I can reach out to help others. It makes me proud and useful.*

3.6 *Physical characteristics and location of the university:* The students explained that the location of the university in the heart of the city, convenient transportation, and proximity to modern shopping centers make it easy to get around. This has a positive impact on the students' happiness and concentration on their academic work. At the same time, they can keep up with fashion or movies.

- *At the heart of the city, only being in this university, I can get nearly everything. Just a few steps, I reach Chamchuri Square, Siam, MBK Center.*
- *Good environment, near many attractions like shopping centers with various facilities like fitness and many more*
- *I admit that the university location makes us happy. First, it's convenient to commute, easy to get around. And the campus isn't too vast.*

Theme 4: Ranking the Importance of Happiness

4.1 *Characteristics of happiness: mental and physical happiness:* When asked to define mental and physical happiness, the students reported that mental happiness was more important. They defined both types as follows:

4.1.1 Mental happiness was ranked first by most of the students, explaining that whatever a person does is motivated by mental comfort, passion, and happiness from doing it. This is reflected in the proverb "a happy hut is better than a gloomy castle." Therefore, the foremost happiness is internal.

4.1.2 Physical happiness is explained by most of the students in terms of good health and plenty of energy.

4.2 *Happy behaviors:* The students rated happiness from relationships and social involvement higher than happiness from studying in the university. They defined both as follows:

4.2.1 *Happiness from relationship with others and social involvement* is formed from interactions and from altruism. Just doing so brings happiness and approval.

4.2.2 *Happiness from studying in an academic institution*, according to the majority of the students, stems from their abilities to do what they want. Thus, they can return many good things to society all along and enjoy their lives, as with the first three types of happiness. However, their primary responsibility is academic work; they have to study hard and pass exams. The subjects reported most students focused on their study but did not give too much importance to grades. Therefore, despite the gravity of academic duties, making friends is more important. They explained when a person has supportive friends, studying and living on the campus can be more enjoyable.

The focus group and interview content analysis revealed two aspects of happiness definitions, psychological and physical aspects, for both "State Happiness" and "Trait Happiness." Most of the students also reported that "they were happy at Chulalongkorn University" (see Table 29.1).

Phase 2 of Project One was the development of the CU Student Happiness Index. The participants in this study were 4,150 graduate and undergraduate students (1,447 males and 2,703 females). These two phases culminated in the CU Student Happiness Index.[2] The Index consisted of the Trait Happiness Scale and the State Happiness Scale. Each scale consisted of forty items. Psychometric properties of the two scales were strongly validated. The results of Cronbach's alpha for the Trait Happiness Scale ranged from 0.75 to 0.90 and that of the State Happiness Scale was 0.92. In addition, convergent validity analyses were conducted between the State Happiness Scale and other scales such as the Oxford Happiness Questionnaire (OHQ; Hills & Argyle, 2002), Life Orientation Test (LOT; Scheier & Carver, 1985), Beck's Depression Inventory (BDI; Beck, Steer, & Garbin, 1988), and State Anxiety Inventory (STAI; Spielberger, 1983). The significantly positive coefficient results were as follows the OHQ ($r = 0.86$) and the LOT($r = 0.61$). Furthermore, divergent validity analyses revealed significantly negative coefficienct results between the State Happiness Scale and BDI ($r = -0.62$), STAI (S-Anxiety) ($r = -0.726$). From these validity results, it was concluded that the State Happiness Scale accurately assesses happiness.

Findings indicated that the students were happy. This result was consistent with their subjective reports during the qualitative interview results previously provided. Confirmatory factor analysis (CFA) identified the five traits of a happy student: positive thinking, intimacy, less pessimism, gratitude, and integrity. Among these, gratitude most increases happiness.

Project Two: CU Happiness Intervention

In Project Two, the happiness intervention aimed to enhance happiness of CU students. The project was cofunded by the Chulalongkorn University Health

Table 29.1 *Psychological and Physical Aspects of State and Trait Happiness*

	State Happiness	Trait Happiness
Psychological Aspects	- Autonomy - Freely expressing of oneself - Having good perspective	- Positive thinking - Good human relations.
Physical Aspects	- Ability to fulfill the basic needs - Having positive relationships with people and society - Having good perspective	- A balanced life

2 www.cuhappiness.com.

Promotion Project and the Thai Health Promotion Foundation. Details of the Buddhist-Ecotherapy intervention and the Buddha Dharma Teaching intervention follow.

The Happiness Enhancement Project Based on Buddhist-Ecotherapy Intervention

Previous research indicated that natural environment decreases distress, increases the sense of unity with nature, and produces a happy mind and a perception of well-being (Kjellgren & Buhrkall, 2010). There are relationships among the sense of dependence, harmony, and timelessness. In addition, depression and anxiety are decreased, but self-esteem increases (Mind, 2007). The Buddhist Dhamma principle teaches individuals to visualize and understand the truth of life and to release *Dukkha,* or suffering. According to Olsen (2003), the Buddhist Dhamma principle develops a peaceful mind. Direct experience with the natural environment helps people to understand the truth of nature and create wisdom (Titmuss, 1995). Connectedness to nature occurs when people realize that they are part of nature (Roszak, 1995).

Previous studies have found that the natural environment increases the sensory experience. Such an environment could be relaxing (Mayer, Frantz, Bruehlman-Senecal, & Dollover, 2009) and make people realize that nature is part of their lives (Mayer & Frantz, 2004). *Panna* in interconnectedness is life wisdom. It teaches that everything depends on everything else and that they must adjust to uncertainty. Previous studies show that having Panna in interconnectedness helps people to perceive the value of everything in relation to them. Moreover, they would be grateful to their family (Proetphan, 2007). The Happiness Enhancement Project, therefore, examines the effectiveness of the Buddhist-Ecotherapy Group in creating connectedness with nature, and of Panna in interconnectedness among undergraduate students.

The Buddhist-Ecotherapy Group has its foundation on the Dharmic principle and the natural environment. The group emphasizes developing and curing the minds of people who misunderstand life, teaching them that wisdom is the main instrument. While the Buddhist-Ecotherapy Group focuses on both Dharmic teaching and the connection between mind and nature, the Ecotherapy group applied group process, and the natural environment is used in the activities and practices in order to cure the body and mind (Mayer et al., 2009).

Twenty-four university students (sixteen females and eight males) from a university in Bangkok, Thailand, were recruited from psychology classes. They voluntarily participated in the study in July and August 2010. Their mean age was 20.17 years (SD = 0.38). The instruments used were the Connectedness to Nature Scale (CNS) and the Panna in Interconnectedness Scale (PIS). The CNS was developed by Mayer and Frantz (2004). Its reliability with Cronbach's alpha is 0.89. The PIS was developed by Proetphan (2007). Its reliability with Cronbach's alpha is 0.86. After receiving approval from the Committee for Human Research, Chulalongkorn University, the researcher contacted the gatekeepers to recruit qualified informants. The researcher selected and randomly assigned twenty-four participants into the three group conditions (Buddhist-Ecotherapy, Ecotherapy, and control). The participants in the Buddhist-Ecotherapy, and Ecotherapy groups participated in the group treatments for about twenty consecutive hours. One-way analysis of variance with repeated measures was used for data analysis.

Findings revealed that the posttest scores on CNS among the three groups were significantly different at $p < 0.01$. This finding suggests that university students can benefit from Buddhist-Ecotherapy for personal growth and subjective well-being. In addition, the findings indicate promising results of the two treatment groups in reducing stress-related concerns such as fatigue, anxiety, and depression, although further investigations are needed. Moreover, the students reported an increased sense of harmony with nature. Such findings corresponded with the research of Kjellgren and Buhrkall (2010), who stated that relaxation in a natural environment enhanced the connectedness to nature. Furthermore, the students who participated in the Buddhist Eco-psychology group reported a stronger sense of connection with nature. This improvement included an increase in self-actualization, sympathy, and adaption. According to Schultz, Shriver, Tabanico, and Khazian (2004), people who are in harmony with nature believe that they are part of nature and understand their dependence upon the environment. This realization would lead to eco-friendly behaviors.

Happiness Enhancement Project Based on Buddha Dharma Teaching

As a result of the findings of the study by Pongvarin et al. (2012), it is recommended to promote happiness among students by creating education programs or activities that promote student personal development. Students should be encouraged to reflect on their lives and duties, to respond to their needs without attachment to other people or external objects. According to the findings, happiness in Buddha Dhamma is a state of mind (satisfied, content, complacent, and peaceful) derived from a life of integrity, a mind that is calm and content, and wisdom and understanding of life. In addition, the findings suggest that the students' happiness depended on doing what they loved, supportive interdependence with others, and faith in right living. Lastly, the students' happiness not only depends on living with integrity but also on a state of mind that is light, relaxed, empty, and tranquil, with the wisdom and understanding of the truth of life that enables them to live with the awareness of present reality with the mind that accepts and understands impermanence without attachment or expectation.

The conceptual framework of happiness in Buddha Dhamma is not limited to a positive psychological state, life satisfaction, or internal characteristics. It is also a mind consisting of wisdom and understanding of the truth of life and faith to the right living that enables a person to live happily and compassionately with others, leading to satisfaction, happiness, and wellness.

In this happiness enhancement project, fifty-one undergraduate and post-graduate students and two CU employees expressed interest in having dharma discourses with a Buddhist monk. The discourses included the following four sessions:

Session 1: "What is life? What causes suffering? How can we lead a happy life?"
Session 2: "Worthwhile life"
Session 3: "Know about suffering...to live happily"
Session 4: "Happy when not being attached"

On the first day of the dharma discourse, the Venerable Buddhist Monk, Bhikku Kanchit Kunavaro, asked us what life is and what it consists of. After discussing a variety of answers, our monk master grouped our answers into the Physical Environment (body, natural environment, people, buildings, places, clothing, wealth, diet, medication); Society and Living Beings (families, friends, teachers, instructors, creatures, religions, cultures); Mind (thoughts, emotions, feelings, beliefs, goodness, boredom, love, happiness); and Wisdom (knowledge, ignorance, attitude).

The students who participated in the project concluded that

> *Our world and lives consist of bodies, minds, societies, and environment: happiness or suffering is in the mind; environments and societies are only components that come in contact with our minds.*
>
> *What makes us suffer are (1) separation from the beloved, the preferred, the liked (2) coming in contact with the disliked, and (3) unmet desires.*

The venerable monk reminded them that

> *Instead of being attached to anything, we should think that a particular thing wouldn't stay with us for long. Remind our minds constantly from the start that everything will leave us, and when things stay with us so briefly, we should do whatever good now with our power, knowledge, ability, and be content with what we have done.*

The venerable monk asked the students why they do everything. The students answered, for happiness. The monk then asked the students where happiness lies and whether the students had looked at it. The monk guided them on how to develop the mind:

(1) *Virtue, which is the quality of mind, includes thinking of and expressing good things, leading to good feelings, and supporting society;*
(2) *Capacity and efficiency of mind, such as determination, perseverance, mindfulness, concentration, and stability;*
(3) *Happiness or health-promoting mental conditions, such as liveliness, elation, purity, satisfaction, content, lightheartedness, and relief. A developed person is happy with everything he or she is doing; when a person is happy, he or she is ready to give.*

During the conversations, the venerable monk showed a few videos with scientific explanations about the world to supplement the discourse related to the mind, which is the cardinal origin of happiness and suffering. The videos recounted stories like "Apple Tree and Little Kid" and "Puifai, the endless miracle of love and caring." The stories reminded us of our parents' unconditional love. Moreover, the venerable monk had the students write letters to their parents, starting with "I'd like to apologize to mom and dad for...," "I'd like to thank mom and dad for...," "I'd like to tell mom and dad that...," and think of "things we can do for our parents," and then to show them to their parents. These exercises made them look at their hearts and at those of the people that they love unconditionally.

Participants in the discourses reported that the dharma discourses helped them to detach from external distractions, to explore their mind and the origin of their happiness and suffering, and to look at people close to them. The students also mentioned that they saw how to develop a happy mind by purifying their mind and radiating kindness.

Conclusions and Future Directions

The research and intervention projects reported in this chapter promoted the happiness of Thai university students. The projects resulted in a Happiness Index (state and trait happiness) and in two interventions for enhancing student happiness. In relation to happiness of CU students, the students' state and trait happiness were moderate to high. Among students' trait happiness (i.e., positive thinking, intimacy, gratitude, integrity, less pessimism), gratitude most enhanced happiness. For psychological interventions, two happiness enhancement projects (Buddhist-Ecotherapy group and Buddha Dharma Teaching) were implemented for students at the CU Wellness Center. These projects demonstrated that counseling and psychological services focusing on happiness can promote student well-being and empower students by integrating them into the university community. In the future, the student happiness projects will become part of the university health services system. Health and happiness campaigns have been created for students and the university community. Although Thai people are familiar with enhancing happiness in a Buddhist context, the prevention psychology interventions to promote happiness and health merit further empirical investigation.

CU recognizes that college and university students are the leaders of tomorrow. These students have academic responsibilities and new social relationships and challenges, which may result in stress (Dwyer & Cummings, 2001; Salami, 2010). Mental health support and prevention efforts are therefore important to provide guidance and services as students are juggling different demands. It is anticipated that CU's Happiness Initiative will maximize students' well-being and success. When discussing happiness in Thai culture, Buddhist philosophy is at the core of the discourse. With more than 90 percent of Thais self-identified as Buddhists, many studies using Thai samples report a significant influence of Buddhist culture on how people perceive and enjoy happiness (Ariyabuddhiphongs & Jaiwong

2010; Wiist, Sullivan, Wayment, & Warren. 2010; Yiengprugsawan, Somboonsook, Seubsman, & Sleigh, 2012). Therefore, targeted well-being promotion initiatives for college students based on Buddhist philosophy are the topic of a recent investigation among CU faculty and administration.

Results from this CU Happiness initiative have implications for university counseling practice and assessment. The themes emerging from the project clarify elements associated with happiness and well-being on which counselors and psychologists can focus. According to the findings from this initiative, students' well-being can be enhanced in the following ways. Students are encouraged to work on identifying clear goals, expressing and living their goals with integrity, and feeling content with their decisions and actions, and learn to overcome life crisis and suffering by seeking support from parents and friends, and mental health professionals on and off campus. They should also be encouraged to learn to develop and maintain calm and smooth relationships through enjoyable activities with families, relatives, and friends. It would also be important for students to cultivate the following characteristics: friendliness and realistic life management with optimism. Students should be encouraged to take pride in themselves and their families. Students also should be encouraged to develop close-knit relationships among students to foster a supportive environment through social involvement at the university and thus enhance their happiness at the university.

References

Ariyabuddhiphongs, V., & Jaiwong, D. (2010). Observance of the Buddhist five precepts, subjective wealth, andhappiness among Buddhists in Bangkok, Thailand. *Archive for the Psychology of Religion* 32(3): 327–44.

Bar-On, R. (2005). The impact of emotional intelligence on subjective well-being. *Perspectives in Education* 23(2): 41–62.

Beck, A. T., Steer, R. A., & Garbin, M. G. (1988) Psychometric properties of the Beck Depression Inventory: twenty-five years of evaluation. *Clinical Psychology Review* 8(1): 77–100.

Becker, D., & Marecek, J. (2008). Dreaming the American dream: individualism and positive psychology.*Social and Personality Psychology Compass* 2(5): 1767–80.

Bergsma, A., Ten Have, M., Veenhoven, R., & De Graaf, R. (2011). Most people with mental disorders are happy; a 3-year follow-up in the Dutch general population. *Journal of Positive Psychology* 6: 253–9.

Bergsma, A., & Veenhoven, R. (2011). The happiness of people with a mental disorder in modern society. *Psychology of Well-Being: Theory, Research and Practice* 1(2): 1–6.

Binkley, S. (2014). *Happiness as Enterprise: An Essay on Neoliberal Life*. Albany: State University of New York Press.

Centreform Commission (2014). The pursuit of happiness: a new ambition for our mental health. www.centreforum.org/assets/pubs/the-pursuit-of-happiness.pdf

Christopher, J. C., & Hickinbottom, S. (2008). Positive psychology, ethnocentrism, and the disguised ideology of individualism. *Theory & Psychology* 18(5): 563–89.

Christopher, M., Skillman, G., Kirkhart, M., & D'Souza, J. (2006). The effect of normative and behavioral persuasion on help seeking in Thai and American college students. *Journal of Multicultural Counseling and Development* 34(2): 80–93.

Dwyer, A. L., & Cummings, A. L. (2001). Stress, self-efficacy, social support, and coping strategies in university students. *Canadian Journal of Counseling* 35(3): 208–20.

Ekman, P., Davidson, R. J., Ricard, M., & Wallace, B. A. (2005). Buddhist and psychological perspectives on emotion and well-being. *Current Directions in Psychological Science* 14(2): 59–63.

Frawley, A. (2015). Happiness research: a reviewof critiques. *Sociology Compass* 9(1): 62–77.

Hills, P., & Argyle, M. (2002). The Oxford Happiness Questionnaire: a compact scale for the measurement of psychological well-being. *Personality and Individual Differences* 33: 1073–82.

Imsupasit, S., Suttiwan, P., Tuicomepee, A., & Loapoonpat, C. (2011). CU Happiness index: Can student's happiness be assessable? Poster presentation at the Association of Pacific Rim Universities (APRU) Convention, March, Mahachulalongkorn Building, Chulalongkorn University, Bangkok, Thailand.

King, K. A., Vidourek, R. A., Merianos, A. L., & Singh, M. (2014). A study of stress, social support, and perceived happiness among college students. *Journal of Happiness and Well-Being* 2(2): 132–44.

Kjellgren, A., & Buhrkall, H. (2010). A comparison of the restorative effect of a natural environment with a simulated environment. *Journal of Environmental Psychology* 30(4): 464–72.

Kobau, R., Seligman, M., Petrson, C., Diener, E., Zack, M., Chapman, D., & Thompson, W. (2011). Mental health promotion in public health: perspectives and strategies from positive psychology. *American Journal of Public Health* 101(8): e1–e9.

Levy, B. R., Slade, M. D., Kunkel, S. R., & Kasl, S. V. (2002). Longevity increased by positive self-perceptions of aging. *Journal of Personality and Social Psychology* 83(2): 261–70.

Mayer, S. F., & Frantz, C. M. (2004). The connectedness to nature scale: a measure of individuals' feeling in community with nature. *Journal of Environmental Psychology*24(4): 503–15.

Mayer, S. F., Frantz, C. M., Bruehlman-Senecal, E., & Dollover, K. (2009). Why is nature beneficial? The role of connectedness to nature. *Environment and Behavior* 41: 607–43.

McDonald, M., & O'Callaghan, J. (2008). Positive psychology: a Foucauldian critique. *Humanistic Psychologist* 36(2): 127–42.

Mind (2007). Ecotherapy: the green agenda for mental health.www.mind.org.uk/cam paigns_and_issues/report_and_resources/835_ecotherapy

National Statistical Office of Thailand (2009). *The 2009 Health and Welfare Survey*. Bangkok: Ministry of Information and Communication Technology.

Newman, I. M., Shell, D. F., Li, T., & Innadda, S. (2006).Buddhism and adolescent alcohol use in Thailand.*Substance Use & Misuse* 41: 1789–1800.

Oswald, A., Proto, E., & Sgroi, D. (2009). Happiness and productivity. Institute for the Study of Labor (IZA) Discussion Paper, 4645. 1–53. Bonn, Germany: IZA.

Page, R. C., Taffel, S., Ruammake, K. C., & Reed, J. (1994). A comparison of Thai and American counseling students' perceptions of counseling. *International Journal for the Advancement of Counseling* 17: 213–23.

Phongvarin, C., Tuicomepee, A., Kotrajaras, S., & Pokaeo, S. (2012). Perceived happiness in the context of Buddha Dharma among undergraduate students: a qualitative investigation. *HRD Journal* 3: 111–19.

Pinyuchon. M., Gray, A., & House, R.M. (2003). The *pa sook* model of counseling Thai families: a culturally mindful approach. *Journal of Family Psychotherapy* 14: 67–93.

Proetphan, D. (2007). Effects of Yonisomanasikara group counseling on Panna in interconnectedness and change. (Doctoral Dissertation). Chulalongkorn University, Bangkok.

PhraphomKhunaphon (P. A. Payutto) (2009). *Buddhadharma*, 11th ed. Bangkok: Mahachulalongkornrajavidhayalaya Press.

Ramasoot, W. (2004).Sources of stress in Chulalongkorn University undergraduate students. (Unpublished master'sthesis).Faculty of Psychology, Chulalongkorn University, Bangkok.

Romano, J. L., & Hage, S. H. (2000). Prevention and counseling psychology: revitalizing commitments for the 21st century. *Counseling Psychologist* 28(6): 733–63.

Romano, J. L., & Netland, J. D. (2008). The application of the theory of reasoned action and planned behavior to prevention science in counseling psychology. *Counseling Psychologist* 36(5): 777–806.

Roszak, T. (1995). Where psyche meets Gaia. In Roszak, T., Gomes, M. E., & Kanner, A. D. (eds.), *Ecotherapy: Restoring the Earth, Healing the Mind.* San Francisco, CA: Sierra Club Books.

Salami, S. O. (2010). Emotional intelligence, self-efficacy, psychological well-being and students' attitudes: implications for quality education. *European Journal of Educational Studies* 2(3): 247–57.

Scheier, M. F., & Carver, C. S. (1985). Optimism, coping, and health: assessment and implications of generalized outcome expectancies. *Health Psychology* 4: 219–47.

Schultz, P. W., Shriver, C., Tabanico, J., & Khazian, A. (2004). Implicit connections with nature. *Journal of Environmental Psychology* 24: 31–42.

Stitmannaithum, B. (2014). *Chulalongkorn University 2013–2014 Sustainability Report. The ISCN-GULF Sustainable Campus Charter*. Boston, MA: International Sustainable Campus Network.

Spielberger, C. D. (1983). *Manual for the State-Trait Anxiety Inventory (Form Y)*. Palo Alto, CA: Consulting Psychologists Press.

Tapanya, S. (2010). Psychology in Thailand. In Weiner, I. B., & Craighead, W. E. (eds.), *The Corsini Encyclopedia of Psychology*. Hoboken, NJ: Wiley, pp.1775–6.

Thai Health Promotion Foundation (2001). *The Annual Report 2001–2010*. Bangkok: Thai Health Promotion Foundation.

Titmuss, C. (1995). *The Green Buddha*. Devon: Insight Book (Totnes).

Tuicomepee, A., Romano, J. L., & Pokaeo, S. (2012). Counseling in Thailand: development from a Buddhist perspective. *Journal of Counseling and Development* 90: 357–61.

Uchida, Y., & Kitayama, S. (2009). Happiness and unhappiness in East and West: themes and variations. *Emotion* 9(4): 441–56.

Wallace, B. A. (2005). *Genuine Happiness: Meditation as the Path to Fulfillment*. Hoboken, NJ: John Wiley and Sons.

Weisz, J. R., McCarty, C. A., Eastman, K. L., Chaiyasit, W., & Suanlert, S. (1997). Developmental psychopathology and culture: ten lessons from Thailand. In Luthar, S. S., Burack, J. A., Cicchetti, D., & Weisz, J. R. (eds.), *Developmental Psychopathology: Perspectives on Adjustment, Risk, and Disorder*. Cambridge, UK: Cambridge University Press, pp. 568–92.

Wiist, W. H., Sullivan, B. M., Wayment, H. A., & Warren, M. (2010). A web-based survey of the relationship between Buddhist religious practices, health, and psychological characteristics: research methods andpreliminary results. *Journal of Religion and Health* 49(1): 18–31.

World Bank (2015). *Thailand Economic Monitor – June 2015: Quality Education for All*. Washington, DC: World Bank. www.worldbank.org/en/country/thailand/publication/thailand-economic-monitor-june-2015

WHO (World Health Organization) (2006). *WHO-MAIS Report on Mental Health System in Thailand*. Geneva, Switzerland: World Health Organization. www.who.int/mental_health/thailand_who_aims_report.pdf

Yiengprugsawan, V., Somboonsook, B., Seubsman, S., & Sleigh, A. C. (2012). Happiness, mental health, and socio-demographic associations among a national cohort of Thai adults. *Journal of Happiness Studies* 13(6): 1019–29.

North, Central, & South America

30 Preventing School Shootings from an American and European Perspective

Robert K. Conyne & Perry Firth

Introduction

This chapter addresses the important, urgent, complex, and challenging goal of preventing school shootings. It presents approaches to school shooting prevention, with special focus on threat assessment within intentional efforts to build healthy, safe, and connected school climates and environments.

The terms "school shooting," "mass shooting," "shooting rampage," and "targeted school violence" (and variations thereof) are used to refer to a school-based event where a young person attacks the children and teachers of a school that he or she currently or used to attend. It specifically underscores that these youth choose the school, or the people within the school, as the target. This definition includes events in which there is typically more than one victim, whether injured or killed. Moreover, despite the number of casualties, the shooter intends to wound many people. It does not include gun-based gang violence or a one-to-one interpersonal event where the school just happened to be the scene of the crime. We also use these terms to describe school attacks that do not utilize a gun but which still meet the other criteria.

The approach in this chapter takes the United States (U.S.) as the primary context but, consistent with this *Handbook*, it also includes a broader perspective, namely referencing the European-international milieu. This expansive scope reflects the global spread of school shootings.

This chapter also contains an introduction to a new theoretical model of wellness and prevention, the *Counseling for Wellness and Prevention Model* (Conyne, 2015), and how it can apply to school shooting prevention. This comprehensive ecological model of wellness and prevention is intended to forestall targeted malfunction while guiding individuals and systems toward optimum levels of wellness. Rather than a specific intervention, it is a framework designed to organize and conceptualize the many different variables and levels involved in well-being and the prevention of dysfunction. Its particular connection to school shootings will be illustrated.

Let us begin by considering prevention in the United States and why applying it against school shootings is challenging.

Some Issues Complicating Prevention Efforts in the United States

Guns have featured prominently in discussions of school shootings in the United States. Therefore, we will first begin with an examination of those factors related to gun policy.

The United States seems to be plagued by a difficult and complicated relationship with guns, contributing to a federal inability to enact gun regulations capable of significantly reducing gun violence. Moreover, masculine norms have tended to connect violence and masculinity with autonomy and access to guns. Not only do these linkages contribute to men being more likely than women to perpetrate violent crime, but to the fact that targeted school violence can become a viable form of problem resolution for a small minority. These relationships also impede gun regulation and legislation.

Moreover, this situation occurs against a larger backdrop of apparent political posturing. That is, because school shootings have been linked inextricably with access to high-capacity weapons, critics assert that school shooting prevention has become another casualty of political maneuvering. In contrast, other countries have strengthened gun laws (e.g., England, Scotland, Australia, Germany, and Finland) (Council on Foreign Relations, 2012; Library of Congress, 2014; McConville & Lawless, 2012). In general, the pain caused by school shootings has proven to be fertile ground for policy change in these countries.

Another issue involves governmental research institutions, which have been prohibited from carrying out public health–style research on gun ownership and injury (IOM & NRC, 2013). The most recent restriction was enacted by the U.S. Congress in 2011, prohibiting the Department of Health and Human Services from collecting data on firearm injury (a restriction already faced by the Centers for Disease Control and Prevention [CDC] since 1996 when Congress denied any funding for CDC research that could be interpreted as promoting gun control). Given that effective prevention involves strong data collection, these measures have seriously retarded the government's ability to understand and act on gun violence.

Prevention of school shootings also is made difficult by the U.S. population's general perception that guns increase personal safety. With high rates of gun ownership (88.8 per 100 residents) (Bangalore & Messerli, 2013), more than six in ten Americans believe guns make homes safer (Gallup, 2014b). This position is held despite research showing that national per-capita gun ownership rates predict gun-related deaths. Because most school shooters have experience with guns, and easy access to them, this situation serves to further obscure prevention. Moreover, if a large number of the U.S. population consider guns crucial to their own personal safety, they may be less willing to regulate them.

School shooting prevention is also compounded due to ambivalence within the United States about prevention, in general. This feeling is reflected across a variety of systems, but most prominently in our medical and mental health care systems. While the U.S. Affordable Care Act has made strides in shifting public will and policy about the importance of thinking preventively, the argument could still be made that Americans are more likely to respond to issues reactively (Conyne, 2015).

Finally, prevention of school shootings is impaired by conceptual and pragmatic oversimplification. It is easy to equate mass shootings solely with mental illness, guns, or bullying, and subsequently focus prevention efforts solely on any of these domains. Yet this reductive approach ignores the interactive nature of these events and artificially restricts preventive efforts. The media, in particular, tend to fuel this type of narrowed interpretation. For instance, as reported by the *Washington Times*, media outlets will frequently make interpretations about the causes of a shooting before the facts are in, or seek facts or interviews that confirm their own hypothesis about a shooting's cause (Harper, 2012).

Brief Overview of School Shootings in the United States and Beyond

Perhaps nothing strikes at the heart of a community like the loss of children's lives. This is especially the case when the loss happens at school. School shootings are powerful because they shake one of our most basic assumptions: *children are safe from murder at school.* They confuse us because of implicit and explicit questions raised about culpability. Is the shooter both victim and villain? To what degree was the shooting facilitated by a national, cultural, community, or school failure?

These questions linger despite the fact that schools continue to be one of the safest places for children and that school crime has been declining, in general (Wike & Fraser, 2009). In 1994, for instance, the school violent crime rate in the United States was thirteen per one thousand students, but by 2007 it had decreased to four per one thousand students (Rocque, 2012), a trend that continued through 2010 (O'Malley & Eklund, 2012). Despite this decrease, students living in urban and suburban areas experienced more nonfatal violence than those in rural areas (Robers, Kemp, Rathbun, & Morgan, 2014), and for the first time in 2012 the total nonfatal victimization rate for children ages twelve to eighteen actually increased to fifty-two students per one thousand from thirty-five per one thousand in 2010 (Robers et al., 2014). However, this more recent increase in nonfatal victimization should still be taken within the context of a general decline in school violence. Importantly, less than 2 percent of homicides take place at school (CDC, 2014).

The extreme violence associated with mass school shootings, coupled with their seemingly random nature, has spurred both academic research and national apprehension (Payne, 2013). Moreover, these events are increasing not only within the United States, but internationally as well (Bockler, Seeger, Sitzer, & Heitmeyer, 2013).

For these reasons, research into school shootings continues to grow. For example, researchers have found that active shooter events (where the perpetrator is attempting to kill as many people as possible) are increasing in the United States (Blair & Martaindale, 2013; FBI, 2014). Moreover, 34 percent of active shooter events have occurred in schools (Blair & Martaindale, 2013).

Although schools are not the leading location for active shooter events (workplaces stand at 37 percent), they come in a close second. Indeed, over the past twenty years an unparalleled number of school shooting rampages have occurred in American schools, despite general school violence declining from the 1990s (Rocque, 2012).

For instance, Blair and Martaindale (2013) report that the rate of active shooter events in the United States (those that occur across a variety of locations) has *increased* since 2008, from an average of five per year to about sixteen per year. Unsurprisingly, as American school shootings continue to dominate the media, nearly a third of parents report that they worry for their children's safety at school (Gallup, 2014a).

The year 1999 especially seemed to mark a school shooting turning point (Bockler et al., 2013). This was the year of the Columbine attack in Littleton, Colorado. Through the Internet's ability to capture and hold information in perpetuity, and its potential to connect isolated and angry young men around violent fantasies (Markward, Cline, & Markward, 2001), Columbine has inspired many other students (Bondü, Cornell, & Scheithauer, 2011; Larkin, 2009). Within the United States itself, of the twelve attacks that Larkin (2009) studied between 1999 and 2007, 66.7 percent of attackers referenced Columbine.

Global Spread of School Shootings

Commonly seen as primarily a problem in the United States, school shootings are instead a global issue. For purposes of this chapter, we have focused our international examination on Europe, with only limited attention to countries beyond.

Even as the United States leads with the highest rate of targeted violence (with Germany following in second place) (Bondü et al., 2011; Leuschner et al., 2011), other countries also cope with school shootings. From a 2007 shooting in an upper secondary school in Finland where an eighteen-year-old man completed a rampage that left eight murdered (Kiilakoski & Oksanen, 2011), to a 2005 incident in Hikari, Japan, where fifty-eight students and teachers were wounded when a student threw bombs containing nails and glass (Bondü et al., 2011), to a 2009 incident in Winnenden, Germany, where a seventeen-year-old former student killed fifteen students, teachers, and three civilians, targeted school violence is a global phenomenon (Bondü et al., 2011; Dougherty, 2009). From 1974 to 2006, researchers counted ninety-nine school shootings internationally (not just within Europe). Since then, with the United States setting the pace, many more have occurred in other countries as well.

European Context

Researchers have started to examine shooting similarities and differences across countries. Certain trends have emerged that transcend borders. For instance, these events are most likely to be perpetrated by young men experiencing interpersonal problems with peers and teachers (Freie Universität Berlin, 2014; Sommer, Leuschner, & Scheithauer, 2014). A German research team analyzed 37 studies examining 126 international cases and found that the vast majority of these young men, regardless of their country of origin, experienced social problems and perceived themselves to be socially marginalized (Freie Universität Berlin, 2014; Sommer et al., 2014). These researchers found evidence of peer rejection in over half of cases, and physical bullying in a third. In just over 40 percent of cases, problems with teachers were identified. Comparing attacks outside of America to those that have occurred within America, Madfis and Levin (2013) note that in non-U.S. attacks, academic failure features more prominently, and school staff are more likely to be targeted.

Moreover, many nations must now deal with elevated threats of violence, even if these threats never translate to an actual rampage. Between 2006 and 2010 in Germany alone, there were 2,600 officially registered threats against schools (Wolfgang, 2012). Since Finland suffered two attacks in 2007 and 2008, it has averaged about 60 threats per year. This stands in stark contrast to pre-attack levels of 5 to 10 threats per year (Lindberg, Sailas, & Kaltiala-Heino, 2012). In the United States, the reporting line that was established in Colorado post-Columbine, "Safe2Tell," logged 361 threats of violence between 2004 and 2010 (Payne & Elliot, 2011), which is about 60 per year. During the 50 days following the Columbine shooting, the State of Pennsylvania reported 354 threats of school violence (Kostinsky, Bixler, & Ketti, 2001). Researchers link these threats to intense media coverage of shootings (Kostinsky et al., 2001). Factors identified by Kostinskey et al. (2001) that increased the likelihood that a Pennsylvania school would receive a threat of violence in the aftermath of Columbine was school size and a greater proportion of White students.

Given ongoing threats, the increase in mass shootings, and parental and school concern about shootings, preventing this type of violence has gained increasing international attention. Researchers and practitioners alike ask two related questions: What causes these events? How do they develop?

School Shootings Evolve from a Long-Term Developmental Pathway

Several challenges converge to blur understanding of the etiology of this particular type of violence. First, school shootings are low-incidence. Their sheer lack of volume complicates developing a working model that describes the type of (mostly) young men who perpetrate them. Second, researchers define these events in various ways and study overlapping case studies. Third, many post-event analyses must occur indirectly because of perpetrator suicide. Finally, school shootings are an inherently complex form of violence, emerging as the eventual product of many factors that interact over a long period of time (Bondü et al., 2011). Contrary to what is often promoted by the media, school shooters do not just suddenly "snap" (O'Toole, 2000).

School Shootings Are Connected to Risk and Protective Factors

In general, acts of violence are influenced by the relationship between the risk and protective factors in a person's life (Office of the Surgeon General, 2001) and how they interact within a developmental framework. Different risk factors gain more predictive power depending on age (Conyne, 2015; Office of the Surgeon General, 2001).

From this perspective, violence can emerge when risk factors overwhelm the positive influence of protective factors, and healthy coping mechanisms fall victim to maladaptive practices. Similarly, school shootings can be conceptualized as failed attempts at coping with long-simmering problems, coupled with increasing hopelessness and personality variables such as narcissism.

School Shootings and Suicide

Many school shooting perpetrators experience depression and suicidal thinking and plan to die in the course of their attack, whether by a self-inflicted gunshot or by police (Lankford, 2015). Parallels between school shooting perpetration and suicide, therefore, deserve specific discussion.

Research conducted on school shooters in the United States (Lankford, 2012) shows that 88 percent attempt suicide following the attack. Many of the factors elevating suicidal risk in general (e.g., social isolation, problems at work or school, hopelessness, and some sort of precipitating crisis) also can be found in the lives of school shooters. From this perspective, school shootings might be conceptualized as a particularly violent and rare form of suicide, described by some as "ceremonial violence" (Rocque, 2012).

It is this desire for revenge and notoriety that may help differentiate the school shooter who completes suicide from the young man who pursues the more typical solitary variety. This difference may be fueled by the real ongoing peer rejection and bullying (Madfis & Levin, 2013; Vossekuil, Fein, Reddy, Borum, & Modzeleski, 2004) that many school shooters face, as well as underlying personality differences, such as a lack of empathy or narcissism (Bondü et al., 2011; Langman, 2009; O'Toole, 2000).

Certain Ecological Factors Associated with School Shootings

The ecology (Bonfenbrenner, 1979) of a school influences school shootings. In this section, we will explore some of these important ecological factors

(Conyne & Mazza, 2006), including the general social and physical environment, prevailing norms and culture, and school climate. We use these terms relatively interchangeably.

School General Environment

Including the role of the environment provides a broader way to approach prevention of school shootings. School officials are unable to significantly change the individual psychology of different students and have less control over what these students do in their free time. However, they can and should change environmental/climate problems such as bullying, student isolation and disconnection from peers and teachers, and inadequate mental health support. Moreover, working on improving environmental conditions provides the added benefit of advancing the overall well-being of the entire school – both at-risk and better-adjusted students can benefit.

While each individual school shooter bears the ultimate responsibility for his or her act, research indicates that in at least some cases there have been contributing environmental factors (Eagan et al., 2014; O'Toole, 2000; Vossekuil et al., 2004). In schools where shootings have occurred, it has been found that rigid social hierarchies tend to be found, punishment is unequally distributed, the school frequently exists in a small town or close-knit suburb, bullying may go unaddressed, and the school's climate may be such that students don't feel connected to teachers (Newman, 2013). There may be an inflexible definition of what "normal" is, especially for boys. Boys who deviate from the school's established masculine gender norms may be picked on, enduring homophobic bullying in particular (Birkett & Espelage, 2010; Kimmel & Mahler, 2003; Newman, 2013).

Given how extreme and destructive shootings are, it may seem hard to conceive that a school's general environment and climate can contribute to such violence. However, a general research base has been established that indicates the school environment influences a range of student behaviors.

Delinquency, dropout rates, substance use, and violence are all at least partially preventable through modifications in the school environment. Moreover, violence rates can be influenced by a school's physical and social environment (Lindstrom-Johnson, Burke, & Gielen, 2011). In particular, positive classroom social interactions, student bonding with the school, favorable student–teacher relationships, and student belief that school rules are fair have all been found to impact the degree to which violence manifests in a school (Lindstrom-Johnson et al., 2011).

School Norms and Culture

School norms can affect violence rates present in a school. Lindstrom-Johnson, (2009) report that though there have been mixed findings around the relationship between school culture and violence, a number of studies have found a relationship between decreasing violence and the degree to which a school emphasizes inclusion, cultural sensitivity, and cooperation. More particularly, clear school rules of which the student population is aware and believes to be fair, a sense of school "ownership" on the part of students, school norms against violence, and an emphasis on student comprehension of these factors have been associated with reductions in violence rates. This information suggests that strong violence prevention programs should attend not only to individual student well-being and behaviors but also to schoolwide policies and climate.

Other research has found that emotional distress, suicide, deviant behavior, and violence can all be reduced when students feel connected to adults in their school (Klein, Cornell, & Konold, 2012), and that a positive, healthy school climate can reduce student aggression and substance use (Klein et al., 2012). Thus, schools that intentionally seek to create and sustain school culture and norms that support healthy and supportive learning environments are more likely to contain well-adjusted students. They also may be less likely to experience a school shooting or threats against the school (Fein et al., 2002).

The following discussion is devoted specifically to bullying (e.g., Birkett & Espelage, 2010; Olweus, 1993; Orpinas & Horne, 2006; Swearer, Espelage, & Napolitano, 2009), as it has been a persistent theme in school shooting research. In fact, bullying has been viewed as a potential precursor to incidents of targeted school violence (Felix & Furlong, 2008).

Bullying as a special case. Bullying and harassment can be described as taunting, peer aggression, physical threats, humiliation, and public ridicule (Juvonen, Nishina, & Graham, 2000). An essential component of bullying is a repetitive imbalance of power (Dill, Redding, Smith, Surette, & Cornell, 2011). As of 2011, 28 percent of twelve-through eighteen-year-old students were reporting frequent bullying (Robers et al., 2014).

Bullying and victimization rates are impacted not only by the schools in which they occur but by neighborhood, family, and gender variables (Dill et al., 2011; Foster & Brooks-Gunn, 2013). As discussed earlier, boys who do not fulfill the requirements of normative masculinity are more likely to experience bullying when their masculinity is called into question.

Individual psychological outcomes of bullying. Bullying is associated with many negative consequences. Students exposed to bullying and peer harassment at school are at higher risk for experiencing psychological difficulties such as low self-esteem, anxiety, loneliness, and depression. Bullying may lead to self-harm behaviors and psychotic symptoms (Dill et al., 2011) and can also lead to suicide (Sommer et al., 2014). Bullied students also may withdraw from peers, and report less positive attitudes toward school, feel helpless, develop psychosomatic problems, and have reduced school attendance and decreased academic achievement (Juvonen et al., 2000; Sommer et al., 2014). Bullying also is associated strongly with social maladjustment (Foster & Brooks-Gunn, 2013), and with poorer school attachment and frustration (Lindstrom-Johnson, 2009).

Clearly, bullying can exert a profoundly negative impact on adolescent development, especially if severe and chronic. However, is it really extreme enough to bring a child to targeted school violence? The answer seems to be a qualified "yes but," or "yes and." Bullying (again with other risk factors) can be a key factor in the development of a shooting.

Research into school shootings has identified that bullying is frequently correlated with school shootings. For instance, bullying was found to be involved in seven of the twelve international non-U.S. shootings examined by Madfis and Levin (2013). Their sample was comprised of events occurring across Finland, Germany, Brazil, Canada, Netherlands, Australia, Brazil, Thailand, and Argentina. Leary, Kowalski, Smith, and Phillips (2003) reviewed fifteen shootings that occurred in the 1990s in the United States, finding that "acute or chronic" rejection in the form of bullying, ostracism, or romantic rejection was an important factor in twelve of these events. In ten cases specifically, bullying, teasing, harassment, and peer rejection were identified as variables. Similarly, research by the American government has identified bullying in 71 percent of cases studied (Vossekuil et al., 2004).

Cumulatively, the research indicates that the school environment and community norms influence bullying, violence, and victimization (Klein et al., 2012; Lindstrom-Johnson, 2009, Lindstrom-Johnson et al., 2011). Experiencing bullying and ongoing social exclusion, in combination with other variables (e.g., access to weapons, suicide ideation, depression, hopelessness, and a desire to "get even" for perceived wrongs) can contribute to the development of school shootings.

Intrapersonal Variables Implicated in School Shootings, U.S. Emphasis

Therefore, it is important to consider the role of the school environment and sociocultural norms (especially as they relate to masculinity, violence, bullying, and power) in contributing to the risk for a school shooting. Attention must also be devoted, however, to the individual psychological factors associated with this type of violence.

For instance, while many perpetrators of targeted school violence report being bullied, the vast majority of students who endure significant peer victimization for years never go on a shooting rampage, though they may suffer serious psychological consequences. Further, many students experience failures, romantic or otherwise, and feel wronged, lonely, and hopeless, but never perpetrate a school shooting.

School shooters emerge from a complex interaction that includes personality, temperament, and behavioral characteristics; adolescent experiences; school structure and climate; family structure and cohesion; parental modeling; and community influences (O'Toole, 2000). Some studies have reported that shooters are more likely to be narcissistic, oversubscribe to masculinity norms, have a history of suicidal ideation, lack empathy, have suffered a significant loss prior to the shooting, possess deficits in social skills and social problem solving, and feel both superior to and victimized by their peers (Kalish & Kimmel, 2010; Langman, 2009; O'Toole, 2000; Vossekuil et al., 2004). The vast majority of them are middle-class young men, and most are White. They may be "injustice collectors," ruminating at length on their victimization experiences (O'Toole, 2000). Within this framework, rage, depression, and substance use may also inhibit the perpetrator's ability to feel empathy, thus further enabling a violent act to be carried out (Mitchell & Brendtro, 2013). Others have noted that contrary to stereotypes, school shooters are not so much "loners" as they are "failed joiners" (Newman, 2012).

Relatedly, evidence suggests that there are different types of school shooters. Langman (2009) reviewed case studies of school shooters in the United States and determined that different shooters could be classified as either traumatized, psychopathic, or psychotic. Others have described school shooters as either antisocial, depressed with personal adjustment problems and coping with stressful conflicts, or as living with a psychotic disorder (Bondü et al., 2011).

That there are different types of shooters is not surprising, but it raises questions about what type of preventive model would be most able equally to reach and defend against the different theorized typologies. For example, creating a healthy school environment (Orpinas & Horne, 2006) may more effectively guard against and reach the traumatized and schizophrenic school shooter than the psychopathic one. Psychopathic shooters may be masters of manipulation and image (Langman, 2009), making them harder to observe. Moreover, for those shooters determined to carry through with an attack and minimize the signs of their attack planning, a responsive school environment alone will be less effective.

School Shooting Prevention Trends

Cumulatively, given the many interacting individual and environmental factors associated with a school shooting, prevention is challenging. The research that has identified trends and risk factors across perpetrators does not necessarily manifest in the ability to prevent these types of attacks.

Profiling or behavior checklists provide a case in point. Profiling has proven to be ineffective and even harmful as school shootings are infrequent and there are too many young men who fit various aspects of any profile who would never perpetrate a shooting (Fein et al., 2002; O'Toole, 2000). Moreover, profiling ignores students who might pose an actual threat (e.g., girls or "popular" kids). Equally ineffective by themselves are checklists of concerning behaviors that could be used to indicate risk (O'Toole, 2000).

However, as intricate as these school shootings are, the possibility exists for effective school-based intervention. If the majority of shootings are months or years in the making, then there is theoretically time to alter a potential perpetrator's trajectory. This reality is something that some schools, both in the

United States and Europe, are grappling with in various ways. Thus, prevention trends have emerged. A brief overview of these trends follows.

Preventive measures have involved strengthening gun control laws (more common outside of the United States), augmenting the physical security of schools, and funding mental health. Calls for and actual funding of mental health treatment increased in the United States after the 2012 Sandy Hook shooting in Newtown, Connecticut (National Alliance on Mental Illness, 2013). However, as of 2014, fewer U.S. states increased mental health funding, and some states experienced significant mental health budget cuts (National Alliance on Mental Illness, 2014).

Strengthening Physical Security

Physical strengthening of schools typically includes random locker checks, metal detectors, security cameras, guest sign-in, funding more school resource officers, and locking classroom doors. Some German schools have proceeded to place alarm buttons in classrooms and hang signs detailing student escape options in the event of a school shooting (Leuschner et al., 2011). Some schools in the United States have implemented tip lines where students can report concerns about bullying or threats against the school (Blad, 2014). However, despite the use of physical strengthening measures, prevention efforts in the United States differ from other countries concerned in one key domain: gun policy.

Gun Policy Related to Control

The United States has adopted relatively weak federal gun laws compared to other developed nations combating school shootings (Council on Foreign Relations, 2012; McConville & Lawless, 2012). There is no federal legislation banning semiautomatic weapons. Even as school shootings internationally have resulted in increased gun restrictions, some states have moved in the other direction, authorizing teachers to carry guns in preparation for a potential attack.

A handful of teachers in Texas now carry guns to school as a rampage shooting preventive measure implemented through their district. These teachers are screened for mental health conditions before going through weapons training. They then teach with a concealed handgun (Shah, 2013). Texas is not the first state to allow teachers to carry guns to school and is part of a larger American trend. The idea of fighting gun violence with guns or "arming the good guys" is a distinctly American approach to preventing school shooting rampages.

Especially after the 2012 Sandy Hook shooting in which twenty-six children and staff died, increased interest has developed in arming teachers. Rural, poorly funded school districts, in particular, have been considering this approach (Severson, 2013).

Officer Training

In response to the Sandy Hook shooting and to research showing that shootings have increased, the U.S. Federal Bureau of Investigation (FBI) developed a two-day training program that thirty thousand officers will receive over the next eighteen months. This is one of the largest training programs undertaken by the FBI. The ultimate goal of the training is to shave seconds off police response and make police response more efficient. This is an important approach because many attacks are over before police arrive (Johnson, 2014).

Threat Assessment

One of the most effective and supported ways to prevent school shootings is to utilize a threat assessment model. Threat assessment should be a component of a school culture that strives to be inclusive, equitable, and responsive to individual student needs (Fein et al., 2002).

Threat assessment was originally developed by the U.S. Secret Service as a way to prevent attacks on public officials (Fein et al., 2002). It involves a systematic approach to identifying, assessing, and managing/helping those who may pose a threat to others (Cornell, Sheras, Gregory, & Fan 2009; Fein et al., 2002).

Since it was originally conceived, threat assessment has been adapted for use in schools. In general, the process asks practitioners to answer systematically and methodically two primary questions: (a) how credible and serious is the threat, and (b) to what extent does the potential perpetrator possess the resources, intent, and motivation to carry out the threat (O'Toole, 2000)?

The process involves assessing threats by evaluating their level of detail as a way to ascertain plausibility and to discover the level of planning and commitment toward the act. Importantly, the "threat" in this case is not necessarily referring to a verbalized warning against the school or a group of people. Rather, analyzing behaviors and actions delivers insight into the mental state of the potential attacker, his or her plans, and commitment to them. In this way, a threat assessment process evaluates more than just a specific verbalized threat and is an essential mechanism for answering the two questions listed earlier (Vossekuil et al., 2004).

These foundational concepts of threat assessment have been codified explicitly in multiple forms, such as the FBI's threat assessment model and the Virginia Model of Threat Assessment (Cornell, 2010; O'Toole, 2000). The U.S. Secret Service also has developed a threat assessment model that has commonalities with the FBI model (Fein, Vossekuil, & Holden, 1995; Vossekuil et al., 2004).

The FBI Threat Assessment Model. This model focuses its exploration on four domains to ensure that risk factors are not overlooked in any key life area. The domains are as follows: (1) student personality, (2) family dynamics, (3) school dynamics and the student's role in these dynamics, and (4) social dynamics. Each of these four areas is examined both individually and in tandem (O'Toole, 2000).

Once a threat has been made, a preliminary examination of the threat is conducted. The conductor may be a school psychologist, counselor, or another specialist who has undergone specific threat assessment training. This person gathers as much information as possible in each of the four previously outlined prongs from other staff, students, parents, or mental health specialists. Threats are sorted into low-, medium-, or high-level category based on information gathered throughout the process. Depending on the severity of the threat, further analysis is done and related action is taken, or the police are immediately notified and existing school safety procedures are undertaken.

Using this model, evaluators are directed to attend to various behaviors, statements, or factors in each prong that may indicate planning toward violence or intrapersonal or environmental conditions that facilitate violence. Examples for what examiners search for within each area follow:

- Personality: Narcissism; low tolerance for frustration; lack of resiliency; injustice collecting (i.e., the student collects and ruminates on perceived slights or experienced injustices); signs of depression and alienation; dehumanization of others; strong attitudes of entitlement and superiority; blame externalizing; low self-esteem and anger management problems; among other considerations.
- Family dynamics: Existence of a turbulent parent–child relationship, parental acceptance of pathological behavior, access to weapons, the student having more power than the parents, and no limits on television and Internet.
- School dynamics: Whether a culture has been established that tolerates bullying, is inflexible, distributes discipline inequitably, has student hierarchy/"pecking order," and a code of silence where students don't feel comfortable reaching out to administration.
- Social dynamics: Whether the student spends significant time with violence-saturated media; whether they use drugs and alcohol, what their interests are; and the role of any recent highly publicized school shootings, as these can spur the copycat effect (O'Toole, 2000).

All of this collected information is systematized within a clear system that is accessible by a well-trained team (O'Toole, 2000). One critique that could be made of this particular model, however, is its vagueness. Many families, for instance, experience "turbulent parent–child" relationships (Ferguson, Coulson, & Barnett, 2011). And, how do practitioners know what is sufficiently turbulent in the parent–child relationship to be considered noteworthy, for example? In this sense, school shooting threat assessment relies on clinical interpretation. It should be used to guide decisions, but cannot provide every answer.

The Virginia Model of Behavioral Threat Assessment. This approach shares similarities with the FBI's four-pronged approach just discussed. It is concerned with identifying whether a student poses a threat (not just whether a concrete threat has been made) and is team-based. The team leader may be the school or assistant principal, and the team might include a school psychologist, counsellor, and resource officer. As this team evaluates a threat, they follow a seven-step decision tree (Cornell, 2010). The steps are summarized as follows:

- Step 1: Use a standard set of questions to interview the student and relevant others.
- Step 2: Determine whether the threat is transient (less serious) or substantive (poses an immediate risk to others or the student of concern). What decisions are made next depend on how the threat is evaluated (transient versus substantive).
- Step 3: Respond to transient threat, or
- Step 4: Decide whether the substantive threat is serious or very serious (this influences whether or not the process goes to Step 5 or Step 6).
- Step 5: Respond to serious substantive threat, or
- Step 6: Conduct safety evaluation.
- Step 7: Implement a safety plan.

Threat assessment may be the best single approach for preventing school shootings, given their developmental nature and the futility of profiling, checklists, and even physical strengthening. Moreover, its methods transfer well across schools and even nations. It can capture a range of threats, from those that are transient and nothing more than inappropriate expressions of passing frustration, to those that reveal ongoing planning, alienation, and revenge seeking. It is a process that guides teams toward the information that should be attended to in crucial life domains, ensuring that they are not distracted by extraneous or unimportant data. Essentially, it guides energies in productive directions. Finally, it provides a framework for analyzing and cataloging severity, guiding decision making and school response.

Threat reporting and school climate. A large determinate of a school's ability to keep itself safe from violence in general and school shootings in particular rests on its ability to communicate its support and caring to students. This is because school climate and connection to teachers influence how willing students are to report bullying, violence, or targeted school violence threats. After all, school personnel can't intervene if they don't know that problems or threats exist. Importantly, in 81 percent of the cases reviewed by the Secret Service, school shooters told at least one other person about their plan of targeted school violence before the attack (Pollack, Modzeleski, & Rooney, 2008; Vossekuil et al., 2004). Of individuals informed of the plan, 93 percent were peers.

Thus, these peers become the first line of defense. Moreover, Centers for Disease Control and Prevention data from the *School Associated Violent Death Study* indicate that prior to completing a homicide, 50 percent of perpetrators leaked or displayed indicators of their intentions prior to the event (CDC, 2014a). This information, referencing school-based homicides in general, suggests the extent to which prevention could be achieved through increased reporting and observation of warning signs.

According to a 2008 study by the U.S. Secret Service and the Department of Education (Pollack et al., 2008), school climate can impact whether students feel comfortable reporting a threat to the administration. Study authors interviewed students who had prior knowledge of a school-based attack (one that either occurred or was successfully averted) to determine what factors influenced reporting or silence. It was found that only 4 percent of students aware of the attackers' plan tried to dissuade them (Pollack et al., 2008).

However, those students who did report did so because they had developed a positive relationship with at least one or more staff member or fellow students, and because they believed that the information they brought forward would be dealt with appropriately. This pattern aligns with research that has found that students with positive relationships with teachers (Orpinas & Horne, 2006; Swearer et al., 2009) are more likely to report threats of violence (Brinkley & Saarnio, 2006; Eliot, Cornell, Gregory, & Fan, 2010) and are less likely to ask teachers for help if they perceive them to be tolerant of bullying or uncaring (Eliot et al., 2010).

Conversely, those students who did not report were influenced by their perception that the school would respond negatively. Other reasons students didn't report threats include the students didn't believe that the attack would occur, the threat in question was "disbelievable," students felt that they had time to decide what to do with their knowledge of the threat, and parental figures influenced against disclosure.

Threat Assessment within a Comprehensive Model

Threat assessment should not stand on its own. For it to be most effective, it should be embedded within a school that specifically emphasizes a healthy and tolerant climate, and the well-being of its students (Fein et al., 2002). As Fein et al. (2002) write, "Environments in which students, teachers and administrators pay attention to students' social and emotional needs – as well as their academic needs – will have fewer situations that require formal threat assessments" (pp. 12–13). A school whose environment projects a climate of trust, respect, and safety and where students are interconnected through positive relationships and a supportive school climate is well positioned for prevention of school shootings; the overall climate both buttresses strengths, and it provides the necessary context for behavioral threat procedures to be successfully enacted.

The U.S. Department of Defense Science Board Task Force report *Predicting Violent Behavior* (Defense Science Board, 2012) further highlights the role of environment in preventing violence, noting that violence prediction is quite difficult, but that prevention can at least be partially achieved through creating environments that minimize isolation and alienation. This research suggests the role of a comprehensive model of school health – one that attends to school culture, environment, community norms, and individual student needs. Threat assessment can become an integral part of this comprehensive paradigm.

Violence prevention must also acknowledge the broader context of neighborhoods and communities in contributing to and sustaining violence. Schools, like any other institution, are at least partially the product of their community. Schools may erect physical walls and boundaries, but they provide no barrier against the flow of community norms and culture across school walls. As discussed earlier in this chapter, community norms can influence violence rates; targeted violence; and, in tight-knit small-town communities, reinforce feelings of alienation when young people feel they don't belong. Therefore, any comprehensive model of school also must be able to account for community influences on school strength and weaknesses and should provide a framework that guides schools toward observing these influencers.

Many of these themes are expressed by a position statement on preventing school shootings, *December 2012 Connecticut School Shooting Position Statement*,[1] signed by individual and organizational leaders across a spectrum of psychological specialties. The position statement emphasizes that the prevention of school shootings must begin long before a shooter approaches his target, and thus must transcend physical strengthening alone – a common preventive approach in America. The authors, much as we ourselves do, suggest that school shooting prevention must involve improving the school environment; improving mental health care; involving the community; using threat assessment; and, most importantly, *integrating* these different factors. They emphasize the importance of fostering wellness and social support for all members of a community, and through increased integration of mental health and other systems, better treatment of mental health conditions. The key words they used to frame this orientation are *balance, communication, connectedness, integration*, and *support.* This position statement reflects the importance of an ecological viewpoint when thinking about preventing violence.

Benefits of a Comprehensive-Ecological Model

Because of the complexity of violence development, there are many benefits to a comprehensive, ecological model of violence prevention, especially in schools (Birkett & Espelage, 2010; CDC, 2014b; Hong, Cho, Allen-Meares, & Espelage, 2011; Orpinas & Horne, 2006; Song & Marth, 2013). Any model intended to prevent violence while increasing the health of the school community will target some of the circumstances that enable a shooting to develop while also providing a framework for a school team to catch struggling students. The FBI acknowledges this point in its report on threat assessment, which stresses that no one factor is decisive in predicting violence (O'Toole, 2000). With threat assessment embedded within a comprehensive, ecological framework, a school can access multiple ways to both prevent and respond to different types of school violence.

1 curry.virginia.edu/articles/sandyhookshooting.

Comprehensive ecological school-based models of violence prevention work to decrease environmental risk, increase environmental supports, and provide individual students the skills they need to be healthy and successful. Further, to drive change that extends across the entire school, programs ideally should target students, teachers, climate, parents, and even interested community partners, and seek to lower the incidence of targeted problems (Conyne, 2015; Furlong, Felix, Sharkley, & Larson, 2005; U.S. Department of Justice, 2004). Such programs also are implemented by a team and can explicitly include a focus on bullying prevention (Furlong et al., 2005).

The Counseling for Wellness and Prevention Model

School shooting incidence could be reduced by integrating strategies within an organized, systemic framework and set of general processes that include threat assessment, physical strengthening, community-school cooperation, and an overarching emphasis on school climate and student well-being (Interdisciplinary Group on Preventing School and Community Violence, 2012). *The Counseling for Wellness and Prevention Model* (Conyne, 2015), described later in this section, offers one approach that seems well suited for school-based work and for violence prevention.

As mentioned at the beginning of the chapter, this model serves as a framework, rather than a specific intervention, something that is no less true when moved into the school environment. Its power derives from the conceptual structure it provides to a team attempting to organize more specific interventions and in its ability to orient a team toward variables known to be related to school shootings.

The Counseling for Wellness and Prevention Model (Conyne, 2015) frames healthy human development and dysfunction in terms of strengths and weaknesses present across ecological levels (personal, relational, and collective) while emphasizing the influence of context in enabling or prohibiting an individual or environment from reaching optimum levels of wellness (psychological and physical well-being). More specifically, the model posits that wellness or dysfunction emerges from the interaction of intrapersonal characteristics and demographic features with unique proximal and broader distal environmental factors. Figure 30.1 summarizes the model.

Key Components of the Model

Risk reduction and strength promotion. Rather than highlighting mitigation of individual human suffering and systems improvement through reducing risks alone, the model emphasizes strengths-based approach to effect tailored and lasting change.

Modal strategies. The model includes seven modal change strategies: education, social competency facilitation, natural caregiving, assistance with

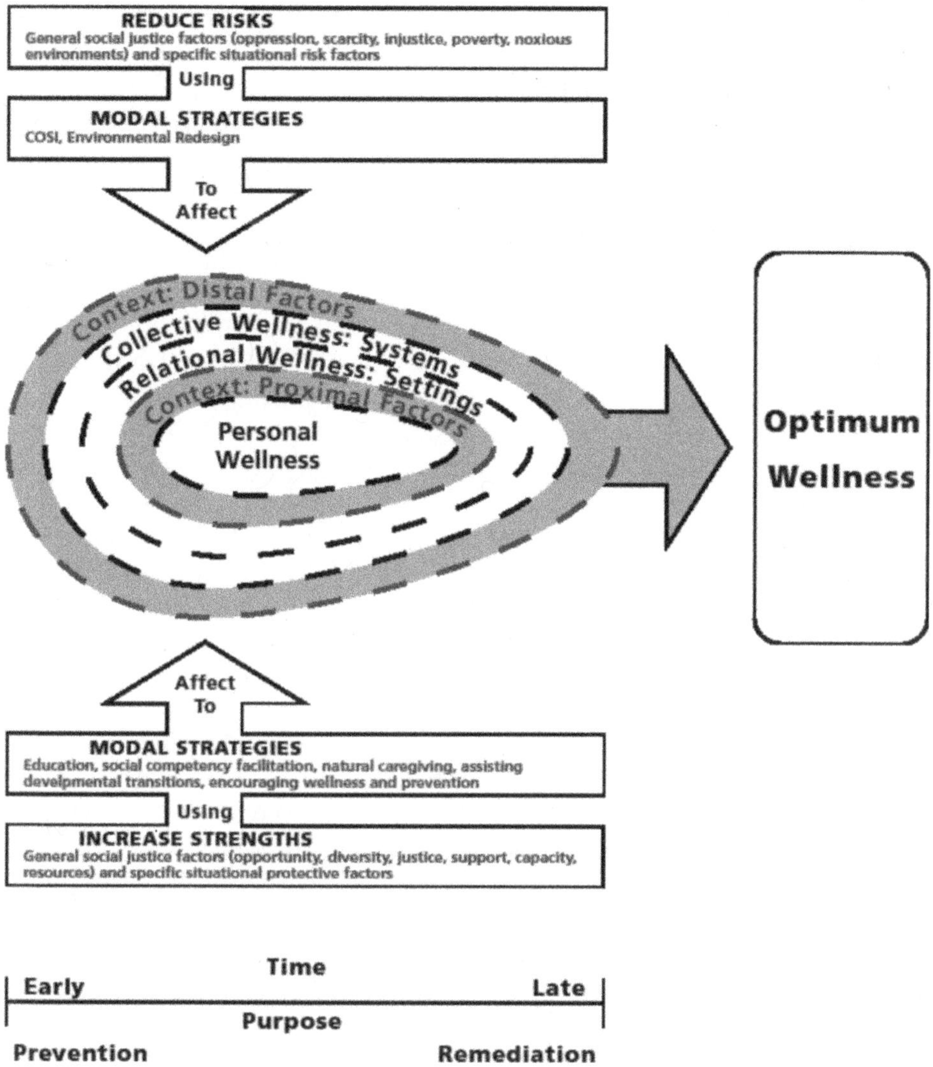

Figure 30.1. *Counseling for Wellness and Prevention Model.*

developmental transitions, encouragement of wellness and prevention, community organization and systems intervention (COSI), and environmental redesign. These broad strategies have been identified across the prevention literature as general methods of prevention, and each one houses more specific approaches (Conyne, 2004; Gullotta & Bloom, 2003).

Cumulatively, these broad strategies are designed not only to orient an individual practitioner to potential change avenues, but also to organize the simultaneous use of multiple applied strategies. Further, using specific programs or preventive measures from the different modal strategies in concert provides the potential for systematic change to be driven in multiple ways.

Context. Another central element of the model (and one that has unique implications when located within the school setting) is its emphasis on how context, or proximal and distal factors, influences the development of pathology or health. Proximal factors are those that affect the individual directly and immediately (e.g., race, gender, sexual orientation, socioeconomic status, community, and family) and can contribute to enhanced or restricted opportunity. Distal factors are broad global, national, or cultural factors (e.g., new legislation or cultural beliefs) or events (e.g., a widely publicized school shooting) that exert a trickle-down effect on the individual.

Social justice factors. Social injustice factors, if present in an ecological system, impede the ability of any one person or organization (e.g., a school) to achieve optimum levels of wellness/functioning. Examples of these factors include oppression and injustice. For instance, shootings are more likely to occur in schools that distribute punishment inequitably and that tolerate bullying (oppression and injustice).

Alternately, the presence of positive social justice factors is essential to well-being for both individuals and systems. These factors include opportunity, support, justice, and diversity. Applying these positive social justice factors within the school might help shape a culture that is tolerant of deviations from strict masculinity norms and would support diversity.

Time frame. The model's elements ideally are applied before the emergence of serious concerns (prevention focus), but its flexibility also permits reactive implementation. Both time frames are important and complementary.

Cumulatively, a model such as this one can be used to guide a team or clinician toward essential points of change. It provides a broad framework to guide thinking about change strategies; acknowledges the role of social justice factors in human, organizational, and national development; and explicitly acknowledges that context, both proximal and distal, can potently influence the capacity to achieve optimal well-being.

Further, the model's ultimate goal is not only to achieve optimum wellness across all levels, but also to achieve incidence reduction – the elimination or the reduction of the rate of new cases of problems, in this case, of school shootings. The prevention of school shootings occurs through positively altering the school environment, increasing the connection of students to the school, and embedding a team-driven threat assessment model.

The Model in International Context

The broad structure and philosophy of this model could be readily applied in different countries or across cultural contexts. Its strength is that practitioners across a variety of environments and cultures use the structure of the model to create change based on their specific needs. For instance, the model includes a focus on social justice factors, such as oppression. Oppression is universally harmful, yet manifests variously in different cultures and nations. Thus, the model can and should be adapted to fit varying circumstances.

Contributions of the Model

The model can be explicitly used as a guide to create a school culture that reduces alienation of student groups and individual students. Students are less likely to lash out violently against the school as an institution or other students if they feel connected to the school. Therefore, increasing positive feelings and connection to school and community (Orpinas & Horne, 2006; Swearer et al., 2009) is an essential component of school shooting prevention. It is also aligned with the *Guidelines for Prevention in Psychology* (APA, 2014), which urge psychologists to pursue interventions adapted to local contexts, that both reduce risks and promote strengths, and that address systemic issues.

Some Positive Prevention Trends in the United States

The adoption of the *Guidelines for Prevention in Psychology* by the American Psychological Association acknowledges the important role that prevention approaches can and ought to play in healthy functioning. It is indicative of a broader movement within the psychological (and, by extension, the mental health) community toward prevention and wellness that includes building positive school climates and environments.

It also aligns with the U.S.'s burgeoning general interest in prevention. For instance, the United States has committed to increased funding of mental health care in schools. As part of President Obama's *Now is the Time Plan*, $99 million in funds has been directed toward training mental health professionals, training teachers around warning signs that a student is struggling, and better connecting young people to mental health care. Of this money, over $48 million is specifically earmarked for use by schools and related community organizations (U.S. Department of Health and Human Services, 2014).

Moreover, some states are working to strengthen gun laws. Washington State, for instance, approved a measure in November 2014 that expands background checks. Now these background checks have been expanded further to include people buying online, from private sellers, and from gun shows (O'Sullivan, 2014). Cumulatively, increased funding for mental health care for young people, the passing of the APA *Prevention Guidelines*, and state-led expansion of background checks indicate the increased concern about youth mental health and pervasive gun violence in our society.

Conclusion and Summary

School shootings, though rare, continue to captivate and worry the nations in which they occur. Researchers are beginning to understand the causes and commonalities between shootings. Yet, because of their very rarity, the high suicide rate of offenders, and their complex developmental pathway, comprehension remains elusive. As such, and because studying school shootings continues to be a specialized research area and is a relatively new development in the psychological field, there are many different frames used to analyze these events. From theorizing that these young men are asserting what they feel to be assaulted masculinity, to bullying, to a school climate that fails to contribute caring in the way it needs to, to personality variables, mental health problems, and suicide, researchers have highlighted different components. Most research emphasizes the contribution of interactional, ecological factors in these attacks and related implications for their possible prevention.

Threat assessment is one of the most promising avenues of school shooting prevention. Especially when embedded within a model of school health designed to create a healthy and connected student body, such as the Counseling for Wellness and Prevention Model (Conyne, 2015), it seems to hold significant potential to diminish the incidence of these attacks.

Many factors conspire to complicate both research in and prevention of school shootings. However, counterbalancing progress is being made to build capacity and avert tragedies in schools. Thus, it appears to be genuinely possible given this positive evolution that school shootings can be reduced, if not substantially eliminated.

References

APA (American Psychological Association) (2014). Guidelines for prevention in psychology. *American Psychologist* 69: 286–96. doi: 10.1037/a0034569

Bangalore, S., & Messerli, F. H. (2013). Gun ownership and firearm-related deaths. *American Journal of Medicine* 126: 873–6. doi: dx.doi.org/10.1016/j.amjmed.2013.04.012

Birkett, M., & Espelage, D. (2010). Homophobic name-calling, peer groups, and masculinity: the socialization of homophobic behavior in adolescents. *Social Development* 24: 184–205.

Blad, E. (2014). Tip lines get a fresh look in school safety initiatives. *Education Week* 33 (20). www.edweek.org/ew/articles/2014/02/05/20tiplines.h33.html

Blair, J. P., & Martaindale, M. H. (2013). Active shooter events from 2000–2010: training and equipment implications. alerrt.org/files/research/ActiveShooterEvents.pdf

Bockler, N., Seeger, T., Sitzer, P., & Heitmeyer, W. (2013). School shootings: conceptual framework and international empirical trends. In Bockler, N., Seeger, T., Sitzer, P., & Heitmeyer, W. (eds.), *School Shootings: International Research, Case Studies, and Concepts for Prevention*. New York: Springer., pp. 1–24.

Bondü, R., Cornell, D. G., & Scheithauer, H. (2011). Student homicidal violence in schools: an international problem. *New Directions for Youth Development* 129: 13–30. doi: 10.1002/yd

Bonfenbrenner, U. (1979). *The Ecology of Human Development*. Cambridge, MA: Harvard University Press.

Brinkley, C. J., & Saarnio, D. A. (2006). Involving students in school violence prevention: are they willing to help? *Journal of School Violence* 5(1): 93–106. doi: 10.1300/J202v05n01_07

CDC (Centers for Disease Control and Prevention) (2014a). School assisted violent death study. www.cdc.gov/violence prevention/youthviolence/schoolviolence/savd.html

CDC (Centers for Disease Control and Prevention) (2014b). The social-ecological model: a framework for violence prevention. www.cdc.gov/violencepreven tion/pdf/sem_framewrk-a.pdf

CDC (Centers for Disease Control and Prevention) (2014c). Suicide: risk and protective factors. www.cdc.gov/violenceprevention/suicide/riskprotectivefactors .html

Conyne, R. (2004). *Preventive Counseling: Helping People to Become Empowered in Systems and Settings*, 2nd ed. New York: Routledge.

Conyne, R. (2015). *Counseling for Wellness and Prevention: Empowering People in Settings and Systems*, 3rd ed. New York: Routledge.

Conyne, R., & Mazza, J. (2006). Ecological group work applied to schools. *Journal for Specialists in Group Work* 32: 19–29. doi: 10.1080/01933920600977499

Cornell, D. (2010). The Virginia Model for Student Threat Assessment. http://curry .virginia.edu/uploads/resourceLibrary/Virginia_Model_for_Student_Threat_Assessment_overview_paper_7-16-10.pdf

Cornell, D., Sheras, P., Gregory, A., & Fan, X. (2009). A retrospective study of school safety conditions in high schools using the Virginia threat assessment guidelines versus alternative approaches. *School Psychology Quarterly* 24(2): 119–29. doi: 10.1037/a0016182

Council on Foreign Relations. (2012). U.S. gun policy: global comparisons. www.pbs.org/newshour/rundown/gun-policy/

Defense Science Board, Department of Defense (2012). Task force report: predicting violent behavior. www.acq.osd.mil/dsb/reports/PredictingViolentBehavior.pdf

Dill, K. E., Redding, R. E., Smith, P. K., Surette, R., & Cornell, D. G. (2011). Recurrent issues in efforts to prevent homicidal youth violence in schools: expert opinions. *New Directions for Youth Development* 129: 113–28. doi: 10.1002/yd.391

Dougherty, C. (2009). Teenage gunman kills 15 at school in Germany. *New York Times*, March 11. www.nytimes.com/2009/03/12/world/europe/12germany .html?_r=1&

Eagan, S. H., VosWinkel, F., Ford, J. D., Lyddy, C., Schwartz, H., & Spencer, A. (2014). Shooting at Sandyhook Elementary School: report of the Office of the Child Advocate. www.ct.gov/oca/site/default.asp

Eliot, M., Cornell, D., Gregory, A., & Fan, X. (2010). Supportive school climate and student willingness to seek help for bullying and threats of violence. *Journal of School Psychology* 48(6): 533–53. doi: 10.1016/j.jsp.2010.07.001

FBI (Federal Bureau of Investigation Law Enforcement Bulletin) (2014). Active shooter events from 2000–2012. leb.fbi.gov/2014/january/active-shooter-events-from-2000-to-2012

Fein, R. A., Vossekuil, B., & Holden, G. A. (1995). Threat assessment: an approach to prevent targeted violence. National Institute of Justice: *Research in Action* (September): 1–7. www.secretservice.gov/ntac.htm

Fein, R. A., Vossekuil, B., Pollack, W. S., Borum, R., Modzeleski, W., & Reddy, M. (2002). *Threat Assessment in Schools: A Guide to Managing Threatening Situations and Creating Safe School Climates*. Washington, DC: U.S. Department of Education, Office of Elementary and Secondary Education, Safe and Drug-Free Schools Program and U.S. Secret Service, National Threat Assessment Center.

Felix, E., & Furlong, M. (2008). Best practices in bullying prevention. In Thomas, A., & Grimes, J. (eds.), *Best Practices in School Psychology*. Bethesda, MD: National Association of School Psychologists, pp. 1279–89.

Ferguson, C. J., Coulson, M., & Barnett, J. (2011). Psychological profiles of school shooters: positive directions and one big wrong turn. *Journal of Police Crisis Negotiations* 11(2): 141–58. doi: 10.1080/15332586.2011.581523

Foster, H., & Brooks-Gunn, J. (2013). Neighborhood, family, and individual influences on school physical victimization. *Journal of Youth and Adolescence* 42: 1586–1610. doi: 10.1007/s10964-012-9890-4

Freie Universität Berlin (2014). Conflicts with teachers are risk factor for school shootings [Press release]. www.fu-berlin.de/en/presse/informationen/fup/2014/fup_14_299-target-forschung-amok-school-shooting/index.html

Furlong, M. J., Felix, E. D., Sharkley, J. D., & Larson, J. (2005). Preventing school violence: a plan for safe and engaging schools. *Student Counseling* 6(1): 11–15. www.nasponline.org. /resources/principals/Student%20Counseling%20Violence%20Prevention.pdf

Gallup (2014a). Fear for child's safety nearly back to pre-Sandy Hook levels. www.gallup.com/poll/174827/fear-child-safety-nearly-back-pre-sandy-hook-levels.aspx

Gallup (2014b). More than 6 in 10 Americans say guns make homes safer. www.gallup.com/poll/179213/six-americans-say-guns-homes-safer.aspx

Gullotta, T., & Bloom, B. (eds.) (2013). *Encyclopedia of Primary Prevention and Health Promotion*. New York: Kluwer.

Harper, J. (2012). Media coverage of Newtown shooting draws criticism. *Washington Times*, December 16. www.washingtontimes.com/blog/watercooler/2012/dec/16/media-coverage-newtown-shootings-draws-criticism/

Hong, J. S., Cho, H., Allen-Meares, P., & Espelage, D. L. (2011). The social ecology of the Columbine High School shootings. *Children and Youth Services Review* 33: 861–8. doi: 10.1016/j.childyouth.2010.12.005

IOM (Institute of Medicine) and NRC (National Research Council) (2013). *Priorities for Research to Reduce the Threat of Firearm-related Violence*. Washington, DC: National Academies Press.

Interdisciplinary Group on Preventing School and Community Violence (2012). December 2012 Connecticut school shooting position statement. curry.virginia.edu/articles/sandyhookshooting

Johnson, K. (2014). FBI trains 30,000 to confront active shooters. *USA Today*, December 22. Retrieved from www.usatoday.com/

Juvonen, J., Nishina, A., & Graham, S. (2000). Peer harassment, psychological adjustment, and school functioning in early adolescence. *Journal of Educational Psychology* 92(2): 349–59. Retrieved from www.apa.org/pubs/journals/edu/

Kalish, R., & Kimmel, M. (2010). Suicide by mass murder: masculinity, aggrieved entitlement, and rampage school shootings. *Health Sociology Review* 9(4): 451–64. doi: 0.5172/hesr.2010.19.4.451

Kiilakoski, T., & Oksanen, A. (2011) Cultural and peer influences on homicidal violence: a Finnish perspective. *New Directions for Youth Development* 33 (129): 31–42. doi: 10.1002/yd.385

Kimmel, M., & Mahler, M. (2003). Adolescent masculinity, homophobia, and violence: random school shootings, 1982–2000. *American Behavioral Scientist* 46. doi: 10.1177/0002764203046010010

Klein, J., Cornell, D., & Konold, T. (2012). Relationships between bullying, school climate, and student risk behaviors. *School Psychology Quarterly* 27: 154–69. doi: 10.1037/a0029350

Kostinsky S., Bixler E. O., & Kettl, P. A. (2001). Threats of school violence in Pennsylvania after media coverage of the Columbine high school massacre: examining the role of imitation. *Archives of Pediatrics and Adolescent Medicine* 155(9): 994–1001. doi: 10.1001/archpedi.155.9.994

Langman, P. (2009). Rampage school shooters: a typology. *Aggression and Violent Behavior* 14: 79–86. doi: 10.1016/j.avb.2008.10.003

Lankford, A. (2012). A comparative analysis of suicide terrorists and rampage, workplace and school shooters in the United States from 1990–2010. *Homicide Studies* 17(3): 255–74. doi: 10.1177/1088767912462033

Lankford, A. (2015). Mass shooters in the USA, 1966–2010: differences between attackers who live and die. *Justice Quarterly* 32(2): 360–79. doi: dx.doi.org/10.1080/07418825.2013.806675

Larkin, R. (2009). The Columbine legacy: rampage shootings as political acts. *American Behavioral Scientist* 52(9): 1309–26. doi: 10.1177/0002764209332548

Leary, M. R., Kowalski, R. M., Smith, L., & Phillips, S. (2003). Teasing, rejection, and violence: case studies of the school shootings. *Aggressive Behavior* 29: 202–14. doi: 10.1002/ab.10061

Leuschner, V., Bondü, R., Shroer-Hippel, M., Panno, J., Neumetzler, K., Fisch, S., Scholl, J., & Scheithauer H. (2011). Prevention of homicidal violence in schools in Germany: the Berlin Leaking Project and the Networks against School Shootings Project (NETWASS). *New Directions for Youth Development* 129: 61–78. doi: 10.1002/yd.387

Library of Congress (2014). Firearms control legislation and policy: Germany. www.loc.gov/law/help/firearms-control/germany.php

Lindberg, N., Sailas, E., & Kaltiala-Heino, R. (2012). The copycat phenomenon after two Finnish school shootings: an adolescent psychiatric perspective. *BMC Psychiatry* 12(91): doi: 10.1186/1471–244X-12–91

Lindstrom-Johnson, S. (2009). Improving the school environment to reduce school violence: a review of the literature. *Journal of School Health* 79(10): 451–65. doi: 10.1111/j.1746-1561.2009.00435.x

Lindstrom-Johnson, S., Burke, J., & Gielen, A. (2011). Prioritizing the school environment in school violence prevention efforts. *Journal of School Health* 81(6): 331–40. doi: 0.1111/j.1746-1561.2011.00598.x

Madfis, E., & Levin, J. (2013). School rampage in international perspective: the salience of cumulative strain theory. In Bockler, N., Seeger, T., Sitzer, P., & Heitmeyer, W. (eds.), *School Shootings: International Research, Case Studies, and Concepts for Prevention*. New York: Springer, pp. 79–104.

Markward, M. J., Cline, S., & Markward, N. J. (2001). Group socialization, the Internet and school shootings. *International Journal of Adolescence and Youth* 10: 135–46. doi: 10.1080/02673843.2001.9747895

McConville, B., & Lawless, J. (2012). Gun control after school shootings: lessons from around the globe. *Christian Science Monitor*, December 18. Retrieved from www.csmonitor.com

Mitchell, M. L., & Brendtro, L. K. (2013). Victories over violence: the quest for safe schools and communities. *Reclaiming Children & Youth* 22(3): 5–11. Retrieved from reclaimingjournal.com/

National Alliance on Mental Illness. (2013). State legislation report 2013: Trends, themes & best practices in state mental health legislation. www.nami.org/Content/NavigationMenu/State_Advocacy/Tools_for_Leaders/2013StateLegislationReportFinal.pdf

National Alliance on Mental Illness. (2014). State mental health legislation 2014: Trends, themes & effective practices. www.nami.org/Template.cfm?Section=Policy_Reports&Template=/Content Management/ContentDisplay.cfm&ContentID=172851

Newman, K. (2012). In school shootings, patterns and warning signs. *CNN*, December 17. www.cnn.com/2012/12/17/opinion/newman-school-shooters/

Newman, K. (2013). Adolescent culture and the tragedy of rampage shootings. In Bockler, N., Seeger, T., Sitzer, P., & Heitmeyer, W. (eds.), *School Shootings: International Research, Case Studies, and Concepts for Prevention*. New York: Springer, pp. 55–77.

Office of the Surgeon General (U.S.); National Center for Injury Prevention and Control (U.S.); National Institute of Mental Health (U.S.); Center for Mental Health Services (U.S.). (2001). *Youth Violence: A Report of the Surgeon General*. Rockville, MD: Office of the Surgeon General (U.S.), ch. 1. www.ncbi.nlm.nih.gov/books/NBK44297/

Olweus, D. (1993). *Bullying at School: What We Know and What We Can Do*. Cambridge, MA: Blackwell.

O'Malley, M., & Eklund, K. (2012). Promoting safe and healthy schools. In Brock, S., & Jimerson, S. (eds.), *Best Practices in Crisis Prevention and Intervention in Schools*. Bethesda, MD: National Association of School Psychologists, pp. 151–76.

Orpinas, P., & Horne, A. H. (2006). *Bullying Prevention: Creating a Positive School Climate and Developing Competence*. Washington, DC: American Psychological Association.

O'Sullivan, J. (2014). Voters approve measure to expand checks for gun buyers. *Seattle Times*, November 4. seattletimes.com/html/localnews/2024953470_elexbackgroundchecksxml.html

O'Toole, M. (2000). *The School Shooter: A Threat Assessment Perspective*. Quantico, VA: National Center for the Analysis of Violent Crime, FBI Academy.

Payne, N. (2013). Dewey Cornell: "schools are safe." *Southwest Times*, February 14. www.southwesttimes.com/2013/02/dewey-cornell-schools-are-safe/

Payne, S. T., & Elliott, D. S. (2011). Safe2Tell. *New Directions for Youth Development* 2011(129): 103–11. doi: 10.1002/yd.390

Pollack, W. S., Modzeleski, W., & Rooney, G. (2008). *Prior Knowledge of Potential School-based Violence: Information Students Learn May Prevent a Targeted Attack*. Washington, DC: United States Department of Education.

Robers, S., Kemp, J., Rathbun, A., & Morgan, R. E. (2014). *Indicators of School Crime and Safety: 2013 (NCES 2014-042/NCJ 243299)*. Washington, DC: National Center for Education Statistics, U.S. Department of Education; and Bureau of Justice Statistics, Office of Justice Programs, U.S. Department of Justice.

Rocque, M. (2012). Exploring school rampage shootings: research, theory, and policy. *Social Science Journal* 49: 304–13. doi: 10.1016/j.soscij.2011.11.001

Severson, K. (2013). Guns at school? If there is a will, there are ways. *New York Times*, September 27. Retrieved from www.nytimes.com/

Shah, N. (2013). Armed teachers a reality in some schools, debated in others. *Education Week*, February 20. www.edweek.org/ew/articles/2013/02/15/21guns_ep.h32.html?tkn=OPVFA LDy452wcD9%2B7piucudTK%2FVFtpv8QqUy&cmp=ENL-EU-NEWS1

Sommer, F., Leuschner, V., & Scheithauer, H. (2014). Bullying, romantic rejection, and conflicts with teachers: the crucial role of social dynamics in the development of school shootings – a systematic review. *International Journal of Developmental Science* 8: 3–24. doi: 10.3233/DEV-140129

Song, S., & Marth, K. (2013). Social justice in the air: school culture and climate. In Shriberg, D., Song, S., Miranda, A. H., & Radliff, K. M. (eds.), *School Psychology and Social Justice: Conceptual Foundations and Tools for Practice*. New York: Routledge.

Swearer, S., Espelage, D., & Napolitano, S. (2009). *Bullying Prevention and Intervention: Realistic Strategies for Schools*. New York: Guilford Press.

United States Department of Health and Human Services (2014). HHS announces $99 million in new grants to improve mental health services for young people [Press release]. www.hhs.gov/news/press/2014pres/09/20140922a.html

United States Department of Justice, Office of Juvenile Justice and Delinquency Prevention (2004). Blueprints for violence prevention (Report No. NCJ 204274). www.ncjrs.gov/pdffiles1/ojjdp/204274.pdf

Vossekuil, B., Fein, R. A., Reddy, M., Borum, R., & Modzeleski, W. (2004). *The Final Report and Findings of the Safe School Initiative: Implications for the Prevention of School Attacks in the United States*. Washington, DC: U.S. Secret Service & United States Department of Education.

Wike, T. L., & Fraser, M. W. (2009). School shootings: making sense of the senseless. *Aggression and Violent Behavior* 14: 162–9. doi: 10.1016/j.avb.2009.01.005

Wolfgang, D. (2012). Study shows increase in school shooting threats. *DW*, July 24. Retrieved from www.dw.de/

31 Ending Child Sexual Abuse

A Look at Prevention Efforts in the United States

Elizabeth J. Letourneau & Ryan T. Shields

Introduction

There is good news about child sexual abuse (CSA) that deserves greater emphasis. First and foremost, in some countries rates of CSA have declined dramatically. For example, United States (U.S.) rates of CSA have declined between 40 percent and 60 percent since 1990 (Finkelhor & Jones, 2006). These declines are evident in a variety of sources, including national victims surveys, child welfare reports, and juvenile and criminal justice records, lending support to the view that these are "real" declines and not attributable to changes in reporting requirements or trends in reporting (Finkelhor & Jones, 2006). It remains unclear to what we should attribute these declines or how to extend these gains so that even fewer boys and girls are sexually abused. But this is where the second piece of good news is relevant. The public has begun to view violence – including CSA – not just as a problem but more specifically as a public health problem. As described in this chapter, CSA victimization increases the risk for myriad serious mental and physical health disorders and behavioral problems across the lifespan. CSA is expensive and entirely preventable. For these and other reasons, the World Health Organization (WHO; Krug, Mercy, Dahlberg, & Zwi, 2002), the Institute of Medicine (IOM, 2013), and other organizations and experts (e.g., Kaufman, 2010) now recognize CSA and other forms of child maltreatment and violence as serious public health problems. Bringing a public health lens to the issue of CSA offers the surest method for developing a scientifically grounded prevention focus. Such a focus can supplement the dominant and largely reactive criminal justice efforts and victim services with which CSA is more typically addressed (Letourneau, Eaton, Bass, Berlin, & Moore, 2014). Moreover, the public health lens expands the reach of interventions from the individual offender or victim to entire populations (Krug et al., 2002).

In this chapter, we describe the epidemiology and burden of CSA, review criminal justice and victim-focused efforts to address CSA, and describe efforts to prevent CSA. CSA is, of course, a global problem. However, we focus primarily (although not exclusively) on U.S.-based efforts to address CSA in part because therein lies our expertise and also because the majority of research on this topic has been conducted in the United States (e.g., see Pereda, Guilaer, Forns, & Gómez-Benito, 2009), and because the breadth of U.S. criminal justice policies designed to address CSA far exceed those of other countries (e.g., see SMART, 2014).

Our conceptualization of CSA is drawn from the WHO Consultation on Child Abuse Prevention (WHO, 1999, pp. 15–16):

> [CSA] is the involvement of a child in sexual activity that he or she does not fully comprehend, is unable to give informed consent to, or for which the child is not developmentally prepared and cannot give consent, or that violates the laws or social taboos of society. [CSA] is evidenced by this activity between a child and an adult or another child who by age or development is in a relationship of responsibility, trust or power, the activity being intended to gratify or satisfy the needs of the other person.

This definition goes on to include specifically commercial sexual exploitation and use of children in pornographic performance and materials and defines "child" as anyone under the age of eighteen except in regions where the legal age of majority is lower than eighteen years. As such, this definition broadly encompasses abuse perpetrated by caregivers (often referred to as sexual abuse) and abuse perpetrated by non-caregivers (often referred to as sexual violence).

Prevalence of CSA

CSA prevalence rates vary markedly, a finding commonly attributed to differences in definitions of abuse, sampling procedures, and data collection methodology (Glasser, Campbell, Glasser, Leitch, & Farrelly, 2001; Krug et al., 2002; Pereda et al., 2009). Results from a meta-analysis of sixty-five prevalence articles in twenty-two countries partly addressed this variation and indicated that 7.9 percent of men and 19.7 percent of women, globally, have experienced CSA (Pereda et al., 2009). By far, most studies were conducted in the United States, whose combined prevalence CSA rate of 15.8 was high relative to European (9.2) and Asian (10.1) countries and low relative to African (34.4) and Oceanian (23.9) countries. The most recent U.S. estimates of lifetime prevalence of exposure to CSA through age seventeen are 26.6 percent for girls and 5.1 percent for boys (Finkelhor, Shattuck, Turner, & Hamby, 2014a). Results from the Violence against Children Surveys (VACS), an ongoing effort to estimate national prevalence rates of CSA and other forms of childhood victimization in low- and middle-income countries (CDC, 2012; VACS, 2015), indicate relatively high rates of CSA exposure, varying from 26 percent to 38 percent among surveyed girls and from 9 percent to 21 percent among surveyed boys. Thus, while news of declining CSA rates is indeed good news, there is much room for improvement, and we should not be satisfied with current rates of CSA or complacent with current prevention efforts.

Negative Sequelae Associated with CSA

Beyond the immediate harm that can accompany CSA, such as emotional pain and fear (e.g., Deblinger & Heflin, 1996) and physical pain, injury, and disease (e.g., Heppenstall-Heger et al., 2003), CSA victimization confers increased risk for severe mental, physical, and behavioral health disorders across the life course (Bedi et al., 2011; Dong et al., 2004; Noll, Horowitz, Bonanno, Trickett, & Putnam, 2003; Noll, Zeller, Trickett, & Putnam, 2007; Putnam, 2003; Sommarin, Kilbane, Mercy, Maloney-Kitts, & Ligiero, 2014). CSA also confers increased risk for subsequent sexual and nonsexual victimization and perpetration (Ogloff, Cutajar, Mann, & Mullen, 2012) and is associated with later relationship and parenting difficulties (Roberts, O'Connor, Dunn, Golding, & ALSPAC Study Team, 2004).

Consequently, the WHO has identified CSA as substantively contributing to the global burden of disease, annually accounting for more than 9 million disability adjusted life years (Mathers, Stevens, & Mascarenhas, 2009). In the United States, CSA ranks twelfth in preventable risk factors and accounts for 0.7 percent of the U.S. burden of disease (U.S. Burden of Disease Collaborators, 2013). The fiscal costs associated with all forms of child abuse and neglect are also high (e.g., Fang, Brown, Florence, & Mercy, 2012), including those attributable specifically to CSA (Hankivsky & Draker, 2003; Miller, Cohen, & Wiersema, 1996; Saied-Tessier, 2014). Thus, effective CSA prevention would avert immediate harm to victims; reduce their risk for an extensive array of severe mental, physical, and behavioral health problems; and reduce their risk of revictimization and of potential perpetration of sexual and nonsexual harm. It would also reduce the monetary and nonmonetary costs borne by victims' families, communities, and society.

Risk and Protective Factors Associated with CSA Perpetration

CSA can be perpetrated by virtually anyone, regardless of relationship, gender, or (almost) age (Berliner, 2011). Nevertheless, the vast majority of offenders are male (Snyder, 2000) and as noted earlier, the majority of victims are female (Finkelhor et al., 2014; Pérez-Fuentes et al., 2013). It is worth emphasizing, however, that offenders can be female and that *male victims are not uncommon and should never be overlooked or excluded from prevention or intervention efforts.* CSA offenders are most commonly acquaintances (e.g., neighbor, friend, peer), followed by family members and then strangers (Berliner, 2011; Finkelhor, Ormrod, Turner, & Hamby, 2005).

The research evidence also tells us that many cases of CSA are perpetrated by *other* children. In U.S. national surveys, more than half of CSA victims indicated that their perpetrators were younger than eighteen years of age (Finkelhor et al., 2014). In analyses involving U.S. law enforcement records, more than one-third of offenders were children or adolescents (Finkelhor, Ormrod, & Chaffin, 2009). In comparison to youth who offend against peers, youth who sexually offend against younger children tend to be young themselves, with offense risk peaking between ages twelve and fourteen years (Finkelhor et al., 2009).

There is a growing literature base regarding risk and (to a much lesser extent) protective factors associated with CSA perpetration. Although risk and protective factors likely exist across the social-ecological spectrum, most research concentrates on individual level factors (e.g., deviant sexual interests) and relationship-level factors (e.g., parental monitoring) with far less attention to community or societal level factors (Letourneau et al., 2014). This is unfortunate because it limits our ability to develop more comprehensive population-level prevention programs.

Factors Associated with Youth CSA Perpetration

Comparisons of youth who have committed sexual versus nonsexual offenses typically find many similarities between these groups. For example, van Wijk and colleagues (2005) reported statistically significant between-groups differences on just two (3 percent) of sixty-six psychosocial characteristics, and a meta-analysis by Seto and Lalumière (2010) including fifty-nine studies reported statistically significant between-groups differences on sixteen (43 percent) of thirty-seven psychosocial factors. Factors that appear to distinguish between these two groups include sexually abused victimization; self- or therapist reported atypical sexual interest; exposure to developmentally inappropriate sexual images; sexual acts or pornography; as well as anxiety, social isolation, and low self-esteem. Relative to youth with nonsexual offenses, youth with sexual offenses had lower odds of interacting with delinquent or gang-involved peers and lower odds of substance abuse. Seto and Lalumière (2010) speculated that in some cases, atypical sexual interests provide the motivation for sexual offending whereas antisocial tendencies influence a youth's willingness to act upon this motivation. However, *many cases of youth-perpetrated CSA do not appear to be motivated by atypical sexual interests* but rather by a host of other, often situational factors (Chaffin, 2008). Factors that appear to influence these more situational adolescent offenses include impulsivity, low sex knowledge, low knowledge of developmental differences between older and younger children, cognitive distortions, and sexual experimentation gone awry (Kwiatkowski, 2012; Letourneau et al., 2009c; Letourneau, Borduin, & Schaeffer, 2008; Letourneau & Schaeffer, 2014).

Parents and other caregivers play a significant role in the healthy development, including sexual development, of youth. Factors such as caregiver monitoring and caregiver–adolescent communication about sex have been consistently linked with safer adolescent sexual behavior (e.g., see Aspy et al., 2007; Baptiste, Tolou-Shams, Miller, McBride, & Paikoff, 2007). Improved parental discipline and reduced association with delinquent peers were two factors found to mediate treatment outcomes for youth who had sexually offended (Henggeler et al., 2009a). Despite the important role families play in protecting adolescents from engaging in sexual risk behaviors, caregivers are often overlooked in CSA prevention efforts (Letourneau et al., 2014; Mendelson & Letourneau, 2015).

While nascent, research is beginning to evaluate protective factors. A recent study on protective factors associated with youth desistence from sexual and nonsexual offending indicated that affective strength (which indicates capacity for emotional intimacy) predicted desistence from sexual offending (Worling & Langton, 2015). Protective factors associated with desistance from nonsexual offending among youth who had sexually offended include school functioning and positive relationships (van der Put & Asscher, 2015; Worling & Langton, 2015).

Factors Associated with Adult Risk for CSA Perpetration

Scholars have focused on identifying risk factors for adult perpetrated CSA. Recent work has examined the genetic underpinnings to sexual interest in children. Alanko, Salo, Mokros, and Santtila (2013) used a sample of 962 monozygotic (i.e., identical) twins and 2,124 dizygotic (i.e., fraternal) Finnish twins and found a weak to moderate genetic influence (approximately 15 percent) on sexual interest in children.

Other research has focused on neurobiological explanations for sexual interest in children. This line of research suggests that pedophilia is related to functional and structural differences in the brain. For example, Cantor et al. (2004) assessed 473 men with problem sexual behavior and found that pedophilia was associated with lower intelligence and decreased memory functioning. Pedophilia was also correlated with non-right-handedness. These findings indicate that pedophilia is associated with what Cantor and colleagues refer to as "neurodevelopmental perturbations" (p. 12). Cantor et al. (2008) also studied brain images and found that men with pedophilia were more likely than nonpedophiles to have lower White matter volume in areas related to responses to sexual cues. They hypothesized that these White matter deficiencies may be linked to the development of or susceptibility to pedophilia. Taken together, these emerging lines of research suggest that sexual interest in children may have, in part, genetic or neurobiological origins.

Other work has focused on environmental conditions that increase risk for CSA perpetration. One commonly identified risk factor is whether a history of physical or sexual victimization increases one's risk for committing physical or sexual abuse during adulthood (e.g., Marshall, Serran, & Cortoni, 2000; Simons, Wurtele, & Heil, 2002). Meta-analyses conclude the sex offenders, and particularly offenders against children, are more likely to have experienced sexual victimizations than non-offenders or nonsexual offenders (Jespersen, Lalumière, & Seto, 2009; Whitaker et al., 2008), a relationship that may be mediated by the development of deviant sexual fantasies (Knight & Simms-Knight, 2003).

Researchers have examined how interpersonal relationships influence risk of CSA perpetration. Much of this research has focused on family dynamics and has found that individuals who perpetrate sexual harm against children are more likely to come from families marked by abuse and dysfunction than offenders who perpetrate against adults (Whitaker et al., 2008).

Scholars have also argued that because sex offenders experience greater deficits in social skills that facilitate the navigation of adult relationships, they may develop coercive social techniques (Tharp et al., 2012). These deficits may be even greater for offenders with child victims. Indeed, research suggests that sex offenders with child victims are more likely than offenders with adult victims to experience difficulty in forming attachments and establishing romantic relationships (Whitaker et al., 2008). Whether this difficulty precedes the abuse of children or is caused by stronger interest in children, relative to adults, is difficult to gauge in the absence of longitudinal research.

Current Approaches in Addressing CSA

The dominant U.S. approach to CSA has been to treat such abuse as a social problem for the victim with a criminal justice solution for the offender (Letourneau et al., 2014). As such, we most often react after abuse has occurred and then intervene by detecting, punishing, monitoring, and (sometimes) treating offenders and by (sometimes) addressing the physical and mental health needs of victims. These activities might serve to prevent CSA if, for example, victims provided with evidence-based treatment are less likely to be revictimized than victims who do not obtain such treatment. They may also be effective to the extent that detection, punishment, monitoring, and/or treatment of offenders lower their recidivism risk. In the following, we review the criminal justice and therapeutic intervention literature with these questions in mind. In addition to a justice-oriented, primarily reactive frame, CSA prevention interventions have been developed over the years, many in the United States. Many of these prevention programs focus on improving children's ability to recognize, resist, and report CSA. As will be seen, while some of these programs are associated with positive outcomes, they appear to be ineffective at reducing children's risk for CSA victimization.

Criminal Justice Interventions for Offenders

In response to growing recognition of the harm caused by sexual assault, U.S. penalties for sex crime convictions were increased, as states' sentencing policy moved from indeterminate sentencing to mandatory minimum sentences (Petrunik, 2003; Spohn, 2000). In the 1990s, several postconviction community sanctions were developed for the purpose of keeping communities safe following sex offender reentry (Meloy, Miller, & Curtis, 2008). These policies include sex offender specific civil commitment, sex offender registration and public notification, and residence restrictions. Other U.S. policies, such as lifetime or intensive supervision, GPS monitoring, and employment and education restrictions, were also implemented but have been less well studied.

Civil commitment. The passage of U.S. sexual violent predator laws in the 1990s marked the reemergence of civil commitment – where sex offenders are evaluated for indefinite commitment to a treatment facility following the completion of their prison term – in the management of sex offenders. The logic of civil commitment is grounded in two key assumptions: (1) that state civil commitment boards are able to identify high-risk sex offenders; and (2) that treatment programs within civil commitment facilities will be effective in addressing offenders' needs to prevent future offending (Mancini, 2014). However, the utility of civil commitment for sex offenders in the prevention of sexual abuse has not been well documented in existing scholarship, making it difficult to assess the robustness of these assumptions (Mancini, 2014). One study using panel data from 1970 to 2002 reported that sex offender civil commitment did not reduce rates of sexual assault (Ackerman, Sacks, & Greenberg, 2012).

Registration and community notification. Following the abduction of Jacob Wetterling (Jacob Wetterling Crimes against Children and Sexually Violent Offender Registration Act, 1994), the death of Megan Kanka (Sample & Evans, 2009), and other high-profile sex crimes and related community action, the U.S. federal government passed legislation requiring states to quickly develop sex offender registries and methods to notify the public about sex offenders living in their neighborhoods. By design, publicly available registries contain many personally identifying elements such as a current photograph, current address and past address history, offense at conviction, correctional status, and license plate number (Sample & Evans, 2009). This information is posted online in all states for purposes of public notification, although additional methods also occur. For example, law enforcement officers and sometimes the actual registered offender may personally notify neighbors (Logan, 2009).

In 2006, the Adam Walsh Child Protection and Safety Act (AWA) was passed to standardize registration practices across the United States (AWA, 2006). With this law, states were required to (1) submit sex offender information to a national registry; (2) classify offenders based on a three-tier system distinguishing lifetime, twenty-five-year, and fifteen-year public notification durations; (3) enact retroactive registration for offenders with a history of registerable offenses; and (4) increase penalties for offenders who fail to register. The AWA was also the first act to require the registration of children. Unlike the Wetterling and Kanka acts, which were quickly adopted by all states, the AWA has been widely decried both as a federal overreach and as anathema to the juvenile justice focus on rehabilitation (see Department of Justice, 2011, p. 1632). Consequently, states have been far less accommodating and, as of this writing, just seventeen states are deemed to be in compliance with this federal statute (SMART, 2015).

A sizable literature finds no relationship between registration policies and sex offender recidivism (Sample & Evans, 2009) suggesting that such policies rarely achieve their intended aim of improved community safety. Moreover, registration and notification policies have deleterious effects on offenders' abilities to find and maintain housing and employment and to develop prosocial relationships (Levenson & Cotter, 2005). Despite this, sex offender registration and notification policies continue to be adopted internationally. A 2014 report from the U.S. agency that oversees federal sex offender registration and notification policies indicated that eighteen countries (e.g., Argentina, Australia, Kenya, South Korea, United Kingdom) have implemented some type of sex offender registration, and more countries are considering doing so, although the scope of these policies is often much narrower than those of the United States (SMART, 2014).

Residence restrictions. U.S. sex offenders may also be subjected to housing restrictions once released into the community (Levenson, 2009). In over thirty states, registered sex offenders are banned from living near places where children gather, such as parks or schools. States typically set restrictions at five hundred to one thousand feet, but local jurisdictions are free to extend the restricted distance (Meloy et al., 2008). These policies are nearly universally supported by the general public (Levenson, 2009; Mancini, Shields, Mears, & Beaver, 2010) but have been repeatedly found to have no effect on community safety (Agan, 2011; Duwe, Donnay, & Tewksbury, 2008; Zandbergen, Levenson, & Hart, 2010). Further, residence restrictions pose a substantial barrier to reentry and may result in homelessness and stress among offenders (Levenson & Cotter, 2005), issues that may contribute to the risk of general and perhaps even sexual recidivism.

Application of Sex Crime Policies to Youth Who Sexually Offend

As with adults, youth adjudicated for sexual offenses have also been subjected to more punitive legislative responses. Since the 1990s, U.S. states have passed legislation to facilitate waivers of juvenile cases to adult court (Kupchik, 2006; Myers, 2005; Torbet et al., 1996), and it appears that youth who commit sex offenses are especially targeted for transfer to adult court (DiCataldo, 2009; Rinehart, Armstrong, Shields, & Letourneau, 2015).

The Adam Walsh Act requires the lifetime registration of at least some youth who have sexually offended (SMART, 2008). As of 2011, thirty-eight U.S. states require registration and eight states require public notification of youth adjudicated for sexual offenses (Pittman & Nguyen, 2011). A growing body of research indicates that these policies are associated with substantial harm to youth and their families (Comartin, Kernsmith, & Miles, 2010; Harris, Walfield, Shields & Letourneau, in press; Pittman, 2013). There is a more robust literature indicating that these policies fail to achieve improved community safety, either via general deterrence (Letourneau, Bandyopadhyay, Armstrong & Sinha, 2010) or via reduced sexual or nonsexual recidivism rates (Batastini, Hunt, Present-Koller, & DeMatteo, 2011; Caldwell, Ziemke, & Vitacco, 2008; Letourneau & Armstrong, 2008; Letourneau, Bandyopadhyay, Sinha, & Armstrong, 2009b). Juvenile registration and notification policies also are associated with the unintended effects of increased dismissal, diversion, and plea bargain from sex to nonsex charges (Letourneau, Bandyopadhyay, Sinha, & Armstrong 2009a; Letourneau,

Armstrong, Bandyopadhyay, & Sinha, 2013). Given concerns about the impact of these policies on youth health and safety and their ineffectiveness at improving community safety, many have argued for the repeal of juvenile registration and notification policies (e.g., DiCataldo, 2009; Garfinkle, 2003; Juvenile Law Center, 2012; Letourneau & Caldwell, 2013; Zimring, 2004).

Youth have also been subjected to residence and other restrictions (Caldwell, 2007) and to civil commitment (Fanniff, Otto, & Petrila, 2010), and such practices have come under increased scrutiny if not outright condemnation in the United States. In the only published evaluation of civil commitment procedures with juveniles, Caldwell (2013) reported that individuals evaluated as meeting one state's civil commitment requirements (but ultimately not committed) and individuals screened out (and also not committed) had statistically similar three-year postevaluation sexual recidivism rates (approximately 12 percent and 17 percent, respectively). This study casts doubt on the feasibility of accurately identifying youth at highest risk of recidivism, not to mention the moral implications of indefinitely confining an individual for an offense committed as a child.

Clinical Interventions for Adult Perpetrators of CSA

There are several treatment approaches available for adults who perpetrate sexual harm, including psychosocial and medical models (Schwartz, 2011). The most common and effective of these approaches is cognitive behavioral therapy (CBT; Hanson et al., 2002; Lösel & Schmucker, 2005; Mancini, 2014; Yates & Kingston, 2011). In CBT, therapists work with clients to identify their problem thinking (i.e., cognitive distortions), devise goals to foster prosocial sexual values, and implement strategies to reach these goals (Mancini, 2014; Yates & Kingston, 2011). Within CBT, treatment providers may select a range of treatment foci, including relapse prevention (CBT-RP; Cortoni, Anderson, & Bright, 2011) as well as cognitive restructuring; anger management; empathy building; and, for clients with deviant sexual interests, arousal reconditioning procedures (LaFond, 2005).

In a review of sixty-nine international studies of sex offender treatment (including studies from the United States, Canada, Germany, Great Britain, and others), Lösel and Schmucker (2005) found that offenders who participated in CBT were significantly less likely to reoffend than offenders who did not participate in treatment or who received non-CBT treatment. Hanson, Bourgon, Helmus, and Hodgson (2009) found that programs that followed a Risk-Needs-Responsivity (RNR) model – where medium- and high-risk offenders are identified, criminogenic needs are targeted, and treatment is tailored to match the abilities of the offender – are also effective. In their meta-analysis of twenty-three studies involving 2,822 offenders, those who participated in RNR-based treatment were less likely to reoffend sexually (10.9 percent versus 19.2 percent) and for any offense (31.8 percent versus 48.3 percent) than the comparison groups (Hanson et al., 2009). In a recent synthesis of eleven international meta-analyses published from 1995 to 2010, Kim, Benekos, and Merlo (2015) concluded that effective treatments are indeed available for perpetrators of sexual abuse, and recent meta-analyses demonstrate significant reductions (22 percent) in recidivism.

Others have cautioned, however, that it may be premature to state definitively that sex offender treatment works (LaFond, 2005), given the variety of treatment programs available, the variation in treatment administration, and the limitations of research evaluation designs. Indeed, Rice and Harris (2003) critiqued earlier evaluations of treatment effectiveness for sex offenders and concluded that the question of whether treatment works remains unanswered.

Treatment interventions for youth who have sexually offended. As summarized by Dwyer and Letourneau (2011), the dominant clinical intervention for youth who have sexually offended is the same as for adult sex offenders: cognitive behavioral therapy with a relapse-prevention framework (CBT-RP). While a meta-analysis supports the effectiveness of CBT-RP relative to alternative interventions in reducing juvenile recidivism rates (Reitzel & Carbonell, 2006), growing recognition of the importance of parents in the treatment of youth behavioral problems (Donohue & Azrin, 2001; McCart, Sheidow, & Letourneau, 2014) has resulted in a shift away from CBT-RP toward more family-focused interventions. A central assumption of these interventions is that parents (or other caregivers) are the key to achieving and sustaining positive youth behavioral change.

The best-validated intervention for youth who have sexually offended is Multisystemic Therapy for Problem Sexual Behavior (MST-PSB). This intervention is based on the original Multisystemic therapy (Henggeler, Schoenwald, Borduin, Rowland, & Cunningham, 2009b), which has been found effective with violent and substance abusing youth across more than one dozen randomized controlled trials, including several conducted outside of the United States (Henggeler & Sheidow, 2012). MST-PSB is a parent-focused, individualized intervention that has been validated across three randomized controlled trials. The first two of these, modest in scope and size, found that significantly fewer youths in the MST condition were rearrested for sexual or nonsexual crimes (Borduin, Henggeler, Blaske, & Stein, 1990; Borduin, Schaeffer, & Heiblum, 2009). A larger trial (N = 127) reported that youth in the MST-PSB condition experienced significantly greater reductions in problem sexual behavior, delinquent behavior, and substance use relative to youth in the control condition over a twelve-month postrecruitment follow-up period and were significantly less likely to have an out-of-home placement (e.g., in detention or residential facilities) through eighteen-months follow-up than were those who received standard community treatment (Letourneau et al., 2009c; Letourneau et al., 2013). Of note, a family-focused CBT intervention designed specifically to address child sexual behavior problems (which are often but not always associated with abuse) has been shown to reduce the likelihood of future illegal sexual behavior relative to a play therapy control condition (Carpentier, Silovsky, & Chaffin, 2006).

Therapeutic interventions for victims. Pollio, Deblinger, and Runyon (2011) summarized the literature on mental health treatment for the effects of CSA. While noting that play therapy, psychodynamic, eclectic, and nonspecific family treatment approaches have been developed for addressing the mental health sequelae of CSA, few well-controlled studies evaluate these interventions. By comparison, adult CBT models adapted for children and adolescents have been well researched. Among these, trauma-focused CBT (TF-CBT; Cohen, Mannarino, & Deblinger, 2006; Deblinger & Heflin, 1996) has been subjected to more than twenty-five evaluation studies, including thirteen randomized controlled trials in at least four countries (Mannarino, Cohen, & Deblinger, 2014; Pollio et al., 2011). Each of these trials supports TF-CBT over comparison treatment conditions or waitlist controls. Importantly, TF-CBT works best when both the child victim and nonoffending parent(s) are included in treatment and works equally well for boys and girls. Improvements have been documented in youth PTSD, depression, anxiety, internalizing and externalizing behaviors, as well as social competence, interpersonal trust, perceived credibility, and shame. Parental distress has also been found to decline with TF-CBT. Moreover, youth treated with TF-CBT demonstrate reductions in sexually inappropriate behavior and improved body safety skills. These latter two findings suggest the promise of TF-CBT in terms of addressing the risk of future revictimization and sexual and nonsexual offending behaviors. However, TF-CBT has not been evaluated for these longer-term outcomes.

Existing CSA Prevention Programs

Criminal justice interventions for offenders and treatment and other services for victims will always be essential to addressing CSA. However, they will also always be reactive. Effective prevention programs hold the promise of protecting children from their first victimization. In 2005, the U.S.-based National Sexual Violence Resource Center (NSVRC) published a comprehensive online directory of CSA prevention-related resources (see NSVRC, 2005). Within its 270 pages are listed approximately twenty-two curricula programs targeting preschoolers, fifty curricula targeting elementary students, fifty targeting middle school students, and about thirty-five targeting high school students. Just three curricula are denoted as targeting "parents/teachers/others" although approximately ninety general parent resources (e.g., pamphlets) are listed. Given the ubiquity of school-based victimization prevention efforts, it is not surprising that research has focused on their effects. These programs are typically designed to teach children how to avoid being victims of sexual assault and what to do if attempts or completed assaults occur, also known as the three Rs: "Recognize, Resist, Report" (NSVRC, 2005; Plummer, 2001; Wurtele, 2009). While some higher-quality programs have been associated with positive outcomes, such as increased disclosure of abuse and decreased self-blame following abuse, exposure to victim-focused prevention programming has not been associated with reduced CSA victimization (Finkelhor, Asdigian, & Dziuba-Leatherman, 1995; Finkelhor, Vanderminden, Turner, Shattuck, & Hamby, 2014b).

To attain measurable reductions in CSA, it may be necessary to alter the focus of prevention programs. Rather than trying to prevent victimization by teaching young children the three Rs, it might be more effective to prevent perpetration through universal and more targeted prevention programs aimed at older children and adolescents (DeGue et al., 2012). Likewise, efforts to ensure that adults are more "capable guardians" who can better protect children are needed (Leclerc, Smallbone, & Wortley, 2015; Mendelson & Letourneau, 2015).

Perpetration prevention efforts targeting teens. Younger teens might be particularly relevant targets for perpetration and bystander-related prevention efforts. As noted earlier, youth who sexually offend against other children and especially against younger children tend to be young themselves, with perpetration rates peaking between the ages of twelve and fourteen (Finkelhor et al., 2009), demonstrating the need to start early. Moreover, youth sexual (mis)behaviors are often transient and modifiable, supporting a universal approach to prevention programming. Regarding transience, the vast majority of youth who sexually offend (90 percent to 95 percent) do not reoffend sexually (Caldwell, 2010; Letourneau et al., 2009b). Such low recidivism rates suggest that many of these offenses were influenced by situational factors rather than deeply rooted deviant sexual interests. Moreover, these incidents often occur in contexts of convenience, such as babysitting (Finkelhor & Ormrod, 2001), suggesting that many adolescent sexual offenses are "crimes of opportunity" (Finkelhor & Ormrod, 2001, p. 5) rather than the acts of incipient sexual predators.

Several factors associated with adolescent sexual offending are good targets for universal prevention efforts. These include low sex knowledge and lack of clear rules about appropriate sexual behavior, low knowledge of developmental differences between older and younger children, cognitive distortions, and inappropriate sexual experimentation (Letourneau et al., 2008, 2009c; Letourneau & Schaeffer, 2014).

Recent reviews of U.S. sexual violence prevention and intimate partner violence prevention concluded that the most effective strategies targeted adolescents (DeGue et al., 2014; Whitaker, Murphy, Eckhardt, Hodges & Cowart, 2013). Three prevention programs have been identified as efficacious. The Safe Dates program is a universal dating violence prevention program delivered via a ten-session curriculum, a poster session, and a student play on dating violence (see Foshee & Langwick, 2010). Safe Dates targets both sexual and nonsexual violence in eighth- and ninth-grade dating relationships and has been shown to reduce both types of violence within the context of randomized controlled trials (Foshee et al., 1998, 2004).

The Shifting Boundaries intervention targets sixth- and seventh-grade students with a six-session curriculum focused on relationship boundaries, laws governing sexual violence and harassment, and bystander behaviors. This curriculum is coupled with a building-level program designed to address school areas identified by students as unsafe and to improve reporting of violent or harassing behaviors (Taylor, Stein, Mumford, & Woods, 2013; for summary, see CrimeSolutions.gov, 2015). Results from a randomized controlled trial that involved thirty U.S. public middle schools indicated that the building intervention alone and the building intervention plus curriculum reduced self-reported sexual harassment, sexual violence victimization by peers or dating partners, and sexual violence perpetration by peers through six-months postintervention.

The "Second Step: Student Success through Prevention" program targets sixth-grader peer aggression, sexual aggression, and victimization (Espelage, Low, Polanin, & Brown, 2013; see Second Step, 2015). This program is associated with reduced physical but not sexual violence, perhaps because program content does not specifically address sexual behavior.

To our knowledge, no evaluations have been conducted on prevention programs that specifically target youth perpetration of sexual abuse against younger children nor have the existing peer prevention programs reviewed in the preceding been evaluated for effects on sexual behavior with younger children. We (Letourneau, Schaeffer, and Bradshaw) have initiated the development of a universal prevention program that will specifically target youth sexual behaviors with younger children (Schaeffer, 2015). The Responsible Behavior with Younger Children program targets sixth- and seventh-grade children and their parents with an eight-session curriculum designed to reduce the likelihood of sexual behavior with younger children. This curriculum incorporates identified best practices of school-based violence prevention programs that have demonstrated positive impacts, including multisession dosage, skills practice, and parent involvement (Bradshaw, 2015; DeGue et al., 2014; Finkelhor et al., 1995).

As noted earlier, few youth are sexually attracted to children. For those who are, there is an almost complete lack of services. In the United States, we (Letourneau, Shields, and colleagues) have initiated a project to develop an intervention for adolescents attracted to young children. Inspired by the Prevention Project Dunkelfeld (discussed later in this chapter), the twin aims of the Help Wanted intervention will be to give adolescents the skills, knowledge and tools they need to (1) avoid the sexual abuse of children and (2) counter the negative self-images many of these youth have internalized and ensure they develop the self-respect and self-esteem needed to navigate adolescence successfully. An initial qualitative study of nonoffending young adults living with sexual attraction to children is under way, the results of which will help inform intervention development and dissemination.

Prevention efforts targeting adults. As noted earlier, parents are critical to the healthy sexual development of children, yet they are often overlooked by CSA prevention efforts (Mendelson & Letourneau, 2015). There is, however, one adult-focused CSA prevention intervention that has been broadly disseminated to adults responsible for the welfare of children, including parents, teachers, childcare professionals, youth services providers, and volunteers. The Stewards of Children (Stewards) program is an adult-focused universal prevention program developed and disseminated by Darkness to Light (D2L.org), a U.S.-based advocacy organization whose mission is to address CSA prevention by targeting adults via education and awareness programming.

An independent multisite randomized controlled trial indicated that Stewards improved knowledge and self-reported preventive behaviors among child care professionals compared to waitlist controls. Effect sizes were generally moderate in size, which is not surprising given the brevity of the training (Rheingold et al., 2014). In a separate study, investigators examined CSA reports in three counties before and after Stewards training efforts were implemented and found that reporting rates increased over time for the targeted counties (Letourneau, Nietert, & Rheingold, 2015). A similar change was not detected between the pre- and post-dissemination period for three counties that had not experienced Stewards training efforts. These results suggest that broad dissemination of the Stewards prevention program might account for increased CSA reports.

Another adult-focused CSA prevention model being implemented across several American states is the Enough Abuse Campaign. Originating in Massachusetts and subsequently implemented in Maryland and New Jersey, the Enough Abuse Campaign currently has a presence in six states. Described as a "statewide education and community mobilization effort to prevent CSA," the emphasis is on the prevention of both adult and youth-perpetrated sexual abuse (Schober et al., 2012, p. 457). Strategies include a twelve-hour "train-the-trainer" curriculum, a single session in-person prevention curriculum for adults, a media strategy to disseminate CSA prevention information, websites with access to prevention information and resources, and strong focus on partnering with state and local agencies to develop resources that support CSA prevention (e.g., revision of CSA-related laws and policies, implementation of statewide helpline numbers). Although empirically rigorous evaluations have not yet been completed with this model, one campaign-supported pre- and postimplementation survey indicated a substantial increase in the percent of respondents who agreed that adults, rather than children, were responsible for preventing CSA (Massachusetts Kids Count, 2003).

Since 1992, the Stop It Now! advocacy organization has conducted media campaigns and other prevention activities to raise CSA awareness and has established online and telephone resources for abusers, those at risk of abusing, and those seeking guidance for responding to CSA in the United States, the United Kingdom, Ireland, and the Netherlands and through partnerships with several agencies in low- and middle-income countries (Tabachnick & Dawson, 2000; see Stop It Now! 2015). A recent summary of Stop It Now!'s phone surveys in six states ($n > 5{,}000$ adults) indicated that CSA knowledge improved since the start of the campaigns in those states, although findings suggest the impact on actually helping adults intervene in CSA situations was limited (Stop It Now! 2014).

In Germany, the Prevention Project Dunkelfeld (PPD; see PPD, 2015) has been under way since 2004. This project includes an extensive media campaign in which commercials, online ads, billboards, and other media encourage CSA offenders and those at risk of offending to contact the project for help (Beier et al., 2009). Those who contact the project are screened, and men assessed as sexually attracted to children are offered free and confidential treatment services. Thousands of men have contacted the project, which has opened seven additional treatment sites to address demand. The project has a strong research focus, although publications to date have primarily described risk factors for offending and have not yet presented data on treatment effectiveness (e.g., Neutze, Grundmann, Scherner, & Beier, 2012).

Numerous youth-serving organizations have taken steps to address the risk of CSA within their ranks. In collaboration with the Boys Scouts of America and the Boys & Girls Clubs of America, the U.S. Centers for Disease Control and Prevention and the National Center for Injury Prevention and Control developed a report to assist youth-serving organizations in preventing CSA (Saul & Audage, 2007). The report included topics such as how to screen and train employees and volunteers to minimize risk of CSA, how to monitor behavior and promote safe environments, and how to respond to suspected CSA (Saul & Audage, 2007). The U.S. Conference of Catholic Bishops (USCCB) instituted similar policies to reduce the likelihood of CSA by clergy (USCCB, 2005), including a code of conduct, training about CSA for adults, and personal safety training for children (Terry & Ackerman, 2008). These policies are based largely on situational crime prevention strategies (Terry & Ackerman, 2008; Wortley & Smallbone, 2006); their impact on CSA incidence has not yet been empirically assessed (Finkelhor, 2009).

Conclusion

In summary, while most resources addressing CSA target after-the-fact, post-abuse interventions, there has been steady growth in the development and dissemination of prevention programs. Unfortunately, the absence of resources has made it difficult to rigorously evaluate existing prevention programs or to develop new ones (Letourneau et al., 2014). To achieve a more comprehensive public health prevention-focused approach to CSA will require substantial investment of resources. Such investment is likely to occur only in the context of the development of comprehensive national public health policy. A national policy could help with overcoming divisions between victim and offender-focused stakeholders, with driving the development and evaluation of new and existing prevention practice and policy efforts, and with support foundational research on risk and protective factors that occur at the community or society level. A cohesive policy could also provide a framework for future sex crime legislation, providing policy makers with a rationale for carefully developing and evaluating new policies and for revising existing ineffective and harmful policies. The development of a national policy will occur only in the context of broad consensus that CSA prevention is both achievable and worthwhile.

References

Ackerman, A. R., Sacks, M., & Greenberg, D. F. (2012). Legislation targeting sex offenders: are recent policies effective in reducing rape? *Justice Quarterly* 29: 858–87.

Agan, A. Y. (2011). Sex offender registries: fear without function. *Journal of Law and Economics* 54: 207–39.

Alanko, K., Salo, B., Mokros, A., & Santtila, P. (2013). Evidence for heritability of adult men's sexual interest in youth under age 16 from a population-based extended twin design. *Journal of Sexual Medicine* 10: 1090–9.

Aspy, C., Vesely, S. K., Oman, R. F., Rodine, S., Marshall, L., & McLeroy, K. (2007). Parental communication and youth sexual behavior. *Journal of Adolescence* 30: 449–66.

AWA (Adam Walsh Child Protection and Safety), H.R. 4472, 109th (2006).

Baptiste, D. R., Tolou-Shams, M., Miller, S. R., Mcbride, C. K., & Paikoff, R. L. (2007). Determinants of parental monitoring and preadolescent sexual risk situations among African American families living in urban public housing. *Journal of Child and Family Studies* 16: 261–74.

Batastini, A. B., Hunt, E., Present-Koller, J., & DeMatteo, D. (2011). Federal standards for community registration of juvenile sex offenders: an evaluation of risk prediction and future implications. *Psychology, Public Policy, and Law* 17: 451–74.

Bedi, S., Nelson, E. C., Lynskey, M. T., McCutcheon, V. V., Heath, A. C., Madden, P. A.F., & Martin, N. G. (2011). Risk for suicidal thoughts and behavior after childhood sexual abuse in women and men. *Suicide and Life-Threatening Behavior* 41(4): 406–15.

Beier, K. M., Neutze, J., Mundt, I. A., Ahlers, C. J., Goecker, D., Konrad, A., & Schaefer, G. A. (2009). Encouraging self-identified pedophiles and hebephiles to seek professional help: first results of the Prevention Project Dunkelfeld (PPD). *Child Abuse & Neglect* 33: 545–9.

Berliner, L. (2011). Child sexual abuse: definitions, prevalence, and consequences. In Myers, J. E. B. (ed.), *The APSAC Handbook on Child Maltreatment*, 3rd ed. Thousand Oaks, CA: Sage, pp. 215–232.

Borduin, C. M., Henggeler, S. W., Blaske, D. M., & Stein, R. J. (1990). Multisystemic treatment of adolescent sexual offenders. *International Journal of Offender Therapy and Comparative Criminology* 996: 105–13.

Borduin, C. M., Schaeffer, C. M., & Heiblum, N. (2009). A randomized clinical trial of multisystemic therapy with juvenile sexual offenders: effects on youth social ecology and criminal activity. *Journal of Consulting and Clinical Psychology* 77: 26–37.

Bradshaw, C. P. (2015). Translating research to practice in bullying prevention. *American Psychologist* 70: 322–32.

Caldwell, M. F. (2007). Sexual offense adjudication and sexual recidivism among juvenile offenders. *Sex Abuse* 19: 107–13.

Caldwell, M. F. (2010). Study characteristics and recidivism base rates in juvenile sex offender recidivism. *International Journal of Offender Therapy and Comparative Criminology* 54: 197–212.

Caldwell, M. F. (2013). Accuracy of sexually violent person assessments of juveniles adjudicated for sexual offenses. *Sexual Abuse: A Journal of Research and Treatment* 25: 516–26.

Caldwell, M. F., Ziemke, M. H., & Vitacco, M. J. (2008). An examination of the Sex Offender Registration and Notification Act as applied to juveniles: evaluating the ability to predict sexual recidivism. *Psychology, Public Policy, and Law* 14: 89–114.

Cantor, J. M., Blanchard, R., Christensen, B. K., Dickey R., Klassen, P.E., Beckstead, A. L., Blak, T., & Kuban, M. E. (2004). Intelligence, handedness, and memory in pedophilia. *Neuropsychology* 18: 3–14.

Cantor, J. M., Kabani, N., Christensen, B. K., Zipursky, R. B., Barbaree, H. E., Dickey, R., et al. (2008). Cerebral white matter deficiencies in pedophilic men. *Journal of Psychiatric Research* 42: 167–83.

Carpentier, M. Y., Silovsky, J. F., & Chaffin, M. (2006). Randomized trial of treatment for children with sexual behavior problems: ten-year follow-up. *Journal of Consulting and Clinical Psychology* 74: 482–8.

CDC (Centers for Disease Control and Prevention) (2012). *Violence against Children in Kenya: Findings from a 2010 National Survey. Summary Report on the Prevalence of Sexual, Physical and Emotional Violence, Context of Sexual Violence, and Health and Behavioral Consequences of Violence Experienced in Childhood.* Nairobi, Kenya: United Nations Children's Fund Kenya Country Office, Division of Violence Prevention, National Center for Injury Prevention and Control, U.S. Centers for Disease Control and Prevention, and the Kenya National Bureau of Statistics.

Chaffin, M. (2008). Our minds are made up – don't confuse us with the facts: commentary on policies concerning children with sexual behavior problems and juvenile sex offenders. *Child Maltreatment* 13: 110–21.

Cohen, J. A., Mannarino, A. P., & Deblinger, E. (2006). *Treating Trauma and Traumatic Grief in Children and Adolescents.* New York: Guilford Press.

Comartin, E. B., Kernsmith, P. D., & Miles, B. W. (2010). Family experiences of young adult sex offender registration. *Journal of Child Sexual Abuse* 19: 204–25.

Cortoni, F., Anderson, D., & Bright, D. A. (2011). Locus of control, coping, and sexual offenders. In Schwartz, B. K. (ed.), *Handbook of Sex Offender Treatment.* Kingston, NJ: Civic Research Institute, pp. 14.1–14.18.

CrimeSolutions.gov. (2015). Shifting boundaries. www.crimesolutions.gov/ProgramDetails.aspx?ID=226

D2L (Darkness 2 Light). (2013). Darkness to light. Retrieved from www.D2L.org

Deblinger, E., & Heflin, A. H. (1996). *Treating Sexually Abused Children and Their Nonoffending Parents: A Cognitive Behavioral Approach.* Thousand Oaks, CA: Sage.

DeGue, S., Simon, T. R., Basile, K. C., Yee, S. L., Lang, K., & Spivak, H. (2012). Moving forward by looking back: reflecting on a decade of CDC's work in sexual violence prevention, 2000–2010. *Journal of Women's Health* 21: 1211–18.

DeGue, S., Valle, L. A., Holt, M. K., Massetti, G. M., Matjasko, J. L., & Tharp, A. T. (2014). A systematic review of primary prevention strategies for sexual violence perpetration. *Aggression and Violent Behavior* 19: 346–62.

Department of Justice (2011). Supplemental guidelines for sex offender registration and notification. *Federal Register* 76: 1630–40.

DiCataldo, F. C. (2009). *The Perversion of Youth.* New York: New York University Press.

Dong, M., Giles, W. H., Felittie, V. J., Dube, S. R. … & Anda, R. F. (2004). Insights into causal pathways for ischemic heart disease: adverse childhood experiences study. *Circulation* 110: 1761–6.

Donohue, B., & Azrin, N. H. (2001). Family behavior therapy. In Wagner, E. F., & Waldron, H. B. (eds.), *Innovations in Adolescent Substance Abuse Interventions*. New York: Pergamon Press, pp. 205–27.

Duwe, G., Donnay, W., & Tewksbury, R. (2008). Does residential proximity matter? A geographic analysis of sex offense recidivism. *Criminal Justice and Behavior* 35: 484–504.

Dwyer, R. G., & Letourneau, E. J. (2011). Juveniles who sexually offend: recommending a treatment program and level of care. *Child and Adolescent Psychiatric Clinics of North America: Special Issue on Forensic Child and Adolescent Psychiatry* 20: 413–29. PMID: 21683910.

Espelage, D. L., Low, S., Polanin, J. R., & Brown, E. C. (2013). The impact of a middle school program to reduce aggression, victimization, and sexual violence. *Journal of Adolescent Health* 53: 180–6.

Fang, X., Brown, D. S., Florence, C. S., & Mercy, J. A. (2012). The economic burden of child maltreatment in the United States and implications for prevention. *Child Abuse & Neglect* 36: 156–65.

Fanniff, A. M., Otto, R. K., & Petrila, J. (2010). Competence to proceed in SVP commitment hearings: irrelevant or fundamental due process right? *Behavioral Sciences and the Law* 28: 646–70.

Finkelhor, D. (2009). The prevention of childhood sexual abuse. *Future of Children* 19: 169–94.

Finkelhor, D., Asdigian, N., & Dziuba-Leatherman, J. (1995). Victimization prevention programs for children: a follow-up. *American Journal of Public Health* 85: 1684–9.

Finkelhor, D., & Jones, L. (2006). Why have child maltreatment and child victimization declined? *Journal of Social Issues* 62: 685–716.

Finkelhor, D., & Ormrod, R. (2001). Crimes against children by babysitters. Crimes against Children Series. *Juvenile Justice Bulletin* NCJ189102: 1–8.

Finkelhor, D., Ormrod, R., & Chaffin, M. (2009). *Juveniles Who Commit Sex Offenses against Minors*. Washington, DC: Office of Juvenile Justice and Delinquency Prevention.

Finkelhor, D., Ormrod, R., Turner, H., & Hamby, S. L. (2005). The victimization of children and youth: a comprehensive, national survey. *Child Maltreatment* 10: 5–25.

Finkelhor, D., Shattuck, A., Turner, H. A., & Hamby, S. L. (2014). The lifetime prevalence of child sexual abuse and sexual assault assessed in late adolescence. *Journal of Adolescent Health*, 55, 329–33.

Finkelhor, D., Shattuck, A., Turner, H. A., & Hamby, S. L. (2014a). The lifetime prevalence of child sexual abuse and sexual assault assessed in late adolescence. *Journal of Adolescent Health* 55: 329–33.

Finkelhor, D., Vanderminden, J., Turner, H., Shattuck, A., & Hamby, S. (2014b). Youth exposure to violence prevention programs in a national sample. *Child Abuse & Neglect* 38: 677–86.

Foshee, V. A., Bauman, K. E., Arrianga, X. B., Helms, R. W., Koch, G. G., & Linder, G. F. (1998). An evaluation of Safe Dates, an adolescent dating violence prevention program. *American Journal of Public Health* 88: 45–50.

Foshee, V. A., Bauman, K. E., Ennett, S. T., Linder, G. F., Benefield, T., & Suchindran, C. (2004). Assessing the long-term effects of the Safe Dates program and a booster in preventing and reducing adolescent dating violence victimization and perpetration. *American Journal of Public Health* 94: 619–24.

Foshee, V. A., & Langwick, S. (2010). Safe Dates. Retrieved from www.hazelden.org/web/public/safedates.page

Garfinkle, E. (2003). Coming of age in America: the misapplication of sex-offender registration and community-notification laws to juveniles. *California Law Review* 91: 163–208.

Glasser, M., Campbell, K. D., Glasser, A., Leitch, I., & Farrelly, S. (2001). Cycle of child sexual abuse: links between being a victim and being a perpetrator. *British Journal of Psychiatry* 179: 482–94.

Hankivsky, O., & Draker, D. A. (2003). The economic costs of child sexual abuse in Canada: a preliminary analysis. *Journal of Health and Social Policy* 17: 1–33.

Hanson, R. K., Bourgon, G., Helmus, L. M., & Hodgson, S. (2009). The principles of effective correctional treatment also apply to sexual offenders: a meta-analysis. *Criminal Justice and Behavior* 9: 865–91.

Hanson, R. K., Gordon, A., Harris, A. J., Marques, J. K., Murphy, W., Quinsey, V. L., et al. (2002). First report of the Collaborative Outcome Data Project on the effectiveness of psychological treatment for sex offenders. *Sexual Abuse: A Journal of Research and Treatment* 14: 169–94.

Harris, A. J., Walfield, S., Shields, R., & Letourneau, E. J. (in press). Collateral consequences of juvenile sex offender registration and notification: results from a survey of treatment providers. *Sexual Abuse: A Journal of Research and Treatment*.

Henggeler, S. W., Letourneau, E. J., Chapman, J. E., Borduin, C. M., Schewe, P. A., & McCart, M. R., (2009a). Mediators of change for multisystemic therapy with juvenile sexual offenders. *Journal of Consulting and Clinical Psychology* 77: 451–62.

Henggeler, S. W., Schoenwald, S. K., Borduin, C. M., Rowland, M. D., & Cunningham, P. B. (2009b). *Multisystemic Therapy of Antisocial Behavior in Children and Adolescents*, 2nd ed. New York: Guilford Press.

Henggeler, S. W. & Sheidow, A. J. (2012). Empirically supported family-based treatments for conduct disorder and delinquency in adolescents. *Journal of Marital and Family Therapy* 38: 30–58.

Heppenstall-Heger, A., McConnell, G., Ticson, L., Guerra, L., Lister, J., & Zaragoza, T. (2003). Healing patterns in anogenital injuries: a longitudinal study of injuries associated with sexual abuse, accidental injuries, or genital surgery in the preadolescent child. *Pediatrics* 112: 829–37.

IOM (Institute of Medicine) (2013). *New Directions in Child Abuse and Neglect Research*. Washington, DC: National Academies.

Jacob Wetterling Crimes against Children and Sexually Violent Offender Registration Act, H. R. 3351, 103rd (1994).

Jespersen, A. F., Lalumière, M. L., & Seto, M. C. (2009) Sexual abuse history among adult sex offenders and non-sex offenders: a meta-analysis. *Child Abuse & Neglect* 33: 179–92.

Juvenile Law Center (2012). Pennsylvania should repeal juvenile sex offender registration law. February 13. www.jlc.org/blog/pennsylvania-should-repeal-juvenile-sex-offender-registration-law

Kaufman, K. (2010). *The Prevention of Sexual Violence and Exploitation: A Sourcebook*. Oklahoma City: Wood & Barnes.

Kim, B., Benekos P. J., & Merlo, A. V. (2015). Sex offender recidivism revisited: review of recent meta-analyses on the effects of sex offender treatment. *Trauma, Violence & Abuse*. doi: 10.1177/1524838014566719

Knight, R. A., & Sims-Knight, J. E. (2003). Developmental antecedents of sexual coercion against women: testing of alternative hypotheses with structural equation modeling. In Prentky, R. A., Janus, E., & Seto, M. (eds.), *Sexual Coercion: Understanding and Management*, New York: New York Academy of Sciences, pp. 72–85.

Krug, E. G., Mercy, J. A., Dahlberg, L. L., & Zwi, A. B. (2002). The world report on violence and health. *Lancet* 360: 1083–8.

Kupchik, A. (2006). *Judging Juveniles: Prosecuting Adolescents in Adult and Juvenile Court*. New York: New York University.

Kwiatkowski, C. (2012). Drivers of youth problem sexual behavior and their relationship to MST treatment outcomes. (Master's thesis). Available upon request from archives@lists.johnshopkins.edu

LaFond, J. Q. (2005). *Preventing Sexual Violence: How Society Should Cope with Sex Offenders*. Washington, DC: American Psychological Association.

Leclerc, B., Smallbone, S., & Wortley, R. (2015). Prevention nearby: the influence of the presence of a potential guardian on the severity of child sexual abuse. *Sexual Abuse: A Journal of Research and Treatment* 27: 189–204.

Letourneau, E. J., & Armstrong, K. S. (2008). Recidivism rates for registered and nonregistered juvenile sexual offenders. *Sexual Abuse: A Journal of Research and Treatment* 20: 393–408. doi: 10.1177/1079063208324661

Letourneau, E. J., Armstrong, K. S., Bandyopadhyay, D., & Sinha, D. (2013). Sex offender registration and notification policy increases juvenile plea bargains. *Sexual Abuse: A Journal of Research and Treatment* 25: 189–207. PMID: 22915204.

Letourneau, E. J., Bandyopadhyay, D., Armstrong, K. S., & Sinha, D. (2010). Do sex offender registration and notification requirements deter juvenile sex crimes? *Criminal Justice and Behavior* 37: 553–69.

Letourneau, E. J., Bandyopadhyay, D., Sinha, D., & Armstrong, K. S. (2009a). The effects of sex offender registration policies on juvenile justice decision making. *Sexual Abuse: A Journal of Research and Treatment* 21: 149–65. doi: 10.1177/1079063208328678

Letourneau, E. J., Bandyopadhyay, D., Sinha, D., & Armstrong, K. S. (2009b). The influence of sex offender registration on juvenile sexual recidivism. *Criminal Justice Policy Review* 20: 136–53. doi: 10.1177/0887403408327917

Letourneau, E. J., Borduin, C. M., & Schaeffer, C. M. (2008). Multisystemic therapy for youth with problem sexual behaviors. In Beech, A., Craig, L., & Browne, K. (eds.), *Assessment and Treatment of Sexual Offenders: A Handbook*. London: Wiley, pp. 453–72.

Letourneau, E. J., & Caldwell, M. F. (2013). Expensive, harmful policies that don't work or how juvenile sexual offending is addressed in the U.S. *International Journal of Behavioral Consultation and Therapy* 8: 25–31.

Letourneau, E. J., Eaton, W. W., Bass, J., Berlin, F. S., & Moore, S. G. (2014). The need for a comprehensive public health approach to preventing child sexual abuse. *Public Health Reports* 129: 222–8.

Letourneau, E. J., Henggeler, S. W., Borduin, C. M., Schewe, P. A., McCart, M. R., Chapman, J. E., et al. (2009c). Multisystemic therapy for juvenile sexual offenders: 1-year results from a randomized effectiveness trial. *Journal of Family Psychology* 23(1): 89–102.

Letourneau, E. J., Henggeler, S. W., McCart, M. R., Borduin, C. M., Schewe, P. A., & Armstrong, K. S. (2013). Two-year follow-up of a randomized effectiveness trial evaluating MST for juveniles who sexually offend. *Journal of Family Psychology* 27: 978–85. PMID: 24188082

Letourneau, E. J., Nietert, P. J., & Rheingold, A. A. (2015). Impact of a prevention intervention in selected South Carolina counties. Manuscript in preparation.

Letourneau, E. J., & Schaeffer, C. (2014). Multisystemic therapy for youth problem sexual behavior: a case example. In O'Donohue, W. T. (ed.), *Case Studies in Sexual Deviance*. Cambridge, MA: Academic Press, pp. 17–34.

Levenson, J. (2009). Sex offender residence restrictions. In Wright, R. G. (ed.), *Sex Offender Laws: Failed Policies, New Directions*. New York: Springfield, pp. 267–90.

Levenson, J. S. & Cotter, L. P. (2005). The effect of Megan's Law on sex offender reintegration. *Journal of Contemporary Criminal Justice* 21: 49–66.

Logan, W. A. (2009). *Knowledge as Power: Criminal Registration and Notification Laws in America*. Stanford, CA: Stanford Law Books.

Lösel, F., & Schmucker, M. (2005). The effectiveness of treatment for sex offenders: a comprehensive meta-analysis. *Journal of Experimental Criminology* 1: 117–46.

Mancini, C. (2014). *Sex Crime, Offenders, & Society: A Critical Look at Sexual Offending and Policy*. Durham, NC: Carolina Academic Press.

Mancini, C., Shields, R. T., Mears, D. P., & Beaver, K. M. (2010). Sex offender residence restriction laws: parental perceptions and public policy. *Journal of Criminal Justice* 38: 1022–30.

Mannarino, A. P., Cohen, J. A., & Deblinger, E. (2014). Trauma-focused cognitive-behavioral therapy. In Timmer, S., & Urquiza, A. (eds.), *Evidence-Based Approaches for the Treatment of Maltreated Children: Considering Core Components and Treatment Effectiveness*. New York: Springer, pp. 165–86.

Marshall, W. L., Serran, G. A., & Cortoni, F. A. (2000). Childhood attachments, sexual abuse, and their relationship to adult coping in child molesters. *Sexual Abuse: A Journal of Research and Treatment* 12: 17–26.

Massachusetts Kids Count (2003, April). *Child Sexual Abuse and Public Opinion in Massachusetts: A Report to the Massachusetts Child Sexual Abuse Prevention Partnership*. Amherst: University of Massachusetts Poll. www.aecf.org/upload/publicationfiles/child%20sexual%20abuse%20in%20massachusetts.pdf

Mathers, C., Stevens, G., & Mascarenhas, M. (2009). *Global Health Risks: Mortality and Burden of Disease Attributable to Selected Major Risks*. Geneva, Switzerland: World Health Organization. www.who.int/healthinfo/global_burden_disease/GlobalHealthRisks_report_full.pdf

McCart, M. R., Sheidow, A. J., & Letourneau, E. J. (2014). Risk Reduction Therapy for Adolescents (RRTA): targeting substance use and HIV/STI-risk behaviors. *Cognitive and Behavioral Practice* 21: 161–75.

McMahon, P. M., & Puett, R. C. (1999). Child sexual abuse as a public health issue: recommendations of an expert panel. *Sexual Abuse: A Journal of Research and Treatment, 11*, 257–66.

Meloy, M. L., Miller, S. L., & Curtis, K. M. (2008). Making sense out of nonsense: the deconstruction of state-level sex offender residence restrictions. *American Journal of Criminal Justice* 33: 209–22.

Mendelson, T., & Letourneau, E. J. (2015). Parent-focused prevention of child sexual abuse. *Prevention Science* 16(6): 844–52.

Miller, T. R., Cohen, M. A., & Wiersema, B. (1996). *Victim Costs and Consequences: A New Look*. Washington, DC: National Institute of Justice.

Myers, D. L. (2005). *Boys among Men: Trying and Sentencing Juveniles as Adults*. Westport, CT: Praeger.

Neutze, J., Grundmann, D., Scherner, G., & Beier, K. M. (2012). Undetected and detected child sexual abuse and child pornography offenders. *International Journal of Law and Psychiatry* 35: 168–75.

Noll, J. G., Horowitz, L. A., Bonanno, G. A., Trickett, P. K., & Putnam, F. W. (2003). Revictimization and self-harm in females who experienced childhood sexual abuse: results from a prospective study. *Journal of Interpersonal Violence* 18: 1452–71.

Noll, J. G., Zeller, M. H., Trickett, P. K., & Putnam, F. W. (2007). Obesity risk for female victims of childhood sexual abuse: a prospective study. *Pediatrics* 120: e61–7.

NSVRC (National Sexual Violence Resource Center) (2005). Preventing child sexual abuse: a national resource directory and handbook. nsvrc.org/projects/child-sexual-assault-prevention/preventing-child-sexual-abuse-resources

Ogloff, J. R. P., Cutajar, M. C., Mann, E., & Mullen, P. (2012). Child sexual abuse and subsequent offending and victimisation: a 45 year follow-up study. *Trends & Issues in Crime and Criminal Justice* 440: 1–6. www.aic.gov.au/media_library/publications/tandi_pdf/tandi440.pdf

Pereda, N., Guilera, G., Forns, M., & Gomez-Benito, J. (2009). The prevalence of child sexual abuse in community and student samples: a meta-analysis. *Clinical Psychology Review* 29: 328–38.

Pérez-Fuentes, G., Olfson, M., Villegas, L., Morcillo, C., Wang, S., & Blanco, C. (2013). Prevalence and correlates of child sexual abuse: a national study. *Comprehensive Psychiatry* 54: 16–27.

Petrunik, M. (2003). The hare and the tortoise: dangerousness and sex offender policy in the United States and Canada. *Canadian Journal of Criminology and Criminal Justice* 45: 43–72.

Pittman, N. (2013). *Raised on the Registry: The Irreparable Harm of Placing Children on Sex Offender Registries in the U.S.* Washington, DC: Human Rights Watch. www.hrw.org/sites/default/files/reports/us0513_ForUpload_1.pdf

Pittman, N., & Nguyen, Q. (2011). *A Snapshot of Juvenile Sex Offender Registration and Notification Laws: A Survey of the States*. Philadelphia, PA: Defender Association of Philadelphia. www.njjn.org/uploads/digital-library/SNAPSHOT_web10-28.pdf

PPD (Prevention Project Dunkelfeld). (2015). Do you like children in ways you shouldn't? Retrieved from www.dont-offend.org/

Plummer, C. A. (2001). Prevention of child sexual abuse: a survey of 87 programs. *Violence and Victims* 16: 575–88.

Pollio, E., Deblinger, E., & Runyon, M. (2011). Mental health treatment for the effects of child sexual abuse. *The APSAC Handbook on Child Maltreatment*. Thousand Oaks, CA: Sage, pp. 267–88.

Putnam, F. W. (2003). Ten-year research update review: child sexual abuse. *Journal of the American Academy of Child and Adolescent Psychiatry* 42: 269–78.

Reitzel, L. R., & Carbonell, J. L. (2006). The effectiveness of sexual offender treatment for juveniles as measured by recidivism: a meta-analysis. *Sexual Abuse: A Journal of Research and Treatment* 18: 401–21.

Rheingold, A. A., Zajac, K., Chapman, J. E., Patton, M., de Arellano, M., Saunders, B., & Kilpatrick, D. (2014). Child sexual abuse prevention training for childcare professionals: an independent multi-site randomized controlled trial of stewards of children. *Prevention Science* 16: 374–85.

Rice, M. E., & Harris, G. T. (2003). The size and sign of treatment effects in sex offender therapy. *Annals of the New York Academy of Sciences* 989: 428–40.

Rinehart, J. K., Armstrong, K. S., Shields, R. T., & Letourneau, E. J. (2015). The effects of transfer laws on youth with violent offenses. Manuscript submitted for publication.

Roberts, R., O'Connor, T., Dunn, J., Golding, J., & ALSPAC Study Team. (2004). The effects of child sexual abuse in later family life: mental health, parenting and adjustment of offspring. *Child Abuse & Neglect* 28: 525–45.

Saied-Tessier, A. (2014). *Estimating the Costs of Child Sexual Abuse in the UK*. London: National Society for the Prevention of Cruelty to Children (NSPCC). www.nspcc.org.uk/globalassets/documents/research-reports/estimating-costs-child-sexual-abuse-uk.pdf

Sample, L. L., & Evans, M. K. (2009). Sex offender registration and community notification. In Wright, R. G. (ed.), *Sex Offender Laws: Failed Policies, New Directions*. New York: Springfield, pp. 211–42.

Saul, J., & Audage, N. C. (2007). *Preventing Child Sexual Abuse within Youth-Serving Organizations: Getting Started on Policies and Procedures*. Washington, DC: Centers for Disease Control and Prevention. www.cdc.gov/violenceprevention/pub/preventingchildabuse.html

Schaeffer, C. M. (2015). Primary prevention of child sexual abuse perpetration. Presented at the Child Sexual Abuse: A Public Health Perspective Symposium. Baltimore, MD, April.

Schober, D. J., Fawcett, S. B., & Bernier, J. (2012). The Enough Abuse Campaign: building the movement to prevent child sexual abuse in Massachusetts. *Journal of Child Sexual Abuse* 21: 456–69.

Schwartz, B. K. (2011). *Handbook of Sex Offender Treatment*. Kingston, NJ: Civic Research Institute.

Second Step (2015). Middle school. www.cfchildren.org/second-step/middle-school

Seto, M. C., & Lalumière, M. L. (2010). What is so special about male adolescent sexual offending? A review and test of explanations through meta-analysis. *Psychological Bulletin* 136: 526–75.

Simons, D., Wurtele, S. K., & Heil. P. (2002). Childhood victimization and lack of empathy as predictors of sexual offending against women and children. *Journal of Interpersonal Violence* 17: 1291–1307.

SMART (Stop Mind Control and Ritual Abuse Today) (2008). Significant changes to the SORNA guidelines. www.smart.gov/pdfs/sorna_significant_changes.pdf

SMART (Stop Mind Control and Ritual Abuse Today) (2014). Global overview of sex offender registration and notification systems. www.smart.gov/pdfs/GlobalOverview.pdf

SMART (Stop Mind Control and Ritual Abuse Today) (2015). SORNA. www.smart.gov/sorna.htm

Snyder, H. N. (2000). *Sexual Assault of Young Children as Reported to Law Enforcement: Victim, Incident and Offender Characteristics*. Washington, DC: U.S. Department of Justice, Office of Justice Programs, Bureau of Justice Statistics. www.bjs.gov/content/pub/pdf/saycrle.pdf

Sommarin, C., Kilbane, T., Mercy, J. A., Maloney-Kitts, M., & Ligiero, D. P. (2014). Preventing sexual violence and HIV in children. *Journal of Acquired Immune Deficiency Syndrome* 66: S217–S223.

Spohn, C. C. (2000). Thirty years of sentencing reform: the quest for a racially neutral sentencing process. *Criminal Justice* 3: 427–501.

Stop It Now! (2014). What do US adults think about child sexual abuse? Measures of knowledge and attitudes among six states. Stop It Now! Report, 2010. Retrieved from www.StopItNow.org

Stop It Now! (2015). Stop It Now! Retrieved from www.stopitnow.org/

Tabachnick, J., & Dawson, E. (2000). Stop it now! Vermont: a four year program evaluation (1995–1999). *Offender Programs Report* 1(4): 49.

Taylor, B. G., Stein, N. D., Mumford, E. A., & Woods, D. (2013). Shifting boundaries: an experimental evaluation of a dating violence prevention program in middle schools. *Prevention Science* 14: 64–76.

Terry, K. J., & Ackerman, A. (2008). Child sexual abuse in the Catholic Church: how situational crime prevention strategies can help create safe environments. *Criminal Justice and Behavior* 35: 643–57.

Tharp, A. T., DeGue, S., Valle, L. A., Brookmeyer, K. A., Massetti, G. M., & Matjasko, J. L. (2012). A systematic qualitative review of risk and protective factors for sexual violence perpetration. *Trauma, Violence, & Abuse* 14: 133–67.

Torbet, P., Gable, R., Hurst, H. IV., Montgomery, I., Szymanski, L., & Thomas, D. (1996). *State Responses to Serious and Violent Juvenile Crime*. Washington, DC: Office of Juvenile Justice and Delinquency Prevention.

U.S. Burden of Disease Collaborators (2013). The state of U.S. health, 1990–2010: burden of diseases, injuries, and risk factors. *JAMA* 310: 591–606.

USCCB (Conference of Catholic Bishops) (2005). Safe environment programs. www.usccb.org/ocyp/websafe.shtml

VACS (Violence against Children Surveys) (2015). Towards a violence-free generation: using science to fuel action and end violence against children. www.cdc.gov/violenceprevention/vacs/index.html

van der Put, C. E., & Asscher, J. J. (2015). Protective factors in male adolescents with a history of sexual and/or violent offending: a comparison between three subgroups. *Sexual Abuse: A Journal of Research and Treatment* 27: 109–26.

van Wijk, A., Loeber R., Vermeiren, R., Pardini, D., Bullens, R., & Doreleijers, D. (2005). Violent juvenile sex offenders compared with violent juvenile nonsex offenders: explorative findings from the Pittsburgh Youth Study. *Sexual Abuse: A Journal of Research and Treatment* 17: 333–52.

Whitaker, D. J., Le, B., Hanson, R. K., Baker, C. K., McMahon, P. M., Ryan, G., et al. (2008). Risk factors for the perpetration of child sexual abuse: a review and meta-analysis. *Child Abuse & Neglect* 32: 529–48.

Whitaker, D. J., Murphy, C. M., Eckhardt, C. I., Hodges, A. E., & Cowart, M. (2013). Effectiveness of primary prevention efforts for intimate partner violence. *Partner Abuse* 4: 175–95.

WHO (World Health Organization) (1999). Report of the Consultation on Child Abuse Prevention. Geneva, Switzerland, March 29–31. World Health Organization, Social Change and Mental Health, Violence and Injury Prevention.

Worling, J. R., & Langton, C. M. (2015). A prospective investigation of factors that predict desistance from recidivism for adolescents who have sexually offended. *Sexual Abuse: A Journal of Research and Treatment* 27: 127–42.

Wortley, R. K., & Smallbone, S. (2006). Applying situational principles to sexual offending against children. In Wortley, R., & Smallbone, S. (eds.), *Situational Prevention of Child Sexual Abuse*. Monsey, NY: Criminal Justice Press/Willow Tree Press, pp. 7–35.

Wurtele, S. K. (2009). Preventing sexual abuse of children in the twenty-first century: preparing for challenges and opportunities. *Journal of Child Sexual Abuse* 18: 1–18.

Yates, P. M., & Kingston, D. A. (2011). Pathways to sexual offending. In Schwartz, B. K. (ed.), *Handbook of Sex Offender Treatment*. Kingston, NJ: Civic Research Institute, pp. 17.1–17.16.

Zandbergen, P. A., Levenson, J. S., & Hart, T. C. (2010). Residential proximity to schools and daycares: an empirical analysis of sex offense recidivism. *Criminal Justice and Behavior* 37: 482–502.

Zimring, F.E. (2004). *An American Travesty: Legal Responses to Adolescent Sex Offending*. Chicago, IL: University of Chicago Press.

32 The Evolution of Alcohol and Drug Prevention Strategies in Latin America

Augusto Pérez-Gómez & Juliana Mejía-Trujillo[1]

Introduction

Latin America (LA) is the name currently employed to designate the eighteen Spanish-speaking countries of the region, plus Brazil (Portuguese), Haiti (French), and Puerto Rico. It would be impossible to examine what occurs in all of these countries, therefore nine of them were selected: Argentina, Brazil, Chile, Colombia, Costa Rica, El Salvador, Mexico, Peru, and Uruguay. This chapter was written on the basis of documents provided by experts from the nine participant countries. The topics important to the prevention of alcohol and drugs will be examined in the nine specific countries, representing different areas of the continent, which in spite of similarities, display many significant differences in multiple domains that contribute to making direct comparisons difficult. Although country authors received identical instructions, the country summaries are not identical because each author commented on issues deemed most important and those with which they are most familiar. However, each country section contains some information on public policies, prevention practices, and research, and in some cases local training. Nevertheless, the chapter offers a realistic perspective on developments and events in LA regarding alcohol and drug prevention practices.

The content areas of each country that are discussed as they relate to alcohol and drug prevention are the following:

- Culture: traditions, beliefs, customs, artistic expressions, and values may vary largely within and between countries.
- Language: about one-third of the population of LA speaks Portuguese (Brazil), and the rest Spanish; this creates a barrier for intercountry collaboration that has not been surmounted.

[1] With the collaboration of : Juan Carlos Mansilla and Alberto Calabrese (Argentina); Sheila G. Murta, Samia Abreu and Maria Inês Gandolfo Conceição (Brazil); Felipe Leyton (Chile); Vera Barahona and Julio Bejarano (Costa Rica); Cristina Amaya (El Salvador); María Elena Castro, Nancy Amador, Jorge Amath Villatoro and Jorge Llanes (México); Carmen Masías (Perú); Gabriela Olivera (Uruguay).

- Socioeconomic conditions and education: there are very rich and very poor countries in LA, with some great educational centers in some of them, and very low levels of professional development in others.
- Political systems: LA has developed a process of stabilization of local governments, most of which have adopted democracy; still, there exists a trend toward political polarization between conservative and liberal values that affect decisions regarding alcohol and drug use and prevention.
- Investment: only some countries (Brazil, Costa Rica, Mexico, Chile, Uruguay) have state policies allowing continuous investment for prevention. In most countries, the political decisions and the corresponding investments move up and down, condemning countries to be deprived of long-term planning and sustainability of prevention programs.

The first approaches applied at the beginning of the 1980s to prevention in LA were very simple and narrow-minded, such as the "Just say no" motto and the Drug Abuse Resistance Education (DARE) program, which were quickly adopted. In some countries, these approaches are still used, with disappointing results. Other programs, appearing later (end of the 1980s and first part of the 1990s), were aimed at improving student communication skills, assertiveness, decision making, and knowledge about drugs. These programs were usually implemented by teachers and very often included keeping records about drug incidents, student drug experiences, and plans for the future. These programs were implemented in schools, and they are currently employed almost everywhere in LA, despite poor evaluations and lack of evidence that they produce desired results.

Today it is clear that no literal translation of prevention programs can be implemented directly from one LA country to another. Programs must be adapted to the local context. However, many prevention programs continue to be used in their original version. One of the reasons for this repeated error is the lack of research. However, this has been changing progressively, especially since universities have become interested in supporting and researching issues associated with the alcohol and drug use.

As lead authors of this chapter, we tried to unify substantially different writing styles and perspectives. We organized highly disparate sets of information and tried, as much as possible, to maintain a homogeneous structure in the sections of each country. These sections include a brief presentation of each country, policies and institutions related to prevention, prevention practices, and prevention research and publications. Most countries provided information about prevention policies and institutions, but not all countries provided specific information about prevention programs and some did not report about prevention research and publications. These omissions may imply a gap in prevention work in the country, or they may reflect author's preferences.

Argentina

Argentina is the second-largest Spanish-speaking country in LA, with a population of 42 million people, most of them of European ancestry, especially from Spain, Italy, France, and Germany. Its powerful economic advancement allowed for major development of the sciences and arts, more so than in other countries in LA. The nation was under a military dictatorship for seven years (1976–83). During this period, the Falkland's war with the United Kingdom occurred. Argentina is one of the countries in LA with the highest rates of consumption of marijuana and coca paste (a crude, smokable product, very popular in many LA countries, that exists before cocaine hydrochloride is obtained).

Policies and Institutions

In 1972, as provided by Decree 452 of President's Office, the National Commission for Drug and Narcotics Addiction (CONATON) was created as a branch of the Ministry of Social Welfare, but with an interministerial nature. The government then was military, and the decree creating this first institution of its kind in the country was intended to promote "research, education, prevention, care, legislation, and repression of drug addiction" (Boletín Oficial de Argentina, 1972, p. A372)

The foundational approach to the problem of "drug addiction" in Argentina originated from a repressive military perspective, concentrating on the "drugs menace" rather than on community and consumers. This social control bias, focusing on illegal substances and stigmatizing youth, would for several years negatively color the perception of "addiction prevention."

The CONATON never offered positive results nor performed effectively. Therefore, the commission was dissolved during the first democratic government after the military dictatorship, and in 1985 the National Drug Commission was created. Unlike the CONATON, the National Drug Commission became more involved in the health problem and educational programs than in the social control problem. At this time, the first efforts to bring the concept of prevention to municipal policy appeared. However, the results were limited and focused on the province of Buenos Aires. In addition, the main emphasis was not prevention but rather therapeutic care for drug users.

In 1989, the National Drug Commission was dissolved and followed by the creation of the Secretariat for the Prevention of Narco-traffic and Drug Consumption (Sedronar). Sedronar promoted, for the first time and within a national organization, the idea of "drug use prevention." However, the actions of Sedronar were aimed more toward the financing and development of non-government organizations (NGOs) that worked in treatment, and the "prevention" actions were aimed at the prevention of drug trafficking.

Some drug abuse prevention programs were implemented over the years, but they could not be sustained over time and they were not installed as systematic and consistent public policy. There was a great deficiency of locally produced prevention materials, and those existing had no impact on the population. The NGOs subsidized by Sedronar were mainly focused on assistance to drug users and very rarely on preventive actions. It was only in the decade from 2000 to 2010, when prevention became an activity of properly trained professionals.

In 2006, Sedronar began a nationwide distribution of prevention teaching materials for elementary schools throughout the country using the Chilean program "I Want to Be" *(Quiero Ser)*. This program is implemented by teachers and is aimed at giving information, promoting healthy lifestyles, and teaching refusal skills and coping strategies. The materials were distributed in almost all provinces of Argentina, reaching much of the country, and funded by the national government. Although *Quiero Ser* was evaluated positively, in 2012 Sedronar (with the collaboration of the United Nations) began reviewing the program's materials to make them more suitable for the country's necessities for prevention. At the same time, Sedronar started the development of other prevention materials for young children, such as "The Magic Mirror" *(El Espejo Magico)*. For the first time, Argentina had didactic materials designed and developed by Argentine technicians and implemented transversally within educational curricula in the provinces involved. However, at the end of 2013 there was a change of management in Sedronar that broke the continuity of the programs. The new governance emphasized prevention work within provinces and created Prevention Centers throughout the country. These youth centers are aimed at stimulating creativity, to improve cultural, sport, and art development and strengthen life projects to create protective networks and reduce involvement in risky situations.

Thus, national policy on the prevention of alcohol and drugs progressed from a social control point of view of the 1970s, to an educational institutional perspective, and finally toward a centralized-territorial emphasis. Unfortunately, preventive public policy has been deficient from a socioeducational-health paradigm perspective, making few advances on territorial presence, transversal across educational and community activities, population coverage, and production of locally produced didactic materials.

Prevention

All Argentina provinces began with the information-about-drugs prevention approach, especially during the 1980 and 1990s. Then some psychologistical approaches (self-esteem, imitation, etc.) appeared, as well as those of Generation of Alternatives (suggestion of activities to use creatively in adolescents' free time). Approaches that emphasized resistance skills and life skills arose in 2000 under the umbrella of "nonspecific approaches." This trend from specific to nonspecific approaches continues today.

Prevention of drugs and alcohol has also emerged and has been conducted in other ways, such as (a) warnings and exemplification messages, which generally are inscribed in medical health logic, with the enumeration of punishments applicable to those who infringe upon the rules, coming from the legal framework; (b) messages from therapeutic communities, which initially joined quasireligious references about the problem of relapse to the logic of damage inflicted to family and society; and (c) rational speeches containing different messages accentuated as appropriate to the psychosocial and sociomedical perspective.

At the provincial level, the dynamic has been quite different from the national level, because it is in the provinces that some of the most systematic and sustained actions on prevention have been carried out. Provinces such as La Pampa, Córdoba, Entre Ríos, Buenos Aires, Ciudad Autónoma de Buenos Aires (CABA), Chubut, Mendoza, Tucumán, and Jujuy are the ones that have developed more preventive programs and activities in a sustained manner. They have managed a specific professional team for prevention programs, developed prevention materials, provided financial resources (although limited), and conducted some program evaluations. All of these actions in the provinces began implementation in the decade of 2000 through 2010, except Buenos Aires, which developed preventive actions in the 1990s, although with large fluctuations due to changes in government.

In the twenty-first century, Argentinian universities became leaders and more committed to training "preventers" (although there were university actions before). Training of prevention professionals has been a positive component of the prevention field, as the training has strengthened and begun to systematize prevention actions and better define prevention. The professionals have also encouraged and promoted the development of prevention programs, assessments, and evaluations.

Brazil

Brazil is the largest country in LA, and the fifth worldwide, with an area of 8,515,000 square kilometers and more than 200 million inhabitants. Even though Brazil is one of the wealthiest countries in the world (the sixth-largest world economy), the inequalities are also extreme, and they are related to high rates of drug use, especially in large cities such as São Paulo and Rio de Janeiro. The National Drug Policy in Brazil (PNAD, an acronym in Portuguese, begun in 2005) is committed to promoting a society protected from licit and illicit drug use and is aligned with a harm reduction framework.

Policies and Institutions

The premises of the PNAD policy are (a) clear distinction between the different categories of users and traffickers; (b) priority for prevention over repression; (c) implementation of actions and strategies coordinated and integrated between different organizations and sectors of society for the development of strategies aimed at addressing social problems associated with the trafficking and consumption of illicit drugs; (d) development of a scientific-academic database that includes results obtained by Brazilian and international experiences, with actions aimed at prevention, monitoring, and repression of drug abuse. The PNAD priorities are prevention, treatment, rehabilitation, and social reintegration; harm reduction; supply reduction; and research and evaluation (Conceição & Oliveira, 2008).

The possession of drugs for personal consumption in Brazil is no longer a "crime" (considered infractions) but remains an offense for which penalties other than imprisonment are given.

Prevention

In Brazil there is a close relationship between health and schooling through the project Health and Prevention in the School, supported by the United Nations Educational, Scientific, and Cultural Organization (UNESCO) and United Nations Children's Fund (UNICEF) (Giacomozzi, Itokasu, Luzardo, & Vieira, 2012). Additionally, in 2004, the University of Brasilia, in partnership with government entities, developed the Course of Drug Abuse Prevention for Teachers of Public Schools; more than 190,000 teachers in 31,294 schools across the country have been trained and some pedagogical adjustments have been made using new technologies. By 2010, according to the Multilateral Evaluation Mechanism (CICAD/OAS, 2009), during the period 2006 to 2009 this was the only prevention program used in the country, which reached over 2 million children. Comparison of two surveys on drug use carried out among students in elementary and secondary schools conducted in 2004 (Galduróz, Noto, Fonseca, & Carlini, 2005), and in 2010 (Carlini, Noto, & Sanchez, 2010) showed a decrease in lifetime prevalence of drug use in all age groups.

Significant advances in public policies to prevent drug abuse in Brazil have taken place in recent years. The General Coordination of Mental Health, Alcohol, and Other Drugs of the Ministry of Health, together with the United Nations Office on Drugs and Crime (UNODC), introduced three preventive evidence-based programs: (a) *Strong Families,* aimed at families and adolescents; (b) *The Good Behavior Game*, aimed at children of elementary school, aged from six to ten years; and (c) *Unplugged*, focused on students aged eleven to fourteen years of Basic School II. These programs were implemented in 2013 on a small scale in three Brazilian cities, and based on initial study the programs were culturally adapted for the Brazilian context.

The Strong Families program was subjected to a process evaluation by researchers at the University of Brasilia, and the Good Behavior Game and Unplugged by the Federal University of Sao Paulo and the Federal University of Santa Catarina. Unplugged was subjected to a quasi-experimental study. The results of these studies have not been yet published. Efficiency and effectiveness evaluation of the programs began in 2014 and are currently in process.

Research and Publications

In Brazil, research projects aimed at the prevention of risk factors are few and relatively recent. Abreu (2012) conducted a series of studies to map domestic production in prevention programs and to identify needs for expansion in this field in Brazil. The first study looked at a systematic review of the literature. It was found that Brazilian studies focused on the early stages of the cycle of prevention research in order to identify and describe mental health problems

(N = 132 items), investigate risk factors and protective factors (N = 56 items), and develop pilot studies of preventive interventions (N = 34 articles). There is a marked lack of published studies on the final stages of the research cycle, evaluation of efficacy (N = 4 studies), effectiveness (N = 3 studies), and dissemination of the results (N = 0). The main topics identified related to prevention by Abreu (2012) were antisocial behavior, peer rejection, violent behaviors, and substance abuse. Although research production in prevention programs is small in Brazil, data from the review by Abreu indicated a trend of increasing number of studies in this field.

Chile

Chile is one of three countries in the southern cone of Latin America, populated by about 18 million people, the majority (90 percent) of European origin or mestizos. After a long period of military government (1973–88), the country established a thriving democracy accompanied by a sustained economic development that now makes it one of the richest countries in the region.

Policies and Institutions

The process of economic development has been accompanied by a sustained increase in the use of psychoactive substances among young people. As a result, multiple activities have been developed in the areas of prevention and treatment of drug and alcohol abuse. These were formalized in 1990 with the creation of an Advisory Council of the Presidency (CONACE) dedicated to the prevention, control, and treatment of drug use and alcohol consumption.

In 2011, CONACE became the National Service for Prevention and Rehabilitation of Drug Use and Alcohol (SENDA), under the Ministry of Interior, with greater autonomy and capacity to administer resources. Even though Chile has developed many prevention initiatives linked to NGOs, educational institutions, and the Ministry of Education, among others, it is SENDA that has led the efforts.

To fund this national policy, there has been an increase in resources allocated; thus in 2001 a total of approximately U.S. $2 million for prevention efforts were assigned, and in 2013 the available budget for such initiatives reached U.S. $9 million. In general terms, SENDA (Construyendo Culturas Preventivas; SENDA, 2013) has increased its budget from U.S. $20 million in 2000 to U.S. $90 million in 2013, that is, in thirteen years there has been an increase of 450 percent (DIPRES, 2013).

Prevention

The early prevention initiatives implemented by CONACE were based on community intervention models and mainly intended to be developed around the municipalities with the purpose of running plans and actions that would be valued by the community itself and the existing network. This program is currently on course (Senda Prevents), although it has experienced changes in structure and orientations, and directing its focus to educational settings.

Later there was increased coverage, with annual exponential growth in the number of beneficiaries of the *Previene* (Prevents) program and its various initiatives. For example, in 1999, 683 community projects were financed with grant funds. In 2000, at school levels, the program reached 1.2 million beneficiaries, including parents, caretakers, and teachers, in addition to students (DIPRES, 2001). The local Previene program was implemented to serve seventy-six small communities in 2000, which corresponds to 22 percent of the country (currently the coverage is 62 percent of the country) (Arratia et al., 2013). In the educational realm, twelve universal prevention programs were developed, covering the total number of educational establishments in the country. Several other programs for families, youngsters, and employment settings were developed and implemented as well.

Theoretical models supporting the Previene programs were extremely diverse, at the strategic, programmatic, and action levels, and definitions of each of them were quite vague and sometimes contradictory. In each initiative, community and systemic models, theories of individual development, and even the proposed activities converged, and the definition of the phenomenon and intervention strategies became diffuse. In addition, even if the Previene programs were consolidated, the corresponding evaluation strategies aimed at supporting their implementation were not developed. Currently, no information is available on changes related to risk and protective factors, hindering determination of whether the purpose and objectives of the Previene programs were achieved (DIPRES, 2013).

With SENDA, programs and interventions were modified and restructured. The priority was focused on creating a relevant theoretical base with programs that were understandable, communicable, and unified, to help ensure that the programs were designed with logic that would allow an evaluation based on relevant indicators. For this reason, the Competency Model was chosen, which defines prevention as an active process of implementing initiatives to modify and improve the integral education of individuals (Becoña, 2002). The model aims at improving the quality of life. In this way, prevention work is done with and from beliefs, experiences, and knowledge of individuals and communities, in order to develop skills to make autonomous and responsible self and collective care decisions (Construyendo Culturas Preventivas; SENDA, 2013). This is a critical and reflective exercise that enables participants to read and diagnose their current living conditions and produce necessary changes and adjustments as suitable (Murillo, 2013). Finally, measurement of achievement (still being developed) is not necessarily based on nonconsumption of drugs for an indeterminate period of time but rather on the achievement of personal competences and their implementation over time.

Research and Publications

CONACE had great achievements at the national level, as well as an important interchange with other countries of the region. One such achievement is a series of studies of drug prevalence at the national level, which have been conducted among both the general and school populations since 1994 (Observatorio Chileno de Drogas, 2015); these studies show a remarkable increase of drug use in Chile, especially in the last ten years.

Colombia

Colombia is located in the north of South America and is the only country in this region with coasts both in the Atlantic and Pacific oceans. Its population is 47 million people, most of them mestizo. Due to its cocaine production, for many years Colombia lived in the eye of the hurricane, and in the 1990s it became the country with the highest levels of drug abuse in LA.

Policies and Institutions

In 1986, the political conditions of the country and the development of drug trafficking led to sanction Law 30 and the creation of the National Drug Council. This law, currently in force, focuses on controlling supply, and only four articles out of ninety-seven are related to demand.

In 1998, for the first time in the history of the country, drug abuse was part of a government platform. The RUMBOS Presidential Program was created as a coordinating institution for drug demand reduction at the local, national, and regional levels and also served as a bridge between governmental and nongovernmental institutions. RUMBOS started a new open concept of prevention within the country, with administrative authority for managing international and national resources for the implementation of such policies. However, during the following governmental period (2002–10), RUMBOS was dismantled; there was no action and no investment, and the problem was ignored almost completely. The president and his government considered drug abuse a low-priority problem and acted accordingly.

During the present government period (2010–18), several important situations occurred; first of all, the possibility of legalizing marijuana for medical purposes was a proposal at the Senate and was still being debated as of February 2015; the problem of psychoactive substances (PAS) consumption became a public health issue; and, finally, a government advisory committee was established on drug policy, which aimed to change the state of abandonment (ignoring the drug problem) that had remained in place.

Prevention

The National Plan for Prevention of Drug Abuse began prevention actions in Colombia in 1985. The plan intended to link efforts from different ministries and public agencies, with financial support from the United Nations. The plan's measures were sparse, with poor conceptual support, and it was only from the Ministry of Education that a process of analysis and reflection led to the proposal of "integral prevention." This concept stated that the drug problem should be addressed by considering all its components: illicit crops, production of substances, drug trafficking, and consumption. However, it also should be connected with many other social problems, such as poor distribution of wealth, teenage pregnancy, and low quality of public education. Several Latin American countries adopted this approach (i.e., Peru, Costa Rica, Chile). From a theoretical perspective, the approach looks promising, but it is practically impossible to realize, as there are conflicts of interests between the applicant entities, poor budget allocations, and different beliefs about the meaning and importance of actions to be executed. Indeed, in Colombia from 1985 to the present, the resources allocated by the government to address the drug problem are very unevenly distributed, as 98 percent of resources are used to control supply and 2 percent to control demand. Under these terms, the issue of "integral prevention" becomes impossible to implement.

Colombia reports to have implemented fourteen prevention programs, most of them foreign programs without evaluation or cultural adaptations. Recently, in addition to the classic program Life Skills Training (Botvin & Griffin, 2004), the government undertook the implementation of three other programs, all created in the United States: Strengthening Families (Kumpfer & Alvarado, 2003), Lions Quest (2015), and Communities That Care (Hawkins & Catalano, 1992). The first of the mentioned programs (Life Skills) appears to be without evaluation in Colombia, the second has a positive evaluation, the third has a negative one, and the fourth (Communities That Care) is in process, requiring several years of work. Two other national programs, Anímate and Consentidos, have positive evaluations, but only Animate's results (highly positive) have been published (Aja Eslava & Gómez Avila, 2013).

Research and Publications

Only in the late 1990s was there a significant increase in the amount of research in the drug prevention field in Colombia, especially at universities, and the trend has been strengthened in the twenty-first century. Epidemiological studies of the general and student populations have been developed and carried out more regularly (Ministerios de Justicia, Educación y Salud, 2011, 2014). However, between 1996 and 2008 studies were conducted only among school populations (RUMBOS, 2002).

The following are the main findings from epidemiological research on drug use in Colombia:

- Colombia is ranked first in South America for early start of alcohol consumption. To date, no formal explanation for this has been provided. However, there is a long history of adult tolerance for alcohol and even the use of alcohol at an early age.

- There has been a tendency among women to increase their use of all substances, both legal and illegal, particularly between the ages of sixteen to twenty-four. In the 1980s, the proportion of males to females regarding illegal drug use was eight to one (Pérez-Gómez, 1989); currently, this proportion is barely three to one (Ministerios de Justicia y Salud, 2014).
- The use of tranquilizers among teenagers is the highest in Latin America, and their use is even higher among adult women.
- Heroin use has risen very rapidly in the last few years.
- Compared to other countries, drug use in Colombia is ranked at an intermediate position, similarly to Peru and Mexico. Chile, Uruguay, Argentina, Brazil, and El Salvador are at the upper levels of drug use, and Ecuador and Bolivia are at lower levels (Pérez-Gómez, 2013; UNODC/CICAD, 2009).

There are some additional studies worth mentioning because they help to give a general overview of the drug problem in Colombia:

- The attributable fractions drugs/crime in adults study (Pérez-Gómez, Valencia, & Rodríguez, 2006) is the first study of this category in LA. The study demonstrated a high relative risk in the relationship between drug use and committing an offense or a crime, and moderate attributable fractions between consumption of alcohol, cocaine, and marijuana and offenses such as personal injuries, murder, and crimes against property.
- The transitions in drug use in a Colombia study (Pérez Gómez, 2007) interviewed ninety-six people in treatment, aged fourteen to fifty, in seven Colombian cities. Five kinds of transitions were identified: general, cumulative, substitutive, reverse, and negative, occurring at nine different points. A total of 113 "transitional patterns" (combinations of two substances) were found, 23 common to men and women, 10 exclusive to women, and 80 exclusive to men. The 10 main transitions involved only four substances – marijuana, cocaine, inhalants, and tranquilizers – and are most common among those under age twenty-three.
- The survey regarding consumption of alcohol among minors (under eighteen years) was administered in nine cities of Colombia (Pérez-Gómez & Scoppetta, 2009). It was found that alcohol consumption among adolescents is very high, and that significant percentages of young people drink alcohol weekly (life prevalence, 87 percent; last year prevalence, 68 percent; last month, 30 percent; last week, 13 percent), at school (15 percent), for a period of several days in succession (8 percent), and drink alcohol alone (4 percent).
- Pérez-Gómez (2011) studied the vulnerability to HIV/AIDS in high-risk drug users in the cities of Medellin and Armenia. This study revealed the main characteristics of heroin users in these cities were as follows: mainly males, between seventeen and twenty-five years, incomplete high school, from single-parent families, and most beginning their drug use with a substance different from heroin. In addition, heroin use began with smoking or inhaling it, and the main reason for shifting to injection was economic: a smoked dose allows eight injections (a gram of 40 percent heroin purity makes eight grams of

5 percent injectable heroin). Most stopped using other drugs (except marijuana) and proposed explicit and timely public policy strategies, such as training the police in order to manage the cases better; giving special attention to homeless people; delivering free kits that include condoms, needles, and syringes; and providing outreach activities led by public health services.

- Two studies assessed marijuana use among university students (Andean Epidemiological Study on Drugs Use in the University Population: Colombia's Report [Andean Community of Nations, 2009, 2013]). Comparison of these two studies showed that there was a statistically significant increase of marijuana use among university students over the four-year period (from 11 percent to 15 percent); cocaine and amphetamine stimulant use remained stable (2.2 percent).
- Pérez-Gómez (2010) studied the consumption of PAS by adolescents in conflict with the law. This study compared adolescents deprived of liberty due to crimes (n = 1670) with a national study conducted in 2011 in school populations (n = 95,000) (Ministerios de Justicia, Educación y Salud, 2011). The problematic use (judged from the consumption in the last month) is between seven and twenty times higher in the infringing youth population compared to the school population. Results showed that offenders used substances with higher frequency compared to nonoffending adolescents in proportions varying between ten and thirty-five times greater.

Costa Rica

This small Central American country (51,100 square kilometers) with almost 5 million people developed an affiliation between the universities and the governmental institutions in charge of taking care of the drug abuse problem; as a result, Costa Rica has a rich database on the epidemiology of drug abuse and on therapeutic and prevention services.

Policies and Institutions

In 1972, the government of Costa Rica and the Panamerican Health Organization signed a Letter of Agreement as foundation for a Center for Alcohol Studies. This Letter of Agreement gave greater attention to the problem of alcohol abuse and facilitated the granting of financial and technical assistance from specialized agencies to develop and implement prevention programs and research projects.

In 1973, the National Institute on Alcoholism (INSA; acronym in Spanish) was created, as an agency attached to the Ministry of Health, and was designated tasks related to research, prevention, and treatment, as well as coordination of public and private programs for this purpose. In 1974, Law No. 5489 was referred to as the Law for the Regulation and Control of Alcohol Advertising. This act enabled the institute to regulate and control advertising related to the consumption of alcoholic beverages. On March 12, 1986, with the enactment of Law No. 7035, the Institute on Alcoholism and Drug Dependence (IAFA), successor of INSA and current governing body on the issue of drugs, was established in Costa Rica. IAFA has functions of prevention, research, treatment, rehabilitation of alcoholism and drug addiction, and the coordination of public and private programs aimed at treating patients with problems of alcohol abuse and other drug use.

Prevention

From 2003 to 2005, the IAFA implemented a pilot project for the prevention of drug use in children. The program, called Learn to Fend for Myself, is a curriculum program based on the approach of the Life Skills program (Botvin & Griffin, 2004). Learn to Fend for Myself promotes the development of social and emotional skills in children. The program includes skills to improve self-esteem, assertiveness, communication, decision making, family relationships, handling of group pressure, and social influence and provides information about tobacco, alcohol, and other drugs.

In 2005, an evaluation of the pilot project of Learn to Fend for Myself was carried out in a process that began at the fourth-grade level and concluded the same year with the sixth grade. The evaluation showed a decrease in the consumption of tobacco and alcohol, high scores on the implementation of the acquired social and cognitive skills, and good acceptance of the program by children, parents, and teachers. On the basis of the evaluation, and after developing and validating the necessary teaching materials, Learn to Fend for Myself (www.iafa.go.cr/.../aprendo-a-valerme-por-mi-mismo.html) became a national program in 2007. In 2015, the program was to be evaluated nationwide for all levels of elementary school.

The IAFA also offers a training program for parents based on the Life Skills program. IAFA also offers a program for the work environment to prevent drug use among workers, a program of detection, and early intervention for secondary school students. These are national programs implemented and funded through the Regional Headquarters of IAFA.

Research and Publications

In 1970, the "National Survey on Alcohol Intake Habits" was designed and implemented, functioning as an exploration at the national level to identify the extent of problem alcohol drinking habits in Costa Rica. This survey officially marked the beginning of research on alcohol problems in the country.

In 1990, IAFA implemented the first national survey on drug use in Costa Rica, and it has been administered every five years since then. Research has focused on drug use in different parts of the country, ad campaigns, patient care, and groups at social risk (Bejarano, 1992). This overview of research on the demand for drugs in the early 1990s was complemented by studies, for the first time within a university, on supply and epidemiology (Bejarano, Carvajal, & San Lee, 1992). Some research projects sponsored by other national institutions and the Central American region aimed to assess the demand for drugs in different populations of Costa Rica (Blanco & Sandí, 1993).

Research in primary and secondary schools has been of great interest, and since 2006, with the support of the Organization of American States (OAS) through the International Commission for Drug Abuse Control (CICAD), a survey has been conducted every three years. This survey has allowed the tracking of the evolving drug demand and has facilitated the design of various preventive interventions. During the first decade of the twenty-first century and continuing to present, national studies conducted in previous periods have been replicated, and Costa Rica has participated in multinational studies on smoking and alcohol use (Bejarano, 2005).

For the period 2015 to 2020, IAFA is expected to continue the development of national household and student surveys, conduct studies on smoking among students in health and medical professions, and conduct studies of the social costs of drugs in Costa Rica (Salas, 2014). It is expected that other research projects will be useful for stakeholders, such as developing a drug information system to collect data on substance demand and related issues.

Finally, research strategies that have been used over the past half-century reveal the predominance of quantitative research, particularly cross-sectional studies that are based on the survey method. There is little documentation in Costa Rica about other methods, such as ethnography studies, action research, longitudinal studies, and descriptive data going beyond epidemiological and quantitative studies.

El Salvador

Affected by a long civil war (1979–92) and later by large gangs called *maras* (tightly related to narco-traffic), this Central American country has a significant drug consumption problem that has been addressed mainly by private institutions. The population of El Salvador is approximately 6.3 million people, and about 2 million more live in the United States.

Policies and Institutions

In El Salvador, there are multiple relevant government organizations to manage the problem of drug use. Article 5 of Decree No. 153 of 2003 created the National Drug Commission (CNA, acronym in Spanish). This national authority is responsible for planning, coordinating, monitoring, and evaluating the plans, strategies, and government policies related to the problem of drug use. CNA is composed of the Superior Council of Public Health and delegates from the ministries of Interior, Health, Education, and National Defense. Some crossover areas covered by the national antidrug plan are research, data collection, and statistical reporting.

Different government agencies assume specific responsibilities for implementing preventive tasks. The Department of Toxicology of the Ministry of Justice and Public Safety is responsible for universal and early intervention strategies in schools and government institutions; the Ministry of Health is responsible for prevention in the framework of the National Mental Health Policy; and the Ministry of Education carries out actions of universal prevention within the educational community.

Private institutions conducting prevention programs are faced with several challenges, including (a) lack of standardized programs and the strategies to evaluate the programs, (b) the need to develop human resources for evaluating prevention programs for PAS use, and (c) the need to undertake diagnosis of target populations to guide prevention programs with appropriate approaches.

Several universities and institutions of higher education include in their curricula courses on prevention and treatment for disciplines and professional careers related to drug abuse. Since 2001 the Central American University (UCA) has offered a master's degree in community psychology, specializing in violence prevention and substance dependency.

Between the years 2004 and 2006, teachers, professors, social workers, health workers, police officers, drug treatment counselors, prison guards, community leaders, and pedagogical and technical advisors were offered short training courses on prevention by universities. During the years 2008 and 2009, additional drug prevention courses were conducted, primarily for teachers to strengthen prevention programs. These training opportunities were valuable initiatives, but they have not been sustained. The country does not offer master's or Ph.D. programs in prevention, treatment, or research in drug abuse.

Prevention

El Salvador has adopted some internationally well-accepted programs such as Strengthening Families (Kumpfer & Alvarado, 2003), Life Skills Training (Botvin & Griffin, 2004), Miles de Manos (Thousand Hands) (Centro de la Promoción de Equidad University of Oregon & GIZ, 2014), and Second Step (Committee for Children, 2002). Some other programs were developed locally and are focused on prevention in different domains, such as schools with different age groups and with specific communities such as drivers, women, nonschool communities, marginal groups, and workers. The relevant theoretical approach in these programs is the biopsychosocial comprehensive approach, which deals with the evaluation of the individual within a complex context. These programs are implemented by governmental and nongovernmental institutions such as the Solidarity Fund for Health, Hogares CREA (Comunidad Reeducadora de Adictos: Center for the Re-Education of Addicts), and the Ministry of National Education.

As in some other countries in this region of the world, there are no formal evaluations of these programs. Rather, evaluations are currently focused on compliance and monitoring of the implemented activities. The main constraints regarding program evaluations are low budgets, lack of specialists in evaluation methods, lack of interagency coordination, and limited knowledge and awareness about substance abuse in the general population.

Research and Publications

Since 2004, El Salvador has carried out surveys on drug and alcohol consumption among high school and university students and the general population. The last general population survey was conducted in 2014. These surveys showed that El Salvador has one of the highest rates of drug abuse in Central America.

In 2013, the Evangelical University of El Salvador conducted a study on the limitations and challenges of evaluating prevention programs for psychoactive substance abuse. This study identified the prevention programs currently implemented in El Salvador, the populations for whom they are conceived, the implementation of evaluation mechanisms, the theoretical and basic conceptual approaches, and the limitations and challenges that the government must address in evaluating prevention programs (Juárez, 2013).

As for private institutions, the Center for Comprehensive Addiction Rehabilitation and Psychotherapy evaluates its secondary prevention program. The Foundation against Drugs of El Salvador and Hogares CREA (both therapeutic communities) are engaged in a similar purpose. The results have not been published to date.

Mexico

The area of Mexico is 2 million square kilometers with nearly 120 million people, making it the second largest (after Brazil) and most populated country in LA. Its population is largely mestizo and of Spanish origins, but there are also migrants from many other countries. For unknown reasons, Mexico had for many years some of the lowest rates of drug abuse in LA. Sadly, this situation has been changing during the last decade, partly because of the core drug traffic moving from Colombia to Mexico.

Prevention

Prevention began in Mexico in 1973 with the founding of the Mexican Center for Studies on Drugs. At that time, the first epidemiological studies at national and local levels were also undertaken. Prevention was basically done under the ethical-legal and medical care approach. As time passed and research developed, prevention moved from a risk and protection approach with community participation toward a sociocultural and psychosocial approach. Around 1995, Mexican prevention materials were developed with a vision toward teaching people to change behaviors rather than merely informing and changing attitudes and perceptions about drug use, as was typical at that time. During this period, evaluations of drug prevention programs began. Around 2005, the predominant prevention approaches focused on the development of competencies and life skills, cognitive-behavioral strategies, and the social representations approach (Moscovici, 1976), which is the one currently in use. Currently, information-only programs have been abandoned.

Pre- and post-outcome evaluations of preventive programs, measuring changes in participant attitudes and personal perceptions, have been conducted and led by government institutions. Unfortunately, evaluations have not been completely integrated into most prevention programs, and this is precisely the challenge facing Mexico, despite the belief that evidence-based prevention programs are most appropriate for the field.

Mexico is aware that it is not easy to transpose research procedures that have been tested in small and controlled studies into real-world prevention programs. In addition, more often evaluations with positive results rather than ones with negative results are published, so the published analysis and findings may have a significant bias. These issues may limit dissemination of available research on drug prevention programs.

Twelve major programs or preventive actions based on models of intervention implemented in Mexico and with well-defined strategies have been chosen for inclusion in this chapter. Some have also reported evaluation results. They are summarized as follows:

1. *Leaving Marks in Your Life* (*Dejando Huellitas en tu vida*), aimed at elementary school students between second and fifth grades, reenforces social skills and includes parents, teachers, and health professionals (Gutiérrez, Villatoro, Gaytán, & Álamo, 2009).
2. *Yo Quiero Yo Puedo (I Want, I Can)* is a program for prevention of substance abuse for elementary school students in the fourth through sixth grades. Its goal is to stimulate the global development of individuals and to strengthen personal skills (Pick & Givaudan, 2006).
3. *Safe School Program (Escuela Segura)* provides a guide for teachers of elementary and secondary schools throughout Mexico. The program identifies environmental risks and teaches students how to make good decisions for a healthy life (Secretaría de Educación Pública de México, 2010).
4. *Build Yourself Program (Construye T)* is aimed at middle school children. It is dedicated to the development of childrens' life projects, to help them create protective networks and prevent their involvement in risky situations (UNESCO, 2010).
5. *Model of Education for Life and Work: Be Careful with Addictions (Modelo de educación para la vida y el trabajo: Aguas con las adicciones)* is a program for adults aimed at strengthening attitudes and skills to prevent drug abuse, through the analysis of lifestyles, risks, and structure of relationships (Instituto Nacional de México para la Educación de los Adultos, 2005).

6. *Preventive Model of Psychosocial Risks. Chimalli Knocks at your Door. (Modelo preventivo de riesgos psicosociales Chimalli toca a tu puerta)* is a method for developing new skills for tackling psychosocial risks such as drug use, inappropriate sexuality, and bad health habits among adolescents (INEPAR, 2012).
7. *National Information Campaign for a New Life (Campaña Nacional de información para una nueva vida)* is designed to protect all citizens' health through the definition and implementation of national policies regarding prevention, treatment, and training of professionals working in the field of addictions (Comisión Nacional de Cultura Física y Deporte, 2009).
8. *Model Eco 2 Intervention in Situations of Social Suffering (Modelo Eco 2 de intervención en situaciones de sufrimiento social)* is aimed at reducing harm and developing treatment strategies for drug abuse and the critical situations associated with it among adults (Machín, 2003).
9. *Model for Community Prevention "Wings" (Modelo de prevención comunitaria Alas)* is a system to train community leaders in order to create prevention networks capable of identifying problems, suggesting interventions, and evaluating action plans in high-risk and vulnerable communities, schools, households, and places of employment (Mateos et al., 2011).
10. *Models of Prevention Implemented in Youth Integration Centers (Modelo de prevención en Centros de Integración Juvenil)* has a general goal to diminish or delay drug use in high-risk populations. The overall target population is people between ten and fifty-four years of age, and the priority target group is people between ten and eighteen years (Consejo Nacional contra las Adicciones, 2003).
11. *Model for Prevention of Use of Alcohol, Tobacco, and Other Drugs in the Workplace (Modelo de prevención del uso de alcohol, tabaco y otras drogas en el lugar de trabajo)* has a purpose to develop and carry out prevention and assistance programs aimed at working populations, including families and communities (Consejo Nacional contra las Adicciones, 2003).
12. *National Program for Prevention of Violence and Crime (Programa Nacional de prevención de la violencia y la delincuencia)* is a governmental and national initiative that includes five types of prevention: social, situational, community, psychosocial, and police-based (Secretaría de Gobernación, 2014).

In reviewing the available literature on these twelve programs, there was wide variability in the type of information obtained about them. Some have scientific articles written about them, others are featured in popular articles, and some have developed implementation manuals. Some programs were developed through public institutions nationwide, whereas others were developed through foundations and associations of civil society. But the main issue is that prevention is a high priority in Mexico. The best-evaluated programs were Leaving Marks on Your Life, Chimalli Knocks at Your Door, and Model Eco2; Safe School and the National Campaign were largely acknowledged and accepted, but their evaluations were not very accurate.

Peru

Peru is a country located between Colombia, Equator, Brazil, and Bolivia, with an area of 1,285,000 square kilometers and a population of 30 million. Sharing many similar problems with Colombia, Peru became at one moment a reference center for prevention, and for that reason some private institutions have received international acknowledgment and support for their work in drug prevention.

Policies and Institutions

With the emergence of coca paste in the 1980s and the substantial business growth in coca crops (estimated in 1986 at 150,000 hectares), Peru had to take action in the field of drugs sooner than other countries of the continent. In 1986, the Centro de Información y Educación para la Prevención del Abuso de Drogas (CEDRO) was created as a nongovernment institution responsible for developing a comprehensive drug strategy, including preventive work related to the chain of production, trafficking, and consumption. Peru also began to exchange experiences with other LA countries, such as Bolivia, Brazil, Ecuador, Venezuela, and Colombia. This network of countries created at the time still stands. There also emerged a rich exchange with the United States and Europe, especially Spain (Red Iberoamericano de organización no gubernamental [RIOD], Cooperation Program on Drugs Policy [COPOLAD]) and the European Observatory on Drugs (EMCDDA). In 1996, Peru created a lead agency (originally called CONTRADROGAS, later renamed the National Commission for Development and Life without Drugs [DEVIDA]), which is mainly supported by civil society, including NGOs and the academic sector.

In the 1990s, there was a substantial decline in the production of coca leaves in Peru (associated with the defeat of the guerrilla Sendero Luminoso, international pressure for reducing coca crops, and the improvement of the Colombian coca bush quality). But in recent years, there has been a significant growth in Peruvian production, which has positioned Peru once more as the largest producer of coca leaves (although Colombia continues to be the number one producer of cocaine hydrochloride).

Epidemiologic studies show in recent years an increase of 150 percent of cocaine consumption in the coca leaf production areas (CEDRO, 2013). Prevention efforts made in the past two years have resulted in the development of a Peruvian National Strategy with clear indicators and targets to reduce drug use. The National Strategy (2012–16) was adopted by the Ministers of State, and sectors of the Executive branch provide technical assistance. The strategy, currently in force, suggests the need for shared work between society and the state, and greater interaction between government sectors, as well as with international organizations such as CICAD, OAS, COPOLAD (a collaboration program between the European Union and LA), and the United Nations in order to prevent and reduce drug use. It is important to work together with an aim to achieve greater effectiveness in actions. In Peru, the struggle against drugs, in all its dimensions, requires concrete and systematic actions to fully implement public policies.

Prevention

Twenty-five years ago, Peru began implementing, monitoring, and evaluating prevention programs. These years saw an increase in the systematization that allows for more precise evaluation of what are effective and noneffective practices in the field of prevention. During this time, many prevention programs were developed and implemented, such as Youth Leadership, Young Entrepreneurs, Young Journalists, and Welcome Centers. All these programs were aimed at adolescents in the coca producing areas. In the 1990s, prevention programs created and evaluated in other countries arrived in Peru, with the intention of adapting and evaluating them for their applicability in Peru. The best known is Strengthening Families (Familias Fuertes; Kumpfer & Alvarado, 2003). This program is currently being implemented in both urban and rural areas of Peru, with appropriate adaptations to Peruvian culture. The program is aimed, above all, toward parents, teachers, and tutors, with the purpose of teaching skills of negotiation and current concepts of discipline to replace punitive parenting practices.

Another program, SAVIA (CICAD, 2012), takes into account community settings and cultural diversity. This program looks for integration of local governments, families, and community leaders, giving them knowledge and prevention methods for early intervention. Teenagers are the target group. The program was produced and evaluated (with positive results) by CICAD and is currently in use in Peru and five other LA countries.

It is important to mention the program Cortes y Drogas (Courts and Drugs), which has been implemented since 2013, thanks to the synergy among health, justice, and civil society sectors. This program is aimed at young users of psychoactive substances. The program has proven to be effective, making it possible for young people who have not committed serious offences or a felony and who use substances to be rehabilitated in separate spaces outside prison that offer an alternative with a better prognosis compared to prison. The study by Droppelmann and Rebolledo (2010) in Chile showed that rehabilitation through the program Cortes tends to substantially reduce recidivism in drug-related crimes compared to punishment and penalties.

Three other programs are conducted as strategies of universal, selective, and indicated prevention. The first is similar to the second and is called Lugar de Escucha (Listening Place). This is a CEDRO program, employing face-to-face and virtual counseling as a way to prevent substance use. The second program is called Frank Talk (Habla Franco), an orientation and counseling phone service offered by the government agency of drug policy, DEVIDA. The third is a therapeutic program for adolescents and young adults who break the law and are heavy drug users. This program was developed by Peru's Public

Ministry of prosecutors and judges, and is listed in the National Strategy for Combating Drugs 2012 to 2016 (DEVIDA, 2012).

Uruguay

Uruguay is a small country (176,000 square kilometers) located in the south of the continent, between Argentina and Brazil. It's one of the wealthiest nations in the region, with one of the highest rates of education. Its population (3.3 million) is 90 percent from European origin. After twelve years of dictatorship (1973–85), Uruguay became a solid and advanced democracy. It is the first territory in Latin America (and the only one to date) where marijuana production and use is legal.

Policies and Institutions

The first institutional experiences with prevention and treatment of drug abuse began in Uruguay in 1970, although in isolated ways not only by type of drugs but also by lack of coordination between the agencies involved. Early efforts appeared in the public health sector, particularly from the Division of Mental Health, and with the creation of the Committee on Substance Abuse and the National Drugs Board in 1988 (Olivera, 2012).

The National Drugs Board (JND, by its acronym in Spanish), as established by Uruguay's National Strategy for addressing the drug problem (Infodrogas, 2011), is in the process of reviewing specific drug legislation referring to the law on narcotics (14,294) of October 31, 1974, and all modifications and subsequent regulations (National Council on Drugs, 2011, p. 17). Decree 463 established the creation of the National Drugs Board agency of the Presidency of the Republic in 1988, with interministerial character, to design national policies on drugs. The JND is chaired by the Secretary of the Presidency and composed of the Secretary General and Secretary General of the National Anti-Assets Laundering Secretariat (NAADS) (Junta Nacional de Drogas, 2011).

Prevention

The first formal prevention initiatives in drug prevention arose from the Ministry of Public Health during the 1970s, and were marked especially by the impact of legal drugs, that is, tobacco and alcohol and their involvement in diseases related to smoking and traffic accidents. The first campaigns promoting smoke-free environments appeared as strategies implemented by different institutions, including educational ones, and were related to the prevention of cancer.

In late 1980, several priority programs were created, including the Priority Prevention Program of Acquisition of Toxic Habits and Addictions. This program started from Public Health, working under the framework of the Health Promotion Division, and its emphasis was centered on improving the quality of life. In the mid-1990s, Alter-Actions was implemented, which presented scientific models to cope with drug abuse; and since 2002 another program called Ides is addressing harm reduction through an outreach strategies. More recently, the Department of Statistics of the Ministry of Public Health reported several studies showing that the country had managed to reduce transmissible (communicable) diseases, but showed a high prevalence of health problems related to social habits and behaviors related to lifestyles (Olivera, 2012).

From the creation of the JND (1988), a team of professionals was established whose main function was to provide technical support for the effective execution of the directives of the JND and gradually to generate what would become in 2002 the Uruguayan Observatory on Drugs (OUD, acronym in Spanish). Since the creation of OUD, the first systematic and national research data on local consumption of alcohol and drugs statistics became available. This team also presented rigorous recommendations for populations of higher vulnerability and informed the nation about what the most consumed drugs were and what would be the best preventive practices to follow. Currently, the OUD is a system of information and research on consumption and supply of drugs. The OUD generates data for analysis of trends in drug and alcohol usage, patterns, and drug traffic, and that data serve to improve the effectiveness of policies and programs under the National Strategy for Addressing the Drug Problem. OUD meets information requirements of national and international communities for comparison purposes. Also, the OUD collaborates with the Inter-American Observatory on Drugs of CICAD providing information and enhancing the comparability of data with other countries in the region. This supports the Multilateral Evaluation Mechanism of CICAD in order to analyze the effectiveness of drug policies in the member states of the OAS.

Although in the early 1980s symposia about drugs were organized by different NGOs and other civil society organizations, specialists in prevention and treatment of problematic drug use with expertise about and commitment to this issue were lacking. While Uruguay still has no specific academic training on the subject, conferences and fora allow for dissemination of information about the drug problem. The conferences and fora provide opportunities to listen to different voices, contributing to the creation of a fruitful analysis and an emerging generation of prevention specialists and proposals to combat drug problems. With the various government authorities and the secretary of each government at the head of the National Drugs Board, the first National Plan for the Prevention of Problematic Drug Use was developed in 1988 with two main axes: demand reduction and supply reduction.

In 2000, the press began to take part through the organization of different events, fora, and debates aimed at improving the approach to the drug problem through mass media presentations. This started the first massive public information campaigns, some rigorously designed and promoted by the National Drugs Board. The campaigns utilized studies on risk perception of alcohol and drug consumption in certain population segments.

Conclusions

The nine countries reported represent some of the main advances on alcohol and drug abuse prevention in Latin America. Some of the most relevant findings include the following:

1. Most countries have abandoned programs focused only on information dissemination and attitude change. Generally speaking, countries are looking for evidence-based programs. Even if foreign prevention programs are still largely in use, in some cases they have been validated with local populations. There is also a notable interest in developing local programs that more directly consider the country's needs. This is happening in Mexico and Peru, where local initiatives have been developed and some of them are under evaluation. Chile was one of the first in the region to create programs widely used in Chile and other LA countries. Costa Rica has just one program, but with a national coverage and positive evaluations over several years. Colombia, Argentina, Uruguay, and El Salvador have been implementing foreign programs, sometimes without adequate adaptations, but this situation is changing. Currently, there is a growing awareness about the need for systematic evaluations that has led to the finding that direct translation of prevention activities is not always a good decision. Brazil is developing several prevention initiatives, but because of its huge population, it will need several years before reaching sufficient coverage throughout the country.
2. Because of the increase of drug use in LA since the middle of the 1980s, and the growing interest among the authorities as well as among the general population, many countries created at least one governmental institution in charge of all the issues related to alcohol and drug consumption and abuse. In every country, such institutions (or new ones with similar purposes) are in force. All countries studied have developed national policies on prevention, and international institutions (e.g., United Nations, CICAD/OAS, European Union) have supported these initiatives. In most countries, civil society, universities, and nonprofit organizations also support governmental initiatives.
3. There are no academic training programs on prevention. Those interested in formal academic training in prevention must attend universities in other countries (e.g., the United States, Canada, Spain). However, in some LA countries, symposia, conferences, and workshops are provided as a means to educate about prevention and share information and research.
4. While there are important differences among countries, all have developed research and evaluation structures, although in many cases these structures are weak and poorly funded. In this context, evaluation and assessment must become a priority to advance the prevention field.
5. The main barriers to successful prevention in LA are basically two: the poor knowledge among those in charge of political decisions about what

"prevention" means; and the irregular funding of prevention initiatives, which makes failure more likely because prevention initiatives must, by definition, be sustained long term.

6. The alcohol and drug problem will be present in LA for a long time. It is essential that academic institutions, and particularly universities, become involved in the construction, development, and implementation of preventive programs, as well as in the evaluation processes aimed at demonstrating their effectiveness. It is equally important to articulate all the components of preventive strategies, including developing mass media messages linked to community interventions, teaching child and adolescent skill development, reducing school dropouts, promoting healthy and creative use of leisure time, and promoting youth participation in the planning and implementation of activities that affect their everyday lives.

After many years of a little erratic search of strategies for tackling the alcohol and drug abuse problem among minors, LA seems currently engaged in the right pathway: instead of just importing foreign programs, the process of adapting and evaluating them, as well as the process of creating local programs, has started in several countries almost simultaneously. At the same time, governments are developing modern, evidence-based policies that transform the problem into a public health issue and are replacing the traditional criminal approach. "Preparation of this chapter was done with the collaboration of : Juan Carlos Mansilla and Alberto Calabrese (Argentina); Sheila G. Murta, Samia Abreu and Maria Inês Gandolfo Conceição (Brazil); Felipe Leyton (Chile); Vera Barahona and Julio Bejarano (Costa Rica); Cristina Amaya (El Salvador); María Elena Castro, Nancy Amador, Jorge Amath Villatoro and Jorge Llanes (México); Carmen Masías (Perú); Gabriela Olivera (Uruguay)."

References

Abreu, S. (2012). *Prevenção em saúde mental no Brasil: a perspectiva da literatura e de especialistas da área (Dissertação de Mestrado não publicada)*. Brasília, Brasil: Instituto de Psicologia da Universidade de Brasília.

Aja Eslava, L., & Gómez Avila, J. (2013). Evaluación y seguimiento de un programa de prevención de consumo de SPA y riesgo de suicidio: 1999–2012. *Tipica Boletín Electrónico de Salud Escolar* 9(2).

Arratia, A., Barkan, A., Jimenez, S., Leyton, F., Miroshnick, Z., & Ugarte, F., (2013). *Construyendo Culturas Preventivas: Guía para el abordaje del consumo y tráfico de drogas y alcohol desde las comunidades educativas*, Chile: SENDA.

Becoña, E. (2002). Bases científicas de la prevención de las drogodependencias.

Bejarano, J. (1992). *La evaluación cuantitativa de campañas antidrogas, En Comunicación contra las Drogas*, Quito, Ecuador: Ed. Quipus.

Bejarano, J. (2005). Alcohol, gender and partner aggression: a study in the Greater Metropolitan Area of Costa Rica. En Obot, I., & Room, R. (eds.), *Alcohol, Gender and Drinking Problems: Perspectives from Low and Middle Income Countries*. Geneva, Switzerland: World Health Organization.

Bejarano, J., Carvajal, H., & San Lee, L. (1992). *El fenómeno de la farmacodependencia en el estudiante de primer ingreso a las universidades estatales de Costa Rica: percepciones de riesgo y consumo*. San José, Costa Rica: Instituto sobre Alcoholismo y Farmacodependencia.

Blanco, C., & Sandí, L. (1993). *Proyecto de vigilancia epidemiológica sobre uso indebido de sustancias psicotrópicas*. San José, Costa Rica: Instituto sobre Alcoholismo y Farmacodependencia.

Boletín Oficial de Argentina (1972). *Decreto 452.*

Botvin, G. J., & Griffin, K. W. (2004). Life Skills Training: empirical findings and future directions. *Journal of Primary Prevention* 25 (2): 211–32.

Carlini, E. A., Noto, A. R., & Sanchez, Z. M. (2010). *VI Levantamento Nacional sobre o Consumo de Drogas Psicotrópicas entre Estudantes do Ensino Fundamental e Médio de Ensino das Redes Públicas e Privadas nas 27 Capitais Brasileiras – 2010*. São Paulo: CEBRID – Centro Brasileiro de Informações sobre Drogas Psicotrópicas, Departamento de Psicobiologia, UNIFESP – Universidade Federal de São Paulo.

CEDRO (Centro de Información y Educación para la Prevención del Abuso de Drogas) (2103). *Estudio sobre consumo de drogas*. Lima: CEDRO.

Centro de la Promoción de Equidad University of Oregon & GIZ (2014). Strong Global Communities: International Conferencie on Prevention Implementation. Eugene, Oregon, April 28–29.

CICAD (International Commission for Drug Abuse Control) (2012). Programa SAVIA Drogas. www.adiccionesxxi.info/2012/02/programa-savia-drogascicad.html

CICAD (International Commission for Drug Abuse Control)/OAS (Organization of American States) (2009). *Multilateral Evaluation Mechanism (MEM)*. Washington, DC: Rounds. cicad.oas.org/mem/reports/5/Full_Eval/Brasil%20-%205ta%20Rd%20-%20POR.pdf

Committee for Children (2002). *Second Step: A Violence Prevention Curriculum*. Seattle, WA: Author.

Comisión Nacional de Cultura Física y Deporte (2009). *Campaña Nacional de Información para una Nueva Vida*. deporte.org.mx/af08/ime/26_10_2009/Campana_Nacional_de_Informacion_para_una_Nueva_Vida.pdf

Conceição, M. I. G., & Oliveira, M. C. S. L. (2008). A relação adolescente-drogas e as perspectivas da nova legislação sobre drogas. *Revista de Informação Legislativa*, 45: 253–62.

Consejo Nacional contra las Adicciones (2003). *Modelos preventivos*. www.uade.inpsiquiatria.edu.mx/pagina_contenidos/libros/modelos_preventivos.pdf

DEVIDA (National Commission for Development and Life without Drugs) (2012). *Estrategia Nacional de Lucha contra las Drogas 2012–2016*. Lima: DEVIDA.

DIPRES (Dirección de Presupuestos) (2001), Informe de Programa de Evaluación de Proyectos Gubernamentales. www.dipres.gob.cl/594/w3-propertyvalue-15221.html

DIPRES (Dirección de Presupuestos) (2013), Informe de Programa de Evaluación de Proyectos Gubernamentales. www.dipres.gob.cl/594/w3-propertyvalue-15221.html

Droppelmann, C., & Rebolledo, L. (2010). *Tribunales de tratamiento de drogas: resultados y desafíos*. Santiago, Chile; Fundación Paz Ciudadana, Fiscalía y CONACE.

Galduróz, J. C. F., Noto, A. R., Fonseca, A. M., & Carlini, E. A. (2005). *V Levantamento Nacional sobre o Consumo de Drogas Psicotrópicas entre Estudantes do Ensino*

Fundamental e Médio da Rede Pública de Ensino nas 27 Capitais Brasileiras – 2004. São Paulo: CEBRID – Centro Brasileiro de Informações sobre Drogas Psicotrópicas, Departamento de Psicobiologia, UNIFESP – Universidade Federal de São Paulo.

Giacomozzi, A. I., Itokasu, M. C., Luzardo, A. R., & Vieira, I. (2012). Levantamento sobre Uso de Álcool e Outras Drogas e Vulnerabilidades Relacionadas de Estudantes de Escolas Públicas Participantes do Programa Saúde do Escolar/ Saúde e Prevenção nas Escolas no município de Florianópolis. *Saúde e Sociedade* 21(3): 612–22.

Gutiérrez, M., Villatoro, J., Gaytán, L., & Álamo, A. (2009). Manual del programa de prevención de habilidades sociales "Dejando huellitas en tu vida." Segunda edición. www.uade.inpsiquiatria.edu.mx/pagina_contenidos/libros/huellitas.pdf

Hawkins, J. D., & Catalano, R. (1992). *Communities That Care*. San Francisco, CA: Jossey-Bass.

INEPAR (Instituto de Educación Preventiva y Atención de Riesgos) (2012). *Modelo preventivo de riesgos psicosociales "Chimalli toca a tu puerta."* Retrieved from www.inepar.edu.mx/INEPAR/

Infodrogas (2011). *Estrategia Nacional para el abordaje del problema drogas 2011–2015*. Retrieved from www.infodrogas.gub.uy

Instituto Nacional de México para la Educación de los Adultos (2005). Modelo deEducación para la Vida y el Trabajo. Aguas con las adicciones. www.conevyt.org.mx/cursos/para_asesor/auto_asesores/cd/saber_mas_mevyt/aguas_adicciones_3a/1_AA_libro.pdf

Juárez, C. (2013). Limitaciones y desafíos para la evaluación de programas de prevención del consumo de sustancias psicoactivantes en El Salvador. Retrieved from www.seguridad.gob.sv/observatorio/

Junta Nacional de Drogas, Presidencia de la República Oriental del Uruguay (2011). Estrategia Nacional para el abordaje del problema drogas 2011–2015. Materiales educativo-preventivos para familias, educadores y equipo socio sanitarios. www.infodrogas.gub.uy

Kumpfer, K. L., & Alvarado, R. (2003). Family-dash strengthening approaches for the prevention of youth problem behaviors. *American Psychologist* 58: (6–7): 457–65.

Lions Quest (2015). Lions' Quest history. Retrieved from lions-quest.org/history.php

Machín, J. (2003). La prevención de las farmacodependencias en el Modelo ECO 2. www.liberaddictus.org/Pdf/0799–75.pdf

Mateos, L., González, A., Morales, M., González, A., Trejo, O., Díaz, T., Arguelles, R., & Osorio, R. (2011). El Sistema de Prevención selectiva comunitaria Alas Vivas. www.grupotellso.com/INEPAR/pdf/descargas/articulos%20spsc%20alas%20vivas%2015%20dic.pdf

Ministerios de Justicia, Educación y Salud (2011). *Estudio nacional sobre consumo de sustancias psicoactivas en población escolar*. Bogota: ALVI Impresores.

Ministerios de Justicia y Salud (2014). *Estudio nacional de consumo de sustancias psicoactivas en Colombia 2013*. Bogota: ALVI Impresores.

Moscovici, S. (1976). *Social Influence and Social Change*. London: Academic Press.

Murillo, F., & curso COPOLAD (Cooperation Program on Drugs Policy) (2013). Consumo de alcohol y otras drogas: Prevención basada en la evidencia, Caso estudio. Programa de prevención universal. Unpublished manuscript.

Observatorio Chileno de Drogas (2015). Las principales estadísticas sobre consumo de drogas y alcohol de la serie de Estudios de Población General de SENDA, de 1994a 2012. Retrieved from www.senda.gob.cl/observatorio

Olivera, Gabriela, (2012) *Reseña de los avances y desafíos en Prevención de consumos problemáticos de drogas en Uruguay*. Montevideo, Uruguay Junta Nacional de Drogas.

Pérez Gómez, A. (1989). *Bogotá and the Consumption of Psychoactive Substances: A Study, a Solution*. Bogota: Mayorship of Bogotá.

Pérez Gómez, A. (2007). *Transiciones en el consumo de drogas en Colombia*. Bogota: Dupligráficas Ltda.

Pérez Gómez, A. (2010). *Estudio nacional de consumo de sustancias psicoactivas en adolescentes en conflicto con la ley en Colombia*. Bogota: ICBF, MIJ, DNE.

Pérez Gómez, A. (2011). *Contexto de vulnerabilidad al VIH/Sida en los grupos deconsumidores de drogas de alto riesgo (CODAR) en las ciudades de Medellín y Armenia*. Bogota: Ministerio de la Protección Social.

Pérez Gómez, A. (2013). Colombia fuera del ojo del huracán pero todavía cerca. *Editorial Revista Adicciones* 25(2): 106–8.

Pérez Gómez, A., & Scoppetta D.G. O. (2009). *Consumo de alcohol en menores de 18 años en Colombia*. Bogota: Nuevos Rumbos.

Pérez Gómez, A., Valencia, J. E. & Rodríguez, C. (2006). Fracciones atribuibles drogas/crimen en adultos. Unpublished manuscript.

Pick, S., & Givaudan, M. (2006). "Yo quiero, yo puedo": estrategia para el desarrollo de habilidades y competencias en el sistema escolar. *Psicologia da Educaçao Sao Paulo* 23: 203–21. yoquieroyopuedo.org.mx/app/webroot/pdfs/Yo%20quiero%20Yo%20puedo%20Estrategia%20%28estudios%20pos-grados%20puc-sp%29.pdf

Política Nacional sobre Drogas (2005). Resolução N°3/GSIPR/CH/CONAD. Retrieved from www.senad.gov.br/

RUMBOS (2002). *Juventud y consumo de sustancias psicoactivas: Colombia 2001*. Bogota: Presidencia de la República.

Salas, C. (2014). *Impacto económico del consumo de sustancias psicoactivas en Costa Rica 2011*. San José, Costa Rica: Instituto sobre Alcoholismo y Farmacodependencia.

Secretaria de Educación Pública de México (2010). *Guía para alumnos de tercero y cuartode primaria. Me valoro y aprendo a cuidarme*. basica.sep.gob.mx/escuelasegura/pdf/guias/guiaAlum3y4.pdf.

Secretaría de Gobernación (2014). Programa nacional para la prevención social de la violencia y la delincuencia 2014 – 2018. Retrieved on December 17, 2014, from http://www.dof.gob.mx/nota_detalle.php?codigo=5343087&fecha=30/04/2014.

SENDA (National Service for Prevention and Rehabilitation of Drug Use and Alcoho) (2013). *Construyendo Culturas Preventivas*. Santiago, Chile: Ministerio delInterior.

UNESCO (United Nations Educational, Scientific, and Cultural Organization) (2010). Evaluación del programa Construye T.: informe final de la primera fasede evaluación de procesos. www.unicef.org/evaluation/files/Mexico_2010-007_Informe_final_Octubre_2010_Construye-T.pdf

UNODC (United Nations Office on Drugs and Crime)/CICAD (International Commission for Drug Abuse Control) (2009). *Estudio comparativo sobre consumo de drogas en la población general en seis países sudamericanos*. Washington, DC: OID.

33 Effectiveness of Brief Prevention Programs for Adolescents in Mexico

Susan Pick, Delil Athié, & Anna-Emilia Hietanen

Introduction

Many studies show that prevention programs can make a difference in health outcomes (Álvarez–Alva, 2012; Sumnal, 2014). In many countries, school-based prevention programs have been used as an effective way to reach children and adolescents (e.g., Wang et al., 2008; WHO, 2009a,b). However, for successful implementation of school-based prevention programs in Mexico, it is crucial to understand that the importance of prevention is not widely accepted in Mexico (e.g., Bronfman, Castro, Zúñiga, Miranda, & Oviedo, 1997a). Its acceptance is lacking whether among social, economic, and human development agencies or among the public health or educational sectors. Prevention is also not a widely accepted social norm in households (Lara-Esquivel, Torres-Muñoz, & Moreno-Gómez, 2012). Given this state of affairs, the probability of successful implementation of prevention programs, both in the schools' and the communities' context, is higher if it is of short duration rather than of long duration. Once such a short-term prevention program is successful, it may open the road to more comprehensive and long-term programming.

Many public health issues can be addressed through short-term programs. One key example is the prevention of gender violence. In Mexico, violent romantic relationships start already in adolescence: 15 percent of the fifteen to twenty-four year olds have suffered from at least one violent incident in their current relationship (Encuesta Nacional de la Violencia en las Relaciones de Noviazgo; ENVINOV, 2007). Dating violence is normative among Mexican adolescents, which is why the problem remains invisible (De Jesús, 2011). Adolescents usually do not have enough knowledge regarding violence to enable them to distinguish between love and violent behaviors, for example, resulting from jealousy (ENVINOV, 2007). Because of the perceived normalcy of the violent behaviors, there is also little institutional or family support for the victims (Ramírez Rivera & Núñez Luna, 2010).

In addition to violence, there are other preventable public health problems that affect Mexican adolescents, such as alcohol abuse and health problems related to poor nutrition. Regarding alcohol abuse, it is alarming that in 2011, 4.1 percent of Mexican adolescents showed signs of alcohol dependence (INSP, 2012). Obesity in Mexico among adolescents is enormous: 35.8 percent of girls and 34.1 percent of boys aged twelve to nineteen are overweight or obese in Mexico (ENSANUT, 2012), which puts them at grave risk to develop type 2 diabetes or other diseases early in life. This problem is similar in other countries in Latin America, such as Argentina, Chile, the Dominican Republic, Uruguay, and Venezuela, and even in countries in other regions such as Australia, Canada, Germany, Greece, New Zealand, and the United Kingdom (WHO, 2009b). Preventing these problems in adolescence is important, as many long-term behaviors and lifestyles are developed and established during adolescence, sometimes leading to numerous problems in the future (e.g., Graber, Hill, & Saczawa, 2014).

Social Norms That Affect Prevention Efforts in Mexico

For the implementation of effective prevention programs, it is important to consider cultural factors, as they can create both favorable conditions and barriers to prevention efforts (Nation et al., 2003; González Castro, Barrera, & Martínez, 2004). In Mexico, certain cultural traits, such as paternalism, fatalism, and strong traditional gender roles, are factors that need to be taken into account in developing and implementing prevention programs.

Mexico has traditionally been both a fatalistic and paternalistic society (Pick & Hietanen, 2014). Paternalism refers to the belief that different kinds of authorities, both religious and secular, are supposed to know better what is good or bad for an individual (Pick & Hietanen, 2014). Individuals are not seen as capable of nor allowed to make decisions or take control over their own lives. These kinds of paternalistic attitudes are present in politicians' relationships to citizens, in schools and workplaces and also inside families, as children are not supposed to question their parents (Pick & Sirkin, 2010). Fatalism refers to a feeling of powerlessness, believing that a higher power determines one's destiny, which leads many people to accept passively even harsh conditions instead of trying to change them. Fatalistic ideas – related not only to divine authorities but also to secular and temporal symbols considered unassailable (such as the President) – limit proactiveness and personal initiative and can lead to a sensation of impotency over one's life and environment (Diaz-Guerrero, 1982). Studies show that fatalistic ideas are often risk factors for health, as individuals do not feel that taking control over their behaviors or habits will have an effect on their health (Espinosa de los Monteros & Gallo, 2013; Soto et al., 2011). Latinos are more likely than Anglos to endorse fatalistic statements; for example, a higher proportion of Latinos believed that having cancer is like getting a death sentence (46 percent vs. 26 percent), that cancer is God's punishment (7 percent vs. 2 percent), and that there is very little one can do to prevent getting cancer (26 percent vs. 18 percent) (Pérez-Stable, Sabogal, Otero-Sabogal, Hiatt, & McPhee, 1992).

Traditional gender roles are also a cultural factor that affects many areas of life and can hinder prevention efforts in relation to many public health behaviors, such as sexual and reproductive health, gender violence, and substance use and abuse. In Mexico, traditional gender stereotypes are still strong (Pick & Sirkin, 2010), especially in rural areas. Even though law reforms (e.g., a law approved in 2013 by Congress incorporating obligation of the state to promote the fight against any sort of discrimination based on gender; curiously enough, it does not refer to prevention) have improved women's position in the last decades, traditional gender roles still limit women's and girl's development. Mexico is a masculine society, where men are expected to be tough, assertive, and dominant and women submissive and obedient (Hietanen & Pick, 2015; Safdar & Kosakowska-Berezecka, 2015).

Traditionally, Mexican men are expected constantly to prove their virility and manhood and avoid behaviors that are considered as "feminine" (e.g., not to take risks, depend on other people, express feelings such as fear, and show weakness) and that can cast doubt on a man's virility and masculinity (Badinter, 1993; Mora, 2006). This need to prove one's manhood is visible in many risk behaviors, such as in early sexual initiation, having many sex partners, and not using a condom (having many children, after all, is a sign of a potent man) (Amuchástegui & Rivas, 2004; Szasz, 1998). Young men also often try to prove their courage by recklessness in driving. *Machismo* has also been associated with young men's drug and alcohol use as a way to assert their masculinity and fearlessness (Soto et al., 2011). In addition, taking care of one's health is not seen as an important part of masculine socialization, and talking about health problems is considered as a sign of weakness, which can be an obstacle for prevention programs (De Keijzer, 2001).

In the case of women, *machismo* works in a different way. Women are supposed to be sexually modest and inexperienced and show no sexual desire; condom use is associated with strongly frowned upon occasional sex and promiscuity. Wanting to use a condom or other preventive or contraceptive methods can make a woman look suspicious, easy, and sexually active, thus risking her reputation and social status and even her possibilities of finding a stable romantic relationship and marrying (Szasz, 1998; Villegas, Lemanski, & Valdéz, 2010). In relation to substance abuse, *machismo* is seen as having an opposite effect on women than on men. Traditionally, women are expected to devote themselves to their family, sacrificing their own interests. In this context, women's alcohol use is seen as rebellious and unacceptable (Soto et al., 2011).

Gender stereotypes are related to high levels of gender violence. Women's greater access to education and political power in the last decades has slowly started to change their social position (Mejia-Arauz, Sheets, & Villaseñor, 2012). However, men's gender roles continue to be restrictive, and violence is sometimes used by men to control women and to address this seeming threat to their traditional social roles and power (Jewkes, 2002).

In addition, psychosocial barriers should be taken into account in implementing prevention programs. In Mexico, the pressure to conform to social norms is strong. Individuals, both male and female, are expected to be respectful and obedient of what is socially acceptable, even if it means putting aside one's own interests (Gongora Coronado, Cortes Ayala, & Flores Galaz, 2002; Peterson & Hennon, 2006; Pick & Sirkin, 2010). That is to say that many social norms reinforce gender stereotypes. Emotions are used as an important psychosocial mechanism to maintain and reproduce existing and traditionally accepted social norms. Fear, guilt, and shame regulate behaviors, as people fear to be exposed and scorned if they transgress the social norms or if they do not live up to the community standards. These emotions function as psychosocial barriers and limit an individual's capacity to take autonomous decisions and actions (Pick, Beers, & Grossman-Crist, 2011; Pick & Hietanen, 2014; Pick & Sirkin, 2010).

Life Skills in Prevention

During the last years, the Mexican public health sector has increased efforts to promote healthy habits and prevention of health problems, both in communicable and noncommunicable diseases. However, national statistics show that the prevalence of preventable diseases, such as diabetes mellitus, cardiovascular diseases, breast and cervical cancer, cirrhosis and other liver diseases, and HIV/AIDS, has not diminished; in fact, many have become more frequent (WHO, 2006). Since these diseases are among the most frequent causes of death in Mexico it can be concluded that health promotion and prevention strategies have not been implemented properly, if at all (Lara-Esquival, et al., 2012).

Caballero Hoyosa et al. (2006) have pointed out that one of the reasons for the inefficiency of the prevention programs is the lack of community participation. In Mexico, the official health system has favored vertical prevention programs that do not promote active community participation. In multicultural contexts, such as Mexico, it would be important to integrate the point of the view of the communities and take into account the cultural and social factors that affect health and the values and meanings associated with health and diseases and prevention of and attention to health problems (Caballero Hoyosa et al., 2006). One way of doing this is through the establishment of prevention programs on the basis of extensive diagnostic studies in which the needs of the community are included, thus leading to a higher likelihood of community members' feelings of ownership and sustainability.

In addition, public health prevention strategies in Mexico, such as HIV prevention programs, breast and cervical cancer prevention programs, and diabetes and cardiovascular diseases prevention programs, have concentrated on providing general information on health issues rather than on facilitating specific positive changes in behaviors (Secretaría de Salud, 2007, 2013). In addition, many programs emphasize negative health consequences of certain habits, such as substance abuse and tobacco use, which may be ineffective for those who have fatalistic ideas and do not feel that they have control over their personal health (Soto et al., 2011).

In any case, information on correct and healthy behaviors is not enough to change behaviors; motivation, skills to realize relevant behaviors (planning activities, negotiating to get family support, choosing healthy food, etc.), and a positive attitude toward adopting a different behavior (Fishbein & Ajzen, 1975; Lara-Esquival et al., 2012; Venguer, Pick, & Fishbein, 2007) are also key components in initiating a desirable change. Hence, prevention programs should promote a positive environment that favors positive attitudes and the practice of healthy habits (Lara-Esquival et al., 2012). Moreover, knowing something does not mean that one knows how to do it; it is key to develop the relevant skills, self-efficacy, personal and social norms, and attitudes to change behaviors effectively (Bandura, 2000, 2001; Piña & Robles, 2005; Pick and Sirkin, 2010; Pick et al., 2011). One way of addressing these issues is to promote life skills acquisition – for example, decision making, problem solving, empathy, assertive communication, negotiation, team building, self-knowledge, and management of emotions (Mangrulkar, Whitman, & Posner, 2001; WHO, 1997). The utility of life skills education has been proven in various countries and with regard to the prevention of different kinds of problems, such as violence, substance abuse, sexually transmitted infections (STIs), gender inequality, and disease prevention (Leenen et al., 2008; Pick et al., 2011; Venguer et al., 2007; WHO, 1999).

The Mexican institution Yo quiero Yo puedo ("I want to, I can") programs follow such a line of reasoning. Namely, Yo quiero Yo puedo-IMIFAP was a pioneer in the design and implementation of programs that promote life skills, thus enabling people to overcome psychosocial and cultural factors that can hinder prevention efforts, such as fatalistic ideas and gender stereotypes (Givaudan, Van de Vijver, Poortinga, Leenen, & Pick, 2007; Pick, Givaudan, Sirkin, & Ortega, 2007; Pick & Sirkin, 2010). The Yo quiero Yo puedo programs also address the psychosocial barriers (e.g., fear, shame, guilt, resentment, and prejudice) that affect individuals' capacity to take autonomous decisions and actions. Two examples will be presented here to provide empirical evidence of these programs effectiveness.

The Effectiveness of Short-Term Programs – Two Case Studies

The Mexican nongovernmental organization (NGO) Yo quiero Yo puedo-IMIFAP (originally IMIFAP: Instituto Mexicano de Investigación de Familia y Población, A.C.) has worked since 1985 with life skills–based prevention programs for adolescents in themes related to prevention of violence, school dropout, HIV/AIDS and other sexually transmitted diseases, unplanned pregnancies, alcohol abuse, and tobacco and illegal drug use.

Another feature of Yo quiero Yo puedo-IMIFAP is the commitment to find ways to apply the principles underlying longer-term programs (i.e., at least twenty-four to forty hours in a span of two to twelve weeks) within shorter versions (i.e., two to eight hours in a span of one to three weeks). It should be noted that, generally speaking, we argue that successful brief programs, based on life skills and reduction of psychosocial barriers, can be effective in fostering sensitivity among the relevant population and authorities regarding knowledge, social norms, attitudes, and behaviors being targeted by each prevention program.

The following are the presentations of two short programs that Yo quiero Yo puedo-IMIFAP has adapted for implementation among Mexican adolescents as the target group: the first one is, "I want to, I can … prevent dating violence," and the second one is, "Tracing my own destiny." These two programs present two different strategies for brief preventative programs. The first consists of a two-hour experiential interactive conference intended to directly prevent adolescents dating violence. The latter is a multithematic program that centers on preventing risk behaviors in dating violence and bullying, substance abuse, and nutrition. It consists of eight-hour-long experiential workshops for teachers, who then are expected to administer the program contents and methodology with their students. Also, in the second program, parents participate in the program through interactive talks of two hours.

"I Want to, I Can… Prevent Dating Violence"

Popular conceptions of romantic love often legitimate male dominance, jealousy, and controlling and violent behaviors as something normal in a romantic relationship (Wood, 2001). The objective of the "I want to, I can … prevent dating violence" program is to foster adolescents' sensitization on dating violence by involving them in interactive talks. These talks facilitate the acquisition of knowledge on violence, so that the participants can recognize different forms and types and understand the violence risk factors, both as a victim and as an aggressor, including false beliefs on romantic love.

The program was implemented in middle schools and high schools of five states in Mexico from September 2013 to June 2014. Altogether, forty-six experiential talks were facilitated in an interactive manner by a group dynamics specialist, addressing the total amount of 2,116 adolescents, 47 percent male and 53 percent female, as well as educational materials dealing with identification and prevention of violence. Fifteen talks were given in the State of Chihuahua; twelve in Chiapas; twelve in Hidalgo; six in Coahuila; and one in the capital of the country, Mexico City (Barriga, García, Givaudan, & Pick, 2014).

The two-hour interactive talks were given by a training expert, using a presentation with key messages and specific game activities so that adolescents could analyze their own attitudes, behaviors, and social norms regarding dating violence. The specific contents that were addressed included friendship and dating relationships, gender stereotypes and roles, beliefs about romantic love, dating violence, types and forms of violence, violence consequences, violence prevention strategies, and life skills such as communication and decision making. To analyze the effects of the interactive talks, a pre-post design with two samples was used. A self-report questionnaire was administered consisting of forty-nine questions that are divided into three domains: (1) knowledge on dating violence; (2) attitudes toward violence; and (3) beliefs about romantic love. At the end of the questionnaire, there were two open-ended questions on (a) what the respondent liked most about the program and (b) what the participant considered was the most important information he or she learned about violence. In each talk, the self-report questionnaire was administered to five voluntary participants before the lecture and to five voluntary participants after the talk. Voluntary in this context merely means that we approached a group and asked who would like to answer a few questions on dating violence. Five of those who accepted were chosen at random. In total, 269 questionnaires were administered before and 238 after the talks. The participants were 46.8 percent male and 53.2 percent female. The mean age of the participants was 15.5 years (Barriga et al., 2014).

The evaluation of the results of the interactive talks show that the talks increased participants' knowledge about violence. After the talks, 44 percent of the participants, as compared to 21 percent before the talks ($X^2 = 28.149$, $p = 0.000$), had a level of knowledge on dating violence, its early detection, and prevention considered to be sufficient[1]; and on the concept of violence, its different forms, and risk and protective factors. After the talks, more adolescents knew that the objective of violence is to control or dominate someone (68 percent vs. 57 percent) ($X^2 = 6.613$, $p = 0.010$), that ignoring someone can be a form of violence (67 percent vs. 43 percent) ($X^2 = 29.001$, $p = 0.000$), that the traditionally accepted conception among many Mexican groups demanding the romantic partner to explain his or her use of money is a form of violence (60 percent vs. 33 percent) ($X^2 = 36.841$, $p = 0.000$), that physical violence does not always leave visible marks (28 percent vs. 16 percent) ($X^2 = 10.414$, $p = 0.001$), that life skills help to prevent violence (76 percent vs. 62 percent) ($X^2 = 11.356$, $p = 0.001$), and that being jealous is not a demonstration of love (81 percent vs. 68 percent) ($X^2 = 11.085$, $p = 0.001$) (Barriga et al., 2014).

A comparison between the rates of respondents who were in favor of violence did not change significantly between the pre-talk and the post-talk measurements. However, it should be noted that this rate was low already in the pre-talk measurement. Even before the talks, the participants presented low levels of attitudes that favor violence (e.g., belief that a woman supports violence because she likes it; belief that if someone is violent, you can behave the same way). This shows that certain cultural and gender stereotypes were originally not accepted by participants. However, there were favorable and statistically significant changes in other attitudes that are related to dating violence prevention. After the talks, more adolescents accepted the idea that violence can be prevented (33 percent after the talks compared to 21 percent before the talks) ($X^2 = 16.285$, $p = 0.001$) and that a person can decide to be violent or not (45 percent after the talks compared to 36 percent before the talks) ($X^2 = 14.333$, $p = 0.002$). Fewer participants (14 percent vs. 24 percent) thought

1 Considering the difficulty level of the questions to address knowledge, 6 points or more in a scale from 1 to 10 was established as a sufficient level of knowledge.

that psychological violence is less harmful than physical violence ($X^2 = 8.719$, $p = 0.033$); that love means suffering (26 percent vs. 37 percent) ($X^2 = 9.728$, $p = 0.021$); that it is good to sacrifice oneself for the romantic partner (20 percent vs. 30 percent) ($X^2 = 10.098$, $p = 0.018$); and that to avoid problems, it is best not to say what one feels or thinks (70 percent vs. 82 percent) ($X^2 = 11.148$, $p = 0.011$).

All these changes indicate a greater rejection of violence following the participation in "I want to, I can … prevent dating violence" short-term program (Barriga et al., 2014). Even though the total rate of participants who were holding mistaken beliefs regarding the role of violence in expressing love was relatively low, both before (14.8 percent) and after (20 percent) the talks (Barriga et al., 2014), that significant and positive change in attitudes against dating violence – that is, positive attitudes toward prevention, of what sacrifice entails, of the role of emotional violence, and a better understanding of myths regarding the role of violence in the expression of love – are an important advancement toward better prevention and early detection of dating violence.

The following testimonials exemplify the results:

> My boyfriend does all these things of romantic love and I thought it was ok that he is jealous of me, but I have to think more whether I really want those things for me. – sixteen-year-old female college student in Chiapas (Barriga et al., 2014).
>
> I learned that we need to have healthy relationships in our home and school, that we must not be violent in different ways that exist and that we need to learn to know ourselves and defend our rights. … I liked that we could participate and act because that way I think we learn better. – fifteen-year-old male high school student in Coahuila (Barriga et al., 2014).
>
> In the beginning of the talks I thought it would be boring to talk about violence (we are already fed up with that theme), but when we started to talk about the difference between love and falling in love, violence and aggression, violent behaviors … I realized that it is easy to confuse jealousy with love, (and) how we are living and reproducing violence in our romantic relationship without noticing. I learned a lot. – fifteen-year-old male high school student in Coahuila (Barriga et al., 2014).

These examples show how short-term intervention fosters significant changes in Mexican adolescents' knowledge, attitudes, social norms, and beliefs, thus paving the way for the improvement of prevention efforts of maladaptive and risky behavior.

"Tracing My Own Destiny" – a Comprehensive Program on Violence Prevention, Nutrition, and Substance Abuse Prevention

The general objective of the "Tracing my own destiny" program is to promote healthy lifestyles (preventing risk behaviors of alcohol abuse and facilitating healthy nutrition and exercise habits) and prevention of violence (bullying and dating violence) among adolescents. Practically, changes should come about through programs that impact the following components: (a) life skills and knowledge; (b) reduction of psychosocial barriers to (c) behavior and (d) norm and attitude change; (e) development of personal agency; and (f) intrinsic empowerment. Therefore, upon the development of these six components, the multithematic program is focused on (1) prevention of bullying and dating violence; (2) prevention of alcohol abuse; and (3) promotion of healthy habits, such as nutrition and exercise (Ramírez et al., 2014).

Program implementation includes different strategies: training high school teachers as replicators of the program; follow-up of the teachers during the replication of the program with students; interactive talks with parents; educational fairs; a web page for teachers, students, and parents; and elaboration of electronic bulletins published in the web page. The following is a short description of each strategy. The teachers were trained in eight-hour workshops, in which all the aforementioned themes are covered, so they acquired knowledge on healthy nutrition, prevention of dating violence, bullying, and substance abuse. They also became more aware of the importance of developing their life skills through previously extensively used interactive games (Givaudan, Karakowsky, Villanueva, & Prado, 2009; Pick et al., 1988; Ramírez et al., 2014) and activities in which they are confronted with real situations regarding their knowledge, attitudes, and behaviors. These activities were developed and tested in the past and proved to contribute significantly to HIV and STI's prevention (Pick, Givaudan, & Poortinga, 2003; Givaudan et al., 2007); rejection of alcohol, tobacco, and drugs (Givaudan & Pick, 2004); prevention of school desertion (Pick & Givaudan, 2007); dating violence prevention (Pick, Leenen, Givaudan, & Prado, 2010a); and gender equality promotion (Pick, Romero, de la Parra, & Givaudan, 2010b).

Through this strategy, the workshops serve first the personal development of the teachers. Once the teachers appropriately comprehend the program goals and nature – that is, feel ownership for both their own development as well as for their students' personal development – they are encouraged and taught how to replicate the program with their students. This repeated, closely supervised strategy with accompanying activities, fosters teachers' commitment and efficacy and makes the program more sustainable, as the teachers continue to refer to and discuss the program goals and procedures long after the formal completion of the program (Pick et al., 2011).

The teachers also receive a guidebook with twenty-four lesson plans that they learn to use during the eight-hour training and that they can conduct in either weekly or monthly lessons with their students. Usually, due to school time restriction, the teachers in this case were able to conduct only seven to eight lessons (30 percent) out of the twenty-four lesson plans. All students, parents, and teachers attended the educational fairs (Ramírez et al., 2014). The fairs include educational activities and games that reinforce the learning process and positive attitudes toward prevention and also promote sustainable behavior change within the educational community. During the replication process, facilitators of Yo quiero Yo puedo-IMIFAP accompanied them in group meetings, outside the classroom sessions, to give them feedback and advice. In these group follow-up sessions, the teachers share their experiences, identify successful strategies to realize the program contents with their students, and create synergies between the participants.

The program has been implemented in four states in Mexico: Chihuahua, Coahuila, Nuevo León, and Puebla. In total, 2,487 teachers have participated in eighty-nine workshops and replicated the program with approximately 91,696 high school students during the school year. In addition, they have replicated the program in nine educational fairs with the school community with 5,871 participants. A total of 1,233 parents have participated in interactive talks directed to parents (Ramírez et al., 2014). The fairs consist of large-scale (one hundred to one thousand individuals) events in which the schools and surrounding communities are invited to participate in a series of educational games (such as roleplays and board games in large patios, fields, or gardens, all dealing with the thematic areas of the program).

To evaluate the program impact on teachers, a pre-post design with a self-report questionnaire was used. The questionnaire designed specifically for this program consisted of fifty-four questions divided in three categories to measure: (1) *attitudes* (attitudes related to being agent of change, nutrition and exercise, violence and bullying, and alcohol consumption); (2) *knowledge* (knowledge on skills and values, nutrition and exercise, violence and bullying, and alcohol consumption); and (3) *life skills* (expression of emotions, management of stress, assertive communication and negotiation, empathy, self-knowledge, critical thinking, decision making, and management of social pressure – i.e., identifying pressure from peers and learning to say no to it, either responding verbally, simply ignoring it, or walking away from it) (Ramírez et al., 2014). All the categories evaluated were reviewed as part of the contents of the eight-hour workshop that was given in one training session. In total, 1,936 teachers completed the evaluation measure before the workshops and 1,846 teachers after the training. They came from 681 different schools. Participants were 62.7 percent females and 37.3 percent males (Ramírez et al., 2014). It is important to note that there was no control group to compare the program results among the teachers.

The pre-post comparisons of teachers' responses show that after the workshops the teachers had more positive attitudes and knowledge toward being agents of change, eating in a healthy manner and exercising, preventing violence and bullying, and preventing alcohol consumption (Ramírez et al., 2014). The percentage of teachers with sufficient knowledge also increased for skills and values, nutrition and exercise, violence and bullying, and alcohol consumption. The largest change was related to percentage of teachers who have sufficient knowledge of violence and bullying after the training; before the workshop, only 10.5 percent of the teachers had sufficient knowledge about this theme, and after the workshop that was the case with 67.6 percent of the teachers (t = –46.985, p = 0.000). For skills and values, only 25 percent of the participants had sufficient knowledge after the workshop, which means that it is necessary to strengthen the training on this theme ($t = -11.715$, $p = 0.000$) (Ramírez et al., 2014). These dramatic increases in knowledge of violence and bullying may be related to the very specific contents and key messages that were provided in the eight-hour training that were directed at clarifying misconceptions and false beliefs (e.g., violence and aggression are not the same) and that therefore contributed to these large knowledge increases. The participants also increased their feelings of mastery of life skills after the training. Of the eight skills evaluated, the teachers showed statistically significant changes in four: management of emotions ($t = -3.709$, $p = 0.000$), empathy ($t = -4.082$, $p = 0.000$), critical thinking ($t = -3.493$, $p = 0.000$), and management of social pressure ($t = -2.657$, $p = 0.008$). In self-knowledge, there was a slight decrease ($t = 3.483$, $p = 0.001$), which they attributed themselves to realizing they knew much less than they had thought, and that participation in the program had allowed them to realize and accept this fact. In skills such as stress management, assertive communication and negotiation, decision making, and problem solving, there was no significant change after the training, which was explained as pointing to the need to practice and put into action their learning.

These results indicate that short programs can potentially have a significant effect on specific skills, such as management of emotions, empathy, and critical thinking. Yet, for further impact, more training and follow-up is needed in order to ensure a wider effect on skills development (Ramírez et al., 2014). In addition, it is also important to perform other methodological strategies in order to evaluate the effect of short-term programs, especially those including the incorporation of a control group.

For the evaluation of the intervention impact on the target population, the students, two self-report questionnaires, developed explicitly for the program, were administered after the educational fairs among a sample of students who participated in the activities. The answers of students from this (intervention) group were compared to the answers of another group of students, studying in similar schools that did not participate in the program (the control group). The self-report questionnaire for first-grade high school students consisted of eighty-six questions and the questionnaire for third-grade high school students of one hundred questions. Both questionnaires were divided into five sections: (1) attitudes (toward being an agent of change, nutrition and exercise, violence and bullying, alcohol consumption, and skills and values); (2) knowledge (nutrition and exercise, violence and bullying, alcohol consumption, and skills and values); (3) behaviors (being an agent of change, promoting healthy nutrition and exercise, preventing violence and bullying, and preventing alcohol consumption); (4) life skills (expression of emotions, management of stress, assertive communication and negotiation, empathy, self-knowledge, critical thinking, decision making, and management of social pressure); and (5) the "Tracing my own destiny" program (implementation of the program, the participants' opinions, and activities in which they participated). In total,

653 students participated in the evaluation in the states of Chihuahua, Coahuila, and Nuevo León; 327 were first-grade high school students, and 326 were third-grade students; 266 students participated in the program, and 387 were in the control group.

The first-grade students showed positive attitudes after participating in the program in comparison to the control group. Especially positive were the attitudes toward being an agent of change (X^2 = 14.544, p = 0.001), promoting healthy nutrition and exercise habits (X^2 = 9.211, p = 0.010), and preventing alcohol consumption (X^2 = 9.313, p = 0.009). Also, in knowledge after the program, there was a significant difference between groups: regarding nutrition and exercise habits (X^2 = 24.260, p = 0.000), alcohol consumption (X^2 = 12.031, p = 0.001), and for violence and bullying (X^2 = 45.501, p = 0.000); students who participated in the program had a higher level of knowledge on violence and bullying, on prevention of alcohol consumption, and on nutrition and exercise compared to students in the control group. The majority of the students who participated in the program (87 percent) thought that program activities were fun and interesting, and 84 percent of them mentioned that they had learned important things to take better care of themselves (Ramírez et al., 2014).

Similarly, the third-grade students who participated in the program had significantly more positive attitudes toward healthy nutrition and exercise than the control group (X^2 = 6.065, p = 0.014). They also showed significantly higher rates of knowledge and positive attitudes toward violence prevention: bullying and dating violence (X^2 = 17.311, p = 0.000), and alcohol consumption (X^2 = 37.150, p = 0.000) as well as knowledge regarding healthy nutrition and exercise (X^2 = 31.011, p = 0.000). The life skills that students developed best, compared to control group students, were management of stress, assertive communication and negotiation, critical thinking, and empathy. A large majority of the third-grade students (91 percent) also thought that the program activities were interesting and fun and that they had learned important things (90 percent) (Ramírez et al., 2014).

Parents were also part of this comprehensive program; 1,233 parents participated in a two-hour interactive talk in which the key messages were reviewed and analyzed. After participating in the talks, they answered an open questionnaire in which they provided their perspective regarding the contents of the talks and shared what they learned. Analyses of the qualitative information indicated active participation of the parents regarding the program. This is based on their answers, alongside written testimonies that were collected from facilitators other than those delivering the prevention program. The testimonies of the teachers, parents, and students who participated in the program also show positive results:

> I never had thought that being able to say “no” in time could save us from such huge problems in the future. Thank you for letting me see that. – fourteen-year-old male student.
>
> To me, of all the skills we learned about today, the one that I liked most was critical thinking, because we are at an age when we must learn that we can

> think in a another way, that we can learn to take our own decisions and that makes us grow, right? – fourteen-year-old female student.
>
> When I started to implement the techniques (learned in the workshop) I really didn't believe that the kids would pay attention, but when I implemented the activities, I was surprised with the result, with their desire to participate and open up with us. In my group they even cried in one activity; in addition, I found in the kids virtues and intelligence I actually didn't imagine they had. – forty-nine-year-old female teacher.
>
> "Tracing my own destiny" is a program that really has come to change not only the kids but also us teachers who participate. Really, before talking about how the program has changed my group, I can say how it has changed me, not only as a teacher, but as a father and a husband. I think this is one of those programs that I will thank life for making me participate. – fifty-year-old male teacher.
>
> This exercise made me realize that my son only sees me as a hard, angry, busy woman, because I always go to work and then home; I understand now why he behaves like that, now I will talk to him, approach to him so that he can get to know me in another way. The communication is important so that he doesn't choose the wrong way. – forty-one-year-old mother.

These results suggest that the "Tracing my own destiny" program has influenced participants in a positive manner, in terms of their attitudes and knowledge regarding the four program themes: becoming agents of change, nutrition and exercise, violence and bullying, and alcohol consumption. Thus, it seems that for life skills based programs are able to sensitize students and have specifically significant results on improving positive attitudes and knowledge.

However, obviously, the design of the evaluation used with the students had limitations and our interpretations have to be somewhat tentative, because of lack of information about both groups before the program was implemented. As previously mentioned, future evaluation should include short- and long-term transversal and longitudinal pre- and post-comparisons that would yield more solid empirical evidence about the program impact both on students and teachers. To enhance the evaluation design, including a control group with a pre- and postevaluation, would be recommended. The evaluation strategies recommended include observations and evaluations after three, six, and twelve months to identify whether the results and effects of the program continue as time goes by.

Summary and Conclusions

In Mexico, the culture of prevention is not widely accepted (Bronfman, Castro, Zúñiga, Miranda, & Oviedo, 1997b). Several sociocultural characteristics, such as paternalism, fatalism, and traditional gender roles, can hinder preventative efforts in public health. Also, psychosocial barriers, such as fear, shame, and guilt, that regulate people's actions and often reinforce the accepted social norms can limit the individual's capacity to take independent decisions and actions (Pick & Sirkin, 2010; Pick et al., 2011). These cultural and psychosocial factors should be addressed in the design and implementation of effective prevention programs in Mexico.

In this context, short-term prevention programs can be more easily accepted in communities and schools than longer-term programs. Since time availability to participate in longer-term programs is limited for a series of reasons – including the fact that prevention is not always valued nor are its short-, mid-, and long-term individual, social, and economic effects really understood – short-term programs become an effective strategy to motivate the participation in prevention programs and enhance specific attitudes, knowledge, and behavior changes that are a basis for further changes. If they are successful, they can also justify the need for more comprehensive and broader prevention programs. Thus, short-term programs are the first step along the road to sensitize participants and initiate the change process with regard to specific knowledge, attitudes, norms, and behaviors.

To address this need for brief prevention programs, the Mexican NGO Yo quiero Yo puedo-IMIFAP has developed life skills–based short programs for teachers, parents, and adolescents on themes that are related to dating violence and bullying, substance abuse, healthy nutrition, and exercise. All these are themes that youth in Mexico currently has to deal with.

Two examples of these short prevention programs implemented by Yo quiero Yo puedo-IMIFAP, "I want to, I can... prevent dating violence" and "Tracing my own destiny," have shown positive effects among adolescents. The first program addresses dating violence through interactive talks directed to high school and college students. The evaluation of the program showed positive results in attitudes and knowledge on dating violence. The second program, "Tracing my own destiny," uses a different strategy: first, high school teachers are trained in eight-hour workshops, and afterward they replicate the program with their students both in classrooms and through interactive educational fairs. In this case, its application was even briefer than it was designed to be (eight-hour training for the teachers, and an average eight-hour training – not the originally planned twenty-four-hour training – with the students and an educational fair). The evaluation of this program also showed positive results in knowledge, attitudes, behaviors, and life skills both in teachers and students. However, it is necessary to further evaluate these programs in order to acquire better knowledge of the programs' impact on the students.

The two programs discussed in this chapter offer encouraging information on the possibilities of short prevention programs to change attitudes and knowledge, to develop life skills, and to initiate behavior changes. As there seems to be an increasing pressure from international development agencies and international and national donors for brief and cost-effective prevention programs, we believe that these results can be useful also for other contexts outside of Mexico, while relevant cultural and social factors would also be taken into account in the program design and implementation.

References

Álvarez Alva, R. (2012). *Salud pública y medicina preventiva [Public health and preventive medicine]*, 4th ed. Mexico City: Manual Moderno.

Amuchástegui, A., & Rivas, M. (2004). Los procesos de apropiación subjetiva de los derechos sexuales: notas para la discusión [The process of subjective ownership of sexual rights: notes for discussion]. *Estudios Demográficos y Urbanos* 19:(3): 543–97.

Badinter, E. (1993). *XY. Identidad Masculina. [XY Male identity]*. Mexico City: Alianza.

Bandura, A. (2000). Exercise of human agency through collective efficacy. *Current Directions in Psychological Science* 9(3): 75–8.

Bandura, A. (2001). Social cognitive theory: an agentic perspective. *Annual Review of Psychology* 52: 1–26.

Barriga, M., García, G., Givaudan, M., & Pick, S. (2014). *"Yo quiero, yo puedo... prevenir violencia en el noviazgo": Programa informativo dirigido a jóvenes en escuelas secundarias y nivel medio superior del estado de Chiapas, Chihuahua, Coahuila, Distrito Federal e Hidalgo. ["I want to, I can ... prevent dating violence": Interactive program for mid school and high school students of the Mexican states of Chiapas, Chihuahua, Coahuila, Distrito Federal and Hidalgo]*. Final report presented to Mary Kay. Mexico City: Yo quiero Yo puedo-IMIFAP.

Bronfman, M., Castro, R., Zúñiga, E., Miranda, C., & Oviedo, J. (1997a). Del "cuánto" al "por qué": la utilización de los servicios de salud desde la perspectiva de los usuarios. [From "how much" to "why": the use of health services from the users' perspective]. *Salud Pública de México* 39(5): 442–50.

Bronfman, M., Castro, R., Zúñiga, E., Miranda, C., & Oviedo, J. (1997b). "Hacemos lo que podemos": los prestadores de servicios frente al problema de la utilización. ["We do what we can": the heath service providers face up to the problem of the use of the service]. *Salud Pública de México* 39(6): 546–53.

Caballero Hoyosa, R., Torres López, T., Chong Villarreal, F., Pineda Lucateroc, A., Altuzar González, M., & López Coutiño, B. (2006). Concepciones culturales sobre el dengue en contextos urbanos de México. [Cultural conceptions of dengue fever in urban contexts of Mexico]. *Rev Saúde Pública* 40(1): 126–33.

De Jesús, D. (2011). Manifestación e invisibilidad de la violencia en el noviazgo. Un estudio de sus significados en Monterrey, Nuevo León. [The appearance and invisibility of dating violence. A study of its meanings in Monterrey, Nuevo León]. In Cantú, C., & Kumar, A. (coords), *Sustentabilidad social. Dinámica de la violencia y segregación en la sociedad.*Monterrey, N.L., Mexico: Universidad Autónoma de Nuevo León, pp. 167–98.

De Keijzer, B. (2001). Hasta donde el cuerpo aguante: Género, Cuerpo y Salud Masculina. [Until the body endures: gender, body and health in males]. In Cáceres, C., et al. (eds.), *La salud como derecho ciudadano: perspectivas y propuestas desde América Latina*. Lima: Universidad Peruana Cayetano Heredia.

Díaz-Guerrero, R. (1982). *Psicología Del Mexicano. [The Psychology of Mexicans]*. Mexico City, Mexico: Trillas.

ENSANUT (Encuesta Nacional de Nutrición) (2012). Mexico City, Mexico: Secretaria de Salud y Asistencia Pública.

ENVINOV (Encuesta Nacional de la Violencia en las Relaciones de Noviazgo) (2007). Mexico City, Mexico: Instituto Nacional de Psiquiatría.

Espinosa de los Monteros, K., & Gallo, L. (2013). Fatalism and cardio-metabolic dysfunction in Mexican-American women. *International Journal of Behavioral Medicine* 20(4): 487–94.

Fishbein, M., & Ajzen, I. (1975). *Belief, Attitude, Intention, and Behavior: An introduction to Theory and Research*. Reading, MA: Addison-Wesley.

Givaudan, M., Karakowsky, Y., Villanueva, T., & Prado, A. (2009). *Programa "Yo quiero, yo puedo . . . tener éxito en la escuela", nivel primaria. [Program "I want to, I can . . . be successful in school" elementary school level]*. Mexico City, Mexico: Idéame.

Givaudan, M., & Pick, S. (2004). A preventive program for substance abuse in Mexico: best practice. *Prevention Perspective*. Retrieved from www.mentorfoundation.org

Givaudan, M., Van de Vijver, F., Poortinga, Y. H., Leenen, I., & Pick, S. (2007). Effects of a school-based life skills and HIV prevention program. *Journal of Applied Social Psychology* 37(6): 1141–62.

Gongora Coronado, E., Cortes Ayala, M. d. L., & Flores Galaz, M. M. (2002). Creencias y acciones de los padres en la crianza de los hijos: un estudio exploratorio. [Beliefs and actions of parents in parenting: an exploratory study]. *La Psicología Social en México* 9: 849–55.

González Castro, F., Barrera, M., & Martínez, C. (2004). The cultural adaptation of prevention interventions: resolving tensions between fidelity and fit. *Prevention Science* 5(I): 41–5.

Graber, J., Hill, J., & Saczawa, M. (2014). Childhood and the entry into adolescence: a pivotal period in health-related behaviors and prevention. In Sloboda, Z., & Petras, H. (eds.), *Defining Prevention Science*. New York: Springer, pp. 59–86.

Hietanen, A.-E., & Pick, S. (2015). Gender stereotypes, sexuality and culture in Mexico. In Safdar, S., & Kosakowska-Berezecka, N. (eds.), *Psychology of Gender through the Lens of Culture: Theories and Application*. New York: Springer, pp. 285–305.

INSP (Instituto Nacional de Salud Pública) (2012). *Encuesta Nacional de Salud y Nutrición 2012. Resultados Nacionales. [National Health and Nutrition Survey 2012. National Results]*. Cuernavaca, Mexico: Instituto Nacional de Salud Pública.

Jewkes, R. (2002). Intimate partner violence: causes and prevention. *Lancet* 359: 1423–9.

Lara-Esquival, E. C., Torres-Muñoz Y. C., & Moreno-Gómez, M. (2012). Actitudes y hábitos ante la prevención. [Attitudes and habits for prevention]. *Revista de Enfermería del Instituto Mexicano del Seguro Social* 20(1): 11–17.

Leenen, I., Venguer, T., Vera, J., Givaudan, M., Pick, S., & Poortinga, Y. H. (2008). Effectiveness of a Mexican health education program in a poverty-stricken rural area of Guatemala. *Journal of Cross-Cultural Psychology* 39(2): 198–214.

Mangrulkar, L., Whitman, C. V., & Posner, M. (2001). *Life Skills Approach to Child and Adolescent Human Development*. Washington, DC: Pan American Health Organization.

Mejia-Arauz, R., Sheets, R., & Villaseñor, M. (2012). Mexico. In Arnett, J. J. (ed.), *Adolescent Psychology around the World*. New York: Psychology Press, pp. 195–209.

Mora, L. (coord.). (2006). *Igualdad y equidad de género: aproximación teórico-conceptual. Herramientas de trabajo en género para oficinas y contrapartes del UNFPA, vol. I. [Gender equality and equity: theoretical and conceptual approach. Working tools for gender at UNFPA's office and counterparts].* www.entremundos.org/databases/Herramientas%20de%20trabajo%20en%20genero%20UNFPA.pdf

Nation, M., Crusto, C., Wandersman, A., Kumpfer, K., Seybolt, D., Morrissey-Kane, E., & Davino, K. (2003). What works in prevention: principles of effective prevention programs. *American Psychologist* 58(6–7): 449–56. dx.doi.org/10.1037/0003–066X.58.6–7.449

Pérez-Stable, E. J, Sabogal, F., Otero-Sabogal, R., Hiatt, R. A., & McPhee, S. J. (1992). Misconceptions about cancer among Latinos and Anglos. *Journal of the American Medical Association* 268(22): 3219–23.

Peterson, G. W., & Hennon, C. (2006). Influencias parentales en la competencia social de los adolescentes en dos culturas: Una comparación conceptual entre los Estados Unidos y México. [Parental influence in adolescents' social competences: a conceptual comparison between USA and Mexico]. In Esteinou, R. (ed.), *Fortalezas y desafíos de las familias en dos contextos: Estados Unidos de América y México. [Strengths and challenges of families in two contexts: USA and Mexico].* Mexico City: Publicaciones de La Casa Chata – DIF.

Pick, S., Aguilar, J., Rodríguez, G., Vargas, E., Reyes, J., Collado, M. E., Pier, D., Acevedo, M. P., & Vargas, E. (1988). *Planeando tu Vida: nuevo programa de educación sexual para adolescentes. [Planning your life: new program of sexual education for teenagers]*, 7th ed., 20th printing (2006). Mexico City, Mexico: Editorial Planeta.

Pick, S., Beers, K., & Grossman-Crist, S. (2011). A human basis for sustainable development: how psychosocial change at the individual level promotes development. *Poverty & Public Policy* 3(3): 1–20.

Pick, S., & Givaudan, M. (2007). Yo quiero, yo puedo: Estrategia para el desarrollo de habilidades y competencias en el sistema escolar. [I want to, I can: strategy to develop life skills and competences on the educational system]. *Psicologia da Educação: Revista do Programa de Estudos Pós-Graduados em Psicologia da Educação* 23(2): 203–21.

Pick, S., Givaudan, M., & Poortinga, Y.H. (2003). Sexuality and life skills education: multistrategy interventions in México. *American Psychologist* 58(3): 230–4.

Pick, S., Givaudan, M., Sirkin, J., & Ortega, I. (2007). Communication as a protective factor: evaluation of a life-skills HIV/AIDS prevention program for Mexican elementary school students. *AIDS Education & Prevention* 19(5): 408–21.

Pick, S., & Hietanen, A.-E. (2014). Psychosocial barriers as impediments to the expansion of functioning's and capabilities: the case of Mexico. *Journal of Human Development and Capabilities: A Multi-Disciplinary Journal for People-Centered Development.* doi: 10.1080/19452829.2014.959906

Pick, S., Leenen, I., Givaudan, M., & Prado, A. (2010a). "Yo quiero, yo puedo...prevenir la violencia": Programa breve de sensibilización sobre violencia en el noviazgo. ["I want to, I can ... prevent violence": brief sensitization program of dating violence]. *Revista Salud Mental [Mental Health Journal]* 33(2): 153–60.

Pick, S., Romero, A., de la Parra, A., & Givaudan, M. (2010b). Evaluación del impacto de un programa de prevención de violencia en adolescentes. [Impact evaluation of a violence prevention program with teenagers]. *Revista Interamericana de Psicología* 44(2): 203–12.

Pick, S., & Sirkin, J. (2010). *Breaking the Poverty Cycle: The Human Basis for Sustainable Development*. New York: Oxford University Press.

Piña, J., & Robles, S. (2005). Psicología y VIH/SIDA en México: su prevención con base en un modelo psicológico de salud biológica. [Psychology and HIV/AIDS in Mexico: its prevention based on a psychological model of biological health]. *Revista de Psicopatología y Psicología Clínica* 10(1): 71–83.

Ramírez, M., Estrada, E., García, D., Athié, D., García, G., & Givaudan, M. (2014). Trazando mi propio destino. Actualizado y Operado por Yo quiero Yo puedo-IMIFAP A.C. Informe final. [Tracing my own destiny: Updated and Implemented by I want to, I can, IMIFAP A.C.]. *Final Report Presented to Cuauhtémoc Moctezuma*. Mexico City: Yo quiero Yo puedo-IMIFAP.

Ramírez Rivera, C. A., & Núñez Luna, D. A. (2010). Violencia en la relación de noviazgo en jóvenes universitarios: un estudio exploratorio. [Dating violence in university students: an exploratory study]. *Enseñanza e Investigación en Psicología* 15(2): 273–283.

Safdar, S., & Kosakowska-Berezecka, N. (2015). *Psychology of Gender through the Lens of Culture Theories and Applications*. New York: Springer International, pp. 285–305.

Secretaría de Salud [Ministry of Health] (2007). Estrategia nacional de promoción y prevención para una mejor salud [National strategy of health prevention and promotion]. Secretaría de Salud – Dirección General de Promoción de la Salud. Mexico promocion.salud.gob.mx/dgps/descargas1/estrategia_nacional.pdf

Secretaría de Salud [Ministry of Health] (2013). Estrategia nacional para la prevención y el control del sobrepeso, la obesidad y la diabetes [National strategy for prevention and control of overweight, obesity and diabetes]. promocion.salud.gob.mx/dgps/descargas1/estrategia/Estrategia_con_portada.pdf

Soto, C., Unger, J. B., Ritt-Olson, A., Soto, D. W., Black, D. S., & Baezconde-Garbanati, L. (2011). Cultural values associated with substance use among Hispanic adolescents in southern California. *Substance Abuse & Misuse* 46(10): 1223–33.

Sumnal, H. (2014). Prevention Science: A Global Issue. In Sloboda, Z., & Petras, H. (eds.), *Defining Prevention Science*. New York: Springer, pp. v–vvi.

Szasz, I. (1998). Sexualidad y género: algunas experiencias de investigación en Mexico. *Debate Feminista* 9: 77–104.

Venguer, T., Pick, S., & Fishbein, M. (2007). Health education and agency: a comprehensive program for young women in the Mixteca region of Mexico. *Psychology, Health & Medicine* 12(4): 389–406.

Villegas, J., Lemanski, J., & Valdéz, C. (2010). Marianismo and machismo: the portrayal of females in Mexican TV commercials. *Journal of International Consumer Marketing* 22(4): 327–46. dx.doi.org/10.1080/08961530.2010.505884

Wang, L., Gutin, B., Barbeau, P., Moore, J.B., Hanes, J. Jr., Johnson, M. H., Cavnar, M., Thornburg, J., & Yin, J. (2008). Cost-effectiveness of a school-based obesity prevention program. *Journal of School Health* 78(12): 619–24.

Wood, J. (2001). The normalization of violence in heterosexual romantic relationships: women's narratives of love and violence. *Journal of Social and Personal Relationships* 18(2): 239–61.

WHO (World Health Organization) (1997). Life skills education for children and adolescents in schools: introduction and guidelines to facilitate the development and implementation of life skills programs. WHO/MNH/PSF/93.7A.Rev.2. www.whqlibdoc.who.int/hq/1994/WHO_MNH_PSF_93.7A_Rev.2.pdf

WHO (World Health Organization) (1999). *Partners in Life Skills Education: Conclusions from a United Nations Inter-agency Meeting*. Geneva, Switzerland: World Health Organization.

WHO (World Health Organization) (2006). Resumen de estrategia de cooperación. [Cooperation Strategy Summary]. hwww.who.int/countryfocus/cooperation_strategy/ccsbrief_mex_es.pdf

WHO (World Health Organization) (2009a). Estimated overweight & obesity prevalence. apps.who.int/infobase/Comparisons.aspx?l=&NodeVal=WGIE_BMI_5_cd.0704&DO=1&DDLReg=ALL&DDLSex=1&DDLAgeGrp=15-100&DDLYear=2010&DDLMethod=INTMDCTM&DDLCateNum=6&TxtBxCtmNum=20%2c35%2c50%2c65%2c80&CBLC1=ON&CBLC3=ON&CBLC4=ON&CBLC6=ON&CBLC8=ON&CBLC10=ON&DDLMapsize=800x480&DDLMapLabels=none&DDLTmpRangBK=0&DDLTmpColor=-3342388

WHO (World Health Organization) (2009b). *Preventing Violence by Developing Life Skills in Children and Adolescents*. Series of briefings on violence prevention: the evidence. Malta: World Health Organization.

Europe

34 Paving the Way for Prevention Science in Croatia

History, Development, and Future of Research and Implementation of Evidence-Based Prevention Programs

Josipa Bašić & Darko Roviš

Introduction

The Republic of Croatia became independent by separating from the former Yugoslavia in 1991. In July 2013, Croatia became the twenty-eighth member of the European Union (EU). The Republic of Croatia, with the land area of 56,594 square kilometres, is situated in the southeastern part of Europe, surrounded by Alps in the west, Sava and Drava rivers in the north and east, and the Adriatic Sea in the south. According to the 2013 midyear population estimate, this area was populated by 4.3 million inhabitants and around 800,000 children – 789,387 from zero to seventeen years old.[1] According to the census report from 2011 (Popis stanovništva . . .," 2012), the majority of the population is Croatian (around 90.42 percent), while the rest are minorities such as Serbs, Italians, Muslims, Roma, Hungarians, and many others. Croatia is divided into twenty counties with the capital city of Zagreb as the twenty-first county.

Prevention science and practice in Croatia is not a future idea (Albee & Gullotta, 1997), but an idea that exists and is growing and developing (Bašić, 2009). Following a social and political transition in the 1990s, Croatian society experienced great changes, some of which were quite disruptive (the Homeland War and war-related migrations, the increase in unemployment rates and social inequality, and related changes in societal norms and values). According to some indicators, the registered unemployment rate for February 2015 was 20.3 percent and the at-risk-of-poverty rate was 20.5 percent, while the rate for people at risk of poverty or social exclusion amounted to 32.3 percent.[2] These changes and their impact on the community and the lives of children and families resulted in raising professional and public awareness of the need for efficient prevention of complex and difficult risk behaviors among children and youth. However, raising public awareness was not an easy task. Raising such public awareness and advocating systematic and sustainable solutions for reducing problem behaviors and promoting children's mental health and well-being can largely be attributed to the

1 Croatian Bureau of Statistics, www.dzs.hr/default_e.htm.
2 Full data are available at the Croatian Bureau of Statistics web page (www.dzs.hr/default_e.htm).

efforts made by educational and health professionals as well as local community champions.

In pursuit of an efficient prevention system, it is necessary to monitor the condition and evaluate the needs of children and youth, relevant adults, and key institutions in order to establish practical prevention systems based on scientific principles. For example, past exposure to war consequences, sufferings and traumas, population's displacement and mobility, exile, the separation of parents from children, the death of parents, poverty, and unemployment – all of these contributed to the current state in Croatia. Practically speaking, it can be advocated that as early as the beginning of their lives, up to late adolescence, almost all Croatian children might be vulnerable to behavioral and emotional problems.

This chapter describes the development of prevention science and practice, along with the fundamental institutional and organizational prevention infrastructure in Croatia. The chapter describes preventive and promotional investments, discusses numerous national prevention strategies aimed at reducing risk factors, as well as strengthening protective factors that are all directed toward the promotion of mental health and well-being among Croatian children and youth. Following an overview of what has been done, further investments in prevention policy solutions and evidence-based programs are presented.

Development of Prevention Science and Practice in Croatia

The establishment of prevention practice in Croatia dates to the middle 1970s. In 1975, the Croatian Parliament issued the first document on the prevention of problem behaviors in children and youth (Singer & Mikšaj Todorović, 1989). The first coordinating bodies were established in cities and regions nationwide. This act marked the beginning of prevention practice, but not that of prevention science. Rather, the beginning of prevention science was marked by several scientific projects (Bašić, Ferić, & Kranželic, 2001) which, for the first time, did not aim at studying children and youth who were already exhibiting risk behaviors and undergoing any institutional treatment, and/or the evaluation of treatments/posttreatment outcomes. Building upon previous studies in criminology that clearly emphasized the link between early occurrence of behavioral problems and later risk behaviors during adolescence and adulthood (Tonry & Farrington, 1995), a group of researchers made a decision to direct their scientific, theoretical, and applied research on prevention. This encompassed exploring and assessing the needs of children learning in preschools and schools as well as the needs of local communities. Therefore, it started gradually to advocate the awareness of the need to invest in empowered professionals engaging in prevention as early as possible (developmental prevention) and across the domains (family, school, local community).

Prevention science know-how and results of basic and applied research were scarce in the 1970s and 1980s; therefore, the projects of early 1990s in Croatia can be considered first prevention science research (Bašić, Žižak, & Koller-Trbović, 1998). In the early 2000s, research began into risk and protective factors and other notions as key foundations for the prevention of risk behaviors. Action research aimed at testing programs such as Communities That Care (Bašić & Grozić-Živolić, 2010; Hawkins, 1999) parallel to developing other evidence-based prevention programs (Bašić & Grozić-Živolić, 2010). Thus, from the beginning of 2002, upon entering a new millennium, global trends in prevention science and intervention were followed; recognition and memberships in world and European prevention research societies (e.g., the Society for Prevention Research [SPR], European Society for Prevention Research [EUSPR], and European Network for Social and Emotional Competences [ENSEC]) were obtained, and active participation in European research programs (e.g., the Seventh Framework program, Comenius, and Horizon 2020) was encouraged. As a result of these developments, Croatia's position in the "global village" of prevention science and practice has become significant and secure.

Given the lack of formal institutions that are in charge of prevention, during the 1990s Croatian nongovernmental organizations (NGOs) increasingly focused on prevention of risk behaviors in children and youth to a point that they largely took over the responsibility for prevention practice. These NGOs were financed by various Croatian sources: municipal and regional budgets (meeting citizens' public needs), several ministries, the Office for Cooperation with NGOs, and the National Foundation for Civil Society Development. In times of war, financial support was also received from numerous foreign funds (e.g., the United Nations Development Programme [UNDP], the Academy for Educational Development [AED], etc.), and NGO members were instructed on how to apply for such funds to support prevention programs. Unfortunately, having a motivating NGO sector engaged in prevention does not guarantee the success of implemented prevention programs. Such prevention programs often have difficulties in fulfilling the criteria for effective prevention. For example, an assessment of twenty-four local prevention programs, conducted in Istria County by the health promotion management instrument called Preffi 2.0[3] (created by Molleman [Molleman, Peters, Hosman, & Kok, 2005] and adapted for Croatian use (Mihić, 2013; Novak, 2013), indicated the lack of both a theoretical basis and a follow-up evaluation as the weakest features of these programs. However, it should be

3 Preffi 2.0 is an effectiveness management instrument intended to be used by health promotion and prevention practitioners to improve the effectiveness of their intervention by applying the Preffi criteria (thirty-nine criteria divided into eight clusters: Contextual conditions and feasibility; Problem analysis; Determinants; Target group; Objectives; Intervention development; Implementation; and Evaluation).

noted that some of those programs deserve close attention, as efforts to improve these programs would result in the development of new programs within Croatia, which could serve as a significant resource for wider implementation and dissemination. To do so, a better cooperation between scientists and practitioners is needed (Biglan, Brennan, Foster, & Holder 2004). As Kumar, O'Malley, Johnston, and Laetz, (2013) noted, even though well-established prevention programs are easy to access (for example, over two hundred commercial prevention programs for addictions are available), two-thirds of observed schools in the United States nevertheless implement locally developed programs. Similar is the case in Croatia, where the majority of the programs are locally developed and not comprehensively evaluated. The need for investing in increased knowledge and cooperation between practitioners and scientists is still on the agenda of numerous roundtables, professional debates, and presentations. In order to develop an evidence-based approach in prevention, a strong commitment to raising awareness of the need for better knowledge on planning, implementing, and evaluating prevention programs and building strong links of science and practice is necessary.

At the turn of the millennium, a significant number of national offices and institutions were formed in Croatia and were actively involved in prevention practice: the the Commission of the Croatian Government for the Prevention of Behavioral Disorders of Children and Youth; the Council for Children's' Affairs; the Office for Combating Drug Abuse of the Government of the Republic of Croatia; the Department for the Prevention of the Ministry of Interior of the Republic of Croatia; Ombudsman for Children; the National Network of Healthy Cities and Healthy Counties; family centers; centers for drug prevention and mental health; and more. All of the aforementioned bodies foster recognition in prevention practice and science and have established an organizational framework for sustainable preventive actions.

The present state of prevention science and practice is characterized by the continuing implementation of prevention programs in local communities, preschools and schools, advisory centers, centers organized by local or county institutions, and numerous nongovernmental associations. Relying on existing and new research, prevention science in Croatia widens its comprehension by participating in international research projects. There are several European projects currently carried out by the University of Zagreb's Faculty of Education and Rehabilitation Science and headed by Professor Josipa Bašić. These include comparative research of risk and protective factors, implementation of evidence-based programs in different EU countries (the project Communities That Care [CTC], the CTC European Network, Making CTC Work at the European level[4]) and development of instruments for measuring outcomes of prevention programs of socio-emotional learning (European Assessment

4 Project reference number HOME/2011/ISEC/AG/4000002522.

Protocol for Children's SEL Skills [EAP_SEL][5]). In addition to conducting the research projects, the University of Zagreb participates in a consortium of organizations devoting efforts to map prevention infrastructure in all EU countries (the Science for Prevention Academic Network [SPAN] project[6]). In Croatia (the University of Zagreb), there are additional competitive science projects such as implementation of the evidence-based prevention program of socioemotional learning through science evaluation and its application into Croatian kindergartens and primary schools (PATHS-RASTEM[7]).

Epidemiological Overview

Data on the presence of risk behaviors in children, youth, and adults serve as a basis for planning preventive strategies and programs. Assessment of risk factors, trends, and factors that facilitate them is necessary for planning corresponding strategies, but it also serves as an important threshold for assessing short-term and long-term outcomes of prevention programs and policies. Unfortunately, Croatia lacks systematic and longitudinal epidemiological researches as well as comparable international ones that could give such valuable data. However, there are some valuable epidemiological surveys integrated in the monitoring system of the national public health system.

Following are epidemiological information and results of several studies, trends in risk behavior, and national follow-up studies of the prevalence of risk behaviors among children and youth in Croatia, conducted during the past several years. Mental health indicators, addictions, and peer violence among children and youth are indicated.

Concerning *mental health problems*, mostly hospital data exist regarding more serious clinical conditions of children and adolescents. Hospitalization rates among adolescents are reported to be 5.1–6.6 per 100,000 (Silobrčić Radić, Hrabak-Žerjavić, & Tomić, 2004). For this age group (ten to nineteen years), the most common causes of hospitalization include mixed behavioral and emotional disorders, childhood-related emotional disorders, alcohol abuse–related mental disorders, and stress. Other studies among adolescents (Vulić-Prtorić, 2002) show that up to 12 percent of children and adolescents

5 Project reference number 527206-LLP-1–2012-1-IT-COMENIUS-CMP.

6 The Science for Prevention Academic Network (SPAN), consisting of experts from thirty-two European institutions across twenty-five countries, has been awarded by the European Commission Lifelong Learning Programme (LLP). The SPAN project will map the prevention science sector, improve education and training, build networks, and run workshops with researchers, with a particular focus upon young researchers. In addition, the project will contribute to the integration of prevention science in higher education across Europe and will provide recommendations on how best to align prevention science with the European Credit Transfer and Accumulation System (ECTS) (SPAN Newsletter, February 2015, number 49).

7 Project number: 61/10 financed by the Unity through Knowledge Fund (UKF) and the Croatian Ministry of Science, Education, and Sports through a World Bank loan in cooperation with the Pennsylvania State University (U.S.).

experience intense fears, especially intensified at the age of eleven and at the age of fifteen, in times of social and/or school transitions. Such fears, if left unattended, can lead to serious problems of phobias and anxiety. For adolescents aged fourteen to nineteen, suicide rates have fluctuated in the last two and a half decades – from 5.8 per 100,000 in 1985 to 12.9 per 100,000 in 1999 – and since 2000 rates have constantly been dropping down to 6 per 100,000 in 2010 (Silobrčić Radić & Jelavić, 2011).

In addition to hospital data, some relevant and comparable data on mental health can be derived from the international (the United States and EU) Health Behaviour in School-aged Children (HBSC) study, conducted in 2002, 2006, and 2010 among students aged eleven, thirteen, and fifteen years (Kuzman et al., 2012b). Among Croatian adolescents asked in 2010 about their health, 32 percent of eleven-year-old girls and 40 percent of fifteen-year-old girls reported having two or more symptoms of disturbed health (e.g., stomach pain; back pain; feeling sad, agitated, in a bad mood, anxious, or nervous; problems with falling asleep; vertigo). Interestingly, only in the cohort of fifteen-year-old girls, the number of girls reporting such problems is showing a slow decline (estimates from 2002 show 48 percent of girls reporting such problems). The rates for boys are quite stable across age groups and almost two times lower (23 percent to 26 percent). The same study revealed that fifteen-year-old girls report lower estimates of feeling satisfied with their life (68 percent to 78 percent in 2002 and 2010 samples) than boys (78 percent to 87 percent) or other age groups regardless of their gender (79 percent to 88 percent) and are generally at higher risk in the period of transition into adulthood (Kuzman, Pavić Šimetin, & Pejnović Franelić, 2012a).

According to the Croatian National Institute of Public Health, the demand for addiction treatment has increased from 260 addicts registered for treatment in 1990 to 7,427 in 2006 and 7,857 in 2013 (Katalinić & Huskić, 2014). The average age of drug addicts entering treatment is 26.4 years, while 7.6 percent of all addicts are under the age of nineteen. During the 1990s, the incidence rates were sharply growing, resulting in a drug addiction epidemic. As of 2001, the incidence rates are constantly dropping, resulting in stable prevalence rates for treatment demand in the last few years. According to the European Monitoring Centre for Drugs and Drug Addiction (EMCDDA, 2013a), the incidence rate of 35 per 100,000 for the population aged sixteen to sixty-four is now just below the average rate of 44 per 100,000 among European countries.

Upward trends can be found for alcohol, tobacco, and illegal drug abuse among Croatian adolescents. The European School Survey Project on Alcohol and Other Drugs (ESPAD) conducted in 2003 found that Croatian rates for most risk behaviors for alcohol, tobacco, and drug use were in line with the ESPAD average. However, in the 2007 survey, Croatia reported upward trends in the use of tobacco and illicit drugs (Kuzman, Pejnovi & Franelić, Pavić Šimetin, & Pejak, 2008); and in the 2011 survey (Kuzman et al., 2012a), Croatian fifteen- and sixteen-year-old students reported above average rates for cigarette smoking in the last thirty days (41 percent Croatian rate vs. 28

percent average ESPAD rate), alcohol use in the last thirty days (66 percent vs. 57 percent), heavy episodic drinking in the last thirty days (54 percent vs. 39 percent), lifetime marijuana use (18 percent vs. 17 percent), inhalant use (28 percent vs. 9 percent), and alcohol volume taken on the last drinking day (6.6 vs. 5.1 ccl). Croatian adolescents' smoking and binge-drinking rates are currently the third highest compared to all European countries.

Furthermore, in the last decade, gambling was found to be highly spread among Croatian adolescents. Unfortunately, no systematic monitoring system and data collection for this problem behavior exists. Nevertheless, a couple of studies have been conducted so far, such as the research among high school students in four big Croatian cities (Ricijaš Dodig, Huić, & Kranželi, 2011), in which it was found that 83 percent of urban students reported on being involved in gambling. In that study, 12 percent of the students showed serious psychological, social, and financial symptoms related to gambling, and another 17 percent showed medium severity levels of these symptoms.

In 2004, the UNICEF office for Croatia (United Nations International Children's Emergency Fund) conducted a study (Pregrad, 2010) that included 23,342 Croatian elementary school students. Results show that 33 percent of them reported being exposed to some form of violence, and 22.3 percent reported experiencing violence once to twice "in the past several months," while 10.4 percent were exposed to violent behavior "2–3 or more times a month." In a 2003 Zagreb Child Protection Centre study about school violence in twenty-five elementary schools, located in thirteen Croatian cities (total sample = 4,904; Buljan Flander, Durman Marijanović, & Špoljar Ćorić, 2007), 7 percent of students reported that they experienced at least one form of peer abuse on a daily basis, 8 percent of the children are "provocative victims" (both experiencing and using violence), while 8 percent of students are violent toward other children on a daily basis but do not experience violence themselves. Results of the HBSC research (Kuzman et al., 2012a) indicated that Croatia ranked in the middle of the European chart with regard to the rate of children participating in physical violence. Differentiation between various types of peer violence, in a sample of elementary school children (Vidović, 2005), shows that the most common types of violence are emotional (21 percent to 46 percent), physical (18 percent to 37 percent), and sexual (16 percent). Research on cyber-bullying, conducted among 2,700 elementary and high school students from different Croatian cities (Buljan Flander, 2008), shows that up to 23 percent of children and youth participates in bullying others, for example by taking photos and/or recording on mobile phones peers who are fighting or engaging in other violent acts.

Strategic and Organizational Framework

It took Croatia a relatively long time to establish a strategic framework for the promotion of mental health and prevention of mental and behavioral disorders of children and youth. Currently, this framework includes national strategic offices and institutions (committees, councils, services, centers, etc.) and legislation (conventions, strategies, action plans, procedural protocols, etc.). All of the preceding also exists on the level of counties, local communities, cities, and towns. In addition, several key national committees, acts, councils, or services have been established from 1998 to 2009 that have been working with the purpose of prevention of risk behavior in children and youth (the Council for Children's Affairs of the Government of the Republic of Croatia; Ombudsman for Children of the Republic of Croatia; Law on the Ombudsman for Children; Commission of the Croatian Government for the Prevention of Behavioral Disorders of Children and Youth; Act on Protection Against Domestic Violence; the Department for the Prevention of the Ministry of Interior of the Republic of Croatia; Act on Combating Drug Abuse; the Commission for Prevention and Treatment of Addiction). Some of the key national and/or regional and local institutions/organizations in the fields of health, social welfare, education, and law enforcement whose scope also includes the prevention of risk behaviors (universal, selective, and/or indicative prevention) are the Croatian National Institute of Public Health; the Agency for Education of the "Ministry of Science, Education and Sports of the Republic of Croatia"; the National Network of Healthy Cities and Healthy Counties; Councils for prevention (of addiction or crimes); County Services for Mental Health, Drug Prevention, and Outpatient Treatment; the Center for Social Welfare/branch offices of family centers; educational institutions; and others.

It is important to note that a significant part of preventive practice includes actions by the civil sector, that is, NGOs. The Office for Cooperation with NGOs is an important body that gathers and finances numerous Croatian associations.

National strategies and corresponding action programs and procedure protocols in the field of prevention have been developed and accepted during the past twenty years. Examples include the *2014–2020 National Strategy for the Rights of Children in the Republic of Croatia*[8]; the *2012–2017 National Strategy for Combating Drug Abuse*[9]; the *2009–2012 National Strategy for Prevention of Children and Adolescent Disorders*[10]; the *2008–2010 National Strategy for Protection from Domestic Violence*[11]; and the *Activities Program for Prevention of Violence among Children and Adolescents*[12].

8 *Vlada Republike Hrvatske "Nacionalna strategija za prava djece u Republici Hrvatskoj za razdoblje od 2014. do 2020. godine [2014–2020 National Strategy for the Rights of Children in the Republic of Croatia],"* 2014.

9 *"Nacionalna strategija suzbijanja zlouporabe droga u Republici Hrvatskoj za razdoblje od 2012. do 2017. godine [2012–2017 National Strategy for Combating Drug Abuse],"* 2012.

10 *"Nacionalna strategija za prevenciju poremećaja u ponašanju djece i mladih od 2009. do 2012. [2009–2012 National Strategy for Prevention of Children and Adolescent Disorders],"* 2009.

11 *"Nacionalna strategija zaštite od nasilja u obitelji od 2008. godine do 2010. godine [2008–2010 National Strategy for Protection from Domestic Violence],"* 2007.

12 *"Program aktivnosti za sprječavanje nasilja među djecom i mladima [Activities Program for Prevention of Violence among Children and Adolescents],"* 2004.

The majority of strategies and policy solutions are being implemented in several key organizational systems and work domains, primarily in the educational system, public health and social welfare systems, and the local community.

The *educational system* has taken over the majority of organizational and implementation-related responsibilities for prevention programs through preschools, elementary, secondary, and higher education. Preschool is the least involved in structured programs dealing with mental health promotion and prevention. However, recently there have been several attempts to implement evidence-based programs such as Promoting Alternative Thinking Strategies (PATHS; PATHS-RASTEM in Croatia) and the Child Assault Prevention Program (CAP). Results have been promising (described later in this chapter) (Maljković & Hitrec, 2009; Novak et al., 2012), and a model of sustainable integration of such content in regular activities is still being considered. It is rather well known that schools are the best places for investment on prevention, so great attention is given to prevention programs in Croatian educational systems. There have been several attempts to structure school prevention programs, primarily for addiction prevention, in order to assure consistency and uniformity of such plans (Bezinović, 2014; Bezinović & Roviš, 2009; Nacionalni program prevencije ..." 2010; Sakoman, 2009). Nevertheless, the structure, scope, and contents of the plans vary significantly between schools. Since 2013, a National Health Education Curriculum is being implemented (Mićanović, 2013a, 2013b, 2013c) through an intercurricular time table. Its main aims are educating students about living a healthy lifestyle, maintaining their health and quality of life, improving gender equality, practicing responsible sexual behavior, establishing human relationships between genders, and preventing addiction and bullying. It is a relatively comprehensive curriculum implemented through ten to twelve lessons annually, from the beginning of elementary education until the completion of secondary education. Although there are still no findings on the effectiveness of this curriculum, it seems to be a high-quality organizational model for implementing contents related to the prevention of risk behaviors.

Moreover, the *public health system* has a significant role in the prevention of behavioral problems. The significant spread of the addiction issue caused Croatia to develop a network of services for prevention and outpatient addiction treatment. Mental health and addiction services were integrated into the county institutes of public health, so there is an available nationwide network of outpatient psychological and psychiatric counseling for youth, adolescents, and adults. Following the amendments to the 2008 Health Protection Act, the network of service activities has been extended to the field of mental health protection. The newly established service for mental health promotion, drug prevention, and outpatient treatment focuses on early detection and rehabilitation of mental and behavioral disorders of adolescents and adults. Although working with adolescents at risk takes a significant part of their scope of activities, these services are still largely engaged in outpatient addiction treatment, primarily through pharmacological therapy. This leaves them less time to be involved in initiating other activities in the field of mental health prevention and promotion, for which they are legally competent (health promotion programs, continuous education for doctors and nongovernmental organizations, cooperation with the media and specific risk groups, etc.).

Along with services for mental health, *school medicine services* are important actors of the public health system. As of 1998, school medicine is exclusively a preventive service oriented toward preventive physical examinations, vaccinations, health education, and health counseling focused on individuals, families, schools, and the community. Although this organizational model is consistent with some other European models, implementation is facing challenges in terms of program scope, lack of personnel, and unsatisfactory cooperation with curative doctors (Jureša, 2007).

The *family centers* are social care institutions for providing counselling and helping families and individuals. Their establishment is important because they raise the quality of life of children, youth, and families and promote family values and responsible parenting. Moreover, they engage in various activities (workshops with family members, lectures for families, short leaflets, radio talks, etc.) to encourage participation in community work, such as volunteering and supporting organizations that deal with socially vulnerable groups, parents, families, children, and youth. Unfortunately, the family centers have recently become branch offices of the Social Care Centers, leading to a decrease in their activities. Preventive services for vulnerable groups, especially children and parents/families who need help in raising their children, have been reduced. *Social Care Centers* are located in all major Croatian cities. Although in part these are preventive-oriented institutions, their activities are directed more toward social and material welfare, services of youth courts, implementation of particular educational measures aimed at young delinquents, and so on.

From an organizational point of view, implementation of the prevention programs (school-based programs, counseling services, etc.) is handled at the local level. Moreover, the local community is often the source and generator of different prevention programs. Local organizations are in direct contact with the population and can provide specific and relevant insights into the problems and needs of the community. Cherishing local partnership and building local coalitions and national networks of coalitions are important resources of the prevention system. Organizational capacities, fostered by the local Croatian community, are the National Network of Healthy Cities and Healthy Counties, Councils for Prevention of Crimes, and the Communities That Care project.

The *Croatian Healthy Cities Network* is one of the oldest European national Healthy Cities network and one of the first registered NGOs in Croatia (1992). The 1988 Healthy Cities conference organized in Zagreb is referred to as the zero point, that is, the start of the Healthy Cites project of WHO's Office for Europe.[13] On the European level, 1,200 cities from approximately 30 European

13 More information on the history and the development of the Croatian National Network of Healthy Cities can be found at www.zdravi-gradovi.com.hr/.

countries have participated in the project. The network ensures the support for local communities in gathering and educating local multisector public health teams responsible for analyzing health needs; setting priorities and choosing strategies; analyzing existing resources; and ensuring support for finding financial funds for programs used to address specific needs. This resulted in the development of numerous local strategic documents, the most important being "Plan for Health," a framework for public health that defines local public health policy of investing in health during the mandate. Thus, a large number of local communities included priorities relating to mental health, youth, alcoholism, and other issues among important public health priorities such as cardiovascular diseases, carcinoma, and aging.

A significant advancement in the organization of prevention in a community was achieved during the implementation of the *Police in Community* project, when the Croatian Ministry of the Interior initiated activities to establish the Council for Prevention of Crimes, modeled after similar councils in numerous European cities. The Ministry of Interior of the Republic of Croatia recognized Communities That Care (CTC) as an effective system for the development of the Council for Prevention model that would be relevant for all communities and prevention committees in Croatia. These councils act within municipal administrations as coordination bodies that bring together representatives from different institutions, NGOs, and citizens who cooperate with the aim of prevention of crimes and other risk behaviors and attitudes, and improvement of the quality of life in their own territory. A special research team from the Faculty of Education and Rehabilitation Sciences at the University of Zagreb worked on a project regarding the assessment of efficiency of prevention councils (in two cities: Split and Čakovec). In the analysis of these councils' activities, Borovec (2013) emphasized criteria that contribute to the councils' efficiency: competent community leaders, choice of priorities based on risk and protective factors assessments, a focus on prevention programs proven to be effective, community willingness, organizational resources, and public and local politicians' attitudes. Based on the results of the survey, recommendations for key people and policy makers, regarding prioritizing preventive investments in communities, were prepared. The project resulted in higher awareness among key leaders and professionals of the need for evidence-based programs connected with risk behaviors and their predictors – risk and protective factors – as well as of the need for evaluation of long-term and short-term preventive investment outcomes (Novak, Mihić, & Bašić, 2013).

The *CTC project* (Hawkins, 1999; Hawkins, Catalano, & Arthur, 2002) was one of the first scientific and action projects in Croatia. Its aim was to control functioning and efficiency of the CTC prevention approach in the community. The project was conducted from 2002 to 2013 in twelve local communities in Istria County (with the leadership of Josipa Bašić) and adequately adapted. There was a greater focus on the sensitization, mobilization, and education of local people in the field of prevention; a larger number of associates from the local government, institutions, and NGOs were gathered for project participation; various expert groups with the task of solving specific issues were formed (groups for data collection and ensuring the quality of epidemiological data gathered; groups for developing prevention programs, improving, and evaluating existing prevention programs, etc.). The project followed all the steps of implementation as the original CTC system: (1) mobilization and community readiness for prevention; (2) assessment of needs and resources; (3) definition of preventive investments priorities; (4) implementation of chosen prevention programs; and (5) system (CTC) evaluation in all of the twelve communities. According to the results of the survey among citizen's key people and members of the local coalition for prevention, this project can be implemented in other areas of Croatia. The efficiency of prevention in these communities can be observed in all implementation domains (family, school, and local community) (Bašić & Grozić-Živolić, 2010). Many tools used and adapted in this project can be used in other Croatian communities, and, by expanding the system in several EU countries, results can be compared, which supports further application of the prevention system in Croatian communities.

The *Office for Cooperation with NGOs and the National Foundation for Civil Society Development* (along with local and regional resources for financing public needs in the fields of health care, education and social care, and EU financing annually or multi-annually) are the main financial resources to support prevention programs. Program application protocols are not generally comprehensive and often lack very important criteria, according to which quality and possible outcomes of the programs would be financed and assessed. Unfortunately, financial resources for prevention programs are not sufficient; however, given the possibility of multiple financing resources for promising and efficient programs, prevention programs are generally implemented continually.

The *Office for Combating Drug Abuse* recently conducted an analysis of public expenditure in the field of combating drug abuse in Croatia (Budak, Jurlina Alibegović, Slijepčević, & Švaljek, 2013). The total estimated specified public expenditure for combating drug abuse in national and county budgets and financial plans of public bodies and civil society organizations in 2011 amounted to just over 13 million euros. However, only 13 percent of the funds were specified for addiction prevention programs. Unspecified expenditures amounted to about 86.7 million euros. The majority of funding was directed to public order and security (80 percent) while a minor part to prevention. Such assessments show that annual costs of combating drug abuse in Croatia amount to almost 100 million euros, or 0.25 percent of the gross domestic product. According to the European Monitoring Centre for Drugs and Drug Addiction (EMCDAA, 2013b), Croatia is placed among the countries that spend a relatively large part of public expenditure on combating drug abuse, primarily with regard to wrapping up the social mess that substance abuse is responsible for.

Reports on financing NGOs' projects and programs from public resources (UZUVRH, 2014) show that the overall amount of finances in 2013 amounted to 75 million euros. Between 2009 and 2013, the amounts were not significantly changed and were around 65 million euros. Referring to the Croatian circumstances, it looks like a relatively large amount of funds have been set aside; however, an insight into the distribution of the funds shows that this is not true for the needs of children and youth. A review of general financing areas shows that only 3.1 percent of the aforementioned funds were used for health protection and preservation, mental and physical integrity, and life quality improvement; 2 percent of the funds were used for prevention of all types of addictions and unacceptable behaviors; only 0.3 percent went toward supporting children, and less than 0.1 percent for encouraging and affirmation of creativity and improvement of life skills and abilities of children and the youth. This indicates that, notwithstanding the preceding strategies, sufficient financial support for prevention programs was not forthcoming at the national level in the past and likely cannot be expected in the future.

Therefore, the findings of the analysis of public expenditure in the field of combating drug abuse in Croatia (Budak et al., 2013) are important. Authors emphasize the need to use the outcome indicators in planning, monitoring, and spending of public finances. Furthermore, it is important to provide increased funds to expand programs, activities, and projects that achieve good results, that is, objectives defined in national strategies. A part of funding should be taken from or canceled for programs, activities, and projects not achieving planned outcomes.

Prevention Programs and Implementation

The majority of prevention programs in Croatia are local and implemented on limited localities; moreover, they are being developed and evaluated on a local level. One research (Bašić, Ferić Šlehan, & Kranželić Tavra, 2007) showed that eight localities in Istria County foster thirty-nine prevention programs organized by municipalities/cities, social care centers, kindergartens, elementary schools, secondary schools, schools for special needs children, associations, healthy cities, and experts/individuals. A methodology similar to the one used by the Substance Abuse and Mental Health Services Administration (SAMHSA), a U.S. government agency, was used to assess the program/interventions efficiency (Schinke, Brounstein, & Gardner, 2002). Programs were classified into five categories: positive development programs (fourteen), problem-oriented prevention programs (fifteen), counseling centers (four), comprehensive community initiative (one), and other programs (five). Among fifteen problem-oriented prevention programs, none could be classified as a "model" program – that is, a program that showed positive outcomes in a number of replicated implementations and evaluation studies and that is prepared for dissemination (having technical materials like staff training, booklets, support by authors, etc.). Only three out of the fifteen could supply some positive results and were thus classified as "promising programs." Another research study (mentioned previously) on the quality of prevention program proposals (Mihić, 2013) assessed the quality of program proposals applied for funding from the local community in Istria County. This study found that the overall quality of the twenty-four program proposals that were examined was almost one standard deviation (–0.97 SD) below the chosen quality criterion, the theoretical mean (TM) of the overall quality index. Only four of the twenty-four proposals were found to be of higher quality. These results suggest that the quality level of project proposals is rather low, with the quality of the described evaluation procedures having the lowest mean score.

However, several Croatian organizations and institutions – like universities, public health organizations, and NGOs – do implement some of the world's best model programs, mostly taken from other countries (mostly the United States), such as PATHS (PATHS-RASTEM in Croatia); CAP; NORTHLAND (modified for implementation in Croatia as Clear Mind without Alcohol – BUBA); and Unplugged.

The PATHS program was originally a U.S. prevention program (Kucshé & Greenberg, 1994), voted one of top ten programs in the Blueprints for Violence Prevention[14] (Mihalic, Irwin, Elliott, Fagan, & Hansen, 2001) classification in the United States. Its aim is to promote socioemotional competence and reduce risks of behavioral and mental health problems in preschool and elementary school children with specially designed curricula. Elementary school teachers conduct the program from grades 1 through 4, delivering on average forty lessons per school year, covering emotion regulation, self-control, friendship, and self-esteem. Preschool teachers conduct the preschool intervention program for one year, delivering thirty-seven lessons covering emotion regulation, self-control, friendship, and self-esteem. The pilot implementation of the PATHS program in Croatia was conducted in elementary schools in Poreč and Labin in Istria County from 2007 to 2010 within the Communities That Care: Development, Implementation and Evaluation of Prevention in the Community project. Between 2010 and 2012, PATHS was conducted in fifteen experimental elementary schools (with an additional fifteen control schools) and six preschools in Zagreb, Rijeka, and Istria County. Several organizational and cultural adaptations were made: a number of themes were adjusted to fit the educational system in Croatia; some teaching methods were adjusted to didactic processes of Croatian classes (e.g., spelling was redundant in the Croatian context); and teaching material was adapted (e.g., children stories and character names were locally adapted). A randomized control trial showed an enhancement in learning behaviors, prosocial behaviors, and skills of emotion regulation in school children receiving the intervention and fewer symptoms of withdrawal and depression, a positive impact on reduction of ADHD symptoms, attention deficit, oppositional behavior, and aggressive behavior. Preschool PATHS utilized a quasi-experimental design. Children who finished preschool just as the program implementation started were used as the control group. The PATHS preschool program had a significantly positive impact on the reduction

14 Blueprints for Violence Prevention, www.ncjrs.gov.

of ADHD symptoms, attention deficit, oppositional behavior, and aggressive behavior. After one program year, the children's prosocial behaviors and emotion regulation had been enhanced, and the children showed fewer symptoms of withdrawal and depression and fewer peer problems (Novak et al., 2012).

Given the growing problem of addictive substances abuse among youth, the Teaching Institute for Public Health of Primorsko-goranska County in 2005 started implementing a systematic and comprehensive program of universal prevention for sixth and seventh graders, based on the Life Skills Training Program (Botvin & Griffin, 2005). Cooperation in the local community led to significant program adaptations (additional themes were added in the curriculum [e.g., cyber-violence], the structure of the curriculum was changed, the number of lessons per school year was reduced, and the period of implementation was prolonged) in order to make it an acceptable, long-term, sustainable program for the Croatian educational system (Roviš, 2012). The program has been implemented for ten years in more than fifty schools in the Rijeka region, with approximately ten thousand pupils from third through seventh grade participating in it each year. Mataija Redžović (2014) gives a good example of insistence on quality of this program's implementation. According to the teachers' assessment, the implementation support system was successful and ensures preconditions for quality implementation, as proposed by Domitrovich et al. (2008). Teachers' feedback on the program was positive, as they were satisfied with the quality of working materials and with the level of standardization of implementation as well as the system of support for executors, characterized by availability and quality support provided by the school coordinator, and the quality of provided education. Furthermore, the personal level of program acceptance and efficiency perception has also been positively assessed. A quasi-experimental evaluation design, with intervention and control school groups, was used in the evaluation of results of program implementation with sixth and seventh graders during the period 2005–2010 (all schools at the county level offered to participate in the program; intervention groups consisted of schools accepting participation in the program, while schools refusing to participate in the implementation were used as control group). Results from the 2005–2008 evaluation (Roviš, 2012), conducted in Rijeka's schools, showed up to 50 percent lower substance use rates among students in intervention schools delivering the complete program. The 2008–2010 evaluation regarding psychosocial benefits of the program is still not published, yet some preliminary key findings could be detailed. The 2008–2010 cohorts were evaluated at the county level dealing with a mixed urban and rural population. Results indicate significant psychological effects ($p < 0.05$) for students in the intervention group who received most of the program content. Schools that failed to deliver more than 50 percent of the curriculum were excluded from the study (final sample, $n = 1{,}537$; intervention group, $n = 1{,}268$; control group, $n = 269$; urban, $n = 611$; rural, $n = 926$; male = 789; female = 729). A significant reduction, compared to the control group, was found in attitudes favorable toward substance use ($F = 23.191$, $p = 0.000$), school anxiety ($F = 7.564$, $p = 0.006$), social anxiety

(F = 7.577, p = 0.006), poor self-image (F = 8.916, p = 0.003), emotional instability (F = 6,043, p = 0.014). Results also indicated better antismoking attitudes (F = 3.824, p = 0.051) and anti-alcohol drinking attitudes (F = 8.694, p = 0.003).

In 2010, the Teaching Institute for Public Health of Primorsko-goranska County started implementing the comprehensive program of mental health screening among seventh graders in Rijeka's elementary schools (Krnić & Ćosić, 2012). As a part of regular physical examinations, students filled out a short (ten-minute) questionnaire. The *Strengths and Difficulties Questionnaire* (Goodman, 1997) is suitable for early detection of difficulties related to behavior, emotional states, and/or peer relations. Psychologists, with extensive experience in working with young people at the Institute for Public Health, conducted the screening process, assisted by a school doctor and other professional services of the school. Based on the results of the screening and the synthesis of information collected by the school doctor, the school's expert assistants, and a mental health professional, recommendations were made to 10 percent of children and their parents to consult further with a psychologist and/or school doctor. Parents and students were recommended to enter individual or family counseling or psychotherapy, psychiatric treatment, parent and adolescent groups, or some other form of treatment. For example, the 2011–2012 screening included 1,240 children from a wider city area. The team syntheses led to 220 referrals being recommended to parents. As a result, 61 children and parents visited the counseling center while 26 remained for longer treatment. Previous experience in the implementation of this program showed that most children visit the counseling center due to behavioral problems, learning difficulties or difficulties with fulfilling school obligations, bullying, anxiety disorders, and general anxiety. This public health approach for screening and indicative prevention interventions was originally locally developed in the City of Rijeka and later adopted in Croatia by other local communities.

The *CAP* program[15] is a universal prevention program providing protection against physical abuse by empowering children and preventing attacks by peers, strangers (abduction), or known adults. CAP seeks to integrate the best community sources of support in order to reduce the vulnerability of children and youth to verbal, physical, and sexual abuse. The program was developed in the United States by the International Centre for Assault Prevention (ICAP) who appointed local organization (Parents' Association Step by Step, Croatia[16]) to be the Regional Training Center for CAP in Croatia, meaning it acts under the auspices of ICAP in the delivery of training and copyrighted curricula, and it is the *only agency authorized* to train people for implementing CAP in Croatia. The CAP program utilizes a three-pronged approach to prevention education:

15 More information on the the International Centre for Assault Prevention and CAP programs can be found at www.internationalcap.org.

16 More information on the Parents' Association Step by Step, Croatia, can be found at www.udrugaroditeljakpk.hr.

staff in-service training, parent's workshops, and children workshops. Assault is presented as a violation of basic human rights and the notion that all people and their children deserve to be "Safe, Strong, and Free." A follow-up study (sample: 646 children, 467 parents, 31 teachers), performed thirty-six months after the end of program, showed significantly improved communication about violence between children, as well as between children and adults (parents and teachers). Teachers reported that children speak more often and more openly about personal safety problems that they have; the majority of children remember safety strategies learned in workshops, and some of them (14 percent) have experienced situations in which they applied these strategies (Maljković & Hitrec, 2009).

BUBA is an original U.S. Northland program (Perry et al., 1996), culturally adapted for use in Croatia. This multicomponent program is designed to discourage alcohol use and promote positive development in adolescents. Training sessions or group activities were administered on a weekly basis from fifth through seventh grade and operated on the family, school, peer, and community levels through components such as parent–child communication sessions, administration of a social-behavioral curriculum, peer leadership training, and community organizing. The program lasted three years (eight to ten hours annually, in the fifth through seventh grades). A local study showed that this prevention program can have an influence on alcohol use among children in primary schools.[17] Although the program had no impact for high-risk children, the BUBA experimental group reported significantly more favorable behaviors, such as not drinking alcohol, not getting excessively drunk, not drinking more than one drink at one occasion, and not going to places where peers drink alcohol, as well as fewer intentions to drink alcohol and fewer occurrences of actual alcohol drinking.

Unplugged[18] is a universal prevention program that promotes positive and healthy behavior and is focused on prevention of the use of addictive substances (tobacco, alcohol, and other addictive substances). It has two components: for students and parents. The student component consists of twelve workshops: four on information and attitudes, four on development of students' interpersonal skills, and four on development of students' intrapersonal skills. Student workshops are led by class masters or teachers. The parent component revolves around the following topics: (1) better understanding of teenagers; (2) parenting a teenager means growing up together; and (3) a good relationship with my child also means setting up rules and limits. Parents' meetings are led by school counselors and class masters/teachers. The program has been implemented in Croatia and significantly reduced children's substance abuse alongside strengthening the prosocial attitudes related to substance use (Kranželić Ferić Šlehan, Ricijaš, & Lotar, 2012).

17 More information on the program implementation can be found at www.zzjzdnz.hr.

18 More information on the Unplugged program can be found at www.mentorinternational.org/uk.

Let's Grow Up Together and *Let's Grow Up Together PLUS* are universal/selective prevention programs, with the Croatian program being developed by the United Nations Children's Emergency Fund (UNICEF) office for Croatia.[19] They are programs and media campaigns for parents of toddlers and preschool children. Let's Grow Up Together is for parents of preschool children, and Let's Grow Up Together PLUS is for parents of children with developmental difficulties. The program consists of eleven sessions, with group themes such as parental roles and goals, needs of children, listening skills, boundaries, problem solving. A quasi-experimental design was used several times, and research has significantly shown that involved parents feel more secure in their role, more critical toward their parental behaviors, have changed their behavior toward the child, have better connection with the child, understand better their children's needs, and spend more quality time with them (Pećnik & Starc, 2010; Starc, 2014).

Educating the Next Generation of Prevention Specialists for Research and Implementation of Evidence-Based Prevention Programs

When thinking about prevention science and practice, in addition to all of the aforementioned (knowledge of the prevalence of problems; risk and protective factors; resources for addressing, i.e., implementing evidence-based prevention programs), it is very clear that well-educated prevention practitioners, public leaders, and prevention theoreticians and researchers are required. A cooperation of science and practice is certainly the best solution for both practice and science in the field of promotion and prevention.

According to Saxena, Jane-Llopis, and Hosman (2006), there are evident limitations in prevention practice across the globe, such as the lack of evidence of program effectiveness, lack of any effect or negative effects in some programs, uneven quality of implementation, limited reach in population, (un) availability of policies and resources to support prevention and promotion in mental health, and finally a limited spectrum of available "programs that work." In order to overcome these limitations, a range of capacities should be built: a competent workforce with relevant knowledge and skills, organizational capacity, coalitions and partnerships, leadership, resources, and public support. As most of these rely on having competent individuals engaging in building and strengthening such capacities (advocating, policy making, decision making, etc.), there is an urgent need to focus on education of existing and future professionals. This is true everywhere, both in Croatia as well as other countries. For example, in Australia, one of the objectives of the Australian Health

19 More information on the Let's Grow Up Together and Let's Grow Up Together PLUS programs can be found at www.rastimozajedno.hr.

Promotion Association's Strategic Plan 2009–2012 is the development of an effective and sustainable health promotion workforce (AHPA, 2009).

According to Saxena et al. (2006), educational opportunities need to be integrated into regular educational programs (college, graduate, and postgraduate programs) and into an institutional framework that will guarantee its sustainability and institutionalization. At college and graduate levels, there are some courses connected with prevention and promotion at some universities and faculties in Croatia. However, most of them are held in the University of Zagreb's Faculty of Education and Rehabilitation Sciences as part of the graduate program of social pedagogy. Needless to say, this is not enough.

A good example of how multidisciplinary postgraduate programs can provide an answer to the changing needs of societies can be found in Ireland. Following the national mental health policy recommendations regarding building a competent workforce, Ireland has developed a strong infrastructure for health promotion with more than three hundred dedicated health promotion specialists working in health promotion and mental health promotion (McKenna, Barry, & Friel, 2005).

Based on the capacity analysis (Roviš, 2010) and taking into account guidelines on core competences of (mental) health promotion specialists (AHPA, 2009; Barry, Battel-Kirk, & Dempsey, 2012), the University of Rijeka, Croatia, initiated a European project that resulted in a curriculum being developed for a postgraduate specialist study in health promotion and drug prevention at the Medical Faculty. The study program was piloted and fully established in 2007–2010. The program is intended for practitioners, public administration officers, and NGOs that are working in the field of mental health promotion and prevention and that are in need of this specific knowledge and skills enabling them to engage in more effective prevention efforts. Students are trained in theoretical concepts and applications of knowledge in the field of socioemotional development of children and youth; epidemiology of substance abuse and other risk behaviors; aetiology, early detection and treatment of addiction, and other risk behaviors; physical health promotion and mental health promotion; prevention strategies and evidence-based programs; and development and evaluation of health promotion and prevention programs. The next step for the program is to apply to international students and strengthen collaboration with acknowledged international professors and organizations in the field of mental health promotion and prevention research.

The postgraduate doctoral program "Prevention Science and Disabilities Studies" was envisioned on the basis of the project "Development and Evaluation in the Community with Supported Prevention and Rehabilitation" (2005–2006), supported by the National Foundation for Science, Higher Education, and Technological Development of the Republic of Croatia (Bašić, 2010) at the University of Zagreb's Faculty of Education and Rehabilitation Sciences. This doctoral program is based on a modern interdisciplinary scientific understanding of health promotion, prevention of mental and behavioral disorders, crime, addiction, violence, and other risk behaviors in children and youth. The program provides training in monitoring and describing problems and needs of children and youth at risk of developing various forms of problem behavior; describing and monitoring occurrences and problems in multi-annual research (longitudinal studies); evaluating and constantly modernizing existing forms of prevention interventions (evaluation studies and cost-effectiveness studies); elaborating and implementing overall strategies and policy for health promotion, risk behavior prevention, and quality of life for children, youth, and adults. Collaboration with professors and scientists from Pennsylvania State University (U.S.; College of Health and Human Development, Human Development, and Families Studies and Prevention Research Center) and the Radboud University Nijmegen (the Netherlands) is very important for this doctoral program bringing together experts from several scientific fields from Croatia and abroad. This doctoral program is the first modern postgraduate doctoral program of its kind in Croatia and one of the rare few in European and global contexts.

Final Remarks and Conclusions

Following a fundamental and disruptive social, political, and economic transition in the 1990s, the Republic of Croatia has been facing growing public health issues in adolescent health. As a response to these challenges, the Republic of Croatia has developed a series of national strategies and action plans for the prevention of various behavioral disorders or protection of children, family, and youth.

Due to the comprehensiveness in the scope of the policy documents and limited resources available, there is room for significant variation in what the final implementation will be. A partial or purely superficial declarative implementation of some measures and significant or overemphasized support of other measures may significantly influence the overall policy related to youth, drugs, violence, and other behavior problems. Justified is likewise the question of necessity to have no less than fourteen national programs and strategies that may be characterized as national prevention policies conducted in primary schools ("Nacionalni program prevencije …," 2010). Therefore, it is also justified to pose the question of the need for cooperation in the implementation of existing strategies or integration of strategies (in general parts) in order to ensure savings (duplication of expenses and tasks); improve cooperation between sectors and experts; and achieve more efficient outcomes and the visibility of efficiency of public policies throughout Croatia. Currently, we witness different levels of "preparedness," by various localities and regions, for the implementation of national strategies instead of a uniform prevention policy and practice in Croatia.

Unfortunately, until now no intensive discussion regarding the evaluation of different strategies concerning youth has taken place in Croatia. As a result of that, many strategies and programs are imposed on local communities that cannot and do not know how or when to implement them. The prevention infrastructure and capacities (e.g., human, expert, organizational) do not comply with the strategies. There is a need to increase visibility and accessibility of programs that have proven effective on local and national levels and to integrate them in a comprehensive national prevention policy.

Some good examples do exist. Following the implementation of the National Strategy for Combating Drug Abuse 2006–2012, the Office for Combating Drug Abuse of the government of the Republic of Croatia conducted an external strategy implementation evaluation. Results indicate communication and interinstitutional cooperation as the weakest points in the applicable strategy in Croatia (2012–2017). They point to a lack of a model program as well as a lack of standardized guidelines for different areas of drug demand reduction, research, and, in general, program and project evaluation in all fields of combating drug abuse ("Nacionalna strategija suzbijanja ... ," 2012). The implementation of this type of external evaluation of the national strategy presents a positive step forward with regard to general prevention standards. These evaluations serve as a basis for a new strategy, thus completing the policy circle. The new National Strategy 2012–2017 for the first time clearly emphasizes the commitment to quality, science-based, and sustainable programs of prevention, early detection, treatment and rehabilitation, and damage reduction.

Croatia still lacks a single database of evaluated projects and a database of successful programs, so-called model programs, even though a few years ago efforts were made in that direction by establishing the National Registry of Addiction Prevention Programs.[20] So far, this registry includes only a list of programs being conducted in Croatia and a brief description of key characteristics with no evaluation results provided. This registry certainly contributes to increasing transparency and visibility of local prevention programs. The publication of results of the evaluation of some of those programs and their cataloguing according to evidence-based standards are expected soon. One of the few evaluations of school-based programs in the city of Rijeka and Istria County proved that significant differences exist in school capacities for self-analysis and evidence-based program planning (Bezinović, 2014; Bezinović & Roviš, 2009). Presently, schools are under constant pressure from education authorities and the public. They are often forced to accept and adopt different fragmented initiatives for resolving different problems, which are imposed without real understanding of their purpose, priorities, and the schools' developmental needs. Moreover, the initiatives are not coordinated, monitored, or evaluated, which impedes their improvement, while their effects often remain unknown. Therefore, a successful implementation requires a coherent, coordinated, and economically organized school prevention program.

The experience of the Rijeka Institute of Public Health shows that it is possible to organize and manage universal and indicated prevention programs

20 The National Registry of Addiction Prevention Programs can be found at www.programi.uredzadroge.hr.

in Croatia at the national level when strong support of key local actors (i.e., health, education) is ensured, where a strong organizational infrastructure and resources of program implementers/coordinators exist (personnel, expertise, material, and technical conditions) along with great commitment of program leaders and compliance with limitations and nonderogation from the rules of profession. The aforementioned is also indicated in the findings of the Communities That Care project in Istria County (Bašić & Grozić-Živolić, 2010), while some prevention committees (Novak et al., 2013) stress the great importance of the level of readiness of communities for prevention as well as of efficient mobilization of key actors, experts, and citizens. Moreover, the ever more numerous experiences in the implementation of evidence-based programs in Croatia show that there are individual and organizational capacities to implement serious programs and studies that should be further strengthened. Since there is no doubt that good practice examples exist at the local level, it is important to point to the need for national institutions to apply those examples at the national level. The task of national services is indeed to ensure the availability of local, regional, and international initiatives and to facilitate intersector cooperation, which is widely recognized as being instrumental to achieving more effective and sustainable health outcomes (WHO, 1997).

References

AHPA (Australian Health Promotion Association) (2009). *Core Competencies for Health Promotion Practitioners*. Queensland: Australian Health Promotion Association.

Albee, G. W., & Gullotta, T. P. (1997). *Primary Prevention Works*, 6th ed.. Thousand Oaks, CA; London; New Delhi: Sage.

Barry, M. M., Battel-Kirk, B., & Dempsey, C. (2012). The CompHP core competencies framework for health promotion in Europe. *Health Education and Behavior* 36: 648–62. doi: 10.1177/1090198112465620

Bašić, J. (2009). *Teorije prevencije: Prevencija poremećaja u ponašanju i rizičnih ponašanja djece i mladih*. Zagreb: Školska knjiga.

Bašić, J. (2010). "Prevention science and disability studies": a postgraduate doctoral study overview. *Journal of Public Health* 19: 39–45. doi: 10.1007/s10389-010-0382-2

Bašić, J., Ferić, M., & Kranželic, V. (2001). *Od primarne prevencije do ranih intervencija [From primary prevention to early intervention]*. Zagreb: Edukacijsko-rehabilitacijski fakultet Sveučilišta u Zagrebu.

Bašić, J., & Grozić-Živolić, S. (2010). *Zajednice koje brinu – Model prevencije poremećaja u ponašanju djece i mladih: Razvoj, implementacija i evaluacija prevencije u zajednici [Communities That Care – a model of behavioural disorder prevention: development, implementation and evaluation]*. Pula-Zagreb, Croatia: Istarska županija i Sveuciliste u Zagrebu Edukacijsko-rehabilitacijski fakultet.

Bašić, J., Šlehan Ferić, M., & Kranželić Tavra, V. (2007). *Zajednice koje brinu – model prevencije poremećaja u ponašanju: Strategijska promišljanja, resursi i programi prevencije u Istarskoj županiji [Communities That Care – strategic approach, recourses and preventive programs in Istria County]*. Pula-Zagreb, Croatia: Istarska županija i Sveuciliste u Zagrebu Edukacijsko-rehabilitacijski fakultet.

Bašić, J., Žižak, A., & Koller-Trbović, N. (1998). *Integralna metoda u primjeni [Implementation of integral method]*. Zagreb: Edukacijsko-rehabilitacijski fakultet Sveučilišta u Zagrebu.

Bezinović, P. (2014). *Istraživanje rizičnih ponašanja učenika srednjih škola kao podloga za planiranje školskih preventivnih programa u Istarskoj županiji [Students' risk behaviour survey as a resource for school-based prevention program planning in Istria County]*. Unpublished manuscript.

Bezinović, P., & Roviš, D. (2009). *Vrednovanje školskih preventivnih programa osnovnih škola Grada Rijeke: Samoanaliza i planiranje školskih preventivnih programa [Evaluation of prevention programs' in elementary schools in Rijeka: school self-analysis and prevention planning]*. Unpublished manuscript.

Biglan, A., Brennan, P. A., Foster, S. L., & Holder, H. D. (2004). *Helping Adolescents at Risk.Prevention of Multiple Problem Behaviors*. New York, London: Guilford Press.

Borovec, K. (2013). Razvoj vijeća za prevenciju kriminaliteta u lokalnoj zajednici prema održvim i učinkovitim koalicijama [Development of Crime Prevention Council in the Local Community Towards the Sustainable and Efficient Coalition]. *Policija i sigurnost* 22: 1–25.

Botvin, G. J., & Griffin, K. W. (2005). Prevention science, drug abuse prevention, and Life Skills Training: comments on the state of the science. *Journal of Experimental Criminology* 1: 63–78. doi: 10.1007/s11292-004-6462-y

Budak, J., Jurlina Alibegović, D., Slijepčević, S., & Švaljek, S. (2013). *Analiza javnih rashoda i prijedlog pokazatelja rezultata i ishoda za praćenje ostvarivanja ciljeva u području suzbijanja zlouporabe droga u Republici Hrvatskoj [Analysis of public costs related to drug abuse in Republic of Croatia]*. Zagreb: Ekonomski Institut Zagreb.

Buljan Flander, G. (2008). Internet djeca – trebamo li brinuti? [Children of Internet–Should we worry?]. *Zbornik radova sa skupa Nasilje nad djecom i među djecom [Proceedings from the symposium Violence against Children and among Children]*. Osijek, Croatia: Sveučilište Josipa Jurja Strossmayera u Osijeku Filozofski fakultet.

Buljan Flander, G., Durman Marijanović, Z., & Špoljar Ćorić, R. (2007). Pojava nasilja među djecom s obzirom na spol, dob i prihvaćenost/odbačenost u školi [Violence among children regarding gender, age and peer acceptance/rejection]. *Društvena istraživanja*, 16, 157–174.

Domitrovich, C. E., Bradshaw, C. P., Poduska, J. M., Hoagwood, K., Buckley, J. A., Olin, S., Romanelli, L. H., Leaf, P. J., Greenberg, M. T., & Ialongo, N. S. (2008). Maximizing the implementation quality of evidence-based preventive interventions in schools: a conceptual framework. *Advances in School Mental Health Promotion* 1: 6–28.

EMCDDA (European Monitoring Centre for Drugs and Drug Addiction) (2013a). *Europsko izvješće o drogama. Trendovi i razvoj*. Luxemburg: Europski centar za praćenje droga i ovisnosti o drogama (EMCDDA).

EMCDDA (European Monitoring Centre for Drugs and Drug Addiction) (2013b). *Statistical Bulletin*. Luxemburg: European Monitoring Centre for Drugs and Drug Addiction (EMCDDA).

Goodman, R. (1997). The Strengths and Difficulties Questionnaire: a research note. *Journal of Child Psychology and Psychiatry and Allied Disciplines* 38: 581–6. doi: 10.1111/j.1469-7610.1997.tb01545.x

Hawkins, D. J. (1999). Preventing crime and violence through Communities That Care. *European Journal on Criminal Policy and Research* 7: 443–58. doi: 10.1023/a:1008769321118

Hawkins, D. J., Catalano, R. F., & Arthur, M. W. (2002). Promoting science-based prevention in communities. *Addictive Behaviors* 27: 951–76. doi: 10.1016/S0306-4603(02)00298-8

Jureša, V. (2007). Zdravstvena zaštita školske djece i mladih – školska i sveučilišna medicina – prednost i nedostaci pojedinih modela zdravstvene zaštite [Health protection of school children – school and university medicine – advantages and disadvantages]. *Hrvatski časopis za javno zdravstvo*, 3: N/A.

Katalinić, D., & Huskić, A. (2014). *Izvješće o osobama liječenim zbog zlouporabe psihoaktivnih droga u Hrvatskoj u 2013. godini [2013 Report on people treated for psychoactive drugs abuse in Croatia]*. Zagreb: Hrvatski zavod za javno zdravstvo.

Kranželić, V., Ferić Šlehan, M., Ricijaš, N., & Lotar, M. (2012). Effectiveness evaluation of the Unplugged – substance abuse prevention program in Croatia. Paper presented at the 20th Annual Meeting of Society for prevention research: Promoting Healthy Living through Prevention Science, Washington, DC.

Krnić, D., & Ćosić, S. (2012). Zaštita menatlnog zdravlja u sustavu javnog zdravstva Primorsko-goranske županije [Mental health promotion and prevention in public health system of Primorsko-goranska County]. Paper presented at the 20th Annual Conference of Croatian psychologists: psychological aspects of contemporary family, marriage, and partnership, Dubrovnik, Croatia.

Kucshé, C. A., & Greenberg, M. T. (1994). *PATHS Program: Instructors Manual*. South Deerfield, MA: Channing Bete.

Kumar, R., O'Malley, P. M., Johnston, L. D., & Laetz, V. B. (2013). Alcohol, tobacco, and other drug use prevention programs in U.S. schools: a descriptive summary. *Prevention Science* 14: 581–92. doi: 10.1007/s11121-012-0340-z

Kuzman, M., Pavić Šimetin, I., & Pejnović Franelić, I. (2012a). *Ponašanje u vezi sa zdravljem u djece školske dobi 2009/2010: Djeca i mladi u društvenom okruženju [Behaviour with regard to health of the 2009/2010 school children: children and youth in social environment]*. Zagreb: Hrvatski zavod za javno zdravstvo.

Kuzman, M., Pavić Šimetin, I., Pejnović Franelić, I., Markelić, M., & Hemen, M. (2012b). *ESPAD the European School Survey Project on Alcohol and Other Drugs 2011*. Zagreb: Hrvatski zavod za javno zdravstvo.

Kuzman, M., Pejnović Franelić, I., Pavić Šimetin, I., & Pejak, M. (2008). *ESPAD (European School Survey Project on Alcohol and Other Drugs 2007)*. Zagreb: Hrvatski zavod za javno zdravstvo.

Maljković, M., & Hitrec, G. (2009). Izvještaj o evaluaciji učinaka/posljedica CAP programa prevencije zlostavljanja djece [Report about outcome evaluation of CAP program of children abuse prevention] (Unpublished paper).

Mataija Redžović, A. (2014). Implementation quality of school based prevention program (Unpublished master's thesis). University of Rijeka.

McKenna, V., Barry, M. M., & Friel, S. (2005). *Review of the National Health Promotion Strategy 2004*. Dublin: Department of Health and Children (DOHC).

Mićanović, M. (2013a). *Priručnik za učitelje i stručne suradnike u osnovnoj školi: Kurikulum zdravstvenog odgoja [Handbook for teachers and expert associates in elementary school: health education curriculum].* Zagreb: Ministarstvo znanosti, obrazovanja i sporta/Agencija za odgoj i obrazovanje.

Mićanović, M. (2013b). *Priručnik za učitelje i stručne suradnike u razrednoj nastavi: Kurikulum zdravstvenog odgoja [Handbook for teachers and expert associates in lower elementary teaching: health education curriculum].* Zagreb: Ministarstvo znanosti, obrazovanja i sporta/Agencija za odgoj i obrazovanje.

Mićanović, M. (2013c). *Priručnik za učitelje i stručne suradnike u srednjoj školi: Kurikulum zdravstvenog odgoja [Handbook for teachers and expert associates in secondary school: health education curriculum].* Zagreb: Ministarstvo znanosti, obrazovanja i sporta/Agencija za odgoj i obrazovanje.

Mihalic, S., Irwin, K., Elliott, D., Fagan, A., & Hansen, D. (2001). Blueprints for violence prevention. *Juvenile Justice Bulletin* 7: 1–15.

Mihić, J. (2013). Study of effectiveness of prevention programs. (Unpublished doctoral dissertation). University of Zagreb.

Molleman, G. R., Peters, L. W., Hosman, C. M., & Kok, G. J. (2005). Implementation of a quality assurance instrument (Preffi 1.0) to improve the effectiveness of health promotion in the Netherlands. *Health Education Research* 20: 410–22. doi: 10.1093/her/cyg142

Nacionalna strategija suzbijanja zlouporabe droga u Republici Hrvatskoj za razdoblje od 2012. do 2017. godine [2012–2017 National Strategy for Combating Drug Abuse](2012). Zagreb: Vlada Republike Hrvatske, Ured za suzbijanje zlouporabe droga.

Nacionalna strategija za prava djece u Republici Hrvatskoj za razdoblje od 2014. do 2020. godine [2014–2020 National Strategy for the Rights of Children in the Republic of Croatia] (2014). Zagreb: Ministarstvo socijalne politike i mladih, Vlada Republike Hrvatske.

Nacionalna strategija za prevenciju poremećaja u ponašanju djece i mladih od 2009. do 2012. [2009–2012 National Strategy for Prevention of Children and Adolescent Disorders] (2009). Zagreb: Ministarstvo socijalne politike i mladih, Vlada Republike Hrvatske.

Nacionalna strategija zaštite od nasilja u obitelji od 2008. godine do 2010. godine [2008–2010 National Strategy for Protection from Domestic Violence] (2007). Zagreb: Ministarstvo socijalne politike i mladih, Vlada Republike Hrvatske.

Nacionalni program prevencije … (2010). *Nacionalni program prevencije ovisnosti za djecu i mlade u odgojno – obrazovnom sustavu, te djecu i mlade u sustavu socijalne skrbi [National Addiction Prevention Program for Children in Education and Social Care System]* (2010). Zagreb: Vlada Republike Hrvatske.

Novak, M. (2013). An empirical study on implementation quality in prevention programs (Unpublished doctoral dissertation). University of Zagreb.

Novak, M., Mihić, J., & Bašić, J. (2013). Učinkovita prevencija u zajednici: smjernice za rad vijeća za prevenciju [Effective community-based prevention: implication for the councils for prevention]. *Policija i sigurnost* 2: 26–41.

Novak, M., Mihić, J., Bašić, J., Domitrovich, C., Nix, R., & Greenberg, M. (2012). Study of preschool and school PATHS implementation in Croatia. Paper presented at the 7th International PATHS Learning Conference: PATHS innovation and implementation, Zagreb.

Pećnik, N., & Starc, B. (2010). *Roditeljstvo u najboljem interesu djeteta i podrška roditeljima najmlađe djece [Parenting in best children's interest and supporting parents of toddlers]*. Zagreb: Ured UNICEF-a za Hrvatsku.

Perry, C. L., Williams, C. L., Veblen-Mortenson, S., Toomey, T. L., Komro, K. A., Anstine, P. S., ... Wolfson, M. (1996). Project Northland: outcomes of a communitywide alcohol use prevention program during early adolescence. *American Journal of Public Health* 86(7): 956–65. doi: 10.2105/AJPH.86.7.956

Popis stanovništva ... (2011). *Popis stanovništva, kućanstva i stanova 2011. Stanovništvo prema državljanstvu, narodnosti, vjeri i materinskom jeziku. [Census of Population, Households and Dwellings 2011. Population by Citizenship, Ethnicity, Religion and Mother Tongue]*. Zagreb: Croatian Bureau of Statistics.

Pregrad, J. (2010). *Program prevencije vršnjačkog nasilja – Za sigurno i poticajno okruženje u školama [Peer violence prevention program – for safe and encouraging school environment]*. Zagreb: Ured UNICEF-a za Hrvatsku.

Program aktivnosti za sprječavanje nasilja među djecom i mladima [Activities Program for Prevention of Violence among Children and Adolescents] (2004). Zagreb: Vlada Republike Hrvatske.

Ricijaš, N., Dodig, D., Huić, A., & Kranželic, V. (2011). *Navike i obilježja kockanja adolescenata u urbanim* sredinama - Izvještaj *o rezultatima istraživanja [Habits and characteristics of adolescents' gambling in urban surroundings – research results report]*. Zagreb: Sveučilište u Zagrebu Edukacijsko rehabilitacijski fakultet.

Roviš, D. (2010). Capacity building for health promotion and drug prevention in Croatia. *Journal of Public Health* 19(S1): 57–68. doi: 10.1007/s10389-010–0385-z

Roviš, D. (2012). Public health approach in implementation of evidence-based prevention programs in Primorsko-goranska County. Paper presented at the 8th International Scientific Conference Research in Education and Rehabilitation Sciences, Zagreb.

Sakoman, S. (2009). *Školski programi prevencije ovisnosti [School programs for addiction prevention]*. Zagreb: Agencija za odgoj i obrazovanje.

Saxena, S., Jane-Llopis, E., & Hosman, C. (2006). Prevention of mental and behavioural disorders: implications for policy and practice. *World Psychiatry* 5: 5–14.

Schinke, S., Brounstein, P., & Gardner, S. (2002). *Science Based Prevention Programs and Principles: Effective Substance Abuse and Mental Health Programs for Every Community*. Rockville, MD: Center for Substance Abuse Prevention, Substance Abuse and Mental Health Services Administration.

Silobrčić Radić, M., Hrabak-Žerjavić, V., & Tomić, B. (2004). *Mentalne bolesti i poremećaji u Republici Hrvatskoj [Mental diseases and disorders in the Republic of Croatia]*. Zagreb: Hrvatski zavod za javno zdravstvo.

Silobrčić Radić, M., & Jelavić, M. (2011). *Mentalne bolesti i poremećaji u Republici Hrvatskoj [Mental diseases and disorders in the Republic of Croatia]*. Zagreb: Hrvatski zavod za javno zdravstvo.

Singer, M., & Mikšaj Todorović, L.j. (1989). *Delinkvencija mladih. [Youth delinquency]*. Zagreb: Udružena samoupravna interesna zajednica socijalne zaštite grada Zagreba i Fakultet za defektologiju Sveučilišta u Zagrebu.

Starc, B. (2014). *Roditeljstvo u najboljem interesu djeteta i podrška roditeljima najmlađe djece s teškoćama u razvoju [Parenting in best children's interest and supporting parents of toddlers with special needs]*. Zagreb: Ured UNICEF-a za Hrvatsku.

Tonry, M., & Farrington, D. P. (1995). Strategic approaches to crime prevention. *Crime and Justice* 19: 1–20.

UZUVRH (Ured za Udruge Vlade Republike Hrvatske) (2014). *Izvješće o financiranju projekata i programa organizacija civilnog društva iz javnih izvora u 2013. godini [Report on financing NGOs' projects and programs from public sources in 2013].* Zagreb: Ured za Udruge Vlade Republike Hrvatske (UZUVRH).

Vidović, D. (2005). Abuse among children in schools (Unpublished master's thesis). Zagreb: University of Zagreb.

Vulić-Prtorić, A. (2002). Strahovi u djetinjstvu i adolescenciji [Fears in childhood and adolescence]. *Suvremena psihologija* 5: 271–93.

WHO (World Health Organization) (1997). *Everybody Business: Strengthening Health Systems to Improve Health Outcomes: WHO's Framework for Action.* Geneva, Switzerland: World Health Organization.

35 Stress Prevention among German Teachers

Stefanie Morgenroth, Petra Buchwald, &
Martina Braasch

Introduction

In 2014, Germany had about 80 million inhabitants (deStatis, 2015a). The most populous federal state is North Rhine-Westphalia (NRW), with about 17.5 million inhabitants (Information and Technique in NRW, 2015). In 2013–2014, about 170,000 teachers worked in North Rhine-Westphalia, which accounts for 23 percent of all teachers in Germany (deStatis, 2015b).

The Basic Law (Art. 30, Grundgesetz [GG], Bundestag, 2015) of the Federal Republic of Germany articulates that the responsibility and development of the educational system are tasks of the federal states (Bundesländer). The federal government is involved in only a few areas, such as external cultural policies or publishing and copyright law. To promote cooperation, all the sixteen education ministers – that is, one per state, such as Hessen, Bayern, or North Rhine-Westphalia – meet at the conference of ministers of education (KMK, 2015). Topics are, for example, interregional questions about education or common standards for curricular and school degrees.

Entering kindergarten is a first step in the German educational system. Kindergarten is provided for all children between two and six years of age, after which school attendance is compulsory (European Commission, 2009). Due to the fact that the federal states decide their own educational policies, the educational system varies per state throughout Germany. Yet, within the last few years, all states had to implement the inclusion system (GEW, 2013) as an essential educational objective of the federal government. Current studies show that teachers/schools of different states experience difficulties in how to handle the inclusion (e.g., Morgenroth, S. & Grosche, M. (in the press) Simon & Kruschel, 2013). One consequence of it is the increase of teachers' stress at work. This is a major problem, as previous studies have already indicated that German school development (which requires intensive teacher cooperation) is shaped by German teachers' stress (Rothland, 2013). This corresponds to the traditional structure of German schools, which is characterized by the individual professional culture of teachers. Namely, surveys show that German teachers are not used to considering each other as potential collaborators. Instead, they tend to perceive their peers as autonomous equals or as competitors. In other words, German teachers mainly follow an autonomy-parity principle (Lortie, 1975).

According to Lortie, this principle mirrors relevant cultural norms and values, which determine teachers' behavior. These norms include the following three tenets: (1) no other adult except for the teacher should exert influence on the lesson, (2) teachers should be regarded and treated as equals, and (3) teachers should interact courteously with each other but not interfere with a colleague's business. Contemporary studies often interpret this principle as a reason for the lack of intensive and effective cooperation in German school practice (cf. Altrichter & Eder, 2004; Gräsel, 2010). Only few studies point to the possibility that the autonomy-parity principle does not influence teachers' cooperation patterns (Soltau, Berthe, & Mienert, 2012).

Recently published figures of the Federal Statistics Office (deStatis, 2015c) show a surprising development. In 1999, the reason for 92 percent of early retirements among teachers was health problems (see §44 BBG). However, data in more recent years show a continued decline of early retirement of teachers: in 2007, the number decreased from 65 percent to 45 percent, and in 2006 and in 2010 even to 21 percent. Thus, data today show the lowest level of early retirement of German teachers since the recording of statistics began in 1993. However, these data in total do not support a positive reversal in the trend of stress among teachers, because current studies still show that German teacher's feel very stressed and exhausted (Hillert, Koch, & Lehr, 2013).

The standards for the theoretical teacher training (KMK, 2004) suggest that teachers should be aware of the basic findings of stress research. These standards imply the obligation to develop continuously one's professional competences. Thus, the awareness of stress and burnout is an essential part of German teacher training (KMK, 2004).

This chapter aims at depicting basic tenets of conservation of resources theory (COR theory). Subsequently, current findings regarding resources and coping strategies will be discussed for teachers in Germany. We will introduce the COR theory (Hobfoll, 1989, 1998) as our basic theoretical framework that allows for an analysis of German teachers' well-being and for an identification of resources crucial for preventing stress. Empirical studies based on COR theory will be discussed in terms of developing prevention programs and fostering the professional competence of teachers in Germany.

Theoretical Models of Stress

Organizational stress is mostly a chronic or repeated episode. When threat or loss conditions in a workplace, such as school, continue over a longer period of time, it results in chronic stress. Repeated episodic stress confronts the individual with different stressors at different times occurring frequently or idiosyncratically. All occupations in which the worker is intensively encountering other people, as in a school setting, are prone to be a source of many different stressors. Accordingly, a teacher would almost permanently be confronted with stressful events or stressors. Thus, the teacher profession is likely to establish chronic stress, which is typified by a significant and ongoing draw on resources (Hobfoll & Shirom, 2001). Fatally, this leaves the teacher in a process of ever-decreasing resources to combat the chronic stress situation.

Furthermore, invalidation of resources in chronic stress situations appears where valuable resources (like social skills or competence) are not valued by the professional environment, such as parents, colleagues, or even the entire society. In today's society, the teaching profession suffers from a loss of reputation (Dolton & Marcenaro-Gutierrez, 2013). In a worldwide survey about the status of the teaching profession, results for Germany showed that less than 20 percent of the participants believed that teachers are respected by their students. Furthermore, regarding trust in teachers' abilities to impart knowledge to their students, German teachers were rated at the bottom of all European countries in the survey (Dolton & Marcenaro-Gutierrez, 2013). Especially hard hit are teachers in Germany, concerning their reputation, with less than 20 percent of the participants in the survey saying they would support their children taking up the teaching profession on their own.

Transactional Model of Stress

Stress has been described as a damaging environmental stimulus, often referred to as an *input* or stressor, as an *output* or reaction to a stressor, or as a *transactional process* (Perrez & Reicherts, 1992; Schwarzer, 2000). Lazarus and Folkman (1984) described stress as a transactional process emphasizing the relationship between person and environment. This model takes into account a person's characteristics and the nature of the environmental event, initiating a stress appraisal (Lazarus & Folkman, 1984). In this transactional model, stress not only can be defined by an input or output, but rather it is especially defined by the relation between the concrete situation and a cognitively appraising individual (Schwarzer, 2000). Further, the basic premise in this model is that perceiving stress and coping with stress constitute processes of information processing that trigger appraisals, actions, and emotions. Stress then depends on an individual's appraisal, which may assess a stressful event as challenging or threatening demanding (Jerusalem, 1990). What becomes apparent is that the perception of stress depends on a subjective appraisal of a demanding situation, with stress being a result of cognitive appraisals – of the relationships between the person and the environment – which can then have either positive or negative consequences (Buchwald, 2002). Such an appraisal can result in perceiving a situation as irrelevant, positive, or stress-relevant, with the stress-relevant appraisal being prone to be further appraised as a threat to the self (Jerusalem, 1990). In their model, Lazarus and Folkman (1984) differentiate the processes of stress appraisal into two simultaneous cognitive steps. In a primary appraisal, a categorization of the situation as stress-(ir)relevant takes place, with further following appraisals concerning the kind of threat the situation triggers. The primary appraisal is further divided into the components *relevance* and *coherence* of the aim and the person's *involvement* (Schwarzer, 2000). Thus, personal goals, motivations, and the self-concept are factors integrated in the primary appraisal process (Bossong, 1999). For the secondary appraisal, the individual then assesses one's resources at hand that could be effectively implied in the coping process. Components relevant for the secondary appraisal are *responsibility*, *coping potential,* and future *expectations* (Schwarzer, 2000). A person's self-efficacy is in the focus of this process, with physical and also social or tangible resources relevant for the coping process. Along with this model, there is a simultaneous situation-focused appraisal on the one hand and a resources-focused appraisal on the other called the person-situation model (Buchwald, 2002). According to Lazarus and Folkman (1984), the concrete coping strategies are a derivation of the secondary appraisal of the resources at hand. Therefore, coping strategies comprise all cognitive and behavioral attempts to solve the threatening demands originating from the interrelation of a person and the demanding factors in the environment (Bossong, 1999).

Coping Strategies within the Transactional Stress Model

Lazarus and Folkman (1984) differentiate between problem- and emotion-focused coping. Problem-focused coping refers to a concrete context and aims at reducing or eliminating threats or to initiate a new process of appraising the situation (Bossong, 1999). Emotion-focused coping is directed to an alleviation of the stress symptoms but not to a concrete solution of the problem (Schwarzer, 2000). Emotion-focused coping often means a mastery of affects such as anger, helplessness, and fear resulting from the appraisal process. Such affects need to be reduced in order to enable a shift of attention. If the person's coping results in a new appraisal of the demanding situation, new strategies can be implied to cope successfully with the stressful situation (Bossong, 1999).

Obviously, Lazarus, and Folkman (1984) put the individual and the individual's appraisal prior to environmental factors. Problematic about this transactional approach to stress is that it does not differentiate their definitions of environmental or external demands on the one hand and coping capacities on the other (Buchwald, Schwarzer, & Hobfoll, 2004; Hobfoll, 1989). Coping capacities are defined as a person's ability to compensate for the demands. Demands, though, are defined as something requiring coping capacities (Lazarus & Folkman, 1984). Here, a circular explanation results where none of the definitions can stand on its own. Accordingly, none of the anticipated principles then can be falsified. If one refers back only to individual appraisals, it is difficult to explain which resources are needed for an individual or group in order to imply resources effectively or which common demands of specific risk groups can appear and be coped with.

However, for stress research and job-related stress prevention, it would be helpful to determine resources needed in specific groups, such as teachers, or to figure out what factors hinder an effective resource use. Furthermore, by focusing on the individual appraisal without taking into account the environmental factors objectively, stress-generating factors might remain undetected.

This could, for example, be the case when a teacher feels stressed once his or her laptop is broken. Such an event is not important for objective analysis of the stress-generating factors among the whole group of teachers. Rather, for understanding the stress at the group level, other variables might be important, such as changes in the curriculum, as these changes would affect all the teachers in the same way. Thus, although the transactional model is a useful theoretical framework to understand predictors and outcomes of stress, we have to widen our perspective on stress and coping by taking a more objective approach into account. Such a wider perspective is suggested by Hobfoll's COR theory, which stresses objective elements of threat and loss and puts special emphasis on real circumstances where concrete stressors occur. As COR theory has become a major theory in the field of burnout (Buchwald & Hobfoll, 2004; Hobfoll & Freedy, 1993; Hobfoll & Shirom, 2001; Ito & Brotheridge, 2003; Neveu, 2007), we will now introduce the basic principles of this theory and later proceed by explaining burnout in terms of COR theory.

Principles of COR Theory

In his COR theory, Hobfoll (1989, 1998) argues that the definition of stress as a state that occurs when demands exceed coping resources (as suggested by Lazarus & Folkman, 1984) is misleading. In COR theory, objective elements of threat and loss are accentuated, concentrating on the real circumstances where clear stressors occur. Of special interest regarding teacher stress and its prevention is that COR theory is a motivational stress theory that is useful for the prediction of a person's behavior when facing stressful events. Accordingly, one basic principle of COR theory is the idea that even when stress is not occurring, awareness of possible future stress would motivate the person to be prepared. This is where prevention research needs to start investigating possibilities of preparing the individual to confront stress with best possible resources at hand.

COR theory is based on several principles that constitute the model's understanding of how people respond to stress. People have a basic motivation to obtain, retain, and protect what they essentially value. What people value are resources. COR theory defines four basic categories of resources: (1) objects (e.g., laptop, teaching material); (2) conditions (e.g., good marriage, employment); (3) personal characteristics (e.g., self-efficacy, rhetorical skills, self-esteem); and (4) energies (e.g., time, money, credit). Psychological stress occurs when individuals (1) are threatened with resource loss; (2) experience an actual loss of resources; or (3) fail to gain desirable resources (Hobfoll, 1988, 1989, 1998, 2011).

Building on COR theory, Hobfoll (1998) suggests several key principles that have been evident in many studies of stress within the last twenty-five years and that allow for an even better understanding of stress, its dynamics, and consequences for the individual. The first principle defines the *primacy of resource loss*. Resource loss is disproportionally more salient than resource gain and impacts people at rapid and accelerating speed. The second principle states that people need to *invest resources* in order to protect against resource loss, recover from losses, and be able to gain new resources. The critical point about this principle is that those with fewer resources are more vulnerable to resource loss and suffer from poor conditions for gaining resources. What can be drawn from the second principle here is that people need to build a resource pool on which they can rely when it comes to a situation where resources need to be invested in order to cope with stress or where new resources could be gained. In this context, Hobfoll (2011) further defines *caravans of resources* for those people who live in resource-enriching environments. The third principle states that although resource loss is more potent than resource gain, the salience of gain increases under situations of resource loss (Hobfoll, 1998). This paradoxical increase in resource gain saliency becomes apparent under conditions of loss, when acting leads to small gains that might result in positive expectancy and thereby trigger further goal-directed efforts.

These principles of COR theory lead to two special dynamics called resource *loss spirals* and *gain spirals* (Hobfoll, 1988, 1998). On the one hand, people who lack resources are more vulnerable to resource loss and initial loss results in future loss *(loss spirals)*. On the other hand, people who have resources at their disposal are more capable of gain, and initial resource gain results in further resource gain *(gain spirals)*.

Referring back to the first principle – primacy of resource loss – loss spirals will be more impactful for the individual and accelerate more easily than gain spirals. According to COR theory, loss spirals are initiated due to the primary loss of resources in a stressful event where further resources are needed to cope with the stress and to offset further resource loss. Those spirals primarily occur when facing long-term stress or when key resiliency resources are threatened or lost. Thereby, an establishment of new resource pools is limited (Schumm, Stines, Hobfoll, & Jackson, 2005).

On the other hand, it is extremely difficult to initiate gain spirals, which then demand significant resource investment by the individual's family and social system. Furthermore, COR theory concludes that people strive to build up and accumulate resources in times without stress (Buchwald, 2002), which results in resource reservoirs (Hobfoll, 2001). By building such resource reservoirs, people engage and deal with their hypothetical future stress events in a preventive way. Teacher trainees, for example, could join advanced training in rhetorical or communicative skills in order to be able to cope with hypothetical communication difficulties in their classroom. Thus, they would gain further resources – in this case, personal resources – which are accumulated and can be used in possible future situations. Indeed, it is further possible for people to develop coping skills in order to establish resource gains. Often, people with a success history are prone to have well-established coping skills, whereas people with a history of failure are likely to lack such coping skills and consequently struggle to initiate gain spirals (Hobfoll & Buchwald, 2004). For prevention in terms of this corollary of COR theory, feelings of success have to be facilitated in order to foster personal resources and to initiate gain spirals. A teacher who prepares lessons on the basis of teaching material from his studies and experiences success with these lessons might foster and enhance this coping strategy by asking other fellow students for their material, for example. This dynamic leads not only to an accumulation of objective resources (teaching material) but also to an increase in personal resources such as self-esteem. Thus, the here depicted gain spiral leads to further gains once initiated. COR theory perspective on *burnout* provides a perfect basis for the development of prevention interventions to reduce teachers' stress and burnout (Käser & Wasch, 2009)

Burnout

Approaches and definitions on burnout are numerous, since Freudenberger (1974) implied this to describe a psychological state that has been detected in exploratory studies with employees in health care. Later on, as this phenomenon became more and more important, there was an inflationary stream of definitions, ranging from *anxiety* to *lack of enthusiasm* (Schaufeli, Enzmann, & Girault, 1993). Freudenberger (1974) himself described *burnout* as failing, wearing out, or becoming exhausted by making demands on energy, strength, or resources. Since then, Freudenberger (1983) redefined his conceptualization and defines it as the process of depletion of physical and emotional resources that are appear in different forms depending on the occupational, organizational, and personal context of the individual. The Maslach Burnout Inventory (MBI; Maslach & Jackson, 1981, 1996), the most frequently used scale to measure burnout, defines the construct as consisting of the three components: emotional exhaustion, depersonalization, and lack of personal accomplishment. Regarding the intensity of stress, burnout is a more gradually increasing process, characterized by reduced productivity, alienation to others, and the aforementioned emotional exhaustion (Maslach & Leiter, 1997).

From COR theory perspective, burnout basically results from a lack of resource gain, as a result of the investment of resources that were maybe even borrowed from family resources or social resources in order to cope with stress at work (Hobfoll, 2001). Thus, burnout as a result of chronic stress can be approached from COR theory's perspective by recalling one of COR theory's basic principles, the individual's resource loss circle. When confronting stress, the individual resource net loss of any combination of the individual's physical vigorousness, emotional robustness, and cognitive ability is the consequence (Hobfoll & Shirom, 2001). In accordance with the aforementioned loss spiral principles and the primacy of resource loss (see Figure 35.1), this net loss, in turn, cannot be defeated by investing other resources or by gaining additional resources through an extant investment. What happens is that for individuals suffering stress, their losses make them enter an escalating loss spiral (Wells, Hobfoll, & Lavin, 1997). Entering this loss spiral, they may reach an advanced

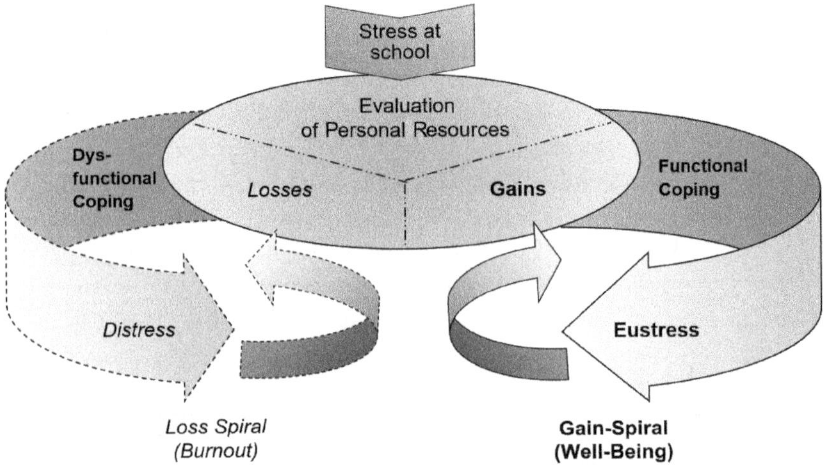

Figure 35.1. *Gains and losses of resources (according to Buchwald & Hobfoll, 2004; Morgenroth, 2015).*

stage of burnout with symptoms of depression or psychological withdrawal. For teachers, this could result in symptoms such as acting with cynicism toward students, parents, or colleagues or dehumanization of their social environment. In early stages of burnout, a depletion of energy resources will be one characteristic. By using up these resources for coping with threatening demands, coping behaviors might become ineffective, and the individual might give up and engage in emotional detachment and defensive behaviors that might lead to depressive symptoms (Ezrahi & Shirom, 1986).

Regarding the burnout process, Hobfoll's (1989, 1998) COR theory may offer further insights into the relations among the different types of intrinsic resources whose depletion is part of the characteristics of burnout. According to COR theory, among object and condition resources there is a distinction between primary and secondary resources (Hobfoll & Shirom, 2001). Primary resources, such as shelter and food or relationships with significant others, are essential for a human being to survive. The reason why Hobfoll defines these resources as secondary lies in their interdependency with primary resources. Secondary resources, such as physical power, mental agility, and emotional capability, determine a person's competitive position with regard to owning and using primary resources. Burnout appears where these secondary resources are lost, depleted, or ineffectively replenished. Furthermore, COR theory states that where individuals overweight the consequences of losses, they need to invest more resources to prevent further losses than the initial threat of losses would actually have demanded. Accordingly, the burnout process is, and remains, inseparably linked with the individual's personal characteristics. In examining the development of burnout at work, one needs to regard the personality type and the individual traits, as always interacting with organizational circumstances.

Based on COR theory's principles Hobfoll predicts that individuals lacking strong resource pools would more likely experience loss spirals of resources. If these loss spirals of resources will not be replenished and a chronic depletion of energy results, which initiates the burnout process. To refer back to our prior example, a teacher who has no own teaching material will have to develop new lessons and put lots of energy into lesson planning. Resources of time and maybe further social resources get lost due to the intensive preparation time, which results in the initiation of a loss spiral. This loss spiral accelerates and aggravates seriously, if the lesson planning does not lead to success or to a lack of recognition from colleagues or pupils, so that a gain of resources could make the investment of time resources worthwhile.

Burnout at School

Chronic stressors may also undermine resources, in and of themselves (Hobfoll & Shirom, 2001). Due to the permanent confrontation, individuals try different strategies to utilize their resources. When the individual experiences coping strategies and the investment of a resource as ineffective, invalidation occurs in the sense that the individual loses faith in the resource. Thus, invalidation of resources can occur on the basis of external but also internal factors.

Episodic stress in school settings as a workplace setting can also occur, but can more easily be handled effectively for those teachers with strong resource pools. Well-prepared teachers with lots of teaching material at hand and social resources can build on their rich resource pool to cope with episodic stress. Because the stress occurs episodic, resources can be invested when demands increase and resources are challenged step by step but can be developed and fostered in a proceeding resource gain. Episodic stress includes phases of relaxation between stressors, which allow a regrouping of resources, analysis of what worked and what did not, and a chance to bolster resources for the future (Hobfoll & Shirom, 2001). Episodic stress, frequently occurring in organizations with periods of peak demand, can be found in the teaching profession toward the end of each term, when demands regarding final exams or school certificates increase. Teachers with a well-established resource pool and experiences and capacities regarding coping skills will be able to invest resources purposely and further grow their coping skills and resource pools due to that challenge. Those teachers, though, who suffered from chronic stress during the whole term feel the urge to invest the last remaining resources for coping with the further increasing stress and will then be highly in danger of deepening their loss spiral or to even pass over into the burnout process.

In a COR theory perspective on burnout, workplace-specific stressors can be regarded in the coping process, such as high workloads (e.g., lesson planning and assessment, social and pedagogical demands in school settings, school community development), difficulties through role conflicts, or the lack of feedback. Teachers confront these stressors with an investment of adequate resources. Object resources for teachers could be the working spaces or material. Condition resources are the teacher's autonomy, participation in decision processes, opportunities for advancement, or security of employment. Self-efficacy, empathy, and social responsibility are important personal resources in the teaching profession. Energy resources, such as methodological or specialized knowledge, time, and money, are typical resources that help to gain further resources. COR theory stresses the relevance of an individual's motivation for the proceeding of burnout and thereby focuses on the premise motivation of people to obtain, retain, and accumulate resources in order to cope with work-specific demands. Emotional exhaustion as one of the three basic components of burnout happens if this motivation is undermined. Thus, when teachers realize that resources such as endurance, empathy, and time are used up to cope with stressors originating from student–teacher interaction, emotional exhaustion may result (Lee & Ashforth, 1996). Depersonalization in the teaching profession occurs if teachers prefer to secure their existing resources in conflicts resulting from social interactions with students, colleagues, or parents. The third dimension of burnout, reduced productivity, may result from a decreasing positive assessment of one's own performance and proficiency. Accordingly, in a longitudinal study, significant negative relations were found between burnout and self-efficacy (Schmitz & Schwarzer, 2000). COR theory does not predict a sequence in which the components of burnout appear, but postulates that the existence of one component triggers the probability of occurrence of the other two. This dynamic process accelerates over time, as the aforementioned loss spirals do. But, with loss spirals in extreme stress situations accelerating within a short period of time, burnout is, more slowly but steadily, a decrease of resources. This gradual, often hardly noticeable process equals in its outcome the severity of extreme stressful events.

This slow, progressive decrease of workplace-specific resources through false investment was proven especially for teachers, who show the highest burnout rate in social professions (Käser & Wasch, 2009). In order to meet their own, students', colleagues', parents', and society's requirements, teachers need to invest an extreme amount of resources in their work with students. In addition to teaching and imparting knowledge, there is a high amount of social work to do in a teacher's profession, with first of all being engaged in positive relationships with one's students. Stressors such as classes with large groups, often high noise levels, and many individual requirements of underachieving children result in a long chain of micro losses on the teacher's side. Teachers' typical isolation aggravates this situation even further (Schmid, 2003). Despite teachers' effort and investments, resource gains are extremely rare. Gains could result from realizing students' growing competence and gaining of new abilities, which were promoted by the teacher. Further, thankfulness of parents, students, the school principal or society would manifest resource gains. Instead, teachers rarely receive clear feedback about their students' progress and only marginal support by colleagues or the school principal (Neuenschwander, 2003).

How teachers cope with these situations was investigated by Schaarschmidt and her team (Schaarschmidt & Fischer, 2003) in the context of Antonovsky's (1987) theory of resources and the transactional model of coping by Lazarus and Folkman (1984). Schaarschmidt investigated the personal resources necessary in the teaching profession to cope with workplace-specific demands. Schaarschmidt and Fischer's (2003) findings suggest a typology of four work-related behavior and experience patterns – types G, S, A, and B. These types were later described by Buchwald and Hobfoll (2004) in terms of COR theory. Teacher type G, which is characterized as healthy, shows a high but not too high engagement and ambition with the ability of alienation and regeneration. In terms of COR theory, this type has the perfect balance between investing and retaining resources but at the same time the ability to distance oneself within one's individual comfort zone to regenerate the personal resources. Schaarschmidt and Fischer (2003) characterize teacher type S as a type sparing oneself. In the COR theory perspective, type S's behavior can be explained as avoidance of stress in order to save resources. As those teachers fear to lose valuable resources through a lack of resource gain after excessive investment, they will cope with problems by strategies of avoidance. Instead of the teacher actively coping with a situation, the fear of losing resources is too dominant and leads to avoiding confrontations. From a pedagogical perspective regarding motivation in one's profession, this behavior is surely questionable, but in terms of the principles of resource dynamics it becomes comprehensible (Buchwald & Hobfoll, 2004). Actually, Schaarschmidt and Fischer (2003) found the reduced pedagogical engagement of the teacher type connected with inner balance, perception of social support, and a positive attitude toward life, but not with resignation.

The two further teacher types need to be in focus of our investigation regarding a potential to suffer from intense stress and/or burnout as they show psychological impairments. Risk type A invests resources with a too high engagement in school and is willing to offer all resources to the profession. Type A lacks the ability to take a healthy distance to work and as such cannot save his or her resources. These teachers' behavior is connected with negative emotions, which means that they step into a loss spiral characterized by a permanent investment of resources with simultaneously lacking a gain or benefit. What follows is a feeling of reduced life satisfaction. Risk type B similarly shows reduced abilities to take distance to work problems and demands. The loss spiral for type B is the most fatal one, as it increases its dynamic and the resulting motivational and emotional constraints to an extremely high extent. This type of teacher is hardly willing to invest resources at all, resigning themselves to showing reduced engagement at work and productivity (Buchwald & Hobfoll, 2004).

Nevertheless, Schaarschmidt and others (e.g., Cherniss, 1995) showed that burnout in the teaching profession did not depend exclusively on specific personal traits and one's personal resources but that the loss of object and condition resources, as conceptualized in COR theory, can also result in burnout. In Schaarschmidt's approach (Schaarschmidt & Fischer, 2003), based on the transactional model (Lazarus, 1999; Lazarus & Folkman, 1984; Lazarus & Launier, 1981), individual differences of burnout were found depending on the teachers' individual appraisal of the extent of demand within individual working groups (e.g., working with problematic students, class size, administrative duties). Accordingly, the subjective appraisal of environmental factors was assessed, but not their objective relevance. COR theory, in contrast, combines objectively and subjectively perceived aspects of one's environment in terms of stress and coping. The former approach bears the risk of leaving objective environmental stressors undetected when strictly focusing on individual perceptions (Buchwald & Hobfoll, 2004). For instance, in a study of Schaarschmidt and Fischer (2003), the perceived state of repair did not correlate significantly with burnout. But, in studies of burnout in kindergarten teachers (Schwarzer, 1999), the objective size of the room was the best predictor of burnout. In this context, it should be stressed that COR theory does not ignore the relevance of subjective perceptions but emphasizes the relevance of subjective and objective resources for investigating stress and burnout processes.

As mentioned previously, from our point of view, this deficit can be confronted by empirical studies that define burnout from a resource-oriented perspective as a consequence of chronic stress accompanied by loss spirals. One of the early studies able to prove COR theory's principles for trainee teachers was launched by Dückers-Klichowski (2005). A study by Klusmann, Kunter, and Trautwein (2009) provided further empirical evidence for the significance of a resource-oriented approach to understand burnout. In a longitudinal study with 158 teachers, Klusmann et al. (2009) examined how Schaarschmidt and Fischer's (2003) professional behavioral characteristics of their four types of burnout, defined by personal resources, actually function as risk or preventive factors for teachers' stress appraisal. Klusmann and colleagues' findings confirmed the correlation between behavioral characteristics of the four burnout types and the stress experience. Furthermore, the findings by Klusmann et al. (2009) confirmed the resource-oriented interpretation of Schaarschmidt and Fischer's (2003) types by Buchwald and Hobfoll (2004) and their relevance for the explanation of a burnout development. Still, by illustrating gain and loss spirals depending on the extent of resource investments (engagement) and resource protection (resilience) in times of stress, Klusmann et al. (2009) looked only at effects on an individual level whereas the social context was neglected.

All in all, there have been many studies analyzing teacher's burnout (e.g., Burke, Greenglass, & Schwarzer, 1996; Morgenroth & Buchwald, 2015; Peters, 2013; Poschkamp, 2008) in which social support was demonstrated to be an effective coping strategy. Yet, it also became clear that the resource management is an important aspect to understand the formation process of burnout (e.g., Böhm-Kasper, 2004; Huber & Wolfgramm, 2011). The following section further describes the relevance of resource management analysis among German teachers, leading to articulate possible stress preventive interventions.

Stress Prevention at School

In pursuit of developing stress prevention strategies for teachers, one needs to investigate what are the specific stressors at the given school. This is due to the need to learn more about the kind of resource demand required for individuals and the school organization, respectively, to cope with stress in this specific workplace setting. Our aim is to shed some light on how different stressors affect teachers' resources, in order to facilitate the conceptualization of stress prevention for teachers. Empirical evidence strongly confirmed that it is of major importance to interrupt or prevent a loss spiral. Hobfoll (1998) describes four basic theoretical assumptions of interventions, which we will discuss in the context of preventing teacher stress: (1) *Change is resource driven, and resources are interrelated.* Thus, teachers need to be provided with resources to bring about changes. Furthermore, personal and social resources can be regarded as interconnected. Hence, major resources are likely to be accompanied by other key resources. In a first step to provide teachers with resources necessary to initiate a change, one should foster a good climate among colleagues and thus increase trust among the teachers. This confidence could then be used for an intervention or for prevention sessions, where teachers could learn about cooperation processes and estimate and assess their resources together. (2) *Empowerment increases resources needed for change.* Within intervention or prevention sessions, teachers should be encouraged in their role as teachers and become aware of their relevance for society's wealth and education. An increasing pride in their own profession is assumed to have direct impact on teachers' personal and social resources. (3) *Increasing the sense of community and attachment helps changing social norms.* There is a need to change the teacher's position as an individual fighter and to break through the isolated position that teachers often hold. Indeed, schools and school principals should be encouraged and supported to develop an atmosphere of openness, trustworthiness, and cooperation among their teaching staff. Potential for constructive and positive feedback, support with the lesson plans, or the ability to seek advice openly without fearing a loss of face fosters teachers' condition, personal, and energy resources. (4) *Multiple sessions provide more opportunity for change.* This theoretical assumption claims that interventions should be spread over multiple sessions (Hobfoll, 1998) as they provide more opportunities to increase teachers' sense of community and empowerment. Such an assumption goes along with the prior assumption, that hours of lessons per week should be reduced in order to arrange prevention sessions on a regular basis. From these assumptions for effective prevention and intervention strategies, one should specifically investigate teachers' stressors in a first step to further identify resources needed and worth promoting in prevention.

Valuable Resources of Teachers

As mentioned before, the COR theory (Hobfoll, 1998) classifies resources into four groups: personal, condition, object, and energy resources. This classification gives consideration to personal and social resources equally. Studies by the research group of Petra Buchwald (e.g. Buchwald, Schorn, & Morgenroth, 2011; Morgenroth & Buchwald, 2015; Ringeisen, Morgenroth, Buchwald, & Schümer, 2013) allow a first adaptation of this resource classification to the school context.

Condition Resources

Social support is one of the most important condition resources. It is claimed that teachers' emotional stress is reduced when they are morally supported by their colleagues and that this support fosters teachers' job-related self-efficacy. However, the positive effect of social support could not be shown consistently. Rothland (2007, 2013) provides an overview of the relevance of social support in school contexts. Schwarzer and Leppin (1989) found that, if unwanted by the recipient, social support even fosters stress. Warner et al. (2011) confirmed this result analyzing the correlation between autonomy and multimorbidity. In a study at a school with two measuring points focusing on teachers' autonomy, similar effects occurred (Morgenroth, Buchwald, & Möller, 2012). The sample of the first and second measuring point included 115 primary German school teachers of North Rhine-Westphalia (88.7 percent female, which is a normal gender distribution of German primary school teachers). The distribution of the age was twenty-nine years or younger = 10 percent, thirty to forty-nine years = 50.9 percent, and fifty years and older = 38.6 percent. Surprisingly, the results of a mediator analysis showed that the gain of competences led to more emotional exhaustion, but this was only true for teachers who did not achieve their competence on their own initiative but were forced into a training program to do so. Other results show that teachers' autonomy correlates with functional coping strategies. Obviously, pedagogical autonomy seems to be a very important condition resource for German teachers.

Another valuable condition resource is performance recognition of teachers in general. A lack of recognition by colleagues, school management, and community enhances teacher stress (van Dick, 2006). This was also confirmed by studies conducted in America and Australia (Needle, Griffin, Svendsen, & Berney, 1980; Punch & Tuettemann, 1990).

Furthermore, teachers appreciate it if there is transparence in decision-making processes. Empirical results show that the transparence in school development processes and a positive participative leadership of school principals reduce teacher stress (Blase, Dedrick, & Strathe, 1986; Stemmer Obrist, 2011).

Personal Resources

Personal resources include personal characteristics and skills. Many studies analyzed the relationship between self-efficacy and teacher stress. Schmitz and Schwarzer (2000) conducted in-depth research in Germany about the effects of self-efficacy on stress and burnout. The results of these studies show that self-efficacy has a strong protective effect on burnout (Dückers-Klichowski, 2005; Käser & Wasch, 2009).

Object Resources

Object resources include material things that teachers need in their job. Deficient capacity of working areas and teaching materials are main stress factors for teachers (Hillert, 2013). Fussangel (2008) attempted to show that the availability and exchange of teaching materials are most important for teachers' health, especially during the implementation of new curricular and other school reforms.

Energy Resources

Energy resources include time, knowledge, and money. Teachers need such resources to gain new resources. Knowledge, for example, fosters self-efficacy as a personal resource, and time, on the other hand, would allow discussions and private talks, which foster a good climate among colleagues.

A teacher's job is extremely diverse, as teachers are often forced to do many things at the same time, which makes energy resources highly valuable for them. Among teachers' tasks are, for example, direct instruction in class, facilitation of understanding and transfer performance, coaching of performance and assessment as well as organizing parents' evenings, school trips, and festivals. All these activities need time, knowledge, and organizing abilities. A study of Buchwald et al. (2011) shows, that time is an important key resource for teachers independent of their age. Trainee teachers and experienced teachers both need an opportunity to concentrate, time and energy for good lesson preparation, and subject didactic knowledge to feel healthy.

Current Prevention of Stress among German Teachers

Prevention programs can be distinguished into three parts of the prevention process, depending on the content and time during the disease process (Lehr, 2011). The aim of the universal prevention is the reduction of stress within the whole teaching staff. Selective prevention is dedicated to a health risk group of teachers. This part of prevention should provide therapeutic activities and thus avoids a manifestation of further health impairment. Indicative prevention includes individual cases of teachers who have a very high health risk. In addition, measures to improve personal health can be valuated separately into changes of working conditions and prevention of behavior (Weiß & Kiel, 2013). In Germany, there is a variety of school stress prevention programs and programs to promote teachers' health. The most popular program is *AGIL* (work and health in the teaching profession; Hillert et al., 2012). The *LeguPan Project* (teacher health: prevention at school; Lehr, Schmitz, & Hillert, 2008) is a co-project of AGIL, with the focus on an effective classroom management for stress prevention.

The central training task of the LeguPan Project is collegial cooperation to foster stress prevention by teachers. This is due to the fact that successful coping with stress at school is not only an individual but a common task. Active, prosocial coping strategies such as seeking and giving social support are central for collegial cooperation (Lehr et al., 2008).

The design of these two projects is based on a three-year evaluation study with the aim of developing an intervention program for teachers on a third prevention level (indicative prevention) including eight training sessions (each ninety minutes long). The input of the training sessions is closely aligned to existing coping strategies such as dealing with social support, employing problem-solving strategies, and relaxing. Analyzing effects of the trainings established instruments of the stress-research context (e.g., Maslach-Burnout-Inventory; Maslach & Jackson, 1981, 1996), and also new concepts of instruments to measure the satisfaction with the training were used at four measuring points. Results of questionnaires (n = 76 teacher) showed a high acceptance of the program. Most teachers who joined the trainings showed an increase in self-efficacy. Moreover, teachers emphasized the recognition of one's individual resource pool and communication techniques as very useful.

In this structured job-related prevention program, teachers obtain a lot of information about stress. The fundamental interest is on individual references, thus on the reflection of the personal strengths and weaknesses to determine what steps can be derived in order to protect the person's health. This ability increases in importance in the context of the debate on professionalization of German teachers. A competent management of demands at school reduces the risk of health problems.

However, the disadvantage of exiting German programs of stress prevention lies in the fact that most interventions are characterized by an individual view on stress (Rothland, 2007; Weiß & Kiel, 2013). Another limitation is that the original goal of the instruments that were developed (e.g., Maslach Burnout Inventory), which were also used for the evaluation of these prevention training programs (i.e., AGIL and LeguPan), was to measure burnout rather than measuring stress. The focus on symptoms of burnout, as a result of chronic stress, makes it difficult to get results about important resources/ stressors of teachers (e.g., time, autonomy) to develop further intervention programs. It is more important to develop effective methods, such as the conservation of resources evaluation scale for teachers (Buchwald et al., 2011) to get more information about resources that are really relevant for teacher health. This practice would also help to identify important prevention factors. Other limitations of existing prevention programs in Germany consist in the negation of pedagogical autonomy as an important key resource and the lack of a differentiated view on the different role of the interaction partners in the process of social support as a relevant coping strategy. Further research about the possibilities of how to foster pedagogical autonomy in the context of interaction at school is necessary to improve teachers' coping strategies and to foster their resilience as competent professional German teachers.

For that reason, it would be important to learn more about teacher-specific resources that particularly lead to resilience against work stress in schools. This would widen the scope from key resources such as robust personal resources, such as autonomy for German teachers (Hobfoll & Lilly, 1993; Schmitz & Schwarzer, 2002) to more particular resources responsible for teachers' stress and burnout. Those specific resources could then be fostered in tailored intervention programs for teachers

As detailed in this chapter, the COR theory and the multiaxial coping model offer a significant contribution to the analysis and management of valuable resources of teachers. Personal as well as social resources and their social transfer could be analyzed based on these theoretical foundations. Preliminary works on the analysis of valuable resources of teachers show that pedagogical autonomy is a key resource of German teachers. When evaluating resources, the cultural background has to be taken into account: pedagogical autonomy might be a key resource within Western cultures but not in communal societies. However, so far little is known about the possibility of fostering pedagogical autonomy through social interaction in Germany. The relationship between pedagogical autonomy and teacher cooperation is mainly discussed in the context of German school development projects. In this context, pedagogical autonomy is considered as an ambivalent factor: too much and too little pedagogical autonomy of teachers are limited factors for teacher cooperation; too much autonomy leads to isolation, whereas too little autonomy leads to stress. Analyses about the relationship between autonomy and social interaction mostly focus on conflicts and not on suitable approaches. Results of a qualitative interview study by Morgenroth (2015) with fourteen German female primary school teachers of North Rhine-Westphalia gave preliminary ideas on how German teachers are able to preserve autonomy in social interaction. In this qualitative study, teachers were asked about their way of cooperation with colleagues, their feelings, and how they are able to beware of their autonomy despite the intensive cooperation that is needed for successful school development. The results indicate that the combination of knowledge/professional expertise and competences of self-reflection and communication is a main factor to preserve autonomy in social interaction at schools in Germany. Additionally, sympathy seems to be an important factor. These complex relations require special efforts by the school principal. How school principals in German schools might proceed and deal with these demands needs to be investigated in further research.

References

Altrichter, H., & Eder, F. (2004). Das "Autonomie-Paritätsmuster" als Innovationsbarriere? [The autonomy-parity-principle as a barrier for innovations?] In Holtappels, H. G. (eds.), *Schulprogramme – Instrumente der Schulentwicklung.* Weinheim: Juventa, pp. 195–221.

Antonovsky, A. (1987). *Unraveling the Mystery of Health: How People Manage Stress and Stay Well.* San Francisco, CA: Jossey-Bass.

Blase, J., Dedrick, C., & Strahe, M. (1986). Leadership behavior of school principals in relation to teacher stress, satisfaction, and performance. *Journal of Humanistic Education and Development* 24: 159–69.

Bossong, B. (1999). *Stress und Handlungskontrolle. [Stress and Regulation of Action].* Motivationsforschung, Bd. 17. Göttingen: Hogrefe.

Buchwald, P. (2002). *Dyadisches Coping in mündlichen Prüfungen. [Dyadic Coping in Oral Exams].* Göttingen: Hogrefe.

Buchwald, P., & Hobfoll, S. E. (2004). Burnout aus ressourcentheoretischer Perspektive [Burnout within the framework of COR-theory]. *Psychologie in Erziehung und Unterricht* 51: 247–57.

Buchwald, P., Schorn, N., & Morgenroth, S. (2011). Resource gains and losses in teachers. In Buchwald P., Moore K. and Ringeisen T. (eds.), *Stress and Anxiety – Application to Education and Health.* Berlin: Logos, pp. 71–81.

Buchwald, P., Schwarzer, C., & Hobfoll, S. E. (eds.) (2004). *Stress gemeinsam bewältigen – Ressourcenmanagement und multiaxiales Coping [Social Coping: Management of Resources and Multiaxial Coping Model].* Göttingen: Hogrefe.

Bundesbeamtengesetz [BBG; Federal Civil Service Act]. §44 Dienstunfähigkeit. www.gesetze-im-internet.de/bundesrecht/bbg_2009/gesamt.pdf

Bundestag (2015). Artikel 30 des Grundgesetzes von Deutschland. [Article 30 of the basic law of Germany]. www.bundestag.de/ bundestag/aufgaben/rechtsgrundla gen /grundgesetz/gg_02/245124

Burke, R. J., Greenglass, E. R., & Schwarzer, R. (1996). Predicting teacher burnout over time: effects of work stress, social support, and self-doubts on burnout and its consequences. *Anxiety, Stress, and Coping* 9: 261–75.

Cherniss, C. (1995). *Beyond Burnout: Helping Teachers, Nurses, Therapists and Lawyers Recover from Stress and Disillusionment.* New York: Routledge.

deStatis (Deutsches Statistisches Bundesamt) (2015a). Bevölkerungsentwicklung in Deutschland [Population development in Germany]. www.destatis.de/DE/ZahlenFakten/GesellschaftStaat/Bevoelkerung/Bevoelkerung.html

deStatis (Deutsches Statistisches Bundesamt) (2015b). Anzahl der teil- und vollzeitbeschäftigten Lehrkräfte allgemeinbildender Schulen in Deutschland im Schuljahr 2013/2014 nach Bundesländern. [Number of teachers per state in Germany]. www.destatis.de/DE/Publikationen /Thematisch/BildungForschungKultur/Schulen/ BroschuereSchulenBlick 0110018149004.pdf?__blob=publicationFile.

deStatis (Deutsches Statistisches Bundesamt) (2015c). National summary sheets in Europe. www.dgstat.be/PortalData/22/Resources/downloads/studien_und_analysen/publikationen/National_summary_sheets_on_education_system_in_Europe_and_ongoing_reforms.pdf

Dolton, P., & Marcenaro-Gutierrez, S. (2013). *Global Teacher Status Index 2013*. www.varkeygemsfoundation.org/sites/default/files/documents/2013GlobalTeacherStatusIndex.pdf

Dückers-Klichowski, S. (2005). *Burnout bei Lehramtsanwärtern im Primarbereich [Burn-out of Trainee Teacher in Primary Schools]*. Berlin: Logos-Verlag.

European Commission (2009). Key data on education in Europe 2009. eacea.ec. europa.eu/education/eurydice/documents/key_data_series/105en.pdf

Ezrahi, Y., & Shirom, A. (1986). Construct validation of burnout. Paper presented at the 21st Congress of the International Association of Applied Psychology, Jerusalem, Israel.

Freudenberger, H. J. (1974). Staff burnout. *Journal of Social Issues* 30: 159–64.

Freudenberger, H. J. (1983). Bumout: contemporary issues, trends, and concerns. In Farber, B. A. (eds.), *Stress and Burnout*. New York: Pergamon, pp. 23–8.

Fussangel, K. (2008). Subjektive Theorien von Lehrkräften zur Kooperation [Subjective theories of teachers in the context of teacher cooperation]. nbn-resolving.de/urn/resolver.pl?urn=urn%3Anbn%3Ade%3Ahbz%3A 468-20080475

GEW (Gewerkschaft Erziehung und Wissenschaft Nordrhein-Westfalen) (2013). Inklusionsgesetz [law of inclusion]. www.gew-nrw.de/uploads/tx_files/Inklusionsgesetz.pdf

Gräsel, C. (2010). Stichwort: Transfer und Transferforschung im Bildungsbereich [Transfer and research on transfer in the field of education]. *Zeitschrift für Erziehungswissenschaft* 13(1): 7–20.

Hillert, A. (2013). Psychische und psychosomatische Erkrankungen von Lehrerinnen und Lehrern [Psychological and psychosomatic illnesses of teachers]. In Rothland, M. (eds.), *Belastung und Beanspruchung im Lehrerberuf*. Wiesbaden: Springer, pp. 140–59.

Hillert, A., Lehr, D., Koch, S., Bracht, M., Ueing, S.. & Sosnowsky-Waschek, N. (2012). *Lehrergesundheit. AGIL – das Präventionsprogramm für Arbeit und Gesundheit im Lehrerberuf [Teacher Health. AGIL – Prevention Program for Work and Health at School]*. Stuttgart: Schattauer.

Hillert, A., Koch, S., & Lehr, S. (2013). *Stressbewältigung am Arbeitsplatz. Trainerhandbuch [Coping at the Office: Trainer Handbook]*. Göttingen: Vandenhoeck & Ruprecht.

Hobfoll, S. E. (1988). *The Ecology of Stress*. Washington, DC: Hemisphere.

Hobfoll, S. E. (1989). Conservation of resources: a new attempt at conceptualizing stress. *American Psychologist* 44: 513–24.

Hobfoll, S. E. (1998). *Stress, Culture, and Community: The Psychology and Philosophy of Stress*. New York: Plenum.

Hobfoll, S. E. (2001). The influence of culture, community, and the nested-self in the stress process: advancing conservation of resources theory. *Applied Psychology: An International Review* 50: 337–421.

Hobfoll, S. E. (2011). Conservation of resource caravans and engaged settings. *Journal of Occupational and Organizational Psychology* 84(1): 116–22.

Hobfoll, S. E. & Buchwald, P. (2004). Die Theorie der Ressourcenerhaltung und das multiaxiale Copingmodell [Conservation of theory and the multiaxial coping model]. In Buchwald, P., Schwarzer, C., & Hobfoll, S. E. (eds.), *Stress gemeinsam bewältigen: Ressourcenmanagement und multiaxiales [Coping Collective coping: Resource Management and Multiaxial Coping]*. Göttingen: Hogrefe, pp. 11–26.

Hobfoll, S. E., & Freedy, J. (1993). Conservation of resources: a general theory applied to burnout. In Schaufeli, W. B., Maslach, C., & Marek, T. (eds.), *Professional Burnout: Recent Developments in Theory and Research*. New York: Taylor & Francis, pp.115–35.

Hobfoll, S. E., & Lilly, R. S. (1993). Resource conservation as a strategy for community psychology. *Journal of Community Psychology* 21: 128–48.

Hobfoll, S. E., & Shirom, A. (2001). Conservation of resources theory: applications to stress and management in the workplace. In Golembiewski, R. T. (ed.), *Handbook of Organizational Behavior*. New York: Marcel Dekker, pp. 57–80.

Huber, S. G., & Wolfgramm, C. (2011). Beanspruchung und Belastung von Schulleitenden. Ergebnisse aus der deutschsprachigen Schulleistungsstudie 2011. www.bildungsmanagement.net/html/projekte/pdf/Huber%20&%20Wolfgramm-TABS-DFGE.pdf

IT NRW (Information and Technique North-Rhine Westphalia) (2015). Primary schools in NRW. www.it.nrw.de/presse/ pressemitteilungen /2015 /pres_042_15.html

Ito, J. K., & Brotheridge, C. M. (2003). Resources, coping strategies, and emotional exhaustion: a conservation of resources perspective. *Journal of Vocational Behavior* 63: 490–509.

Jerusalem, M. (1990). *Persönliche Ressourcen, Vulnerabilität und Streßerleben [Personal Resources, Vulnerability and Stress]*. Göttingen: Hogrefe.

Käser, U., & Wasch, J. (2009). *Burnout bei Lehrerinnen und Lehrern [Burnout of Teachers]*. Berlin: Logos.

Klusmann, U., Kunter, M., & Trautwein, U. (2009). Die Entwicklung des Beanspruchungs-erlebens bei Lehrerinnen und Lehrern in Abhängigkeit beruflicher Verhaltensstile [Development of demands regarding to the professional behavior of teacher]. *Psychologie in Erziehung und Unterricht* 56: 200–12.

KMK (Kultusministerkonferenz) (2004). Standards für die Lehrerbildung: Bildungswissenschaften [Standard for teaching and teacher education]. www.kmk.org/fileadmin/veroeffentlichungen_beschluesse/2004/2004_12_16-Standards-Lehrerbildung.pdf

KMK (Kultusministerkonferenz) (2015). Responsibilities of KMK. www.kmk.org/wir-ueber-uns/aufgaben-der-kmk.html

Lazarus, R. S. (1999). *Stress and Emotion: A New Synthesis*. New York: Springer.

Lazarus, R. S., & Folkman, S. (1984). *Stress, Appraisal and Coping*. New York: Springer Verlag.

Lazarus, R. S., & Launier, R. (1981). Stressbezogene Transaktion zwischen Person und Umwelt [Stress-related transaction between individual and environment]. In Nitsch, J. R. (ed.), *Stress, Theorien, Untersuchungen, Maßnahmen [Stress, Theories, Analyses, Actions*]. Bern: Huber, pp. 213–60.

Lee, R., & Ashforth, B. E. (1996). A meta-analytic examination of the correlates of the three dimensions of job burnout. *Journal of Applied Psychology* 81: 123–33.

Lehr, D. (2011). Belastung und Beanspruchung im Lehrerberuf. Prävention und Intervention der personenbezogenen Forschung [Stress and demands at school. Prevention and intevention]. In Terhart, E., Bennewitz, H., & Rothland, M. (eds.), *Handbuch der Forschung zum Lehrerberuf [Handbook of Research on the Teaching Profession]*. Münster: Waxmann, pp. 774 –87.

Lehr, D., Schmitz, E., & Hillert, A. (2008). Bewältigungsmuster und psychische Gesundheit [Coping and health]. *Zeitschrift für Arbeits- und Organisationspsychologie* 52(1): 3–16.

Lortie, D. C. (1975). *Schoolteacher – a Sociological Study*. Chicago: University Press.

Maslach, C., & Jackson, S. (1981). The measurement of experienced burnout. *Journal of Occupational Behaviour* 2: 99–113.

Maslach, C., & Jackson, S. (1996). *Maslach Burnout Inventory*. Mountain View, CA: CPP.

Maslach, C., & Leiter, M. P. (1997). *The Truth about Burnout: How Organizations Cause Personal Stress and What to Do about It*. San Francisco, CA: Jossey-Bass.

Morgenroth, S. (2015). *Lehrerkooperation unter Innovationsstress [Teacher Cooperation and Innovation Stress]*. Wiesbaden: Springer.

Morgenroth, S., & Buchwald, P. (2015). Burnout und Ressourcenerhaltung bei Lehrkräften [Burnout and conservation of resources of teachers]. *Unterrichtswissenschaft* 2: 136–49.

Morgenroth, S., Buchwald, P., & Möller, C. (2012). Innovationsstress bei Grundschullehrkräften – Welche Rolle spielt das Autonomieerleben? [Innovation stress among elementary teachers – which role plays autonomy?]. In Hellmich, F., Hoya, F., & Förster, S. (eds.), *Bedingungen des Lehrens und Lernens in der Grundschule: Bilanz und Perspektiven [Conditions of Teaching and Learning in Primary School: Results and Perspectives]*. Wiesbaden: Verlag für Sozialwissenschaften, pp. 161–4.

Morgenroth, S. & Grosche, M. (in the press). Inklusion durch interdisziplinäre Kooperation. Erweiterung des Modells "response-to-intervention" um Aspekte von Kokonstruktion und Co-Teaching. [Inclusion through interdisciplinary cooperation]. In S. Barsch, N. Glutsch & M. Massumi (Hrsg.), Blickwechsel Diversity. Internationale Perspektiven der LehrerInnenbildung. Münster: Waxmann.

Needle, R. H., Griffin, T., Svendsen, R., & Berney, C. (1980). Teacher stress: sources and consequences. *Journal of School Health* 50: 96–9.

Neuenschwander, M. P. (2003). Belastungen und Ressourcen bei Burnout von Lehrkräften der Sekundarstufe I und II [Demands and resources in the context of teachers burnout]. *Psychologie in Erziehung und Unterricht* 50: 210–19.

Neveu, J.-P. (2007). Jailed resources: conservation of resources theory as applied to burnout among prison guards. *Journal of Organizational Behavior* 28: 21–42.

Perrez, M., & Reicherts, N. (1992). *Stress, Coping and Health: A Situation-Behavior Approach: Theory, Methods, Applications*. Seattle, WA: Hogrefe & Huber.

Peters, J. (2013). *Arbeitsbezogene Verhaltens- und Erlebensmuster von Waldorflehrern im Zusammenhang mit Arbeitsbelastung und Berufszufriedenheit. Eine empirische Untersuchung. [Work-related Behavior and Patterns of Behavior of Waldorf Teachers in the Relation with Job Demands and Job Satisfaction: An Empirical Analysis]*. Alfter: Alanus Hochschule. alanus.edu/publikationen/

Poschkamp, T. (2008). Lehrergesundheit. Belastungsmuster, Burnout und Social Support bei dienstunfähigen Lehrkräften (Band 1) [Teachers health, coping, burnout and social support of disabled teachers]. In Buchwald, P., & Ringeisen, T. (eds.), *Angewandte Stress- und Bewältigungsforschung [Applied Research of Stress and Coping]*. Berlin: Logos Verlag.

Punch, K. F., & Tuettemann, E. (1990). Correlates of psychological distress among secondary school teachers. *British Educational Research Journal* 16: 369–82.

Ringeisen, T., Morgenroth, S., Buchwald, P., & Schümer, M. (2013). How does social support foster the development of teacher cooperation? Disentangling the differential relations over time. In Moore, K.A., Kaniasty, K., Buchwald, P., & Sesé, A. (eds.), *Stress and Anxiety – Application to Health and Well-being, Work Stressors, and Anxiety Assessment*. Berlin: Logos, pp. 103–15.

Rothland, M. (2007). Soziale Unterstützung bei Lehrkräften [Social support and teacher]. In Rothland, M. (ed.), *Belastung und Beanspruchung im Lehrerberuf. Modelle, Befunde, Interventionen [Stress of Teachers: Models, Results and Intervention]*. Wiesbaden: VS Verlag für Sozialwissenschaften, pp. 249–66.

Rothland, M. (ed.) (2013). *Belastung und Beanspruchung im Lehrerberuf [Stress and Demands among Teachers]*. Wiesbaden: VS Verlag für Sozialwissenschaften.

Schaarschmidt, U., & Fischer, A. (2003). *AVEM – Arbeitsbezogenes Verhaltens- und Erlebensmuster [Patterns of Professional Behavior and Experience of Teachers]*. Frankfurt: Swets & Zeitlinger.

Schaufeli, W. B., Enzmann, D., & Girault, N. (1993). Measurement of burnout: a review. In Schaufeli, W. B., Maslach, C., & Marek, T. (eds.), *Professional Burnout: Recent Developments in Theory and Research*. Washington, DC: Taylor & Francis, pp. 199–215.

Schmid, A. C. (2003). *Stress, Burnout und Coping [Stress, Burnout and Coping]*. Bad Heilbrunn: Klinkhardt.

Schmitz, G. S., & Schwarzer, R. (2000). Selbstwirksamkeitserwartung von Lehrern [Self-efficacy of teachers]. *Zeitschrift für Pädagogische Psychologie* 14: 12–25.

Schmitz, G. S., & Schwarzer, R. (2002). Individuelle und kollektive Selbstwirksamkeitserwartung von Lehrern [Individual and collective self-efficacy of teachers]. Beiheft: Selbstwirksamkeit und Motivationsprozesse in Bildungsinstitutionen [Self-efficacy and motivation in educational institutions]. *Zeitschrift für Pädagogik* 44: 192–214.

Schumm, J. A., Stines, L. R., Hobfoll, S. E., & Jackson, A. P. (2005). The double-barreled burden of child abuse and current stressful circumstances on adult women. *Journal of Traumatic Stress* 18: 467–76.

Schwarzer, C. (1999). Kindergärten als lernende Organisationen. [Kindergarden as learning organization]. In Caritas (eds.), *Jahrbuch der Caritas: Berichte aus der Praxis [Annual Book of Caritas. Reports of the Practice]*. Aachen: Caritas Verlag, pp. 271–4.

Schwarzer, R. (2000). *Streß, Angst und Handlungsregulation [Stress, Anxiety and Regulation of Action]*. Stuttgart: Kohlhammer.

Schwarzer, R., & Leppin, A. (1989). *Sozialer Rückhalt und Gesundheit [Social Support and Health]*. Göttingen: Hogrefe.

Simon, T., & Kruschel, R. (2013). Gesundheitsförderung mithilfe des Index für Inklusion? [Health promotion with the help of the index of the inclusion?] *Zeitschrift für Inklusion 2*. www.inklusion-online.net/index.php/inklusion-online/article/view/13/13

Soltau, A., Berthe, S., & Mienert, M. (2012). Das Autonomie-Paritäts-Muster [The autonomy-parity-principle]. In Huber, S., & Ahlgrimm, F. (eds.), *Kooperation*. New York: Waxmann, pp. 89–102.

Stemmer Obrist, G. (2011). Schulleiterinnen und Schulleiter in der Aargauer Volksschule [School manager of the Aargauer school]. (Doctoral dissertation). University Zürich/Institut für Erziehungswissenschaft. Ms. Baden.

van Dick, R. (2006). *Stress und Arbeitszufriedenheit bei Lehrerinnen und Lehrern [Stress and Job Satisfaction of Teachers]*. Marburg: Tectum Verlag.

Warner, L. M., Ziegelmann, J. P., Schüz, B., Wurm, S., Tesch-Römer, C., & Schwarzer, R. (2011). Maintaining autonomy despite multimorbidity: self-efficacy and the two faces of social support. *European Journal of Aging* 8: 3–12.

Weiß, S., & Kiel, E. (2013). Lehrergesundheit – Belastung, Ressourcen und Prävention. [Teacher health – demands, resources and prevention]. In Marchwacka, M. A. (ed.), *Gesundheitsförderung im Setting Schule [Health Promotion in the School Context]*. Wiesbaden: Springer, pp. 347–63.

Wells, J. D., Hobfoll, S. E., & Lavin, J. (1997). Resource loss, resource gain, and communal coping during pregnancy among women with multiple roles. *Psychology of Women Quarterly* 21: 645–62.

36 Prevention and Schooling in Italy

From Past and Present to the Future

Laura Nota, Lea Ferrari, Teresa Maria Sgaramella, & Salvatore Soresi

Introduction

The dramatic changes experienced by Western countries are occurring so fast that it is increasingly more difficult to develop a clear awareness of them and accordingly modulate the rhythms of our existence. In Italy, as in several other Western countries, many individuals are experiencing frustration in aspirations due to the lack of adequate income, the inadequacy of social safety nets, and the difficult access to the labor market, each of which requires sophisticated coping strategies because, besides work and future perspectives, individual well-being and quality of life are at risk (Nota, Soresi, Ferrari, & Ginevra, 2014b; Soresi, Nota, Ferrari, & Sgaramella, 2013a).

At the same time our life contexts present such high levels of complexity that even sophisticated methods of scientific analysis, to which scholars used to refer, now appear weak and unable to fully understand what is happening and what future consequences will be. Thanks to the contributions of theories of complexity, such as chaos theory (Cambel, 1993; Robertson & Combs, 2014), in Italy we also are becoming more aware that reality is mostly made of systems characterized by a high number of elements that in turn influence each other through micro-influences whose consequences are difficult to predict (Parisi, 2013). The idea is also emerging that management of complex phenomena requires sophisticated knowledge modalities and skills that constantly evolve and, in any case, are quite different from those used in the past (Savickas et al., 2009).

New modalities are then required to face negative feelings, discomfort, frustration, insecurity, and widespread feelings of depression shown by increasingly larger groups of the population. Additionally, it is worth remembering that there is an increasing number of publications, both in the medical and psychological fields, focused on the effects of the socioeconomic crisis, the spread of helplessness feelings, the increase in suicide rates, alcohol and drugs abuse, and the spread of the discrimination phenomenon against the most at-risk individuals (see, for instance, Kiosses, Szanto, & Alexopoulos, 2014; Mounteney, & Griffiths, 2014). The World Health Organization (WHO) is also so aware of this situation that it launched a warning concerning the need to undertake actions to address the aforementioned problems in Western countries; Italy is certainly one of them, hitherto considered as not particularly at risk, at least for some specific health problems, when compared with other countries (WHO, 2011).

Besides involving a larger number of individuals, the increase in risky behaviors, the complexity, the hardships, and negative feelings are relevant for and permeate several life domains, from health to education and training, from work to social and community life. They are also increasing the need for wide-ranging, universal, selective and indicated, preventive projects and plans. School can be considered as a "privileged place" for developing effective prevention initiatives. This statement is consistent with the ecologic-educational view, according to which health outcomes are determined by the interaction between the characteristics of individuals and environments (Green, & Kreuter, 2005), and with the Interactive Domain Model (IDM), which suggests that health is based on the interaction among underpinnings, understanding of the environment, and practice within the context of the immediate and broader environments (Kahan, & Goodstadt, 2005). Additionally, both approaches received a particular consensus in Europe from governmental, education, and sanitary authorities (WHO, 2009). Additionally, school can be considered as a gym for strengthening a series of psychosocial resources crucial when dealing with twenty-first century challenges (De Santi, Guerra, & Morosini, 2008). In our opinion, research and interventions in educational contexts – especially during the earliest years –besides having a high level of ecological validity because they occur in a setting that can be characterized as "natural" for individuals of schooling age, assume social relevance because of the issues they are dealing with, such as healthy and adaptive behaviors. These issues might, in fact, promote changes and innovation and foster an increase in well-being experienced by the most consistent number of individuals (Nota, Ginevra, & Santilli, 2015a; Ridley, 2010). To prepare youth for a satisfying life and for resiliency in the future is strictly related to what prevention means in the context of this chapter.

In this chapter, we will provide evidence about the role school played in the history of our country in developing a cultural background and giving careful attention to issues related to prevention. This has increased the sensitivity to prevention issues and openness to prevention and to difficulties experienced in current times, which, in turn, require a specific emphasis on new ideas in prevention programs. In order to highlight some crucial ideas for preventive action for the present and for the future, we will describe efforts that our colleagues and our laboratory have made to implement prevention programs in public institutions and in schools.

School in Italy: From Past to Present

As in many countries, in Italy school is a privileged context for studying conditions that either positively or negatively influence the development of children and adolescents. Education in Italy is compulsory from six to sixteen years of age and is divided into five stages: kindergarten *(scuola dell'infanzia)*, primary school *(scuola primaria* or *scuola elementare)*; lower secondary school (*scuola secondaria di primo grado*, lasting three years) and upper secondary school (*scuola secondaria di secondo grado*, lasting five years), which correspond to high school; and university *(università)*. Scuola primaria (primary school) lasts five years, and students are given a basic education in Italian, mathematics, natural sciences, history, geography, English, social studies, physical education, and visual and musical arts. The goals of lower secondary school are to facilitate the development of basic academic skills and foster academic skills relevant for secondary education. Upper secondary school has, in turn, the task of preparing youths for university studies (Liceo [lyceum]) or for work (Istituto Tecnico [technical institute] or Istituto Professionale [vocational institute]). However, independent of the secondary school attended, every student can have access to university. Fortunately, and probably due to Italy's troubled history and increased attention devoted to the inclusion process, no barriers have been set for university enrollment, and students are aware that obtaining a diploma also opens the doors to university and to new professional trajectories.

This asset of the Italian schooling system, with further refinements, started with the Italian Unification process (Risorgimento) during the first half of the nineteenth century and developed during the second half of the century. The first task undertaken by schools pertained to transmitting knowledge about Italy and about Italy's past rich and strongly nuanced cultures, which new generations should master in order to understand better and in a more comprehensive way their present life and future actions. At that time, in fact, backgrounds, habits, and development of health and social services were characterized differently across the regions of Italy. For example, the availability of water in the Piemonte region in the Northwest spurred the development of agriculture, and earthquake-proof rules were implemented in Campania in the South (Petraccone, 2005; Segre, 1983; Vecchi, 2012). The second task of schooling, given the heterogeneity of traditions characterizing Italy during that period, dealt with promoting personal and group participation in civil and social development of the country, that is, the development of citizenship. From 1860 and during the following decades, school was ascribed the task of "making Italians," as in a very popular saying of that period, by fighting against illiteracy and both linguistic and cultural fragmentation.[1] These differences, additionally

1 The sentence Massimo d'Azeglio pronounced, "We have made Italy now we are asked to make Italians," was from early beginnings "sponsored" by several intellectuals and philosophers (see, for instance, Mazzini) and by highly influential politicians, such as Cavour, who suggested that the march toward democracy goes necessarily through public schools and citizen education in order to remove Italians' barriers due to the geopolitical differences that characterized previous conditions (Romeo, 1984), as underlined by the number of states existing at that time (the Reign of Sardegna, the Dukedom of Parma, the Dukedom of Modena, the Dukedom of Lombardo Veneto, the Grand Duchy of Toscana, the Papal States, the Reign of Due Sicilie).

and unfortunately, sustained thereafter enduring prejudices against people from the South of Italy and their different habits.

Educational services in Italy are still required to address these two demanding tasks. Also required is the active participation of family members, whose role in schools has been explicitly set by a decree of the President of the Italian Republic (Decreto del Presidente della Repubblica; DPR 416) in 1974. Social inclusion and well-being may depend on these two tasks. But dealing with these tasks in the current complex conditions of Italy can influence the adequacy and satisfaction that many teachers experience. Taking into account teacher satisfaction, the International Hope Research Team at the University of Padova involved five hundred Italian teachers in a research study. Their mean age was approximately forty-two years; 45 percent were women. In similar proportions, the teachers worked with students attending different school grades. Teachers were presented with a series of questionnaires that addressed their positive psychological resources. More specifically, they were asked to complete the Design My Future Questionnaire (Soresi, Nota, Ferrari, & Sgaramella, 2013b) which focused on their resilience and future time perspective. In addition, they completed the About Work Questionnaire (Soresi et al., 2013b) concerning their ability to instill in students the same values as their teacher. From a cluster analysis conducted on data collected, four groups of teachers emerged, characterized by different attitudes toward teaching. The first group of teachers was defined as "pessimist and deluded" (35 percent) and included teachers who consider themselves unable to instill confidence and hope in others, and in particular to deal with complex situations that students experience. The second group included teachers "moderately supportive, optimistic and realistic" (27 percent) and are characterized by sufficient professional self-efficacy beliefs. The third group is composed of teachers who are "very positive, optimistic and resilient" (21 percent); these teachers expect that more positive than negative events will happen. The fourth group includes individuals "definitely not happy and pessimists" (17 percent). These teachers have limited self-efficacy beliefs, consider themselves unable to help students who are experiencing difficult situations, and are not capable of instilling feelings of hope and confidence in students. These teachers attach low social prestige to the activities they carry out as teachers. Students who are taught by teachers belonging to either the first or last group, regardless of deficits or "special needs," we expect will experience more learning difficulties, low motivation, low self-efficacy, and self-regulation (Soresi et al., 2013c). Although until now anecdotal, evidence for this relationship is expected from research and suggested by studies in the literature. For instance, results from one study have shown that individuals with intellectual disabilities and characterized by low self-determination, quality of life, and social skills are cared for by practitioners with low self-efficacy (Nota, Ferrari, & Soresi, 2007). In order to instill hope and optimism, and promote resiliency in students, teachers need to possess strong self-esteem and confidence (Hoy, Tarter, & Hoy, 2006).

Prevention in Schools

There are four "emergencies" that need to be taken into account and carefully considered in order to identify goals and guide priorities for preventive actions in twenty-first century Italian schools.

1. *Values and economic crisis.* Over the last two decades, globalization, the labor market crisis, models offered from media fostering individualistic and meritocratic values, competition, and self-entrepreneurship have made it difficult for schools to cope with the second task, that is, pursuing the development of participation, by promoting, for instance, cooperation, inclusion, and solidarity. Today, Italian schools are capable of dealing with the task of transmitting present and past cultures, but they experience difficulties in preparing youths for a satisfying present life and to face the future with resiliency. It seems that school is mainly devoted to accomplishing the first task and surrendering the second one, which is perceived as difficult, and requiring competencies that teachers are not always ready to use. Discrepancies among past, present, and future have been experienced between mainly cognitive and social goals, academic and professional success, and what happens inside and outside school (Parisi, 2013). These inconsistencies produce discomfort and ill-feelings in all main "players" involved: teachers, students, counselors, and administrators. It is not surprising, then, the "disinvestment" shown by families and youths who do not support teachers' work and reduce efforts to promote a sense of student responsibility that motivates school success (Center for Studies on Social Investments [CENSIS], 2014). Consider school attendance as an example. According to a recent survey conducted within the Programme for International Student Assessment promoted by the Organization for Economic Cooperation and Development (OECD-PISA), only 57.6 percent of youths declared they never missed a school day in the two previous weeks (OECD, 2014). The disinvestment from education and school is also evidenced and supported by data provided by the Istituto Nazionale di Statistica (National Statistics Institute; Istat, 2014). These data show that 45 percent of Italians, whose age ranges from twenty-five to sixty-four years, do not have an upper secondary school diploma, while for the same age range the percentage of individuals who do not invest in secondary education reached 25 percent in Europe; 18 percent of Italian students from fifteen to nineteen years drop out of school; individuals not in education, employment, and training (NEET) was 19.2 percent in 2008 and increased to 24.6 percent in 2012; additionally, the number of students enrolling at university has significantly been reduced over the same time period (Istat, 2014).

2. *Resources reduction, job insecurity, and aging of teachers.* According to professionals, especially those involved in prevention activities in schools, there are additional warning signs as a result of the substantial reduction (about 5 percent) of total public investments allocated in the last ten years to improving the quality of school services (OECD, 2014). In order to provide adequate and safe facilities, information and didactic supports, and increase in

professionalism, large investments are required. On the other hand, when there is a reduction in financial resource investments, there is, at the same time, an additional increase in job insecurity. Starting from 2009, this condition has been seen in many teachers. Job insecurity characterizes 22 percent of the Italian teaching workforce, and this profoundly influences quality of teaching because every year some teachers work in a different school and with a different group of students, at the cost of limited continuity in education and didactics. The impact of this is mainly evidenced in students who for various reasons experience marked difficulties in adapting to school proposals and curricula (Istat, 2014).

As a consequence, the number of students in each class has shown an increase up to thirty students rather than ranging from fifteen to twenty-four. This is particularly relevant for first-grade pupils. These students, in fact, should be provided higher educational attention given the novelty of the transition they are experiencing. However, there is an increased difficulty in implementing personalized actions with potentially significant effects, for instance, on the prevention of learning difficulties. More working hours are required by teachers, who less and less can rely on shared teaching and cooperation from other colleagues because those colleagues are experiencing similar difficulties, and because almost 20 percent of them are temporary workers and only partially involved in school activities. For several reasons, then, recruitment of new teachers has been reduced, with an increase in age of remaining teachers, as more than 60 percent of teachers are over fifty years old (OECD, 2014). Thus students have a reduced possibility to benefit from recently educated teachers who have been trained to face complexity and use dynamic and multidisciplinary approaches, such as flexible learning approaches and teaching processes that require extended times for teaching, having specific places to carry out laboratory activities, and using personalized teaching modalities that are different from traditional ones (Parisi, 2013).

3. *Progressive deterioration of school "human capital."* The third emergency refers to the awareness of the degree of commitment and difficulty teaching requires today. Education is involved with complex contexts that more frequently leave to schools the responsibility of managing heterogeneous and problematic situations; additionally, and differently from what happened only a few years ago, the teaching profession is often attributed as low in social prestige, especially when referring to secondary school teachers. Teachers themselves think the prestige of their profession is reduced (nearly 80 percent of them), and nearly half of them expect that the prestige of teachers will be further reduced in the future; additionally, these views have shown an increase of about 15 percent in the last ten years (Cavalli, & Argentin, 2010).

4. *Threats to inclusion from medicalization of heterogeneity (variability).* Finally, from 2012 a problem in the Italian schools, mainly cultural and ideological in nature, has been raised in relevance and potential impact. There are new forms of "medicalization" deriving from new "diagnoses" introduced

into the school context. We refer here, for instance, to the "Special Education Needs" label. Based on a recently introduced Italian law, this label, besides identifying the traditional learning difficulties, has been also used to label sociocultural disadvantage and immigrant children who have not mastered the Italian language. As a consequence, there is an increase in the use of "diagnostic labels" that become attached throughout life to these individuals; in sharp contrast with the International Classification of Functions suggestions (WHO, 2013), school professionals are encouraged to ask for a specialized analysis of student deficits carried out by a team of experts in a sanitary setting outside of school and to implement special interventions in "special" times (e.g., after school time) and often in separate spaces, that is, outside the room where their classmates are working (Soresi et al., 2013c). These issues interfere with the educational development of students who so early in life are labeled and require specific attention. Being considered "different" facilitates a dramatic reduction in self-efficacy beliefs and in professional achievement (Soresi et al., 2008).

We have until now taken into account and described factors which in school contexts negatively affect the development of conditions that can facilitate inclusion of all students in those situations requiring major supports and help. These factors interfere with the investment in prevention and with the successful experiences we will shortly describe. At the same time, these issues underscore the need to undertake new routes and facilitate preventive actions more deeply involving the entire school community.

School: A Privileged Context for Prevention Programs

From the preceding outlined analysis, it follows that school can be considered in Italy as a "mandatory place," a touchstone for serious and concrete programs aimed at achieving a large and positive impact on the health of the entire country. More than any other institution, in fact, schools can help not only in preventing appearance of disturbances but, more crucially, in developing a more healthy, satisfying, and productive way of living (De Santi et al., 2008). As prevention programs show, educational contexts can easily take charge of (1) promoting knowledge about health and well-being; (2) producing change in cognitive and emotional variables, and change in dimensions responsible for activating risk behaviors and facilitating changes in relational, cultural, and environmental determinants that can support and reinforce the reduction of deviant behaviors; and (3) removing risk behaviors, thus fostering the acquisition of new healthy information, attitudes, and lifestyle.

Early on, initiatives undertaken have focused on preventing learning difficulties in reading and writing and in math. These initiatives, developed by Soresi (1988) and shared by several Italian scholars (Moderato, & Pino, 1990; Perini, Benedetto, & Ingrassia, 1991; Perini, 1992) consisted mainly in instructing teachers on conducting psychoeducational activities involving five- to six-year-old children and aimed at developing and strengthening prerequisites of the specific academic skills. Alternatively, some programs were devoted to promoting the development of student social skills or collaborative behaviors (Moderato, & Moderato, 2004; Nota, & Soresi, 1997).

In the last decade, however, there has been an increase in the number of school-based prevention programs that have been supported by the central government (Ministero della Salute and Ministero dell'Istruzione) and from local cultural and social organizations. Their efficacy has been verified in specific areas across Italy. For instance, in a study conducted in Stradella, a town in the Northwest of Italy, five teachers were trained to teach their students adaptive habits. The intervention (two hours a week for eight weeks) addressed how to improve blood cholesterol levels by changing dietary habits. The 150 participants (ages six to eleven years) showed better lipid profiles than the control group six months after the end of the activity (Aquilani et al., 2007).

In another study, La Torre and colleagues (2010) involved 534 children and 308 adolescents attending grades 4 through 6 (ages nine to eleven years) and grade 9 (ages fourteen to fifteen years) respectively. More than two hundred students attended a one-year training program to prevent tobacco use. The program was carried out by teachers working on participants' knowledge about health issues and smoking consequences, understanding of mechanisms underlying initiation of smoking, and skills to refuse the social pressures to smoke. Posttest and a follow-up two years later showed that trained teachers can effectively work on cognitive and behavioral aspects of tobacco use and thereby reduce the risk of smoking in children and adolescents.

Several programs on nonadaptive behaviors have focused on preventing addictive behaviors. Camoni, Colucci, and Lombardi (2004), for instance, using a three-factor model (Information-Motivation-Behavioral Skills), developed a health education course for the prevention of drug use that involved 417 students in two high schools. The study showed that efforts to prevent drug use in young people need to focus on more than just content, because young people already seem to possess basic information concerning the risks connected to substance abuse; the study, instead, supports the relevance of referring to specific theoretical choices in prevention, in particular taking into account the role of information, motivation, and adults providing role models for correct behaviors. More recent programs have focused on emerging addictions. Capitanucci (2012), for example, focused on gambling and analyzed several programs promoted and realized by different institutions from 2006 al 2011. The analysis showed that the most effective program was based on working with narratives (e.g., Lucky's video), together with a workbook guide, and was helpful in addressing basic ideas and developing awareness of cognitive errors leading to losing control and to addiction. In several consecutive implementations of the program, "Il caso Lucky non si può influenzare" (Lucky case cannot be influenced), a development of knowledge was observed together with changes in erroneous thinking that persisted over six months. The author underscored the relevance of results obtained from programs implemented at school with respect to editions proposed outside school and school time.

With regard to school-based bullying problems and their prevention, which have been given attention in schools, Menesini, Nocentini, and Palladino (2012) provide an example of a successful prevention program tackling bullying and cyber-bullying in secondary schools in Toscana, a region in central Italy. They involved more than seven hundred high school students in a six-month web-based program, which included designing and developing a website to promote peer-to-peer content against bullying and cyber-bullying. After an awareness-raising step, each of the involved students worked as an online educator in the forum for two weeks, each day controlling the forum and posting new threads and answering questions. A face-to-face peer educator activity was also conducted with a different school class. This consisted of organizing a meeting with local school administrators to ask for specific help and preparing a related TV program for a local network. Peer educators acted as agents of change. Eight high schools were involved. Over a six-month interval, a reduction was observed in the frequency of behaviors experienced among those analyzed by bullying and cyber-bullying measures, thus underscoring the relevance of direct active involvement of participants in prevention programs with age-appropriate materials and modalities.

Besides these programs, there are prevention programs by the Istituto Superiore della Sanità (National Health Institute) structured and provided to schools; the programs disseminate information and awareness about the relevance of targeted problems. The prevention programs use media to educate about bullying, obesity prevention, and physical activity promotion (De Santi et al., 2008). Other Italian-based prevention programs have focused on road safety, which should be offered during early school years (first- to third-grade levels) because there is a general agreement that more satisfying outcomes are expected as a result of long, sufficiently focused, and systematic interventions on perception of risks and personal vulnerabilities (Brunello, & De Martis, 2009). By starting in the early school years, there is more time to develop awareness and to give positive feedback for positive behaviors. As an example of a prevention program taking into account and addressing goals at different developmental steps, the Road Safety Education Program (De Santi, Zuccaro, Filipponi, Minutillo, & Guerra, 2010) is presented. This program has been developed for children from primary (five years) through secondary school (eighteen years). It is a school-based program, delivered by teachers. Knowledge, attitudes, and behaviors are the dimensions taken into account in this prevention program. For primary school, the goals are developing knowledge about security, commitment, and responsibility toward acting in a safe way and using safety supports. For secondary school students, goals are developing knowledge about sources of risks and consequences, awareness of safe behaviors, and modifying risk behaviors.

In order to develop awareness of the role of prevention and facilitate implementation of prevention programs in schools, guidelines and detailed materials for realizing school activities are provided by the Ministero dell'Istruzione (Ministry of Education) to schools interested in prevention. These actions are worth mentioning because they are common in the Italian context, although their efficacy has not been verified. Research on prevention in Italy should then deal also with these programs.

Over time, school-based prevention programs in Italy have widened, moving from programs more related to socioemotional dimensions to those focused on more health-related issues. Suggestions provided by the World Health Organization (WHO, 2009) have been taken into account. These suggestions include proposing and developing prevention programs as early as possible during the life cycle and sharing the vision that more consistent development of adequate behaviors is expected, with actions taking place during the developmental window devoted to personality organization, that is, during infancy and pre-adolescence. This vision has led to defining and sharing in a systematic way basic principles for realizing effective prevention programs. They are (a) the notion of "age-specific prevention goals" for primary or secondary schools, or even for different classes within both primary and secondary schools; (b) the role of cognitive and executive development, and propensity to engage in risk behaviors that are more pronounced in adolescence; (c) the relevance of skills characterized by specific timing in development, such as the ability to anticipate consequences that occur throughout adolescence; and finally, (d) the relevance of fostering the engagement of positive role models among peers, thus developing civic commitment in youth.

We are proud of the path that prevention has taken in Italian schools; however, we hope that economic threats will not be a barrier to fully realize prevention programs such as those describe in this section or to their dissemination across Italy. New conditions are needed and new themes should be faced in order to realize more completely prevention science moving forward in Italy.

Strengthening Prevention: The Role of Teachers, Students, and Parent Involvement

We are strongly convinced that the probability of implementing successful prevention programs depends on the possibility of promoting consensus and active participation from specialists involved in the program and also from teachers, parents, and students. It is important that schools realize and benefit as soon as possible and give attention to sufficient resources and health-promoting attitudes and skills so that young people can benefit and cope with our difficult times. We refer to solidarity and an inclusive vision of school, as well as hope, optimism, resilience, career adaptability, reflexivity, and argumentation (Cattani et al., 2014). Thus, in this section we aim to share examples of preventive activities conducted at the Larios Laboratory, which is the laboratory for research and intervention in career counseling at the University of Padova.

Research and Interventions That Focus on Teachers, Parents, and Students

As far as *teachers* are concerned, both those actively working in schools and preservice teachers, they suffer from changes Italy is currently facing. Teachers complain that they are unable to understand how they can help students face their future challenges with confidence. About 34 percent of school principals, for example, assert that their school staff lacks motivation and is discouraged (Censis, 2014). Specific and upgraded educational actions, such as postgraduate university master courses, are needed to help teachers master a series of new and heterogeneous competencies that can be useful to implement preventive actions and to sustain them in schools. These competencies and attitudes include the following:

1. Recognizing the uniqueness of persons and using verbal and narrative modalities is necessary to overcome the trend toward using labels and stereotyped visions.
2. Heterogeneity, disability, and vulnerability should be used and managed as richness and not as a threat from which we should defend ourselves. Teachers must become aware that words such as "special," "disability," "special needs," and so on, have such strong negative connotations that teachers are induced to generalize problems and difficulties, encouraging the co-construction of a marginalized identity (Ben-Yehuda, Lavy, Linchevski, & Sfard, 2005; Nota & Soresi, 2009; Sgaramella, Nota, Ferrari, & Soresi, in press). They should be prepared to accept the idea that their professional role requires them to deal at the same time with diverse challenges ranging from more school learning related to challenges related to personality development of their students and to managing nonadaptive risky behaviors.
3. Teachers of the future will be required to work increasingly as a team with other professionals operating in schools, including those with different competencies (e.g., social service providers, technology specialists). As reported by the "Key Data on Learning and Innovation through ICT at School in Europe 2011" (Eurydice, 2011), online safety modules should immediately be included in training programs for Italian teachers in order to increase their skills coping with new technological problems such as cyber-bullying.

These improvements in teacher education will lead to an increase in quality and efficacy of teacher skills and help to strengthen student relationships. Teachers will take the responsibility of actions that are closer to tutorial activity, counseling, and coaching (Parisi, 2013; Soresi, & Nota, 2013). They should coordinate learning activities during school time with other teachers but also with community agencies and adopt a highly personalized teaching style that allows students to become more self-regulated in deciding their learning goals. In addition, teacher training should include problem-solving strategies in order to help them face unexpected difficulties and use their skills to solve negative events occurring in school. It is hoped that improvements in teacher training will help overcome the propensity to avoid responsibilities, delegate tasks to others, and ultimately resign. Thus, the tendency to be passive and give up will be overcome. National reports (i.e., Censis, 2011) in fact depict Italian teachers as "disappointed." While 53 percent chose their job for personal aspiration, more than one-third (50 percent of secondary school teachers) would not choose the profession again. About 69 percent believe teaching suffers from poor social recognition and about 53 percent from a lack of economic progression, and 82 percent believe that school goals of valuing education and civil coexistence are not achieved.

One example of a university course that shows it is possible to facilitate changes and improvements in school professionals was developed by the Larios Laboratory in 2013 in the field of career education. This one-year postgraduate master course involved nearly fifty participants for 120 hours of lessons that focused on theoretical models, qualitative and quantitative assessment, efficacy verification, and observation. Teaching activities included lectures by national and international experts, discussions, individual and small-group exercises, case studies, out-of-class homework, and the design and implementation of a project that was supervised by teaching staff and presented to all the participants at the end of the course. Pre- and posttest measures included Working Today with Persons (Soresi et al., 2013b), which evaluates self-efficacy beliefs about work; the About Work Questionnaire (Soresi et al., 2013b), which evaluates job attitude; and the Hope Centered Career Inventory (Niles, Yoon, Balin, & Amundson, 2010), which evaluates hope and goal setting. Repeated analyses of variance showed that the involved psychologists, teachers, and other professionals working with schools showed an increase in their self-efficacy (toward their professional skills $F [1, 48] = 7.887$, $p = 0.009$ and achievement, $F [1, 48] = 6.498$, $p = 0.016$); in their job attitude (optimism, $F [1, 48] = 7{,}020$, $p = 0.014$, resilience, $F [1, 48] = 30.986$, $p = 0.001$ and positive representation of the job $F [1, 48] = 7{,}890$, $p = 0.009$); and finally in hope and goal setting (hope, $F [1, 48] = 13.003$, $p = 0.001$, self-reflection, $F [1, 48] = 13.248$, $p = 0.001$, goal setting and planning skills, $F [1, 48] = 12.771$, $p = 0.001$, implementing skills, $F [1, 48] = 17.565$, $p = 0.005$, and adapting skills, $F [1, 48] = 5.694$, $p = 0.024$).

As far as parents are concerned, evidence (Ginevra, Nota, & Ferrari, 2015; Soresi, Nota, Ferrari, & Ginevra, 2014) suggests that dimensions such as hope, optimism, emotional stability, and commitment to school and the future are important characteristics to promote among parents in order for youth to face difficulties that characterize Italian society. These play an important role in the parent–child relationship, and schools, with the involvement of parents, become the place to facilitate the development of these strengths. Parent training programs that were carried out in the year 2000 confirmed that it is possible to increase parents' ability to develop supporting and positive relationships with their children, acquire strategies to educate their children to help others, and respect individuals' needs and differences (Nota, Soresi, & Ferrari, 2014a; Soresi, & Nota, 2001). Themes of the parent training included knowledge on disability, how to promote positive child behaviors, and the teaching of social skills and helping behaviors. According to recent literature (Larsen, Edey, & Lemay, 2007; Nota, & Rossier, 2015), however, parent training should dedicate more attention to storytelling and facilitating hope and positive changes using narrative strategies, such as thinking of the multitude of ways the word "hope" is used, asking questions about hope and reflecting on its antecedents and consequences, or creating a collage of pictures that may provide access to a client's stories of hope (Larsen et al., 2007). Narratives and stories talking about hope and positive actions should be encouraged with the potential result of increasing the probability that parents will produce more hopeful narratives within their family context (Larsen et al., 2007). Following these suggestions and referring to Life Design approach, a group of twenty parents who had an active role in school with children aged eleven to fourteen years old, and living in a northern Italian underprivileged area, were involved in a program called "The Life Design Project on the Parents' Side: A Shared Pathway" (developed by the authors of this chapter). These parents were elected by school parents to represent families and children' interests in school and to take part in school representative bodies. They represent a unique group of parents who can influence "school and social policy" in the school attended by their children and enjoy prestige among other parents, and, when properly educated, they may in turn facilitate further engagement of other parents and support the idea of school as a place for their participation and for strengthening other parents' competencies. The program emphasizes the parents' role, given that career construction is considered the result not only of intrapersonal but also contextually built processes. Parents can actively contribute to co-construct a better future and foster career adaptability in children before difficulties in constructing positive career options for the future arise (Nota, & Rossier, 2015; Savickas et al., 2009). The training program consists of ten meetings, two hours each, once a week, and is conducted by two doctoral students in psychology under the supervision of one of the authors of this chapter. A trainer manual was developed for each session that included a detailed description of the session goals, session activities, and teaching strategies to be used (i.e., instruction, discussions, modeling, exercises, homework, feedback, and reinforcements). The meetings focused on (1) an overview of the course; (2) how to support children's interests, especially career interest development; (3) how to sustain self-efficacy beliefs, especially in math and decisions about the future; (4) how to control irrational ideas and increase open-mindedness and appreciate changes; (5) how and when to speak of vocational guidance in the family, using negotiation and compromise; (6) how to help children focus on their career goals with creativity and consider the idea of goals and planning for the future by connecting past and present; (7) how to help children get information about career options and to stimulate novel exploration through interviews of workers and their direct observation; (8) how to help children choose among options, focusing on adaptive and maladaptive decisional styles; (9) how to facilitate children's transitions and the journey "toward" the future; and (10) how to support children's self-determination. To verify the efficacy of the training program, quantitative and qualitative measures at pre- and posttest were used. As a quantitative measure, we used the *How Much Confidence Do I Have in Myself? Parents' Questionnaire* (Soresi & Nota, 2007), which assesses self-efficacy beliefs about one's parenting abilities, one's ability to handle difficult situations, and one's ability to support his or her children; *My Life as a Parent* (Soresi & Nota, 2007), which measures satisfaction with family relations, sense of well-being, job satisfaction, relations with one's own children, free time, support and parental backup available, and self-determination opportunities associated with self-development. Drawing on McAdams's (1995) and Rehfuss's (2009) work, qualitative procedures were also used for co-constructing stories of life, linking past, present, and future events and exploring multiple future perspectives. At pre- and posttest, parents were asked the following questions: (1) "Could you please write down a few lines or a brief paragraph about what you hope for your son's/daughter's future?" (2) "Could you please write down a few lines or a brief paragraph about what you hope for your own future?" (3) "Across the lifespan, people have to set different goals for their future. Some may be short-term, like saving money to buy something that is needed or desired; others may be long-term, like choosing a study course, training for a new job, starting a family, etc. Currently, what is your most important goal? Please describe a recent event or fact which illustrates what you have done or are doing to achieve your important goal." (4) "'I think Vocational Guidance is. . ..'." The R-Manova on data collected at pre- and posttest underlined that parents showed higher self-efficacy beliefs in their ability to support their children (Pre: M = 24.0; SD = 3.89; Post: M = 26.80; SD = 3.46; $F[1, 9] = 13{,}674$; $p = 0.005$) and higher levels of satisfaction with relations they experience with their children (Pre: M = 21.60; SD = 4.30; Post: M = 24.20; SD = 3.71; $F[1, 9] = 10{,}418$; $p = 0.01$) and with self-determination opportunities (Pre: M = 15.80; SD = 2.44; Post: M = 17.20; SD = 2.39; $F[1, 9] = 5{,}128$; $p = 0.05$).

With regard to the qualitative analysis of the Life Design intervention, each parent's initial and subsequent narrative responses were paired off for comparison, conducted by a triangulation of researchers (Eisner, 1991). The narrative content was examined directly on the documents (circling verbs, underlining phrases, highlighting themes) searching for similarities and changes in the content, specifically noting whether statements about occupations changed or not. The analysis at the end of the training showed that parents' narratives were more organized and detailed and included "new" issues. This showed that in-depth thinking and reappraisal had taken place and that some issues had been better mastered and more greatly reflected on. Regarding the first question that asked parents to tell their hopes about their son's or daughter's future, answers changed from making a conscious choice (i.e., "I would like him to make a conscious choice when he will leave school") to making a conscious choice following exploration of several possibilities and options (i.e., "I would like my son to make a decision about the future after wholly understanding what it means to do different jobs"); from making a choice in line with interests and aspirations (i.e., "I hope my daughter will make a choice based on her interests") to making a choice in line with their interests and aspirations by getting rid of irrational career beliefs (i.e., "I hope my daughter will think about her future and take full advantage of her abilities because, even if she is a woman, she will have to get along by herself"); from chances of job placement (i.e., "I would like him to find a job, given the crunch we are experiencing these days") to job satisfaction (i.e., "I would like my daughter to find a job that will enable her to grow and find satisfaction in her work as a person and also to pursue her career goals"); from economic security (i.e., "I hope she can find a job that will enable her to make a living") to ability to cope with transitions (i.e., "I hope he will be able to exploit the opportunities that will come his way and also be satisfied"). Moreover, a new category emerged that authors called "Relationships: Having a family life and developing abilities to play different roles" (i.e., "I wouldn't like it if he were appreciated only for the way he does his job ... I would like him to be also a good husband and father").

With regard to the question four that asked parents about the meaning of vocational guidance, answers changed from vocational guidance understood as proper advice (i.e., "A good piece of advice for my child") to vocational guidance concerning the ability to plan one's own future (i.e., "Vocational guidance doesn't mean giving advice on this or that profession. It means learning to see the different aspects of this or that profession and set one's own professional goals"); from vocational guidance understood as support to one's children's decisions (i.e., "It is above all a way to help youths make a decision") to vocational guidance is a constructive dialogue between parents and children that must be properly supported (i.e., "As a parent, I think it means thinking when they ask for support and helping them realize their dreams"). Moreover, the theme of vocational guidance as the action of experts (i.e., "It is a difficult issue that should be left up to counselors or teachers") disappeared at posttest.

The Life Design program suggests that parents can be actively involved in a demanding project, and that some Life Design key concepts can be understood and used by them to better support their children's career development. First of all, parents can experience the importance of offering opportunities to explore environment and career options; discussing career issues, giving feedback, and offering suggestions; and making them feel more efficacious and satisfied. In doing this, they can co-construct a positive future and stimulate reflexivity and investment in a career before the urgency of school career transitions emerge. Secondly, thanks to this type of involvement, parents strengthen their parenting skills and can increase their self-efficacy beliefs and perceive higher satisfaction from discussing career issues with their children. Thirdly, these parents represent role models, and through their behaviors and testimony can stimulate other parents to think about career development as a process that takes place over time and that can enrich their own and their children's lives.

When thinking about children and the development of important skills in a multi-ethnic and globalized society, it is a priority to teach them to be inclusive and to behave with solidarity (i.e., giving help, sustaining people's efforts, and promoting advocacy for people rights) as soon as possible, together with teaching them to be able to invest in their future. Taking inspiration from the work carried out by Soresi (1989) during 1980s, and the recent emphasis on the need to increase inclusion and solidarity (i.e., European Commission, 2014), the authors of this chapter implemented the training program called "The Good Actions" involving children younger than six years. The following components were emphasized: (a) the ability to highlight peer differences; (b) the ability to emphasize their own and others' strengths (with or without disability); (c) the ability to involve, help, and support peers; and (d) the ability to rely on their own positive aspects to establish positive relationships. This intervention program was implemented by a psychologist and included eight meetings, half an hour each, once a week, with the aim of teaching the targeted behaviors. Experimental and control groups included respectively twelve children randomly selected. No children with disabilities were included. The meetings focused on the following:

1. The *good actions,* that is, the eight positive actions that can be taken within and outside school: saying nice things to others, smiling, thanking, asking please, taking turns, asking for something with kindness, helping, and playing together.
2. The *good actions for helping each other,* that is, the advantages obtained from assisting people in need and how to implement helping behaviors toward their mates.
3. *Making our friends happy,* that is, taking positive actions toward classmates.
4. *I can do so many things and so many I can learn,* that is, how to introduce themselves and the benefits arising from this positive presentation.
5. *Introducing others,* that is, how to introduce people they know emphasizing activities and actions they are able to do.
6. *Introducing our classmates,* that is, positively introducing their classmates.
7. *We play and we can teach how to do it,* that is, how to behave as a model for peers who experience difficulties in performing some activities
8. *Learning new good actions,* a diploma of "friendly child" is delivered to each participant together with the book of all the "good actions," consisting of pictures and drawings made during training and a DVD containing all the movies recorded during the intervention.

Some clips of cartoons very popular among children were used to show targeted behaviors throughout the training. These were selected from free online movies, cartoons, and pictures for a reduction of costs, and were also edited using free and user-friendly apps and programs. All materials were recorded on a DVD and in a book delivered to all parents and teachers with simple instructions. Parents and teachers were then encouraged during a two-hour meeting to implement similar activities in familiar contexts in order to stimulate children positively to behave and express solidarity. Additionally, to exercise and reinforce the target behaviors, two generalization meetings were carried out by the psychologist in regular classes. The psychologist stimulated children from the experimental group to exercise the good actions they learned during the previous session with other children in the experimental and control groups. An iPad was used to record these behaviors and all the target behaviors children spontaneously produced. These videos were later used to praise children in front of teachers, parents, and other children. This procedure allowed the researchers to reinforce the children who executed the target behavior to have good role models, foster the salience of positive behaviors, and address also the children from the control group who could benefit from the intervention with no additional cost. The training effectiveness was analyzed by applying direct observations by two doctoral students working at the Larios Laboratory. For the experimental and control groups, frequency of positive and negative social behaviors toward classmates with disability were assessed for three twenty-minute observation sessions during play activities both in the classroom and in the school garden. For direct observations, the following behavioral categories were assessed: positive behaviors exhibited by classmates toward students with a disability; and negative behaviors exhibited by classmates toward students with a disability. At posttest, results showed that experimental group children showed more positive behaviors toward peers with disabilities than did the control group (Wilcoxon test $z = -1.84$, $p = 0.05$).

Finally, a training implemented by the authors of this chapter that they consider innovative and interesting for contemporary times is summarized. It is called *Palestra di Botta e Risposta* ("The Questions & Answers Gym"; Cattani, 2012) and was launched by a group of university scholars in philosophy with the aim of increasing high school students' abilities to argue and counterargue, that is, to debate. Developing these skills is considered crucial to realize youth's identity, promote self-determination and sustain their rights, prepare for the many transitions they will encounter in life, and foster their skills to manage many contextual requests and succeed in complex societies. It is especially in the first years of high school that all of this acquires a preventive role (Eurydice, 2011). High schools from diverse Italian regions select students to be trained by philosophers, experts on argumentation and communication, on how to identify, set out and neutralize errors and fallacies in discussions, and propose arguments that are free of errors and fallacies. Immediately after these four meetings, about five to eight students from every school are selected by their peers to participate in the "Question & Answer Gym" tournament to compete for the "title" of Magnificent Disputant of the year. Cattani (2012) reports that the use of principles of argumentation increased during the intervention while the number of fallacies decreased. In the 2014 edition of the project, the Larios Laboratory was involved with the aim of making debating skills a valuable tool for building positive relationships in the classroom and constructing abilities to face their own future challenges. Reflections about resilience, future time perspective, and courage to build a future of quality were included for this purpose. Qualitative and quantitative procedures assessing the efficacy of the project included a questionnaire on argumentative skills (*Le mie ragioni e quelle degli altri;* My reasons and the others ones; Cattani et al., 2014); the Scale for Interpersonal Behavior (Nota, Arrindell, Soresi, van der Ende, & Sanavio, 2011), for assessing frequency of assertive behaviors and perceived discomfort, the Courage Scale (Norton, & Weiss, 2009), for assessing courage. The R-Manova comparing pre- and posttest measures found that at posttest participants rated themselves higher on argumentativeness (Pre: M = 15.60; SD = 4.85; Post: M = 17.25; SD = 3.04; $F[1,62] = 26.72$; $p = 0.001$) and assertiveness (Pre: M = 13.17; SD = 4.94; Post: M = 15.47; SD = 3.27; $F[1,62] = 44.092$; $p = 0.001$], and on thinking with hope and courage about the future [Pre: M = 46.26 ; SD = 7.75 ; Post: M = 48.19; SD = 6.22; $F[1, 62] = 30.23$; $p = 0.001$) (Di Maggio, 2015). To support the preventive role of this program, the multidisciplinary group is planning an intervention involving middle schools, whose students, at least in Italy, have to manage at fourteen years old their school career choice and cope with many pressures from parents, teachers, and peers. Increasing their argumentative skills could be particularly helpful in clarifying pros and cons of making a choice and sustaining their career decisions in front of significant others. This could reduce the probability of unweighted choices and the tendency to follow decisions made by others and experience future frustration and dissatisfaction.

Conclusions

Prevention for the twenty-first century will be an important tool to give boosts to new strengths and energies and to facilitate a process of social renovation useful in improving human conditions and getting benefits from current changes. As suggested by Romano (2012) and, in Italy, by the Italian Network for Counseling (Network Universitario per il Counselling, Uni.Co.[2]) born in 2014, prevention is aimed at reinforcing individuals' strengths in the interest of people's health and well-being, in academic and work success and in active and generous participation in community life.

These are very important tasks that cannot be put off any longer. Researchers and professionals must face up to the challenges of postmodernity characterized by increasing complexity and unpredictability, innovate their intervention strategies, and offer high-quality services. Actions and prevention programs that the authors of this chapter have described are examples of a new trend in Italy and support the need to renovate and add new goals to traditional ones. The rapid changes Italy is currently witnessing are in fact challenging prevention and counseling models and older practices that need to move from theories, instruments, and actions based on predominantly linear principles and equations to

2 larios.psy.unipd.it/.

new and promising ones that explicitly aim to help people reflect and face the multiplicity of career and life transitions and the unpredictability of the future that characterizes our societies. The Life Design approach, for example, aims to equip people in managing career and life transitions before they occur. Sustaining solidarity, inclusion, hope, optimism, resilience, career adaptability, reflexivity, and argumentation to encourage new changes and improvements is expected to be useful to innovate and capitalize on the collective intelligence that humanity has achieved (Nota et al., 2015b).

In conclusion, the authors wish[1] to underscore that those who promote prevention programs in schools, now more than ever, should make their voices heard and work with policy makers and institutions to facilitate the realization of high-quality schools. Fortunately, in Italy we are in the process of approving a new school reform *La buona scuola* ("the good school"[3]). This reform started with the largest public consultation in Europe, from September 15 to November 15, 2014, in which more than 1,800,000 individuals participated. Several suggested goals are in line with programs and reflections discussed in this chapter, such as strengthening students' skills with flexibility in academic programs, inclusion and integration of all students, school-to-work transitions, and innovation in teacher training and competences, while at the same time making teachers more capable of preparing and equipping children and adolescents to be citizens of a global world. The debate about this educational reform in Italy is continuing, and we hope that the participation of many people, including researchers, teachers, and prevention and counseling scholars, can lead to the development of new trajectories for more inclusive schools that focus on prevention, and teachers who are able to teach students the necessary skills to live successfully in the twenty-first century.

References

Aquilani, R., Parisi, U., Bigoni, N., Maggi, L., Ghioni, G., Zucchella, M., . . . & Boschi, F. (2007). School teachers can effectively manage primary prevention of adult cardiovascular disease: the Stradella Project. *Preventive Medicine* 45: 290–4.

Ben-Yehuda, M., Lavy, I., Linchevski, L., & Sfard, A. (2005). Doing wrong with words: what bars students' access to arithmetical discourses. *Journal for Research in Mathematics Education* 36: 176–247.

Brunello, G., & De Martis, G. (2009). *Le stragi del sabato sera [Saturday Night Massacres]*. Venezia: Marsilio Editore.

Cambel, A. B. (1993). *Applied chaos theory: a paradigm for complexity*. San Diego: Academic Press.

Camoni, L., Colucci, A., & Lombardi, R. (2004). Un'esperienza di educazione alla salute per i giovani della scuola media superiore [An experience of health education with high school students]. *Annali dell'Istituto Superiore di Sanità* 40(2): 245–50.

3 labuonascuola.gov.it.

Capitanucci, D. (2012). Strategie di prevenzione del gioco d'azzardo patologico tra gli adolescenti in Italia. L'utilizzo di strumenti evidence-based per distinguere tra promozione e prevenzione [Prevention strategies for pathological gambling among adolescents in Italy. The use of evidence-based tools to distinguish promotion and prevention]. *Italian Journal on Addiction* 2: 3–4.

Cattani, A. (2012). *Dibattito. Doveri e diritti, regole e mosse [Debate, Duties and Rights, Rules and Moves]*. Naples: Loffredo.

Cattani, A., Ferrari, L., Ginevra, M. C., Di Maggio, I., Nota, L., Santilli, S., Sgaramella, T. M., & Soresi, S. (2014). Le mie ragioni e quelle degli altri [My reasons and the others ones]. Paper presented at the 8th meeting of the network Uni.Co., Rome.

Cavalli, E., & Argentin, G. (eds) (2010). *Gli insegnanti italiani: come cambia il modo di fare scuola [Teachers in Italy: How Teaching Is Changing]*. Bologna: Il Mulino

Censis (2011). *Fenomenologia di una crisi antropologica. I miti che non funzionano più [Phenomenology of an Anthropological Crisis: The Myths That No Longer Work]*. Rome: Censis.

Censis (2014). *I vuoti che crescono [The growing absence]*. Milano: Franco Angeli.

De Santi, A., Guerra, R., & Morosini, P. (eds.) (2008). *La promozione della salute nelle scuole: Obiettivi di insegnamento e competenze comuni [Health Promotion in Schools: Teaching Goals and Common Competences]*. Rapporti ISTISAN 08/1. Rome: Istituto Superiore di Sanità.

De Santi, A., Zuccaro, P., Filipponi, F., Minutillo, A., & Guerra, R. (2010). *La promozione della salute nelle scuole. Prevenzione degli incidenti stradali e domestici. [Health Promotion in Schools. Preventing Road and Domestic Accidents]* Rapporti ISTISAN 10/3. Rome: Istituto Superiore di Sanità.

Di Maggio, I. (2015). *Preliminary results of 'the Q & A Gym'*. Internal report. Padova: Larios Laboratory.

Eisner, E. W. (1991). *The Enlightened Eye: Qualitative Inquiry and the Enhancement of Educational Practice*. New York: Macmillan.

European Commission (2014). *Erasmus + Inclusion and Diversity Strategy*. Brussels: European Commission.

Eurydice (2011). *Key Data on Learning and Innovation through ICT at School in Europe 2011*. Brussels: EACEA.

Ginevra, M. C., Nota, L., & Ferrari, L. (2015). Parental support in adolescents' career development: Parents' and children's perceptions. *Career Development Quarterly* 63: 2–15.

Green, L. W., & Kreuter, M. W. (2005). *Health Program Planning: An Educational and Ecological Approach*. New York: McGraw-Hill.

Hoy, W. K., Tarter, C. J., & A. W. (2006). Academic optimism of schools: a force for student achievement. *American Educational Research Journal* 43(3): 425–46.

Istat (2014). *Rapporto Annuale 2014. La situazione del Paese [Annual Report 2014: The National Situation]*. Rome: Istat.

Kahan, B., & Goodstadt, M. (2005). *The IDM Manual*. University of Toronto: Centre for Health Promotion.

Kiosses, D. N., Szanto, K., & Alexopoulos, G. S. (2014). Suicide in older adults: the role of emotions and cognition. *Current Psychiatry Reports*, 16: 1–8.

La Torre, G., Chiaradia, G., Monte, L., Moretti, C., Mannocci, A., Capitanio, D., . . . & Boccia, A. (2010). A randomised controlled trial of a school-based intervention to prevent tobacco use among children and adolescents in Italy. *Journal of Public Health* 18: 533–42.

Larsen, D., Edey, W., & Lemay, L. (2007). Understanding the role of hope in counselling: exploring the intentional uses of hope. *Counselling Psychology Quarterly* 20: 401–16.

McAdams, D. P. (1995). What do we know when we know a person? *Journal of Personality* 63: 365–96.

Menesini, E., Nocentini, A., & Palladino, B. E. (2012). Empowering students against bullying and cyberbullying: evaluation of an Italian peer-led model. *International Journal of Conflict and Violence* 6: 313–20.

Moderato, L., & Moderato, P. (2004). *CAPIRE: Checklist per l'Analisi e la Programmazione Informatizzata del Ritardo Evolutivo [CAPIRE: Checklist fot the Computerized Analysis and Planning in Mental Retardation]*. Firenze: O.S. Organizzazioni Speciali

Moderato, P., & Pino, O. (1990). Effetti del contesto e delle caratteristiche del materiale sulla rievocazione in soggetti di 7 anni [Effects of context and characteristics of material on seven-year-old subjects' recall]. *Ricerche di Psicologia* 3: 35–54.

Mounteney, J., & Griffiths, P. (2014). Increasing complexity in European drug use: highlights from the EMCDDA's 2014 European drug report. *Drugs: Education, Prevention and Policy* 21: 482–3.

Niles, S. G., Yoon, H. J., Balin, E., & Amundson, N. E., (2010). Using a hope-centered model of career development in challenging times. *Turkish Psychological Counseling & Guidance Journal* 4: 101–8.

Norton, P. J., & Weiss, B. J. (2009). The role of courage on behavioral approach in a fear-eliciting situation: a proof-of-concept pilot study. *Journal of Anxiety Disorders* 23: 212–17.

Nota, L., Arrindell, W. A., Soresi, S., van der Ende, J., & Sanavio, E. (2011). Cross-cultural validity of the scale for interpersonal behavior. *International Journal of Adolescent Medicine and Health* 23: 39–44.

Nota, L., Ferrari, L., & Soresi, S. (2007). Self-efficacy and quality of life of professionals caring for individuals with intellectual disability. *Journal of Policy & Practice in Intellectual Disabilities* 4: 129–40.

Nota, L., Ginevra, M. C., & Santilli, S. (2015a). Life Design and prevention. In Nota, L., & Rossier, J. (eds.), *Life Design and Career Counseling*. Göttingen: Hogrefe, pp. 183–99.

Nota, L., Ginevra, M. C., & Soresi, S. (2015). An intervention program to influence attitudes of elementary school students towards classmates with developmental disability. Paper presented at the annual conference of the Italian Society of Vocational Guidance, Pavia.

Nota, L., & Rossier, J. (2015). *Life Design and Career Counseling*. Göttingen: Hogrefe.

Nota, L., Sgaramella, T. M., Ferrari, L., Santilli, S., Ginevra, M. C., & Soresi, S. (2015b). Counseling for the future. Paper presented at the annual conference of the Italian Society of Vocational Guidance, Pavia.

Nota, L., & Soresi, S. (1997). *I comportamenti sociali: Dall'osservazione all'intervento [Social Behaviors: From Observation to Intervention]*. Pordenone: ERIP Editrice.

Nota, L., & Soresi, S. (2009). Ideas and thoughts of Italian teachers on the professional future of persons with disability. *Journal of Intellectual Disability Research* 53: 65–77.

Nota, L., Soresi, S., & Ferrari, L. (2014a). School inclusion in Italy: emerging trends and future directions. In McLeskey, J., Waldron, N. L., Spooner, F., & Algozzine, B. (eds.), *Handbook of Research and Practice for Effective Inclusive Schools*. London: Routledge, pp. 521–30.

Nota, L., Soresi, S., Ferrari, L., & Ginevra, M. C. (2014b). Vocational designing and career counseling in Europe. *European Psychologist* 19: 248–59.

OECD (Organization for Economic Cooperation and Development) (2014). *Education at a Glance 2014: OECD Indicators*. Paris: OECD.

Parisi, D. (2013). Articolo bersaglio: Gli psicologi e l'apprendimento a scuola [Target article: psychologists and learning at school]. *Ricerche di Psicologia* 1: 107–19.

Perini, S. (1992). *La tecnologia dell'educazione nella prevenzione del ritardo cognitivo: Modelli teorici e verifiche empiriche. [Technology in education for preventing cognitive delay: models and empirical testing]*. In Di Nuovo, S., & Moderato, P. (eds), *La Psicologia oggi [Psychology Today]*. Catania: CUECM.

Perini, S., Benedetto, L., & Ingrassia, M. (1991). *Procedure di apprendimento senza errori nella prevenzione del ritardo cognitivo: Una comparazione metanalitica [Errorless learning procedures in preventing cognitive delay: a metanalytical comparison]. Bollettino di Psicologia Applicata [Bulletin of Applied Psychology]* 199: 13–23.

Petraccone, C. (2005). *Le "due Italie": La questione meridionale tra realtà e rappresentazione ["Two Italys": Reality and Representations of the South Issue Question]*. Bari: Laterza.

Rehfuss, M. C. (2009). The future career autobiography: a narrative measure of career intervention effectiveness. *Career Development Quarterly* 58: 82–90.

Ridley, M. (2010). *The Rational Optimist: How Prosperity Evolves*. London: Fourth Estate.

Robertson, R., & Combs, A. (eds.) (2014). *Chaos Theory in Psychology and the Life Sciences*. New York: Psychology Press.

Romano, J. L. (2012). Prevention in the 21st century. In Vera, E. M. (ed.), *The Oxford Handbook of Prevention in Counseling Psychology*. Oxford: Oxford University Press, pp. 36–50.

Romeo, R. (1984). *Cavour e il suo tempo [Cavour and His Times]*, vol. 3. Bari: Laterza.

Savickas, M. L., Nota, L., Rossier, J., Dauwalder, J.-P., Duarte, M. E., Guichard, J., … van Vianen, A. E. M. (2009). Life designing: a paradigm for career construction in the 21st century. *Journal of Vocational Behavior* 75: 239–50.

Segre, L. (1983). *Agricoltura e costruzione di un sistema idraulico nella pianura piemontese (1800–1880) [Agriculture and a New Idraulic System in Piedmontese Lowlands]*. Milan: Banca Commerciale Italiana.

Sgaramella, T. M., Nota, L., Ferrari, L., & Soresi, S. (in press). The Italian path to school and social inclusion: problems, strengths and perspectives. In Hanes, R. (ed.), *International Histories of Disabilities*. Toronto: Toronto Press.

Soresi, S. (1988). *Comunità, prevenzione e apprendimento [Community, Prevention, and Learning]*. Bergamo: Editrice Ferrari.

Soresi, S. (1989). *Psicologia dell'handicap e della riabilitazione [Psychology of Handicap and Rehabilitation]*. Bologna: Il Mulino.

Soresi, S., & Nota, L. (2001). *La facilitazione dell'integrazione scolastica [Facilitating school inclusion]*. Pordenone: Erip Editrice.

Soresi, S., & Nota, L. (2007). *ASTRID Portfolio per l'assessment, il trattamento e l'integrazione delle disabilità [ASTRID Portfolio for the Assessment, Intervention, and Inclusion of Disabilities]*. Firenze: Giunti-Organizzazioni Speciali.

Soresi, S., & Nota, L. (2011). *Inclusione senza se e senza ma [Inclusion without if and but]*. Paper presented at the seminar "The Future of Inclusion," Padova.

Soresi, S., & Nota, L. (2013). Developing resilience and instilling hope in time of crisis. Paper presented at the annual conference of the Italian Society of Vocational Guidance, Milan.

Soresi, S., Nota, L., Ferrari, L., & Ginevra, M. C. (2014). Parental influences on youths' career construction. In Arulmani, G., Bakshi, A., Leong, F., & Watts, T. (eds.), *Handbook of Career Development: International Perspectives*. New York: Springer, pp. 149–72.

Soresi, S., Nota, L., Ferrari, L., & Sgaramella, T. M. (2013a). The IHRT survey. Presentation at the Symposium on the International Hope Research Team at the International Conference on Life Design and Career Counseling Building Hope and Resilience, June, Padova.

Soresi, S., Nota, L., Ferrari, L., & Sgaramella, T. M. (2013b). Career development and career thoughts. In Wehmeyer, M. L. (ed.), *The Oxford Handbook of Positive Psychology and Disability*. New York: Oxford University Press, pp. 239–64.

Soresi, S., Nota, L., Ferrari, L., & Sgaramella, T. M., Ginevra, M. C., & Santilli, S. (2013c). Inclusion in Italy: from numbers to ideas … that is from "special" visions to the promotion of inclusion for all persons. *Life Span and Disability* 16: 187–217.

Soresi, S., Nota, L., Ferrari, L., & Solberg, S. (2008). Career guidance for persons with disabilities. In Athanasou, J. A., & Van Esbroeck, R. (eds.), *International Handbook of Career Guidance*. Dordrecht: Springer Science, pp. 405–17.

Vecchi, G. (2012). *Sviluppo economico, benessere e disuguaglianza: Italia, 1861–2011 [Economic development, well-being and dysequity: Italy, 1861–2011]. Rivista di Storia Economica [Review of Economic History]* 28: 177–96.

WHO (World Health Organization) (2009). *Global Status Report on Road Safety: Time for Action*. Geneva, Switzerland: World Health Organization.

WHO (World Health Organization) (2011). *Impact of Economic Crises on Mental Health*. Copenhagen: WHO Regional Office for Europe.

WHO (World Health Organization) (2013). *How to Use the ICF: A Practical Manual for Using the International Classification of Functioning, Disability and Health (ICF). Exposure Draft for Comment*. Geneva, Switzerland: World Health Organization.

37 Cultural Adaptation of Family Evidence-Based Drug Prevention Programs in Spain

Carmen Orte, Lluís Ballester, Marga Vives, Joan Amer, & Martí X. March

Introduction

Parental and family factors are key elements with regard to substance abuse prevention. The main objectives of this chapter are twofold: firstly, to outline the important role that the family has when dealing with drug prevention; secondly, to emphasize the relevance of cultural adaptation for evidence-based programs. The findings in this chapter are supported by a case study in Spain, that examined the use of the Family Competence Program (FCP) – known in Spanish as the Programa de Competencia Familiar (PCF). The FCP is a cultural adaption of the U.S. Strengthening Families Program (SFP).

This chapter is divided into six parts. First, the main facts about teen drug use in Spain are examined. Second, the role of the family in drug prevention is emphasized. Third, a general overview of at-risk families in Spain is presented. Fourth, a description of the cultural adaptation process used to make the selective U.S. Strengthening Families Program relevant to Spain. Fifth, an evaluation of the FCP and its results are listed. Finally, there is a description of new implementation models as well as practical implications and potential future research subjects for family prevention programs and their cultural adaptations.

Drug Use among Adolescents in Spain

In Spain, drug prevention is structured through the Plan Nacional sobre Drogas (PNSD, the National Strategy On Drugs), a governmental initiative created in 1985 to coordinate and empower drug policies carried out by various levels of government and care agencies. Since 1994, the PNSD has conducted a national survey every two years, named ESTUDES (Encuesta Estatal sobre Uso de Drogas en Enseñanzas Secundarias)[1] on the consumption of alcohol, tobacco, and other drugs among high-school students between ages fourteen and eighteen. The most recent study was conducted in 2012 with 27,503 students from 747 private and public schools. Results of this survey

1 www.pnsd.msc.es/Categoria2/observa/estudios/home.htm.

indicated that the average age of first consumption of any psychoactive substance was between thirteen and sixteen years old. While there are regional differences in the age of first consumption of psychoactive substances, the general mean age for first tobacco consumption among Spanish teenagers is 13.6 years old; 13.9 years old for first alcohol consumption; and 14.9 years old for first cannabis consumption. The most consumed drugs in the 2012 survey were: alcohol (81.95 percent), tobacco (35.3 percent), and cannabis (26.6 percent). The data described in ESTUDES 2012 indicate that alcohol consumption is especially higher among young teenagers (fourteen and fifteen year olds); intensive consumption, drunkenness, and binge drinking are more common among those who use illegal drugs (polyconsumption). For intensive consumption, the study's findings on teen drunkenness were as follows: 60.7 percent had been very drunk at some point in their life; 52.0 percent during the last year: and 30.8 percent in the last month. More than half of the adolescents got drunk during the last year, especially younger girls (fourteen to sixteen years old), whose intensive consumption patterns were higher than previously reported. Regarding binge drinking (i.e., five or more glasses in approximately two hours), a similar pattern of drunkenness was observed: half of the seventeen year olds were engaged in binge drinking during the last month. Generally speaking, intensive consumption (drunkenness and binge drinking) was more frequent among those participating in open-air drinking sessions. Open-air binge drinkers also consume – in higher percentages – other substances such as cannabis and cocaine.

According to PNSD (2012), 43.8 percent of the students surveyed in Spain smoked tobacco at least once in their life; 35.3 percent in the last year; and 12.5 percent smoke tobacco on a daily basis (30 percent of European students according to 2011 European School Survey Project on Alcohol and Other Drugs [ESPAD] research). For cannabis consumption among fourteen to eighteen year olds in Spain, 33.6 percent had consumed it at least once in their life (24 percent for European students [ESPAD 2011]); 26.6 percent in the last year (20 percent for European students [ESPAD 2011]); and 16.1 percent in the last month (12 percent for European students [ESPAD 2011]); and 2.7 percent of Spanish students consume cannabis daily. Polyconsumption is even more frequent among adolescents, both in Spain and Europe, with four out of every ten Spaniard students.

Importance of Family in Drug Prevention

Globally speaking, evidence shows that teenagers are prone to risk behaviors such as smoking, alcohol consumption, antisocial behaviors, and unprotected sexual intercourse (Steinberg, 2008); these risk behaviors are related to a higher risk of deficient educational results, morbidity, and premature death (Biglan, Brennan, Foster, & Holder, 2004). Hence, preventive interventions can play a major role in reducing preliminary tendencies toward risk behaviors and are also more efficient in limiting possible damage once risk behaviors have become habitual (MacArthur et al., 2012).

The quality of a child's upbringing and family life has an important influence on the child's development (Waller, Gardner, Dishion, & Sitn, 2014). Families can influence their children's prosocial behaviors in a way that can reduce their vulnerability to problem behaviors. Competent parenting includes a wide array of tasks and functions, such as communication and family cohesion, that should be adapted to a child's developmental stage and cultural context (Leidiy, Guerra, & Toro, 2010). Effective parent–child relationships are characterized by high levels of protection, care, and education, defined as basic needs fulfillment; emotional and economic security (Amato, 2005; McCoy, Cummings, & Davies, 2009); appropriate guidance and limits; supervision; stimulation and stability; use of effective control strategies; and support through the various developmental stages (Nanninga, Jansen, Knorth, & Reijneveld, 2015). Accordingly, in a review of forty-six longitudinal studies of prevention programs that promote effective parenting, Sandler, Schoenfelder, Wolchik, and McKinnon (2011) indicated that some of the most frequently cited factors that have the most influence on positive child development are bonding; self-control; positive parent–child relationships; and positive discipline.

Parental and family factors play a major role in adolescent's decision-making process with regards to substance abuse (Dishion & Kavanagh, 2003; Whitesell, Bachand, Peel, & Brown, 2013; Wood, Read, Mitchell, & Brand, 2004). In a similar vein, the United Nations Office on Drugs and Crime (UNODC, 2009) describes the key family factors associated with drug prevention as reliable and healthy parent–children attachment; parental monitoring; follow-up and effective discipline; transmission of prosocial family values; parental involvement in a child's life; and parental support (emotional, cognitive, social, and financial support) of children.

Parental factors are assembled under the concept of positive parenting, a general term that covers different parental behaviors, including warmth and sensitivity; a structured environment; and setting limits. Positive parenting is a robust factor that has repeatedly shown its influence on teenagers' risk behavior in many investigations with rigorous research designs. These data have their origin in Baumrind's classic works (Baumrind, 1966, 1967, 1975, 1991) on the concept of positive parenting. Baumrind investigated parenting styles, demonstrating a link between parental behavior and the development of instrumental competencies in children. According to the Baumrind theorem with regard to setting limits, the emphasis should be an authoritative – but not authoritarian – manner, as opposed to a permissive style (see also Stephenson, Rápida, Atkinson, & Tschida, 2005).

Data also indicate that mental health and social problems are the consequences of disruptive family relationships (Repetti, Taylor, & Seeman, 2002; Sanders & Duncan, 1995); thus, a disruptive family relationship is a risk factor. These authors outlined some important points, both in educational models used in the parenting process and those found in the context of family dynamics involving child development. Family risk factors can have important consequences regarding the development and maintenance of antisocial behaviors (e.g., drug use) also among Spaniard youth (Llorens, Barrio, Sánchez, & Suelves, 2011; Estévez & Emler, 2011). Due to family disruption and its effect on problematic behaviors, when parents use drugs, children have a higher probability of repeating family conflicts, violence, and drug use (CSAT, 2004). The United Nations Office for Drugs and Crime (UNODC, 2010) lists the key family risk factors associated with youth drug use as (a) lack of connection and an insecure relationship with their parents; (b) lack of a meaningful relationship with an adult; (c) ineffective parenting skills; (d) chaotic family setting; (e) parents or siblings suffering from drug abuse, a mental illness, or involvement in illegal activities; and (f) social isolation of children.

Evidence points to the effectiveness of family prevention programs in dealing with drug abuse and other problematic behaviors (Foxcroft & Tsertsvadze, 2011; Kumpfer & Alvarado 2003; Kumpfer, Xie, & Magalhães, 2012). Prevention programs that focus on the family include skills-learning programs that cover key factors such as the role of the family in child development and the prevention of drug use. These programs aim to create and/or reinforce family protection factors, such as positive family relationships, supervision of children, and family communication. These programs are multicomponent; they include (1) parental training to strengthen parenting skills; (2) personal and social skills training for children; and (3) family practice sessions.

Families at risk are those that are associated with adolescent alcohol and drug consumption and antisocial behavior. Teenage risk probability is increased by living with families at risk and having friends involved in antisocial behaviors (Sandler, Ingram, Wolchik, Tein, & Winslow, 2015).

Families at Risk in Spain

Recent reports by the FOESSA Foundation (2014) and UNICEF (2014), based on an analysis of several indicators, demonstrate the reality of family and childhood circumstances in Spain. The reports highlight the following points:

1. According to FOESSA (2014), 25 percent of the Spanish population is at risk of social exclusion – that is, more than 11.7 million people. Out of this 11.7 million, 5 million people are in extreme risk situations.
2. Due to the economic recession, the percentage of homes simultaneously affected by a lack of material goods and financial poverty has increased by almost 50 percent (FOESSA, 2014).
3. One out of ten families in Spain is now a single-parent family, a situation associated with a risk of poverty (FOESSA, 2014).
4. The economic recession and its policies have increased the rate of child poverty while causing a reduction in the funding available for basic services

intended for at-risk groups to deal with issues such as malnutrition; "energy poverty" (e.g., being unable to pay for heating or hot water); and school absenteeism (UNICEF, 2014).

5. The vast majority of social indicators imply that the well-being of Spanish children has deteriorated. This is due to the ever-increasing risk of poverty, along with an increase in unemployment among families with children (UNICEF, 2014).

Spain's 2009–2016 National Strategy on Drugs (PNSD, 2008) takes into account that the family continues to be a very important societal unit in Spain. It is one of the most solid reference points for teenagers who consider family, along with friends, among the most important spheres in their life. That is why, to better protect young people against exposure and consumption of drugs, the 2008 PNSD encouraged the implementation of actions to improve family competences and family management, as well as actions that facilitated an increase in family cohesion and reinforced family resilience.

Family Prevention Programs in Spain

The Exchange on Drug Demand Reduction Action (EDDDRA) database compiles information on evaluated prevention practices in the European Union[2]. The EDDRA database belongs to the European Union's European Monitoring Centre for Drugs and Drug Addiction. In order to obtain a high-quality family prevention program for Spain, this database was used to search for indexed programs that had families as the target group. Three of the programs listed in the EDDRA database are described in this section: Entre Todos, Hirusta, and Building Health.

According to EDDRA, the family prevention program Entre Todos (All Together) was developed by the Proyecto Hombre organization to provide an effective intervention model that could be used in the Proyecto Hombre centers throughout Spain. The Entre Todos program aims at influencing the risk and protection factors related to drug consumption among teenagers between ages twelve and fourteen.

EDDRA describes Hirusta as a prevention program for families with teenagers who demonstrate risk behaviors. The program is based on a preventive intervention model that contemplates both universal and selective prevention. Hirusta developed two fields of activity: one that included actions focused on community education and the training of all those agents who might act preventively with teenagers (parents, teachers, and social mediators); and a second activity field in which specific preventive interventions were carried out with teenagers and families that experienced concrete behavior problems.

2 www.emcdda.europa.eu/themes/best-practice/examples.

Building Health is another prevention program included in EDDRA. The general objective of Building Health is to teach parents how to enhance family environmental factors that protect their children against drug use and antisocial behavior. The specific objectives of Building Health are to (1) provide a realistic view of adolescence and the problem of drug use; (2) further the establishment of adequate parenting styles characterized by good communication between parents and their children, cooperative conflict resolution, and suitable supervision of adolescent behavior; and (3) encourage parents to establish household rules about drug use.

However, these programs haven't yet been empirically evaluated. Namely, currently in Spain, there is a lack of validated universal family prevention programs (Díaz-Aguado, Martínez-Arias, & Ordóñez, 2013; Lloret, Espada, Cabrera, & Burkhart, 2013). Rather, the only evidence-based program that is currently implemented in Spain is a selective prevention program called the Programa de Competencia Familiar (Family Competence Program, FCP). This program is an adaptation of the U.S. Strengthening Families Program (SFP) for use in Spain. The FCP was designed by the Grupo de Investigación y Formación Educativa y Social (GIFES) at the Universidad de las Islas Baleares; between 2005 and 2011, the FCP was used on forty-five occasions in three different contexts:

1. Families in a drug rehabilitation program: Proyecto Hombre (PH)
2. Families at risk of social marginalization that were using social services
3. Families involved with child protection services (Orte, Ballester, & March, 2013a)

Two methods were used in adaptation of the U.S. Strengthening Families Program to the Spanish culture and circumstances: a pretest and posttest evaluation, design with control groups, and a process evaluation (Orte et al., 2015a).

Cultural Adaptation of the Selective Strengthening Families Program in Spain: The Programa de Competencia Familiar

Over time, there have been different European adaptations of both the original Strengthening Families Program (Kumpfer, DeMarsh, & Child, 1989) and the SFP-IOWA-version.[3] However, only the SFP 12–16 adaption in Ireland and the SFP 6–11 and 12–16 adaptions in Spain opted to create cultural adaptations of the SFP. In Spain's case, the cultural adaptation also included a longitudinal (i.e., follow-up) analysis of the application results.

The Spanish adaption of the Strengthening Families Program began in 2003. The Strengthening Families Program was selected because it was recommended

3 www.extension.iastate.edu/sfp/.

by the U.S. government agency Substance Abuse and Mental Health Services Administration (SAMSHA). SAMSHA recommended this program because of the intervention fidelity; the rigorous evaluation process; the validity of the measuring procedures; and the positive behavioral changes (Orte & Amer, 2014).

The cultural adaptation created by the GIFES group (Orte & GIFES, 2005) was done using a pretest/posttest design with control groups, complemented by process evaluations (Orte et al., 2013a), as well as the aforementioned longitudinal follow-up study. For the 2009 application, the follow-up study was done in 2011; and for the 2010 application, the follow-up was done in 2012.

The cultural adaptations mainly focused on:

A. *Formal elements*
   1. Language elements (ways of addressing people; name adaptation; game adaptation; incorporation of icons in the manuals; and the use of a nonsexist language).
   2. Presentation aspects (i.e., educational standards for the preparation of material).

B. *Structural elements*
   1. Session-monitoring and session-opening intervals (formal sessions and break periods were considered to be family-monitoring moments).
   2. Session duration (most sessions were extended by five to fifteen more minutes).
   3. Group management (more information was given to trainers, especially in their instruction manuals).

C. *Session contents*
   1. Objectives: objective details and/or the creation of subobjectives were included in order to give more information.
   2. Focus on certain issues (especially those liable to generate a certain degree of disagreement, e.g., corporal punishment).
   3. Modification of activities and creation of material (e.g., a DVD to facilitate technique and skill acquisition, a relaxation CD, or a CD and content support guide for families with reading and writing difficulties).
   4. Creation of new activities (e.g., communication techniques were included in the problem solving sessions).

Implementation and Long-Term Results: The Family Competence Program in Spain

The Family Competence Program designed by GIFES for use in Spain is based on a cognitive-emotional perspective, using a multicomponent format, that is, it is implemented simultaneously among children, parents, and other family members, allowing for a systematic family focus (Orte et al., 2013a). In the FCP, key components for establishing family competence are family cohesion and organization, communication, and cooperative problem solving. These factors interact and are mutually synergic. For example, better family organization is linked to better cohesion among core family members, as well as better communication between family members and more cooperative problem solving. Effective strategies were developed based on the premise that family issues can be resolved by focusing on positive family elements as a means of problem solving.

Between 2005 and 2011, the Spanish version of the Family Competence Program was deployed forty-five times in Spain, reaching a total of 335 families (Orte et al., 2015a). The program was used in two contexts: a drug treatment program (Proyecto Hombre) and within public social services (Orte et al., 2013a). The FCP′s objectives include prevention of substance abuse and behavioral problems and improved family dynamics.

The Family Competence Program aim was to achieve learning objectives and behavior change in parents, their children, and the family as a whole. Accordingly, family members, working in different groups over fourteen weeks, learned different types of skills that are listed in Table 37.1.

Implementation of the Family Competence Program

The Family Competence Program application began with facilitators' training that included a web tool for doubt consultation during the applications and for uploading session self-reports (Orte & Amer, 2014). In order to evaluate the program design, a quasi-experimental and multigroup design was used, with pretest and posttest measures as well as a control group. The process evaluation consisted of (1) a trainer self-report after every session and (2) a fidelity evaluation by external evaluators. The results were evaluated using two surveys: the original parent and child surveys that Kumpfer used in the original Strengthening Families Program (Kumpfer et al., 1989) and the Behavior Assessment System for Children (BASC) questionnaire (Reynolds & Kamphaus, 2004). For the BASC questionnaires, only the scales for the assessment system (validated specifically for the Spanish population) were used.

The KK-Parent Questionnaire (Kumpfer, 1998) uses thirteen scales with 135 items (approximately thirty minutes duration). The scales are positive parenting and parental involvement; family conflict; family organization; clear rules about drugs; drug consumption; parental supervision; parental effectiveness; communication and parenting skills; family cohesion and strength; learning skills and social skills; impulsivity; concentration problems/depression and aggressiveness. In the questionnaire, there are 135 items about the following:

1. The family's sociodemographic profile and family relationships
2. Forty items on parental self-evaluation and the parent–child relationship
3. Five options about parental alcohol and drug consumption (SAMHSA GPRA/NIDA)

Table 37.1 *Family Competence Program Contents*

	Parental competence program	Social skills program for children	Program for improving family relationships
1	Introduction and group formation	Greeting and rules	Introduction and group formation
2	Expectations, development, and stress management	Social skills I: active listening skills	Game of sons and daughters
3	Rewards	Social skills II: conversation skills	Game of sons and daughters: rewards
4	Goals and objectives	Learning good behavior	Goals and objectives
5	Differential attention: paying attention and ignoring	How to say "NO" to stay out of trouble	Differential attention: tables and roulette
6	Communication I: relationship improvement	Communication I: better relationships	Communication I: introduction to the family game
7	Communication II: family meetings	Communication II: family meetings	Communication II: consolidation of the family game
8	Drugs and family: risk factors	Alcohol and drugs	Learning from fathers and mothers
9	Solving problems and giving instructions	Solving problems	Solving problems and giving instructions
10	Setting limits I: redirecting misbehavior	Introduction to the game of fathers and mothers	The game of fathers and mothers I
11	Setting limits II: practice	Confrontation skills I: recognizing feelings	The game of fathers and mothers II
12	Setting limits III: solving behavioral problems	Confrontation skills II: facing criticism	The game of fathers and mothers III
13	Building and using behavioral programs	Confrontation skills III: facing anger	Remembering what helps us and why it helps us
14	Achieving and maintaining good behavior	Graduation, resources, and review	End of program and graduation party

4. Twelve items about family strengths and family resilience (Kumpfer, 1998)
5. Items about potential shared family activities, indicating frequency and duration
6. Forty-four parental observations about the children's activities

The KK-Children Questionnaire (Kumpfer, 1998) is designed for children aged seven or older; it contains ten scales with 134 items and is approximately thirty minutes in length and is done in the presence of an evaluator. The scales are positive parenting; communication; parental supervision; parental follow-up of school issues; disruptive behavior; lack of self-control; drug abuse; social skills for prosocial behavior, empathy, and assertiveness. The questionnaire for children contains 134 items:

1. Twenty-two items about their relationship with their father, and twenty-two items (same items, taking into account gender variation) about their relationship with their mother
2. Five items about family dynamics (meetings, quarrels, etc.); three items about school difficulties; and two items about tobacco and alcohol consumption
3. Forty items on behavior self-evaluation
4. Eighteen items about the children's social skills
5. As in the parents' questionnaire, items about potential shared family activities, indicating frequency and duration

BASC (Reynolds & Kamphaus, 2004) is a multidimensional evaluation system that measures several behavior and personality aspects. There is a self-report for children and then a report about the children done by parents and teachers. The children's self-report provides information about the following scales: negative attitudes toward school; negative attitudes toward teachers; social stress; anxiety; depression; interpersonal relationships; relations with parents; and self-esteem. The questionnaires for parents and teachers measure aggressiveness; hyperactivity; behavior disorders; attention problems; learning problems; depression; anxiety; adaptability; social skills; and study skills. The duration of the questionnaire is about thirty minutes for the children (self-report) and twenty minutes for parents and teachers.

With regard to results, 74.6 percent of the families reported positive changes (Orte et al., 2013a). An improvement in family competence was also observed, that is, an improvement in family communication and in parent–children relationships. The evaluated items were selected from the Kumpfer, BASC and ESFA questionnaires. Improvements were also seen in family organization and cohesion (Orte et al., 2013a).

A longitudinal follow-up analysis of the results was also carried out. Of the 335 families that fully collaborated with the Family Competence Program, 63 families from the Proyecto Hombre (PH) implementation (the application was offered at the end of the PH treatment) and 92 families using social services participated in this longitudinal analysis.

The FCP obtained good results (in consistency and quality) in families with a variety of difficult situations over time, demonstrating a considerable maintenance of results (Orte et al., 2015a, 2015b).

Table 37.2 summarizes the most relevant data from the sample analyzed. The analysis is based on 155 families (53.45 percent) out of the experiment's original number of 355 families.

The mean ages and standard deviations (SDs) for the various subgroups that participated in the follow-up study are presented in Table 37.3.

The first set of factors analyzed in the follow-up study refers to the family group or to the parents. The six factors under consideration represent the results from the factor analysis of the parents' questionnaire. The results of the PH families and the social support groups are presented in Table 37.4.

Table 37.2 *Monitoring of the Participant Families*

	Starting PCF	Ending PCF	%	Completion	% (Final PCF)
PH - Families	87	73	83.91	63	86.30
SS - Families	292	217	74.32	92	42.40
Total	379	290	76.52	155	53.45

Table 37.3 *Mean Age and SD of Parents and Children (Proyecto Hombre and Social Services)*

	Mean Age – Parents	Mean Age – Children
Proyecto Hombre (EG)	40.28 (SD 3.98)	12.38 (SD 2.47)
Proyecto Hombre (CG)	41.11 (SD 5.64)	12 (SD 2.17)
Social Services (EG)	41.46 (SD 7.95)	11.25 (SD 1.94)
Social Services (CG)	38.82 (SD 13.22)	9.65 (SD 1.53)

About PH families and parents results, in Table 37.4, Factor 1 deals with family resilience, meaning the family's capacity to deal with challenges (health, affective relationships, family support, etc.). The results show a small increase in the values observed at the end of the FCP program. The difference is not significant ($p > 0.05$).

Factor 2 deals with the parent–child relationship within the family context. This factor includes a wide variety of significant information, as it is a principal component in the following factors: communication, quality time, and learning relationships. The results show a significant increase in the values observed at the end of the FCP ($p = 0.001$).

Factor 3 deals with family cohesion. In the parents' questionnaire, this factor refers to low conflict levels and healthy relationships (respect, family atmosphere). The results also show a moderate increase in the observed values at the end of the FCP ($p < 0.05$), confirming the maintenance of effects.

Factor 4 focused on family organization. As with the previously mentioned factors, this factor received special attention in the FCP, to the extent that a series of actions specifically aimed at improving family organization were included. The results show a nonsignificant reduction ($p > 0.05$) in the observed values at the end of the FCP.

Factor 5 deals with positive parenting, based on positive discipline, as well as efficient supervision and other parenting elements. The results show a significant improvement after the end of the FCP ($p = 0.001$).

Finally, Factor 6, parenting skills, refers to one of the family competency components, that is, the capacity to give efficient guidance, to set limits, to motivate children, and so on. The results show a small – but not significant ($p > 0.05$) – improvement noted by the parents, maintaining the reasonably good results observed at the end of the FCP.

Table 37.4 *Mean, SD and Pre-post T-tests on Family Factors*

among PROYECTO HOMBRE (PH)						
KK-Parent questionnaire (N = 63)						
		FCP Completion		**Follow-up**		
		Mean	SD	Mean	SD	t test
Factor 1	Family resilience	37.11	10.72	38.41	12.36	–0.62
Factor 2	Parent–child relationship	83.11	14.84	88.90	11.25	–3.35**
Factor 3	Family cohesion	21.43	4.79	21.95	4.35	–0.89
Factor 4	Family organization	19.05	3.40	18.19	3.13	1.99*
Factor 5	Positive parenting	9.78	2.37	10.78	2.04	–3.47**
Factor 6	Parenting skills	8.94	3.41	9.24	3.62	–0.54
KK-Children Questionnaire (N = 44)						
		FCP Completion		**Follow-up**		
		Mean	SD	Mean	SD	t test
Factor 1	Family involvement	46.32	8.28	49.33	7.18	–3.48**
Factor 2	Family cohesion	15.48	4.14	15.76	4.20	-0.74
Factor 3	Management of school problems	11.87	2.21	12.22	2.10	–1.78
Factor 4	Social skills	46.33	9.27	50.08	8.69	–3.61**
Factor 5	Setting limits	8.05	1.83	8.67	1.51	–2.94*
among SOCIAL SERVICES						
KK-Parent Questionnaire (N = 92)						
		FCP Completion		Follow-up		
		Mean	SD	Mean	SD	t test
Factor 1	Family resilience	37.76	7.90	40.49	12.57	–2.13*
Factor 2	Parent–child relationship	86.50	13.56	90.02	12.45	–2.36*
Factor 3	Family cohesion	22.30	3.90	23.15	3.50	–3.51**
Factor 4	Family organization	20.03	2.88	19.74	2.70	1.20
Factor 5	Positive parenting	10.38	2.21	11.42	1.95	–4.35**
Factor 6	Parenting skills	9.47	2.78	10.25	3.62	–2.19*
KK-Children Questionnaire (N = 92)						
		FCP Completion		Follow-up		
		SD	Mean	SD	Mean	SD
Factor 1	Family involvement	49.34	11.32	51.15	13.50	–2.31
Factor 2	Family cohesion	15.40	4.39	15.80	4.05	–1.48
Factor 3	Management of school problems	10.37	2.65	10.62	2.55	–1.32
Factor 4	Social skills	48.35	9.32	49.76	9.43	–2.29*
Factor 5	Setting limits	48.35	9.32	49.76	9.43	–1.32

$p < 0.05$
$^{**}p < 0.00$

About PH families, the second set of factors analyzed deals with the family and children. Under consideration are the five factors obtained from the factorization of the children's questionnaire.

Factor 1 deals with family involvement, meaning active parental involvement in the children's psychosocial development processes. The results show a moderate increase in the observed values at the end of the FCP. The difference is significant ($p = 0.001$).

Factor 2 deals with family cohesion (as did the third factor in the parents' questionnaire). In the children's questionnaire, this factor also referred to low conflict levels and good relationships (respect, family atmosphere). The results show maintenance of the values observed at the end of the FCP ($p > 0.05$); it should be noted that the parents evaluated this factor in a similar manner.

Factor 3, management of school issues, refers to conflict issues in addition to academic problems. A moderate ($p = 0.080$) but not significant improvement was observed, indicating a maintenance of effects.

Factor 4 deals with a wide set of strategic social skills for children: speaking, listening, auto-control, establishing relationships, assertiveness, and so on. The data show a significant improvement ($p = 0.001$).

Finally, Factor 5 (referring to the capacity to set limits) also showed a significant improvement ($p = 0.005$).

Table 37.4 shows also the results of the family and parental factors analyzed for the SS families; the results are similar to those of the PH families, although the SS family results show a more notable improvement.

In Table 37.4, the Factor 1 deals with family resilience. The results show a significant difference ($p = 0.035$), in favor of the two-year follow-up time frame. It appears that, in the families participating in the longitudinal study, family resilience improved over the two-year interval.

Factor 2 deals with the parent–child relationship within the family context. The results show a significant increase in the values observed at the end of the FCP ($p = 0.020$), similar to the evolution observed in the PH families.

Factor 3 deals with family cohesion. The results also show a significant increase in the values observed at the end of the FCP ($p = 0.001$); in this case, there is better behavior than that observed in the PH families.

Factor 4 focuses on family organization. The results show a nonsignificant reduction ($p > 0.05$) in the values observed at the end of the FCP, similar to the results of the PH families.

Factor 5 deals with positive parenting. The results show a significant improvement in the period under consideration since the end of the FCP ($p = 0.00$), similar to the results of the PH families.

Finally, Factor 6 deals with parenting skills. The results show a moderate increase in the good results observed at the end of the FCP ($p = 0.031$).

Next, Table 37.4 shows also the results of the SS family and children factors. The Factor 1 deals with family involvement. The results show a moderate increase in the values observed at the end of the FCP. The difference is significant ($p = 0.023$), with a result similar to the PH families.

The Factor 2 deals with family cohesion. The results show a maintenance of the values observed at the end of the FCP ($p > 0.05$), similar to those of the PH families.

The Factor 3 deals with management of school issues. The values obtained at the end of the FCP ($p > 0.05$) were maintained.

Factor 4 deals with a wide set of social skills. The data show a significant improvement ($p < 0.024$) similar to that of the PH families.

Finally, the Factor 5 (referring to the capacity to place limits) shows maintenance of the values observed at the end of the FCP ($p > 0.05$).

One of the relevant research questions for this case study was based on differences in family vulnerability levels. The research hypothesis was that greater vulnerability leads to a worsened family dynamic. In order to test this hypothesis, a Family Vulnerability Index was used.

The Family Vulnerability Index (FVI) was calculated based on three indicators from the information provided by all the families: job circumstances; parental education level; and family structure. The family situation was evaluated in 2009–2010 and 2012–2013, as the economic recession had changed family circumstances after 2009.

To calculate the FVI, a variable with a range from 0 to 20 points was used, based on mean scores from the three indicators. The indicators were treated with the following relative weights: job circumstances = 40 percent; parental education level = 30 percent; family structure = 30 percent. When vulnerability situations were added up, a higher score indicated higher relative vulnerability; thus, the indicator had a negative implication.

A family with unemployed parents who had very low education levels and didn't live with their children (the latter being in institutional care or temporarily with relatives) obtained the highest scores in the Family Vulnerability Index. A family with parents holding permanent jobs, university studies, and a stable family unit obtained a much lower Family Vulnerability Index score.

The 2009–2010 circumstances of families that participated in both the FCP applications (2009–10) and the longitudinal evaluations two years later (2011–12) were analyzed. A higher level of vulnerability was observed among the SS families (mean = 12,44), in comparison with the PH families (mean = 11,71). The differences were not statistically significant, but they confirm a premise established in the work sessions. This was without taking into account that often families with greater vulnerability, usually SS families, might have left Spain during 2009–2010.

Based on the FVI (2012–13), a correlation analysis was carried out (Spearman's rho) using all the factors and scales that were studied. With regard to the PH families that participated in the FCP (Table 37.5), there was no significant influence in the factor and scale results.

There was also no significant influence in the factor and scale results for the data from the SS families that participated in the FCP (Table 37.5). Only one of the scales (the capacity to set limits) shows correlation with the FVI.

In order to better explain and understand the study results over the long term, a typology analysis of the families was done, using cluster analysis (conglomerates). The analysis was done using the PH and SS families. The typology was studied at the end of the FCP and at the end of the follow-up study. The typology was not exactly the same at both moments, given that the factors had also changed.

Table 37.5 *Spearman's Rho Correlation between the Evaluated Factors and the Family Vulnerability Index (FVI) as Measured Two Years Later*

Proyecto Hombre (PH) Group (N = 44)		
Among parents		
Factor 1	Family resilience	0.065
Factor 2	Parent–child relationship	–0.130
Factor 3	Family cohesion	–0.079
Factor 4	Family organization	0.155
Factor 5	Positive parenting	0.030
Factor 6	Parenting skills	–0.010
Among children		
Factor 1	Family involvement	0.077
Factor 2	Family cohesion	0.147
Factor 3	Management of school problems	0.199
Factor 4	Social skills	–0.035
Factor 5	Setting limits	–0.107
Social Services Group (N = 92)		
Among parents		
Factor 1	Family resilience	–0.027
Factor 2	Parent–child relationship	–0.062
Factor 3	Family cohesion	0.096
Factor 4	Family organization	0.099
Factor 5	Positive parenting	0.036
Factor 6	Parenting skills	–0.040
Among children		
Factor 1	Family involvement	0.184
Factor 2	Family cohesion	0.040
Factor 3	Management of school problems	0.084
Factor 4	Social skills	0.177
Factor 5	Setting limits	0.294*

*p = 0.005

Based on the information obtained at the end of the FCP, combined with the findings of the 155 families from the longitudinal study, three family types were designated, which accounted for 94.84 percent of families studied (see Table 37.6).

The first type represents the families that obtained the best results (33.55 percent of families obtained high-to-good results); the second type represents families that obtained medium-level results for children and slightly lower results in parents (29.68 percent of families); the third type is for families that had medium-level results for the parents and slightly lower results for children (31.61 percent of families).

Table 37.6 *Family Typology Analysis*

Proyecto Hombre (PH) and Social Services (SS) (FCP Completion) (N = 155)			
	Family Type Identification	**Number of Families**	**%**
Type 1	Best result	52	33.55
Type 2	Medium results for children and lower for parents	46	29.68
Type 3	Medium results for parents and lower for children	49	31.61
No classification	No classification	8	5.16
	Total	155	100.00

Table 37.7 *Family Typology Analysis: Factors Considered*

Proyecto Hombre (PH) and Social Services (SS) (FCP Completion) (N = 155)		
Variance analysis between Types	**F**	**Significance**
Family resilience	35.45	0.00
Parent–children relationships	123.95	0.00
Family cohesion	6.16	0.00
Positive parenting	31.63	0.00
Family involvement	56.12	0.00
Management of the school problems	3.25	0.04
Children's social skills	38.81	0.00
Setting limits	7.30	0.00

A variance analysis (Table 37.7) was used to select the seven factors that were significant for differentiating among family typologies. It is interesting to note how, at the end of the FCP, family vulnerability had not yet become significant in distinguishing between family types. In 2012–2013, family vulnerability would be a very significant factor among the families participating in the longitudinal study.

A variance analysis (Table 37.8) was also used to select the ten factors significant in differentiating between family types in the follow-up study.

The follow-up analysis was based on 155 families who had participated in the FCP study, of which 91.61 percent of families were classified according to three family types (see Table 37.9). Type 1 in Table 37.9 shows families with the best results (24.52 percent of families); Type 2 shows families with medium children results and somewhat lower results for the parents (47.74 percent of families); and for Type 3, families with medium results in the parents and somewhat lower children results (19.35 percent of families).

Table 37.10 shows the distribution of families according to which agency they were involved with (i.e., Proyecto Hombre or social services). In both agencies, families showed considerable improvement. Table 37.10 also shows a high presence of families with medium results in PH (50.79 percent), as opposed to SS families with medium results (45.65 percent). Finally, a small number of

Table 37.8 *Family Typology Analysis: Factors Considered*

Proyecto Hombre (PH) and Social Services (SS) (Follow-up Two Years Later) (N = 155)		
Variance Analysis between Types	**F**	**Significance**
Family vulnerability synthetic index	3.72	0.02
Valuation of the change achieved through PCF	6.96	0.00
Family resilience	45.03	0.00
Parent–children relationships	62.76	0.00
Family cohesion	6.73	0.00
Positive parenting	17.35	0.00
Family involvement	60.88	0.00
Management of the school problems	10.85	0.00
Children's social skills	38.58	0.00
Setting limits	6.32	0.00

Table 37.9 *Family Typology Analysis*

Proyecto Hombre (PH) and Social Services (SS) (Follow-up Two Years Later) (N = 136)			
	Family Type Identification	**Number of Families**	**%**
Type 1	Best results – good PCF valuation – FVI medium level	38	24.52
Type 2	Medium results for children and lower for parents	74	47.74
Type 3	Medium results for parents and lower for children	30	19.35
No classification	No classification	13	8.39
	Total	155	100.00

Table 37.10 *Family Typology Analysis per Agency (Proyecto Hombre and Social Services)*

Proyecto Hombre (PH) and Social Services (SS) (Follow-up Two Years Later) (N = 155)				
	Proyecto Hombre (PH)		Social Services (SS SS)	
	Number of families	%	Number of families	%
Type1	13	20.63	25	27.17
Type 2	32	50.79	42	45.65
Type 3	13	20.63	17	18.48
No classification	5	7.94	8	8.70
Total	63	100.00	92	100.00
Pearson's Chi-square			0.975 (p = 0.807)	
Association contingency coefficient			0.079	

families with low results and a high vulnerability index were noted in both groups (20.63 percent and 18.48 percent).

The majority of the changes identified in this case study, based on the factors investigated, continued to be relevant for the majority of families. Largely positive results were obtained from a wide range of relevant factors related to family dynamics:

Family factors (parental analysis): the maintenance of results obtained at the end of the FCP was confirmed, as well as a difference in comparison with the control group family results. The evolution of families using social services seems more positive than that of the PH families.

Family factors (child analysis): the maintenance of the good results observed at the end of the FCP was also confirmed. Furthermore, is should be noted that the children underwent a significant developmental change, as the two-year difference represents a significant psychosocial maturation in some cases.

Summary of Evaluation Studies Results

The results described in this chapter give rise to a series of observations and questions:

1. The evaluation of result maintenance over a long term (two years) is especially difficult with families in vulnerable situations. Within the FCP setting, in the general focus on family competence, there is a great variety of factors that are relevant to maintenance (changes in family structure, a child´s developmental processes, participation in other social programs, etc.).
2. The FCP has shown its effectiveness in maintaining the participants' commitment over time, obtaining an important sample level. The family members understood what they were doing; they understood the benefits of the process in which they were participating and saw improvements in the issues addressed by the program.
3. Despite difficulties, the FCP has demonstrated its effectiveness in maintaining positive results in the majority of factors studied.
4. As with all socioeducational family programs, various important questions present themselves during follow-up studies; in the case of the FCP, the longitudinal studies already under way are beginning to shed light on the following issues:
   a. What are the long-term effects of the programs and what are the most significant factors in the maintenance or loss of effects?
   b. How does the FCP deal with the changes that occur in families?
   c. Are the results of the FCP applications (as applied to Proyecto Hombre and social services) as consistent as the results of the original U.S. Strengthening Families Program and its international adaptions (Kumpfer & Alvarado, 2003; Kumpfer, Pinyuchon, de Melo, & Whiteside, 2008)?

In conclusion, the use of the Family Competence Program for families with social and educational difficulties has shown quite considerable results in the medium and long term. The maintenance of effects has been consistent with the original Strengthening Families Program model used to develop the FCP program, as well as consistent with the SFP's other international program versions. This positive feedback confirms the FCP's efficacy in achieving the majority of its objectives for use in Spain, in both the short and medium-long term.

Suggestions Regarding Policy, Research, and Future Practice

With regard to the political implications of the subject matter discussed in this chapter, the findings for Spain indicate a situation with a high measure of demographic mobility associated with new population scenarios and issues of cultural diversity. The cultural adaptation of family evidence-based programs represents a valuable tool for social cohesion policies.

Regarding recommendations or comments for future research, the experience gained in designing and applying the Family Competence Program indicates that there are three things that need to be examined more closely: age groups, formats, and session dynamics. For age range, the adaptations for the characteristic elements of every age group should be revised. Especially for programs targeting teenagers, cultural adaptions need to incorporate a focus on adolescent personal identity (with different nuances depending on cultural differences). For formats, research needs to be done to evaluate the efficiency and effectiveness of emerging audiovisual formats (evaluating their suitability for cultural adaptation, as well as their results). It is also important to explore combined implementation formats that mix universal modes with selective modes. Finally, regarding session dynamics, it is important to do more research in two areas: the role of trainers (their importance regarding the families' involvement in the program); and in evaluating session dynamics and activities (in order to emphasize those that provide deeper understanding, motivation, and maximized benefits for the families). A process evaluation would allow for a better understanding of the applications' functioning and prevent these operations from becoming a "black box," that is, a closed entity whose functioning is unknown.

With regard to the practical implications, the following considerations have arisen from the application and evaluation of the culturally adapted Family Competence Program in Spain:

1. In addition to the importance of fidelity, cultural adaptations need to include session activities and debates that enhance the different family members' involvement and motivation. This requires good session planning and well-chosen trainers with strong leadership who are able to manage different situations.

2. An increase in quality family time results in better family dynamics and better communication.
3. Evidence-based family prevention allows for positive changes in family dynamics: family members have a better understanding of their roles and the consequences of their thoughts and actions.

All in all, drug prevention family evidence-based programs work effectively in developing different skills that are essential in child development and drug use prevention. These programs are good for the long haul, cost-effective, and scientifically robust, and they can be adapted to different family typologies and cultural contexts. That is why it is important to develop proper cultural adaptations that will contribute to maintaining fidelity and effectiveness.

Acknowledgments

The writing, translation, and proofreading of this chapter has been funded by the Spanish government (Research Project EDU2013-42412-R). The Family Competence Program (family evidence-based prevention program) described here has been funded by the following Spanish government research projects: projects EDU2013-42412-R, EDU 2010–20336, and SEJ2007-67306.

References

Amato, P. (2005). The impact of family formation change on the cognitive, social and emotional well-being of the next generation. *Future of Children* 15: 75–96.

Baumrind, D. (1966). Effects of authoritative parental control on child behavior. *Child Development* 37: 887–907.

Baumrind, D. (1967). Child care practices anteceding three patterns of preschool behavior. *Genetic Psychology Monographs* 75: 43–88.

Baumrind, D. (1975). Early socialization and adolescent competence: adolescence in the life cycle. In Dragastin, S. E., & Elder, G. H. (eds.), *Adolescence in the Life Cycle: Psychological Change and Social Context*. Washington, DC: Hemisphere, pp. 117–43.

Baumrind, D. (1991). The influence of parenting style on adolescent competence and substance use. *Journal of Early Adolescence* 11: 56–95.

Biglan, A., Brennan, P. A., Foster, S. L., & Holder, H. (2004). *Helping Adolescents at Risk: Prevention of Multiple Problem Behaviors*. London: Guilford Press.

Center for Substance Abuse Treatment (2004). *Substance Abuse Treatment and Family Therapy*. Treatment Improvement Protocol (TIP) Series, No. 39. Rockville, MD: Substance Abuse and Mental Health Services Administration (U.S.), ch. 2. Retrieved from www.ncbi.nlm.nih.gov/books/NBK64258/

Díaz-Aguado, M. J., Martínez-Arias, M. D. R., & Ordóñez, A. (2013). Prevenir la drogodependencia en adolescentes y mejorar la convivencia desde una perspectiva escolar ecológica. *Revista de educación* 1 (N° extra 2013): 338–62.

Dishion, T., & Kavanagh, K. (2003). *Adolescent Problem Behavior: A Family-centered Approach*. New York: Guilford Press.

Estévez, E., & Emler, N. (2011). Assessing the links among adolescent and youth offending, antisocial behavior, victimization, drug uses and gender. *International Journal of Clinical and Health Psychology* 11: 269–89.

FOESSA (2014). *VII Informe sobre exclusión y desarrollo social en España 2014*. Madrid, España: Fundación Foessa & Cáritas Española.

Foxcroft, D., & Tsertsvadze, A. (2011). Universal multi-component prevention programs for alcohol misuse in young people (review). *Cochrane Library* 2011: 9.

Foxcroft, D., & Tsertsvadze, A. (2012). Universal alcohol misuse prevention programmes for children and adolescents: Cochrane systematic reviews. *Perspectives of Public Health* 132: 128–34.

Kumpfer, K. L. (1998). Selective prevention interventions: the strengthening families program. In Ashery, E. R. S., Robertson, E. B., & Kumpfer, K. L. (eds.), *Drug Abuse Prevention through Family Interventions* (NIDA Research Monograph, 177, NIH Publication 99-4135. Washington, DC: U.S. Government Printing Office, pp. 160–217.

Kumpfer, K. L., & Alvarado, R. (2003). Family strengthening approaches for the prevention of youth problem behaviors, *American Psychologist* 5: 457–65.

Kumpfer, K. L., DeMarsh, J. P., & Child, W. (1989). *Strengthening Families Program: Children's Skills Training Curriculum Manual, Parent Training Manual, Children's Skill Training Manual, and Family Skills Training Manual*. Salt Lake City: University of Utah.

Kumpfer, K. L., Pinyuchon, M., de Melo, A., & Whiteside, H. (2008). Cultural adaptation process for international dissemination of the Strengthening Families Program (SFP). *Evaluation and Health Professions* 33: 226–39.

Kumpfer, K. L., Xie, J., & Magalhães, C. (2012). Cultural adaptations of evidence-based family interventions to strengthen families and improve children's outcomes. *European Journal of Developmental Psychology* 9: 104–16.

Leidiy, M., Guerra, N., & Toro, R. (2010). Positive parenting, family cohesion and child social competence among immigrant Latino families. *Journal of Family Psychology* 24: 252–60.

Llorens, N., Barrio, G., Sánchez, A., & Suelves, J. M. (2011). Effects of socialization and family factors on adolescent excessive drinking in Spain. *Prevention Science* 12: 150–61.

Lloret, D., Espada, J. P., Cabrera, V., & Burkhart, G. (2013). Prevención familiar del consumo de drogas en Europa: una revisión crítica de los programas contenidos en EDDRA. *Adicciones: Revista de socidrogalcohol* 25: 226–34.

MacArthur, G., Kipping, R., White, J., Chittleborough, C., Lingam, R,. Pasch, K., Gunnell, D., Hickman, M., & Campbell, R. (2012). Individual-, family-, and school-level interventions for preventing multiple risk behaviours in individuals aged 8 to 25 years. *Cochrane Database of Systematic Reviews* 6: Art No: Cd009927. doi: 10.1002/14651858.CD009927

McCoy, K., Cummings, M., & Davies, P. (2009). Constructive and destructive marital conflict, emotional security and children's prosocial behavior. *Journal of Child Psychology and Psychiatry* 50: 270–9.

Nanninga, M., Jansen, D., Knorth, E., & Reijneveld, S. (2015). Enrolment of children and adolescents in psychosocial care: more likely with low family social support and poor parenting skills. *European Child & Adolescent Psychiatry* 24: 407–16.

Orte, C., & Amer, J. (2014). Las adaptaciones culturales del Strengthening Families Program en Europa. *Un ejemplo de programa de educación familiar basado en evidencia. Estudios sobre educación* 26: 175–95.

Orte, C., Ballester, L., & March, M. (2013a). The family competence approach, an experience of socio-educational work with families. *Pedagogía Social. Revista interuniversitaria* 21: 3–27.

Orte, C., Ballester, L., March, M. X., Amer, J., Vives, M., & Pozo, R. (2015a). The Strengthening Families Program in Spain: a long-term evaluation. *Journal of Children's Services* 10: 101–19.

Orte, C., Ballester, L., March, M. X., Oliver, J. L., Pascual, B., & Gomila, M. A. (2015b). Development of prosocial behaviour in children after the improvement of family competences. *Journal of Children's Services* 10: 161–72.

Orte, C., & GIFES (Grupo de Investigación y Formación Educativa y Social) (2005). Los programas de prevención de drogas centrados en la familia: una visión desde la investigación y la práctica. *Revista Proyecto* 53: 14–17.

PNSD (Plan Nacional Sobre Drogas) (2008). *Estrategia Nacional sobre Drogas 2009–2016*. Madrid: Delegación del Gobierno para el Plan Nacional sobre Drogas.

PNSD (Plan Nacional Sobre Drogas) (2012). *Encuesta estatal sobre uso de drogas en enseñanzas secundarias (ESTUDES)*. Madrid: Plan Nacional Sobre Drogas.

Repetti, R., Taylor, S., & Seeman, T. (2002). Risky families: family social environments and the mental and physical health of offspring. *Psychological Bulletin* 128: 330–66.

Reynolds, C., & Kamphaus, R. (2004). *BASC. Sistema de evaluación de la conducta de niños y adolescentes*. Madrid: TEA Ediciones.

Sanders, M. R., & Duncan, S. B. (1995). Empowering families: policy, training, and research issues in promoting family mental health in Australia. *Behaviour Change* 12: 109–21.

Sandler, I., Ingram, A., Wolchik, S., Tein, J.-Y., & Winslow, E. (2015). Long-term effects of parenting-focused preventive interventions to promote resilience of children and adolescents. *Child Development Perspectives* 9: 164–71. doi: 10.1111/cdep.12126

Sandler, I., Schoenfelder, E. N., Wolchik, S. A., & McKinnon, D. P. (2011). Long-term impact of prevention programs to promote effective parenting: lasting effects but uncertain processes. *Annual Review of Psychology* 62: 299–329.

Steinberg, L. (2008). A social neuroscience perspective on adolescent risk-taking. *Developmental Review* 28: 78–106.

Stephenson, M. T., Rápida, B. L., Atkinson, J., & Tschida, D. A. (2005). Authoritative parenting and drug prevention practices implications for antidrug ads for parents. *Health Communication* 17: 301–21.

UNICEF (United Nations Childrens' Fund) (2014). *La infancia en España. El valor social de los niños: hacia un Pacto de Estado por la Infancia*. Madrid: Author. Retrieved from www.unicef.es/sites/www.unicef.es/files/infancia-espana/unicef_informe_la_infancia_en_espana_2014.pdf

UNODC (United Nations Office on Drugs and Crime) (2009). *Guide to Implementing Family Skills Training Programs for Drug Abuse Prevention*. New York: Author. www.unodc.org/documents/prevention/family-guidelines-E.pdf

UNODC (United Nations Office on Drugs and Crime) (2010). *International Standards on Drug Use Prevention*. New York: Author. Retrieved from www.unodc.org/documents/drug-prevention-and-treatment/PreventionStandards/prevention_standards_january_meeting_report_final_120322.pdf

Waller, R., Gardner, F., Dishion, T., & Sitn, S. L. (2014). Early parental positive behavior support and childhood adjustment: addressing enduring questions with new methods. *Social Development* 24: 304–22. doi: 10.1111/sode.12103

Whitesell, M., Bachand, A., Peel, J., & Brown, M. (2013). Familial, social, and individual factors contributing to risk for adolescent substance use. *Journal of Addiction* 2013: 1–9. doi: 10.1155/2013/579310, Article ID 579310

Wood, M., Read, J., Mitchell, R., & Brand, N. (2004). Do parents still matter? Parent and peer influences on alcohol involvement among recent high school graduates. *Psychology of Addictive Behaviors* 18: 19–30.

38 Youth Risk Behavior Prevention Based on Positive Relationships

Warsaw Adolescent Study

Krzysztof Ostaszewski & Agnieszka Pisarska

Introduction

The main goal of this chapter is to present theoretical and empirical background of prevention efforts, among Polish youth, based on positive relationship building in the context of a positive youth development concept. Positive relationships with important adults (parents, teachers, natural mentors) and social relationships associated with youth participation in constructive leisure time activities are connected with lower risk of a variety of problem behaviors such as substance use, violence, delinquency, school problems, and sexual risky behaviors (Nation et al., 2003; Zimmerman et al., 2013).

The content of the chapter builds upon research that explores the protective factors associated with adolescent problem behaviors. The importance of positive factors in prevention research is evidenced by the burgeoning research on resilience (Borucka & Ostaszewski, 2008; Fergus & Zimmerman, 2005; Luthar, 2006; Mazur et al., 2008; Rutter, 2012; Werner, 2005) and the positive youth development movement (Catalano, Berglund, Ryan, Lonczak, & Hawkins, 2004a; Lerner, Von Eye, Lerner, Lewin-Bizan, & Bowers, 2010). Contrary to this direction, until recently in Poland most research on aetiology of youth risk/problem behaviors was focused on risk factors associated with substance use and abuse. Only a few researchers in Poland have studied relationships between positive factors and adolescent risk behaviors (Bobrowski, 2002; 2003; Kwiatkowski, 2009; Mazur et al. 2008, 2009; Okulicz-Kozaryn, 2010; Ostaszewski, 2009, 2014; Ostaszewski, Bobrowski, Borucka & Pisarska, 2002; Pyżalski, 2012).

Results of the Warsaw Adolescent Study (Ostaszewski, 2014), presented in this chapter, address an existing gap in prevention science as observed in Poland. While doing so, the chapter provides a review of the current status of prevention science in Poland by exploring the role of positive youth relationships in preventing risky behaviors. The chapter is organized in three sections: section 1 discusses barriers to implementing well-informed prevention activities and current challenges of science-based prevention in Poland; section 2 contains a literature review that explores the associations between positive relationships and youth risk behaviors; and section 3 presents results of Warsaw Adolescent Study with a focus on associations between youth risk behavior and psychosocial positive factors.

Barriers to, and Challenges of, Science-Based Prevention in Poland

Poland is a central European country with a rich culture and population of more than 38 million. Although of strong democratic traditions, the country only relatively recently (during the early 1990s) has become a democracy with new freedoms after years of totalitarian/authoritarian rule in the former Eastern Bloc of the Soviet Union. The major democratic political and social changes began in 1989, when Poland started a transformation to a market economy and multiparty parliamentary system. As a result of these political and economic changes, Poland joined North Atlantic Treaty Organization (NATO) in 1999, the European Union (EU) in 2004, and the Schengen Area[1] in 2007.

Young people currently growing up in Poland represent one of the first generations of youth under the new democratic rule. Although the transition from socialism to capitalism has brought clear benefits to the society, it also has created some new risks that have had a strong negative effect on health-related behaviors among youth population. The opening of borders and the resulting influence of Western culture created and reinforced alcohol and other substances use among Polish youth (Anderson & Baumberg, 2006; Wojtyniak, Moskalewicz, Stokwiszewski, & Rabczenko, 2005). Economic changes, especially privatization processes, have brought a rapid increase in availability of alcohol and cigarettes (Świątkiewicz, 1997). In the first decade of transformation (1989–99), insufficient funding resulted in the closure of organizations and reduction in services that traditionally offered extracurricular activities for children and youth (e.g., sport clubs, youth organizations, and small cinemas). It took several years to create and implement new financial mechanisms at the local community level that would support extracurricular activities in Poland.

During these uncertain times, psychoactive substance use became a source of entertainment for youth as they had few other outlets in their free time. It is demonstrated by a rapid increase in youth psychoactive substance use at the first decade of political transformation in Poland (Centrum Badania Opinii Społecznej, 2003; Ostaszewski & Pisarska, 2008; Szymański, Woynarowska, & Mazur, 2001). Results of school surveys indicate, for example, that last year prevalence of any illicit drug use among fifteen to sixteen year olds increased from 3 percent in 1988 to 20 percent in 2000 (Ostaszewski, 2001) and among eighteen to nineteen year olds from 5 percent in 1992 to 23 percent in 2003 (Centrum Badania Opinii Społecznej, 2003). Alcohol drinking among underage youth also increased rapidly in the 1990s. Beer became the most popular drinking beverage among youth. According to the World Health Organization's Health Behavior in School-Aged Children (WHO-HBSC) 1990–1998 project results, the percentage of eleven- to fifteen-year-old teenagers who drank beer regularly increased from 5 percent in 1990 to 10 percent in 1998

1 The Schengen Area is the area comprising twenty-six European countries that have abolished passport and any other type of border control at their common borders.

(Szymański et al., 2001), and according to the Warsaw school survey the percentage of fifteen- to sixteen-year-old students who drank beer in the past thirty days increased from 18 percent in 1988 to 45 percent in 2000 (Okulicz-Kozaryn & Borucka, 2001). The Warsaw school surveys have also shown that between 1988 and 2000 regular cigarette use among fifteen to sixteen year olds had increased from 7 percent to 14 percent (Ostaszewski & Pisarska, 2008).

Alcohol and other psychoactive substance use, violence, and delinquency constitute a great risk for healthy development among Polish youth. The WHO-HBSC survey conducted in Poland in a school year 2013–2014 indicated that among fifteen and sixteen year olds, 10 percent smoked cigarettes regularly, 39 percent drank alcohol, 15 percent got drunk at least once during last thirty days, about 24 percent used marijuana or hashish at least once in their life, and 35 percent were involved in peer-to-peer direct or indirect aggression during last two months (Mazur, 2015). In a 2011 nationwide survey conducted within the European School Survey Project on Alcohol and Other Drugs (ESPAD), 58 percent, 30 percent, and 10.5 percent of the Polish ninth graders (fifteen and sixteen year olds) and 80 percent, 42 percent, and 15 percent of the Polish eleventh graders (seventeen and eighteen year olds) reported drinking, smoking cigarettes, and using marijuana/hashish (respectively) at least once in the last thirty days (Sierosławski, 2011). Current youth risk/problem behavior rates in Poland shadow the sudden rise in drinking, smoking, and drug taking seen in the 1990s (Okulicz-Kozaryn & Borucka, 2001; Ostaszewski & Pisarska, 2008; Szymański et al. 2001), juvenile delinquency (Kirwil, 2004), and school violent behavior (Mazur & Małkowska, 2003). At that time, for example, the percentage of school bullying perpetrators increased from 32.5 percent in 1994 to 37 percent in 2002 (Mazur & Małkowska, 2003), and juvenile delinquency rates rose significantly in all types of crime (Kirwil, 2004).

In response to these growing problems, a number of prevention programs have been implemented in Poland over the last twenty years. The use of evidence-based prevention programs, whether universal, selective, or indicative, is limited. These kinds of programs are more challenging for schools, more expensive for local authorities, more time-consuming for teachers or other school staff. However, some local authorities in Poland invested in well-informed prevention activities, including the program for parents and teachers, Szkoła dla Rodziców i Wychowawców (Sochocki, 2008)[2] (eighty-nine local communities); the program of integrated prevention, Archipelag skarbów (Grzelak, 2006)[3] (sixty-two local communities); programs for youth at risk, such as Fred Goes Net (Chojecki, 2011)[4] (forty-seven local communities) and Szkolna Interwencja Profilaktyczna[5] (Borucka, Pisarska, & Okulicz-Kozaryn,

2 www.ore.edu.pl/programy-i-projekty-98419/szkoa-dla-rodzicow-i-wychowawcow/o-szkole-dla-rodzicow-i-wychowawcow

3 www.program.archipelagskarbow.eu/progas:info:ogolnie

4 www.kbpn.gov.pl/portal?id=106315

5 www.ore.edu.pl/index.php?option=com_content&view=article&id=447&Itemid=1024

2003); and the Polish version of the EU Drug Abuse Prevention program Unplugged (Borkowska, 2011; Van der Kreeft et al., 2009)[6] (thirty-seven local communities) (Malczewski, 2015). Two other evidence-based alcohol prevention programs have been taking place in Poland since the early 2000s: Program Domowych Detektywów (PDD) and Program Fantastyczne Możliwości (Bobrowski, Pisarska, Ostaszewski, & Borucka, 2014 Ostaszewski, Bobrowski, Borucka, Okulicz-Kozaryn, & Pisarska, 2000). It is estimated that more than one hundred thousand students participated in these two programs in the past decade. Since the early 1990s, Spójrz inaczej[7] (Kołodziejczyk, Czemierowska, & Kołodziejczyk, 2007), a well-informed program based on social-emotional learning, has been implemented in Polish primary schools. According to the State Agency for Prevention of Alcohol Related Problems (PARPA), in 2009 this program was implemented in 161 local communities in Poland (about 2,500 local communities exist in Poland).

In Poland, a lot of prevention efforts are directed at children and youth at risk. Most of them are based on sociotherapy. This approach can also be considered as a well-informed prevention, although its evaluation has brought mixed results (Junik, 2007). Elements of sociotherapy are widely used by schools and other organizations working with school-age children. Sociotherapy is a concept combining group therapy techniques, social support, life skills training, and counseling. It is offered for children and youth with conduct problems, school failures, and families at risk, especially for families facing alcohol problems. In 2013, about 1,239 child/youth-care facilities provided these kinds of preventive activities in all regions of Poland for more than forty thousand children/youth at risk (Państwowa Agencja Rozwiązywania Problemów Alkoholowych, 2013).

Besides, there is a big number of child care facilities that provide an ordinary day care for children whose parents are working. Some of these children/youth belong to high-risk groups for substance abuse or other problem behaviors. These places are supported by local governments and treated as a kind of prevention activity. In 2013, in all regions in Poland about 4,448 of this type of facility provided day care activities for about 150,000 children/youth at risk. Altogether, about 200,000 of children and youth were covered by sociotherapy or ordinary child care service. Among them, about 35 percent were identified as children facing alcohol problems at home (Państwowa Agencja Rozwiązywania Problemów Alkoholowych, 2013).

As mentioned, development and dissemination of effective, evidence-based prevention programs have faced several barriers in Poland (Ostaszewski, 2015). The most important barriers are related to the changing political and sociocultural backdrop. By the end of the 1990s, Poland's Alcohol Law was amended, shifting responsibility for alcohol prevention funding from the government to local municipalities. A few years later (in 2002), the Minister of Education

6 www.kbpn.gov.pl/portal?id=1681804 7 www.spojrzinaczej.pl/index.php/opis-programu

signed an ordinance obliging schools to prepare and implement their own youth problem behavior prevention programs. These changes were obviously elements of democratization processes that shifted responsibility for social policy to local communities and the nongovernmental organization (NGO) sector. However, these reforms were implemented without sufficient preparation, training, and resources. As a result, in youth risk behavior prevention, school and community-based financial mechanisms support bottom-up initiatives conducted by local NGOs and prevention leaders who are often competent to market their products but less competent in prevention programming and evaluation. Mainstream practices in the field of prevention consist of ad hoc developed programs and actions. Most implemented activities are school-based programs/actions prepared by teachers and are a compilation of previous ideas and scenarios, one-time initiatives, theater productions in schools, special events in the local communities (picnics, family parties), competitions, sport events, and other leisure time alternatives (Terlikowska & Okulicz-Kozaryn, 2015).

These initiatives are mainly based on personal believes rather than on knowledge about social needs and effective prevention strategies. Needs assessment of the problems specific to a particular community of children/adolescents and adult populations is rarely conducted. Most of the prevention programs and activities are implemented without relevant evaluation. Moreover, in most cases prevention is treated as nonprofessional activity that does not require any special qualification. In practice, everyone who has "some promising ideas" and is able to promote them effectively can be funded by the local community and become a prevention leader. The number of well-educated prevention specialists is insufficient to respond to growing wave of problems.

Proper education is fundamental for successful implementation of any social policy based on knowledge. This is where we currently face a major problem in prevention science in Poland. Prevention studies are not officially or practically related to pedagogical sciences, psychology, or sociology. There are only a few scientific centers dealing with prevention and undertaking research on prevention programs' effectiveness. Moreover, there is no scientific journal devoted to prevention of children/adolescent risk behaviors. Therefore, articles on this issue are published in different journals related to medicine, psychology, or pedagogical science, which impedes flow of the knowledge between scientists and practitioners interested in evidence-based prevention. As a consequence these limitations, there is no nationwide training system or core curriculum that provides high-quality education in risk behaviors prevention for teachers, school principals, representatives of local authorities, representatives of NGOs, family physicians, journalists, and so on. Only recently (in 2014), an initiative aimed at developing a core curriculum for prevention specialists' training course was launched (Bukowska, 2014).

The use of evidence-based prevention is currently limited to a small group of researchers and experts only and has little impact on policy makers and prevention practice at the national and local level. Due to several limitations, including the absence of significant grants, the efficacy/effectiveness prevention studies based on randomized controlled trials are very limited in Poland. There is no distinct institution at the state level established to support development of well-informed prevention programs or fund serious prevention research. Governmental agencies assigned for national drug and alcohol policy implementation such as the PARPA and the National Bureau for Drug Prevention (KBPN) lack sufficient funds to support longitudinal studies on prevention. They invest their limited funds on research projects on epidemiology or related issues that are necessary for shaping national policy and international exchange. Research methods have been broadly used to determine risk factors, patterns of use, social and health consequences of substance abuse; define populations at risk; and so on. These studies provide data, but only a few scientific centers have been using research strategies to develop and evaluate prevention programs. This creates a gap between existing research efforts and prevention programming.

The development of evidence-based prevention of youth risky behaviors is not among the state priorities (Ostaszewski, 2015). There is a lack of integrated social milieu to form a lobby for a new system that would be established on a comprehensive and cohesive vision of contemporary knowledge on health promotion and prevention. Prevention science around substance use and other risk behaviors does not have high prestige in Poland and loses a race for funding against a strong and well organized lobby supporting research on cardiology, oncology, and other salient public health problems. In reality, most of the substance use and other risk behavior prevention programming is expected from people working outside research community, such as teachers, school pedagogues/psychologists, police officers, and NGOs. Politicians responsible for social policy and public health issues believe that substance use/risk behaviors prevention programming does not require research methods. The concept of evidence-based methods commonly used in clinical medical practice is almost unknown area in prevention reality. As a consequence, research infrastructure working for prevention science is insufficient.

Nevertheless, some efforts are being made to improve the quality of prevention programs. A Group for Prevention Programs Assessment and Recommendation was established to recommend relevant, best-practice prevention programs to schools and local communities. The expert group consists of representatives of PARPA, the KBPN, the Center for Education Development (ORE), and the Institute of Psychiatry and Neurology (IPiN). These nation-level institutions play important roles in the public health area by supervising substance use/risk behavior prevention activities in Poland. The improvement of prevention quality is a shared priority for all institutions involved in this project. New prevention programs are recommended for use at three levels: promising, good practice, and effective (a model program). To date, eighteen programs[8] (twelve promising programs, five good practice programs, and one

8 www.ore.edu.pl/programy-profilaktyczne/bank-programow-profilaktycznych/bank-programow-profilaktycznych-22811; www.parpa.pl/index.php/profilaktyka-system-rekomendacji/rekomendowane-programy-profilaktyczne

model program) received recommendation based on their well-informed concept and good or promising evaluation results, but this number does not correspond to the needs (Radomska, 2014). The Polish system of prevention programs recommendation is based on both the prevention standards developed within the European project titled Exchange on Drug Demand Reduction Action (EDDRA[9]) and the Polish prevention experts' knowledge and experience.

Establishing the Stage for Connecting Positive Relationships and Youth Risk Behaviors

Positive relationship building is a promising science-based prevention strategy that, once implemented properly, may increase effectiveness of youth risk behavior prevention programs (Nation et al., 2003; Ostaszewski, 2014; Zimmerman et al., 2013). Two types of relationships drew the attention of prevention specialists. These are primarily the relationships between an adolescent and important adults, including parents, teachers, and other adults who care and often serve youth as natural mentors (grandparents, youth leaders, coaches, priests, counselors, and others) (Hurd, Zimmerman, & Xue, 2009; Kumpfer & Alvarado, 2003; Lee, 2012; Tabak, 2008). The second important source of positive influence are the relations with peers established during extracurricular activities (Kołoło & Mazur, 2008; Rose-Kranor, Busseri, Willoughby, & Chalmers, 2006). Organized leisure time activities help to establish communication and interactions with positive peer and community leaders who model healthy behaviors. Moreover, organized activities supervised by adults might also serve as a social mechanism that filters negative peer/neighborhood influences. In this sense, organized extracurricular activities offer a number of significant advantages over adolescent unstructured use of time (Barnes, Hoffman, Welte, Farrell, & Dintcheff, 2007). Experts in adolescents' social life underline that peers, more often than parents or other significant adults, are the source of negative behavior, through influence and modeling (Ary et al. 1999; Hawkins & Wies, 1985; Jessor, 1998; Oettting & Donnemeyer, 1998).

The importance of positive relationships in youth risk behaviors prevention is further evident from the progress in adolescent resilience research (Fergus & Zimmerman, 2005; Masten, 2004; Masten & Powell 2003; Werner, 2000; 2005) and positive youth development movement (Bernat & Resnick, 2006; Catalano et al., 2004a). The resilience concept provides a framework for understanding why some children and adolescents who are exposed to a number of risk factors do not develop negative health and social outcomes. In other words, it focuses on those factors that help children and youth avoid the negative consequences of risk exposure (Fergus & Zimmerman, 2005; Luthar, 2006; Masten & Powell, 2003;

9 www.emcdda.europa.eu/themes/best-practice/examples

Rutter, 2012; Werner, 2005). The research on adolescent resilience and the concept of positive youth development radically changed the perspectives on the role of activity in the area of youth risk behavior prevention (Ostaszewski, 2014; Zimmerman et al., 2013). These two concepts have influenced school/local community policies toward adolescent risky behaviors (Bernat & Resnick, 2006). Prevention activities have become more positive and attractive to young people. Strength-based prevention concentrates on supporting youth social relations and on care to provide access to pro-developmental resources. Its promising directions include strengthening constructive child–parent relations, building a positive school climate, and mentoring and developing constructive forms of extracurricular activity.

Parent–Child Relationships: The Role of Effective Monitoring

Several studies indicate that positive parent–child relationships and effective parenting are the most influential protective factors in the context of youth risk behaviors (Lee, 2012; Pico & Kovacs, 2010; Resnick et al., 1997; Salem, Zimmerman, & Notaro, 1998; Tabak, 2008; Tabak & Mazur, 2008; Willoughby & Hamza, 2011). Effective parenting during adolescence includes supervision and monitoring, emotional support, communication, and positive modeling. Among many manifestations of positive parenting, monitoring seems to be the key element to strengthen family-based protection during the childhood and adolescent years (DiClemente et al., 2001; Dishion & McMahon, 1998; Lee, 2012). Monitoring has been found to be one of the most powerful protective mechanisms that help parents to reduce the incidence of psychoactive substance use (Dever et al., 2012; Griffin, Botvin, Scheier, Doyle, & Williams, 2003; Lee, 2012; Pico & Kovacs, 2010; Rai et al., 2003; Salem et al., 1998), antisocial behaviors (Griffin et al., 2003; Salem et al, 1998), sexual high-risk behaviors (DiClemente et al., 2001; Elkington, Bauermeister, & Zimmerman, 2011; Rai et al., 2003), and in general a range of youth problem/risk behaviors (DiClemente et al., 2001; Ostaszewski, 2014; Willoughby & Hamza, 2011).

In the literature, parental monitoring is characterized in two slightly different ways. Some authors pay more attention to a set of correlated behaviors intentionally directed to track and supervise children's whereabouts, activities, and adaptation (Dishion & McMahon, 1998), while others underline the crucial role of adequate child–parent communications and adolescent child willingness to disclose information about their outside activities to parents (Stattin & Kerr, 2000; Willoughby & Hamza, 2011). Despite some differences, there is a consensus around important components of parental monitoring; these are supervision, parent–child communication, and parental knowledge of children's whereabouts (Lee, 2012; Rai et al., 2003). These parental rearing practices decrease the likelihood of substance use/violence exposure, sexual violence and abuse, association with problematic peers, or involvement in antisocial/delinquent behaviors. Mutual communication and parental attention create for parents favorable conditions that allow them to recognize child's stressful or traumatic experiences and if necessary help to cope with them (Lee, 2012).

Positive child–parent relationships are critical conditions for effective monitoring, especially in adolescent years. Parental emotional support may elicit adolescent disclosure, and such disclosure may facilitate opportunities for parents to engage in stronger and deeper interaction with an adolescent child. Strong family bonding and open communication with adolescents tend to play a central facilitating role in effective parental monitoring (Stattin & Kerr, 2000; Willoughby & Hamza, 2011). Parental knowledge about their adolescent's activities is usually the result of both child-driven and parental monitoring-driven processes. That point of view has been emphasized in the literature on youth development and risk behaviors in adolescence and is supported by a growing number of research studies (Dishion & McMahon, 1998; Lee, 2012; Stattin & Kerr, 2000; Willoughby & Hamza, 2011). On the other hand, investigators indicated that a high level of family conflicts, harsh and inconsistent discipline, and lack of support lead to low levels of parent–child involvement, and such family conditions result in less effective or just poor parental monitoring (Ary et al. 1999; Willoughby & Hamza, 2011).

The scientific knowledge on parental monitoring has significant implications for prevention programs. Namely, it seems that prevention programs and activities designed for youth may benefit from targeting positive parenting practices, family processes, and specifically parental monitoring. The Strengthening Families Program is among the most internationally known example of a successful family-based prevention program, both at the universal prevention level (targeting teenagers aged ten to fourteen and their parents; Spoth, Clair, Shin, & Redmond, 2006; Trudeau, Spoth, Randall, & Azevedo, 2007) and for selective/indicated levels of prevention (families facing alcohol/drug problems; Kumpfer, 1998). A Polish adaptation of this program showed positive outcomes – improved parental skills and practices (Okulicz-Kozaryn, 2015).

Parental skills and relationships factors are universal, so the preventive intervention based on their improvement should be applicable for low- and high-risk children and families. Generally speaking, family-centered intervention that includes parental monitoring is a well-informed strategy aimed at improving developmental outcomes among adolescents. Parental motivation building – to monitor, set clear family rules, and strengthen communication with their adolescents – is the critical component of family-based prevention approaches (Ashery, Robertson, & Kumpfer, 1998; Kumpfer & Alvarado, 2003). Several prevention programs that properly address parent–child communication and rule setting have proven to be effective (Bobrowski et al., 2014; Ostaszewski et al., 2000; Rohrbach et al. 1995; Williams & Perry, 1998).

The alcohol use prevention program called PDD is a good example (Ostaszewski et al., 2000). The program aims to prevent underage drinking and consists of five teacher- and peer-led sessions combined with parent–child activities to be undertaken at home. Four booklets, one to be worked through each week, provide information on underage drinking, alcohol advertising and modeling, peer pressure, and the consequences of alcohol consumption. The activities in the booklets are designed to facilitate parent–child communication about alcohol and other substance use and to establish effective family rules to deal with underage drinking. At the end of the program, a family evening is organized where pupils present posters to their parents and participate in other fun activities. PDD is a Polish adaptation of the American Slick Tracy Home Team Program (Ostaszewski et al., 1998; Williams et al., 1995). The outcome evaluation showed that the program was effective in reducing alcohol use and intention to use. It was also demonstrated that participation in the program was associated with increased parent–child communication about the effects of both alcohol and cigarette use (Ostaszewski et al. 2000). Rohrbach et al. (1995) and Okulicz-Kozaryn & Foxcroft (2012) argue that improvement in parental practices is a key protective mechanism underlying students' behavioral changes.

Relationships with Teachers and Bonds with School

There is a growing body of evidence from different cultures and countries indicating that supporting teacher–student relationships and a sense of belonging to school is consistently associated with positive school adjustment and achievements and lower levels of students problem and risk behaviors (Catalano, Haggerty, Oesterle, Fleming, & Hawkins, 2004b; Khoury-Kassabri, Benbenishty, Astor, & Zeira, 2004, 2004; Kulesza, 2007; Ostaszewski, 2014; Resnick et al. 1997; Wingspread Declaration on School Connections, 2004). Caring and supportive relationships with adults in school and feeling connected to students attending the same class and/or school provide youth with the social support and emotional security needed to achieve a variety of school and developmental outcomes. In contrast, having poor relationships with teachers and poor bonds with school is associated with emotional distress, violence, substance use, delinquency, conduct problems, and poorer school achievements (Baker, 2006; Murray & Greenberg, 2000). Quality of student–teacher relationships has a powerful impact on youth social and emotional development and is one of the critical components of positive school climate (Anderson, 1982; Brand, Felner, Shim, Seitsinger, & Dumas, 2003; Cohen & Geier, 2010). Teachers' fair behaviors and their supportive attitudes decrease students' antisocial behaviors, including substance use, violence, and gang involvement (Voisin et al., 2005).

The importance of supportive school environment in youth positive development is emphasized by the social development model that integrates control and social learning theories (Hawkins & Wies, 1985). According to this model, the formation of youth positive social bonds to family, and then to school and teachers, reduces the likelihood of risky relationships with delinquent peers, because the behaviors rewarded by caring families and schools and deviant youth are opposite. These assumptions were supported by findings from number of studies that examined the associations between school bonding/teacher connectedness and youth problem/risk behaviors. For example, students who reported stronger school bonding and better relationships with teachers had generally lower rates of substance use (Aspy et al., 2012; Dever et al., 2012; McNeely & Falci, 2004; Ostaszewski, Rustecka-Krawczyk, & Wójcik, 2011; Resnick et al., 1997; Shears, Edwards, & Stanley, 2006; Simons-Morton, Crump, Haynie & Saylor, 1999; Voisin et al., 2005), aggressive behaviors and violence (Loukas, Suzuki & Horton, 2006; McNeely & Falci, 2004; Resnick et al., 1997; Wilson, 2004), sexual risky behaviors (Aspy et al., 2012; McNeely & Falci, 2004; Resnick et al., 1997; Voisin et al., 2005), and emotional and conduct problems (Loukas et al., 2006; Resnick et al., 1997).

The aforementioned social development model guided the development of Seattle Social Development Project (U.S.). This multicomponent intervention was designed to affect school bonding during elementary grades and promote children's healthy development (Catalano et al., 2004b). The six-year intervention, implemented in the United States, consisted of classroom management, proactive classroom instruction, parent intervention, and student skill development. Long-term results indicated that students who participated in the program were significantly more bonded to school, compared to the control group, at ages thirteen and eighteen (Hawkins, Guo, Hill, Battin-Pearson, & Abbott, 2001). Students in the intervention group reported less substance use, antisocial involvement, and school dropout during secondary grades (Catalano et al., 2004b) and better school/work and emotional functioning in early adulthood (Hawkins, Kosterman, Catalano, Hill, & Abbott, 2005). These and other results provide a clear support for the preventive intervention and polices that strengthen school bonding and positive youth relationship with teachers (Cohen & Geier, 2010; Wingspread Declaration on School Connections, 2004).

Social Relations: The Role of Extracurricular Activities

Research findings have provided quite consistent evidence that youth active involvement in extracurricular activities, after-school programs, and youth organizations contribute to positive development (Denault & Poulin, 2009; Feldman Farb, & Matjasko, 2012; Mahoney, Harris, & Eccles, 2006). Constructive time use has been shown to produce positive effects on youth development in three important areas. First, youth extracurricular involvement is positively related to academic achievements, school bonding, and educational aspirations (Darling, 2005; Denault & Poulin, 2009; Eccles, Barber, Stone, & Hunt, 2003; Feldman et al., 2012; Fredricks & Eccles, 2006; Rose-Krasnor, Busseri, Willoughby, & Chalmers, 2006). Second, such involvement contributes toward psychosocial well-being during adolescent years, including establishing positive relations with peers of similar interests and positive relations with community leaders and other significant adults and building competences, self-esteem, and prosocial attitudes (Denault & Poulin, 2009; Frederics & Eccles, 2006; Hansen,

Larson, & Dworkin, 2003; Rose-Krasnor et al., 2006). Third, organized activities are often linked to reduced levels of youth problem/risk behaviors, such as substance use, aggression, and delinquency (Barnes et al., 2007; Darling, 2005; Habbib, Zimmerman, & Ostaszewski, 2014; Kołoło & Mazur, 2008; Ostaszewski, 2014; Rose-Krasnor et al., 2006).

The majority of youth organized activity types except organized sport has proved to have positive impact on social and personal youth development (Feldman et al., 2012). The effects of extracurricular activities may depend upon structure, whether they are school-based or community-based, or the activity itself. As participation in two or more different activities, called "breadth of participation," may have cumulative effects on youth, some researchers examined associations between a number of organized activities and youth development. Breadth of participation reflects the number of different types of activities in which the youth are involved (Rose-Krasnor et al., 2006). The concept of breadth of participation is useful because different types of activities may offer different beneficial effects. Results of the breadth of participation examination suggest that any involvement greater than one organized activity has a positive effect on youth development (Denault & Poulin, 2009; Feldman et al., 2012; Frederics & Eccles, 2006; Rose-Krasnor et al., 2006). With various types of youth activity, youth involved in prosocial activities and participation in faith-based programs seem to have the most beneficial effects (Eccles et al., 2003; Hansen et al., 2003; Rose-Krasnor et al., 2006).

Extracurricular activities offer an outlet for adolescents to learn social roles, life skills, and competencies. They provide opportunities for youth to practice leadership, teamwork, cooperation, and decision making; give assistance to others; and acquire other important social skills. Getting involved in organized voluntary activity, youth can also gain autonomy from their family, develop new interests, and explore identity. In other words, these activities help youth navigate through adolescent-specific developmental needs and tasks (Denault & Poulin, 2009). Extracurricular involvement may help youth overcome the risk of negative social influences because they expose youth to adults and other youth engaging in positive behaviors as role models. This is true, especially, if the organized activities are meaningful for youth and provide them with opportunities to develop skills, a sense of competence and worth, and a sense of environmental mastery (Maton, 1990: Ostaszewski, 2011; Zimmerman & Maton, 1992). Recognizing the value of extracurricular activities, we believe that different types of organized activities may have significant effects for youth positive development and protect them against a variety of risk behaviors. This view has been supported by growing scientific evidences (Feldman et al., 2012; Kołoło & Mazur, 2008; Ostaszewski, 2014).

The concept of resilience and the important role of youth-positive relationships in prevention have been further shaped in Poland research on adolescent risk behaviors. In this context, a four-year research project titled the Warsaw Adolescent Study was implemented. This particular project contributes to the process of strengthening science-based prevention by providing scientific evidence on positive factors in salient adolescent problem behaviors.

A Longitudinal Analysis of Positive Relationships and Youth Risk Behaviors: The Warsaw Adolescent Study

Background

The Warsaw Adolescent Study[10] builds upon research that explores the protective factors associated with adolescent risk behaviors.[11] Until recently, in Poland, most research on the etiology of youth risk/problem behaviors was focused on risk factors associated with substance use and abuse. Until the late 2000s, there were only a few studies in Poland that examined relationship between protective factors and adolescent risk behaviors (Bobrowski, 2002, 2003; Kwiatkowski, 2009; Ostaszewski et al. 2002). These studies, however, were limited to cross-sectional analyses only. Even recently, researchers who have applied the concept of positive factors to their studies are lacking in collecting longitudinal data (Mazur et al. 2008, 2009; Pyżalski, 2012).

Our research (Ostaszewski et al. 2011; Ostaszewski, 2014) addresses these gaps in prevention research by including three waves of observation over three years of Polish middle school youth (grades 7, 8, and 9, thirteen to sixteen year olds). This longitudinal study was originated with reference to an ecological model of resilience, according to which multiple psychosocial factors (individual, family, school, and peer level) should be explored in pursuing better understanding of adolescent problem behaviors, including substance use, violence, delinquency, and school problems (Fergus & Zimmerman, 2005). The model utilizes the growing recognition that many adolescent problem behaviors have a common root (Biglan, Brennan, Foster, & Holder, 2004; Jessor, 1998). Thus, by including a broad socioecological perspective (Bronfenbrenner, 1994), this study helps to overcome another limitation of youth problem behavior research in Poland, which is typically focused on individual or family-level risk factors.

Study Objectives

The original aim of the study was to explore what are psychosocial determinants (risk and protective factors) of youth risk behaviors. The study was conducted in a sample of middle school graders (thirteen to sixteen year olds) from Warsaw, the capital and largest urban center in Poland. It was hoped that the study

10 grantome.com/grant/NIH/R01-TW007647-02.

11 This study was supported by both the Fogarty International Center grant number 5R01TW007647 from the U.S. National Institute of Health and the grant number N N106 366540 from the Polish National Science Center.

findings would supply information that would be useful for the development of prevention activities among Polish youth (Ostaszewski et al., 2011).

From the methodological point of view, the study longitudinal design enabled the test of two theoretical submodels regarding the psychosocial factors that might influence youth risk behaviors. These submodels are presented Figure 38.1.

The first submodel focuses on family relationships and specifies a series of links among family relationships/parental practices, meaningful activities, social negative influences, and engagement in problem behavior. This model is derived from theoretical approach that emphasizes the role of family risk factors in shaping the development of youth's problem behaviors, such as parental conflicts, poor family relationships, ineffective parental monitoring, and problematic peer group influences (Ary et al. 1999; Patterson, DeBaryshe, & Ramsey 1989). In completion to these concepts, it was posited that positive family relationships in grade 7 would foster effective parental monitoring in grade 8, which in turn would have a direct mitigating effect on risk behaviors in grade 9. It was also hypothesized that parental monitoring would lessen social negative influences that constitute the most powerful risk factor (Griffin et al., 2003; Hair, Park, Ling, & Moore, 2009) and would strengthen youth engagement in meaningful extracurricular activities that have been proved to be associated with lower levels of risky behaviors (Feldman et al., 2012).

The second submodel, as presented in Figure 38.1, specifies a series of links between social relationships/school bonding, meaningful activities, social negative influences, and engagement in risk behaviors. This model is derived from the social development model (Hawkins & Weis, 1985) and a growing number

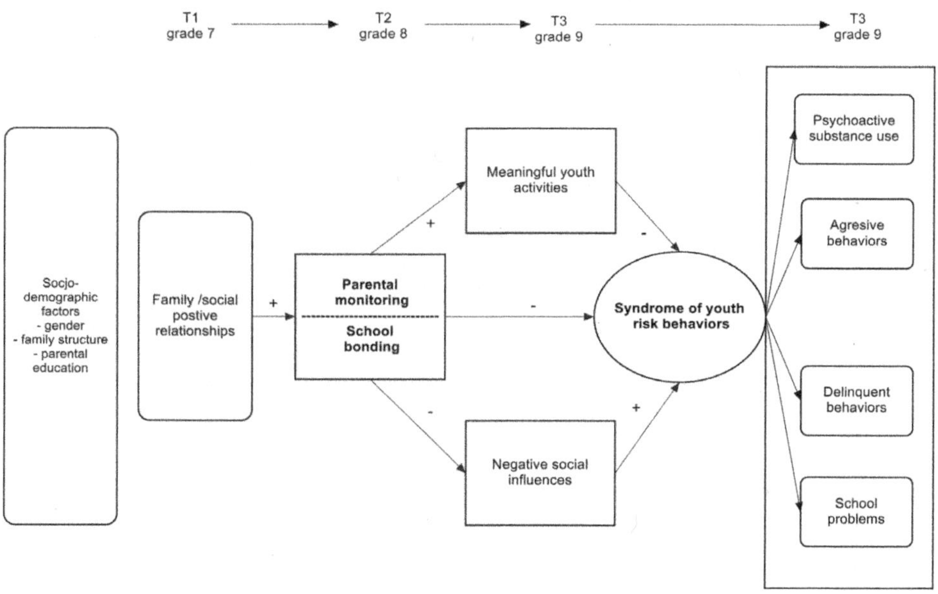

Figure 38.1. *Model of association between parental practices/school bonding, meaningful activities, negative social influences, and adolescent risk behaviors.*

of research studies (Aspy et al., 2012; Dever et al., 2012; McNeely & Falci, 2004; Resnick et al., 1997; Simons-Morton et al., 1999; Shears et al., 2006; Voisin et al., 2005) that emphasizes the role of social bonds to conventional society in positive versus negative socialization. In this context, it was posited that positive social relations in grade 7 would foster positive school bonding in grade 8, which in turn would have a direct mitigating effect on risk behaviors in grade 9. Similarly to the family relationship (first) submodel, it was also hypothesized that positive school bonding would lessen negative social influences and would strengthen youth engagement in meaningful extracurricular activities.

Both submodels, described in the preceding, utilize the concepts of meaningful instrumental behavior (MIB) (Maton, 1990; Zimmerman & Maton, 1992) and of involvement in multiple extracurricular activities, described in the literature as breadth of participation (Barnes et al., 2007; Feldman et al., 2012; Rose-Krasnor et al., 2006). These two concepts refer to involvement in activities that provide youth with opportunities to develop skills, a sense of competence and worth, and a sense of environmental mastery. Usually, these extracurricular activities include participation in community service organizations, organized sports teams, youth programs, and church activities.

Method

Sample. The study sample includes 1,841 adolescents (56 percent females, 83 percent living with both parents) who participated in Wave 1 (seventh grade), Wave 2 (eighth grade), and Wave 3 (ninth grade) of a three-wave longitudinal study conducted in public and nonpublic middle schools in Warsaw (61 percent response rate from Wave 1 to Wave 3). The Wave 1 data were collected from a sample of seventh graders (thirteen and fourteen years old) who began middle school in the school year 2006–2007. A class was the unit of randomization and the final sample of 158 classes was selected from the sample frame of 600 seventh-grade classes from all public and nonpublic Warsaw middle schools (Ostaszewski, 2014).

Procedure. Students answered the self-administered questionnaire during school lessons. They were asked by trained data collectors to participate in the study and were informed about the voluntary and anonymous nature of their involvement. Informed consent was attained from school principals, parents, and teachers and an assent from the youth. Participating students were asked to create a special ID code, which was used to track the same person over a three-year period of study, but they never used their names. To ensure participants anonymity, after completing the questionnaire, students were asked to return it in a sealed envelope.[12]

12 The Bioethical Committee of the Institute of Psychiatry and Neurology in Warsaw, Poland, as well as the Human Subject Protection in the Fogarty International Center of the National Institute of Health, approved this study.

Measures. All measures were based on previously validated items or scales, and most of them were adapted from the Longitudinal Study of School Dropout and Substance Use,[13] also known as Flint Adolescent Study.[14] The risk behaviors variables included measures of substance use – alcohol, nicotine, and illegal drugs (Johnston, O'Malley, & Bachman, 2003) – as well as aggressive behaviors (Stoddard, Zimmerman, & Bauermeister, 2012; Zimmerman, 2014), delinquent behaviors (Salem et al., 1998; Zimmerman, 2014), and school problems (Bryant & Zimmerman, 2002; Zimmerman, 2014).

The measures used as psychosocial factors represent multiple levels of influence (family, school, peers, and neighborhood) described in social ecological theory (Bronfenbrenner, 1994). Parental and friends support scales were based on prior work by Procidano and Heller (1983). Parental monitoring, school bonding, importance of school to students, alcohol abuse by nonfamilial adults, negative peer influences, and natural mentor support were adopted from Flint Adolescent Questionnaire (1997). The family rituals scale was taken from the EMCDDA bank of instruments, and meaningful activities were based on our previous work (Bobrowski, Pisarska, & Ostaszewski, 2007). Table 38.1 presents the study variables, along with the number of items in each scale, the scales means, the standard deviations, Cronbach's Alphas if appropriate, and a sample item from each scale.

Demographic variables included gender, father and mother education, family structure, and type of middle school. Gender and type of school became dummy-coded to 1 = males, 2 = females; and 1 = public school, 2 = nonpublic school. Family structure responses were "with parents," "only with father," "only with mother," "with one of parents and with stepmother/stepfather," and "with another person," to a dichotomous variable: 1 = those who lived with both parents, and 2 = those who did not. Possible answers for maternal and paternal education ranged from 1 = "completed elementary school" to 4 = "completed college or university." The highest reported education level between mother and the father was used in the analyses.

Model testing. Structural equation modeling (SEM) with asymptotic distribution-free (ADF) estimation was conducted to test the two complementing submodels and compare their parameters (using SPSS software AMOS 5). An ADF estimator was used because all risk behavior variables demonstrated notable departure from normality. In assessing model fit, chi square statistics were used, but because of the large sample size and correlations between variables, a significant chi-square statistic was expected. Hence, model fit was assessed also on the basis of multiple fit indices: the standardized root-mean-square residual (SRMR), the comparative fit index (CFI), and the root-mean-square error of approximation (RMSEA). As recommended by Hu and Bentler (1998), SRMR supplemented by CFI or RMSEA is the best solution for the ADF estimation method. Although cutoff values for ADF-based indices are not clear,

13 grantome.com/grant/NIH/R01-DA007484-01A2
14 prc.sph.umich.edu/projects/flint-adolescent-study/

Table 38.1 *Measures Used in the Structural Equation Models and Their Descriptive Statistics*

Factors (no of items)	$\bar{X}$	SD	α	Sample item (type of scale used)
				Parental/familial
Mother support (5)	4.23	0.84	0.90	I rely on my mother for emotional support (5-pt Likert, 1 = not true, 5 = very true)
Father support (5)	3,80	1,16	0,95	I rely on my father for emotional support (5-pt Likert, 1 = not true, 5 = very true)
Parental monitoring (9)	4,07	0,75	0,89	When I go out in the evening my parents know where I am (5-pt Likert, 1 = never, 5 = always)
Family rituals (7)	2,76	0,55	0,73	During an average week, how often do you get involved in each of these activities with your mother or father? Eat dinner together (4-pt Likert, 1 = never, 4 = almost every day)
				Peer
Peer negative influences (12)	1.63	0.56	0.59	How many of your peers: cut class – just don't go? How many of your friends drink beer or wine at least once a month? (5-pt Likert 1 = none, 5 = all)
Friends support (4)	3,77	0,93	0,87	I rely on my friends for emotional support (help, comfort, advise) (5-pt Likert 1 = not true, 5 = very true)
				School
School bonding (4)	2.80	0.67	0.83	I like school (4-pt Likert 1 = completely not true, 4 = completely true)
Importance of school to student (4)	4,36	0,68	0,86	Grades are very important to me (5pt-Likert 1 = not true, 5 = completely true)
				Neighborhood
Alcohol abuse by nonfamilial adults (3)	1.52	0.63	0.80	Not including your parents or the important adults you live with how many adults do you know who get drunk at least once a week? (6-pt Likert 0 = don't know, 1 = none, 5 = all)
Natural mentor support (5)	2,63	1,78	0,98	To what degree this person encourages you and cheers you up when you need it? (5-pt Likert, 1 = not at all, 5 = to very large extent)
				Individual /behavioral
Meaningful extracurricular activities index (5)	1.66	1.13	NA	How many hours per week (in your free time) you usually spend on? A list of five activities were included: reading for pleasure, private lessons to learn foreign language, church or scout groups, volunteering and other organized activities like dance or playing instrument (5-pt Likert, 1 = 0 hours, 5 = 8 hours or more)
				Risk behaviors
Substance use (4)	2,17	3,17	0,82	How often have you smoked cigarettes during the last 30 days? (5-pt Likert, 0 = not at all, 4 = about one pack per day or more)

Table 38.1 (*cont.*)

Factors (no of items)	$\bar{X}$	SD	α	Sample item (type of scale used)
Aggressive behaviors (4)	1,09	2,24	0,78	During the last 12 months, how often have you gotten in a fight in school? (5-pt Likert, 0 = never, 4 = four times or more)
Delinquent behaviors (4)	0,69	1,78	0,71	During the last 12 months, how often have you gotten into trouble with police because of something you did? (5-pt Likert, 0 = never, 4 = four times or more)
School problems (4)	3,08	2,48	0,72	How many whole days of school have you skipped because of truancy? (5-pt Likert, 0 = 0 days, 4 = eleven days or more)

conservative criteria of cutoff values with SRMR value < 0.08, CFI < 0.90, and RMSEA < 0.06 were used (Schreiber, Stage, King, Nora, & Barlow, 2006).

Additionally, a confirmatory factor analysis (CFA) was conducted to determine whether the risk behaviors loaded onto a single factor, called a "latent" or "hidden" variable, which is not directly observed and not directly measured. It is inferred through a mathematical model from other variables that are directly measured (observed). For the fit of the syndrome of youth risk behaviors, the latent variable was quite good, chi-squared (2) = 19.93; $p < 0.001$, SRMR = 0.046, CFI = 0.92, and RMSEA = 0.07. The fit of the measurement model can be enhanced by allowing just one correlation among residuals variances to be estimated from the data chi-squared (1) = 1.03; $p < 0.31$, SRMR = 0.006, CFI = 1.00, RMSEA = 0.004. The enhanced model is shown in Figure 38.2. Each factor loaded significantly and greater than 0.50 showing that the latent variable is reliably assessed.

Missing data. Multiple imputation (MI) was used to handle missing data. A missing values analysis indicated that data were missing at random. Amount of missing data ranged from 0.3 percent to 5.5 percent for each variable. Using MI, missing data for a participant is imputed using information from a participant's other known characteristics. Statisticians suggest that MI may result in less biased estimates of associations than using techniques such as complete case analyses and mean imputation (Graham, 2009; Schafer & Graham, 2002). As suggested by Graham (2009), all variables, including both predictors and dependent variables used in the final analysis, were incorporated in the MI model. It was assumed that MI options enhance the quality of the data.

Findings

Family relationships model. The hypothesized model is presented in Figure 38.3 and the standardized estimates for the parameters are displayed. The overall model indicated an adequate fit. We used the SRMR value as the primary fit index, which indicated good model fit (SRMR = 0.051). Two other fit indices

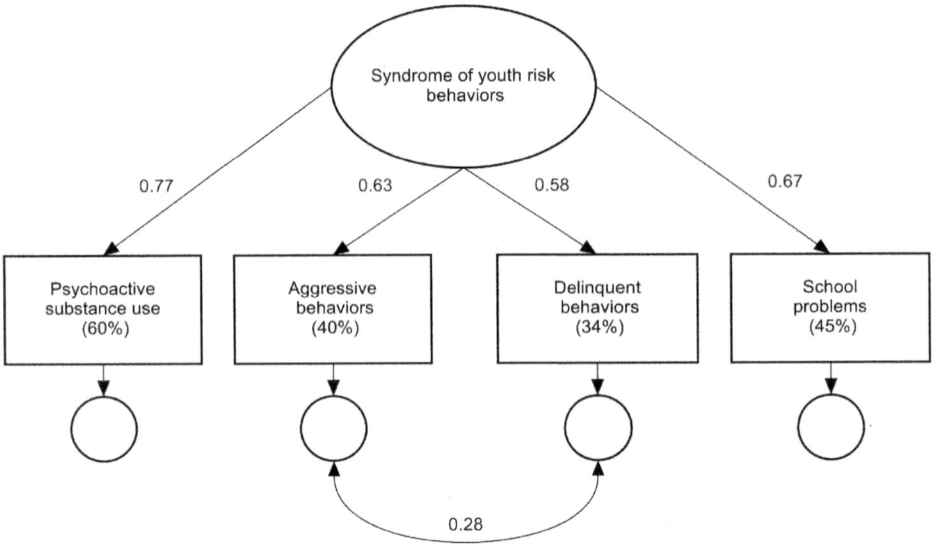

Figure 38.2 *Structure and standardized factor loadings for the measurement model of the syndrome of youth risk behaviors.*
Note. A large oval is a latent variable; rectangles are measured indicators; small ovals are residual variances; a curved arrow is a correlation; straight arrows are standardized regression weights

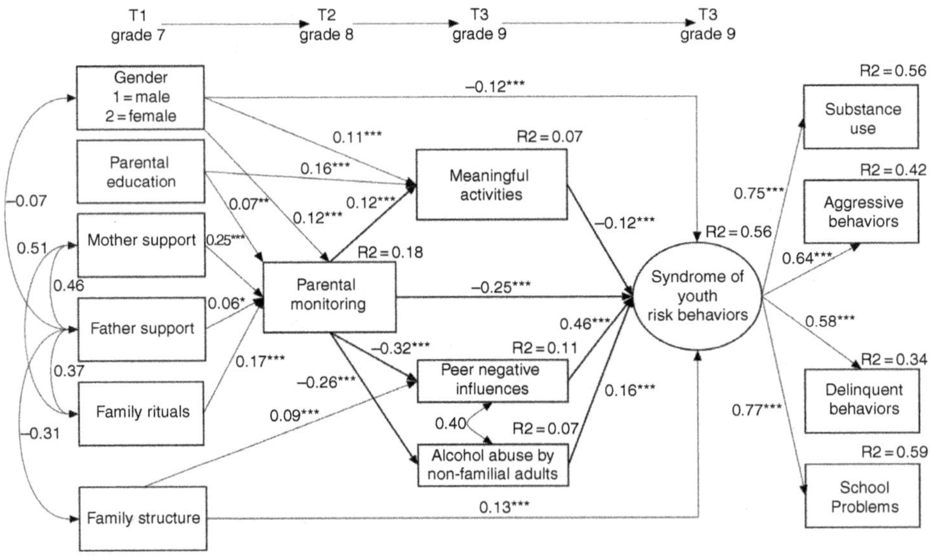

Figure 38.3. *Structural model of association among positive family relationships/parental practices, meaningful activities, negative social influences, and adolescent risk behaviors, chi^2 (63) = 309.16, $p < 0.001$; $chi^2/d.f. = 4.91$, SRMR = 0.051, CFI = 0.814, RMSEA = 0.046.*
*Note. A large oval is a latent variable; rectangles are measured indicators; curved arrows are correlations; straight arrows are standardized regression weights; r-squared are percentage of explained variances, * < 0.05, ** $p < 0.01$, *** $p < 0.001$.*

values were not consistent: CFI (0.814) was below the expected level of 0.90, and the RMSEA value (0.046) was adequate. This model accounted for 56 percent of the variance in adolescent risk behaviors, which can be consider satisfactory in longitudinal analyses.

Parental monitoring had significant direct effect, $\beta = -0.25$, $p < 0.001$ on later adolescent risk behaviors. In addition, the indirect effect of monitoring on risk behaviors mediated through meaningful activities and negative social influences was significant $\beta = -0.21$, $p < 0.001$. As expected, parental monitoring predicted higher levels of meaningful activities and lower levels of negative social influences. Thus, the total effect on risk behaviors for monitoring was $\beta = -0.46$, $p < 0.001$.

As hypothesized, family relationships had significant effects for effective parental monitoring. Although mother and father support were correlated ($r = 0.46$), the direct effect of mother support ($\beta = 0.25$, $p < 0.001$) on later parental monitoring was much higher than the direct effect of father support ($\beta = 0.06$, $p < 0.05$). In addition, indirect effects of mother support on risk behaviors mediated through monitoring was significant ($\beta = -0.11$, $p < 0.001$), whereas the indirect effect of father support on risk behaviors reached only the 0.05 level of significance ($\beta = -0.03$, $p < 0.05$). The direct effects of family rituals on monitoring was also significant, $\beta = 0.17$, $p < 0.001$.

Social relationships model. The hypothesized model is presented in Figure 38.4, and the standardized estimates for the parameters are displayed. The overall model indicated quite adequate fit. We used the SRMR value as the primary fit index, which indicated good model fit (SRMR = 0.065). Two other fit indices values were not consistent: CFI (0.794) was below the expected level of 0.90, and the RMSEA value (0.052) was adequate. This model accounted for 49 percent of the variance in adolescent risk behaviors, which can be considered satisfactory in longitudinal analyses.

School bonding had significant direct effect, $\beta = -0.21$, $p < 0.001$ on later adolescent risk behaviors. In addition, the indirect effect of school bonding on risk behaviors mediated through meaningful activities and negative social influences was significant: $\beta = -0.19$, $p < 0.001$. As expected, school positive bonding predicted higher levels of meaningful activities and lower levels of negative social influences. Thus, the total effect on risk behaviors for school bonding was $\beta = -0.40$, $p < 0.001$.

As hypothesized, social relationships had significant effects for positive school bonding. Both natural mentor and friends support predicted positive school bonding. The direct effects of these relationships on later school bonding were similar: $\beta = 0.09$, $p < 0.001$ (for friends support) and $\beta = 0.12$, $p < 0.001$ (for mentor support). However, importance of school to student indicated the highest direct effect on later school bonding ($\beta = 0.29$, $p < 0.001$). This individual-level factor had also significant direct ($\beta = -0.10$, $p < 0.001$) and indirect effects mediated through school bonding ($\beta = -0.12$, $p < 0.001$) on later risk behaviors. Thus, the total effect on risk behaviors for importance of school was $\beta = -0.22$, $p < 0.001$.

Both models. In both models, being female (versus being male) and living with both parents (versus not living with both parents) were found to significantly

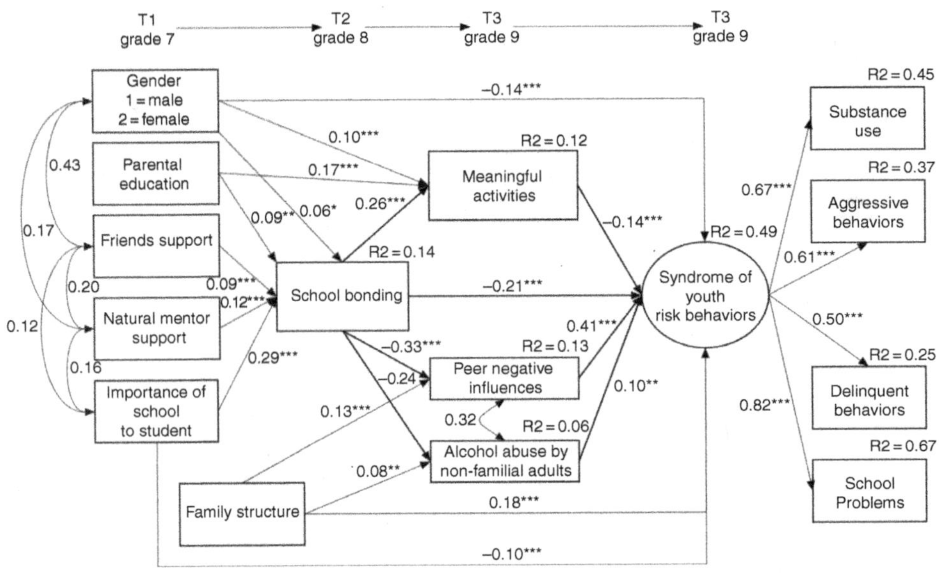

Figure 38.4. *Structural model of association between positive social relationships/school bonding, meaningful activities, negative social influences, and adolescent risk behaviors,* $chi^2(62) = 364.77$, $p < 0.001$; $chi^2/d.f. = 5.88$, $SRMR = 0.065$, $CFI = 0.794$, $RMSEA = 0.052$.

*Note. A large oval is a latent variable; rectangles are measured indicators; curved arrows are correlations; straight arrows are standardized regression weights; r-squared are percentage of explained variances, * < 0.05, ** p < 0.01, *** p < 0.001.*

predict a lower level of adolescent involvement in risky behaviors (see Figures 38.3 and 38.4). Moreover, in both models higher parental education predicted higher involvement in meaningful activities ($\beta = 0.16$ and 0.17, $p < 0.001$). As expected, in both models students' involvement in meaningful activities were associated with lower level of risk behaviors ($\beta = -0.12$ and -0.14, $p < 0.001$), and negative social influences were associated with higher level of risk behaviors, especially peer negative influences ($\beta = 0.46$ and 0.41, $p < 0.001$).

Both models fit to a great extent to empirical data (have similar fitting parameters). This suggests that in relation to the Warsaw population of middle school youth, both models have a similar accuracy in explaining the association between psychosocial risk and protective factors and youth risk behavior. However, it is worth mentioning that the family relationships model was slightly better than the other model in explaining youth risk behaviors. After including sociodemographic factors, the family relationships model explained 56 percent of youth risk behaviors syndrome variance, while the social relationships model explained 49 percent of variance.

Discussion

The model of family relationships provides clear support for the influence of familial/parental practices on the development of adolescent risk behaviors.

The results have extended the evidence, which indicates that parental monitoring plays a crucial role in preventing the entire range of adolescent unhealthy and risky behaviors (Dever et al., 2012; DiClemente et al., 2001; Elkington et al., 2011; Griffin et al., 2003; Lee, 2012; Pico & Kovacs, 2010; Rai et al., 2003; Salem et al.,1998; Willoughby & Hamza, 2011). Generally speaking, the more effective parents are in monitoring practices, the lower their adolescent children's level of involvement in risk behaviors would be. However, the study findings indicate that positive influence of parental monitoring is associated with two specific developmental processes that lead to a lower level of risky behaviors. First, parental practices would decrease exposure to negative social influences, especially peer negative influences, which constitute the most powerful risk factors of later problem and risk behaviors (Ary et al., 1999; Griffin et al., 2003; Hair et al., 2009). Second, parental supervision strengthens children engagement in meaningful activities that helps adolescents to use free time in constructive ways and develop psychosocial skills. Thus, these two processes could protect Polish youth from risky choices.

These research findings further explain how familial processes contribute to the development of effective monitoring. Namely, two aspects of family life seem to be important: mother and father emotional support and family common rituals (Fiese et al., 2002; Tabak, 2008). Monitoring is based on good communication and positive relationships with the parents' adolescent child, leading to their child's willingness to share with the parent information about one's activities and experiences outside of the home. These observations are consistent with findings of other researchers that underlined the role of positive parenting and adolescent disclosure in effective monitoring (e.g., Lee, 2012; Stattin & Kerr, 2000; Willoughby & Hamza, 2011).

The findings suggest that mothers play a leading role in positive parental practices among Warsaw adolescents. Traditional socializing roles that mothers play in Polish society seem to be resistant to change, despite rapid social changes that Polish society has been facing since late 1980. Despite official governmental policy promoting equality between men and women in parenting, women look after their children and their home while working at the same time. Moreover, mothers in Poland (like many other places in world) are more active than fathers in helping children' management of school life; for example, they more often attend parent–teacher meetings, help with homework, and coordinate children's extracurricular activities (Okulicz-Kozaryn & Raduj, 2012). Teenagers more often communicate with mothers about their school achievements, friends and peer relationships, interests, and everyday life events (Tabak & Mazur, 2008). Positive relationships result with better maternal knowledge of children's whereabouts, which in turn facilitates mothers' ability to monitor their children. The father's lower involvement in positive parenting is culturally conditioned in Polish society but also is associated with poor emotional support of fathers who are not living in the same home.

The model of social relationships provides further support for the importance of school bonding in adolescent good adjustment. The results of the Warsaw study (Ostaszewski, 2014) have extended the evidence, which indicates that positive social relationships and school bonding contribute toward youth healthy development and the prevention of adolescent risk behaviors (Aspy et al., 2012; Dever et al., 2012; Hurd, Zimmerman, & Xue, 2009; Resnick et al., 1997). The more positive student relationships with teachers and school are, the lower student risk behavior involvement is. Similarly to the family model, the positive influence of social relationships is associated with two protective processes: lesser exposure to negative social influences and higher engagement in meaningful activities.

The findings also indicate that social and individual-level factors contribute to the development of positive school bonding, and positive school connectedness is associated with student attitudes toward school and learning. Positive school attitudes are associated with school learning by Warsaw adolescents. Taking this into account, successful primary education that motivates children to learn and develop curiosity for the world is crucial for developing attitudes that are positive toward school. As indicated by Hawkins at al. (2001), positive school bonding in primary school predicts more positive student attitudes toward school in later stages of education.

The longitudinal analyses also contribute in clarifying the role of friends' support in youth development. Contrary to family support, in previous research, friends' emotional support was found to be associated with higher levels of adolescent alcohol and cigarette use (Okulicz-Kozaryn, 2010; Wills, Resko, Ainette, & Mendoza, 2004). The Warsaw study findings suggest that friends' emotional support helped to create a protective environment for adolescents by facilitating positive school bonding. Friends' support along with natural mentor support constitutes proper social conditions for positive school adjustment. The results are consistent with previous resilience research that underlines the positive effects of social support, including natural mentoring and friends' support, in youth lives (Werner, 2000; Zimmerman, Bingenheimer, & Notoro, 2002).

Closing Remarks

The development of science-based prevention requires conducting longitudinal studies, which are the more reliable source of knowledge on antecedents of positive youth development. This is of enormous significance for the building of effective prevention programs. The research on Warsaw middle school students was one of the first longitudinal studies in Poland devoted to prevention. Most of existing research on Polish youth behavior was concentrated on risk factors. The current study, however, was conducted among Warsaw middle school students and focused on identification of protective factors. Yet, the concept of positive youth development does pose further demands on youth researchers. Namely, future studies of positive development require the expansion of variables that would be taken into account, such as psychosocial skills, positive relations with others, successes in various aspects of life, a sense of one's own value, and respect of social norms. In addition, in future studies we are planning to mutually explore determinants of youth problem behavior together with those related to positive youth development.

Acknowledgments

The authors would like to thank Professor Marc Zimmerman from the University of Michigan for his great mentoring work on the Warsaw Adolescent Study, and members of the research team who participated in that study at various stages: Krzysztof Bobrowski, Anna Borucka, Katarzyna Kocoń-Rychter, Katarzyna Okulicz-Kozaryn, Anna Rustecka-Krawczyk, and Magdalena Wójcik.

References

Anderson, C. (1982). The search for school climate: a review of the research. *Review of Educational Research* 52: 368–420.

Anderson, P., & Baumberg, B. (2006). *Alcohol in Europe*. London: Institute of Alcohol Studies.

Ary, D., Duncan T., Biglan, A., Meltzer, C., Noell, J., & Smolkowski, K. (1999). Development of adolescent problem behavior. *Journal of Abnormal Child Psychology* 27: 141–50.

Ashery, R., Robertson, E., & Kumpfer, K. (eds.) (1998). *Drug Abuse Prevention through Family Interventions*. NIDA Research Monograph 177. Washington, DC: U.S. Department of Health and Human Services.

Aspy, C., Vesely, S., Oman, R., Tolma, E., Rodine, S., Marshall, L., & Fluhr, J. (2012). School-related assets and youth risk behaviors: alcohol consumption and sexual activity. *Journal of School Health* 82: 3–10.

Baker, J. (2006). Contributions of teacher–child relationships to positive school adjustment during elementary school. *Journal of School Psychology* 44: 211–29.

Barnes, G., Hoffman, J., Welte, J., Farrell, M., & Dintcheff, B. (2007). Adolescents' time use: effects on substance use, delinquency and sexual activity, *Journal of Youth and Adolescence* 36: 697–710.

Bernat, D., & Resnick, M. (2006). Healthy youth development: science and strategies. *Journal of Public Health Management Practice* (November; Suppl.): S10–S16.

Biglan, A., Brennan, P., Foster, S., & Holder, H. (2004). *Helping Adolescents at Risk: Prevention of Multiple Problem Behaviors*. New York: Guilford Press.

Bobrowski, K. (2002). Poczucie koherencji oraz inne zasoby odpornosciowe a uzywanie substancji psychoaktywnych przez mlodziez [Sense of coherence, other resistance resources and adolescent substance use]. *Alkoholizm i Narkomania* 15: 221–39.

Bobrowski, K. (2003). Sposoby spedzania wolnego czasu przez mlodziez a uzywanie substancji psychoaktywnych [Adolescents' free time activities and substance use]. *Medycyna Wieku Rozwojowego* 1: 91–104.

Bobrowski, K., Pisarska, A., & Ostaszewski, K. (2007). *Rekomendacje narzedzi do oceny zagrożeń zdrowia psychicznego mlodziezy do dalszego stosowania w badaniach mokotowskich oraz w innych badaniach ankietowych mlodziezy szkolnej [Recommendations on self-report instruments for assessing mental health and behavioral problems in school surveys]*, Warsaw: Instytut Psychiatrii i Neurologii.

Bobrowski, K., Pisarska, A,, Ostaszewski, K., & Borucka, A. (2014). Skuteczność programu profilaktyki alkoholowej dla dzieci na progu dojrzewania [Effectiveness of alcohol prevention program for pre-adolescents], *Psychiatria Polska* 48: 527–39.

Borkowska, A. (2011). Program profilaktyki uzależnień "Unplugged" [Drug use prevention program "Unplugged"]. *Remedium* 10: 8–9.

Borucka, A., & Ostaszewski, K. (2008). Koncepcja resilience. Kluczowe pojęcia i wybrane zagadnienia [Concept of resilience: key terms and chosen aspects]. *Medycyna Wieku Rozwojowego* 12: 587–97.

Borucka, A., Pisarska, A., & Okulicz-Kozarn K. (2003). Ocena przydatności i funkcjonowania metody interwencji profilaktycznej w szkole [Process and outcome evaluation of the preventive intervention method at school]. *Medycyna Wieku Rozwojowego* 7: 157–72.

Brand, S., Felner, R., Shim, M., Seitsinger, A., & Dumas, T. (2003). Middle school improvement and reform: development and validation of a school-level assessment of climate, cultural pluralism, and school safety. *Journal of Educational Psychology* 95: 570–88.

Bronfenbrenner, U. (1994). Ecological models of human development. In *International Encyclopedia of Education 2(3)*, 2nd ed. Oxford: Elsevier, pp. 1643–7.

Bryant, A., & Zimmerman, M. (2002). Examining the effects of academic beliefs and behaviors on changes in substance use among urban adolescents. *Journal of Educational Psychology* 94: 621–37.

Bukowska, B. (2014). Refleksje i rekomendacje dotyczace podstawy programowej szkolenia w zakresie profilaktyki uzależnień [Recommendations for the core curriculum training course in drug use prevention], *Serwis Informacyjny Narkomania* 67: 6–8.

Catalano, R., Berglund, L., Ryan, J., Lonczak, H., & Hawkins, D. (2004a). Positive youth development in the United States: research findings on evaluation of positive youth development programs. *Annals of the American Academy of Political and Social Science* 591: 98–124.

Catalano, R., Haggerty, K., Oesterle, A., Fleming, C., & Hawkins, D. (2004b). The importance of bonding to school for healthy development: findings from the social development research group. *Journal of School Health* 74: 252–61.

Centrum Badania Opinii Społecznej, (2003). *Młodzież 2003 (Youth 2003)*. Raport z realizacji badania ankietowego dla Krajowego Biura Przeciwdziałania Narkomanii. Warsaw: Centrum Badania Opinii Sołecznej. www.cinn.gov.pl/portal?id=166545

Chojecki, D. (2011). Ewaluacja europejskiego programu wczesnej interwencji wobec młodych użytkowników substancji psychoaktywnych ["Fred Goes Net": evaluation of the European program of early preventive intervention toward young psychoactive substance users]. *Serwis Informacyjny Narkomania* 53: 4–7.

Cohen, J., & Geier, V. (2010). *School Climate Research Summary – January 2010*. New York: Center for Social and Emotional Education. www.schoolclimate.org/climate/documents/SCBrief_v1n1_Jan2010.pdf

Darling, N. (2005). Participation in extracurricular activities and adolescent adjustment: crosssectional and longitudinal findings. *Journal of Youth and Adolescence* 34: 493–505.

Denault, A., & Poulin, F. (2009). Intensity and breadth of participation in organized activities during the adolescent years: multiple associations with youth outcomes. *Journal of Youth and Adolescence* 38: 1199–1213.

Dever, B., Schulenberg, J., Dworkin,J., O'Malley, P., Kloska, D., & Bachman, J. (2012). Predicting risk-taking with and without substance use: the effects of parental monitoring, school bonding and sport participation. *Prevention Science* 13: 605–15.

DiClemente, R., Wingood, G., Crosby, R., Sionean, C., Cobb, B., Harrington, K., Davies, S., Hook, E., & Kim, M. (2001). Parental monitoring: association with adolescents' risk behaviors, *Pediatrics* 107: 1363–8.

Dishion, T., & McMahon, R. (1998). Parental monitoring and the prevention of child and adolescent problem behaviors: a conceptual and empirical formulation. *Clinical Child and Family Psychology Review* 1: 61–75.

Eccles, J., Barber B., Stone M., & Hunt J. (2003). Extracurricular activities and adolescent development. *Journal of Social Issues* 59: 865–89.

Elkington, K., Bauermeister, J., & Zimmerman, M. (2011). Do parents and peers matter? A prospective socio-ecological examination of substance use and sexual risk among African American youth. *Journal of Adolescence* 34: 1035–47.

Feldman Farb, A., & Matjasko, J. (2012). Recent advances in research on school-based extracurricular activities and adolescent development. *Developmental Review* 32: 1–48.

Fergus, S., & Zimmerman, M. (2005). Adolescent resilience: a framework for understanding healthy development in the face of risk. *Annual Review of Public Health* 26: 399–419.

Fiese, B., Tomcho, T., Douglas, M., Josephs, K., Poltrock, S., & Baker, T. (2002). A review of 50 years of research on naturally occurring family routines and rituals: cause for celebration? *Journal of Family Psychology* 16: 381–90.

Fredricks, J., & Eccles, J. (2006). Extracurricular involvement and adolescent adjustment: impact of duration, number of activities, and breadth of participation. *Applied Developmental Science* 10: 132–46.

Graham, J. (2009). Missing data analysis: making it work in the real word. *Annual Review of Psychology* 60: 549–76.

Griffin, K., Botvin, G., Scheier, L., Doyle, M., & Williams, C. (2003). Common predictors of cigarette smoking, alcohol use, aggression, and delinquency among inner-city minority youth. *Addictive Behaviors* 28: 1141–8.

Grzelak, S. (2006). *Profilaktyka ryzykownych zachowań seksualnych młodzieży. Aktualny stan badań na świecie i w Polsce [Prevention of youth risky sexual behaviors: current research in Poland and in the world]*. Warsaw: Wydawnictwo Naukowe Scholar.

Habbib, E., Zimmerman, M. A., & Ostaszewski, K. (2014). International note: prevailing with extracurricular activities in an alcohol-dominated environment: sex differences in resilience among middle school. *Journal of Adolescence* 29: 81–100.

Hair, E., Park, M., Ling, T., & Moore, K. (2009). Risky behaviors in late adolescence: co-occurrence, predictors, and consequences. *Journal of Adolescent Health* 45: 253–61.

Hansen, D., Larson, R., & Dworkin, J. (2003). What adolescents learn in organized youth activities: a survey of self-reported developmental experiences. *Journal of Research on Adolescence* 13: 25–55.

Hawkins, D., Guo, J., Hill, K., Battin-Pearson, S., & Abbott, R. (2001). Long-term effects of the Seattle Social Development Intervention on school bonding trajectories. *Applied Developmental Science* 5: 225–36.

Hawkins, D., Kosterman, R., Catalano, R., Hill, K., & Abbott, R. (2005). Promoting positive adult functioning through social development intervention in childhood. *Archives of Pediatrics and Adolescent Medicine* 159: 25–31.

Hawkins, D., & Weis, J. (1985). The social development model: an integrated approach to delinquency prevention. *Journal of Primary Prevention* 6: 73–97.

Hu, L., & Bentler, P. (1998). Fit indices in covariance structure modeling: sensitivity to underparameterized model misspecification. *Psychological Methods* 3: 424–53.

Hurd, N., Zimmerman, M., & Xue, Y. (2009). Negative adult influence and the protective effects of role models: a study of urban adolescents. *Journal of Youth and Adolescence* 38: 777–89.

Jessor, R. (1998). New perspectives on adolescent risk behavior. In Jessor, R. (ed.), *New Perspectives on Adolescent Risk Behavior*. New York: Cambridge University Press, pp. 1–10.

Johnston, L. D., O'Malley, P. M., & Bachman, J. G. (2003). *Monitoring the Future National Survey Results on Drug Use, 1975–2002,* vol. I, *Secondary School Students* (NIH Publication No. 03–5375). Bethesda, MD: National Institute on Drug Abuse.

Junik, W. (2007). Ewaluacja działalności świetlic socjoterapeutycznych – cz. IV [Outcome evaluation of the sociotherapy child care facilities, part IV]. *Remedium* 10: 30–1.

Khoury-Kassabri, M., Benbenishty, R., Avi Astor R., & Zeira, A. (2004). The contributions of community, family, and school variables to student victimization. *American Journal of Community Psychology* 34: 187–204.

Kirwil, L. (2004). Changes in the structure of crime during the transition period in Poland. *International Journal of Sociology* 34: 48–82.

Kołodziejczyk, A., Czemierowska, E., & Kołodziejczyk, T. (2007), Spójrz inaczej. *Program zajęć wychowawczo-profilaktycznych dla klas 1–3 szkół podstawowych [Have a second look, a program for primary school 1–3 grades].* Starachowice: Wydawnictwo ATE s.c.

Kołoło, H., & Mazur, J. (2008). Zaangażowanie w konstruktywną działalność oraz wybrane zasoby osobiste jako czynniki chroniące w grupie posiadanych kompetencji [Extracurriculum activities and chosen personal assets as protective factors]. In Mazur, J., Tabak, I., Małkowska-Szkutnik, A., Ostaszewski, K., Kołoło, H., Dzielska, A., & Kowalewska, A. (eds.), *Czynniki chroniące młodzież 15-letnią przed podejmowaniem zachowań ryzykownych.* Warsaw: Instytut Matki i Dziecka, pp. 130–44.

Kulesza, M. (2007). Klimat szkoły a zachowania przemocowe uczniów w świetle wybranych badań empirycznych [School climate and students' aggressive behaviors – chosen empirical data]. *Seminare* 24: 261–77.

Kumpfer, K. (1998). Selective prevention interventions. the Strengthening Families Program. In Ashery, R., Robertson E., & Kumpfer, K. (eds.), *Drug Abuse*

Prevention through Family Interventions. NIDA Research Monograph 177. Washington, DC: U.S. Department of Health and Human Services.

Kumpfer, K., & Alvarado, R. (2003). Family-strengthening approaches for the prevention of youth problem behavior, *American Psychologist* 58: 457–65.

Kwiatkowski, P. (2009). Poczucie koherencji a eksperymentowanie młodzieży z narkotykami (perspektywa ryzyka i ochrony) [Sense of coherence and youth experiments with drugs]. In Borecka-Biernat, D. (ed.), *Poszukiwanie uwarunkowań zaburzeń w zachowaniu młodzieży w interakcjach społecznych*. Wałbrzych: Wałbrzyska Wyższa Szkoła Zarządzania i Przedsiębiorczości, pp. 133–48.

Lee, R. (2012). Community violence exposure and adolescent substance use: does monitoring and positive parenting moderate risk in urban communities? *Journal of Community Psychology* 40: 406–21.

Lerner, R., Von Eye, A., Lerner, J., Lewin-Bizan, S., & Bowers, E. (2010). Special Issue Introduction: the meaning and measurement of thriving: a view of the issues, *Journal of Youth and Adolescence* 39: 707–19.

Loukas, A., Suzuki, R., & Horton, K. (2006). Examining school connectedness as a mediator of school climate effects. *Journal of Research on Adolescence* 16: 491–502.

Luthar, S. (2006). Resilience in development: a synthesis of research across five decades. In Cicchetti, D., & Cohen, D. (eds.), *Developmenthal Psychopatology: Risk, Disorder, and Adaptation*, 2nd ed., vol. 3. New York: Wiley, pp. 740–95.

Mahoney, J., Harris, A., & Eccles, J. (2006). Organized activity participation, positive youth development, and the over-scheduling hypothesis. *Social Policy Report* 20: 3–32.

Malczewski, A. (2015). Działania dużych miast w przeciwdziałaniu narkomanii w 2013 roku – cześć II [Drug prevention activities conducted in big cities in 2003, part II]. *Serwis Informacyjny Narkomania* 69: 44–8.

Masten, A. (2004). Regulatory processes, risk, and resilience in adolescent development. *Annals of the New York Academy of Sciences* 1021: 310–19.

Masten, A. S., & Powell, J. L. (2003). A Resilience Framework for Research Policy and Practice. In Luthar, S. (ed.), *Resilience and Vulnerability*. New York: Cambridge University Press, pp. 1–28.

Maton, K. (1990). Meaningful involvement in instrumental activity and well-being: studies of older adolescents and at risk urban teen-agers. *American Journal of Community Psychology* 18: 297–320.

Mazur, J. (ed.) (2015). *Zdrowie i zachowania zdrowotne młodzieży szkolnej w Polsce w kontekście uwarunkowań socjodemograficznych. Wyniki badań HBSC 2013/14 [School children health and health-related behaviors in Poland in the context of socio-demographic conditions. Results of the HBSC Study 2013/14]*. Warsaw: Instytut Matki i Dziecka.

Mazur, J., & Malkowska, A. (2003). Sprawcy i ofiary przemocy wśród uczniow w Polsce [Bullies and victims among Polish school-aged children]. *Medycyna Wieku Rozwojowego* 7: 121–34.

Mazur, J., Tabak, I., Małkowska-Szkutnik, A., Dzielska, A., Kołoło, H., & Kowalewska, A. (2009). Risk and protective factors among determinants of risk behavior syndrome R(BS) in 15-year-old Polish adolescents. Results from HBSC 2006 Survey. In *Determinants of Health and Health Behaviors in Polish Adolescents: Review of Studies Conducted in 2005–2008*. Warsaw: Institute of Mother and Child, pp. 33–57.

Mazur, J., Tabak, I., Małkowska-Szkutnik, A., Ostaszewski, K., Kołoło, H., Dzielska, A., & Kowalewska, A. (2008). *Czynniki chroniące młodzież 15-letnią przed podejmowaniem zachowań ryzykownych [Factors that protect 15-year-old youth from risk behaviors]*. Warsaw: Instytut Matki i Dziecka. Zakład Ochrony i Promocji Zdrowia Dzieci i Młodzieży.

McNeely, C., & Falci, C. (2004). School connectedness and the transition into and out of health-risk behavior among adolescents: a comparison of social belonging and teacher support. *Journal of School Health* 74: 284–92.

Murray, C., & Greenberg, M. (2000). Children's relationship with teachers and bonds with school: an Investigation of patterns and correlates in middle childhood. *Journal of School Psychology* 38: 423–45.

Nation, M., Crusto, C., Wandersman, A., Kumpfer, K,. Seybolt, D., Morrissey-Kane, E., & Davino, K. (2003). What works in prevention. principles of effective prevention programs. *American Psychologist* 58: 449–56.

Oetting, E. R., & Donnermeyer, J. F. (1998). Primary Socialization Theory: the etiology of drug use and deviance. I. *Substance Use and Misuse* 33: 995–1026.

Okulicz-Kozaryn, K. (2010). School as a risk factor for psychoactive substance use by middle school students. *Procedia – Social and Behavioral Sciences* 2: 1620–4. doi: 10.1016/j.sbspro.2010.03.247

Okulicz-Kozaryn, K. (2015). Skuteczność polskiej adaptacji Strengthening Families Program (SFP10-14) [Effectiveness of the Polish version of Strengthening Families Program (SFP10-14)]. *Polskie Forum Psychologiczne* 20: 78–100.

Okulicz-Kozaryn, K., & Borucka, A. (2001). Picie alkoholu przez młodzież z mokotowskich szkół średnich w latach 1984–2000 [Alcohol use among Mokotów high schools youth in 1984–2000]. *Alkoholizm i Narkomania* 14: 245–59.

Okulicz-Kozaryn, K., & Foxcroft, D. (2012). Effectiveness of the Strengthening Families Programme 10–14 in Poland for the prevention of alcohol and drug misuse: protocol for a randomized controlled trial. *BMC Public Health* 12: 319.

Okulicz-Kozaryn, K., & Raduj, J. (2012). Skuteczność Programu Wzmacniania Rodziny po roku od jego realizacji [Effectiveness of Strengthening Family Program: one year after implementation]. *Serwis Informacyjny Narkomania* 58: 18–22.

Ostaszewski, K. (2001). Trendy w używaniu przez młodzież substancji psychoaktywnych. Badania mokotowskie – kontynuacja [Trends in youth substance use – the Mokotów Study]. *Alkoholizm i Narkomania* 14: 387–406.

Ostaszewski, K. (2009). Risk/protective factors in salient adolescent problem behaviors: the Warsaw Adolescent Study. In *Determinants of Health and Health Behaviors in Polish Adolescents: Review of Studies Conducted in 2005–2008*. Warsaw: Institute of Mother and Child, pp. 33–57.

Ostaszewski, K. (2011). Meaningful instrumental behaviors and youth risky behaviors: Warsaw adolescent study, Poster presented at II Meeting EUSPR "Synergy in prevention and health promotion: individual, community, and environmental approaches," December 8–9, Lisbon.

Ostaszewski, K. (2014). *Zachowania ryzykowne młodzieży w perspektywie mechanizmów resilience [Youth risk behaviors from resilience mechanisms perspective]*. Warsaw, Instytut Psychiatrii i Neurologii.

Ostaszewski, K. (2015). Bariery i wyzwania profilaktyki zachowań ryzykownych młodzieży [Barriers and challenges of youth risk behaviors prevention]. *Świat Problemów* 1: 5–11.

Ostaszewski, K., Bobrowski, K., Borucka, A., Okulicz-Kozaryn, K., Pisarska, A., Perry, C.,. & Williams, C. (1998). Program Domowych Detektywów. Adaptacja amerykańskiego programu profilaktyki alkoholowej dla młodzieży we wczesnym okresie dojrzewania [Program Domowych Detektywow; a Polish adaptation of American alcohol use prevention program for pre-adolescents]. *Alkoholizm i Narkomania* 32: 339–60.

Ostaszewski, K., Bobrowski, K., Borucka, A., Okulicz-Kozaryn, K., & Pisarska, A. (2000). Evaluating innovative drug-prevention programmes: lessons learned. In *Evaluation – a Key Tool for Improving Drug Prevention.* EMCDDA Scientific Monograph Series No 5, European Commission. Lisbon: EMCDDA, pp. 75–85.

Ostaszewski, K., Bobrowski, K., Borucka, A., & Pisarska, A. (2002). Subiektywne normy a intencja używania substancji psychoaktywnych przez nastolatków [Teenagers' subjective norms and their intention to substance use]. *Alkoholizm i Narkomania* 15: 305–25.

Ostaszewski, K., & Pisarska, A. (2008). Trends in adolescent substance use: the Mokotow study 1988–2004. *Drugs: Education, Prevention and Policy* 15: 378–94.

Ostaszewski, K., Rustecka-Krawczyk, A., & Wójcik, M. (2011). *Czynniki chroniące i czynniki ryzyka związane z zachowaniami problemowymi warszawskich gimnazjalistów: klasy I –III [Risk and protective factors associated with youth risk behaviors among Warsaw middle school students].* Warsaw: Wydawnictwo Instytutu Psychiatrii i Neurologii.

Państwowa Agencja Rozwiązywania Problemów Alkoholowych (2013). Profilaktyka i rozwiązywanie problemów alkoholowych w Polsce w samorządach gminnych [Prevention and solving of alcohol problems in local communities in Poland]. Retrieved from www.parpa.pl/index.php/analizy-badania-raporty/statystyki

Patterson, G., DeBaryshe, D., & Ramsey, E., (1989). A developmental perspective on antisocial behaviour. *American Psychologist* 44: 329–35.

Pico, B., & Kovacs, E. (2010). Do parents and school matter? Protective factors for adolescent substance use. *Addictive Behaviors* 35; 53–6.

Procidano, M., & Heller, K. (1983). Measures of perceived social support from friends and from family: three validation studies. *American Journal of Community Psychology* 11: 1–24.

Pyżalski, J. (2012). *Agresja elektroniczna i cyberbullying jako nowe ryzykowne zachowania młodzieży [Electronic aggression and cyber-bullying as new youth risk behaviors]*, Kraków: Oficyna Wydawnicza Impuls.

Radomska, A. (2014). Rekomendowane programy profilaktyczne i promocji zdrowia psychicznego [Best practice mental health promotion and prevention programs]. *Serwis Informacyjny Narkomania* 65: 2–3.

Rai, A., Stanton, B., Wu, Y., Li, X., Galbraith, J., Cottrell, L., Pack, R., Harris, C., D'Alessandri, D., & Burns, J. (2003). Relative influences of perceived parental monitoring and perceived peer involvement on adolescent risk behaviors: an analysis of six cross-sectional data sets. *Journal of Adolescent Health* 33: 108–18.

Resnick, M. D., Bearman, P. S., Blum, R. W., Bauman, K. E., Harris, K. M., Jones, J., Tabor, J., Beuhring, T., Sieving, R. E., Shew, M., Ireland, M., Bearinger, L. H., & Udry, J. R. (1997). Protecting adolescents from harm: findings from the

National Longitudinal Study on Adolescent Health. *Journal of the American Medical Association* 278: 823–32.

Rohrbach, L., Hodgson, C., Broder, B., Montgomery, S., Flay, B., Hansen, W., & Pentz, M. (1995). Parental participation in drug abuse prevention: results from the Midwestern Prevention Project. In Boyd, G.. Howard J., & Zucker R. (eds.), *Alcohol Problems among Adolescents: Current Directions in Prevention Research.* Hillsdale, NJ; Erlbaum, pp. 173–95

Rose-Kranor, L., Busseri, M., Willoughby, T., & Chalmers, H. (2006). Breadth and intensity of youth activity involvement as contexts for positive development. *Journal of Youth and Adolescence* 35: 385–499.

Rutter, M. (2012). Resilience as a dynamic concept. *Development and Psychopathology* 24: 335–44.

Salem, D., Zimmerman, M. A., & Notaro, P. (1998). Effects of family structure, family process, and father involvement on psychological outcomes among African American adolescents. *Family Relations* 47: 331–41.

Schafer, J., & Graham, J. (2002). Missing data: our view of the state of the art. *Psychological Methods* 7: 147–77.

Schreiber, J., Stage, F., King, J., Nora, A., & Barlow, E. (2006). Reporting structural equation modeling and confirmatory factor analysis results: a review. *Journal of Educational Research* 99(6): 323–37.

Shears, J., Edwards, R. & Stanley, L. (2006). School bonding and substance use in rural communities. *Social Work Research* 30: 6–18.

Sierosławski, J. (2011). *Używanie alkoholu i narkotyków przez młodzież szkolną. Raport z ogólnopolskich badań ankietowych zrealizowanych w 2011 r.* [Alcohol and drug use among youth: a report from a Poland-wide self-report survey]. Warsaw: Instytut Psychiatrii i Neurologii, Warszawa. www.parpa.pl/images/file/Raport%20ESPAD.pdf

Simons-Morton, B. G., Crump, A. D., Haynie, D. L., & Saylor, K. E. (1999). Student-school bonding and adolescent problem behavior. *Health Education Research* 14: 99–107.

Sochocki, M. (2008). Szkoła dla rodziców i wychowawców w badaniach ewaluacyjnych [Evaluation of a school for parents and teachers]. *Remedium* 4: 1–3

Spoth, R. L., Clair, S., Shin, C., & Redmond, C. (2006). Long-term effects of universal preventive interventions on methamphetamine use among adolescents. *Archivés of Pediatrics and Adolescent Medicine* 160: 876–82.

Stattin, H., & Kerr, M. (2000). Parental monitoring: a reinterpretation. *Child Development* 71: 1072–85.

Stoddard, S., Zimmerman, M., & Bauermeister, J. (2012). A longitudinal analysis of cumulative risk, cumulative promotive factors, and adolescent violent behaviour. *Journal of Research on Adolescence* 22: 542–55.

Szymański, J., Woynarowska, B., & Mazur, J. (2001). Picie napojów alkoholowych przez młodzież szkolną w Polsce i w innych krajach. Tendencje zmian w latach 1990–1998 [Alcohol use among youth in Poland and other countries: changes in 1990–1998]. *Alkoholizm i Narkomania* 14: 213–28.

Świątkiewicz, G. (1997). Regulating unregulated markets. *Addiction* 92(suppl. 1): 67–72.

Tabak, I. (2008). Dobre relacje w rodzinie jako czynnik chroniący w grupie uwarunkowań związanych ze środowiskiem rodzinnym [Positive family relationships as a protective factor in family factors domain]. In Mazur, J., Tabak, I.,

Małkowska-Szkutnik, A., Ostaszewski, K., Kołoło, H., Dzielska, A., & Kowalewska, A. (eds.), *Czynniki chroniące młodzież 15-letnią przed podejmowaniem zachowań ryzykownych*. Warsaw: Instytut Matki i Dziecka. Zakład Ochrony i Promocji Zdrowia Dzieci i Młodzieży, pp. 85–97.

Tabak, I., & Mazur, J. (2008). Współczesna rodzina a zdrowie psychiczne i zadowolenie z życia polskich nastolatków [Contemporary family and mental health of Polish teenagers]. In Okulicz-Kozaryn, K., & Ostaszewski, O. (eds.), *Promocja Zdrowia Psychicznego – badania i działania w Polsce*. Warsaw: Wydawnictwo Instytutu Psychiatrii i Neurologii, pp. 101–17.

Terlikowska, J. & Okulicz-Kozaryn, K. (2015). Jakie działania profilaktyczne realizują i finansują gminy? [What kind of preventive activities are implemented and funded by local communities?]. Oral presentation at the Conference Promocja zdrowia i profilaktyka – inwestycją w lokalny kapitał społeczny, March 23–24, Warsaw. Ośrodek Rozwoju Edukacji.

Trudeau, L., Spoth, R., Randall, G. K., & Azevedo, K. (2007). Longitudinal effects of a universal family-focused intervention on growth patterns of adolescent internalizing symptoms and polysubstance use: Gender comparisons. *Journal of Youth and Adolescence* 36: 725–40.

Van Der Kreeft, P., Wiborg, G., Galanti, M., Siliquini, R., Bohrn, K., Scatigna, M., Lindahl, A., Melero, J., Vassara, M., Faggiano, F., & Eu-Dap Study Group "Unplugged" (2009). A new European school programme against substance abuse. *Drugs: Prevention, Education and Policy* 16: 167–81.

Voisin, D., Salazar, L., Crosby, R., Diclemente, R., Yarber, W., & Staples-Horne, M. (2005). Teacher connectedness and health-related outcomes among detained adolescents. *Journal of Adolescent Health* 37: 337–53.

Werner, E. (2000). Protective factors and individual resilience. In Shonkoff, J. P., & Meisels, S. J. (eds.), *Handbook of Early Childhood Intervention*. New York: Cambridge University Press, pp. 115–32.

Werner, E. (2005). What can we learn about resilience from large-scale longitudinal studies? In Goldstein, W. S., & Brooks, R. (eds.). *Handbook of Resilience in Children*, New York: Springer Science + Business Media, pp. 91–105.

Williams, C., & Perry, C. (1998). Lessons from Project Northland: preventing alcohol problems during adolescence. *Alcohol Health & Research World* 22: 107–16.

Williams, C., Perry, C., Dudovitz, B., Veblen-Mortenson, S., Anstine, P., Komro, K. A., & Toomey, T. L. (1995), A home-based prevention program for sixth-grade alcohol use: Results from Project Northland, *Journal of Primary Prevention* 16: 125–47.

Willoughby, T., & Hamza, C. (2011). A longitudinal examination of the bidirectional associations among perceived parenting behaviors, adolescent disclosure and problem behavior across high school years. *Journal of Youth and Adolescence* 40: 463–78.

Wills, T., Resko, J., Ainette, M., & Mendoza, D. (2004). Role of parent support and peer support in adolescent substance use: a test of mediated effects, *Psychology of Addctive Behaviors* 18: 122–34.

Wilson, D. (2004). The interface of school climate and school connectedness and relationship with aggression and victimization. *Journal of School Health* 74: 293–9.

Wingspread Declaration on School Connections (2004). *Journal of School Health* 74: 233–4.

Wojtyniak, B., Moskalewicz, J., Stokwiszewski, J., & Rabczenko, D. (2005). Gender-specific mortality associated with alcohol consumption in Poland in transition. *Addiction* 100: 1779–89.

Zimmerman, M. (2014). Flint [Michigan] Adolescent Study (FAS): a longitudinal study of school dropout and substance use, 1994–1997. ICPSR34598-v1. Ann Arbor, MI: Inter-university Consortium for Political and Social Research [distributor], 2014-11-07. doi.org/10.3886/ICPSR34598.v1

Zimmerman, M., Bingenheimer, J., & Notaro, P. (2002). Natural mentors and adolescent resiliency: a study with urban youth. *American Journal of Community Psychology* 30: 221–43.

Zimmerman, M., & Maton, K. (1992). Life-style and substance use among male African-American urban adolescents: a cluster analytic approach. *American Journal of Community Psychology* 20: 121–38.

Zimmerman, M., Stoddard, S., Eisman, A., Caldwell, C., Aiyer,,S., & Miller, A. (2013). Adolescent resilience: promotive factors that inform prevention. *Child Development Perspectives* 7: 215–20.

39 Interventions to Promote Positive Parenting in Spain

María José Rodrigo, Sonia Byrne, & Miriam Álvarez

Introduction

The main objective of this chapter is to present a contemporary view of the progress that has been achieved in the parenting domain in Spain, referring to the evolution of family and parenting policies, the scope of parental support initiatives, and the implementation of evidence-based parent education programs that may have an impact on child and family well-being. This broader view is necessary to properly understand the political, social, and practical context in which interventions to promote positive parenting are delivered in Spain.

As part of this broader scope, some relevant information about the Spanish population, living conditions, and children's well-being is briefly presented to characterize the prevention context. Spain has been a member of the European Union (EU) since 1986 and is ranked as the fifth-largest economy in the EU. As of January 1, 2014, according to the Spanish National Statistics Institute (INE), the resident population of Spain is 46.5 million (with 17.9 percent of the population under seventeen years of age and 18.2 percent over the age of sixty-five). The population is aging due to the low fertility rate (1.27), women's high average age at childbirth (31.7 years of age), and life expectancy at birth (79.9 years for males and 85.6 years for females). Traditionally, as in other southern European countries such as Portugal, Italy, and Greece, the Spanish family has been characterized by strong bonds of affection and a supportive role in caring for young and dependent members. There are signs of modernity, however, in the growing diversity of family forms, the more democratic parent–child relationships enjoyed in the family, and an increasing awareness in favor of the protection of children's rights, the promotion of gender equality, and the prosecution of any form of family violence (Delgado, Meil, & Zamora, 2008).

Spain's national public health and educational systems offer extended and free coverage for the population. The outcomes of the Spanish health care system compare favorably with those of other European health care systems. However, even though Spanish legislation recognizes the importance of prevention, health practice has traditionally focused mainly on the treatment of already established illness and much less on prevention. This means that, within the large population of parents, particularly important groups such as vulnerable parents at points of transition – those in the perinatal period and parents of adolescents, for instance – do not receive any preventive support other than for the treatment of established illness.

For its part, the public education system (free of charge to all children aged between three and eighteen years) has brought about great improvements in the training and educational attainment of the Spanish population. However, the educational system needs to be strengthened in at least three important ways: (a) to ensure that the greatest possible number of students obtain the school leaving certificate (the rate of early school leavers is 21.9 percent on average in Spain); (b) to foster higher enrollment in formal professional training; and (c) to improve the level of educational attainment, which is currently below the average scores according to the Organization for Economic Cooperation and Development (OECD) (PISA, 2012). All these aspects account for the high proportion of the adult population aged twenty-five to sixty-four years with no more than a primary education (19 percent), a figure that highly conditions the probability of being unemployed.

According to a comprehensive assessment of the lives and well-being of children and young people in twenty-nine nations of the industrialized world, Spanish children compare reasonably well in terms of health and safety, lifestyle behaviors and risks, and housing and environmental safety (UNICEF, 2013). However, they rate much lower in material well-being (due to monetary and material deprivation) and educational attainment (with below-average academic grades and a higher chance of leaving school early). Spain has slipped down the rankings from fifth out of twenty-one countries in the early years of the last decade (2000–10) to nineteenth out of twenty-nine countries in 2009–2010. This is largely due to the fact that since 2008, Spain – like other world economies – has been in the throes of an economic crisis that has had a huge impact on household income, particularly among families with dependent children. The most vulnerable sectors (e.g., households where parents have low levels of education and are immigrants) have been disproportionately affected by cuts in social, health, and educational budgets and shrinking family benefits. Consequently, child poverty is closely linked to the rising unemployment of parents and limited social protection. In 2008, 28.2 percent of children in Spain lived below the poverty threshold, which is far above that of the EU (20.4 percent). In 2012, the child poverty risk rate reached 29.9 percent (2.2 million children), a 1.7 percent rise from 2008. In the EU, the rise in this rate between 2008 and 2012 was half of that in Spain (0.8 percent). In fact, children now represent in Spain the age group with the highest social exclusion rates (e.g., the progressive loss of integration or participation of people in different economic, political, and social settings), thus overtaking the elderly as the most affected; the latter are more economically covered by the pension system, which has remained unaffected.

Against the backdrop of the Spanish context depicted in the preceding, the following two sections of this chapter describe how family policy in Spain has evolved from its former approach into a new one focused on child and family well-being, inspired by the Council of Europe's positive parenting framework.

The impact of this European initiative has also led to a clear recognition in Spain of the importance of adopting a prevention focus for family intervention, as well as the need to strengthen parental capacities and empower communities, along with the adoption of codes of professional best practices to improve prevention work with families. The chapter continues by addressing the common features that characterize service provision to families in Spain, developed under the umbrella of the Council of Europe's positive parenting framework, providing an overview of the main types of services and programs. It concludes with a description of the implementation and evaluation of evidence-based positive parenting programs in Spain, along with an illustration of some of the program results.

Rise of Family Support Policies in Spain

Spanish family policy played a prominent political and social role during the dictatorship regime (1936–75). Traditionally, family policy translated, on the one hand, into very restrictive legal provisions to reinforce traditional family relationships based on authoritarian and paternalist child-rearing and, on the other hand, into a relatively generous policy of income transfers designed to keep women at home, caring for their families, and also to raise birth rates (Meil & Iglesias de Ussel, 2001). With the transition to democracy, social policy priorities were radically redesigned, fueled by profound changes in gender roles, lifestyles, and the economic growth model. Providing decent and sufficient pensions, thereby ensuring financial independence for each generation, became a priority objective, together with the development of social protection for the unemployed. The pursuit of these objectives left a very narrow margin for the development of other social welfare policies, particularly family policies; moreover, family policies were deeply discredited, as they were associated with social protection for the traditional family.

The past two decades (since 1995) have seen the construction of a modern social protection system in Spain, with the promotion of public policies for income, health, education, housing, and social services (Delgado et al., 2008; Meil, 2006). The country's main political and social stakeholders have begun to express the need for an active family policy, and certain measures have been taken in this regard. Family support policies today address issues related to housing (promoting easier access to ownership), the labor market (reducing temporary employment), old age (offering more public support for the elderly), and gender equality (seen, for instance, in measures promoting the presence of women in the workplace, the balance between work and family life, and parental leave).

In the last six years, the ongoing economic and unemployment crisis has threatened the Spanish welfare state, jeopardizing the sustainability and viability of the social protection system. However, the critical situation in Spain has been accompanied by a renewed political impetus toward the promotion of family policies, with a specific emphasis on those ensuring child and family well-being. In this political context, four national action plans should be mentioned. First, the *II National Strategic Plan for Childhood and Adolescence* (2013–16), approved in April 2013, aims to promote the well-being of children and adolescents, taking into consideration their needs and interests in order to increase their quality of life and foster the full development of their capabilities as active subjects of their rights.

Second, the *Comprehensive Plan for Family Support* (2015–17) was approved in April 2015, with the aim of structuring a family policy explicitly as a coherent set of standard measures involving the action of several Spanish ministries. Thus, the plan covers not only social aspects but also health, education, and justice aspects, among others, with impact on family policies. In particular, one of the strategies involves a set of measures with developments in reconciliation and joint responsibility for personal, family, and working life, in reinforcement of the intergenerational solidarity and in improvement of the parental competences to promote positive parenting.

A third political measure, the *National Action Plan for Social Inclusion* (2013–16), approved in December 2013, aims to provide a response to needs related to poverty and social exclusion, all under the framework of the EU targets set out in the Europe 2020 Strategy for smart, sustainable, and inclusive growth (European Commission, 2010). Specifically, the fight against child poverty relies on the following three points: (a) access to suitable resources and home support, which involves supporting parents' participation in the labor market, allowing for greater work, family, and personal life balance as well as providing suitable income in harmony with social benefits; (b) access to quality services, which means investing in early childhood education and care to reduce inequalities and in the development of educational systems that make an impact on equal opportunities; preventing health inequality through early intervention; providing suitable housing and a risk-free environment; and fostering social services that protect children and support their parents; and (c) child participation, with suggestions to support the inclusion of children in social, cultural, leisure, and civic activities, as well as establishing mechanisms to ensure their implication in decisions that affect their lives.

Finally, it is worth mentioning the *Prevention and Health Promotion Strategy of the National Health System*, approved in December 2013, aimed at health promotion and universal prevention of major risk of illness at all stages of life, with a special focus on promoting healthy lifestyles during pregnancy, children's emotional well-being in the first three years of life, and healthy and active lifestyles in the ageing population. This strategy involves training professionals not only in treating disorders, as was previously the case, but in prevention as well. All these national strategic plans have enrolled stakeholders (e.g., the Platform of Childhood Organizations, Cáritas Española, the Spanish branch of SOS Children's Villages, the Federation of Associations to Prevent Child Abuse, the Spanish Red Cross, and UNICEF Spain) in their design and implementation and have been welcomed as important developments to help overcome the negative impact of the economic crisis on children and their families.

Impact of the European Positive Parenting Framework in Spain

The recent developments in family policy in Spain have been inspired in part by the positive parenting framework emanating from the Council of Europe's Recommendation 19 (2006) of the Committee of Ministers of the Member States, which provides guidance on how governments can support positive parenting. As a major intergovernmental organization that currently includes forty-seven member states, the Council of Europe has a long record in the area of children's rights and has made efforts to reach a broad consensus among member states to include positive parenting under the umbrella of public policies. In the Council of Europe's Recommendation 19 (2006), positive parenting is defined "as parental behavior based on the best interest of the child that is nurturing, empowering, non-violent and provides recognition and guidance, which involves setting boundaries to enable the full development of the child" (see Table 39.1).

The concept of positive parenting entails a view of children as active subjects who contribute to shaping their own development (Daly, 2007; Rodrigo, 2010; Rodrigo, Byrne, & Rodríguez, 2014). The role of parents is to facilitate the child's exercising of his or her rights, by providing direction and guidance appropriate to the child's evolving capacities. When translated into the family setting, values of mutual respect, equal dignity, authenticity, integrity, and responsibility are the foundations for developing parent–child relationships that promote children's rights.

The Council of Europe's Recommendation also aims to encourage parents to strengthen their parenting capacities and to seek assistance if they encounter

Table 39.1 *Child's and Parent's Needs According to the Positive Parenting Framework (Daly, 2007)*

Child's needs	Parent's needs
Nurturing: Experience positive feelings of love, acceptance, and joy.	*Guidance*: Having access to information and advice.
Structuring and Stimulation: Live in an environment with routines, norms, and learning opportunities.	*Time* for their children, for themselves, and to spend on family leisure.
Empowerment: Acquire the capacity to grow up as an active and competent family member.	*Self-confidence* in the parental capacities to perform the parenting role well.
Free from violence: Do not experience any form of verbal and physical violence in the family.	*Informal and formal support* to overcome difficulties and reduce stress on the family.

difficulties in bringing up their children. Parents should be provided with sufficient support mechanisms to meet their important responsibilities in bringing up their children, in keeping with the following principles: (a) adequate family governmental policies must be put into place that create the necessary legislative, administrative, and financial frameworks; (b) services must be provided to support parents, such as local counseling services, help lines, online parent support, and therapeutic and psychoeducational programs; (c) services must support parents from a broad variety of family situations, but especially those parents and children facing adverse circumstances (e.g., marital violence, low educational background, poverty, lack of social support, substance abuse); and (d) diversity must be recognized and respected in relation to family patterns and cultural and gender differences, while keeping in mind the best interest of the child. In sum, the Council of Europe's Recommendation endorses the importance to children of growing up in a positive family environment and emphasizes the responsibility of the state to create the best conditions for this by providing parents with sufficient and adequate support.

The Council of Europe's guidance has been widely disseminated in Europe (Rodrigo, Almeida & Reichle, 2016). Spain is one of the southern European countries where the initiative has received the greatest support due to the political involvement in the dissemination of this European initiative at the national level. In particular, Spain has adopted the prevention approach to family intervention and recognized that strengthening parental capacities and empowering communities are the best ways to protect children, preserve their rights, and promote their development. To this end, in 2009 a partnership was created that brings together the Spanish Ministry of Health, Social Services, and Equality; the State Federation of Towns and Provinces (FEMP in Spanish); and a consortium of six Spanish Universities (Universidad Autónoma de Madrid, Universidad de Barcelona, Universidad de La Laguna, Universidad de Las Palmas de Gran Canaria, Universidad del País Vasco, and Universidad de Oviedo). It is difficult to build up this type of collaborative venture involving policy makers, researchers, and professionals as well as public and private agencies and corporations, but when successful, it represents a fertile ground for promoting prevention work with families.

The first objective of this collaborative venture is to disseminate the positive parenting framework described in the preceding among professionals working in child and family services and to the network of social, health, and community services in both printed and online versions (Rodrigo, Máiquez, & Martín, 2010a, 2010b, 2011). Taking a preventive stance to family intervention involves a profound shift in the way professionals understand their work with families, moving from a deficit approach to one based on prevention and promotion (Kumpfer & Alvarado, 2003; Rodrigo, Byrne, & Álvarez, 2012). According to this view, prevention efforts should be directed at diminishing the impact of the risk factors and promoting the protective factors present in the family and the neighborhood. Focus should be placed on the promotion of parental capacities, which means moving toward a strengthening approach that identifies parents' existing skills and strengths and builds on these capacities. Professionals should avoid making decisions for families, which can lead to excessive dependency on the services, but instead increase their self-confidence through a collaborative alliance. Interventions should be based on empowering children by promoting their strengths and resources and helping them to communicate their feelings and needs. And finally, there should be cooperation and interdisciplinary coordination between entities, facilitating means of sharing and working in an interdisciplinary network.

The second objective of the collaborative venture has been to draft a *Guide of Best Practices in Positive Parenting (Guía de Buenas prácticas en Parentalidad positiva,* Rodrigo et al., 2016), meant as a resource to support professional practice with families. The main objective is to introduce the positive parenting framework into family support services, enhancing the innovative and quality assurance processes by means of changes to the organizational cultures and professional practices. The *Guide* is not only the fruit of the work undertaken by the panel of experts from the aforementioned consortium of universities but also the result of the collaborative efforts of many professionals working in public and private agencies in Spain, who provided feedback from the field throughout the drafting process. The *Guide* includes an online protocol that provides a detailed explanation of the best practices to be followed in preventive work with families around three topics: (a) characteristics of the family support services and organizational culture; (b) the intervention process with the family (i.e.. reception, assessment, intervention, and supervision); and (c) the use of evidence-based preventive psychoeducational and community programs targeted at the child and the family. In this regard, the *Guide* is directed at the professionals, service users, and policy makers involved in the process of improving the services offered to families.

Parental Support Initiatives in Spain

Under the impetus of the focus on the Council of Europe's positive parenting recommendation, the services and resources specifically addressing parents' needs in bringing up children have undergone rapid expansion across the country. A common schema has been followed in the way parenting support is delivered through three levels of responsibility. The development of parental support policies is generally the responsibility of the central government. The central authorities are responsible for the legislative framework and regulations, the drafting of national action plans, and part of the financial support. In turn, the governments of the Autonomous Communities (Spain is made up of seventeen Autonomous Communities and the Autonomous Cities of Ceuta and Melilla situated in the north of Africa) are responsible for specific legislative regulations, co-funding, and the general organization of services within their territories. The implementation of the programs through the provision of parenting support activities is, in most cases, a responsibility of the local administrations, involving public and private agencies and organizations from the voluntary sector, with different degrees of coordination and funding.

A detailed account of the child and family support services in Spain is beyond the scope of this chapter. Instead, the chapter describes three common features that characterize the prevention focus in Spanish service provision to families: (a) the families targeted come from a broad variety of situations with different levels of parental needs and requiring a continuum of support measures; (b) there is a trend to reinforce community and specialized services to support families at the local level; and (c) there is a clear recognition of the importance of promoting intersectoral (social, education, health, and justice) work and introducing the positive parenting framework into prevention efforts in each area. Each of these features is described in turn in the following.

Targeting a wide-ranging population. Many parents are doing reasonably well in their parenting task; they have created a caring and nurturing environment for their children, are sensitive to their needs, are able to set up flexible norms, and are ready to provide learning opportunities to their children, in keeping with positive parenting principles. They are aware of their needs as parents, and can easily fulfill them by reading books, attending lectures, or searching for online or peer support from other parents. However, there are families in which the parents' needs are not easily perceived and fulfilled, as they are multiple and acute and not primarily focused on the child's well-being. Between the two extremes, there is a gradient of parental needs that could be categorized into different levels, as suggested by the professional practice in the child and family services (see Table 39.2) (Asmussen, 2011).

Targeting a wide-ranging population requires dealing with families of various levels of need who require the provision of increasing levels of support (information, education, training, counseling/therapy, and other measures or services), as illustrated in Table 39.2.

Reinforcing community and specialized services at the local level. Another important feature of service provision in Spain is the reinforcement of community and specialized services at the local/municipal level. There is a reasonably well-resourced and systematically organized public sector engaged in the delivery of family and social services throughout the country. Community services are the gateway to the social protection system, as they provide information and guidance to the population regarding the social resources available to satisfy their needs (e.g., housing, employment, aid for dependent people), collaborate in the management of social actions carried out in the community, and refer people to specialized services, among other functions. In turn, the specialized social services in charge of family matters are aimed at promoting child and family well-being in vulnerable families experiencing a range of circumstances that may produce child protection concerns.

The municipal and regional (i.e., Autonomous Community) levels of government have complementary roles in child protection, according to the Spanish System for the Protection of Minors, which is regulated under a national Child Protection Law dating from 1996. The main responsibilities of local councils lie

Table 39.2 *Levels of Parental Need and Continuum of Support Measures (Asmussen, 2011)*

Level	Description	Support
Low need	Parents seeking support for stresses and difficulties experienced by most families at some points in their life transitions or in their child's development.	Occasional orientation, lectures, peer support, online support.
Moderate need	Parents requiring support for issues (e.g., couple or child problems) that could potentially develop into serious problems, but are usually of recent onset.	Guidance, group intervention.
Complex needs	Parents living in families with numerous needs that may have persisted over time, multiple family problems, ongoing child conduct issues and antisocial behavior, and child protection concerns.	Family counseling/therapy, and group intervention.
High needs	Parents living in families facing crisis and at risk of dissolution, with gender violence, mental health problems, child maltreatment, child's delinquent behavior, substance abuse, or child being under protection measures.	Home visits, intensive therapeutic help, crisis intervention.

in the areas of prevention, early detection, and family preservation in families at psychosocial risk, with the goal of preventing unnecessary placement of children into foster care. In turn, the regional government intervenes when the preventive actions taken at the municipal level fail and it is necessary to separate the minor from his family and provide residential child care, foster care, or adoption services (del Valle, Canali, Bravo, & Vecchioto, 2013; del Valle, López, Montserrat, & Bravo, 2009; Palacios & Amorós, 2006).

The current focus on prevention work with families has produced important changes in the specialized social services offered at the municipal level. In the past, the tendency was that these services were mostly attending to high-need families with resources exclusively tailored for them (see Table 39.2). Nowadays, these services tend to provide support to a greater variety of families in the context of community-based psycho-educational interventions involving the full range of family needs described in Table 39.2. The focus is on increasing parenting skills and social support in order to improve parents' autonomous functioning. There is also a promotion of a collaborative framework in the context of family-service partnerships involving children, families, professionals, and communities, with a clear focus on the wishes, feelings, safety, and well-being of children (Dolan, Pinkerton, & Canavan, 2006). The view is also promoted that the most effective interventions are those that strengthen informal support networks, as these are natural sources of help that increase parents' sense of confidence in their own capabilities (Rodrigo & Byrne, 2011). Finally, there is a clear emphasis on empowering the community, creating participation

Table 39.3. *Examples of Child and Family Support Services and Programs in the Municipal Services in Spain (Rodrigo et al., 2010b).*

Services	Programs
Family mediation and meeting points	Workshops to promote co-parenting and co-responsibility in the organization of family life
Day care centers and PC labs for children and adolescents	Out-of-school educational activities to promote children's positive development
Sports and leisure centers	Leisure and recreation programs to promote healthy lifestyles in the family
Civic centers	Community programs to promote family-school-neighbor collaboration
Community social services	Time banks to facilitate work–family balance
Youth centers	Street education for young people from vulnerable families at psychosocial risk

platforms involving local stakeholders in many communities to strengthen and coordinate the networks of local resources available to families and to the population in general. As a result, a broad variety of preventive services and programs are now implemented at the local social services level, as illustrated in Table 39.3 (Rodrigo, Máiquez, & Martin, 2010b).

Promoting intersectoral work. Another important feature of service provision in Spain is that the positive parenting framework has moved beyond the social domain and is having a progressively larger impact on the educational, health, and justice sectors in Spain. In each of these sectors, there is a clear recognition of the importance of including the positive parenting framework in prevention efforts. Some ongoing experiences involving national and regional initiatives, but still without formal evaluations, are provided here to illustrate this emerging trend toward intersectoral action.

- *Implementation of group-based positive parenting programs to prevent early abandonment of secondary schooling.* To address the high school dropout rate, the Consejeria de Educacion Universidades y Sostenibilidad (2014) of the Autonomous Community of Canarias, has implemented since 2014 positive parenting programs targeted at parents of secondary school children to increase parents' skills and enhance their involvement in promoting the child's school motivation and academic performance to prevent early school leaving. The novelty is that teachers are being trained as facilitators of parent groups, resulting in the strengthening of family–school relationships and their greater involvement in family matters. Rate of early school leaving has dropped from 26 percent to 22.9 percent in the Community of Canarias in the last year, suggesting a positive contribution, among other factors, of the parenting programs implemented at the secondary schools.
- *Inclusion of parenting support into the Prevention and Health Promotion Strategy of the National Health System at national and regional levels.* The Department of Health of the Spanish Ministry of Health, Social Services, and

Equality is designing a program on positive parenting to provide universal online support to parents of young children under the age of three, with the aim of diminishing risk factors in the family context and promoting the child's physical and emotional well-being (Ministerio de Sanidad, Servicios Sociales e Igualdad, 2016). In turn, the Department of Health of the Autonomous Community of Andalusia is ready to implement its universal Infant and Adolescent Health Program targeting all families with children under the age of fourteen (Proyecto Apego, 2014). This program provides family counseling and parental psychoeducational support through the health care system by trained health professionals at specific points in time: prenatal and perinatal checkups, mandatory and voluntary child health visits, and urgent consultations.

- *Family support dimension in the juvenile justice services.* The Department of Justice of the Autonomous Community of Catalonia provides psychosocial support to families of convicted juveniles who are avoiding imprisonment through their engagement in social activities on behalf of the community, among other actions (Projecte Tècnic de Medi Overt, 2013). Providing psychoeducational support to these families is seen as the most important part of the intervention process carried out with juvenile offenders. As such, families are strongly encouraged to attend positive parenting workshops to enhance their parenting skills (i.e., monitoring, supervision, affective relations) in order to facilitate key changes in the juveniles' social networks to better promote their positive development.

The preceding examples offer an idea of the depth and breadth of the impact of the European positive parenting framework on intersectoral prevention policies directed at ensuring child and family well-being in Spain. The scope of these and other initiatives represent a further step toward promoting a wider culture of family-based prevention and promotion across these sectors.

Implementation and Evaluation of Evidence-Based Positive Parenting Programs

Of all the prevention work inspired by the positive parenting framework in Spain, the flagship initiative involves the implementation and evaluation of evidence-based positive parenting programs. The term "evidence-based programs" refers to a specific subset of programs that are theoretically based, with their contents fully described and structured in a manual, their effectiveness evaluated according to standards of evidence, and the factors that influence the implementation process identified and taken into account to explore variations in program results (e.g., Fixsen, Naoom, Blase, Friedman, & Wallace, 2005; Flay et al., 2005; Kellam & Langevin, 2003).

There are still difficulties in Spain, however, in applying what constitutes "best evidence" to practice and policy in the field of child and family services.

This is a very controversial issue even in countries with a longer tradition in applying the evidence-based movement to social domains (e.g., United States and United Kingdom). Some researchers and practitioners consider that other standards of evidence, besides the use of randomized controlled trials (RCTs), should be taken into account when moving from clinical trials to multi-agency delivery of practice in community settings based on prevention and strength-based approaches (Boddy, Smith, & Statham, 2011; Eurochild, 2013; Johnson & Austin, 2005). Some examples of suggestions for potential indicators of best evidence include adapting the program to make it acceptable to a wide range of socioeconomic/cultural groups (Davis, McDonald, & Axford, 2012), ensuring that the program is implemented with fidelity by agencies and staff (Durlak & DuPre, 2008), and assuring sustainability by integrating the program into the network of community resources (Rodrigo et al., 2012).

Despite the absence of international consensus on what is meant by "best evidence" in the field of positive parenting, Spanish regional and municipal administrations are strongly committed to supporting the implementation of evidence-based positive parenting programs at local levels to support parents in their parenting role. Traditionally, support for parents delivered by public administrations has been developed mainly with the aim of preventing child maltreatment in at-risk families. The typical profile of targeted parents attending parenting programs includes low-income parents who have had poor models of parenting, lack personal empowerment, have inadequate life management skills, are punitive in managing children's behavior or provide inadequate supervision of children and neglect of their basic needs (Menéndez, Hidalgo, Jiménez, Lorence, & Sánchez, 2010). Progressively, the services' exclusive focus on child protection/child safety issues has changed to also include general concerns about parenting issues and family well-being in a wider range of family situations.

Table 39.4 shows some examples of evidence-based positive parenting programs implemented in Spain, arranged by children's age. The institution that supported the program, the target population, intervention focus, dose of the program, and outcome measures are provided. This is a highly selective list of the programs that best represent the spirit of the European positive parenting framework. The parent education programs listed in Table 39.4 (e.g., Family Competence Program) are generally meant to help parents develop and enhance their parenting skills by trying alternative approaches to child-rearing, improving the family learning environment, fostering their sense of personal competence, and strengthening their capability to draw upon available resources, among informal and formal support networks, for their own well-being and the well-being of their young and adolescent children (Kaminski, Valle, Filene, & Boyle, 2008). The programs summarized in Table 39.4 are grounded in solid theories and research on attachment, parental cognition, child-rearing practices, social learning, parental self-efficacy, family communication and conflicts, life transitions, family stress, and social support. Accordingly, the core contents of these programs are very diverse, including affectional bonds

Table 39.4 *Examples of Evidence-Based Positive Parenting Programs Implemented in Spain*

Program	Institutions	Target population	Intervention focus	Dose	Outcome measures
Programa de Apoyo Psicológico P/Materno-Infantil Parent–Child Psychological Support (PCPS) program (adapted from Cerezo (1992) original program) www.pcpsparenting.org/consists-of/	Child and family services, health clinics	Parents and infants aged 3 to 18 months	Support parenting and promote protective adaptive systems in children to prevent mental health problems	6 office-based appointments at 3, 6, 9, 12, 15, and 18 months	Quality of the child's attachment; parental sense of competence; distress, rigidity, unhappiness, problems with the child, the family, and other people.
Crecer Felices en Familia Growing Up Happily in the Family group-based program (Rodrigo et al., 2008) portal.asociacionhestia.org/	Social services, educational centers, NGOs	At-risk and non-at-risk parents of children aged 0 to 5 years	Promotion of parental warmth, sensitivity, positive expectations of child development, strategies for child's self-regulation and family-school support as protection factors for child development	22 weekly group sessions of 1.5 hours	Parental child-rearing attitudes, parental sense of competence; parenting stress; knowledge of child's developmental timetable and perceived parental influence; knowledge of child's needs
Crecer Felices en Familia Growing Up Happily in the Family home-visiting program	Social services	At-risk parents of children aged 0 to 5 years	Provide information, guidance, practical help and emotional	12 weekly sessions of 1.5 hours	Parental child-rearing attitudes, parental sense of competence;

Table 39.4 (*cont.*)

Program	Institutions	Target population	Intervention focus	Dose	Outcome measures
(Máiquez et al., 2009) portal.asociacionhestia.org/			support to families to improve psychoeducational home conditions, promote family well-being and prevent child abuse and neglect		parenting stress; knowledge of child's developmental timetable and perceived parental influence; quality of home environment
Aprender Juntos, Crecer en Familia Learning Together, Growing Up in the Family group-based program (Amorós et al., 2011) obrasocial.lacaixa.es/ambitos/caixaproinfancia/caixaproinfancia_es.html	Network of NGOs participating in the Caixa Proinfancia Program	Vulnerable families from disadvantaged backgrounds with children aged 6 to 12 years	Promotion of positive parent–child affection bonds, compromise about rules and values, shared family organization, communication and conflict resolution and participation in family leisure	14 sessions of two hours: parent and child separated, and parent–child together	Parents' child-rearing strategies; child's perception of family discipline; parental sense of competence; family leisure activities; and parent and child family satisfaction
Construir lo cotidiano. Un programa de educación parental Building the Everyday parent education program (Torío et al., 2013) www.uniovi.es/asoced	Educational centers	Parents with children aged 2 to 11 years	Family dynamics to reconstruct the frame of relations, the division of tasks and redistribution of responsibilities, so	10 weekly group sessions of 2 hours, plus other sessions presented in	Families' attitudes, preferences, and beliefs about gender roles and housework; families'

			that habits of equality, solidarity, and shared responsibility are promoted in mothers and fathers.	each topic area	cooperation and children's participation in family responsibilities
Programa de Competencia Familiar (PCF) Family Competence Program (FCP) (Kumpfer et al., 2006) www.competenciafamiliar.com/pags/en/family-competence-program.html	Proyecto Hombre centers for drug abuse treatment, social services	High-risk parents in treatment for drug abuse or in vulnerable situations that might induce 8- to 17-year-old children to engage in addictive and antisocial behavior	Spanish adaptation of the Strengthening Families Program, a multicomponent program of proven efficiency in preventing drug use and other behavioral problems in children	14 sessions of 2 hours: parent and child separated, and parent–child together	Parenting skills (e.g., supervision and monitoring, involvement, self-efficacy), family relationships (cohesion, communication, conflicts, resilience) and children's social competence and behavior (peer resistance, substance abuse)
Vivir la Adolescencia en Familia Living Adolescence in the Family group-based program (Rodrigo et al., 2010c) portal.asociacionhestia.org/	Social services, educational centers, NGOs	At-risk and non-at-risk parents of adolescent children aged 11 to 17 years	Promotion of parental supervision, communication, and conflict resolution	21 weekly group sessions of 1.5 hours	Parental conceptions of adolescence; parental monitoring and supervision;

Table 39.4 (*cont.*)

Program	Institutions	Target population	Intervention focus	Dose	Outcome measures
			strategies to improve family life, healthy lifestyles, Internet regulation, and family-school relationships		conflict resolution strategies in the family
Apoyo Personal y Familiar (APF) Personal and Family Support group-based program (Rodrigo et al., 2000) www.jcyl.es/web/jcyl/binarios/735/585/PROGRAMA%20EDUCAR%20EN%20FAMILIA-evaluacion%20final.pdf?blobheader=application/pdf;charset%3DUTF-8	Social services	At-risk and non-at-risk parents of children of any age for prevention and family preservation purposes	Promotion of parental competences to face their parenting role with a sense of agency and satisfaction according to the child's developmental needs	32 weekly group sessions of 1.5 hours	Parental beliefs on child development and education, positive and negative child-rearing practices, personal agency (self-efficacy, locus of control, couple agreement, and role difficulty) and informal and formal support networks
Programa de Formación y Apoyo Familiar (FAF) Family Training and Support group-based program (Hidalgo, Menéndez, López, Sánchez, & Lorence, 2011) institucional.us.es/programafaf/	Social services	At-risk parents of children of any age for prevention and family	Promotion of parental psychoeducational competences to fulfill children's needs and to	16 to 20 weekly group sessions per year (two years);	Knowledge about developmental-educational needs of children and adolescents;

		preservation purposes	promote positive child development from an ecological system approach	sessions of 1.5 hours	ideas about parental practices; perceived quality of life of children and adolescents in physical, psychological, school, and family areas; self-esteem, self-efficacy, and satisfaction perceived as a parent; social support networks
Programa-Guía para el Desarrollo de Competencias Emocionales, Educativas y Parentales Program-Guide to Develop Emotional, Educational and Parental Competences group-based program (Martínez, 2009) www.observatoriodelainfancia.msssi.gob.es/	Social services, educational centers	At-risk and non-at-risk parents of children aged 2 to 17 years	Promotion of personal, emotional and educational strategies to help parents develop their role properly and to promote positive family relationships	11 weekly group sessions of 2 hours	Awareness of children's developmental characteristics; self-regulation abilities; self-esteem and assertiveness; emotions and communication strategies; abilities to listen and express themselves;

Table 39.4 (*cont.*)

Program	Institutions	Target population	Intervention focus	Dose	Outcome measures
					strategies to solve conflicts and to negotiate; and norms, limits, and consequences to promote discipline
Entrenamiento familiar en habilidades educativas para la prevención de la drogodependencia (PROTEGO) Family training in educational skills for drug abuse prevention (Larriba, Durán, & Suelvez, 2004) www.pdsweb.org	Social services, educational centers, health centers, community programs for drug abuse prevention	Parents of 9- to 13-year-old children and adolescents at risk of drug abuse	Modifying the exposure to family risk and protective factors for drug abuse among high-risk children and adolescents by improving parenting skills (communication, limits, norms, monitoring)	Eight 2-hour sessions for groups	Family communication; family relationships and family conflict; family norms and limits related to drug use
Educar en positivo Positive Parenting, online program (Torres et al., 2015) educarenpositivo.es/	Website available to Spanish-speaking parents	Families with children at any age	Providing information, and online support to families and promoting positive parenting	Five training modules with web-interactive activities	Level of Internet expertise, online support, positive parenting, parental sense of competence, satisfaction with activities and modules

in the family, family norms and values, stimulation and joint leisure activities, emotional regulation, communication and conflicts, healthy peer relationships, methods for coping with daily stress, social support, family-school collaboration, and regulation of Internet use.

Most of parenting programs in Table 39.4 are developed from the ground up. Some of them, however, are culturally adapted from well-known international programs that researchers from Spanish universities endorsed as examples of evidence-based practices (e.g., the Family Competence Program). Most of the programs in Table 39.4 received public financial support for their development, implementation, and evaluation. In some cases, it has been possible to obtain funding from nongovernmental organizations (NGOs); in another (Caixa Pro-Infancia program), support is provided by a banking foundation. This financial support ensures rigorous evaluation and sustained support for the large-scale implementation of the programs. In all the group-based programs in Table 39.4, group facilitators are professionals working in public or private services who are well trained by the program staff in the program principles and content, group management, and the implementation and evaluation of the program. Finally, in all the programs in Table 39.4 quality assurance and program fidelity are enhanced by training workshops, site visits by the program staff, and online supervision.

The majority of the programs listed in Table 39.4 are delivered in a format of prevention-oriented groups (from eight to twelve participants on average), given that this approach is more cost-effective and user-friendly than individual interventions (Kumpfer, Whiteside, Greene, & Allen, 2010). Group discussions can also be a strong opportunity for nonstigmatizing support for vulnerable parents. Group interactions are aimed at constructing a joint discourse among the participants and the group facilitator, avoiding lecturing and dependency on the professional, and depend very much on the facilitator's knowledge, personal attitudes and values, and interpersonal skills (Martínez, 2009; Orte, Ballester, Amer, & Vives, 2014). The most effective parental groups are those in which the facilitator helps parents better verbalize their interpretations of family situations; enrich their interpretations by thinking about others' views; reflect upon the consequences of their own actions on family life, especially on the child's development; and promote a sense of parental competence (Rodrigo, Correa, Máiquez, Martín, & Rodríguez, 2006). There is also an increasing use of web resources in Spanish that provide online support to parents (Torres et al., 2015).

Considerable evidence indicates that variability in the implementation of prevention programs in large-scale interventions has an impact on the outcomes achieved by these programs (Berkel, Mauricio, Schoenfelder, & Sandler, 2011; Fixsen et al., 2005). Accordingly, the Spanish parenting programs in Table 39.4 have placed special emphasis on establishing the conditions that must be met to successfully implement group-based programs across sites: advertised properly as a support for positive parenting; careful group selection; training and continuity of the facilitators, coordinated with the service and program staff; transport facilities; refreshments and parallel activities for the children; cultural group activities offered alongside the program; and assurance of program fidelity in the implementation and rigorous evaluation, coordination, and integration of the program into the network of social resources when possible (Rodrigo, 2016).

The Spanish evidence-based programs presented in Table 39.4 use a variety of evaluation designs to test their effectiveness. In the following paragraphs, we select a few of the programs in Table 39.4, named by their English title, to illustrate some of the evaluation studies performed. All programs employed designs consisting of pre-post comparisons. Longitudinal designs and RCT trials are less frequently used, as they involve greater complexity and organizational support. However, an example of each one of them will be presented. Accumulating participants of several trials attending the Family Competence Program (Kumpfer et al., 2006), significant positive changes of parental outcomes after program completion were obtained in a sample of 217 families facing psychosocial risks. Positive changes included increased parental supervision and monitoring, parental involvement, parenting efficacy, parenting skills, parenting confidence, improved family relationships (e.g., communication, cohesion, organization, family conflict, and resilience), and improved children's behavioral outcomes (e.g., social skills) (Orte, Pascual, & Ballester, 2013). Longer-term positive effects on parental, family, and child outcomes have also been shown, suggesting sustained effects of the program over two years (Orte et al., 2015).

In the second example, an RCT design was applied for the evaluation of the program Learning Together, Growing Up in the Family (Amorós et al., 2011) carried out within a network of NGOs with 1,834 people, of whom 1,270 (609 parents and 661 children) completed the program, and 564 (296 parents and 268 children) were randomly assigned to the control group. The results showed that immediately after the program, and in comparison with the control group, the strict (authoritarian) style, the permissive style, and the use of criticism and rejection had significantly decreased and parental affection and communication had increased. There was also an increase in family leisure activities, satisfaction with family life improved, and greater community integration for the families, as self-reported by parents and children and by focus groups performed with parents, children, and professionals (Amorós, Balsells, Buisan, Byrne, & Fuentes-Pelaez, 2013).

There are also evaluation studies performed with the parenting programs in Table 39.4 searching for moderation effects in pretest and posttest comparisons. For example, results from the Family Education and Support program (Hidalgo et al., 2011) have shown, in a sample of 168 parents at psychosocial risk (88 in the program group and 80 in the control group) referred by social services, significant increases in parental knowledge of child development, more positive child-rearing practices, higher emotional and family self-esteem, increasing feelings of parental competence, greater perceived support, higher family cohesion and adaptability, and better children's quality of life (emotional, family and peer domains) in comparison with the control group

(Hidalgo et al., 2015). Additional analyses aimed at revealing the participant profile that most benefited from the program showed that mothers facing more negative life events experienced greater improvement in the quality of family life; also, participants with higher expectations about the program had better results in parental sense of competence, family adaptability, and size of the emotional support network. Finally, mothers with less social support showed greater improvement in emotional self-esteem, family cohesion, and parenting practices upon program completion.

Some evaluation studies for the programs in Table 39.4 are aimed at exploring patterns of individual change, for instance, those performed with the Personal and Family Support program (Rodrigo et al., 2000) in a sample of 496 parents at psychosocial risk referred by social services (Byrne, Rodrigo, & Máiquez, 2014). Cluster analyses revealed that the program worked well for 46 percent of the parents (total or partial positive changes on parental conceptions, child-rearing practices, and parental sense of competence), achieved mixed improvement for 30 percent of the parents (positive and negative changes), and worked poorly for 24 percent of the parents (negative changes). Those clusters with participants attending mixed groups (of at-risk and non-at-risk parents) benefited more from the program, suggesting that this aspect of the implementation process should be included in the analysis of program effectiveness in intervention studies (Byrne, Salmela-Aro, Read, & Rodrigo, 2013).

It is also worth noting that many programs identified in Table 39.4 use qualitative methods to complement the use of self-reported questionnaires for the evaluation and to evaluate the process during the sessions. For instance, the *Program-Guide to Develop Emotional, Educational, and Parental Competences* (Martínez, 2009) uses a variety of methods as part of data collection, such as parents' discussion groups, individual parental self-reports after the sessions, participant observation, and focus groups with parents and facilitators, to give a comprehensive picture of what is going on during the sessions and the extent to which program fidelity is achieved. The evaluation design of the program also includes quantitative self-reports obtained on parental outcomes after the program completion.

Finally, according to the standards of evidence-based programs (Fixsen et al., 2005), some intervention studies explore the impact of the quality of implementation on program results in the programs identified in Table 39.4. In the evaluation of the Parent–Child Psychological Support Program (Cerezo, 1992) performed with 594 families from the community, an impact of dose effects was found for the parental sense of competence (parental self-efficacy dimension) and the proportion of securely attached children, both of which were significantly higher in groups with medium and high program dose (Cerezo, Dasi, & Ruiz, 2013). In another study performed with the Growing Up Happily in the Family program (Rodrigo et al., 2008), which was run with 196 parents attending municipal social services, it was found that the best predictors of participants' attendance and several parental outcomes were the application of a complete program dose; adequate session duration; higher levels of interest and participation in the group dynamics; and the presence of fewer obstacles to participant adaptation to the program contents, in the logistics of the sessions, and in coordination with the services (Álvarez, Rodrigo, & Byrne, 2016). These findings illustrate the importance of identifying the optimal conditions of implementation to better adapt the program to the variety of local conditions in Spain without losing effectiveness.

Conclusions

Spain is a modern European country with a long cultural tradition of strong family bonds, high endorsement of family values, and a great investment by the family in supporting children and dependent members. Notably, these views have strongly supported the Spanish people moving firmly toward adopting a modern view of the family, as revealed in their attitudes of respect for family diversity, the promotion of more horizontal parent–child relationships, the observance of children's rights, the achievement of more gender equality and firm opposition to any form of gender violence.

For much of its history, family policy in Spain has not kept pace with the psychological and economic investment of families in child and family well-being, having favored a traditional view of the family during the dictatorship regime and moved the focus away from the family scene following the transition to democracy. The national strategic plans currently undertaken to promote child and family well-being represent a new line of family policies, underscoring the important role that positive parenting plays as a protective factor for child development and recognizing the need to provide more preventive and integrated support to families. In this regard, it is expected that the preliminary intersectoral actions described in this chapter may increase in the future, providing more comprehensive and coordinated support to families.

In the context of recent policy developments, the establishment of a framework for collaboration among policy makers, researchers, and professionals under the umbrella of the European positive parenting initiative is an important achievement. For the first time, multiple agents coming from previously disconnected areas have raised their voices in favor of the promotion of universal, selective, and indicated prevention actions in the domain of child and family services. Thanks to the active dissemination of the positive parenting framework, stakeholders now share a common language for communication about these issues, and a broad consensus has been reached on the importance of promoting preventive work with families following the "road map" provided by the positive parenting framework.

The existing network of basic and specialized municipal social services in Spain offers a promising launch pad for family-based prevention initiatives. Well-trained, motivated professionals working in multidisciplinary teams are the force that will guarantee positive results for these initiatives. Spain is also fortunate to have a robust network of NGOs and volunteer movements providing support to families facing adverse circumstances or with special needs. In fact, the fast and efficient reaction of the entire network of public and private support to families has been a real protective factor for Spanish children suffering the recent economic crisis. However, a focus on prevention activities to promote positive parenting and local community development has not (yet) been uniformly adopted in the municipal social services. For instance, there are still some services oriented solely at supporting high-need families, with the result being that multi-assisted families are targeted while the wider communities remain underresourced and underserved.

The increasing implementation of evidence-based programs in Spain under partnership schemes is an important step toward introducing the evidence-based movement in the domains of child and family services. In this regard, it is good news to see quality assurance in the provision of services increasingly being placed at the forefront of efforts by policy makers, researchers, and professionals to deliver the best evidence-based programs aimed at supporting parents. Ironically, the current economic crisis has been a positive force for the introduction of the evidence-based movement in Spain. Facing a growing emphasis on accountability for achieving results in times of funding restrictions for child and family services, decision makers such as funders and service providers are increasingly making programming choices based on the best evidence from research.

The flip side of the coin is that irrational cuts to prevention initiatives may put the entire social protection system in Spain at risk. Among other measures, it is important to guarantee the sustainability of evidence-based programs as a prevention resource for family intervention at the local level. A key element for promoting these programs' sustainability is to demonstrate that the incorporation of evidence-based programs not only produces changes in child and family well-being but also leads to positive changes in professionals' work with families and contributes to the better organization of the services.

One source of concern is the fact that there is still a weak evaluative culture in the child and family services in Spain. There is a need to better identify the Spanish parenting programs that work in different regions. In fact, we provide in this chapter the first collection of evidence-based positive parenting programs implemented in Spain. It is also important to promote more rigorous research on effective parenting programs that not only provides information about the quality of the programs but is also useful in informing social actions and social policies. In turn, professionals should be trained in the use of those best practices that are strongly supported by scientific knowledge and the professional consensus, and there must be sustained efforts to continue introducing and adapting the evidence-based approach in the child and family services. In this regard, it is also important to identify the competences required to work with families under this prevention framework, for training purposes. Finally, the family's perspective should be incorporated into the services' quality-assurance process. In sum, the introduction of a preventive approach into work with families is no longer a distant outcome in Spain but a real achievement that should be preserved and enhanced to serve all families and empower communities.

Acknowledgments

We are especially grateful to the professionals and the families who participated in the positive parenting programs. Part of the results reported was funded by the Spanish Ministry of Economy and Competitivity grants (EDU2012-38588; PSI 2012–32879).

References

II National Strategic Plan for Childhood and Adolescence (2013–16). www.observatoriodelainfancia.msssi.gob.es/documentos/pdf/II_PLAN_ESTRATEGICO_INFANCIA_English.pdf

Álvarez, M., Rodrigo, M. J., & Byrne, S. (2016). What implementation components predict positive outcomes in a parenting program? *Research on Social Work Practice*. doi: 10.1177/1049731516640903

Amorós, P., Balsells, M. A., Buisan, M., Byrne, S., & Fuentes-Pelaez, N. (2013). Implementation and evaluation of the "learning together, growing in family programme": the impact on the families. *Revista de Cercetare si Interventie Sociala* 42: 120–44.

Amorós, P., Mateos, A., Fuentes, N., Pastor, C., Rodrigo, M. J., Byrne, S., . . . Guerra, M. (2011). *Aprender Juntos, Crecer en Familia.* Barcelona: Obra Social "La Caixa."

Asmussen, K. (2011). *The Evidence-Based Parenting Practitioner's Handbook*. Abingdon, UK: Routledge.

Berkel, C., Mauricio, A. M., Schoenfelder, E., & Sandler, I. N. (2011). Putting the pieces together: an integrated model of program implementation. *Prevention Science* 12: 23–33.

Boddy, J., Smith, M., & Statham, J. (2011). Understandings of efficacy: cross-national perspectives on "what works" in supporting parents and families. *Ethics and Education* 6: 181–96.

Byrne, S., Rodrigo, M. J., & Máiquez, M. L. (2014). Patterns of individual change in a parenting program for child maltreatment and their relation to family and professional environments. *Child Abuse & Neglect* 38: 457–67.

Byrne, S., Salmela-Aro, K., Read, S., & Rodrigo, M. J. (2013). Individual and group effects in a community-Based implementation of a positive parenting program. *Research on Social Work Practice* 23: 46–56.

Cerezo, M. A. (1992). *Programa de Apoyo Psicológico Materno-Infantil (Unpublished manuscript)*. Valencia: Universitat Valéncia.

Cerezo, M. A., Dasi, C., & Ruiz, J. C. (2013). Supporting parenting infants: evaluating outcomes for parents and children in a community-based program. *Evaluation and Program Planning* 37: 12–20.

Comprehensive Plan for Family Support (2015–17). National Social Report Spain. www.google.com/?gws_rd=ssl#q=Integral+PLan+for+family+support+in+Spain

Consejería de Educación, Universidades y Sostenibilidad de Canarias (2014). Parentalidad positiva. www.gobiernodecanarias.org/noticias/Educacion_Uni

versidades_Sostenibilidad/57411/educacion-pone-marcha-programa-fomentar-competencias-parentales-desarrollo-personal

Council of Europe (2006). Recommendation Rec(2006)19 of the Committee of Ministers to member states on policy to support positive parenting. wcd.coe.int/ViewDoc.jsp?id=1073507

Daly, M. (2007). *Parenting in Contemporary Europe: A Positive Approach*. Strasbourg, France: Council of Europe.

Davis, F., McDonald, L., & Axford, N. (2012). *Technique Is Not Enough: A Framework for Ensuring That Evidence-Based Parenting Programmes Are Socially Inclusive*. Discussion Paper. Leicester, UK: British Psychological Society. www.bps.org.uk/system/files/images/tine.pdf

Del Valle, J., Canali, C., Bravo, A., & Vecchiato, T. (2013). Child protection in Italy and Spain: influence of the family supported society. *Psychosocial Intervention* 22: 227–37.

Del Valle, J. F., López, M., Montserrat, C., & Bravo, A. (2009). Twenty years of foster care in Spain: profiles, patterns and outcomes. *Children and Youth Services Review* 31: 847–53.

Delgado, M., Meil, G., & Zamora López, F. (2008). Spain: short on children and short on family policies. *Demographic Research* 19: 1059–1104.

Dolan, P., Pinkerton, J., & Canavan, J. (2006). Family support: from description to reflection. In Dolan, P., Canavan, J., & Pinkerton, J. (eds.), *Family Support as Reflective Practice*. London: Jessica Kingsley, pp. 11–26.

Durlak, J. A., & DuPre, E. P. (2008). Implementation matters: a review of research on the influence of implementation on program outcomes and the factors affecting implementation. *American Journal of Community Psychology* 41: 327–50.

Eurochild (2013). Family and parenting support in challenging times. *Round Table Report 7*. Brussels: Eurochild. www.eurochild.org/fileadmin/Events/2013/05_FPS_roundtable/Eurochild_FPS_round_table_7_May_2013_Report.pdf

European Commission (2010). EUROPE 2020: a strategy for smart, sustainable and inclusive growth. ec.europa.eu/eu2020/pdf/COMPLET%20EN%20BARROSO%20%20%20007%20-%20Europe%202020%20-%20EN%20version.pdf

Fixsen, D. L., Naoom, S. F., Blase, K. A., Friedman, R. M., & Wallace, F. (2005). *Implementation Research: A Synthesis of the Literature*. Tampa: Louis de la Parte Florida Mental Health Institute Publication.

Flay, B. R., Biglan, A., Boruch, R. F., Castro, F. G., Gottfredson, D., Kellam, S., . . . Ji, P. (2005). Standards of evidence: criteria for efficacy, effectiveness and dissemination. *Prevention Science* 6: 151–75.

Hidalgo, M. V., Menéndez, S., López, I., Sánchez, J., & Lorence, B. (2011). *Programa de Formación y Apoyo Familiar*. Sevilla: Ayuntamiento de Sevilla.

Hidalgo, M. V., Menéndez, S., López-Verdugo, I., Sánchez, J., Lorence, B., & Jiménez, L. (2015). Programa de formación y apoyo familiar. In Rodrigo, M. J. (ed.), *Manual práctico de parentalidad positiva*. Madrid: Síntesis.

Johnson, M., & Austin, M. J. (2005). *Evidence-Based Practice in the Social Services*. Berkeley: University of California, Berkeley, School of Social Welfare.

Kaminski, J. W., Valle, L., Filene, J., & Boyle, C. (2008). A meta-analytic review of components associated with parent training program effectiveness. *Journal of Abnormal Child Psychology* 36: 567–89.

Kellam, S. G., & Langevin, D. J. (2003). A framework for understanding "evidence" in prevention research and programs. *Prevention Science* 4: 137–53.

Kumpfer, K. L., & Alvarado, R. (2003). Family-strengthening approaches for the prevention of youth problem behaviors. *American Psychologist* 58: 457–65.

Kumpfer, K. L., Orte, C., March, M. X., Ballester, L., Touza, C., Fernández, C., Oliver, J. L., Fernández, M. C., & Mestre, L. (2006). *Programa de competencia familiar: Manuel de implementación del formador y de la formadora*. Palma de Mallorca: Universitat de les Illes Balears.

Kumpfer, K. L., Whiteside, H. O., Greene, J. A., & Allen, K. C. (2010). Effectiveness outcomes of four age versions of the Strengthening Families Program in statewide field sites. *Group Dynamics: Theory, Research, and Practice* 14: 211–29.

Larriba, J., Duran, A., & Suelves, J. M. (2004). *PROTEGO: Entrenamiento familiar en habilidades educativas para prevenir conductas de riesgo en la adolescencia*. Barcelona: Promoción y Desarrollo social.

Máiquez, M. L., Rodrigo, M. J., Padilla, S., Rodríguez, B., Byrne, S., & Pérez, L. (2009). *Programa domiciliario Crecer Felices en Familia*. Valladolid: Junta de Castilla y León.

Martínez, R. A. (2009). *Programa-Guía para el desarrollo de competencias emocionales, educativas y parentales*. Madrid: Ministerio de Sanidad, Política Social e Igualdad.

Meil, G. (2006). Welfare policies, work and family lives in modern Spain. In Rossi, G. (ed), *Reconciling Family and Work: New Challenges for Social Policies in Europe*. Milan: Franco Angeli, pp. 37–58.

Meil, G., & Iglesias de Ussel, J. (2001). *La política familiar en España*. Barcelona: Ariel.

Menéndez, S., Hidalgo, M. V., Jiménez, L., Lorence, B., & Sánchez, J. (2010). Perfil psicosocial de familias en situación de riesgo. *Un estudio de necesidades con usuarias de los Servicios Sociales Comunitarios por razones de preservación familiar.* Anales de Psicología 26: 378–89.

Ministerio de Sanidad, Servicios Sociales e Igualdad. Gobierno de España (2016). Parentalidad positiva: Ganar salud y bienestar de 0-3 años. www.msssi.gob.es/profesionales/saludPublica/prevPromocion/Estrategia/Parentalidad_Positiva.htm

National Action Plan on Social Inclusion for the Kingdom of Spain (2013–16). www.msssi.gob.es/destacados/docs/PNAIN_2013_2016_EN.pdf

Orte, C., Ballester, L., Amer, J., & Vives, M. (2014). Assessing the role of facilitators in evidence-based family prevention programs via Delphi technique. *Families in Society, the Journal of Contemporary Social Services* 95: 236–44.

Orte, C., Ballester, L., March, M. X., Amer, J., Vives, M., & Pozo, R. (2015). The Strengthening Families Program in Spain: a long-term evaluation. *Journal of Children's Services* 10: 101–19.

Orte, C., Pascual, B., & Ballester, L. (2013). Educación para la prevención. *Resultados de un programa de competencias familiares*. Revista Iberoamericana de Educación 61(3): 1–8.

Palacios, J., & Amorós, P. (2006). Recent changes in adoption and fostering in Spain. *British Journal of Social Work* 36: 921–35.

PISA (Programme for International Student Assessment) (2012). www.oecd.org/pisa/keyfindings/PISA-2012-results-spain-ESP.pdf

Prevention and Health Promotion Strategy of the Spanish National Health System (2013). www.msssi.gob.es/profesionales/saludPublica/prevPromocion/Estrategia/docs/ExecutiveSummary.pdf

Projecte tècnic de Medi Obert de Justícia Juvenil (2013). Department de Justícia de la Generalitat de Catalunya. justicia.gencat.cat/web/.content/home/ambits/formacio__recerca_i_docum/formacio/gestcon/comunitats_de_practica/medi_obert_de_justicia_juvenil/projecte_tecnic_medi_obert.pdf

Proyecto apego (2014). Promoción de la parentalidad positiva en el sistema sanitario público de la Comunidad Autónoma de Andalucía. www.janela-aberta-familia.org/es/content/apego-promocion-de-la-parentalidad-positiva-en-el-sistema-sanitario-publico-andaluz

Rodrigo, M. J. (2010). Promoting positive parenting in Europe: new challenges for the European Society for Developmental Psychology. *European Journal of Developmental Psychology* 7: 281–94.

Rodrigo, M. J. (2016). Quality of implementation in evidence-based positive parenting programs in Spain: introduction to the special issue. Psychosocial Intervention, 25: 63–68. doi.org/10.1016/j.psi.2016.02.004

Rodrigo, M. J., Almeida, A., & Reichle, B. (2016). Evidence-based parent education programs: a European perspective. In Ponzetti, J. (ed.), *Evidence-Based Parenting Education: A Global Perspective*. London: Routledge, pp. 85–104.

Rodrigo, M. J., Amorós, P., Arranz, E., Hidalgo, V., Máiquez, M. L., Martín, J. C., Martínez, R. A., & Ochaita, E. (2016). *Guía de Buenas Prácticas en Parentalidad Positiva.* Madrid: Federación Española de Municipios y Provincias (FEMP). www.familiasenpositivo.es/es/system/files/guia_de_buenas_practicas_2015.pdf

Rodrigo, M. J., & Byrne, S. (2011). Social support and personal agency in at-risk mothers. *Psychosocial Intervention* 20: 13–24.

Rodrigo, M. J., Byrne, S., & Álvarez, M. (2012). Preventing child maltreatment through parenting programmes implemented at the local social services level. *European Journal of Developmental Psychology* 9: 89–103.

Rodrigo, M. J., Byrne, S., & Rodríguez, B. (2014). Parenting styles and child well-being. In Ben-Arieh, A., Casas, F., Frønes, I., & Korbin, J. E. (eds.), *Handbook of Child Well-Being,* vol. 4. New York: Springer, pp. 2173–96.

Rodrigo, M. J., Capote, C., Máiquez, M. L., Martín, J. C., Rodríguez, G., Guimerá, P., & Peña, M. (2000). *Programa Educar en Familia.* Valladolid: Junta de Castilla y León.

Rodrigo, M. J., Correa, A. D., Máiquez, M. L., Martín, J. C., & Rodríguez, G. (2006). Family preservation services in Canary Islands: predictors of the efficacy of a parenting program for families at-risk of social exclusion. *European Psychologist* 11: 57–70.

Rodrigo, M. J., Máiquez, M. L., & Martín, J. C. (2010a). *La educación parental como recurso psicoeducativo para el apoyo de la parentalidad positiva.* Madrid: Federación Española de Municipios y Provincias (FEMP). www.msssi.gob.es/ssi/familiasInfancia/docs/eduParentalRecEducativo.pdf

Rodrigo, M. J., Máiquez, M. L., & Martín, J. C. (2010b). *Parentalidad positiva y políticas locales de Apoyo a las familias. Orientaciones para favorecer el ejercicio de las responsabilidades parentales desde las corporaciones locales.* Madrid: Federación Española de Municipios y Provincias (FEMP). www.msssi.gob.es/ssi/familiasInfancia/docs/folletoParentalidad.pdf

Rodrigo, M. J., Máiquez, M. L., & Martín, J. C. (2011). *Buenas prácticas profesionales para el apoyo a la parentalidad positiva.* Madrid: Federación Española de

Municipios y Provincias (FEMP). www.msssi.gob.es/ssi/familiasInfancia/docs/BuenasPractParentalidadPosit iva.pdf

Rodrigo, M. J., Máiquez, M. L., Byrne, S., Rodríguez, B., Martín, J.C., Rodríguez, G., & Pérez, L. (2008). *Programa Crecer Felices en Familia. Programa de apoyo psicoeducativo para promover el desarrollo infantil.* Valladolid: Junta de Castilla y León.

Rodrigo, M. J., Martín, J. C., Máiquez, M. L., Álvarez, M., Byrne, S., González, A., Guerra, M., Montesdeoca, M. A., & Rodríguez, B. (2010c). *Programa Vivir la adolescencia en familia. Programa de apoyo psicoeducativo para promover la convivencia familiar.* Toledo: Junta de Comunidades de Castilla La Mancha.

Torío, S., Peña, J. V., Rodríguez, M. C., Fernández, C. M., Molina, S., Hernández, J., & Inda, M. M. (2013). *Programa de Educación Parental "Construir lo cotidiano."* Barcelona: Octaedro.

Torres, A., Suarez, A., Álvarez, M., Padilla, S., Rodríguez, E., & Rodrigo, M. J. (2015). Apoyo parental online. In Rodrigo, M. J. (ed.), *Manual práctico de parentalidad positiva.* Madrid: Síntesis.

UNICEF (2013). *Child Wellbeing in Rich Countries: A Comparative Overview.* Innocenti Report Card 11. Florence, Italy: UNICEF Office of Research.

Africa & the Middle East

40 An Investigation of HIV/AIDS-Related Stigma, Blame, and Shame in Swaziland

Adebowale Akande, Bolanle E. Adetoun, Modupe Adewuyi, Titilola Akande, M. M. Tserere, K. A. Bates, & K. M. Nyama

Introduction

> No human destruction on the face of earth has been more devastating than HIV/AIDS global crisis
>
> (Oranyan, 2005).

> A hospital administrator spoke with a man known to be infected with HIV. Throughout their conversation, the man continually played with a pencil lying on the administrator's desk. Afterwards, the administrator was reluctant to use this pencil and finally threw it away. She admitted that the pencil evoked negative feelings despite her realization that there was no possible danger of contracting HIV/AIDS from it
>
> (Pryor & Reeder, 1993).

> Now Adam slept with his wife, Eve, and she became pregnant. . ...
>
> (Genesis 4:1).

It is universally accepted that two people can enjoy sexual relations for pleasure and love, but pleasure always come with all its associated risks. The aftermath of relations may be the possibility of getting a sexually transmitted infection (STI), a kind of which may be human immunodeficiency syndrome (HIV) – the most insidious disease or pandemic in this period of human history. The current chapter will describe stigma and shame related to HIV/AIDS and mental illness in southern Africa and report on a survey study dealing with HIV-related stigma, as conducted in Swaziland.

Current Situation in Swaziland (Southern Africa)

Swaziland (eSwatini) is a kingdom and a small landlocked nation in the southern African region, which is still experiencing an epidemic of HIV infection where one in four adults is living with HIV. Its capitals are Mbabane (administration) and Lombanba (government) as the legislative and royal capital. The population is about 1.4 million people, most of whom see the Swazi royal family as their spiritual authority. Swazi ethnic group is the majority in the population, which also consists of a few Zulu and White people of British and Afrikaner origin.

The Swazis are part of the four Nguni family of South African tribes, which also speak four major languages that include the siSwati, isiZulu, isiXhosa, and isiNdebele. In the early days, more than 1.5 million members of the Nguni group known as the Swazi, with almost one million in Swaziland and the rest in South Africa, were settled around the KaNgwane homestead. However, after the beheading of their king, Dingiswayo (Ngwane I), in a bitter war (1817), the mainstream Swazis withdrew and fled into the mountainous terrain that today is known as the Kingdom of Swaziland.

Swaziland probably has the highest prevalence rates of HIV and tuberculosis (TB) in the world. More than 30 percent of Swaziland's able-bodied adult population (aged eighteen to forty-nine years) is infected with HIV. Of these adults, more than 85 percent of the transmission occurred through heterosexual contact (UNAIDS, 2010). Migration and poverty are rampant in the Kingdom as well as in many other countries in southern Africa. While AIDS is bad and has wreaked havoc on the entire sub-Saharan African continent (see Figure 40.1), it is much worse in the southern African region, mostly in Swaziland, South Africa, and Botswana (see Figure 40.1). This is due to a set of factors that include much younger populations, small rates of male circumcision, fewer sexual partners using condoms, more ulcerative STIs, cultural taboos, slow access to antiretroviral treatment (ARVs), and more prostitutes who create sexual network epicenters that are efficacious at spreading infection as a result of sexual relations. Historical facts, while useful as a backdrop to appreciate current circumstances, are equally useful with new efforts to understand the migration to South Africa's *egoli* goldmines and reduce poverty in southern Africa. Since the formation of an economic community named, SADC, southern Africa is a new geo-entity with a new vision and mission to promote regional integration and trade, with goals of playing a key role not only in Africa but in the entire world.

Swaziland invariably has one of the highest global rates of HIV. There is still misperception and miscommunication about the transmission and prevention of HIV/AIDS, as polygamy is common. There is a concomitant increase in the public health problem in Swaziland, as physical and moral appearances are crucial to being accepted in society. Shame, stigmatization, prejudice, and fears are still common among people living with HIV/AIDS (PLWHA) given the alarming rate of increase of HIV cases. Ever since the first diagnosis of the disease in the mid-1980s, there has been overt discrimination and different reactions against PLWHA among families, at workplaces, and in the communities. It has been argued that due to low socioeconomic status and gender inequalities, Swazi women have been disempowered and unable to insist on condom use, hence becoming extremely vulnerable to HIV and other STIs. Among women in the world, African women from patriarchal structures and societies (e.g., Swaziland) have the highest risk for contracting HIV (Ramjee & Daniels, 2013). Paradoxically, these women never see themselves to be at risk nor perceive the necessity to engage in safe-sex practices.

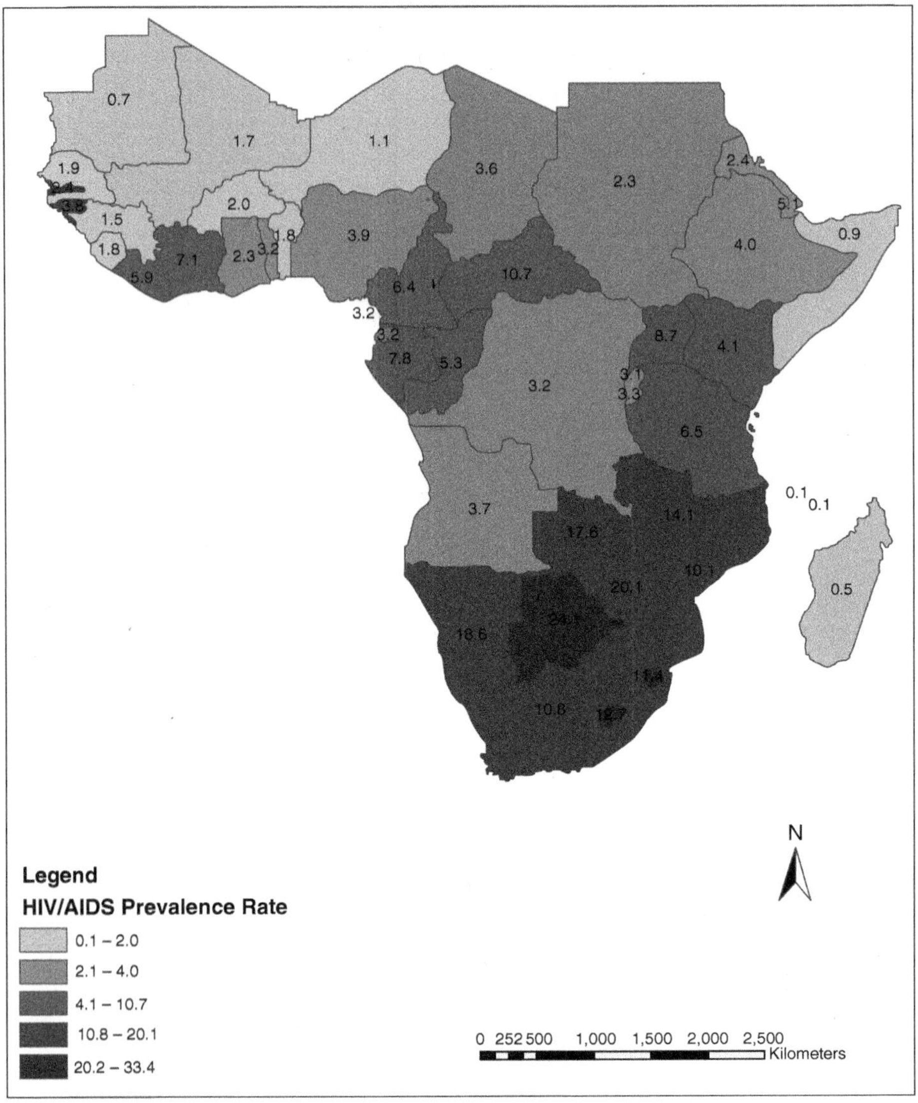

Figure 40.1. *Adapted Africa continental HIV prevalence rate.*

HIV/AIDS-Related Stigma and Its Measurement

Some theorists have stated that AIDS has certain traits that spark and ignite a high level of stigma (Baral, Karki, & Newell, 2007; Parker & Aggleton, 2003). It also carries a high level of fear, as AIDS contraction is associated with risky sexual behavior and the fear of psychological and somatic consequences of catching the noncurable disease (Akande & Ross, 1994; Amuri, Mitchell, Cockroft, & Andersson, 2011). In sub-Saharan Africa, heterosexual sex is the main route of HIV infection (the ticking time bomb). In recent history, no other health or medical event has caused such personal and public fear and stigma as HIV/AIDS. The reduction of stigma and discrimination is a prerequisite for effective prevention and care and reaffirms that discrimination on the grounds of one's HIV status is a stigma. The firsthand experience of HIV/AIDS stigma and discrimination is ubiquitous across individuals and cultures; in fact, it exists worldwide. The differences are simply manifested in different ways across geopolitical entities, cultures, societies, religious groups, and people.

AIDS-related stigma, or AIDS stigma, is the feeling of prejudice, discounting, discrediting, and discrimination directed at people living with HIV/AIDS (PLWHA). Stigma, a human reaction, is the extreme disapproval of, or discontent with, individuals on the grounds of characteristics that distinguish them from other members of a community. Stigma is also a mark of disgrace associated to a particular circumstance, person, or event (Piot, Bartos, Ghys, Walker, & Schwartlander, 2002). One way to elucidate more fully how a priori attitudes are like a "retrograde force" that can subvert prevention goals is to know how PLWHA are dehumanized and devalued. Throughout history, many diseases have carried considerable stigma, including leprosy, TB, cancer, mental illness, and many sexually transmitted diseases. HIV/AIDS is only the latest disease to be stigmatized. Hence innumerable PLWHA live in a shadow world, unwilling or unable to go public with their infections because they fear losing their jobs, their friends, or the new acquaintances. They also fear being labeled, negatively stereotyped, and rejected by negative discrimination, and experience status loss, compulsory HIV testing without prior consent, and the devaluing of their social identity (Awofeso, 2011; Decety, Echols, & Correll, 2009). The stigma that still surrounds the disease "can affect behavior, including delayed HIV testing, putting off needed care, and not disclosing status to medical providers" (Adeokun, Okonkwo, & Ladipo, 2006). HIV stigma is often layered on top of many other stigmas associated with such specific groups as homosexuals and commercial sex workers and such behaviors as drug abuse using needles and casual sex. These behaviors are perceived as controllable, and therefore such groups are assigned more blame and receive less sympathy, and instead arouse more anger; such groups are also less likely to receive assistance than people with AIDS who were infected through circumstances where there was no control, such as through a blood transfusion. Myths still abound about how HIV is transmitted.

Stigma and discrimination are as old as the pandemic itself. The experience of AIDS is not limited to the symptoms of the killer disease. It is officially accompanied by what Novick (1997) called a "second epidemic" or likened to what is termed a "second illness," that is, the reactions of the social milleu, the stigma associated with the pandemic. This strangely stigma-sensitive syndrome is also encapsulated by the "layers of stigma" it is made of (Jurgensen, 2013; Sandelowski, Barrosso, & Volls, 2009). There is evidence from the onset that stigma, silence, fear, and discrimination have fueled the transmission of HIV and have greatly increased the negative impact associated with the epidemic. Stigmatization is "a dimension of suffering added to the pandemic experience," and has been observed to also lead to social isolation, limited life changes, and delayed help-seeking behavior (Schulze & Angermeyer, 2003).

The current picture of the AIDS stigma panorama is that it is rampant on the African, Asian, and Latin American continents (the Southern hemisphere); looms large in the entire (southern) African society; and continues to be manifested in every geopolitical entity of the world, layering with gender, race, ethnicity, sexual-orientation, and class. The epidemic has decimated entire communities, and communities and societies around the globe are paralyzed by it every day. Activists claimed governments were "fiddling while Rome burned," thus posing major challenges to preventing further infection, alleviating impact, and providing adequate care, support, and treatment.

In addition to this observation, stigma has silenced open, free, and unhindered discussions about the cause and appropriate interventions necessary. Visibility and candor are necessary for successful mobilization of the citizenry, societies, and governments to respond effectively to the pandemic. A similar line of reasoning guided researchers such as Arrindell and van der Ende (1986) and Decety, Echols, and Correll (2009) to suggest that stigma promotes concealment, which in turn leads people to a sense of denial of a problem (unjustified overgeneralizations or misleading undergeneralizations), which consequently causes unnecessary delays in taking action. Hence, PLWHA are looked at as a problem rather than being part of the solution to achieve public health goals to overcome the epidemic.

Responses to the AIDS epidemic can be placed along a continuum of prevention, lifesaving care, and treatment, with each side of the response resulting in stigmatization, underpinned by many factors. These include misperceptions of and misconceptions about the transmission of HIV, among others. This state of affairs has led to various human rights violations, discrimination, and prejudice, which in turn affect the well-being of PLWHA and cause fears, which affect socially sensitive issues such as sexuality, disease and death, and drug use.

With the aforementioned facts, there is strong evidence to suggest that over the past decades, prevention experts have shied away from interventions targeting people living with HIV/AIDS because of a strong concern about further stigmatization of this already socially devalued and dehumanized group. UNAIDS (2010) estimated that in 2008 more than 33 million people were living with this lethal disease, and more than 2.4 million people had been killed by the disease in that one year. Today, with the face of the pandemic changing the world over, and with the availability of highly active antiretroviral therapy (HAART) to take care of people living with the disease, AIDS is no longer a subacute and fatal lethal weapon; it is a manageable, but chronic, disease (Thorpe, 2009).

The frantic threat of AIDS has triggered a worrying stress response to the perceived threat of catching the disease (CDC, 2011). Key behaviors characterizing the stress response are avoidance, extreme precautions, and verbal expression of fear concerning HIV/AIDS. Regardless of the scientific evidence for the low risk of exposure to this infection, many individuals and professionals still demonstrate terrible stigma.

At the present, suggestive evidence shows that stigma has been a sufficiently complex construct to make any simple hypothesis unsustainable, that is, a "mark" on an individual's identity (prejudice, discounting, discrediting, and overt discrimination) that glues PLWA, their loved ones, their affiliations, and their neighborhoods to undesirable characteristics and labels (Markowitz, 2005). Stigmatizing attitudes can turn to public stigma, perceived illegitimacy, and a strong sense of negativity or devalued social identity toward individuals suffering in a stigmatizing condition (Herek & Capitanio, 1998; Rusch, Angermeyer, & Corrigan, 2005). Of course, in this case, this "socially constructed experience," misinformation, and incorrect conceptualizations about HIV/AIDS and the disease's wrongly assumed association with marginalized and morally bankrupt people of the society have led to negativity and stigmatizing attitudes, thoughts, and behaviors toward PLWHA. Indeed, PLWA are judged with anger and blame and are stigmatized and socially rejected. In Africa, mental illness is believed to have a genetic or biological cause, and people with mental illness are perceived as dangerous. Likewise, AIDS is perceived as a disease of shame, punishment, or judgment from God, and PLWA are seen to be solely responsible for their "sins or misfortune" and as such the societal people are more likely to keep their distance from them (Rao, Angell, Lam, & Corrigan, 2008; Tsai & Venkataramani, 2015). The discrimination or ostracism against this group of people may include verbal and physical abuse; rape; denial of public utilities; refusal of medical care and social services; and total rejection by spouse, families, and friends (Dlamini, 2007). PLWA may even be murdered (e.g., a South African woman was butchered by her community for AIDS activism and overt disclosure of her HIV positive status, and another African woman shared her view about her HIV+ serostatus status rather than keep it private and was gang-raped and later killed by a vicious group of eight women haters).

Research Study of PLWA and Stigma in Swaziland

Discrimination may occur when attention is focused on a group of people who become potential targets for prejudice (Gibbons & Ashdown, 2010). Stigma is often associated with concepts such as discrimination, secrecy, ignorance, fear, and lack of human rights, and there is interdependence among these concepts (Arrindell & van der Ende, 1986; Brown, Macintyre, & Tujillo, 2003; Kalipeni, 2012; Yeboah, 2007). However, for the purpose of the study described in this chapter, the focus will be on fear, discrimination, and stigma.

Many studies conducted by Ollendick along with other researchers (Akande, Adewuyi, Akande, & Adetoun, 2016; Akande & Ollendick, 1997; Akande & Ross, 1994; Bastian & Haslam, 2006; Downing, 2008; Garrett, Smith, Chiu, & Young, 2016; Godlonton & Thornton, 2012; Ingman, Ollendick, & Akande, 1999; Polansky, M., Teti, M., Chengappa, R., & Aaron, E., 2015; Rao et al., 2008; Sabone, 2015) have shown that attitudes (especially stigmatizing attitudes) are influenced by societal, cultural, and psychological factors. In addition, inaccurate understanding about HIV transmission, misinformation, misperceptions, and folk conceptualizations about HIV can distort educating the public about the illness and thus lead to stigmatizing behaviors (Goffman, 1963). PLWA are often perceived to be morally flawed. Ollendick, Yang, King, Dong, and Akande (1996) concluded that, "although such global cross-cultural differences fail to attend to potentially important ethnic and geographic influences within ... these countries, they do demonstrate the overall influence of culture – the person-made part of the human environment – on behavior problems (i.e. fear, stigma, discrimination, anxiety, worries, and depression of AIDS or HIV infection)" (p. 213).

Health education models such as the Health Belief Model (Janz & Becker, 1984), protection-motivation theory (Floyds, Prentice-Dunns, & Rogers, 2000), and Theory of Planned Behavior (Ajzen & Madden, 1986) emphasize the importance of attitudes and beliefs in health promotion and the prevention of disease, such as HIV/AIDS. Such models require that for effective risk reduction, individuals must see the disease as being serious and avoidable, themselves as being at risk, and the benefits of preventive actions as overweighing the costs.

Link, Feingold, Charap, Freeman, and Shevlov (1988) put emphasis on measurement of HIV stigma to be also important in the provision of health educational services to PLWA, as there have been reports of services being refused or inferior care being given. In health care contexts, particularly in situations where HIV is epidemic, this may have profound implications for both health care and health education (Neal et al., 2012).

The *Fear of AIDS Scale* (FAIDSS) was developed by Arrindell et al. (1989) to measure level and dimensionality of personal concerns about acquiring AIDS. FAIDSS items were derived from the Fear Survey Schedule and based on previous research on the content of AIDS fears, stigma, and discrimination. The scale was developed and tested in three Western societies (the Netherlands, the United States, and Australia). Although there has been a plethora of studies examining AIDS stigma, most studies have examined the zero-order relation between behavior and AIDS stigma without examining in detail the exact behavior and the mediating effects of participants' perception of their behavior. In our research, we sought first to compare the results of the earlier studies with the results obtained from a substantially different population of participants. Second, we investigated the cross-cultural experience of stigmatization, measurement of current attitudes (stigma), and degree and dimensions of personal concern about acquiring HIV among southern African participants. Of specific interest are the participants in Swaziland.

Comparability factors are a necessity for valid cross-cultural comparison, and this may be done by showing the equivalence of psychological concepts and data across geopolitical entities to attain what Frijda and Jahoda (1966) called dimensional identity (termed comparative dimensionality by Eysenck and Eysenck, (1983). In order to eschew "bias" or "lack of equivalence" of our scores, the logic of comparison required dimensional identity of which a comparison is made. Violating this condition is termed as qualitative bias

(Bijnen, Van der Net, & Poortinga, 1986). Hence, in the study we provided evidence of the metric identity of our data and concepts across the nations, in order to test our generalizability and applicability (Arrindell et al., 1989). We conducted our local (emic) study from within a culture – that is, Swaziland – and then integrate the results until a valid and usable framework for comparison was attained (named a derived etic). We avoided external, culturally inappropriate concepts, tests, or methods. As different cultures "cut their pie of experience somewhat differently," we integrate the local data from the cultures we are comparing to each other, on a common baseline, in order to ensure we attained "evidence of data equivalence across cultural groups" (Arrindell et al., 1989; Earnshaw & Quinn, 2011).

Research Methods

Review material. We gathered germane information for the study from many sources and undertook a review of reports that were available as of October 2015. First, we conducted a computerized search of most major academic databases (e.g., Bielefeld Academic Search Engine [BASE], Ebsco, PubMed, Springlink Web of Science, Embase, Medline, PsycINFO, ERIC, Social Science Citation Index, local SABINET, and Dissertation Abstracts International using key words such as *HIV [social aspects of AIDS-related stigma], HIV [AIDS] discrimination/stigma*, and *blame*). Consequently, we further searched all available years of all journals/periodicals relevant to the topic. Thereafter, we checked cross-references in the obtained reports and sent requests for information and technical assistance to all of our research collaborators to assess relevant seminal and well-respected materials relevant to the topic. In addition, we used authors' own experience in previous related studies

Participants. Participants were all students at three institutions in Mbabani, Matsapha, and Manzini, Swaziland. The colleges were chosen to be typical of the ethnic, religious, and socioeconomic mix of these major centers of the population. Different methods were employed to recruit participants. These included visiting dormitories to recruit students, distributing questionnaires during and after laboratory class time, and attending student meetings. Completing the questionnaire took each participant ten to fifeen minutes. More than 290 computer studies, commerce, nursing, and health-related students completed the questionnaire, but only 248 met the criteria for selection and only their data were analyzed. The criteria for selection was only students enrolled full-time first semester of 2009 or earlier. These students were included in the sample on the premise that students who had been enrolled less than one semester would not have had adequate exposure for a valid evaluation of the questionnaire distributed. The participants were composed of 111 male and 127 female (data on gender were missing for the remainder). Their ages range from twenty-one to twenty-three years old (M = 22.3 years). All participants were volunteers, and almost all those approached agreed to complete the scale. Just like in most cities of the world, most people in Mbabani, Manzini, and

Matsapha, have heard about the HIV/AIDS epidemic, but their knowledge about the transmission of the disease is misperceived and not comprehensive. With few known prior studies in Swaziland's four regional geographic strata or districts (Hhohho, Manzini, Lubombo, and Shiselweni) to assess the dimensions of AIDS stigma, Swaziland regions appear a good choice for a pioneering research on AIDS stigma. In addition, all participants personally knew someone with HIV/AIDS, and each of them gave informed consent but was not paid for his or her participation.

Measures. Participants were given the adapted FAIDSS adapted from Arrindell et al, (1989), which gave attention to the tripartite model of attitude structure (e.g., Rosenber & Howland, 1960) before judging the conceptual validity of the scale. The FAIDSS was originally based on Wolpe and Lang's Fear Survey Schedule (FSS-III) in order to get "responses of fear to experiences related to the existence of HIV/AIDS" (Arrindell et al., 1989; Wolpe & Lang, 1977). The scale is a measure of current attitudes (stigma), things and experiences that may cause fear or other unpleasant feelings, and the degree and dimensions of personal concern about acquiring AIDS/HIV. The items covered a wide range of fears, for example, fears of stigma and discrimination; sex or extramarital sexual contact; frequent anonymous sexual contacts; death and medical intervention; loss of physical attractiveness; contact with outgroups or outsiders (and other variables of stigma); loss of self-respect/control; and, of course, fear of HIV infection via blood or illness (symbolic prejudice). Existing explorations of FAIDSS reliability (Bell, Molitor, & Flynn, 1999; Starks, Rendina, Breslow, Parsons, & Golub, 2013) indicate that it is adequately valid and reliable statistically as well as straightforward and quick to administer.

Procedure. Students were given brief instructions on how to complete the questionnaire. It was made clear that the questionnaires were anonymous, that there were no right or wrong answers, and that they were asked to answer questions honestly. They were assured that the anonymous questionnaires would be analyzed by a team of international researchers. Attempts were made to debrief students about the study immediately after they completed the questionnaire.

Analytic strategy. Analysis of quantitative data was conducted using the SPSS^{X}PC package (version 15). Factor analysis was carried out using maximum-likelihood extraction followed by oblique rotation (direct oblimin, delta = 0). Because cutoffs of eigenvalues of > 1 lead to overextraction, decisions were based on scree test and rotating to the maximum number of factor,s which provided factors with three or more loadings ≥ 0.30 as suggested by Arrindell et al. (1989). Based on this criterion, five factors were extracted. Bartlett's test of sphericity indicted that the population correlation matrix was not an identity (33689.6, $p < 0.00001$), and the Kaiser-Meyer-Otkin measure of sampling adequacy (0.95) was extremely high, with only 3.7 percent of elements of the anti-image correlation matrix being > 0.09, indicating that factor analysis was appropriate for these data (see Akande & Ross, 1994).

Factor-scored scales were constructed by multiplying the item score by the loading, and compared across gender and age (split into two groups at the median) using *t*-test. Reliabilities of these scales were computed by Cronbach's Alpha coefficient. Factor comparison was carried out using the FACTOREP program (Walkey & McCormick, 1985), which computes Cattell's s index (Boyle, 1984; Cattell, Balcar, Horn, & Nesselrode, 1969) between the factor solution for different samples. This statistic enables an examination of the similarities between factor solutions to be computed for different samples by comparing the loadings above a predetermined hyperplane cutoff point for the items in the scale across the number of factors obtained. The three FAIDSS samples used for comparison were two samples for Australian health professionals (ns = 134 and 66) and one of the Australian nursing students (n = 220), previously reported by Ross and Hunter (1992) and compared using the *s* index with an identical methodology. In the present study, hyperplane cutoffs of 0.35 were used as the most appropriate based on the experience of Ross and Hunter (1992), who found that for the FAIDSS there was little difference between hyperplane cutoffs of 0.40 and 0.37, apart from a finer degree of discrimination between rotated matrices for the 0.35 hyperplane cutoff.

Results

Results of the factor analysis are shown in Table 40.1. The first factor extracted was described as a Loss of Control factor; the second as a Fear of Sex factor; and the third as a Contact with Outsiders or Stigmatized Groups factor. The fourth factor was described as Fear of Infection or symbolic prejudice and context and variables associated with HIV stigma, and the final factor was a Fear of Death and dying factor. Factor intercorrelations are presented in Table 40.2, and illustrate that the factor solution was moderately correlated.

Factor scores on the five scales are shown in Table 40.3. There were significant differences on the factor scale measuring Fear of Sex, with females and younger respondents having significantly greater fear, and on the scale measuring Fear of Outsiders, males scored significantly higher than females. Table 40.3 also indicates that reliabilities of the five scales were Factor 1, 0.83; Factor 2, 0.68; Factor 3, 0.61; Factor 4, 0.77; and Factor 5, 0.68.

Results of the comparison of the rotated matrix of the Swazi sample with the three sample matrices of Ross and Hunter (1992) are presented in Table 40.4. There are accurate and significant matches for factors with the first Australian sample of health workers and, with the exception of one split match for each of the respective samples, also accurate and significant matches. These two exceptions out of a possible fifteen accurate matches illustrate the high level of comparability between the factor structures of the Swazi and three Melbourne samples.

Discussion

These data are based on a large proportional sample and on an analytic technique for which there is evidence of appropriate robustness for the sample.

Table 40.1 *Factor Structure of FAIDDS in Swaziland*

Item	Loading
Factor I: Loss of control	
Helplessness	0.64
Hopelessness	0.62
Loss of self-respect	0.61
Becoming dependent on others (not financially)	0.71
Infecting others with one's illness	0.62
Becoming mentally ill	0.61
Display of physical suffering of others	0.61
Becoming physically unattractive	0.61
Inadequate (abnormal) behavior	0.52
Infection through blood	0.41
Infection through someone's illness	0.40
Infection through sexual contact	0.40
Having contact with blood of other human beings	0.32
Drugs or chemicals	0.31
(28.1% of variance)	
Factor 2: Fear of infection or symbolic prejudice	
Sexual contact with different partners	0.71
Frequent anonymous sexual contacts	0.61
Having extramarital sexual contacts	0.62
Sexual intercourse	0.47
Having sexual contact with a prostitute	0.48
Having sexual contact with bisexual men or women	0.34
(4.5% of variance)	
Factor 3: Context with outsiders and variables associated with HIV stigma	
Having nonintimate contact (e.g., talking to a prostitute)	0.51
Having nonintimate contact (e.g., talking with homosexual men or women)	0.50
Intimate contact (e.g., kissing on the cheek) with acquaintances, family members or friends	0.51
Having nonintimate contact (e.g., talking to) with bisexual men or women	0.52
Having physical contact with sick patients (medically ill people)	0.50
Anxiety over being HIV+	0.61
Depressive symptoms over being HIV+	0.61
CD4 count and viral load	0.61
Judged negatively by a health caregiver for trying to have baby	0.62
Judged negatively by a heath caregiver for trying to fall pregnant	0.61
Judged negatively by a friend or colleague	0.59
Judged negatively by an extended family member	0.61
Risk of disclosing HIV status	0.59

Table 40.1 (*cont.*)

Item	Loading
Being HIV+ and pregnant	0.62
Being underestimated because of HIV status	0.61
Foreigners	–0.63
Taking medical tests	0.51
Having physical contact with people who you know are addicted to drugs	0.44
Getting an injection	0.24
(5.1% of variance)	
Factor 4: Infection and contact with infected people	
Contracting AIDS	–0.61
Contracting venereal disease	–0.70
Having physical contact with a person with AIDS	–0.63
Viruses	–053
Undergoing blood transfusions	–0.41
Having sexual contact with homosexual men or women	–0.41
(2.4% of variance)	
Factor 5: Death	
Death	–0.72
Dying	–0.61
Growing ill	–0.31
(1.0% of variance)	

Table 40.2 *Intercorrelations between FAIDSS Factors*

	Factor 1	Factor 2	Factor 3	Factor 4
Factor 2	0.37			
Factor 3	0.41	0.31		
Factor 4	0.52	0.37	0.37	
Factor 5	0.41	0.23	0.33	0.37

All $p < 0.001$.

While it is difficult to generalize to nontertiary (community) educated Swazi people, there are nevertheless some clear implications both for the use of the FAIDSS cross-culturally and for the targeting of HIV prevention programs in Swaziland's four regions.

First, the factor structure is very similar to that obtained by Ross and Hunter (1992) in Melbourne health professionals (a group with a education level similar to the present sample) in both the number of factors extracted using the same rotational approach and the factor content. The factor comparison analysis indicates that there is a significant and very accurate match between the factor solutions obtained with three previously reported Australian samples on the

Table 40.3. *Factor Scores by Sex and Age Groups*

	Male	Female	< 22	≥ 22
Factor 1. Loss of control	22.1 ± 8.1	22.3 ± 8.2	22.1 ± 9.4	22.4 ± 7.1
Factor 2. Fear of infection or symbolic prejudice	9.1 ± 4.2	10.1 ± 4.7 **	10.2 ± 4.5	10.2 ± 4.4**
Factor 3: Contact with outsiders & Variables associated with HIV stigma	9.1 ± 3.3	9.1 ± 3.8*	9.1 ± 4.1	19.1 ±3.8
Factor 4: Infection and contact with infected people	10.3 ± 4.3	11.1 ± 4.3	10.1 ± 4.3	10.1 ± 4.1
Factor 5: Death	4.1 ± 2.1	5.2 ± 2.4	5.1 ± 2.1	5.1 ± 2.1

* $p \leq 0.01$
** ≤ 0.001

FAIDSS (Ross & Hunter, 1992) and the South African metropolitan factor solution. Second, these data have implications for prevention of HIV transmission in Swazi cities and in other African cities with similar cultural backgrounds. These data indicate that a major fear is of loss of control and becoming dependent. This factor has over 43 percent of its variance in common with the fear of infection or symbolic prejudice and over 16 percent of this variance in common with fear of death and contact with outsiders, variables associated with HIV stigma. The close association between fear of loss of control and fear of AIDS suggests that concern about the discriminating, stigmatizing, socially dislocating, and disabling aspects of HIV disease are a major concern. Of more immediate interest, however, is the association of the item measuring fear of infection or symbolic prejudice with fear of blood transfusions and contact with outsiders and other variables associated with HIV stigma. These data suggest that heterosexual sexual contact is not seen as a means of HIV transmission in the four regions of Swaziland studied in this research.

These data must be interpreted with southern African (Swaziland) attitudes toward mental illness, leprosy, or other diseases in mind; there are both traditional and modern attitudes that may be relevant. In an ideal society, all persons would have access to voluntary and confidential counseling and testing to learn about their HIV status without fear of repercussions or regrets. HIV-negative result holders should be given appropriate and detailed prevention counseling and be encouraged to stay HIV-negative. However, those who test

Table 40.4 *S indices between Swazi Student Factors and Melbourne Factors on the FAIDSS*

	Swazi factors				
Australian sample factors	1	2	3	4	5
Health workers (1) (n =134)					
Factor 1	0.58*	0.00	0.00	0.00	–0.13
Factor 2	0.11	0.54*	0.00	0.00	0.00
Factor 3	0.33	0.00	0.29	–0.54*	0.00
Factor 4	0.33	0.00	0.51*	0.00	0.00
Nursing students (n = 220)					
Factor 1	0.31	0.38*	0.00	–0.33	0.00
Factor 2	0.68*	0.00	0.00	0.00	–0.11
Factor 3	0.13	0.11	0.62*	0.00	0.00
Factor 4	0.34	0.00	0.11	0.31*	–0.31*
Factor 5	0.00	0.00	0.41	-0.43*	0.00
Health workers/teachers (2) (n = 66)					
Factor 1	0.52*	0.21	0.33	0.21	–0.13
Factor 2	0.51*	0.21	0.21	0.00	0.00
Factor 3	–0.04	0.00	0.23	0.00	–0.14
Factor 4	0.00	0.00	0.41*	–0.21	0.00
Factor 5	0.13	0.00	0.00	0.21	0.41*

* $p < 0.01$.

HIV-positive must not be ostracized or labeled, but provided with regular treatment and care and prevention counseling to guard against them spreading the disease or becoming reinfected. The establishment of effective prevention interventions against the disease is needed globally. In prevention, we should explore traditional sources of support and "connectedness" – such as is provided by the community, church, and extended family – to encourage people to achieve "spiritual connectedness." This will enable leaders and followers alike to gain personal insight and informed analysis into applying spiritual qualities such as justice, fortitude, and prudence into understanding the dangers of stigma and discrimination while incorporating ways to reduce such dangers into HIV/AIDS prevention programming. The southern African society, or the so-called epicenter of AIDS, has a major role to play in demonstrating to the world how a very diverse (inclusive of PLWA) population can live, work, and play together; win the compassion and support of members of the community in which they live; and thus lift prevention planning to new heights.

Traditional attitudes include those which encourage able-bodied dominance and a subservient role for those with disabilities or who are "physically challenged" within society, and which discourage the participation of those with disabilities in social, political, and economic activities. Although modern attitudes encourage participation of people with mental illness, PLWA in southern Africa are not fully accepted within the home and to a lesser extent outside. Southern Africans with a more "modern" attitude are most likely to be those from urban backgrounds, be better educated, and have a greater religious commitment. PLWA may be isolated and entrapped since the developments of effective social supports are not well developed. HIV stigma as studied in this sample addresses both traditional and modern attitudes toward HIV/AIDS and other health problems (e.g., mental illness, leprosy, disability) in southern Africa, with the implication that the level of stigma may be higher than in higher-income countries given the lower level of support and acceptance in southern African society to people living with these and other disabilities. However, this study found that the structure of fears and stigma does not appear to be appreciably different in Swaziland compared to Melbourne, Australia.

The results of the current study are in agreement with the conclusions from previous small cohort studies, and the obtained factor structure was very close to that obtained in the Melbourne sample. This conclusion is buttressed by evidence that AIDS is conceptualized as being associated with homosexual persons and blood transfusions and that preventive education of a comprehensive package of interventions, tailored to the local context, will be needed to address the multiple causes of discrimination. Such interventions will also need to emphasize the risk of heterosexual HIV transmission and deemphasize the perception that only particular classes of people are at risk. One goal for future research will be to investigate the factors that can influence a shared "resonance and empathic accuracy" to facilitate caring behaviors for in-and outgroup members of a society (see Decety, Echols, & Correll, 2009).

It must be emphasized that the present study was specifically an investigation of AIDS stigma in Swaziland as part of an ongoing project on HIV stigmatization in subcultures in Africa. This study's findings may not apply equally to all cohort studies conducted in South Africa, Botswana, and Nigeria.

It is tempting, however, to point attention to the possible reassurance that the present findings will provide for future research to consider, that is, the role of certain individual variables "social construction of individual realities," as mediating and moderating influences of attitudes toward HIV/AIDS. The personal and emotional meaning of one's "social identity," as well as other attributes, may depend upon one's cultural and psychological values. After all, "fear (anxiety)"or discrimination or "stigma" are more accurately a cultural construct than a biogenetic one, and interracial variation greatly surpasses interracial differences (Downing, 2008). This study suggests both a gap and a disparity in noninclusion of stigma and discrimination in the prevention planning related to HIV/AIDS. It also indicates the feasibility of and need for a large, representative population-based study on contextual issues constructed at the societal level and pertinent to HIV-related stigma/discrimination among PLWHA. Such a large-scale study would address one of the limitations of this study, limited generalizability due to a small sample size and little information on socioeconomic status.

In closing, studying health-related beliefs of other geopolitical cultures in our quest for a universality thesis, by way of applying a hybrid "personality-social psychology" strategy to the study of AIDS-stigma, very well may have the potential to awaken the functional theories of behavioral change, AIDS stigma, discrimination, human emotion, and social influence from their long winter of hibernation (Russell, 1994). Specifically, it is our hope, however, that this study will act as a springboard to further clear new paths to our understanding of the development of cross-cultural intimate social relationships and stigma associated with HIV/AIDS. Yet we must advance beyond just theories to understand why differences in people and cultures lead to immense misperception and misinformation, and why AIDS stigma, violence, abuse, conflict, prejudice, discrimination, and insensitivity exist in the first place.

Within this context, structural approaches with an interdisciplinary perspective, that recognize that cultural, social, physical, economic, legal, political, or policy-related and environmental factors that directly affect HIV risk and vulnerability must revolve around the reduction of stigma and anxiety (fear) within a context of community identity and community values, not just simply on "overly simplistic magic bullets" and individual-level behavior interventions. It is hoped that clear evidence for a multidimensionality of stigma found in this project hereinafter will stimulate further research into hierarchical ordering of these dimensions and further consideration of how (and/or whether) different components of stigma should be combined to obtain higher-order components (Cooley, 1902; Marsh, Relich, & Smith, 1983). Serious efforts must be made to define, identify, and build capacity to reduce stigma. In addition, we must strongly endorse community strength, full empowerment for all members, social mobilization, emotional support, and cross-current models for advocacy and social change. We need to facilitate morally courageous actions subject to automatic self-regulatory mechanisms based on values and virtues, so that as AIDS becomes a nonfatal disease it can be both treated and prevented, with hope that attitudes will change and all its associated stigmas will end (Bagozzi, 2003; Bagozzi, Wong, & Yi, 1999).

Exclusion of stigma and discrimination reduction in prevention planning represents a missed opportunity for HIV prevention. Not only is a replication (with extension) of this research or study seriously warranted, but its repetition with professional and nonprofessional samples or the general population also is very much needed. Stigma is still alive and well, and there is always room for more research to better understand it. As HIV/AIDS becomes a subacute disease that can be both prevented and treated, it is hoped that attitudes will change, and denial, stigma, and discrimination will rapidly be reduced.

Acknowledgments

We express our sincere gratitude to all the participants who took part in this Swaziland phase of our Africa project for their time and knowledge.

We thank the Swazi students at the international office who enabled us to carry out the project in Swaziland. We also thank our Swazi colleagues who have contributed to make this project possible, and our eminent professors Ti. Laviza, Moshe Banai, David Watkins, Gregory J. Boyle, C. Kagitcibasi, T. H. Ollendick, R. P. Bagozzi, and Mike Ross, whose thoughts and words we cited, for their suggestions and comments. Finally, we thank our editors, for their stoic endurance, help, and brilliance in reading over the chapter proposal several times.

References

Adeokun, L., Okonkwo, P., & Ladipo, O. A. (2006). The stigmatization of people living with HIV/AIDS. In Adeyi, O., Kanki, P., Odutolu, O., & Idoko, J. A. (eds.), *AIDS in Nigeria: A Nation on the Threshold*. Cambridge, MA: Harvard University Press, pp. 213–33.

Ajzen, I., & Madden, T. J. (1986). Prediction of goal-directed behaviour: attitudes, intentions, and perceived behavioral control. *Journal of Experimental Social Psychology* 22: 453–74.

Akande, A., Adewuyi, M., Akande, T., & Adetoun, B. (2016). If one goes up one must come down: understanding gender and learning style – a non-western perspective. *Social Indicators Research (USA)*: 1–13.

Akande, D., & Ollendick, T. H. (1997). Dimensions of fears in African children. (Unpublished paper). Virginia State University and Polytechnic, Blacksburg.

Akande, D., & Ross, M. W. (1994). Fears of AIDS/HIV in Nigerian students. *Social Science & Medicine* 38: 330–42.

Amuri, M., Mitchell, S., Cockcroft, A., & Andersson, N. (2011). Socio-economic status and HIV/AIDS stigma in Tanzania. *AIDS Care: Psychological and Socio-medical Aspects of AIDS/HIV* 23: 378–92.

Arrindell, W. A., Ross, M. W., Bridges, K. R., van Hout, W., Hofman, A., & Sanderman, R. (1989). Fear of AIDS: are there replicable, invariant questionnaire dimension? *Advanced Behavior Research* 11: 69–115.

Arrindell, W. A., & van der Ende, J. (1986). Further evidence for cross-sample invariance of phobic factors: psychiatric impatient ratings on the Fear Survey Schedule III. *Behavior Research Therapy* 24: 289–97.

Awofeso, N. (2011). Leprosy control, public health paradigms and stigma. *Australian and New Zealand Journal of Public Health* 35: 9–11.

Bagozzi, R. P. (2003). Positive and negative emotions in organizations. In Cameron, K. S., Dutton, J. E., & Quinn, R. E. (eds.), *Positive Organizational Scholarship: Foundations of a New Discipline*. San Francisco, CA: Berrett-Koehler, pp. 176–93.

Bagozzi, R. P., Wong, N., & Yi, Y. (1999). The role of culture and gender in the relationship between positive and negative affect. *Cognition and Emotion*, 13: 641–72.

Baral, S. C., Karki, D. K., & Newell, J. (2007). Causes of stigma and discrimination associated with tuberculosis in Nepal: a qualitative study. *BMC Public Health* 7: 211–21.

Bastian, B., & Haslam, N. (2006). Psychological essentialism and stereotype endorsement. *Journal of Experimental Social Psychology* 42: 228–35.

Bell, R. A., Molitor, F., & Flynn, N. M. (1999). Fear of AIDS: assessment and implications for promoting safer sex. *AIDS and Behavior* 3: 135–47. doi: dx.doi.org/10.1023/A:1025488007373

Bijnen, E. J., Van der Net, T. J., & Poortinga, Y. H. (1986). On cross-cultural comparative studies with the Eysenck Personality Questionnaire. *Journal of Cross-Cultural Psychology* 17: 3–16.

Boyle, G. J. (1984). Reliability and validity of Izard's Differential Emotions Scale. *Personality* 56: 747–50.

Brown, L., Macintyre, K., & Trujillo, L. (2003). Interventions to reduce HIV/AIDS stigma: what have we learned? *AIDS Education and Prevention* 15: 49–69.

Cattell, R. B., Balcar, K. R., Horn, J. L., & Nesselrode, J. R. (1969). Factor matching procedures: an improvement of the s index, with tables. *Educational Psychology Measurement* 29: 781–92.

Centers for Disease Control, Divisions of HIV/AIDS Prevention CDC semi-annual HIV/AIDS surveillance report 2011. www.cdc.gov/hiv/stats.htm.

Cooley, C. H. (1902). *Human Nature and Social Order*. New York: Scribner's.

Decety, J., Echols, J., & Correll, J. (2009). The blame game: the effect of responsibility and social stigma on empathy for pain. *Journal of Cognitive Neuroscience* 22: 917–50.

Dlamini, P. S. (2007). Verbal and physical abuse and neglect as manifestations of HIV/AIDS stigma in five African countries. *Public Health Nursing* 24: 389–99.

Downing, M. J. (2008). The role of home in HIV/AIDS: a visual approach to understanding human–environment interactions in the context of long-term illness. *Health & Place* 14: 313–22.

Earnshaw, V. A., & Quinn, D. M. (2011). The impact of stigma in healthcare on people living with chronic illnesses. *AIDS Care: Psychological and Socio-Medical Aspects of AIDS/HIV* 23: 16–45.

Eysenck, H. J., & Eysenck, S. B. G. (1983). Recent advances in the cross-cultural study of personality. In. Butcher, J. N., & Spielberger, C.D. (eds), *Advances in Personality Assessment*, vol. 2. Hillsdale, N.J.: Lawrence Erlbaum, pp. 41–69.

Floyd, D. L., Prentice-Dunn, S., & Rogers, R. W. (2000). A meta-analysis of research on protection motivation theory. *Journal of Applied Social Psychology* 30: 407–29.

Frijda, N., & Jahoda, G. (1966). On the scope and methods of cross-cultural research. *International Journal of Psychology* 1: 109–27.

Garrett, R., Smith, J., Chiu, J., & Young, S.D. (2016). HIV/AIDS stigma among a sample of primarily African-American and Latino men who have sex with men social media users. *AIDS Care* 28(6): 731–5. doi: 10.1080/09540121.2016.1146395

Gibbons, J. L., & Ashdown, B. K. (2010). Ethnic identification, attitudes, and group relations in Guatemala. *Psychology* 1: 116–27.

Godlonton, S., & Thornton, R. (2012). Peers effect in learning HIV results. *Journal of Developmental Economics* 97: 118–27.

Goffman, E. (1963). *Stigma: Notes on the Management of Spoiled Identity*. New York: Simon and Schuster.

Herek, G. M, & Capitanio, J. P. (1998). Symbolic prejudice or fear of infection? A functional analysis of AIDS-related stigma among heterosexual. *Basic Applied Social Psychology* 20: 230–41.

Ingman, K. A., Ollendick, T. H., & Akande, A. (1999). Cross-cultural aspects of fears in African children and adolescents. *Behavior Research and Therapy* 37: 337–45.

Janz, N. K., & Becker, M. H. (1984). The health belief model: a decade later. *Health Education Quarterly* 11: 1–47.

Jurgensen, M. (2013). Effects of home-based voluntary counselling and testing on HIV-related stigma: findings from a cluster-randomized trial in Zambia. *Social Science & Medicine* 81: 16–25.

Kalipeni, E. (2012). HIV/AIDS in women: stigma, and gender empowerment. *Malawi. Future Medicine* 2: 142–53.

Link, R. N., Feingold, A. R., Charap, M. H., Freeman, K., & Shevlov, S. P. (1988). Concerns of medical and pediatric house officers about acquiring AIDS from the patients. *American Journal of Public Health* 78: 455–9.

Markowitz, F. E. (2005). Sociological models of mental illness stigma: progress and prospects. In Corrigan, P. (ed.), *On the Stigma of Mental Illness*, Washington, DC: American Psychological Association, pp. 129–44.

Marsh, H. W., Relich, J. D., & Smith, I. D. (1983). Self-concept: the construct validity of interpretations based upon the SDQ. *Journal of Personality and Social Psychology* 45: 173–87.

Neal, J., Nemser, B., Cumming, R., Lelerai, E. Amor, Y. B., & Pronyk, P. (2012). HIV attitudes, awareness and testing among older adults in Africa. *AIDS and Behavior* 50: 663–8.

Novick, A. (1997). Stigma and AIDS: three layers of damage. *Journal of the Gay and Lesbian Medical Association* 1: 53–60.

Ollendick, T. H., Yang, B., King, N. J., Dong, Q., & Akande, A. (1996). Fears in American, Australian, Chinese and African children. *Journal of Child Psychology & Psychiatry* 37: 213–20.

Oranyan, B. A. A. (2005). Words of encouragement. (Unpublished manuscript), DTS Institute.

Parker, R., & Aggleton, P. (2003). HIV and AIDS-related stigma and discrimination: a conceptual framework and implications for action. *Social Science & Medicine* 57: 13–24.

Piot, P., Bartos, M., Ghys, P. D., Walker, N., & Schwartlander, B. (2002). The global impact of HIV/AIDS. *Nature* 410 (April 14): 968–73.

Polansky, M., Teti, M., Chengappa, R., & Aaron, E. (2015). Risk and protective factors for HIV self-disclosure among poor African-American women living with HIV/AIDS. *Issues in Mental Health Nursing* 36: 171–81.

Pryor, J. B., & Reeder, J. D. (1993). Collective and independent representation of HIV/AIDS stigma. In Pryor, J. B., & Reeder, G. D. (eds), *The Social Psychology of HIV Infection*. Hillsdale, NJ: Lawrence Erlbaum, pp. 263–86.

Ramjee, G., & Daniels, B. (2013). Women and HIV in sub-Saharan Africa. *AIDS Research and Therapy* 10: 30. doi: doi.org/10.1186/1742–6405-10–30

Rao, D., Angell, B., Lam, C., & Corrigan, P. (2008). Stigma in the workplace: employer attitudes about people with HIV in Beijing, Hong Kong, and Chicago. *Social Science & Medicine* 67: 1541–9. doi; 10.1016/j.socscimed. 2008.07.024

Rosenberg, M. J., & Hovland, C. I. (1960). Cognitive, affective, and behavioral components of attitudes. In Hovland, C. I., & Rosenberg, M. J. (eds.), *Attitude Organization and Change: An Analysis of Consistency among Attitude Components*. New Haven, CT: Yale University Press, pp. 1–14.

Ross, M. W., & Hunter, C. E. (1992). Replication of the factor structure of the Fear of AIDS Schedule (FAIDSS) across samples. *Psychology and Health* 6: 39–44.

Rusch, N., Angermeyer, M., & Corrigan, P. (2005). Mental illness stigma: concepts, consequences, and initiative to reduce stigma. *European Psychiatry* 20: 529–39.

Russel, J. A. (1994). Is there universal recognition of emotion from facial expression? A review of the cross-cultural studies. *Psychological Bulletin* 115: 102–41.

Sabone, M. B. (2015). The dynamics, dilemmas and complexities of AIDS: the cultural context of Botswana. *Issues in Mental Health Nursing* 36: 118–26.

Sandelowski, M., Barrosso, J., & Volls, C. I. (2009). Gender, race/ethnicity, and social class in research reports on stigma in HIV-positive women. *Health Care for Women International* 30: 273–88.

Schulze, B., & Angermeyer, M. C. (2003). Subjective experience of stigma: a focus group study of schizophrenic patients, their relatives and mental health professionals. *Social Science & Medicine* 56: 299–312.

Starks, T. J., Rendina, H. J., Breslow, A. S., Parsons, J. T., & Golub, S. A. (2013). The psychological cost of anticipating HIV stigma for HIV-negative gay and bisexual men. *AIDS and Behavior* 17: 2732–41. doi: dx.doi.org/10.1007/s10461-013-0425-0

Thorpe, R. D. (2009). "Doing" chronic illness? Complementary medicine use among people living with HIV/AIDS in Australia. *Sociology of Health & Illness* 31: 375–89. doi: dx.doi.org/10.1111/j.1467-9566.2008.01137.x

Tsai, A. C., & Venkataramani, A. S. (2015). The causal effect of education on HIV stigma in Uganda: evidence from a natural experiment. *Social Science & Medicine* 142: 37–46.

UNAIDS (2010). Report on the Global AIDS Epidemic: a UNAIDS 12th anniversary special edition. data.unaids.org/[ub/GlobalReport/2010/2010_CH02_en.pdf)

Walkey, F. H., & McCormick, I. A. (1985). FACTOREP: a Pascal program to examine factor replications. *Educational Psychology Measurement* 45: 147–50.

Wolpe, J., & Lang, P. J. (1977). *Manual for the Fear Survey Schedule*, San Diego, CA: Educational and Industrial Testing Service.

Yeboah, I. E. A. (2007). HIV/AIDS and the construction of sub-Saharan Africa: heuristic lessons from the social sciences for policy. *Social Sciences & Medicine* 64: 1128–50.

41 What Intensifies Governmental Support of Prevention? Lessons from Israel

Moshe Israelashvili

The State of Israel is located on the coast of Mediterranean Sea, on the edge of the Middle East. Israel is a small country; the entire land area of the State of Israel is smaller than Yosemite Park (United States [U.S.]). It was established in 1948, based on the United Nations resolution after the World War II massive killing of Jews (the Holocaust). However, according to Jewish tradition, Jews were living on this ground for many years, dating back to about three thousand years ago. Yet, the relatively recent memories of the World War II Holocaust, and the awareness that another holocaust must be prevented – that is, by having a free state for the Jews, with its own army and capacity of self-defense – is a vital component to all (not only Israeli) Jews.

Thus, to some degree it could be said that the idea of prevention lies in the very heart of every Israeli-Jew; however, on the same token, the almost absolute helplessness of the Jews living in Europe during the Holocaust time and the repeated attacks against Jews reported in history are well known to every Israeli-Jew as well.

The current chapter will introduce several of current Israel's essential characteristics, shortly describe the position of prevention activities in Israel, explain the extensive governmental support to three prevention programs (substance abuse, suicide prevention, and school-to-army transition), and conclude by suggesting that the reader take home a message regarding a possible way to increase (any) decision makers' collaboration in the development and implementation of prevention programs.

Living in Israel

Many travelers experience a kind of acculturation shock when they confront the reality of daily living in Israeli. Far from its "armed" image, travelers generally find Israel to be a mixture of modern and ancient places, a land that has both snow in the North and desert in the South, endless shopping centers and merchants' stands almost everywhere, and crowded streets in which people of all colors and ethnicities sit side by side in numerous coffee shops or along the Mediterranean Sea beach; a state where one meets soldiers carrying guns and security at the entrance to every mall and yet people feel completely safe walking in most places and feel bad for tourists who may complain about not feeling safe in their own homeland or place of residence (abroad). Such positive experiences would justify "Lonely Planet's top 10 cities for 2011" nomination of Tel Aviv as being "a modern Sin City on the sea ... a truly diverse 21st-century Mediterranean hub ...," as well as TripAdvisor's nomination of Jerusalem as one of 2011's "Top 25 Destinations in the World" (based on travelers' choice) for its "profound cultural and historical significance."

The truth about Israel is that both images are true, depending on the circumstances. Israel was established in 1948, with less than 1 million Jewish people. Gradually it has become a vibrant, well-developed, and modern home for about 8 million people. This has happened even though during the sixty-seven years of its existence, Israel has been involved in more than a dozen major armed conflicts with the Arab nations that surround Israel, as well as endless security problems on a daily basis. However, in spite of – and maybe due to – the endless stream of security problems, Israel has become a well-developed and modern state, very Westernized, with an advanced academic and industrial life that truly justifies its label as a "start-up nation" (Senor & Singer, 2009). Israel is essentially an immigrant society, as many immigrated and still immigrate to Israel due to their connection to Judaism. However, the Israeli society includes people of all ethnicities, religions, and values. Generally speaking, the Israeli society is composed of three major groups: Jews (75 percent), Arabs (20 percent), and others (5 percent). Yet, it should be noted that within each of the aforementioned groups there are several subgroups, such as the differentiation within the group of Orthodox Jews, between national-religious and ultra-Orthodox, the subdivision between ex–Soviet-born (15 percent of the Israeli population) and others, or the subdivision within the Arab population between the Muslim-Arab (81 percent of the Arab people) who are divided into the Falach (landowners) and Bedouin (originally the wondering tribes), the Christian-Arab (10 percent), and others (9 percent; i.e., Druze, Adyghe-Sharkas, Bahá'í). Taking into account the many countries of origin of Jewish people who immigrated to Israel in order to feel safe (after the Holocaust) and the diversity within the non-Jewish population, it is evident why Israel's society represents a kaleidoscope of many ethnic and social groups (Israelashvili & Benjamin, 2009).

In 2011, Israel led the Western world birth rate, with the average of 18.71 births per 1,000 – in comparison to 12.26 for the United Kingdom, 10.28 for Canada, and 10.14 for Spain. However, gradually the Israeli population follows the Western trends, in terms of suspension of marital age (currently, 29.5 years among the Jewish grooms) and an increase in the divorce rate (currently about 33 percent for Jews, 12 percent for Muslims, and 4 percent for Christians). According to a World Health Organization (WHO) report, the average life expectancy of Israeli men is 80.2 years, the fourth highest in the world after Iceland (81.2), Switzerland (80.7), and Australia (80.5). Thus, Israel's demography is slightly changing, from a young society with many of the Jewish population having no grandparents (as a result of the Holocaust), to a society that has to devote growing attention to the elders' population.

The Israeli–Arab conflict has protracted for more than a hundred years and developed on a territory that both Arabs and Jews have perceived as exclusively their own (the same land of conflict was labeled either as Palestine by Arabs or as Israel by Jews). The Israeli–Arab conflict violently erupted as a local conflict between Jews and Arabs who lived together under British mandate and developed to an interstate conflict during the 1948 war between Israel and its surrounding countries. Following the 1948 war, several additional wars occurred along with occasional armed encounters, almost on a weekly basis. As the conflict proceeded, many lives were taken, and literally all Israelis (Jews and non-Jews) are personally acquainted, directly or indirectly, with victims of this seemingly endless armed conflict. Accordingly, an extremely significant trajectory for all Jewish and several other non-Jewish (e.g., the Druze) youth and their development is the mandatory military service. Due to its existential security problems, high school graduates are routinely enlisted into compulsory military service. The Israeli army (IDF) enlists (Jewish) adolescents for two years (females) or three years (males). Those who are medically unable to serve, along with many who are not obliged to serve (e.g., Christian-Arabs), voluntarily choose to join the civil service, as a kind of developmental milestone and a way to be related to the majority of the Israeli youth.

Resilience in Israel

In light of the continuing armed conflict and its significant implications for daily living, not a few people are wondering how the Israelis get along with such a situation. Moreover, there is evidence that an increase in the Arab–Israel conflict reduces, rather than increases, the emigration rate from Israel abroad (Cohen, 1988). While detailed discussion of this question is out of the scope of the current chapter, three complementing answers can be suggested:

1. *Meaningful life.* Living in Israel forces its inhabitants to think about the meaning of life, as well as to think about their own goals and values in life. The almost daily encounter with an actual death – for example, due to a terrorist attack – or with the possibility of death – such as the recent "reminder" issued by Supreme Leader Ayatollah Ali Khamenai on September 9, 2015: "... God willing, there will be no such thing as a Zionist regime (i.e., Israel) in 25 years. Until then, struggling, heroic and jihadi morale will leave no moment of serenity for Zionists"– leave no option but to think (internally) and discuss (with other people) one's attitudes toward the state, toward one's family, toward relatives and friends who live abroad, toward the inner voice saying "why do you need to risk yourself?" and to search and find a meaning in current life that would justify staying in such an abnormal corner of the world (Israelashvili, 2005). The answers to these internal/external debates vary – be it a religious, social, cultural, practical, or other nature of reason – but the conclusion is the same: that is, many Israelis hold

a good reason for living here, and that answer articulates the ability to perceive life as meaningful. This is true not only for the Jewish citizen but also for the Arab–Israeli citizen whose *Arab* village was under missile attacks directed at them from Lebanon (even though they were originally was meant to hit the neighboring *Jewish* villages, such as during 2007), or the Arab–Israeli citizen whose children might equally be exposed to a sudden terrorist attack on their school bus. Thus, people living in Israel don't have the privilege of ignoring questions that are related to the meaning of their life and the values in which they believe. Those who do not approach good answers to such questions and debates *are* willing to immigrate abroad.

2. *Social support.* It's well established in the Jewish religion, and hence in Jewish history, that Jews must take care of other Jews. Judaism is a collectivistic religion, not only a religion of the individual versus God. The same goes for the Arab people living in Israel, as the traditional collectivistic-oriented nature of their lives still connects people strongly to their family and tribe. Hence, both Jewish and non-Jewish people in Israel intensively interact with each other as well as with strangers. Hence, many Israelis feel connected to people around them and truly believe that in times of need they'll get support from family, friends, and also complete strangers (who occasionally realized that they are in need). Accordingly, charity is extremely developed in all segments of the Israeli society.
3. *A feeling that there is no alternative* – Relatively speaking, the majority of the Jews who live in Israel are convinced that should they move abroad, their situation – as Jews – might be worsen, in comparison to their current situation. The *Holocaust* is perceived not only as an historical event but rather as a potential threat that might repeat itself. Moreover, the repeated waves of Jewish people who immigrate to Israel, while saying that they felt insecure in their previous countries (e.g., the recent waves of French Jews who have immigrated to Israel) further strengthen the common feeling among Israelis, who complain about everything in Israel but usually end up by saying that "Israel is not the best place to live in, but for sure not the worse one." While thinking about these and other issues, the Israelis are well-known for their willingness to travel abroad; according to figures published recently by the Israeli Central Bureau of Statistics (CBS), 777,500 Israelis – that is, 10 percent of the Israel population – departed on vacations abroad in July 2015 only, by air, land, and sea. Interestingly, in times of war many Israelis who immigrated several years ago (or occasionally stay abroad) return back to Israel, in order "to protect our home." Namely, there are two types of Israel and Israelis, the one in peacetime and the one in wartime: while the first is gradually more selfish and Westernized, the other remains the same person of 1948 who is ready to scarify his or her life for the shake of "the only land we (the Jewish people) have got."

To sum up, Israel security and survival are the top issues to both the Israel government as well as ordinary citizens of Israel. Thus, somehow a short visit to

Israel is misleading, as on a regular day it all looks like a sunny and pleasurable Mediterranean country, highly developed and vibrant, where everyone is minding one's own business. Yet, the government and people are constantly searching, on a daily basis, for any indication of a potential threat to Israel's survival – and, unfortunately, occasionally do identify one (e.g., a bomb left in a bus; a rocket hitting a near-border village; a coordinated attack on Israeli posts, started at once by armies of three neighboring countries as in 1973) – and collectively try to address it once such a threat has been identified. Accordingly, all matters that are related to security gain top priority in Israel. The same goes for issues related to mental health and well-being; that is, in times of national security crisis (e.g., war), many national health institutions offer counseling and psychotherapy free of charge. This is their way to contribute to the collective efforts in pursuit of preventing war-related maladjustment and major psychopathology. The difference between the free access to counseling and mental health services in times of war and peace is so evident that sometimes it leads to the public impression that in times of crisis Israeli counselors and psychologists are reaching out for patients (Raviv & Weiner, 1995).

Prevention in Israel

Prevention in the School System

Since the establishment of the State of Israel, the school has had a major role in times of war and trauma. Not surprisingly, following a review of the literature on mental health and war trauma among children in Israeli schools, Abel and Friedman (2009) acknowledged the school, in addition to the children's parents, as a major source of social support and a facilitator of recovery. School counselors in Israel are in charge of support of those children who are in need of help in times of (personal and/or community) crisis, as well as guiding the school team about how to manage in times of difficulty. In Israel, school psychologists provide intensive individual therapy to students who are already suffering from psychopathology (but still attend school). Hence, it should be noted that in Israel, the role of the school mental health team is not limited to academic and guidance problems alone, but to a great extent to the students' socioemotional state and well-being as well (Israelashvili, 2015a).

Currently, in most Israeli schools – elementary, secondary, and high schools – students can receive counseling from school counselors. In some areas in Israel, educational counseling starts in kindergarten, where the counselor guides kindergarten teachers and parents on how to foster children's optimal development. A meeting between a student and the school counselor might be initiated by a teacher who notices that a student is in need of guidance, or by the school counselor who follows students' social and emotional development using observations, questionnaires, and consultations, or by the student's family who requests assistance. In all of these cases, the school counselor would first explore the origins of the student's difficulties. Usually the school counselor would try to help those students whose problems stem from temporary or environmental difficulties rather than major and chronic mental health problems. Students with major mental health problems would be directed to the school or clinical psychologist either inside (if available) or outside of the school system. Unfortunately, many students (approximately 70 percent; Tatar, 2001) perceive the school counselor as "a member of the teachers' team" and hence will resist seeking the counselor's help even in times of a major crisis unless they are very distressed (Israelashvili, 1999).

Activities of school counselors and school psychologists are directed by a special counseling wing that exists in the Israel Ministry of Education, named the *Psychological-Counseling Department*. This wing has several subunits. The *Psychological Unit*, which supervises educational psychologists who work on a municipal basis, mainly in conducting educational and psychological diagnoses, short-term psychological interventions, school team consultations, and crisis interventions. The *School Counseling Unit* is responsible for developing the policy and practice of the counseling services in all Israeli educational institutions. The School Counseling Unit deals with the establishment of guidelines for the promotion of a positive school climate, promotion and maintenance of preliminary and posteriori interventions to reduce the problems caused by stressful situations, and the planning and guidance of school counselors' professional development. Another unit is the *Prevention and Development Programs Unit*. This unit is responsible for developing programs related to health and wellness with special attention to cultural issues (e.g., Jewish vs. Arab). The list of programs includes developing life skills, preventing substance abuse and sexual vulnerability, and preventing aggression and maladjustment. The fourth unit is the *Learning Disabilities Unit*, which is responsible for promoting an optimal educational environment for children with learning disabilities. Lastly, the *Emergency Counseling and Psychological Services Section* is responsible for the preparation of the educational system for stressful situations and emergencies, such as missile attacks, wars, evacuations, and suicidal behavior.

Practically speaking, the Prevention and Development Programs Unit and the Emergency Counseling and the Psychological Services Section, within the Ministry of Education, are the leading formal governmental organizations that develop and implement K–12 prevention programs in Israel.

Additional Governmental Units Dealing with Prevention

The following are other official organizations to initiate and supply prevention programs:

1. The Ministry of Health, which focuses on both disease prevention as well as development of children's health and positive nutrition.
2. The IDF, which initiates, develops, and implements prevention programs to support the well-being of all soldiers and military personnel (e.g., substance

abuse prevention, stress management, prevention of intercultural conflicts, and individual preventive counseling).

3. The Israel Anti-Drugs and Alcohol Authority (IADA), which recently moved from the Prime Minister's Office to the Ministry of Interior Security.
4. The Authority for Traffic-Accident Prevention, which is related to the Ministry of Transportation.

It should be noted that many small private companies offer specific services that are related to prevention, especially with regard to substance abuse prevention (e.g., using sports/movies to deliver messages to prevent substance abuse). Finally, there are many groups of volunteers, most of them with no formal training, who are dedicated to the prevention of a specific problem, such as HIV/AIDS prevention.

Naturally, while each of these organizations is taking care of its interest, collaborations do exists in various contexts. One example is prevention intervention in early childhood. In this context, it should be noted that one of the more developed activities in Israel, initially supported by the Israeli Ministries of Health and Education, is early-age education. In Israel, about 20 percent of all children are already in a kind of kindergarten by the age of two years. The roots of this situation can be traced back to the time of the establishment of Israel, when parents were obliged and willing to work, either for a living and/or for "building the kibbutz/nations/etc." However, in light of the many immigrants who approached Israel during the 1950s, many of them with no formal education, a need for training parents how to become "a good parent" emerged. This need was true also for not a few of those who were born and living in Israel, but had problematic childhoods themselves, sometimes as children whose parents passed away (e.g., during wars).

Hence, in these years a well-known promotion program for effective parenting was developed in Israel, later known as Home Instruction for Parents of Preschool Youngsters (HIPPY). HIPPY (www.hippy-international.org/) was developed in the late 1960s at the Hebrew University in Jerusalem (Israel) and later imported (in 1986) to the United States by then-Governor and the First Lady of Arkansas, Bill and Hillary Clinton, who believed that HIPPY is the right intervention for empowering parenting, and consequently children's development, among low-income families (see www.arhomevisiting.org/app-programs/hippyusa). Several studies explored the impact of HIPPY on children's development and achievements; for example, a recent U.S. study by Brown and Lee (2014) followed the school performance of children who participated in the HIPPY program as three, four, or five year olds for about ten years, that is, during the third, fifth, seventh, and ninth grades. Data analyses indicated that in all four grades HIPPY children had significantly higher rates of school attendance, lower rates of retain, fewer repeat discipline referrals, higher scores, and higher pass rates on the Reading and Math tests in comparison to matching children without HIPPY experience (see also Bradley & Gilkey, 2002). Currently, HIPPY is still implemented in Israel, as well as in various countries around the world, such as twenty-two states in the United States, Australia, South Africa, Sweden, Italy, New Zealand, and others (e.g., Nievar, Jacobson, Chen, Johnson, & Dier, 2011).

Another example of interorganizational collaboration in prevention efforts is the recent initiation of the IADA to establish standards for universal prevention intervention in the field of substance abuse prevention. The committee that has been established includes members of all the relevant ministries and organizations, such as ministries of Health, Education, Law, Interior Security, and Immigration. The committee checked more than seventy mostly universal prevention programs that have been submitted for evaluation and outlined eight standards that were adopted by the IADA (2015) as guidelines for future approval of universal prevention activities in schools, youth centers, and such. It is worth mentioning that at first glance, none of the submitted seventy prevention programs met the eight Standards of Prevention; the major limitation was the lack of robust evaluation studies to support the effectiveness of the programs. Nevertheless, sixteen of the programs were ranked as more recommended for implementation (e.g., in schools) than others (for more details, see Israelashvili, 2015b), with the definite announcement that this label might be changed in the future should these programs will fail to meet all the eight standards.

Thus, altogether it can be concluded that prevention efforts are prominent in Israel, especially among school graders, and that several government offices and other formal organizations have made efforts to prevent risk behaviors and disease. The prevention efforts are implemented with programs that have been especially developed for Israeli people, as well as with programs that have been imported from other nations.

Yet, there is a significant gap between the intensity of prevention efforts and the evidence of either efficacy and/or effectiveness. In a recent survey of academic publications on prevention programs that was conducted in Israel between the years 2001 and 2012, Nakash, Razon, and Levav (2015) report that on only 5 percent of the academic manuscripts in Israeli behavioral science referred journals and 6 percent of Ph.D. and M.A. thesis research were based on prevention program research or evaluation studies. Moreover, it seems that the main reason for the lack of prevention research is the lack of prevention education and training in Israel, as well as lack of funding for prevention research. For example, in spite of the widespread and intensive prevention efforts that are implemented by the aforementioned organizations as well as others, currently none of the research universities in Israel offers a graduate program in prevention. According to Nakash et al. (2015), only 5 percent of elective courses in Israeli universities' graduate programs addressed primary prevention.

When Do Prevention Efforts Gain Extensive Governmental Support?

The need for cultural adaptation of prevention programs, as well as the need to adapt a given preventive program to the special characteristics of a given group (e.g., a class in school), is well documented in international prevention literature (e.g., van Weel, Roberts, De Maeseneer, & van der Velden, 2011; Wang, et al., 2016). Another notion that is well documented is the need to coordinate the development and future implementation of prevention programs with the relevant decision makers and stockholders (e.g., Kilburn & Cannon, 2015; Sucaldito et al., 2014). Yet, addressing these two needs should be done while finding the right balance between the scientific knowledge of what should be prevented and how, and those environmental, social, and personal characteristics that exist in the given environment in which the prevention program is to be implemented (e.g., Abelin, 2006; Bruhn, Hirsch, & Lloyd, 2015). These three notions – that is, adaptation, coordination, and fidelity (or integration) – are among the major challenges for any prevention initiation that is going to scale (e.g., Romano, 2015). Within this process, a major component for success is the acquiring of policy-maker collaboration and readiness to support, both financially and publicly, the prevention activities (e.g., Milat, King, Bauman, & Redman, 2013). Notably, all of the suggestions, as detailed in this paragraph, can be applied to prevention efforts anywhere in the world.

A review of the common dynamic of prevention interventions in Israel indicates a dual approach of both decentralized along with recentralized prevention efforts in Israel. Namely, on several issues the government encourages local, community-oriented prevention efforts, while on other issues – and sometimes when the circumstances are changed – the government encourages broader, governmental-directed prevention initiations and implementations. The term "local prevention" refers to those cases where the Israeli government, through the relevant ministry, encourages every municipality and community to initiate intervention programs that fit into the specific community circumstance, such as in the case of HIV prevention. However, sometimes the opposite happens, when the government is intensively involved in the initiation and promotion of prevention programs on a certain topic, including intensive involvement and resource devotion until the strategic picture seemed to be change. Not surprisingly, the general differentiation between these two kinds of behaviors is related to the Israel government perception of the given topic as (un)related to security; that is, intensive governmental prevention efforts will emerge whenever the government is convinced that a certain topic/behavior (to be prevented) is a potential risk to Israel's security. The term "local consideration" represents the opposite situation, where the government turns over control and funding to the local community. Following are descriptions of three cases in which the special security circumstances in Israel led to relatively intensive governmental prevention efforts.

Substance Abuse Prevention. The IADA routinely follows trends of substance abuse in the Israel population, especially Israeli youth. Data from the IADA 2011 report indicate that 21 percent of all Israeli youth have already experienced cigarette smoking by the age of sixteen years, with 6.2 percent smoking on a weekly basis; the average rate of weekly use of any alcohol (not for religious reasons; the *Kiddush*) was 15 percent, ranging between 17 percent drinking beer and 9 percent drinking soft alcoholic drinks; for high school students (ages sixteen to eighteen years), the average rate of drug abuse was about 4 percent, ranging between 6 percent using inhalants to 2.5 percent using heroin, crack, and opium. While significant differences exist between the religions (Jews vs. non-Jews), the genders, and school relatedness (school dropouts vs. those who attend regular [i.e., academic-oriented] schools), it should be noted that these rates are relatively low in comparison to the findings in most of the Western countries, as presented in Figure 41.1. Figure 41.1 presents the 2008 substance abuse rate of Israel youth versus several Western countries (retrieved from the IADA website on September 2015).

What is interesting about substance abuse prevention in Israel is that until recently the IADA was related to the Prime Minister's office, rather than being related to either the ministries of Health, Education, or Interior or being an independent and unrelated government organization. The reason for this act refers to issues of security. Back to the 1970s, when the IADA was established, there were – and still are – indications that Israel's enemies are intensively and purposely trying to smuggle drugs into Israel, seeing it as a strategic weapon to weaken the Israeli society, and especially the IDF. Some people believe that Israel's enemies were inspired by the major drug problem that the U.S. army encountered (see Bentel & Smith, 1971) during the Vietnam War (1963–73). Others believe it has to do with the intensive drug business of several terrorist groups in the Middle East. Be it this inspiration or another, the IDF and other security organizations found it essential to try to prevent substance abuse among Israel's population while at the same time trying to prevent substance smuggling into Israel. Practically speaking, as mentioned previously, while IADA is very active in dealing with all matters that are related to substance abuse, most of the prevention work is carried out in the school system, mostly by the school counselors. Currently, substance abuse prevention and support of the school-to-army transition are the only two mandatory prevention activities in all Israeli high schools. Several prevention programs have been explored by the Ministry of Education experts, and currently none of them have been widely adopted. However, according to existing data, as published by the Psychological Counseling Department (2015), the most popular prevention activities – that is, those preferred most by school counselors – are peer-led intervention (Sheppard, Golonka, & Costanzo, 2012); life skills promotion (Botvin & Griffin, 2004); school climate improvement (Ryabov, 2015); and the incorporation of an ex-addict (Israelashvili, 2011). While none of these, as well as other prevention programs, has been extensively evaluated with Israeli adolescents, it is hope that future research will yield evidence-based interventions, perhaps motivated by the new IADA standards for prevention programs.

Suicidal Behavior Prevention. In 2013, the Israel government announced that suicidal behavior is a national problem, and the government established the National Program for the Prevention of Suicidality and Suicide as a permanent counsel within the Ministry of Health (www.health.gov.il/English/MinistryUnits/HealthDivision/MedicalAdministration/Psychology/Pages/suicide-prev.aspx).

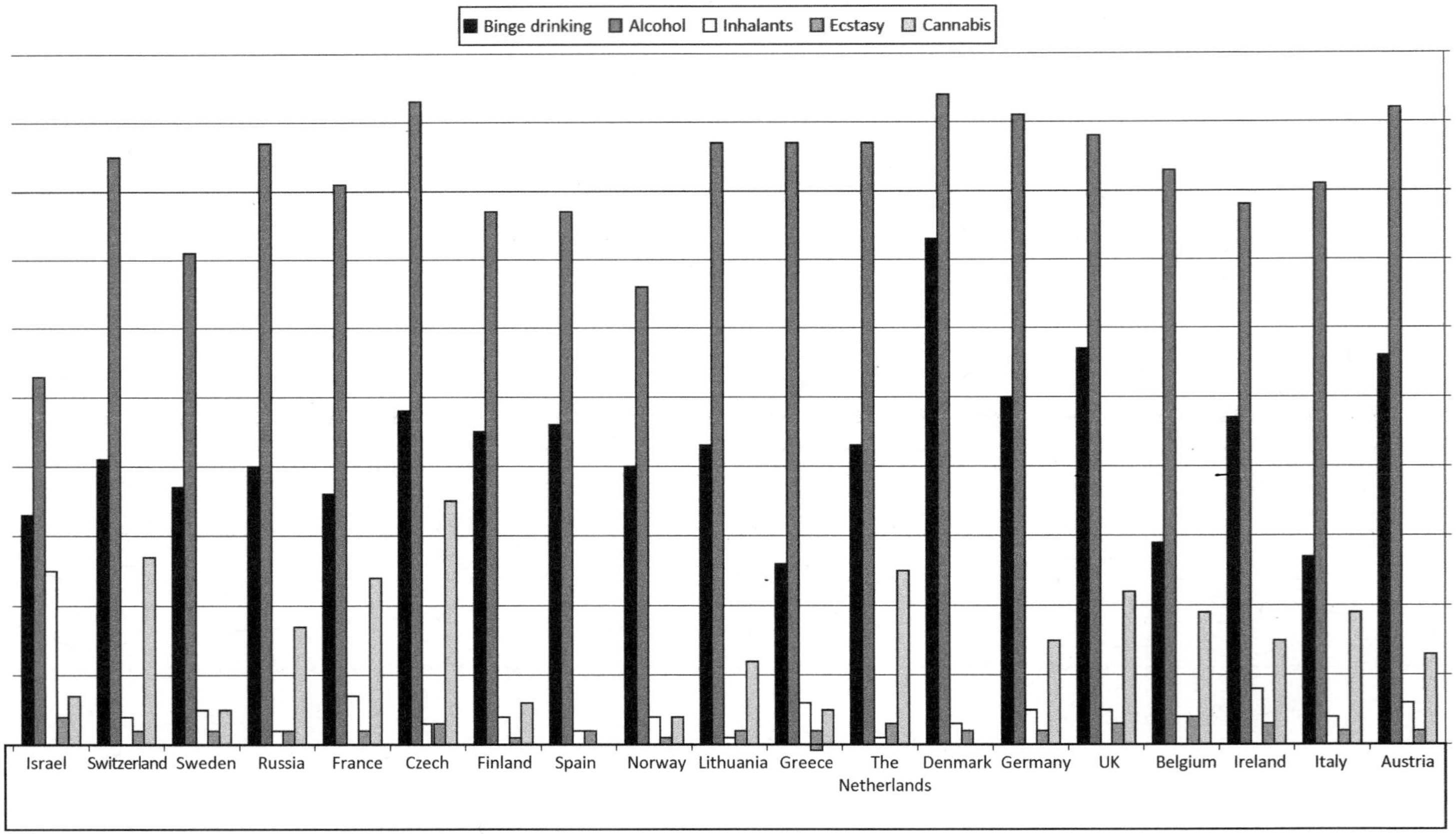

Figure 41.1. *Adolescents' substance and alcohol use in recent years – 2007.*
Source: IADA: www.antidrugs.gov.il/template/default.aspx?catid=120

Currently, the annual number of Israelis who commit suicide is five hundred and an additional six thousand are labeled (e.g., by hospital emergency rooms) as people who have tried to commit suicide. Yet, the total rate of suicidal behavior in Israel is relatively low in comparison to most Organization for Economic Cooperation and Development (OECD) countries, as illustrated in Figure 41.2. Hence, the reasons for the establishment of such a national program deserve clarification. In this context, a first note should be mentioned regarding the at-risk populations for suicidal behavior. Suicidal behavior in Israel is the second reason for death among ages fifteen to twenty-four years and among new immigrants. Thus, these two groups of (mostly) young people are of interest for the (gradually becoming older) Israel population. However, what seems to be more significant in explaining the government's decision is its acceptance of the scientifically long-lasting notion regarding the negative correlation between the salience of the Israel–Arab conflict and the suicide rate in Israel (Kimmerling, 1974) – that is, when the conflict escalates, there is a temporary decrease in suicidal behavior until it seems that the (Israeli) state gains control over the conflict (see also Andriessen, 2007; Durkheim, 1897). In addition, there was an increased awareness of the possible implications of exposure to the emerging suicidal bomber phenomenon (i.e., a terrorist attack in which the attacker intends to kill other people and expects to die in the process), especially indications that many who later became suicidal bombers expressed preliminary suicidal tendencies (Khan, 2012; Perry & Hasisi, 2015). There was also increased awareness of ordinary citizens' readiness either to imitate such suicidal bomber behavior or, preferably, to ask for help in times of personal need. Currently, most of the government attention is given to indicative prevention (those most at risk), by reaching out to people who are served by one of the health institutions in Israel (either general or mental health hospitals or clinics). Yet, universal prevention (for the entire population) programs have occasionally been initiated (Orbach, 2003), and increased attention is given to this issue by the Ministry of Education. Similarly, too many global interventions to prevent suicidal behavior (see Barzilay et al., 2015) and explorations of suicidal prevention interventions in Israel focused mainly on the following three components: (1) normalization of stress and depression feelings, (2) teaching coping skills, and (3) encouraging the take and give of social support when (someone is) in need.

School-to-Army Transition. As mentioned previously, in Israel, every Jewish adolescent is obliged to join the army for at least two years (females) or three years (males). Surveys among Israeli adolescents have shown that most of them welcome their enlistment into the IDF. This occurs for two reasons (Israelashvili & Karisa, 2014; Liblich, 1990): (a) they feel that there is a real public need for their military service; and (b) they expect military service to contribute highly to their preparation for adulthood. Confirmatory support for the validity of these two reasons emerges from studies conducted among Israeli emerging adults who have completed their military service, in which most ex-soldiers indicated that their military service was important and fostered their

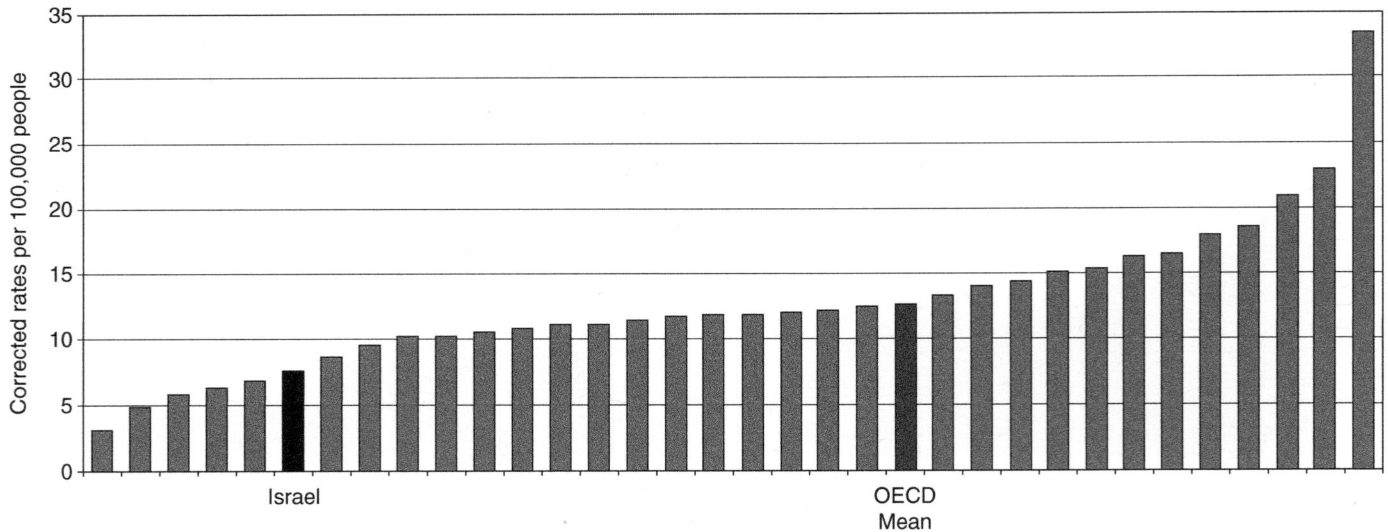

Figure 41.2. *2011 suicide rate in OECD countries.*
Source: www.health.gov.il/NewsAndEvents/SpokemanMesseges/PublishingImages/24112013_3.jpg

preparedness for adulthood (Dar & Kimchi, 2000). Nevertheless, since military service is mandatory and approaching, many Israeli high school students search for guidance and preparation to support their adjustment to their upcoming military service (Israelashvili & Karisa, 2014; Mayseless, 1993). In view of these findings, and in light of the importance of student preparation for the school to life transition, a preparatory intervention was designed for twelfth graders – boys and girls – facing military enlistment (Israelashvili, 2006). The program, known as the School-to-Army (STA) preparation, is a prevention program that aims to foster enlistees' self-efficacy and ability to adjust well to basic training. The program does not intend to serve the army's needs but rather to serve the needs of the adolescents who depart from school, home, and civilian life and move to compulsory military service. The STA program is intended to improve recruits' mental health and well-being by supplying the recruit with knowledge, skills, and training of the adjustment process to the military service. However, though the program targets the recruit's wellness, the army benefits also from the expected lower rate of maladaptive behavior in basic training.

The STA program was gradually developed, on a trial-and-error basis. Namely, three parallel actions were made in order to learn the problem to be prevented and to articulate the way to do it. First, in the school system, data on adolescents' needs were collected. Second, an analysis of what can practically be done while adolescents are still learning in high schools was conducted. Third, in the military system, several action studies of basic training were carried out in order to analyze exactly what the critical events are in basic training and what helps new recruits to adjust better to military life. The STA program was established based on information that was gathered along these explorations, and fit well into Meichenbaum's Stress Inoculation Training (SIT) model (Meichenbaum, 1993; Novaco, Cook, & Sarson, 1983)

In practice, the sequential order of the STA components is as follows:

1. The importance of transition from high school
2. The recruitment office – the "what," "when," and "why"
3. The "how" of vocational decision making
4. Physical training
5. The parents' meeting – how to support a child in transition
6. Mapping of stress in the course of organizational entry
7. Study day for familiarization with future military options
8. Coping and adjustment techniques
9. Meeting with soldiers who graduated from the student's high school
10. Simulated basic training
11. Conclusions following training
12. Consideration of what the student has currently has that will help the student cope in the future
13. Separate meetings with male and female students to answer their questions
14. Reflections on the preparation program and summing up

15. Broad view on the place of the newcomer within the IDF
16. Indicative prevention interventions to address current and future individual problems

Evaluative research has established the significant short-term impact of participation in military preparation programs, both on participants' subjective feelings of preparedness for military enlistment (Israelashvili & Taubman, 1997; Israelashvili & Wegman-Rozi, 2007) and on their behavior during basic training (Carmeli, 1999). In their study, Israelashvili and Wegman-Rozi (2007) explored the short-term and long-term effects of participation in the STA program, designed to foster students' transition from high school to compulsory military service in Israel. A multivariate longitudinal study of 247 male and female twelfth graders, divided into an intervention group and a control group, was conducted. The intervention group participated in a ten-meeting preparation program, focusing on the enhancement of empowerment feelings regarding entrance into military service. Measurements were conducted at three points in time: (1) before exposure to the preparation program, (2) after exposure to the preparation program, and (3) six to twelve months after military enlistment. Results of this study indicated that participants' preliminary feelings of general adjustment to life, as measured during their twelfth grade in high school, was a powerful predictor of their later adjustment to military life. Namely, the STA program served as a universal prevention program and did not meet the needs of those who are in need of more comprehensive support and counseling to help them better manage their life before military enlistment.

The point to be highlighted here is that the IDF's collaboration and investment in establishing the program and implementing it was significant, from the very first moment, and this was followed by the Ministry of Education's acceptance of the program as a mandatory intervention in all regular high schools in Israel. The motivation of both the IDF as well as the Ministry of Education to support the STA program stemmed from their realization of the program's contribution not only to the well-being of the enlisted individuals but also to improvement in Israel's security, due to a better adjustment of new recruits into the army.

Take-Home Message

In these three prevention program examples, security problems have led to intensive governmental intervention in contexts that are not trivial. This is a unique phenomenon, as it could be expected that in face of the increasing security problems the government might limit, rather than extend, its investment in prevention activity due to the limited resources and the need to address immediate security problems (Price & Bohara, 2013). The opposite has happened in Israel, for two reasons:

1. The government understands that security needs will not be solved by massive reaction to the immediate security problems. Rather, the government and

people of Israel assume that the security problems in which Israel is engaged will be an integral and lasting part of Israel's location in the Middle East.

2. Israeli governments over the years have accepted the basic notions that there are strong links between the intensity and characteristics of the security problems and the Israeli public's resilience. Moreover, the Israeli government has accepted the idea that prevention interventions could contribute to lessening problem behaviors and might promote the population's resilience and well-being.

Security is the major issue for any Israeli government, and seems that it will continue to be in the coming years. Hence, connecting other problem behavior (e.g., substance abuse) to security was an efficient path to gain governmental recognition and support. Similarly, in every country there are issues that seem to be essential for the population, as the government perceives it. Hence, this chapter aimed to highlight these two notions, as take-home messages from the case of Israel; that is, decision makers and politicians would be much more willing to cooperate and support prevention programs initiation and implementation once two conditions exist: (1) they are convinced that a well-established connection exists between a specific problem behavior and other regional/national parameters of survival and well-being; (2) they are convinced that a problem behavior can be prevented via the implementation of a proper intervention. The challenge that every prevention scholar faces is, firstly, to identify those issues that policy makers, and the public, perceived as major to their community life and existence, followed by finding the links between this (specific) issue and the problem to be prevented and the suggested prevention program.

Summary

Although geographically located in the Middle East, Israel has many characteristics of a typical Western society. As such, prevention programs are conducted on a regular basis. However, Israel is atypical in its awareness of issues related to national and personal security. Hence, those prevention programs that could be linked – directly or indirectly – to topics that are related to security gain extensive governmental support. Three examples have been outlined in this chapter: substance abuse prevention; suicidal behavior prevention; and STA promotion. It is suggested that many countries and states have similar major topics of concern that can get the government's attention. Thus, it is suggested that prevention specialists devote special efforts to the three following steps: (1) identify the priorities of the leadership and stakeholders; (2) explore data about the (negative) impact of the problem to be prevention on that priority topic; and (3) help leadership and stakeholders comprehend the connections between the behavior to be prevented and leadership/stakeholder priorities. While the first step is familiar to prevention scholars, such as

Communities that Care (Fagan & Hawkins, 2015; Oesterle et al., 2015), the other steps are less familiar and hence are suggested for implementation globally.

References

Abel, R. M., & Friedman, H. A. (2009). Israeli school and community response to war trauma: a review of selected literature. *School Psychology International* 30: 265–81. doi: 10.1177/0143034309106493

Abelin, T. (2006). Legal measures in support of prevention in Switzerland. *Journal of Public Health Policy* 27: 355–65. doi: dx.doi.org/10.1057/palgrave.jphp.3200093

Andriessen, K. (2007). Two further comments on Durkheim's *Le Suicide*. *Crisis: The Journal of Crisis Intervention and Suicide Prevention* 28: 44–5. doi: dx.doi.org/10.1027/0227–5910.28.1.44

Barzilay, S., Feldman, D., Snir, A., Apter, A., Carli, V., Hoven, C. W., & Wasserman, D. (2015). The interpersonal theory of suicide and adolescent suicidal behavior. *Journal of Affective Disorders* 183: 68–74. doi: dx.doi.org/10.1016/j.jad.2015.04.047

Bentel D. R. & Smith D. E. (1971). Drug abuse in combat: the crisis of drugs and addiction among American troops in Vietnam. *Journal of Psychedelic Drugs* 4: 118–22.

Botvin, G. J., & Griffin, K. W. (2004). Life skills training: empirical findings and future directions. *Journal of Primary Prevention* 25: 211–32. doi: dx.doi.org/10.1023/B:JOPP.0000042391.58573.5b

Bradley, R. H., & Gilkey, B. (2002). The impact of the Home Instructional Program for Preschool Youngsters (HIPPY) on school performance in 3rd and 6th grades. *Early Education and Development* 13: 301–11. doi: dx.doi.org/10.1207/s15566935eed1303_4

Brown, A., & Lee, J. (2014). School performance in elementary, middle, and high school: a comparison of children based on HIPPY participation during the preschool years. *School Community Journal* 24: 83–106.

Bruhn, A. L., Hirsch, S. E., & Lloyd, J. W. (2015). Treatment integrity in school-wide programs: a review of the literature (1993–2012). *Journal of Primary Prevention* 36: 335–49. doi: dx.doi.org/10.1007/s10935-015–0400-9

Carmeli, A. (1999). Follow-up of preparation program effectiveness in supporting recruits to I.D.F. (Unpublished research report).

Cohen, Y. (1988). War and social integration: the effects of the Israeli–Arab conflict on Jewish emigration from Israel. *American Sociological Review* 53: 908–18.

Dar, Y., & Kimchi, S. (2000). Self perception of maturation following the military service (Hebrew). *Megamot* 40: 612–23.

Durkheim, E. (1897). *Le Suicide: Étude de sociologie*, Paris: Félix Alcan.

Fagan, A. A., & Hawkins, J. D. (2015). Enacting preventive interventions at the community level: the Communities that Care Prevention System. In Scheier, L. M. (ed.), *Handbook of Adolescent Drug Use Prevention: Research, Intervention Strategies, and Practice.* Washington, DC: American Psychological Association, pp. 343–60. doi: dx.doi.org/10.1037/14550-020

IADA (Israel Anti-Drugs & Alcohol Authority) (2015). Prevention guidelines. www.antidrugs.org.il/template/default.aspx?catid=395

Israelashvili, M. (1999). Adolescents' help-seeking behaviour in times of community crisis. *International Journal for the Advancement of Counselling* 21: 87–96.

Israelashvili, M. (2011). The paradox of realism in exposing students to ex-addict. Paper presented in EUSPR Conference, Lisbon, Portugal.

Israelashvili, M. (2005). Staying normal in an abnormal world: reflections on mental health counseling from an Israeli point of view. *Journal of Mental Health Counseling* 27: 238–47.

Israelashvili, M. (2015a). School mental health in Israel: background, services and challenges. In Kutcher, S., Weist, M., & Wei, Y. (eds.), *School Mental Health: Global Challenges and Opportunities*. Cambridge, UK: Cambridge University Press, pp. 125–38.

Israelashvili, M. (2015b). The unspoken shift from quality to quantity standards in substance use(r) treatment and prevention: a challenge to unfinished intervention business. *Substance Use & Misuse* 50: 1079–82.

Israelashvili, M. (2006). The school-to-army transition: interventions for high-school students and their families. In Buchwald, P. (ed.), *Stress and Anxiety: Application to Health, Community, Work Place, and Education.* Cambridge, UK: Cambridge Scholar Press Ltd., pp. 325–46.

Israelashvili, M., & Benjamin, B. A. (2009). Context and diversity in the provision of counseling services in Israel. In Heppner, P., Ægisdóttir, S., Leung, A., Norsworthy, K., & Greenstein, L. (eds.), *Handbook of Cross-Cultural Counseling: Cultural Assumptions and Practices Worldwide*. Thousand Oaks, CA: Sage, pp. 449–64.

Israelashvili, M., & Karisa, L. (2014). Occupational preferences during the military compulsory enlistment: a comparison between new recruits and released soldiers. Research Report, Tel Aviv University.

Israelashvili, M., & Taubamn, O. (1997). Adolescents' preparation for military service: a preliminary evaluation. *Megamot* 38: 408–20.

Israelashvili, M., & Wegman-Rozi, O. (2007). Effectiveness of preparing 12th graders for mandatory military service. *Military Psychology* 19: 175–96.

Khan, A. (2012). Psychological makeup of a Pakistani Muslim suicide bomber: an observation-based perspective. *International Journal of Cultic Studies* 3: 25–34.

Kilburn, M. R., & Cannon, J. S. (2015). Home visiting start-up: lessons learned from program replication in New Mexico. *Journal of Primary Prevention* 36: 275–9. doi: dx.doi.org/10.1007/s10935-015–0392-5

Kimmerling, B. (1974). Anomie and integration in Israeli society and the salience of the Israeli–Arab conflict. *Studies in Comparative International Development* 9: 64–89.

Liblich, A. (1990). Transition to adulthood during compulsory service in the I.D.F. In Benyamini, K., Dolev, A., Amir, M., Cohen, E., & Schlesinger, I. M. (eds.), *Theory and Application in Psychology* (Hebrew). Jerusalem: Magnes Press, pp. 271–82.

Mayseless, O. (1993). Attitudes toward military service among Israeli youth. In Ashkenazy, D. (ed.), *The Military in the Service of Society and Democracy*. Westport, CT: Greenwood Press, pp. 32–5.

Meichenbaum, D. (1993). Stress inoculation training: a twenty-year update. In Woolfolk, R. L., & Lehre, P. M. (eds.), *Principles and Practice of Stress Management.* New York: Guilford Press, pp. 373–406.

Milat, A. J., King, L., Bauman, A. E., & Redman, S. (2013). The concept of scalability: increasing the scale and potential adoption of health promotion interventions into policy and practice. *Health Promotion International* 28: 285–98. doi: dx.doi.org/10.1093/heapro/dar097

Nakash, O., Razon, L., & Levav, Y. (2015). Primary mental health prevention themes in published research and academic programs in Israel. *Israel Journal of Health Policy Research* 4: 3. doi: 10.1186/2045–4015-4-3

Nievar, A. M., Jacobson, A., Chen, Q., Johnson, U., & Dier, S. (2011). Impact of HIPPY on home learning environments of Latino families. *Early Childhood Research Quarterly* 26: 268–77.

Novaco, R. W., Cook, T. M., & Sarson, I. G. (1983). Military recruit training. In Meichenbaum, D., & Jaremko, M. (eds.), *Stress Prevention and Management*. New York: Plenum, pp. 377–419.

Oesterle, S., Hawkins, J. D., Kuklinski, M. R., Fagan, A. A., Fleming, C., Rhew, I. C., & Catalano, R. F. (2015). Effects of communities that care on males' and females' drug use and delinquency 9 years after baseline in a community-randomized trial. *American Journal of Community Psychology* 56: 217–28. doi: dx.doi.org/10.1007/s10464-015–9749-4

Orbach, I. (2003). Suicide prevention for adolescents. In King, R. A. & Apter, A. (eds.), *Suicide in Children and Adolescents.* New York: Cambridge University Press, pp. 227–50.

Perry, S., & Hasisi, B. (2015). Rational choice rewards and the jihadist suicide bomber. *Terrorism and Political Violence* 27: 53–80. doi: dx.doi.org/10.1080/09546553.2014.962991

Price, J. I., & Bohara, A. K. (2013). Maternal health care amid political unrest: the effect of armed conflict on antenatal care utilization in Nepal. *Health Policy and Planning* 28: 309–19. doi: dx.doi.org/10.1093/heapol/czs062

Psychological-Counseling Department, Israel Ministry of Education (2015). Publications on substance abuse: cms.education.gov.il/EducationCMS/UNITS/Shefi/Templates/RegularText.aspx?NRMODE=Published&NRNODEGUID=%7b6F0C753D-9C12-409F–9EE2-6E450430A6FF%7d&NRORIGINALURL=%2fEducationCMS%2fUnits%2fShefi%2fSamimTabakAlcohol%2f&NRCACHEHINT=NoModifyGuest#5

Raviv, A., & Weiner, I. (1995). Why don't they like us? Psychologists' public image in Israel during the Persian Gulf War. *Professional Psychology: Research and Practice* 26: 88–94.

Romano, J. L. (2015). *Prevention Psychology: Enhancing Personal and Social Well-Being.* Washington, DC: American Psychological Association. doi: dx.doi.org/10.1037/14442-008

Ryabov, I. (2015). Relation of peer effects and school climate to substance use among Asian American adolescents. *Journal of Adolescence* 42: 115–27. doi: dx.doi.org/10.1016/j.adolescence.2015.04.007

Senor, D., & Singer, S. (2009). *Start-Up Nation: The Story of Israel's Economic Miracle*. New York: Twelve.

Sheppard, C. S., Golonka, M., & Costanzo, P. R. (2012). Evaluating the impact of a substance use intervention program on the peer status and influence of adolescent peer leaders. *Prevention Science* 13: 75–85. doi: dx.doi.org/10.1007/s11121-011–0248-z

Sucaldito, N. L., Tayag, E. A., Roces, M. C. R., Malison, M. D., Robie, B. D., & Howze, E. H. (2014). The Philippines Field Management Training Program (FMTP): strengthening management capacity in a decentralized public health system. *International Journal of Public Health* 59: 897–903. doi: dx.doi.org/10.1007/s00038-014-0603-5

Tatar, M. (2001). Comparing adolescents' considerations for self-referral and counsellors' perceptions of these considerations: an exploratory study. *Journal of Adolescence* 24: 171–81.

van Weel, C., Roberts, R., De Maeseneer, J., & van der Velden, K. (2011). Public health: profession, health system, government control. *Lancet* 378: 468–9. doi: dx.doi.org/10.1016/S0140-6736(11)60275-4

Wang, B., Stanton, B., Lunn, S., Rolle, G., Poitier, M., Adderley, R., … Deveaux, L. (2016). The impact of teachers' modifications of an evidenced-based HIV prevention intervention on program outcomes. *Prevention Science* 17: 122–33. doi: dx.doi.org/10.1007/s11121-015-0592-5

42 Preventing the Spread of HIV/AIDS in Botswana

Rex Stockton, Daniel Goldberg, Tebatso Paul, & Barbara De Larm

This chapter examines prevention methods for human immunodeficiency virus/acquired immune deficiency syndrome (HIV/AIDS) in a specific southern African country, Botswana. AIDS is a worldwide problem and, like all epidemics, has social, economic, and cultural implications. While the chapter focuses on Botswana, it is important to understand it in a global context. Thus, examples from other countries are included. As Murphy, Greene, Mihailovic, & Olupot-Olupot (2006) noted, "The sooner we confront HIV/AIDS as the multifaceted complex issue it is, the sooner we can make important steps towards progress in HIV prevention" (p. 379).

Economic, Social, and Cultural Make-Up of Botswana

To understand the impact of AIDS in Botswana, it is crucial to understand something about the country's economic, social, and cultural make-up. Botswana occupies a large landmass of 5,800 square kilometers (the majority is located in the Kalahari Desert), but is thinly populated, with an overall population of 2,045,752 (Ministry of Health, 2013). The bulk of the population, estimated at 600,000, is in the capital city of Gaborone (Ministry of Health, 2013). Botswana is located in southern Africa, surrounded by Namibia, South Africa, and Zimbabwe. The country is divided into ten regions. Botswana gained independence from Britain in 1966. It is unique in its part of the world, in that it began with a constitutional democracy. At that time (1966), it was among the twenty-five poorest and least developed countries in the world, with a gross domestic product (GDP) of $300 per capita (Hanemann, 2005).

Botswana has the good fortune of being mineral rich, and with the discovery after independence of the world's largest diamond mines, the country negotiated a 50–50 ownership of the mines with the De Beers Diamond Company in South Africa. Unlike many other African countries, Botswana has been able to translate these resources into infrastructure and a solid governmental body (Stegling, 2004). The government is centralized, and decision making is relatively top-down. The official governmental system is paralleled by a traditional *dikgotla* system of chiefs and councils. This system has been somewhat absorbed into the centralized government; however, much of its influence over decision making has been greatly decreased (Allen & Heald, 2004). The lack of inclusion of indigenous beliefs and traditional leaders in the decision-making process had real implications in how the country mobilized to combat the AIDS epidemic, specifically in the exclusive use of Euro-American medical practices as opposed to including traditional healing practices and healers (Levers, 2006).

With a 2013 GDP of $7,315 (World Bank, 2013), Botswana has made phenomenal economic progress with a relatively noncorrupt governmental and business structure. Fueled by its mineral resources, Botswana has moved from one of the poorest nations in the world (1966) to a middle-income country. Infrastructure such as hospitals and clinics, highway development, and water access has improved from almost nothing to being readily accessible. Literacy was almost nonexistent in 1966, and, as of 2003, adult literacy was estimated at 78 percent (Stegling, 2004). The government has been democratic since its beginning, so in many ways Botswana has been a model country in the African continent. Even with all of this material progress, however, the country has been severely affected by the AIDS epidemic.

The History of the AIDS Epidemic

The problem of AIDS in Botswana is extremely serious, with one of the highest incidence rates in Africa. The average life expectancy was close to sixty-five years in the early 1990s in Botswana but dramatically decreased in 2002 to an average of thirty-six years (Mahajan et al., 2008). This was in large part due to HIV/AIDS (Mahajan et al., 2008). The AIDS problem in Botswana is just a microcosm of the AIDS epidemic that rapidly became worldwide. It has progressed to the point that every country in the world is affected. In addition to the high rate of deaths associated with untreated AIDS, it has ramifications on sociological, cultural, biological, psychological, and other areas of one's life. Therefore, it is not surprising that great fear and irrational behavior have been associated with AIDS since its inception. This has resulted in extreme stigma and violence, including death, against those who are infected.

The first reports of a mysterious new disease began in medical centers in the 1950s that had dire effects on the human immune system. This often led to death from a host of other diseases, most notably pneumonia, Kaposi's sarcoma (a malignant skin cancer), and candidiasis (a fungus appearing on various parts of the body) (Jennings, 2012). These typically led to the death of a patient within a two-year period. While there has been much discussion as to the origin of AIDS, the first diagnosed AIDS cases were reportedly assessed in New York City in 1979 (Jennings, 2012). Other reports have the first reported cases of HIV/AIDS happening in Los Angeles (Jennings, 1988; Merson, O'Malley, Serwadda, & Apisuk, 2008.) However the case may be, AIDS as an epidemic is a relatively recent development that rapidly grew to epidemic proportions.

The current (2014) hysteria and fear related to the Ebola epidemic in Africa brings to mind a similar response when AIDS first appeared in an ever increasing amount in the 1980s. Before it was known why people were contracting a previously unknown disease with death as inevitable, HIV/AIDS brought forth much anxiety and stigma to those affected by the disease. HIV-related stigma is the process of degrading and dehumanizing people living with HIV/AIDS (PLWHA), and HIV-related discrimination is a behavioral manifestation of mistreatment based on one's HIV/AIDS status (Ogden & Nyblade, 2005). HIV/AIDS infection is often associated with already previously stigmatized behaviors in many societies (e.g., sharing needles for drug use, homosexual acts, and promiscuous sex) and is often considered to be the infected individual's fault (Ogden & Nyblade, 2005). It was not until "innocent individuals" contracted AIDS through blood transfusions that the stigma associated with AIDS as being regarded as a disease of homosexuals was mitigated.

Take for instance the case of Ryan White in the 1980s. Ryan was a young boy attending middle school in Kokomo, Indiana (United States [U.S.]), who contracted AIDS after receiving contaminated blood in treatment for his haemophilia. Parents and teachers affiliated with Ryan's school petitioned to ban Ryan. Hysteria was rampant as people feared he would infect others. Ryan and his family experienced hostile threats, including a gunshot through a window in his home, and lawsuits from those in the community who were ignorant of the nature of HIV and how it is contracted. After a difficult battle with the disease and enduring hostility from the school and the Kokomo community, Ryan and his family moved to another small town that was much more welcoming. As information regarding the nature of AIDS and how it is contracted became more widely recognized, Ryan became a kind of "poster boy" for AIDS in the United States. Ryan became nationally known through the media and served as a symbol of innocence for a highly stigmatized disease. After battling with this disease for several years, Ryan passed away. Shortly after his death, the United States put into action the Ryan White Act, which would continue to help HIV/AIDS-positive individuals without resources receive care through federal funding. AIDS has certainly not gone away, but the stigma attached to it has been greatly reduced as the information and treatment of the disease has been well established. This holds true in other countries as well.

Ryan's case is a prime example of the negative effects of stigma and a lack of information and understanding that is so prevalent in the current Ebola epidemic. HIV/AIDS has presented a monumental health challenge, beginning with a small number of individuals in the late 1970s and 1980s, and has spread throughout the world as a pandemic. Sub-Saharan Africa, especially Botswana, has been hard hit. For several years, it held the distinction of being the epicenter of the AIDS epidemic. In the early stages of the epidemic, Botswana's National AIDS Coordinating Agency reported a 73.2 percent increase in the mortality rate across all diseases, 10 percent of the overall rate being attributed to HIV/AIDS (Stegling, 2004). As of 2013, the World Health Organization (WHO) estimated that 35 million people were living with HIV/AIDS, of which 2.1 million were newly infected. In addition, 1.5 million deaths were attributable to AIDS. However, these statistics have been questioned by Chris Jennings (2012), a prominent scholar and writer, as he concluded that WHO is overestimating the number of individuals with HIV. Whatever the actual figures, this disease remains a very serious public health epidemic. While the disease has spread worldwide, sub-Saharan Africa currently holds 68 percent of the global population of HIV (WHO, 2011). In Botswana specifically, the rate of HIV/AIDS is estimated at 18.5 percent by the Office of Central Statistics (BAIS-IV, 2013).

Reminiscent of other pandemics, the disease spread in an almost hypergeometric fashion, and countries were overwhelmed with the number of individuals who became HIV-positive. To put this in human terms, when the first author of this chapter began his work in Botswana in 2002, AIDS patients did not have access to the antiretroviral medication that dramatically lengthens life expectancy of those infected. When conducting a weeklong group counseling workshop in 2002, he was struck by the number of times participants talked about funerals they were attending on Saturdays. It seemed that every Saturday was consumed by attending funerals for those who had died of AIDS.

Unlike in the United States, where the preponderance of AIDS victims initially were male, in Botswana females were also early causalities of AIDS. According to the Department of HIV/AIDS Prevention and Care in the Botswana Ministry of Health (2012), "women now account for almost 52% of global adult prevalence (60% of prevalence in sub-Saharan Africa)." Thus, it is especially important to provide prevention services to this and other high-risk populations, such as men who have sex with men, young people aged fifteen to twenty-four, drug users who share needles, and sex workers (WHO, 2011). However, these are not the only populations at risk, and prevention needs to be available for the entire population. The good news is that the rate of new infections and deaths in sub-Saharan Africa attributed to AIDS has dropped 19 percent from 2004 to 2009 (WHO, 2011). Specifically, the incidence rate in Botswana has significantly decreased since 2008 (Statistics Botswana, 2013). This is not to say that AIDS is not a continuing problem. There are multiple reasons why this is so, such as culture; lack of knowledge concerning prevention and treatment; and, high on the list, a lack of resources (WHO, 2011). Unlike medical problems such as heart disease, cancer, and so forth, the stigma attached to AIDS is a major problem, as this represents a leading factor for individuals avoiding treatment (Wolfe et al., 2006).

Botswana's Governmental Response to the HIV/AIDS Epidemic

The WHO recommends four strategic steps for the health sectors response to this epidemic:

> Strategic direction 1: Optimize HIV prevention, diagnosis, treatment and care outcomes.
>
> Strategic direction 2: Leverage broader health outcomes through HIV responses.
>
> Strategic direction 3: Build strong and sustainable systems.
>
> Strategic direction 4: Reduce vulnerability and remove structural barriers to accessing services
>
> (WHO, 2011).

This chapter focuses on strategic direction 1, specifically prevention. Since 1987, prevention efforts have taken on many forms. The chapter examines the history of these efforts, largely focusing on Botswana. This began with Botswana's Ministry of Health (MOH) National AIDS Control Program (NACP). The program consisted of both short- and medium-term plans. The short-term plan was designed, in collaboration with the WHO, to address the HIV/AIDS crisis and utilized a single-sector approach (Stegling, 2004).

The medium-term plan was put into action over a five-year period, where it focused on the HIV/AIDS problem, first in terms of public health and then as a multipronged approach, with several different government offices getting involved. These changes were in line with what was happening in general in the AIDS world. Because of the complex nature of the HIV/AIDS epidemic, prevention strategies changed to be much more comprehensive.

In the early 1990s, prevention approaches emphasized abstinence, faithfulness to one's partner, and the use of condoms, commonly known as the "ABC" approach (Singh, Darrock, & Bankole, 2004). The approach focused on sex education for those who were unmarried. "A" stood for abstinence. The government encouraged young people to wait until marriage before engaging in sexual intercourse. Since one of the primary modes of contracting AIDS is through the transmission of bodily fluids, the government believed by encouraging people to limit their contact, they could limit the spread of the disease. The commitment to be faithful to one's partner was part "B" of the approach. It was clear that if one was faithful to his or her partner, and both partners were HIV-negative, the two would not contract the disease. However, many individuals (especially males), participated in extramarital sex. The "C" represented utilization of condoms for those who did not remain abstinent. This recommendation was put in place to minimize risk of contraction through safer sexual contact. Theoretically, it was a very sound program. Practically, it did not take into account that women, especially African women, could be faithful to their husbands, but their husbands might well have outside sexual affairs. It is very difficult for a wife to refuse to have sex with a husband, even though he is having sex outside of the marriage. Thus the widely adopted approach had mixed results.

For comparison purposes, it is instructive to compare Botswana's approach to HIV/AIDS with Uganda's. In the 1980s, Uganda was regarded as having the highest HIV/AIDS rate in the world. Despite this, Uganda was able to reduce the numbers of those affected with AIDS using the ABC approach (Singh et al., 2004). As noted, the "ABC" approach failed to take into account that a substantial number of males in many societies are not monogamous. Of course, the same can also be true with females. The success of the ABC method is attributed to individuals reducing their number of sex partners. While the lowered rate in Uganda was particularly hailed as evidence that the ABC technique was effective, as Singh et al. (2004) pointed out that this was not necessarily the case, as there was strong governmental commitment (particularly by the President of Uganda) to reduce HIV/AIDS, efforts were made to destigmatize people living with HIV/AIDS, and there were intensive campaigns in the areas of sexual activity and the promotion of condom use; all of these factors had important roles to play in reducing HIV/AIDS. Additionally, the method of measuring AIDS incidence in Uganda was skewed since only urban areas were surveyed, and a large portion of the overall population lives in a rural setting (Murphy et al., 2006). While the reduction of the incidents of AIDS was good news, the AIDS problem remained severe across sub-Saharan Africa.

Ironically, while the AIDS incidence rate seemed to be stabilizing in Uganda, it was on the rise in Botswana. As Allen and Heald (2004) point out, Botswana and Uganda began their HIV/AIDS prevention campaigns in roughly the same time period. While Uganda's AIDS rates diminished, Botswana's were on a rapid increase, despite the countries' use of similar prevention techniques (Allen & Heald, 2004). This is especially ironic considering the rapid economic progress in Botswana during this time. Allen and Heald (2004) attribute this in part to the lack of involvement of key individuals at the grassroots levels as well as significant cultural factors.

Botswana benefited from a stable government and an economic growth that continued to rise. In both countries, the governments responded swiftly, and both welcomed outside aid from international entities. Botswana made good use of its resources in developing a universal, primary, and secondary education system, and a health care system of hospitals and clinics was developed. This was paralleled by a welfare system that provided for orphans, the elderly, and other needy individuals. In many ways, the country has had an effective and thoughtful leadership. So the question as to why the AIDS rate was continuing to increase, despite the various plans, was very real. The anthropologists Allen and Heald (2004) noted that in the earliest days of Botswana's governmental response to AIDS, decisions were made from the top down, that is, the local authorities (e.g., tribal chiefs, village elders, and others) were not involved as decision makers. A campaign for AIDS prevention began with the ABC model and was publicized using posters that were placed in governmental offices and other public places. The results were only partially successful. In particular, the campaign to utilize condoms did not seem to be effective. Allen and Heald (2004) advanced the idea that the promotion of condom use at an early stage backfired for cultural reasons. The lack of involvement of individuals at the grassroots, failure to enlist local healers, and other cultural reasons resulted in a lack of compliance of the Botswana population, which resulted in increasing AIDS rates.

The first national campaign in Botswana against AIDS in 1988 used radio messages, car bumper stickers, and T-shirts as a medium for prevention messages. Allen and Heald (2004) believe that the fact that the government response was so swift and depended on trust in the message before the population had a great deal of experience with AIDS and its severe consequences meant that the message was easily disregarded. This was not the case in Uganda since the population was already aware of the severity of the disease and its consequences due to the epidemic occurring earlier than in Botswana. It was not surprising that the Botswana population was sceptical at first about the prevention messages. AIDS became known as the "radio disease" because the earliest advertising campaign was done via the radio. For the local population, condom promotion was seen as encouraging "immorality," and in a perverse twist of logic there was a widely held belief that condoms were not useful to control the disease, but were in fact spreading the disease. In Setswana culture, sexual intercourse has special properties due to the belief that it engages *a flow of bloods between partners*, which promotes health, as well as being procreative. Given this belief, many locals viewed condom use as counterproductive. This was especially true in rural regions of Botswana. Thus, ironically, the initial Botswana HIV/AIDS rate continued to climb while Uganda's rate declined.

The Setswana cultural beliefs are deeply held, and the AIDS prevention campaign was easily disregarded until the death rate became so high that it became obvious to all that the country had a significant problem. It was only after the government began to involve the grassroots population, including the tribal chiefs, their associated councils, and local healers, that the public realized the importance of testing and knowing one's status, as well as not having casual sex. At this point, the campaigns had become more effective at spreading prevention messages. Also, in a helpful act in 2003, the then–Botswana President Mogae gave his full support to the testing program as well as the antiretroviral (ARV) program.

However, eventually a need for a more comprehensive approach became apparent. Following the "ABC" approach, a newly revised approach was put into place by the Botswana government and reflected what was going on internationally. The new approach was multipronged and focused on several key problem areas such as location, resource availability, and high-risk populations.

The new approach was termed the Botswana Medium Term Plan (MTPII – 1997–2002) and included the development of the National AIDS Council, which was charged with coordinating the national response with the National AIDS Coordination Agency (NACA) serving as its secretariat.

This first phase is now over and Botswana is well under way in its Second National Strategic Framework created for 2010–2016 (NACA, 2009). During the First National Strategic Framework's midimplementation review, the recommenders advocated the need for prevention of HIV as a primary concern. In addition, serious challenges obstructing Botswana's efforts to eliminate HIV/AIDS have been found. Some of these obstacles include decreased condom use, lack of funds, stigma and discrimination, male circumcision practices, gender issues, and data collection issues. Many of these issues can be handled with preventive measures. Thus, as part of Botswana's Second National Strategic Framework, the first priority is to focus on prevention methods. While zero new infections is a lofty goal, according to the latest Botswana AIDS Impact Survey (BAIS IV), Botswana has decreased the incidence rate of HIV/AIDS infection from 1.45 percent in 2008 to 1.35 percent in 2013 (Statistics Botswana, 2013).

According to NACA (2009), there are a number of objectives and strategies in place to reach these goals. Some of the strategies for prevention in the Second

National Strategic Framework include increasing efforts in interventions advocating for the reduction of multiple and concurrent sexual partners; increasing national communication for HIV prevention programs; increasing gender-specific HIV/AIDS knowledge and knowledge related to substance use, condom use, and male circumcision; increasing the quality of HIV testing and counseling services; increasing medicinal treatment for all members of the population, but specifically for pregnant women; and increasing access to prevention services in hard-to-reach populations. These strategies are designed to increase utilization of health care for HIV prevention and reduce the incidence of HIV transmission.

HIV/AIDS and Stigma

As in other cultures, Botswanan society has many negative beliefs about individuals infected with HIV/AIDS. For instance, research has shown that people living with HIV/AIDS experience stigma physically, mentally, and emotionally (Ogden & Nyblade, 2005). Culture has a great deal to do with how those individuals living with HIV/AIDS are perceived and the amount of associated stigma. For example, in order to be fully masculine or feminine in Botswana society, one must be a reproductive individual (Upton & Dolan, 2011). Thus, risky sexual practices, such as having multiple partners, must be weighed against the need to prove one's gender identity. One can assume that not being able to have children is stigmatized on a level similar with a HIV diagnosis, in terms of self-worth of both genders.

The NACA has conducted numerous survey studies assessing the population's overall knowledge and perceptions about HIV/AIDS. Its first survey in 2001 found that while the population knew that HIV/AIDS posed a serious risk to their communities, and that prevention measures existed to avoid the virus, there was a distinct lack of knowledge regarding the specifics of HIV/AIDS (Stegling, 2004). Additionally, many of the previous efforts to reduce HIV/AIDS transmission in Botswana (e.g., fear-based campaigns) resulted in perpetuating stigma without decreasing the prevalence rates. Furthermore, these campaigns often did not provide education about the disease and made clear distinctions between PLWHA and those not infected, which led to PLWHA feeling isolated and alone.

There are a number of ill effects stigma can have on an individual's well-being. Elford et al. (2005) stated that stigmatizing beliefs can become engrained in an individual's self-perception and may cause detrimental outcomes. This is not only true for one's psychology, but also for one's biology. Logie and Gadalla (2009) conducted a meta-analysis on the impact of HIV stigma on the health of PLWHA in North America, which also has significance for Botswana. The analysis reported that high stigma was related to a variety of negative health effects, such as meager social support, reduced physical health, and poor mental health. More precisely, high stigma was associated with poor mental health by a correlation effect of $r = -0.4$ (Logie & Gadalla 2009). Peltzer and Ramagan (2011) explored how stigma affected a large sample of South Africa's HIV/AIDS patients in a quantitative study. They found depression and low quality-of-life scores were related to internalized stigma, and that perceived stigma levels were high when the patients began treatment but lowered slightly over the course of the following year. The authors concluded that HIV treatment should include counseling and support for stigma-related issues, and that AIDS education mediated this relationship (Peltzer & Ramagan, 2011).

HIV/AIDS stigma has also been shown to be a barrier to receiving medicinal treatment for PLWHA (Mahajan et al., 2008; Wolfe et al., 2006). In Wolfe et al.'s study, 15 percent of the participants directly attributed HIV-related stigma to be a barrier for them in following their medication regime. Mahajan et al. (2008) stated from their meta-analysis utilizing UNAIDS and WHO studies that, "in addition to devastating the familial, social, and economic lives of individuals, H/A (HIV/AIDS) stigma is cited as a major barrier to accessing prevention, care, and treatment services."

While stigma clearly has a strong negative effect on PLWHA, there are some hopeful signs that stigma can be reduced. For example, a South African study surveyed town members before and three years after implementing an antiretroviral therapy program and a community-based HIV program seeking to increase awareness and educate the town (Mal, Middelkoop, Mark, Wood, & Bekker, 2013). The researchers found that upon the program's completion, the knowledge of HIV/AIDS increased, HIV/AIDS testing increased, and surveyed stigma scores were significantly lower compared to the first survey (Mall et al., 2013).

Botswana's Current Prevention Methods: An Overview

As HIV/AIDS still has no cure, behavioral change is hailed as playing a vital role in preventing the epidemic for the foreseeable future (NACA, 2009). Methods that may have the greatest likelihood to have positive preventive effects consider cultural and systematic predictors of vulnerability. Some predictors are geographical prevalence and high-risk populations (e.g., children, young women, males who have sex with males, and people who inject drugs; Gerson, 2014). It is important to know where to target resources.

As outlined in the preceding, HIV/AIDS prevention is a topic of national importance in Botswana, given its high prevalence rate. Prevention efforts are in place, but it is critical that these efforts are utilizing methods that have a high likelihood of success. While the following studies did not take place in Botswana, the recommendations for effective prevention efforts have significance for Botswana as well as globally. Merson et al. (2008) discuss the aspects of successful prevention techniques. The researchers suggest that a combination of prevention techniques that utilize behavioral, biomedical, and structural approaches have the best chance for success. The Rural HIV/AIDS Prevention Work Group (2009) in the United States notes three important factors for successful HIV/AIDS prevention programs: (1) educational programs must be interactive rather than directive in nature in order to effect actual behavior change (such as changing safe sex habits); (2) prevention efforts need to be targeted to specific audiences, taking cultural and social beliefs/values into consideration as well as other factors such as literacy level; (3) HIV/AIDS prevention education treads on extremely personal topics, such as safe sex practices/sexual behaviors, and needs to be non-judgmental and encourage participants to choose to make behavioral changes rather than instructing them to do so. While these tenets hold true for community-level interventions, in order for national prevention techniques to be successful, governmental leadership, especially intergovernmental, is necessary alongside community activism (Merson et al., 2008).

One study that took place in northwestern Zimbabwe found that individuals are more receptive to utilizing prevention methods when they are knowledgeable about the AIDS virus and the consequences of infection (Anderson et al., 1990, as cited by Bekalu & Eggermont, 2014). It is important to point out that while knowledge about AIDS and preventive methods are linked, there is not a one-to-one ratio (Bekalu & Eggermont, 2014). Additional measures are needed to promote behavior change beside knowledge about the virus. For example, a study of HIV/AIDS in Nigeria illustrates that, while participants had a high knowledge level concerning HIV/AIDS, were willing to be tested, and knew where testing sites were located, overall testing levels remained low (Abiodun, Sotunsa, Ani, & Jaiyesimi, 2014). Kanekar (2011) notes that in order for participants' engagement in preventive methods, such as increased use of condoms, counseling efforts need to focus on risk/harm reduction, and realize that education-related programs do not necessarily produce changes in participant behavior. The next sections of the chapter summarize specific prevention methods utilized in Botswana and details their effectiveness, as well as discussing specific interventions targeted toward at-risk populations.

Male Circumcision

Male circumcision is one important strategy. It is a highly advocated preventive measure to help minimize the transfer of HIV. Wamai et al. (2011) discussed the role of male circumcision as an important and extremely effective practice in HIV prevention. Biologically, removal of the male foreskin is thought to decrease risk of contracting HIV. The inner area of the foreskin lacks protective keratin in the skin and also contains T cells, which are more likely to be capable of taking in HIV cells. Male circumcision has been incorporated into prevention plans in Botswana, with estimated net savings by 2025 predicted at close to $250 million U.S. dollars. However, it is reported that only 11 percent of males in Botswana are circumcised, but there is a goal in place to circumcise 80 percent of males ages zero to forty-nine by 2014 (Wamai et al., 2011). Part of Botswana's new strategy is to increase male circumcision in the coming years by adding this into national responses due to its demonstrated effectiveness (NACA, 2009). As reported in the

WHO Global HIV/AIDS Response Epidemic Update, this strategy has been employed by thirteen priority countries, including Botswana, utilizing various methods such as mobile services and stand-alone clinics, as well as being made less time consuming with research focusing on developing nonsurgical devices for the procedure (WHO, 2011).

Condom Use

Condom use is another well-regarded strategy that the country has been attempting to focus on. It is a difficult to remember proper safe sex practices when one is emotionally and physically aroused. Thus, it is not surprising that reported condom use among the general population has fallen from 90.2 percent in 2008 to 81.9 percent in 2012 in Botswana (Statistics Botswana, 2013). Efforts to inform the population at large about the effectiveness of condom use in preventing HIV/AIDS are in place, specifically the "ABC" approach discussed earlier in the chapter. However, Merson et al. (2008) noted that the "ABC" approach was "naively simple" and had only partial success.

Biomedical Preventions

Behavioral change is the only guaranteed approach for eliminating one's potential to contract HIV/AIDS. For the past thirty years, scientists and researchers across the globe have put considerable effort into finding a way to eliminate and prevent AIDS via medicine. The scientific community has not found success for a cure or vaccine to prevent it. However, biomedical treatment of HIV/AIDS has become one of the most prominent issues in medical research, and many drugs to help treat the disease have been created. This chapter is focused on the preventive behavioral intervention in the battle with HIV/AIDS, but the focus on pharmaceuticals cannot be ignored for their role in prevention, especially in Botswana, where the use of drugs in treatment and prevention of HIV/AIDS is free.

Immediately upon recognition of the virus and how HIV functions as the precursor to AIDS in the early 1980s, scientists began clinical trials to find drugs to treat and cure the virus. HIV was found to deplete the body's CD4+ T cells (white blood cells of the immune system), which send signals to other important cells within the immune system to fight off infection (Palmisano & Vella, 2011). HIV does this by binding to host cells and then replicating itself by attaching to the host cell's DNA. This process enables HIV to copy itself in order to infect other cells, which in effect neutralizes the host cell's ability to protect the body. Palmisano and Vella (2011) discussed the history of antiretroviral therapy (ART), which is now the leading treatment in Botswana for PLWHA. ARV drugs began to be tested in the 1980s as a way to inhibit HIV cells from spreading. ARV drugs work by blocking HIV from entering cells and also by stopping them from replicating. This neutralizes HIV's ability to continue damaging the host's cells. ART has been shown in many clinical studies to reduce levels of HIV in blood, semen, and other genital fluids that have been found to be the key in the transmission process (Kanters, Mills, Thorlund, Bucher, & Ioannidis, 2014). Currently, there are twenty-eight classes of ARV drugs, and many are now used in combination to halt the spread of HIV within the body.

Given the preventive qualities of ARV drugs, ARV therapy was intended to be used postcontraction of HIV. However, many doctors in Botswana, as well as other countries, believe that treatment could be used as a preventive method due to the function of the drugs PLWHA were taking. Due to lowering the viral load in PLWHA, doctors believed that over time it could decrease the risk of transmission because there were lower levels of the virus and the transmission risk was lower. In Cohen et al.'s (2011) monumental study, antiretroviral therapy was distributed to over 1,700 individuals across nine countries, including Botswana. The study's participants were all couples in serodiscordant relationships (in which only one partner is HIV-positive), and they were randomly placed in an early initiation-therapy trial or a delayed-therapy trial. After giving ART to partners who were HIV-positive, rates of transmission were reduced by 96 percent. This study showed beyond reasonable doubt the effectiveness of ARV therapy in preventing transmission. As discussed earlier, antiretroviral therapy was found to be instrumental in preventing transmission from a mother to her child through this process as well.

While PLWHA can take ARV medication to lower their HIV viral load, ARV medication can also be used as a preventive measure for individuals with a high risk of contracting the virus. In essence, there are two ways to decrease the risk of spreading AIDS through medicine: either pre- or post-exposure. Antiretroviral post-exposure prophylaxis (PEP) is a preventative strategy to decrease the risk of transmission. In Roland et al.'s (2005) study, composed of over seven hundred participants who were recently exposed to HIV through needles or sexual activity and who were given ARV PEP within seventy-two hours of exposure, only 1 percent (seven subjects) were seroconverted after twelve weeks of treatment. Each of the seven subjects also had exposure to HIV six months prior to the study. Providing PEP to individuals can be a significant strategy to decrease the risk of HIV infection and transmission.

In further support of ARV's use among individuals at risk, a study in Botswana by Thigpen et al. (2012) found that in over 1,200 heterosexual sexually active participants, HIV transmission was decreased by 62 percent in individuals taking pre-exposure prophylaxis (PrEP). This percentage was increased when accounting for individuals who strongly adhered to the daily regimen of the PrEP. Other studies have found these strategies to be an effective approach as well (Baeten et al., 2012; Grant et al., 2010; Haberer et al., 2013). Although PEP and PrEP have not been found to be 100 percent effective, this regimen is promising for individuals who were recently exposed to the virus or who may be at serious risk for contracting HIV. Biomedical approaches should be considered as treatment *and* prevention.

AIDS is no longer considered a death warrant but a chronic disease in Botswana. Continued adherence of ARV treatment and healthy behavioral change can help PLWHA live satisfying lives while lowering the risk of transmission; thus, prevention of the disease can be obtained through active treatment. However, Palmisano and Vella (2011, p. 14) wrote, "treated people have to maintain lifelong adherence and face the risk of delayed drug toxic effects." Consequentially, the long-term consequences of taking a difficult medicinal regimen can have its own complications via treatment fatigue and side effects.

Preventing Mother to Child Transmissions: An Early Success

An early success story was a program in Botswana to prevent transmission of AIDS to unborn children, titled Prevention of Mother to Child Transmission Programme (PMTCT). Before this program began, HIV-positive women were very likely to bear a child with AIDS. There was a lack of knowledge on how to prevent such an occurrence besides using abstinence. At this point, however, abstinence was too late. In 1999, a large-scale program was launched to prevent transmission of HIV to unborn children as part of the new approach (NACA, 2014). Fortunately, funding at the international level through both foundations and the U.S. President's fund for President's Emergency Plan for AIDS Relief (PEPFAR) became available, and the program was well funded (NACA, 2014).

PMTCT focused on four areas of prevention and care in Botswana. The first area focused on preventing HIV in women who were at an age and ability to have children. The second focused on preventing unplanned pregnancies in women with HIV. The third focused on stopping the transmission of HIV from mothers to their children. Finally, the fourth area focused on giving continuing care to mothers, children, and other family members who have HIV/AIDS (Luo et al., 2007). The fourth area is particularly important due to the moral beliefs regarding gender norms that often depict women as deviant and responsible for HIV/AIDS transmission (Ogden & Nyblade, 2005).

Matambo et al. (2014) conducted a study of the effectiveness of the PMTCT program in Botswana. Between the 2008 and 2012, nearly twenty thousand women visited clinics and received triple antiretroviral therapy. The effect of this medication combined with other components of the PMTCT program helped to reduce the percent of mother-to-child transmission from 3 percent to 1 percent. So even though the mother has the disease and must have treatment for the duration of her life, the child is HIV free and can live a life without the dreadful effects of HIV/AIDS. While 3 percent may not seem large, the social consequences of being born with HIV/AIDS are severe. Thus, any prevention approach, biological or social, that reduces the impact of HIV/AIDS is meritorious.

Voluntary Counseling and Testing

Counseling is a risk reduction prevention technique that utilizes psychoeducation to prevent individuals already infected from transmitting the disease to others. In Botswana, it is provided on a voluntary basis immediately following a positive HIV test result. Sessions can continue on an extended basis. In addition to addressing the emotions involved with a positive diagnosis, HIV/AIDS counseling encourages clients to practice safe sex, eat a balanced diet, adhere to medication regimes, and be aware of secondary infections and risks associated with substance use (Stockton, Nitza, Ntinda, & Ncube, 2015b). Furthermore, HIV/AIDS counseling facilitates these individuals to live positively and build their personal relationships in a society that is highly stigmatizing. Without proper medication, these individuals would have died within a relatively short time period. However, now that the medicine extends the life period drastically, with counseling, these individuals can focus on learning how to live with a chronic disease. Counseling services help patients learn how to accept their positive status, thereby lessening the negative effect of stigma. Counseling acts as a behavioral intervention that focuses on decreasing disease transmission through pre- and posttest sessions by integrating medical, social, and psychological perspectives (Kanekar, 2011). In one study, Botswanan men showed increased risk reduction skills, had fewer sexually transmitted infections, and reported less unprotected sex over a six-month period after undergoing counseling (Kalichman, Rompa, & Cage, 2005).

In an effort to continue improving counseling training, and education, Stockton et al. (2015b) reviewed preliminary data from the qualitative section of a countrywide survey that sought to elicit HIV/AIDS clients' perceptions of counseling services in Botswana. The goal of this study is to discover areas of focus for current counselors and to improve counselor education and training throughout the country. Most of the respondents reported that their counseling sessions focused on psychoeducational pieces regarding treatment adherence, safe sex, avoidance of substance use while on antiretroviral medication, physical health (nutrition and exercise), and general HIV prevention. However, many respondents also stated that their counselors helped them deal with accepting their positive status, helping them disclose their status to significant people in their lives, and also helping them to learn to live positive lives. For example, one respondent wrote, "Through counseling I was able to accept myself and make better plans for my future and family." A significant number of individuals also reported that counseling helped them deal with the stigma and discrimination they faced as a result of their positive status. One individual wrote, "(Counseling) has helped me to face stigma and discrimination, even when people label me I contain myself, and not be intimidated in most cases."

At-Risk Populations: Substance Abusers

In a population struggling to maintain healthy bodies and minds in its battle with HIV/AIDS, substance use is a serious issue. Years of research have shown that using substances can cause a number of negative physical effects and have lasting negative social consequences. There are a number of risks involved when PLWHA use drugs. HIV can be transmitted when individuals share needles they use to inject drugs. Individuals therefore can be susceptible to becoming infected with HIV or risk infecting another person if they are HIV-positive already. Furthermore, drug use has been shown to increase the likelihood of a person engaging in risky behaviors that could potentially compromise one's general health or even HIV treatment.

In a longitudinal study by Hinkin et al. (2007), conducted in the United States, PLWHA who used drugs showed worse rates of highly active antiretroviral treatment medication adherence, known as HAART. In the study, current drug users (measured through urine samples) were four times more likely to have adherence rates that were less than ideal. More so, individuals who used stimulants were seven times more likely to have low levels of medication adherence than those who did not test positive for stimulants. The authors concluded that drug use can often lead to an unstructured lifestyle and cognitive impairment, which can make it difficult to follow the strict and coordinated effort of medication management. The willingness of drug abusers to participate in unprotected sexual activity with others is also a risk factor. Thus HIV/AIDS patients who abuse drugs and have unprotected sex may transmit AIDS to their sexual partner, through this means as well as by needle sharing.

Other research, interestingly, has shown that taking HIV medication can influence drug-injecting behaviors and unsafe sex practices among PLWHA. Tun, Celentano, Vlahov, and Strathdee (2003) measured attitudes of PLWHA taking HAART with regard to sexual and drug-injecting behaviors. They found that nearly two-thirds of participants who were sexually active did not use condoms, and nearly half of those who injected drugs through needles shared those same needles with others. The authors concluded that these correlations could be explained by a belief among HAART adherers that taking HAART decreases risk of transmitting HIV. Thus, individuals who were on medication may believe that they are less likely to transmit the disease and may forgo protective drug and sexual behaviors. Although the Tun et al. (2003) study was conducted in the United States, the conclusions can be generalized across cultures. The authors stressed that PLWHA may become fatigued of practicing risk reduction behaviors as it becomes a lifelong practice. As PLWHA live longer due to medication, their beliefs may begin to change regarding the risk of transmitting if they are healthy because of their medication. Clearly, education on the limits of HAART medication should be considered as a prevention method for safe sex and safe drug use behaviors as well as informing PLWHA about the likelihood of fatigue in their battle with HIV/AIDS.

Using drugs risks infecting yourself or another person with HIV, may lead to decreases in one's medication adherence, and could compromise treatment for HIV. This being said, why would someone living with HIV/AIDS turn to drug use? There are a number of reasons that are not so different from the reasons anyone would turn to using substances. Underlying all of these is a desire to escape one's current reality. Loss of family/friends, fear, and pain (both physical and emotional) are all reasons one may turn to substance use. Another serious issue to consider is the pain that ensues from a chronic disease such as AIDS. The virus suppresses the immune system, which may lead to a number of painful infections that could easily persuade someone to desire an escape from their painful life. Thus, another strategy in preventing HIV/AIDS transmission should be to inform the public about the dangers of using drugs in terms of preventing the spread of the disease and the dangers associated with drug use while HIV/AIDS-positive.

Sexual Orientation

There are strong cultural taboos against homosexuality in Botswana, and homosexual activity is illegal, making this population virtually unserved and highly marginalized. The very existence of the orientation is denied by the majority of the population; however, that does not mean that the orientation does not exist or that men who have sex with men are not at a high risk of contracting HIV/AIDS (Stockton et al., 2015a).

Summary and Recommendations

This chapter serves as a review of the history of HIV/AIDS and the measures that Botswana has taken to prevent this disease from spreading. Summarizing previous efforts, the original Botswana response to the AIDS epidemic had been largely medical in nature (NACA, 2009). This original response included the Short-Term Plan and the First Medium-Term Plan, which had a larger focus on the reactive care of those diagnosed. With the implementation of the Second Medium-Term Plan (during 1997–2002), the country became aware of the need to provide a multifaceted approach that included more preventive strategies. This included programs such as the antiretroviral program (MASA); Preventing Mother-to-Child Transmission (PMTCT); voluntary HIV testing and counseling; and the first Botswana AIDS Impact Survey (BAIS I), which was piloted in 2001. In 2003, the First National Strategic Framework for HIV and AIDS was created and then implemented in 2003 through 2009. This framework was built to address the weaknesses in the original responses, such as insufficient coordination efforts (including more emphasis on grassroots inclusion), education, legislation, and guidance for each sector attending to the epidemic. The goal of this effort in Botswana was to eliminate new occurrences of HIV and reduce the negative impact resulting from HIV/AIDS.

A number of recommendations for prevention emerge from these discussions. There are multiple levels at which HIV prevention can be implemented. Systematic, local, and individual levels have similar methods to prevention but are facilitated in different ways. HIV is transmitted mainly through sexual acts, blood, and mother-to-child during pregnancy, and there are behavioral measures to help reduce the risk of transmission. Behavioral change may be needed in order to do this, but individuals must be knowledgeable about the rationale needed to change their behavior. Education must be a primary prevention method used at every level.

Systematically, public education about HIV/AIDS awareness can be utilized through schools and media campaigns by the government. By passing on knowledge to the young and adult populations about realistic consequences and risks of both safe and unsafe sex, education can have a positive impact. A U.S. study by Kirby (2007) reviewed sex education programs in communities, schools, and clinics. In the review, comprehensive sex education programs were much more likely to have a positive impact than abstinence-only programs, which may do little to inform people of real sexual behaviors and risks. In 71 percent of these comprehensive programs, a positive effect on reducing partners and frequency of unprotected sex acts was realized, and none of the programs increased sexual behavior (which some people believed could happen). In addition, Kirby found that 66 percent of programs had a positive impact on at least one sexual behavior, and 48 percent had a positive impact on two or more behaviors. These comprehensive programs consisted of focusing on clear behavioral health goals (e.g., HIV prevention), teaching and giving clear advice on specific behaviors that could lead to attaining these goals (e.g., using condoms), and discussing physical and psychological risk factors that can influence sexual behavior. These programs also included interactive activities and teaching methods that engaged participants. Education programs should consider including these components to help communicate effectively to participants in the community. Those who develop prevention interventions at systematic levels can use comprehensive programs to increase the effectiveness of the programs they design. We believe these findings have direct relevance to Botswana as well as other countries.

The International Antiviral (formerly AIDS) Society–USA HIV Prevention Recommendations Panel reviewed studies reported at scientific conferences over a seventeen-year period. They conducted a literature review and identified behavioral and biomedical prevention measures to implement in clinical settings (Marrazzo et al., 2014). Offering HIV testing for all is one of the foremost suggestions from this review. Mazzarro et al. (2014) stated that close to 50 percent of PLWHA worldwide do not know of their positive status. People say that knowing is half the battle, but perhaps it is even more in this serious case, where individuals can now reduce their risk of contracting HIV after a possible exposure through pre exposure and post exposure prophylaxis medication. HIV testing is especially critical in populations who are more likely to contract the disease through their work or risky behaviors. Individuals who are at risk should get tested often in order to increase awareness of their ability to spread HIV/AIDS and also to begin treatment to lead a healthy life with HIV/AIDS. Marrazzo et al. (2014) also discusses the importance of education in clinical settings. Clinicians need to provide education both to uninfected populations and PLWHA about the transmission process, the importance of ARV therapy, and how to prepare for a life with HIV/AIDS. Furthermore, Marrazzo et al. (2014) stress that HIV counseling is important to aid in harm reduction upon acknowledgment of a positive status. Thus, through education, counseling, and testing at a local level, individuals can increase their awareness of safety measures. Marrazzo et al. (2014) recommend that community clinics and health care sites offer free testing periodically and be supported by knowledgeable staff who can clearly explain to individuals preventive measures and direct them to proper resources if their status is positive.

It is important to consider social and cultural contexts of a community when implementing at both the systematic and local levels. The cultural traditions and beliefs of a community can drastically shape how they view education, sex, and health care professionals. The implementers of comprehensive programs need to take into account the culture of the community or country in which these programs are being implemented so that the audience will be receptive. To do otherwise is to risk valuable efforts for naught. For example, educators must consider that it is part of the culture of Botswana to have sex with many different partners. Therefore, educators should consider focusing on safe sex. Leaders in education may find it useful to provide multicultural education to the individuals who are educating others about HIV prevention so that they can consider important factors that may put an individual at higher risk. Some cultures make it easier to justify having sex with multiple partners or, conversely, it may not be socially acceptable to discuss sex in the home. Some cultures talk openly about sex, and some consider it taboo to speak of it in the open. In an article relating to underrepresented populations globally, Schoorman, Baxley, Acosta, and Sena Sister (2012) advocated for an approach where educators and their audience are in a dialogic partnership to open up communication as opposed to an expert–student relationship that solely focuses on transmitting information. This approach consists of using stories to facilitate discussion, using symbols familiar in the audience's culture, and using roleplays or dramas. The approach aims for educators to learn from their audience about the specific context in which they live and tailor knowledge about HIV prevention to their situation. The authors recommend that these and similar educational strategies be tailored culturally to the group so that their audience feels safe to ask questions and is open to dialogue and learning.

At an individual level, people can become concerned with their own status and regularly get tested, be more aware of risky behaviors, and volunteer to help test others and spread knowledge about preventive measures others can take. Finally, individuals can take up arms against HIV/AIDS attitudes and not stigmatize those who are infected. PLWHA are not solely the behavior they have engaged in to contract the disease. A young child with HIV/AIDS whose mother transmitted the disease should not be socially ostracized for infections passed down to them. Similarly, an individual who is unaware of how HIV is transmitted should not be discriminated against in the workplace because a sexual partner did not tell that he or she was HIV-positive and passed along the virus. No one wants to contract this virus. It is up to individuals afforded the privilege of education on the matter and those who are knowledgeable of HIV prevention to help change the culture of society and its treatment of these individuals who are suffering.

References

Abiodun, O., Sotunsa, J., Ani, F., & Jaiyesimi, E. (2014). Knowledge of HIV/AIDS and predictors of uptake of HIV counseling and testing among undergraduate students of a privately owned university in Nigeria. *BMC Research Notes* 7(1): 639.

Allen, T., & Heald, S. (2004). HIV/AIDS policy in Africa: what has worked in Uganda and what has failed in Botswana? *Journal of International Development* 16(8): 1141–54.

Anderson, J. E., Kann, L., Holtzman, D., Arday, S., Truman, B., & Kolbe, L. (1990). HIV/AIDS knowledge and sexual behavior among high school students. *Family Planning Perspectives* 22: 252–5.

Baeten, J. M., Donnell, D., Ndase, P., Mugo, N. R., Campbell, J. D., Wangisi, J., . . . & Celum, C. (2012). Antiretroviral prophylaxis for HIV prevention in heterosexual men and women. *New England Journal of Medicine* 367: 399–410. doi: 10.1056/NEJMoa1108524

Bekalu, M. A., & Eggermont, S. (2014). Media use and HIV/AIDS knowledge: a knowledge gap perspective. *Health Promotion International* 29(4): 739–50. doi: 10.1093/heapro/dat030dat030

Cohen, M. S., Chen, Y. Q., McCauley, M., Gamble, T., Hosseinipour, M. C., Kumarasamy, N., & . . . Fleming, T. R. (2011). Prevention of HIV-1 infection with early antiretroviral therapy. *New England Journal of Medicine* 365: 493–505. doi: 10.1056/NEJMoa1105243

Department of HIV/AIDS Prevention and Care, Ministry of Health (2012). MASA ARV Programme. www.hiv.gov.bw/content/masa-arv-programme

Elford, J., Bucher H. C., Rawstorne, P., Fogarty, A., Van de Ven, P., kippax, S., Ekstrand, M., Bharat, S., Ramakrishna, J., Simbayi, L. C., & Kalichman, S. C. (2005). International perspectives. In Kalichman, S. C. (ed.), *Positive Prevention: Reducing HIV Transmission among People Living with HIV/AIDS.* New York: Kluwer Academic/Plenum, pp. 245–77.

Gerson, M. (2014). Progress, still deep challenges on AIDS. *Indianapolis Star*, December 3, p. A11.

Grant, R. M., Lama, J. R., Anderson, P. L., McMahan, V., Liu, A. Y., Vargas, L., . . . & Glidden, D. V. (2010). Preexposure chemoprophylaxis for HIV prevention in men who have sex with men. *New England Journal of Medicine* 27: 2587–99.

Haberer, J., Baeten, J., Campbell, J., Wangisi, J., Katabira, E., Ronald, A., &. . . Bangsberg, D. (2013). Adherence to antiretroviral prophylaxis for HIV prevention: a substudy cohort within a clinical trial of serodiscordant couples in East Africa. *Plos Medicine* 10 (9).

Hanemann, U., (2005). *Literacy in Botswana.* Hamburg: UNESCO Institute of Education. unesdoc.unesco.org/images/0014/001460/146005e.pdf

Hinkin, C., Barclay, T., Castellon, S., Levine, A., Durvasula, R., Marion, S., . . . & Longshore, D. (2007). Drug use and medication adherence among HIV-1 infected individuals. *AIDS & Behavior* 11(2): 185–94.

Jennings, C. (1988). *Understanding and Preventing AIDS: A Book for Everyone.* Health Alert Press.

Jennings, C. (2012). *HIV-AIDS in South Africa: The Facts and Fiction.* Hudson, NH: Health Alert Communications.

Kalichman, S. C., Rompa, D., & Cage, M. (2005). Group intervention to reduce HIV transmission risk behavior among persons living with HIV/AIDS. *Behavior Modification* 29(2): 256–85.

Kanekar, A. S. (2011). HIV/AIDS counseling skills and strategies: can testing and counseling curb the epidemic? *International Journal of Preventive Medicine* 2(1): 10.

Kanters, S., Mills, E. J., Thorlund, K., Bucher, H. C., & Ioannidis, J. A. (2014). Antiretroviral therapy for initial human immunodeficiency virus/AIDS treatment: critical appraisal of the evidence from over 100 randomized trials and 400 systematic reviews and meta analyses. *Clinical Microbiology and Infection* 20(2): 114–22. doi: 10.1111/1469 0691.12475

Kirby, D. (2007). Abstinence, sex, and STD/HIV education programs for teens: their impact on sexual behavior, pregnancy, and sexually transmitted disease. *Annual Review of Sex Research* 18: 143–77.

Levers, L. L. (2006). Traditional healing as indigenous knowledge: its relevance to HIV/AIDS in southern Africa and the implications for counselors. *Journal of Psychology in Africa* 16(1): 87–100.

Logie, C., & Gadalla, T. M. (2009). Meta-analysis of health and demographic correlates of stigma towards people living with HIV. *AIDS Care* 21(6): 742–53.

Luo, C., Akwara, P., Ngongo, N., Doughty, P., Gass, R., Ekpini, R., . . . & Hayashi, C. (2007). Global progress in PMTCT and paediatric HIV care and treatment in low-and middle income countries in 2004–2005. *Reproductive Health Matters* 15(30): 179–89.

Mahajan, A. P., Sayles, J. N., Patel, V. A., Remien, R. H., Ortiz, D., Szekeres, G., & Coates, T. J. (2008). Stigma in the HIV/AIDS epidemic: a review of the literature and recommendations for the way forward. *AIDS (London, England)* 22(Suppl 2): S67.

Mall, S., Middelkoop, K., Mark, D., Wood, R., & Bekker, L. G. (2013). Changing patterns in HIV/AIDS stigma and uptake of voluntary counselling and testing services: the results of two consecutive community surveys conducted in the Western Cape, South Africa. *AIDS Care* 25(2): 194–201.

Marrazzo, J. M., del Rio, C., Holtgrave, D. R., Cohen, M. S., Kalichman, S. C., Mayer, K. H., & Benson, C. A. (2014). HIV prevention in clinical care settings: 2014 recommendations of the International Antiretroviral Society–USA Panel. *JAMA, The Journal of the American Medical Association* 312(4): 390–409.

Matambo, S., Machakaire, E., Motswere-Chirwa, C., Legwaila, K., Letsholathebe, V., Dintwa, E., & Glenshaw, M. (2014). Quality assurance of prevention of mother-to-child transmission of HIV in Botswana. *African Journal of Midwifery and Women's Health* 8: 130–3.

Merson, M. H., O'Malley, J., Serwadda, D., & Apisuk, C. (2008). The history and challenge of HIV prevention. *Lancet* 372(9637): 475–88.

Ministry of Health (2013). *Botswana: AIDS Impact Survey IV (BAIS IV) 2013, Summary Results*. Gaborone, Botswana: Statistics Botswana.

Murphy, E. M., Greene, M. E., Mihailovic, A., & Olupot-Olupot, P. (2006). Was the "ABC" approach (abstinence, being faithful, using condoms) responsible for Uganda's decline in HIV? *PLoS Med* 3(9): e379.

NACA (National AIDS Coordinating Agency) (2009). *The Second National Strategic Framework for HIV and AIDS: 2010–2016*. Gaborone, Botswana: NACA.

NACA (National AIDS Coordinating Agency) (2014). Botswana 2013 global AIDS response report. www.unaids.org/en/dataanalysis/knowyourresponse/country progressreports/2014c untries/BWA_narrative_report_2014

Palmisano, L., & Vella, S. (2011). A brief history of antiretroviral therapy of HIV infection: success and challenges. *Annali Dell'istituto Superiore Di Sanita* 47(1): 44–8. doi: 10.4415/ANN-11-01-10

Peltzer, K., & Ramlagan, S. (2011). Perceived stigma among patients receiving antiretroviral therapy: a prospective study in KwaZulu-Natal, South Africa. *AIDS Care* 23(1): 60–8.

Ogden, J., & Nyblade, L. (2005). Common at its core: HIV-related stigma across contexts. www.icrw.org/files/publications/Common-at-its-Core-HIV-Related-Stigma-Across-Contexts.pdf

Roland, M. E., Neilands, T. B., Krone, M. R., Katz, M. H., Franses, K., Grant, R. M., . . . & Martin, J. N. (2005). Seroconversion following nonoccupational postexposure prophylaxis against HIV. *Clinical Infectious Diseases* 41(10): 1507–13.

Rural HIV/AIDS Prevention Workgroup (2009). Tearing Down Fences: HIV/STD Prevention in Rural America. www.indiana.edu/~aids/TearingDownFencesBook.pdf

Schoorman, D., Baxley, T., Acosta, M. C., & Sena Sister, R. (2012). Critical pedagogy in HIV-AIDS education for a Maya immigrant community. *Multicultural Perspectives* 14(4): 194–200. doi: 10.1080/15210960.2012.725317

Singh, S., Darroch, J. E., & Bankole, A. (2004). A, B and C in Uganda: the roles of abstinence, monogamy and condom use in HIV decline. *Reproductive Health Matters* 12(23): 129–35.

Statistics Botswana. (2013). *Botswana AIDS Impact Survey IV (BAIS IV), 2013, Summary Results*. Gaborone, Botswana: Republic of Botswana

Stegling, C. (2004). Botswanas HIV/AIDS programme: a model for SADC? *Development Update* 5(3): 225–44.

Stockton, R., Nitza, A., Ntinda, K., & Ncube, P. (2015a). Counseling in Botswana. In Hohenshil, T. H., Amundson, N. E., & Niles, S. G. (eds.), *Counseling around the World: An International Handbook*. New York: Wiley, pp. 21–30.

Stockton, R., Paul, T., Voils-Levenda, A., Robbins, M., Li, P., & Zaitsoff, A. (2015b). Counselors' perceptions of HIV/AIDS counseling in Botswana: professional identity, practice, and training issues. *International Journal for the Advancement of Counselling* 37(2): 143–54.

Thigpen, M. C., Rose, C. E., Chillag, K. L., Buliva, E., Hart, C., Kebaabetswe, P. M., & . . . Brooks, J. T. (2012). Antiretroviral preexposure prophylaxis for heterosexual HIV transmission in Botswana. *New England Journal of Medicine* 367(5): 423–34.

Tun, W., Celentano, D. D., Vlahov, D., & Strathdee, S. A. (2003). Attitudes toward HIV treatments influence unsafe sexual and injection practices among injecting drug users. *AIDS* 17(13): 1953–62. doi: 10.1097/00002030-200309050-00014

Upton, R. L., & Dolan, E. M. (2011). Sterility and stigma in an era of HIV/AIDS: narratives of risk assessment among men and women in Botswana: original research article. *African Journal of Reproductive Health* 15(1): 95–100.

Wamai, R. G., Morris, B. J., Bailis, S. A., Sokal, D., Klausner, J. D., Appleton, R., . . . & Banerjee, J. (2011). Male circumcision for HIV prevention: current evidence and implementation in sub-Saharan Africa. *Journal of the International AIDS Society* 14: 49.

Wolfe, W. R., Weiser, S. D., Bangsberg, D. R., Thior, I., Makhema, J. M., Dickinson, D. B., … & Marlink, R. G. (2006). Effects of HIV-related stigma among an early sample of patients receiving antiretroviral therapy in Botswana. *AIDS Care* 18(8): 931–3.

World Bank (2013). Global economic prospects. www.worldbank.org/en/publication/global-economic-prospects#data

WHO (World Health Organization) (2011). *New Global Strategy on HIV Set to Prevent Millions of Infections, Deaths.* Geneva, Switzerland: World Health Organization. www.who.int/hiv/mediacentre/feature_story/hiv_strategy/en/

The Future of Prevention Science

43 Prevention Science

A Call for Global Action

John L. Romano & Moshe Israelashvili

This *Cambridge Handbook of International Prevention Science* is the first of its kind to address prevention science from an international perspective. The *Handbook* is a rich collection of prevention science activities, research, and scholarship from twenty-seven different countries, offering a global snapshot of prevention throughout the world. In addition to country-specific chapters from Asia and Australia, North and South and Latin America, Europe, the Middle East, and Africa, the *Handbook* includes chapters on the foundational areas of prevention such as costs and benefits of prevention, prevention ethics, research methods, and implementation of prevention initiatives. In this concluding chapter, we will present the major themes that emanated from the chapters included in the *Handbook;* discuss challenges associated with prevention science applications and research from different areas of the world; and make a call for major global initiatives, highlighted by a Global Summit, to advance prevention science in the twenty-first century.

Country Contributors and Major Themes

The number of contributors to the *Handbook* is large, especially since most chapters have more than one author and therefore represent the work of more than one hundred different authors. However, the large majority of the chapters were written by authors from four regions of the world: Asia, Australia, Europe, and North America. All but five of the forty-one invited chapters (not including the first and last chapters of the *Handbook,* written by the coeditors) were written by authors from these regions. There were two chapters from sub-Saharan Africa (i.e., Stockton, Goldberg, Paul, & DeLarm, 2017, on prevention of HIV in Botswana, and Akande, Adetoun, Adewuyi, & Akandi, 2017 on HIV prevention in sub-Sahara Africa) and one chapter from South and Latin America (with contributors from several Latin American countries; see Pérez-Gómez & Méjía-Truillo, 2017), a chapter focused exclusively on Mexico (see Pick, Athie, & Hietanen, 2017), and one from Israel (see Israelashvili, 2017). Authors from the United States (U.S.) and European countries contributed to more than half of the chapters. Some chapters were written by authors and coauthors who identified with more than one country. To solicit chapter authors during the development of this *Handbook*, the editors used several resources to invite chapter proposals, including professional databases, their own and colleagues' professional networks, and professional organizations. However, despite these efforts, the editors were successful in attracting only a few proposals from Central and South America, Africa, and the Middle East. A few authors from these regions whose proposals were accepted withdrew from the process, some due to difficulties in meeting the editorial requests and others due to lack of time to complete their demanding proposal because of previous commitments to other projects. English is a second language for many authors, and therefore lack of English written fluency also contributed to time demands made on the authors completing chapters, and for this reason some withdrew from writing a chapter.

Despite the imbalanced representation of authors from some regions of the world, the chapters represented in the *Handbook* cover vast areas of the globe. The following highlights major impressions and themes from these authors.

Prevention topics. The author contributions represent a variety of prevention topics from across the globe, including several topics that have not previously received much attention among prevention scholars in the professional literature. These unique topics include (a) a large-scale, countrywide system of activities and initiatives to prevent Internet and smart phone addiction in South Korea; (b) prevention of problems associated with recreational night life in Spain and other European countries; (c) prevention associated with the impact of natural and man-made disasters; (d) prevention of school gun violence and shootings; (e) the potential of neuroscience to address underlying mechanisms in the prevention of sleep disorders; (f) suicide prevention in India and Israel; and (g) forgiveness interventions to enhance health and interpersonal relationships. The chapter on the impact of natural and human-made disasters and their relationship to prevention science is enlightening, as the authors show through case studies how prevention science can be applied when disasters occur (see Shultz, Espinola, Rechkemmer, Cohen, & Espinel, 2017). Other topics of the chapters focused on populations that have previously received more attention in the literature, such as prevention science related to children and youth and college student well-being (e.g., see Toumbourou, 2017; and Tuiceomepee & Sirikantraporn, 2017). The traditional prevention topics focusing on the prevention of alcohol and drug use among youth was a prominent area of intervention in many of the countries represented in this *Handbook*, as were topics on the prevention of school bullying and school violence. While younger age groups were often targeted for prevention activities in the chapters, there was no or little attention given to adults from middle- to older-age groups, despite the fact that the World Health Organization (WHO) reports that in almost all countries, the fastest growing segment of the population is adults sixty years and older. Certainly, this age group merits attention in the prevention science literature across the globe.

In addition to the lack of attention to prevention interventions for an aging population worldwide, there was also a lack of topics covered in this *Handbook* on the prevention of disease and health promotion interventions. The omission of these topics is important since the WHO reports that noncommunicable diseases (NCD) kill 38 million people per year worldwide, and nearly three-quarters of these deaths occur in middle- and low-income countries.[1] According to the WHO, 82 percent of NCD deaths are caused by four diseases – cardiovascular diseases, cancers, respiratory diseases, and diabetes – and lifestyle behaviors increase a person's risk of dying from an NCD. These behaviors of lifestyle are tobacco use, physical inactivity, abuse of alcohol, and unhealthy diets. All of these lifestyle risk factors can be reduced through education and behavioral interventions. While some of the chapters in the *Handbook* addressed prevention related to alcohol and drug prevention (e.g., Shek's chapter on the prevention of alcohol and drug use in Hong Kong, 2017; and Pérez-Goméz & Mejía-Trujillo's chapter on prevention initiatives in Latin America, 2017), none of them directly addressed the prevention of NCD in their country or region, although some chapters in the *Handbook* are related to the prevention of NCD (e.g., Morgenroth, Buchwald, & Braasch, 2017, on stress prevention among teachers in Germany; Worthington, Griffin, Lavelock, Wade, & Kulick, 2017, on forgiveness). Given the importance of reducing NCD in countries across the globe, NCD as a focus of prevention work is critically important. While the majority of scholars who contributed chapters to the *Handbook* have careers in affiliation with educational and mental health organizations, their expertise, when utilized in partnership with scholars from the health sciences, have potential to strengthen prevention initiatives significantly to reduce NCD and other disorders (e.g., see Krigbaum & Wigton's chapter on addressing insomnia with biofeedback technology, 2017). Psychologists, counselors, and mental health professionals are skilled in assisting people in making behavioral changes, which are needed to reduce lifestyle problem behaviors as risk factors of NCD. Educators and mental health professionals, working in partnership with public health professionals, can impact universal prevention mass media messages to increase awareness of risk factors across a population.

One of the strengths of several chapters was the focus on promoting health and well-being along with emphasizing the prevention of problems, that is, promoting positive behaviors that serve as protections against problems as well as preventing specific problem(s) (e.g., Ostaszewski & Pisaraka, 2017, Poland; Tourmbourou, 2017, Australia; Solomon & Solomon, 2017, India; Humayun & Scott, 2017). In recent definitions of prevention, the promotion of protective behaviors, along with the prevention of problem behaviors, has been included as important in conceptualizations of prevention (National Research Council and Institute of Medicine, 2009; Romano & Hage, 2000). Therefore, it is important that authors addressed not only the reduction or elimination of risk behaviors but also the promotion of behaviors that are protective. This balance was noted in several chapters of the *Handbook*. For example, the "Mission: I'm Possible" project in Singapore (see Chong, Tang, Koh, & Choo, 2017)

1 www.who.int/mediacentre/factsheets/fs355/en/.

emphasizes an ecological systemic approach addressing both risk and protective factors to meet the needs of children; and the chapter by DiFabio, Kenny, and Claudius (2017) addresses risk and protective factors in their career development interventions in Italy. Similarly, Frydenberg (2017) discusses the promotion of coping skills with children, adolescents, and parents in Australia. In their literature review, Humayun and Scott (2017) write about the importance of addressing protective factors in the prevention of childhood antisocial behavior. These are only a few examples from the *Handbook*, and the attention to protective behaviors is significant in the body of scholarship displayed in the *Handbook* chapters.

Cultural adaptations. Some of the most interesting observations made by the *Handbook* editors were the cultural adaptations (or lack of them) made by authors who cited or used prevention programs developed in other countries but implemented as interventions in their own country. While authors noted the prevention interventions implemented in different countries from where they were initially developed, and made adaptations to the country where they were delivered, others did not report any cultural adaptation to the local context. This issue is an important one, as noted in the chapter by Orte, Ballester, Vives, Amer, and March (2017), which addresses cultural adaptations for family drug prevention programs, and the chapter by Tuicompee and Sirikantraporn (2017), who write about Buddhism as integral to their prevention initiatives with university students in Thailand.

A critical yet neglected aspect of cultural adaptation is the need to use culturally adequate measurements (scales) that would properly evaluate either the efficacy or the effectiveness of a prevention intervention. This topic, mentioned by Tein (2017), is further complicated by the fact that pursuing reliable, culturally relevant scales as part of a prevention intervention puts further pressure on the usually limited financial and professional resources that exist in many nations, including the more developed ones (see discussion on funding later in this chapter). The ability to develop culturally adapted evaluation tools is currently one of the major obstacles to the wider global implementation of already existing prevention programs that have been developed and validated in only one nation (culture).

It is critically important that prevention interventions developed for one cultural context also be assessed for suitability in another cultural context, especially if the two cultures are quite different from each other. Cultural differences are also relevant for areas of prevention science not directly related to interventions, such as prevention ethics and costs and benefits of prevention applications. For example, ethics of prevention may be addressed differently depending on the cultural context of the country where a prevention intervention is implemented (see Hage, Schwartz, & DeMartino, 2017).

Several authors directly focused on multicultural issues and their relationship to prevention science (see Hong, Peguero, Espelage, & Allen-Mercer, 2017; Navsaria & Hong; Suzuki, Hasan, & Rundles, 2017; Wong, Vaughan, & Klann, 2017). These chapters are important as they highlight the need to attend to multicultural considerations when developing and implementing prevention interventions and research. Wong, Vaughan, and Klann (2017) further extend their discussion of multicultural issues in the support of social justice, which has been intimately connected to prevention for many years and was instrumental in the development of prevention science as a specialty (Albee, 1983; Kenny & Hage, 2009; Kenny, Horne, Orpinas, & Reese, 2009; Romano, 2015). Wong et al. (2017) discuss specifically a multicultural social justice framework for prevention and address several cultural and social justice principles important to prevention science. Nota, Ferrari, Sgaramella, and Soresi (2017) also discuss prevention in relation to special needs children and youth in Italian schools. Calafat and Juan (2017) also address the importance of understanding the cultural context in relationship to alcohol and drug abuse associated with recreational night life, as does Stockton et al. (2017) in their discussion of the stigma attached to the treatment and prevention of HIV/AIDS in Botswana. Similarly, Akande, Adetoun, Adewuyi, and Akande (2017) provide an extensive discussion of social stigma associated with HIV/AIDS treatment in sub-Sahara Africa. Stigma associated with receiving mental health services in their country were also discussed in the chapters on student well-being in Thailand (see Tuicomepee & Sirikantrporn, 2017) and on the incidence of suicides and suicide prevention in India (see Solomon & Solomon, 2017). Thus, several authors of the *Handbook* chapters directly incorporate cultural issues as important components of prevention in their country and setting.

Empirically supported interventions. Most of the authors were quite cognizant of using empirically supported interventions for their prevention applications. However, the authors tended to rely on research of the interventions that were carried out in locales and regions of the world different from their own. Empirically supported prevention interventions relevant for one culture may not be applicable to other cultures or countries. Therefore, prevention applications that are adapted for a different cultural context than that for which it was originally developed and intended should be evaluated for their suitability in the different culture. Gewirtz and Youssef (2017) address this issue, as they report that empirical evidence for parent training that they reviewed was concentrated in higher-income, Western countries, but empirically supported evidence was lacking in lower-income countries. Therefore, prevention specialists need to become skilled, either through their own training or in collaboration with specialists in research methods and statistics, in applying research methodologies to their prevention interventions. Galanti, Engström, Forsell, Månsdotter, and Möller (2017) and Tein (2017) have provided very useful information about research methods and statistics related to prevention science interventions. In addition, Campello, Heikila, and Maalouf (2017) describe the International Standards on Drug Abuse Prevention, a review of policies and interventions found to be effective for the prevention of drug abuse. Similarly, Israelashvili (2017) discusses the recently created standards for universal prevention programs in Israel and noted that few of the existing Israeli programs meet empirically supported evaluation criteria based on these standards.

Prevention specialists may also consider qualitative methods to assess their prevention activities, especially during the early stages of prevention activities. Qualitative and mixed methods research have been used in some of the prevention activities reviewed in this volume (e. g., see Tuicomepee & Sirikantraporn's research conducted with university students in Thailand, 2017; and Nota et al.'s chapter on Italian youth, 2017). Other research methodologies may be especially helpful to prevention specialists as they make cultural adaptations to prevention programs that were developed in other countries. These research methods include participatory research methods (Kidd & Kral, 2005). See Wong, Vaughan, and Klann (2017) and Hage, Schwartz, and DeMartino (2017) for examples. Elicitation research is another method to assess variables important to the group targeted for prevention programs. Elicitation research has been most used in conjunction with the Theory of Reasoned Action and Planned Behavior (Ajzen, 1991; Ajzen & Fishbein, 1980; Fishbein, 1967). However, elicitation research is also applicable for prevention initiatives based on other prevention science frameworks and theories (Romano & Netland, 2008).

Funding and resources for prevention science. Several authors commented on the various government agencies and nongovernmental organizations (NGOs) that support prevention initiatives in their country (e.g., see Cho's chapter on Korea's Internet and smart phone addiction program, 2017). However, in many countries, the financial and resource demands of meeting the needs of crisis conditions and events give these needs priority over prevention applications (e.g., see Dolkar's chapter on Bhutan, 2017). Thus, funding for prevention is limited in many countries. Pérez-Gómez and Méjía-Truillo (2017) noted a similar financial and resource issue for some countries in Latin America, similarly for India (see Solomon & Solomon, 2017). In addition, even in high-income countries, such as the United States, Letourneau and Shields (2017) lament about the lack of funding to evaluate child sexual abuse prevention programs rigorously, commenting that most resources are expended on interventions for child sexual abuse after the abuse has occurred. Israelashvili (2017) shows how prevention science initiatives in Israel have been directly connected to security issues in the country and how this association has created funding for prevention interventions. Solomon and Solomon (2017) have called for a national suicide prevention strategy in India to reduce the suicides in the country. Corrective interventions (regardless of the target behavior) are costly in terms of the monetary resources needed and the emotional suffering that people and their loved ones must endure (see Romano, 2015, for a review of the economics of prevention; and Temple & Reynolds, 2017).

Temple and Reynolds (2017) assert financial and social gains in their cost-benefit analyses of prevention interventions. However, the analyses were conducted in higher-income countries, and economic benefits may not apply similarly to middle- and lower-income countries. Prevention scholars in low- and middle-income countries are encouraged to conduct their own cost-benefit analyses of prevention interventions to demonstrate the benefits of prevention to major stakeholders, government agencies, and funding entities. Temple and Reynolds (2017) provide an excellent summary of steps necessary to conduct a cost-benefit analysis, and they provide an example from Child–Parent Centers in the United States.

Education and training for prevention science. In all countries and regions of the world represented in this volume, there is limited evidence of formal degree training and education of prevention scientists and practitioners across the globe. Most prevention specialists seem to gain their prevention education through less formal means, such as through professional conferences and workshops and "on-the-job training" after degree completion. One international training innovation is described by Campello et al. (2017). Under the auspices of the United Nations Office on Drugs and Crime, an innovative series of seminars designed for prevention policy makers from many countries is summarized. This type of training not only builds capacity for prevention work internationally, but also provides a network of policy makers to support prevention and health promotion initiatives globally.

The lack of formal training and education of prevention scientists is a reality across countries (e.g., see Ostaszewski & Pisaraka, 2017, about the lack of systematic prevention training in Poland). Conyne, Newmeyer, Kenny, Romano, and Matthews (2008) and Eddy, Smith, Brown, and Reid (2005) report on prevention training and needs in the United States. In addition, a small number of U.S. universities are offering more formal academic programs in prevention, such as at the University of Minnesota (see www.preventionscience.umn.edu) and the University of Wisconsin (see www.preventionscience.wisc.edu). In addition, the first author of one of the chapters in the *Handbook* has a long history of training prevention researchers at Arizona State University (U.S.) (see Sandler, Wolchik, Berkel, Jones, Mauricio, Tein, & Winslow, 2017). As noted, there are some prevention training and education programs in a few countries. However, it is important to publicize these programs widely, especially within the global region, where the program is offered to encourage the exchange of cross-national training and education in prevention science.

Prevention science research and scholarship primarily focused in higher-income and Western countries. As summarized in the preceding, the majority of chapters in this *Handbook* were authored by scholars in four areas of the world, despite the editors' efforts to solicit authors from other regions. Only five chapters were contributed by scholars from sub-Sahara Africa, the Middle East, Mexico, and Central and South America. It may be that the editors' professional networks were not sufficiently large enough to reach scholars in some of the areas of the world, but it is more likely that prevention scholarship is limited in low- and middle-income countries. This is a challenge to prevention scholars as the need for preventive interventions is often greater in lower- and middle-income countries in comparison to the homelands of scholars who are intensively researching prevention issues in higher-income countries. However, even in higher-income countries prevention science represents a relatively small population of scholars as discussed by Fowler (2015). Ostaszewski and Pisaraka (2017) commented on the lack of evidence-based prevention interventions in Poland, and the research that does exist has had little impact on national and local policy makers. There is certainly need for greater attention to prevention science among professionals across disciplines as diverse as education, psychology, policy, economics, and health professions. It also behooves countries, especially those with limited resources and personnel, to collaborate with other countries in their region to address societal problems using the science of prevention. These partnerships and collaborations are currently occurring in some South American countries (see Pérez-Gómez & Mejía-Trujillo, 2017).

Cross-national guidelines and standards begin to emerge. Recently, the American Psychological Association (APA) approved a set of aspirational guidelines to advance prevention science among psychologists worldwide. See Conyne and Firth (2017) as to their incorporation of the guidelines into their chapter. The guidelines, titled "Guidelines for Prevention in Psychology" (APA, 2014), offer nine aspirational guidelines to strengthen prevention within psychology. While the guidelines received approval from the American Psychological Association after a lengthy process of review and comments from major stakeholders with APA and outside of APA, they are very applicable to prevention specialists who do not affiliate or identify with psychology. Prevention is an interdisciplinary specialty, and thus the guidelines were written to be useful and important to prevention professionals within and outside the profession of .psychology. The nine guidelines are as follows: (1) select and implement theory- and evidence-based prevention interventions; (2) use socially and culturally relevant preventive practices adapted to the context when implemented; (3) develop and implement interventions that reduce risks and promote human strengths; (4) incorporate research and evaluation as integral to prevention program development and implementation; (5) consider ethical issues in prevention research and practice; (6) attend to contextual issues of social disparities that inform prevention practice and research; (7) increase one's knowledge and skills essential to prevention through various avenues such as continuing education, training, and consultation; (8) engage in systemic and institutional change interventions that strengthen the health of individuals, families, and communities and that prevent psychological and physical distress and disability; and (9) inform the deliberation of public policies that promote health and well-being when relevant prevention science findings are available. Within the full document of the guidelines is a rationale for each guideline and how it might be applied to prevention science. While most authors of the *Handbook* chapters did not mention the guidelines directly, their chapters reflected in many cases the goals of the guidelines. For example, see McQueen's chapter (2017) on policy development and decision making in prevention science;

Cho's chapter (2017) on systemic, countrywide change to prevent Internet and smart phone addiction; and Koch and Knutson's chapter (2017) on comprehensive school counseling programs, especially as they implement systemic prevention and health promotion programs across schools and school districts. In addition, Campello et al. (2017) provided some detail about the development of the United Nations supported International Standards on Drug Use Prevention. Israelashvili (2017) also discussed the newly developed standards for prevention programs in Israel.

Thus, it seems timely to use the approved APA Guidelines for Prevention in Psychology (APA, 2014), along with relevant consideration from the *Handbook*'s chapters and other related documents, such as the Society for Prevention Research's Advocacy Statement of scientific advances and principles (www.preventionscience.org/advocacy/) and pursue formal adoption of a set of cross-national guidelines and standards to serve as cornerstones for the advancement of prevention science globally.

The Accumulating Generic Knowledge on Prevention Science

In spite of the many differences that exist between the countries that are represented in this *Handbook*, a review of all the chapters in the *Handbook* leads to the acknowledgment of several common cross-cultural denominators (or notions) that need to be highlighted. The major ones are summarized as follows:

1. Prevention activities are taking place in many countries.
2. Across the globe, there is acceptance of the idea that prevention and health/wellness promotion are complementary terms.
3. The educational systems are major contexts where prevention efforts are taking place.
4. The family is another context to implement prevention. Increasing importance is given to effective parenting, not only to prevent problems but also to enhance health and well-being.
5. It is widely accepted that prevention programs should be comprehensive, that is, they should address the person, the family, and the community (e.g., school, organization) and engage government and political entities to support prevention.
6. There is wide agreement that cultural adaptation is crucial and critically important, no matter how much evidence a prevention program has already received in other countries or cultural contexts.
7. There is a growing tendency to develop and implement local prevention programs, even though there is little or no evidence to support their effectiveness.
8. In most countries, central governmental contributions to prevention are limited. Most often, prevention interventions are supported and implemented by local administration, educational institutions, and NGOs.

9. Democracy "invades" into prevention, that is, prevention programs are developed while taking into account both financial and political realities alongside matters of social justice and ethics.

While the need for cultural awareness in prevention is evident, this partial list of general notions is in line with the *Handbook*'s respect of the universal knowledge on prevention that has been accumulated, as represented by its two major sections, that is, (1) general knowledge and (2) country-based interventions. Thus, in spite of the cultural and local differences that need consideration, there is a growing body of common knowledge on prevention that can serve as a basic theorem for prevention science. Hence, the future challenge of prevention science is not only to promote it internationally, with awareness of existing differences around the globe, but also to identify the common knowledge and standards that can be drawn from achievements in prevention that have been learned from across the world.

Major Challenges to Advance Prevention Science Globally

The number of international scholars and the prevention science themes that are represented in this *Handbook* are impressive. There is important scholarship occurring in many regions of the world, and it is satisfying to learn about this work. However, there remain several challenges to advance prevention science globally. These challenges are summarized as follows.

Funding for prevention and lack of mental health and prevention personnel. The WHO has identified four major objectives in its 2013–2020 action plan for mental health at its May 2013 World Health Assembly, which was attended by nearly two thousand delegates of WHO member states (see www.who.int/mediacentre/news/releases/2013/world_health_assembly_20130527/en/). Each objective is relevant to prevention science and reflects some of the goals and objectives discussed in the chapters of the *Handbook*. WHO four objectives for mental health are strengthen mental health leadership and governance; provide comprehensive, integrated, and responsive mental health and social care services in community settings; implement strategies for health promotion and prevention in mental health; and strengthen information systems, evidence, and research for mental health. The WHO action plan places emphasis on human rights and empowerment to people with mental disabilities, and sets implementation, progress, and impact targets for 2020. While the goals are laudable and important to promote mental health and prevention worldwide, in reality, many countries face serious financial problems due to increasing budget needs related to many social, environmental, health, and security needs in their country, such as funding for educational improvements, health care (e.g., chronic illness, epidemics, infectious diseases), military resources, reduction of poverty, resources to address needs of immigrants, and improvements of the environment, to name only a few. All too often, prevention, especially to promote mental health and prevent mental and behavioral disabilities, takes a "back-seat" and receives much less funding support. A comprehensive WHO report, *Investing in Mental Health* (WHO, 2003), reports the great disparities between country budgets for mental health. In high-income countries, 6.89 percent of the health budget is provided for mental health, while in low-income countries it is 1.54 percent of the total health budget. These public expenditures have not changed very much, as a more recent WHO report shows that in low- and middle-income countries, less than $2.00 (U.S.) per capita is spent, and much of these expeditures are for inpatient mental health care (WHO, 2014). And, these percentages represent all of mental health treatment and care, including prevention. Therefore, prevention is given even a smaller percentage of the total budgets. Complicating the budget problems, there are a lack of mental health workers in many countries of the world (see Hage et al., 2017 and Solomon & Solomon, 2017). For example, the WHO reports that in high-income countries there is one mental health worker per one thousand people, but in middle- and low-income countries the ratio increases tremendously, to one mental health worker per one hundred thousand people (Bulletin of the World Health Organization, 2015).

Training of prevention specialists. As indicated previously, the training and education of prevention specialists are critically important to advance the specialty. The training and education are important across the globe, in both higher- and lower-income countries. In the United States, Eddy et al. (2005) surveyed groups of prevention specialists about their training and needs for additional training. The survey included graduate students, early career professionals, and later career professionals. The authors found differences among the three groups surveyed in terms of the importance they attached to different training areas and their need for additional training. For example, while established professionals rated themselves high on more traditional areas of prevention training, such as research design and evaluation, graduate students and early professionals rated themselves low in these areas. All three groups rated themselves low in the areas of ethics and economic analysis. One of the chapters in the *Handbook* (see Pérez-Gómez & Mejía-Trujillo, 2017) noted the lack of training in prevention in their region, and those interested in prevention need to travel to other countries (e.g., United States, Canada, Spain) to receive prevention education and training by attending seminars, workshops, and conferences. However, at least one country in Latin America (i.e., El Salvador) offers a master's degree program in community psychology with a specialization in prevention (see Pérez-Gómez & Mejía-Trujillo, 2017). While some noted specialized training for people involved in specific initiatives (e.g., see Pick et al. 2017; Cho, 2017), there appears to be a lack of comprehensive prevention education and training of professionals engaged in (or desiring to engage in) prevention work. However, one exception noted in the *Handbook* is the chapter written by Basic and Rovõs (2017), who describe the innovative and interdisciplinary doctoral degree program in prevention science and disabilities studies in Croatia.

Romano and Hage (2000) identified eight areas and skills important to the training of prevention specialists: (a) developing community and multidisciplinary partnerships, (b) understanding the history of social and public policies related to a topic targeted for prevention, (c) knowledge of risk and protective factors as they relate to a prevention topic, (d) implementation of prevention interventions, (e) understanding of current social and political issues surrounding a prevention topic, (f) psychoeducational group skills, (g) research and evaluation, and (h) prevention ethics. In addition, prevention specialists should be knowledgeable about theoretical frameworks or theories that can form a foundation for a prevention intervention(s). Romano (2015) has summarized several of these theories, including the Transtheoretical Model of Behavior Change (Prochaska, Johnson, & Lee, 2009), the Theory of Reasoned Action and Planned Behavior (Ajzen, 1991; Fishbein & Ajzen, 1975), the Health Belief Model (Rosenstock, 1974), and Motivational Interviewing (Miller & Rollnick, 2002). Koch, Eye, Ellison, and Gourley (2017) cited motivational enhancement therapy as one strategy to strengthen preventive interventions for people at risk for anxiety sensitivity. In their review of literature on childhood antisocial behavior, Humayun and Scott (2017) identified several theories (e.g., attachment theory and social learning theory) that have been cited as important to understanding antisocial behavior.

While there are multiple ways to gain training in prevention, and some degree programs offer some training, many programs, especially those in the mental health fields, offer limited if any training. Public health degrees likely offer the most comprehensive prevention training, as prevention science is a foundation of the field. However, regardless of the ways that training is delivered, it is important that pre-service and in-service professionals who wish to engage with prevention science receive training in the specialty. This *Handbook* provides one avenue for such training by exposing the reader to important areas of study, as well as specific prevention training activities in various countries and regions, such as that described by Campello et al. (2017).

Regional collaboration and partnerships. The development of regional partnerships to support prevention efforts across countries is challenging, but, if achieved, it has the potential to enhance significantly prevention applications and research. However, intercountry collaborations can also pose challenges, such as language differences; limited financial resources; and lack of awareness of prevention activities being developed, implemented, and researched in the region that can encourage intercountry partnerships. It is hoped that this *Handbook* increases awareness among prevention specialists to promote increased collaborations across countries and regions. Few chapter authors in this *Handbook* reported that they were engaged in intercountry partnerships, although chapter authors cited literature and research conducted in other countries to aid in the development and implementation of their own prevention activities. For example, Rodrigo, Byrne, and Álvarez (2017) discuss the Council of Europe's Recommendation 19, on the support of positive parenting, and how this Recommendation guides their prevention interventions to promote positive parenting in Spain. It is likely that prevention specialists are primarily focused on developing partnerships within their own country (e.g., local communities, schools, government agencies, and NGOs), and thus reaching out to specialists beyond their borders is challenging. However, it is hoped that this *Handbook* provides an impetus to begin the process of establishing professional networks and collaborations to strengthen prevention applications and research across the globe.

Call for Major Global Initiatives to Advance Prevention Science in the Twenty-first Century

There are exciting prevention science activities occurring across the globe, as shown by the authors of the chapters in this *Handbook*. However, as noted previously, there is a lack of awareness, and not enough exchange, of what prevention specialists are doing in different parts of the world, as well as the common challenges and solutions that all of us share. Therefore, the editors of the *Handbook* are proposing a call for several global initiatives to advance prevention science in the twenty-first century. These initiatives would bring together prevention science leaders (researchers, practitioners, and policy makers) from different countries (many of whom are authors of chapters in this *Handbook*) for intensive and continuing dialogue related to furthering the goals of prevention science. While such initiatives can take several forms, one example to expand the global dialogue is a call for an international summit (or perhaps regional summits) on prevention science. The summit can take the form of a conference of several days with commitment to following up and staying engaged with participants once the summit ends. In addition to prevention scholars taking part, a summit may include representatives from prominent international organizations that have major interests in prevention science, such as representatives from the WHO, United Nations (e.g., UNICEF), and Centers for Disease Control and Prevention (CDC). Other international organizations that are major stakeholders in the advancement of prevention science would also be invited, such as representatives from professional organizations (e.g., the Society for Prevention Research, the European Society for Prevention Research, and the Clifford-Beers Foundation) and regional governmental agencies (e.g., the European Monitoring Centre on Drugs and Drug Addiction). While this type of summit is similar to the policy decision makers workshops described by Campello et al. (2017), invitees to the proposed summit would include a broader range of prevention specialists and the summit agenda would be more comprehensive than the United Nations Office on Drugs and Crime workshops (see Campello et al., 2017). The goals of the summit would include the following:

1. To provide a forum for prevention scientists from across the globe to share their expertise, needs within their own country/region, and explore possible areas for collaboration.

2. To explore with major organizational stakeholders (e.g., WHO) how they might support prevention activities within a country or region. The support could be in the form of financial resources and grants, training opportunities, and material resources (e.g., technical support).
3. To develop a network of prevention scientists from all parts of the world for the purposes of sharing information and technical tools, research collaborations, and supportive interactions through electronic and/or in-person communication and discussion.
4. To encourage conference attendance by regions that were not well represented in the *Handbook*, such as scholars from the Middle East, sub-Sahara Africa, Eastern Europe and Russia, and Central and South America. Efforts would be made to offer financial incentives to attend the summit, if financial concern was a major barrier to attendance.
5. To continue working on the goals of the summit once the summit ends through focused electronic dialogues and regional meetings of summit delegates. Examples of post-summit goals may include intercountry collaborations on developing professional conference symposia proposals, development of scholarly papers for publication, opportunities to share expertise across countries to promote prevention education, and intercountry comparative research projects. Therefore, the summit would not be a "one and done" activity, but it would mirror strong prevention interventions, that is, continue efforts to promote partnerships and collaborations across countries once the formal summit ends. The summit could be reconvened periodically, such as every two years, to further evaluate the impact of the summit and support new and ongoing collaborations. Thus, it is hoped that such a summit or series of summits would provide an impetus for the development of other international initiatives to strengthen the specialty of prevention science across the globe.

Summary and Conclusions

This *Handbook*, the first of its kind, attracted many authors from across the globe. While some regions and continents were better represented than others, the authors presented a wide range of prevention topics and methodologies. The authors described not only behaviors to be prevented (e.g., drug and alcohol abuse) but also behaviors to be enhanced and strengthened (e.g., promoting health and well-being). Thus, the authors presented interventions to reduce risk behaviors as well as those to enhance protective behaviors of individuals and communities. Several authors noted challenges associated with prevention work in their country, most notably the lack of funding for prevention activities, limited training opportunities, and the need to validate empirically prevention interventions implemented in their country. To address some of the challenges noted by the chapter authors, the *Handbook* editors propose, as one example, an international prevention science summit, or series of summits, to advance prevention science in the twenty-first century. The summit would bring together prevention leaders from countries across the globe and/or region as well as representatives from major organizations that are important stakeholders in prevention science (e.g., WHO) to share knowledge and expertise and to facilitate professional networks and collaborations.

The editors of the *Handbook* thank all of the scholars who contributed to this volume and hope that these scholars' work is an inspiration to others, including students, new professionals, as well as established professionals, who are engaged in prevention science. It is hoped that the *Handbook* can serve as a major resource and enriching challenge as students and scholars advance the field of prevention science.

References+

+ Citations in this chapter that refer to chapters in the *Handbook* are not referenced below.

Ajzen, I. (1991). The theory of planned behavior. *Organizational Behavior and Human Decision Processes* 50: 179–211. doi: 10.1016/0749-5978(91)90020-T

Ajzen, I., & Fishbein, M. (1980). *Understanding Attitudes and Predicting Social Behavior*. Englewood Cliffs, NJ: Prentice Hall.

Albee, G. W. (1983). Psychopathology, prevention, and the just society. *Journal of Primary Prevention* 4: 5–40. doi: 10.1007/BFO1359083

APA (American Psychologicial Association) (2014). Guidelines for prevention in psychology. *American Psychologist* 69: 285–96. doi: 10.1037/a0034569

Bulletin of the World Health Organization (2015). *Public Health Round-Up* 93: 515–16. doi: dx.doi.org/10.2471/BLT.15.010815

Conyne, R. K., Newmeyer, M. D., Kenny, M., Romano, J. L., & Matthews, C. R. (2008). Two key strategies for teaching prevention. *Specialized Course and Infusion: The Journal of Primary Prevention* 29: 375–401. doi: 10.1007/s10935-008-0146-8

Eddy, J. M., Smith, P., Brown, C. H., & Reid, J. B. (2005). A survey of prevention science training: implications for educating the next generation. *Prevention Science* 6: 59–71. doi: 10.1007/s11121-005-1253-x

Fishbein, M. (ed.) (1967). *Readings in Attitude Theory and Measurement*. New York: Wiley.

Fishbein, M., & Ajzen, I. (1975). *Belief, Attitude, Intention, and Behavior: An Introduction to Theory and Research*. Reading, MA: Addison-Wesley.

Fowler, P. J. (2015). Prevention psychology: aptly timed referendum or just more of the same? *PsycCRITIQUES* 60(10): Article 1.

Kenny, M. E., & Hage, S. M. (2009). The next frontier: prevention as an instrument of social justice. *Journal of Primary Prevention* 30: 1–10.

Kenny, M. E., Horne, A. M., Orpinas, P., & Reese, L. E. (eds.) (2009). *Realizing Social Justice: The Challenge of Preventive Interventions*. Washington, DC: American Psychological Association.

Kidd, S. A., & Kral, M. J. (2005). Practicing participatory action research. *Journal of Counseling Psychology* 52: 187–95.

Miller, W. R., & Rollnick, S. (2002). *Motivational Interviewing*, 2nd ed. New York: Guilford Press.

National Research Council and Institute of Medicine (2009). *Preventing Mental, Emotional, and Behavioral Disorders among Young People: Progress and Possibilities.* Washington, DC: National Academic Press.

Prochaska, J. O., Johnson, S., & Lee, P. (2009). The transtheoretical model of behavior change. In Shumaker, S. A., Ockene, J. K., & Riekert, A. (eds.), *The Handbook of Behavior Change*, 3rd ed. New York: Springer, pp. 59–83.

Romano, J. L. (2015). *Prevention Psychology: Enhancing Personal and Social Well-Being.* Washington, DC: American Psychological Association.

Romano, J. L. & Hage, S. M. (2000). Prevention and counseling psychology: revitalizing commitments for the 21st century. *Counseling Psychologist* 28: 733–63. doi: 10.1177/0011000000286001

Romano, J. L. & Netland, J. D. (2008). The application of the theory of reasoned action and planned behavior to prevention science in counseling psychology. *Counseling Psychologist* 36: 777–806. doi: 10.1177/0011000007301670

Rosenstock, I. M. (1974). Historical origins of the health belief model. *Health Education Monograph* 2: 328–35.

WHO (World Health Organization) (2003). *Investing in Mental Health.* Geneva, Switzerland: World Health Organization.

WHO (World Health Organization) (2014). *Mental Health Atlas 2014.* Geneva, Switzerland: World Health Organization.

Index